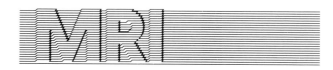

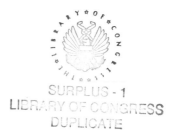

Magnetic Resonance Imaging of Children

Mervyn D. Cohen, M.B., Ch.B
Professor of Radiology
Director, Pediatric Radiology

Mary K. Edwards, M.D.
Associate Professor of Radiology
Chief, Section of Neuroradiology

James Whitcomb Riley Hospital for Children
Indiana University Medical Center
Indianapolis, Indiana

Magnetic Resonance Imaging *of* CHILDREN

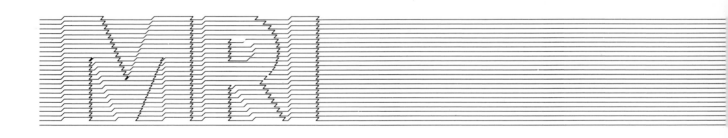

1990•B.C. Decker, Inc.
PHILADELPHIA
TORONTO

Publisher

B.C. Decker Inc.
3228 South Service Road
Burlington, Ontario L7N 3H8

B.C. Decker Inc.
320 Walnut Street
Suite 400
Philadelphia, Pennsylvania 19106

Sales and Distribution

United States and Puerto Rico
Mosby-Year Book Inc.
11830 Westline Industrial Drive
Saint Louis, Missouri 63146

Canada
Mosby-Year Book Limited
5240 Finch Ave. E., Unit 1
Scarborough, Ontario M1S 5A2

Australia
**McGraw-Hill Book Company
Australia Pty. Ltd.**
4 Barcoo Street
Roseville East 2069
New South Wales, Australia

Brazil
**Editora McGraw-Hill do Brasil,
Ltda.**
rua Tabapua, 1.105, Itaim-Bibi
Sao Paulo, S.P. Brasil

Colombia
**Interamericana/McGraw-Hill de
Colombia, S.A.**
Apartado Aereo 81078
Bogota, D.E. Colombia

Europe
McGraw-Hill Book Company GmbH
Lademannbogen 136
D-2000 Hamburg 63
West Germany

France
MEDSI/McGraw-Hill
6, avenue Daniel Lesueur
75007 Paris, France

Hong Kong and China
McGraw-Hill Book Company
Suite 618, Ocean Centre
5 Canton Road
Tsimshatsui, Kowloon
Hong Kong

India
**Tata McGraw-Hill Publishing
Company, Ltd.**
12/4 Asaf Ali Road, 3rd Floor
New Delhi 110002, India

Indonesia
P.O. Box 122/JAT
Jakarta, 1300 Indonesia

Italy
McGraw-Hill Libri Italia, s.r.l.
Piazza Emilia, 5
I-20129 Milano MI
Italy

Japan
Igaku-Shoin Ltd.
Tokyo International P.O. Box 5063
1-28-36 Hongo, Bunkyo-ku,
Tokyo 113, Japan

Korea
C.P.O. Box 10583
Seoul, Korea

Malaysia
No. 8 Jalan SS 7/6B
Kelana Jaya
47301 Petaling Jaya
Selangor, Malaysia

Mexico
**Interamericana/McGraw-Hill de
Mexico, S.A. de C.V.**
Cedro 512, Colonia Atlamp
(Apartado Postal 26370)
06450 Mexico, D.F., Mexico

New Zealand
**McGraw-Hill Book Co. New Zealand
Ltd.**
5 Joval Place, Wiri
Manukau City, New Zealand

Panama
**Editorial McGraw-Hill
Latinoamericana, S.A.**
Apartado Postal 2036
Zona Libre de Colon
Colon, Republica de Panama

Portugal
**Editora McGraw-Hill de Portugal,
Ltda.**
Rua Rosa Damasceno 11A-B
1900 Lisboa, Portugal

South Africa
Libriger Book Distributors
Warehouse Number 8
"Die Ou Looiery"
Tannery Road
Hamilton, Bloemfontein 9300

Southwest Asia
McGraw-Hill Book Co.
348 Jalan Boon Lay
Jurong, Singapore 2261

Spain
**McGraw-Hill/Interamericana de
Espana, S.A.**
Manuel Ferrero, 13
28020 Madrid, Spain

Taiwan
P.O. Box 87-601
Taipei, Taiwan

Thailand
632/5 Phaholyothin Road
Sapan Kwai
Bangkok 10400
Thailand

*United Kingdom, Middle East
and Africa*
**McGraw-Hill Book Company (U.K.)
Ltd.**
Shoppenhangers Road
Maidenhead, Berkshire
SL6 2QL England

Venezuela
McGraw-Hill/Interamericana, C.A.
2da. calle Bello Monte
(entre avenida Casanova y Sabana
Grande)
Apartado Aereo 50785
Caracas 1050, Venezuela

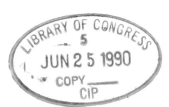

Magnetic Resonance Imaging of Children

ISBN 1-55664-166-4

© 1990 by B.C. Decker Incorporated under the International Copyright Union. All rights reserved. No part of this publication may be reused or republished in any form without written permission of the publisher.

Library of Congress catalog card number: 89-51061

10 9 8 7 6 5 4 3 2 1

Dedication

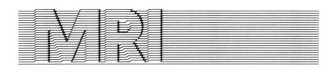

To Eugene Klatte, M.D., chairman of the department
of Radiology, and all our clinical colleagues at Indiana
University Medical Center.

Contributors

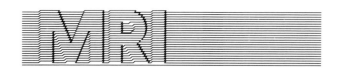

JAMES ABRAHAMS, M.D.
Assistant Professor, Department of Radiology,
Yale University School of Medicine, New Haven,
Connecticut

A. JAMES BARKOVICH
Assistant Professor of Radiology, Neurosurgery,
and Pediatrics, University of California, San
Francisco, School of Medicine, San Francisco,
California

PAUL BERGER, M.D.
Director, Department of Radiology, Long Beach
Memorial Medical Center, Long Beach, California

GEORGE S. BISSET III, M.D.
Associate Professor of Radiology and Pediatrics,
University of Cincinnati College of Medicine;
Chief, Section of Body Imaging, Children's
Hospital, Cincinnati, Ohio

JAMES R. BOGNANNO, M.D.
Lecturer, Indiana University School of Medicine;
Neuroradiology Fellow, Indiana University
Medical Center, Indianapolis, Indiana

SHARON E. BYRD, M.D.
Associate Professor, Department of Radiology,
Northwestern University Medical School; Head,
Division of Neuroimaging, Department of
Radiology, Children's Memorial Hospital,
Chicago, Illinois

JOSEPH W. CARLSON, Ph.D.
Assistant Professor in Residence, University of
California, San Francisco, School of Medicine,
San Francisco, California

GORDON CHEUNG, M.D.
Lecturer, University of Toronto Faculty of
Medicine; Neuroradiologist, Sunnybrook Medical
Centre, Toronto, Ontario, Canada

H. SYLVESTER CHUANG, M.D.C.M.
Associate Professor, University of Toronto Faculty
of Medicine; Head, Division of Special
Procedures, The Hospital for Sick Children,
Toronto, Ontario, Canada

MERVYN D. COHEN, M.B., Ch.B., B.Sc.(hon)
Professor of Radiology, Indiana University School
of Medicine; Chief of Pediatric Radiology, James
Whitcomb Riley Hospital for Children,
Indianapolis, Indiana

PATRICIA C. DAVIS, M.D.
Associate Professor, Department of Radiology,
Emory University School of Medicine, Atlanta,
Georgia

KAREN L. DAWSON, M.B., B.S.
Clinical Fellow, Department of Diagnostic
Radiology, Stanford University School of
Medicine, Stanford, California

ROSALIND B. DIETRICH, M.B., Ch.B.
Assistant Professor, Section of Pediatric
Radiology, Department of Radiological Sciences,
University of California, Los Angeles, School of
Medicine, Los Angeles, California

JEFFREY L. DUERK, Ph.D.
Assistant Professor of Radiology and Biomedical
Engineering, Case Western Reserve University
School of Medicine; MRI Research Scientist,
MetroHealth Medical Center, Cleveland, Ohio

MARY K. EDWARDS, M.D.
Associate Professor of Radiology, Indiana
University School of Medicine; Chief,
Neuroradiology Section, Indiana University
Medical Center, Indianapolis, Indiana

STEVEN J. FAGAN, D.O.
Assistant Professor of Radiology, Uniformed
Services University of the Health Sciences; Head,
Diagnostic Radiology, National Naval Medical
Center, Bethesda, Maryland

THEODORE R. HALL, M.D.
Assistant Professor in Residence, University of California, Los Angeles, School of Medicine, Los Angeles, California

TODD M. HARRIS, M.D.
Instructor, Department of Radiology, Indiana University School of Medicine; Fellow, Neuroradiology, Indiana University Medical Center, Indianapolis, Indiana

MICHAEL A. KUHARIK, M.D.
Neuroradiologist, St. Vincent Hospital and Health Care Center, Indianapolis, Indiana

PAUL L. MOLINA, M.D.
Assistant Professor of Radiology, Mallinckrodt Institute of Radiology, Washington University School of Medicine, St. Louis, Missouri

SHEILA G. MOORE, M.D.
Assistant Professor, Department of Diagnostic Radiology, Stanford University School of Medicine, Stanford, California

PETER A. ROTHSCHILD, M.D.
Assistant Professor in Residence, University of California, San Francisco, School of Medicine, San Francisco, California

GUY H. SEBAG, Med. Doc.
Pediatric Radiologist, Service de Radiologie, Hôpital des Enfants Malades, Paris, France; Formerly Fellow, Department of Radiology, Stanford University School of Medicine, Stanford, California

MELVIN SENAC, M.D.
Associate Professor of Radiology, University of Southern California School of Medicine; Staff Radiologist, Children's Hospital, Los Angeles, California

MARILYN J. SIEGEL, M.D.
Professor of Radiology, Mallinckrodt Institute of Radiology, Washington University School of Medicine, St. Louis, Missouri

RICHARD R. SMITH, M.D.
Assistant Professor of Radiology and Neurology, Indiana University School of Medicine; Staff Neuroradiologist, Indiana University Medical Center, Indianapolis, Indiana

MURRAY A. SOLOMON, M.D.
Clinical Director, Peninsula Imaging Center, Burlingame; Clinical Director, Los Gatos Imaging Center, Los Gatos, California

PHILIP STANLEY, M.D.
Professor of Radiology, University of Southern California School of Medicine; Pediatric Radiologist, Children's Hospital, Los Angeles, California

GORDON SZE, M.D.
Associate Professor of Radiology and Chief, Section of Radiology, Yale University School of Medicine, New Haven, Connecticut

MICHAEL TWOHIG, M.D.
Clinical Instructor of Radiology, Yale University School of Medicine, New Haven, Connecticut

Foreword

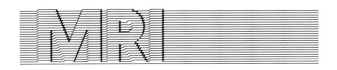

It is now almost exactly ten years since the first MR examination of a child and five years since the publication of Dr. Cohen's first book, *Pediatric Magnetic Resonance Imaging*. There could be no more fitting way to mark these events than by the publication of *Magnetic Resonance Imaging of Children*.

In the last chapter of his earlier book, Dr. Cohen made six predictions about the future development of MRI. These were reduction in scan times, optimization of pulse sequences, increased use of surface coils, reduction in slice thickness, wider use of spectroscopy, and licensing of contrast agents for general use. All of these developments have now come to pass, and a great deal more are in prospect including new forms of chemical shift imaging, perfusion and diffusion imaging, applications of solid state techniques, and more specific contrast agents. We are also likely to see much more use of three-dimensional techniques and ultrafast forms of imaging.

While this rapid development is exhilarating in many ways, it may also be a source of great confusion. Articles and chapters that explain new principles and concepts are therefore particularly welcome in MRI. We are fortunate that in this book, chapter after chapter clarifies and elucidates the principles and applications of MRI, and that much of this refers to advances that have just occurred within the last two years.

Even practitioners of general radiology can expect 20 percent of their workload to involve children, so a text of this type is of value not only to specialists in pediatric radiology, but also to the radiologic community as a whole.

On a personal level, I first saw Dr. Cohen's outstanding work on MRI of the body in children in Washington in 1983. The hundred cases he had studied was an incredible number for that time, but his work was also particularly notable for his ingenious use of the adult head coil of a 0.15T resistive system for pediatric body imaging. When this was combined with his astute radiologic interpretation it was clear that something of major importance was happening in pediatric radiology. It is heartening to see how far pediatric MRI has progressed since these early days.

Apart from the important advantage of lack of ionizing radiation, MRI offers other features that are especially important in pediatrics. The smaller size of the infant is no handicap; in fact smaller receiver coils are often more efficient than larger ones and lead to better image quality. The long T2 of the neonatal brain allows greater time for data collection, the smaller nasal sinuses cause less susceptibility artifact than in adults, and the low level of fat in the abdomen in children may lead to less motion artifact than in adults. The end result is that there are quite significant technical advantages to imaging children with MRI when compared with adults.

In spite of these advantages, the cost of MRI is still high, and pediatric examinations generally take longer than those of adults. It is therefore important to choose the patients for MR examinations carefully and integrate their work-up into protocols that best exploit the strengths of all available diagnostic techniques. This book culls together the best advice currently available on these issues. Radiologists throughout the world owe a debt of gratitude to Dr. Cohen and his fellow authors for the effort they have put into this book and the great success they have made of it.

Graeme M. Bydder, M.B., Ch.B.
Professor of Diagnostic Radiology
Royal Postgraduate Medical School
London
Past President, Society of Magnetic
Resonance in Medicine

Preface

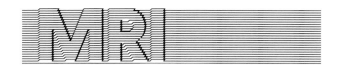

The 1980s witnessed the introduction, maturation, and coming of age of MRI. As we forge ahead toward the next century, we have already seen early predictions that MRI would have a major impact on pediatric radiology become reality. *Magnetic Resonance Imaging of Children* is intended as a comprehensive reference work on the current applications of MRI in children. We hope that pediatric radiologists, general radiologists who devote some of their time to pediatric imaging, and pediatricians will all find it a valuable, comprehensive sourcebook on pediatric MRI. Those seeking a brief introduction to the technology and basic application should see *Pediatric Magnetic Resonance Imaging,* Cohen, published by W.B. Saunders.

The book begins with a section that covers the physics behind image creation and interpretation, and safety considerations in using this technology. It is written for the practicing physician, rather than the basic scientist, to provide the information required to interpret MR images accurately and to improve one's own radiologic techniques. The second and third sections describe clinical applications of MRI; the second section focuses on the central nervous system, and the third deals with the rest of the body.

The clinical sections follow a logical format. Initial classification of disease is by anatomic location. For each anatomic region, the disorders are classified by major underlying etiologic categories: congenital, inflammation and infection, tumor, trauma and mechanical, vascular, degenerative and connective tissue, endocrine and metabolic, iatrogenic, and miscellaneous.

Common disorders and those in which MRI can play a major role in clinical care have received the greatest emphasis. However, to be comprehensive, we have also included MR descriptions of all disorders that have been published in the literature. Some of these disorders may be found incidentally on MR images and knowledge of their appearance is, therefore, important. For completeness, we have included clinical, pathologic, and therapeutic descriptions of the more significant disorders.

For each disease, the specific role of MRI and its comparison with other imaging modalities is discussed in as much depth as current knowledge permits. Where MRI has a unique role to play, this is emphasized. The literature review of MR publications pertaining to pediatrics is comprehensive. In order to present the full spectrum of the MR appearance of various disorders, we have included a vast number of images. On occasion, when the appearance of a particular disorder is expected to be similar in adults and children and no pediatric images have been available, we have borrowed from the adult world.

We are extremely grateful to all of our contributing authors who have worked hard to provide state-of-the-art presentations. Without exception, the authors accepted our guidelines and editorial revisions so that we could achieve a uniformity of presentation and balance throughout the book. Thank you authors!

Finally, our sincere gratitude is given to our secretary, Barbara Smith. Her name is not listed with the contributing authors, but without her contribution this book would not exist.

Mervyn D. Cohen, M.B., Ch.B.
Mary K. Edwards, M.D.

Contents

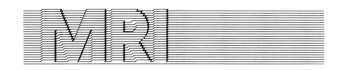

S E C T I O N

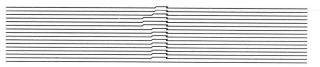

FUNDAMENTALS OF MAGNETIC RESONANCE IMAGING

Basic Physics: Constructing the Magnetic Resonance Image

JEFFREY L. DUERK, Ph.D.

BASIC PHYSICS OF NUCLEAR MAGNETIC RESONANCE

While the role of magnetic resonance imaging (MRI) in future diagnostic imaging appears secure, its growth and development continue at a rapid pace. This growth varies from new detector coils to new pulse sequences, to ever higher field strengths and beyond. Unfortunately, these rapid changes and modifications can cloud both the basic physics of MRI and the underlying principles of image interpretation. This chapter reviews, albeit in a cursory manner, the basic physics involved in generating a nuclear magnetic resonance (NMR) signal, and how this signal is used in constructing an image.

Simplified Review

The hydrogen nucleus may be considered as a tiny magnetic needle (magnetic moment).[1,2] If the body is placed in a very strong uniform magnetic field, a small fraction of its tiny hydrogen magnets will tend to align themselves along the axis of the magnetic field.[3,4] They precess (or wobble) around this axis at a fixed frequency proportional to the magnetic field strength. If the aligned hydrogen nuclei are bombarded with radiowaves of the same frequency as the wobble frequency, they will *absorb energy* and flip to a higher energy level, tipping off their equilibrium alignment along the axis of the field. When the radiowaves are turned off, the hydrogen nuclei will return to their resting state. Prior to returning to their initial alignment, they precess about the magnetic field and release energy of radiowave frequency by inducing a voltage in a receiving coil of wire (an antenna). It is this signal that is used to generate images.

Like computed tomography (CT), MR images are "slices" through the body. Also like CT, each slice is made up of a number of image volume elements (voxels) or picture elements (pixels), each of which is typically assigned a shade of gray between white and black. The intensity of the pixel is dependent on the amount of energy that is detected from each spatial location.[5]

Magnetic Nuclei and their Behavior in a Magnetic Field

The nuclei of all atoms is made up of protons (positive charge) and neutrons (no net charge). Both particles can be shown to have angular momentum that arises out of their possessing "spin," a quantum characteristic. Specifically, those nuclei with an odd number of protons and an even number of neutrons (or vice versa) or an odd number of both have quantum spin, which causes them to possess angular momentum and a magnetic moment. The atoms we are most interested in biologically are 1H, 13C, 19F, 23Na, and 31P.[6]

3

The magnetic moment of these nuclei will attempt to align with the axis of an applied magnetic field owing to the interaction between the magnetic moment and the magnetic field.[7]

This may seem rather complicated, but we have all experienced the alignment of a magnetic moment in a magnetic field through the bar magnet in a compass orienting itself with the earth's magnetic field. Unfortunately, the analogy between the compass needle and the magnetic moment of the nucleus breaks down, since the compass needle has only a magnetic moment, and no angular momentum.

The external magnetic field applies a torque (twisting energy) that attempts to align the magnetic moment with the field. However, torque is equal to the rate of change of angular momentum of the object. In our early physics training, we all learned that an object's momentum varies only if acted on by some external force. In this case, the change in angular momentum of the nucleus is equal to the torque on the magnetic moment by the magnetic field. The net result is that the magnetic moment of the spin precesses about the axis of direction of the field, yet does not align with it, as the forces, torques, and angular momentum interact (Fig. 1–1).[2,7,8]

Fortunately, there is a simple analogy to the nuclear gyrations just described. Imagine a child's toy, the top.

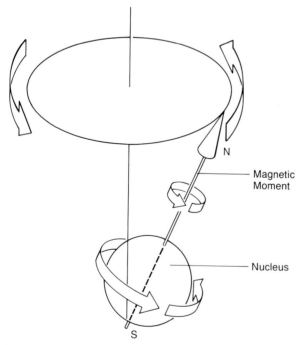

Figure 1–1. Biologically relevant nuclei, such as 1H, 31P, 19F, and 23Na, have quantum spin and therefore an inherent magnetic moment. This magnetic moment acts like a magnetic dipole (compass needle) in a magnetic field. However, interaction between the torque trying to align the moment and the angular momentum causes the magnetic moment to precess about the magnetic field. (From Harms SE, Morgan TJ, Yamanashi WS, et al. Principles of magnetic resonance. Radiographics 1984; 4:25–38.)

If the top is not spinning, it has a moment of inertia yet no angular momentum. When placed in a gravitational field, the top simply falls over, aligning with the field. However, once the top is spinning, its response in a gravitational field is very different. The gravitational forces on the spinning top produce a torque on the top, identical to the torque exerted on the magnetic moment of the nucleus when placed in a magnetic field. This torque causes the top's angular momentum to change, forcing it to precess about the gravitational field in the shape of a cone. If there were no friction, the top would spin forever at its initial angle relative to the gravitational field. Again, the magnetic moment precesses about the applied field identically to the precession of the top, at a fixed angle Θ to the magnetic field if not disturbed by external forces.[9]

It is important to remember that the frequency of precession is not the frequency with which the magnetic moment (or top) is spinning about its own axis. It is, instead, the frequency with which it rotates about the magnetic (or gravitational) field. Spin and precession are different, as seen in the example of the top. The top spins about its own axis at some fixed frequency, and precesses about the field at a different rate. If one were to work through the various equations governing the motion of the magnetic moment of the nucleus in an applied static magnetic field, it could be shown that the frequency of precession, or Larmor frequency, of the magnetic moment is equal to the magnetic field strength times a constant (the gyromagnetic ratio).

The gyromagnetic ratio is a scale factor that relates the magnetic moment and the angular momentum of the nucleus, and is unique for different nuclei. For most biologically relevant nuclei, the Larmor frequencies are in the range of megahertz (MHz, millions of cycles per second) in magnetic field strengths available from current magnet technology. For the most part, we will be dealing with hydrogen, with a Larmor frequency of 64 MHz at 1.5 Tesla (T). (Tesla is a unit of magnetic field strength equal to 10,000 Gauss such that 1.5T is about 30,000 times the strength of the earth's magnetic field at Washington, DC.)[4,9]

The analogies that have been used so far have dealt with classical mechanics. The presence of a net magnetic moment and precession can also be pursued from a purely quantum mechanical analysis. Basically, we first have to determine the number of quantum spin states of the nuclei of interest. In the case of 1H, 13C, and 19F, there are two possible states. These correspond to having a precessional axis pointed antiparallel or parallel to the magnetic field. The energy level associated with each state depends on the strength of the magnetic moment and the strength of the magnetic field. There are thus two possible energy levels for the nuclear spins, corresponding to being aligned with or opposed to the axis of the magnetic field. Thus, a spin must absorb some amount of energy to go from the lower energy state (aligned with the field) to being opposed to it in the higher energy state. Alternatively, a spin that loses a specific amount of energy can go from the higher energy level (opposed to the field) to the lower state (aligned with the field). Quantum theory, as described in Planck's law, allows us to determine the frequency of the quantum amount of energy that must be supplied or given off in moving from one energy level to another. Solving the various equations, the frequency of energy that must be supplied to or removed from the system is exactly equal to the Larmor frequency described earlier with regard to classical mechanics. The implications of this result will be described shortly.[4,7–9]

If one looks at the electromagnetic spectrum (Fig. 1–2) and the range of energies and frequencies associated with traditional imaging modalities, such as x-ray, two facts about nuclear magnetic resonance (NMR) are apparent. The first is that the wavelength of energy used is quite long (corresponding to radiowaves), ranging from a few to several hundred meters. Therefore, the resolution in MRI will not be the result of traditional photon wavelength effects. Second, the energy level of the NMR spin state transition is approximately a factor of 10^{10} below x-ray energy and about 10^7 below normal infrared energy (heat) associated with the molecular vibrations and translations in the human body. Therefore, NMR is inherently a low signal energy level modality.[9]

While the spins are trying to line up with an applied magnetic field, thermal vibrations and microscopic local magnetic field variations add sufficient energy to prevent alignment of all the spins or protons in our body. In fact, at typical body temperatures and in typical magnetic fields associated with MRI, a *net alignment* of only about one proton in 100,000 occurs.[10,11] The number of protons aligning with the magnetic field is proportional to *magnetic field strength* and inversely proportional to the temperature of the sample.[7,8] With only one in 100,000 spins producing any net alignment along the magnetic field, one might be concerned that a sufficient net magnetic moment (the sum of all the individual magnetic moments of the protons in our body) required to produce a discernible

signal above background noise could not be obtained. Fortunately, our body is composed of about 90 percent water, each molecule with two protons. Thus, in 1 g of tissue, about 10^{19} protons align with the magnetic field, providing the source for a net magnetic moment in the body. Up to this point, a single spin (or proton for 1H) had been considered. Fortunately, the large number with a net alignment along the magnetic field forces us to generate and use a concept called the net magnetic moment, which is simply the sum of all the magnetic moments of all the spins in our sample (or patient). Only the net aligned protons need be considered, since all others are cancelled by one opposed to it.

It is imprecise to say that the spins are "aligned" with or opposed to the field. Instead, they have a net tendency to precess about the field, at a fixed angle Θ. Each spin stays at its initial angle relative to the field. However, with a net alignment of one in 100,000 and with the large number of protons available, it can be shown that any values of Θ are possible, none being preferred. Similarly, the spins have no preferred position on the surface of their precessional cone about the field.[6] Therefore, the net aligned spins all have a component of their magnetization along the axis of the field in common. Components perpendicular to the field are cancelled by other aligned spins that are at the same angle but at an opposite point on the precessional cone. The only thing both have in common is a component pointed along the field. Thus, summing over all spins produces a net bulk magnetic moment along the axis of the field only. *This net magnetic moment can be shown to act as a single spin, albeit with a much stronger moment.*

$$N(\text{aligned})/N(\text{opposed}) = e^{(\gamma H/kT)}$$
$$= 1 + (\gamma H/kT)$$
(H is field strength and T is temperature)

The equation above represents the basic source of motivation to use higher field strengths in MRI. In order to get more signal, corresponding to a greater net magnetic moment, we must either increase the

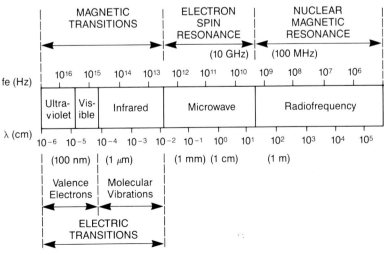

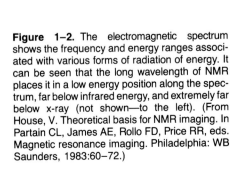

Figure 1–2. The electromagnetic spectrum shows the frequency and energy ranges associated with various forms of radiation of energy. It can be seen that the long wavelength of NMR places it in a low energy position along the spectrum, far below infrared energy, and extremely far below x-ray (not shown—to the left). (From House, V. Theoretical basis for NMR imaging. In Partain CL, James AE, Rollo FD, Price RR, eds. Magnetic resonance imaging. Philadelphia: WB Saunders, 1983:60–72.)

strength of the magnetic field or lower the temperature of the patient. Ideally, we would obtain a tremendously strong signal from a patient at absolute zero ($-458°F$, $-273°C$), with catastrophic results to the health of the patient. Therefore, the only convenient way to get more spins (protons) aligned with the magnetic field in MRI is to increase the magnetic field strength.

Radiofrequency Pulses

Unfortunately, the production of a net magnetic moment for the sample does not ensure that a signal or technique is available that can be used for imaging or spectroscopy. In fact, it is difficult to detect the magnetization along the Z-axis (the axis of the magnetic field). Therefore, something must be done to the magnetization that will allow a useful signal to be generated. It can be shown that a radiofrequency (RF) pulse of energy, applied at the Larmor frequency, exerts a torque on the net magnetic moment, causing it to tip away from the Z-axis toward the X-Y plane.[1,7-11]

Once the RF pulse is complete, the net (bulk) magnetization has been tipped away from the Z-axis by an angle given by:

$$\text{angle of tip} = \text{gyromagnetic constant} \\ \times \text{strength of radiowave pulse} \\ \times \text{duration of radiowave pulse.}$$

Before the initial RF pulse, the bulk magnetization was totally along the Z-axis. The RF pulse converted Z-magnetization into magnetization in the X-Y plane. Once there, it precesses about the axis of the main magnetic field and leads to oscillating magnetization along the X- and Y-axes. Eventually, this magnetization disappears owing to T2 decay, as discussed shortly, and because the spin system will attempt to return to equilibrium by T1 (spin lattice) recovery through the loss of energy from the spins to the lattice. The oscillating magnetization along the X- and Y-axes can be detected and used to generate a signal in a detector coil, and then finally to reconstruct the MR image.

Generation of a Detectable Signal

At first glance, it is not apparent that the RF pulse has done anything constructive for us. Before the pulse, there was no magnetization along the X- and Y-axes. Yet, after the pulse, there was an oscillating magnetization in the X-Y plane. Fortunately, Faraday's law of induction states that the induced electromotive force (EMF in units of volts) in a circuit is proportional to (except for a minus sign) the rate of change of the magnetic flux through the circuit. In translation, the law states that a voltage will be produced in a fixed coil of wire that is proportional to the rate of change of the magnetic flux linking the coil and the magnetic moment. Specifically, this indicates that

the oscillating magnetization in the X-Y plane will induce a voltage in a coil of wire. Thus, we can use coils or resonant circuits to detect a voltage from the sample in the magnetic field after the application of an RF pulse because of coupling that exists between the time-varying magnetization and the coil. The frequency of the oscillating electric voltage will be equal to the Larmor frequency of the magnetization.

SIGNAL LOCALIZATION: CREATING IMAGE SLICES, ALTERING SLICE THICKNESS, AND LOCALIZING POINTS IN AN IMAGE SLICE

For most MRI applications, the hydrogen nuclei must be localized along three axes in the body. For this discussion, assume that the slice selection is defined along the Z-axis and points within a slice in the X- and Y-planes. In most imaging systems the axis of the main magnetic field is along the Z-axes. The scenario to be discussed will produce a slice in the transverse plane of the body. For other imaging planes, see Table 1–1.

Simplified Review

The American College of Radiology asserts that MR images should all be viewed in a standard position. Transverse images should be positioned so that one is viewing the anatomic area from the patient's feet, coronal images should be positioned so that one is viewing them from the patient's front, and sagittal images should be viewed as if standing on the patient's left side.

In a uniform magnetic field, all hydrogen atoms precess at the same frequency. If a weak magnetic field gradient is applied along the Z-axis, the hydrogen atoms along the line of the gradient will all be at slightly different magnetic field strengths and therefore precess at slightly different frequencies. If a band of radiowaves covering all the wobbling frequencies is applied, each hydrogen will be tipped off the axis of the main magnetic field toward the X-Y plane by the portion of the radiowave of the corresponding precessional frequency. Once the RF pulse is completed, the slice select gradient is turned off and all spins in the X-Y plane precess at the Larmor frequency associated with the main field alone (since no gradients are applied).

A short time later, a second gradient oriented along one of the imaging axes is applied, forcing the spins to

Table 1–1. IMAGING PLANES AND ROLE OF EACH AXIS GRADIENT (TYPICAL)

Plane	Slice Selection	Frequency Encoding	Phase Encoding
Transverse	Z	X or Y	Y or X
Sagittal	X	Z (typically)	Y (typically)
Coronal	Y	Z (typically)	X (typically)

precess at a frequency determined by their position along it. If the rate of change of the magnetic field strength along the gradient is known and the frequencies of the detected radiofrequency signal can be determined, the position and amount of the magnetization are very easily obtained.

Applying varying RF bandwidth pulses or using variable slice select gradient strength will allow variable width slices to be nutated into the X-Y plane. Localization along the slice-select axis is performed by varying the center frequency of the RF pulse to correspond to that of the desired location along the slice-select axis. Therefore, frequency encoding is used to localize along two axes (along the Z-axis for slice selection and along either the X or Y axis within the imaging plane). Localizing in the third plane is achieved by using a transient magnetic field gradient to place precessing hydrogen atoms at different phases. A small gradient is applied for a brief time following the RF pulse, but before the signal is detected by the imager. Protons at different positions along the gradient precess at different speeds and go out of phase. When the gradient is turned off, all the protons continue spinning at the same speed but out of phase. The degree by which a proton is out of phase is directly related to its position along the line of the gradient field.

Slice Selection

To cover the process of slice selection in more depth, consider a patient inside a perfectly homogenous magnetic field. If an RF pulse at the Larmor frequency were applied, all spins would be tipped by the same amount regardless of their spatial position. If this was a 90-degree pulse, all spins from the patient would be tipped completely into the X-Y plane from their initial position oriented along the axis of the main magnetic field (typically, the Z-axis). Unfortunately, imaging at a specific spatial location is desired, requiring the use of some technique for spatially selecting spins at the imaging plane desired. That is, some technique is required that will enable the spins from one location to be nutated into the X-Y plane, leaving others undisturbed along the Z-axis.

The most common technique for performing this spatial localization is to apply a linear variation of the magnetic field (linear magnetic field gradient) along the axis perpendicular to the imaging plane desired. For an axial image from a conventional superconducting magnet, the Z-axis is perpendicular to the desired imaging plane, as shown in Figure 1–3. Here, spins at each point along the long axis of the body resonate at a slightly different Larmor frequency since each is at a different magnetic field strength, and as previously shown, the frequency of precession is dependent on magnetic field strength. Common gradient strengths on present imagers are from 1 to 15 milli-Tesla per meter (mT/m), or about 2,000 times weaker than the main field over the usable volume of the imager.

Once an RF pulse is applied at some frequency, there is only one spatial location along the Z-axis with that resonant frequency. Therefore, only spins at that spatial location along the slice-select axis will be affected by the RF pulse, and nutated away from the Z-axis toward the X-Y plane. Transmitting a second

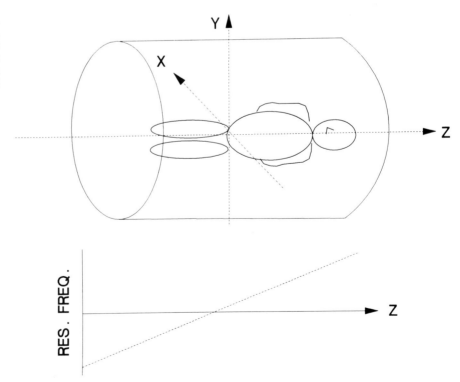

Figure 1–3. A patient in an MR imager typically lies along the Z-axis. A slice-select gradient applied along this axis varies the strength of B_0 at each spatial location so that there is a unique resonant frequency for all spins along the axis.

pulse at a different frequency will excite spins at a different spatial location (Fig. 1–4).

The imaging plane selected without the use of a magnetic field gradient produced all spins nutated away from the Z-axis, corresponding to an infinite slice thickness with no spatial localization. With the application of the magnetic field gradient and appropriate selection of the pulse frequency, it was possible to perform spatial localization. Unfortunately, the slices were almost infinitely thin, since only one specific spatial location was at the same (resonant) frequency as the RF pulse. Spatial localization has been achieved at the expense of infinitely thin slices. Fortunately, there is a way around this problem.

Nonzero slice thickness can be obtained by applying an RF pulse that has some bandwidth, or distribution of frequencies, within it. In this way, a range of spatial locations is excited. By narrowing the bandwidth, the range of spatial locations can also be narrowed. Alternatively, the bandwidth can be increased, corresponding to a greater spatial distribution experiencing excitation. Figure 1–5 shows how the slice thickness could conceivably be varied along the Z-axis at location "f" in the abdomen by applying an RF pulse centered at a Larmor frequency f_{abd} and whose bandwidth changes from BW1 to BW2. However, specific bandwidth pulses would be required for each slice thickness for the fixed value of G_z.

The most common means of changing the slice thickness is by simply changing the gradient strength along the Z-axis for a fixed bandwidth pulse. Increasing the gradient strength by a factor of 2, for example, decreases the slice thickness to one-half its previous

value, as shown in Figure 1–6. Similarly, it can be seen in this illustration that the resonant frequency of the spatial location varies as well. Thus, spatial localization and varying slice thickness over the entire usable volume of the imager can be obtained by scaling the magnetic field gradient (slice thickness) along the slice-select axis, and changing the center frequency of the RF pulse (slice position). The bandwidth of the pulse is the same for all slices and all slice thicknesses. The only factors varied are the center frequency and the gradient strength. Table 1–2 lists techniques used to perform slice thickness selection and localization.

It can be shown that the bandwidth of a pulse is defined, to a first approximation, by the Fourier transform of its envelope.[10] Imagine a uniform slice profile, corresponding to all spins from the front to the back of the slice being excited equally, and all having the same initial phase in the rotating reference frame. A pulse

Table 1–2. METHODS FOR VARYING SLICE THICKESS AND LOCATION IN MRI

Gradient	RF	Net Thickness
Constant	Increase bandwidth, constant frequency offset	Increased
Constant	Decrease bandwidth, constant frequency offset	Decreased
Increased	Fixed bandwidth, increased frequency offset	Decreased
Decreased	Fixed bandwidth, decreased frequency offset	Increased

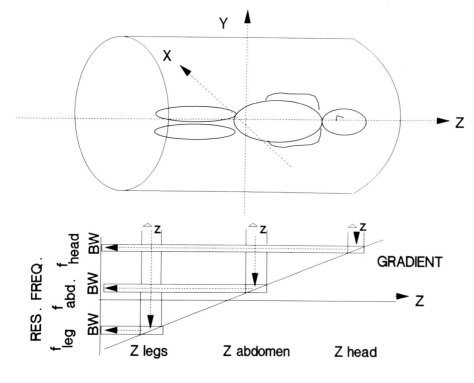

Figure 1–4. To select a specific location during the application of the slice-select gradient, the center frequency of the RF pulse is varied. This figure shows how different slice positions can be obtained in the presence of the magnetic field gradient by applying pulses centered at the resonant frequency of the legs, abdomen, and head. The bandwidth (BW) of the pulse determines the slice thickness. In this case, the same bandwidth was used for all slices, so that all had the same slice thickness.

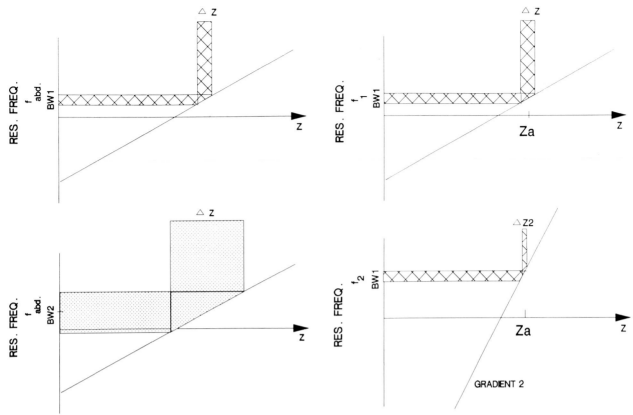

Figure 1–5. Application of an RF pulse at the resonant frequency of the abdomen in the presence of the slice-select gradient nutates spins in the abdomen into the X-Y plane for detection. The thickness of the excited slice could conceivably be varied by changing the bandwidth of the pulse, from BW1 to BW2 in this case, producing the differences in the slice thicknesses.

Figure 1–6. An alternate approach to varying the slice thickness is to vary the strength of the slice-select gradient, using the same bandwidth pulse for all applications. This figure shows how the slice thickness can be varied by changing the gradient strength from 1 to 2. However, this forces the resonant frequency of the location of interest to change. Fortunately the relationships governing the resonant frequency and the gradient strength are known, so that gradient strength and frequency offset alone can be varied to perform variable width slice selection.

with a uniform bandwidth over the frequency range of interest is needed. The inverse Fourier transform of this frequency distribution would produce an RF pulse amplitude that would vary as shown in Figure 1–7. However, since this function would last forever in time, it must be truncated, with corresponding reductions in the slice profile.

Two-Dimensional Localization within a Slice

During slice selection, it was possible to encode each position along the axis perpendicular to the imaging plane by applying a linear magnetic field gradient. This made each position resonate at a slightly different frequency, allowing us to select specific spatial locations by applying RF pulses at specific frequencies. Once the pulse was completed, the magnetization in the X-Y plane precessed about the static magnetic field. Unfortunately, all spins are at the same frequency, with no known spatial dependence other than that associated with inhomogeneities in the magnetic field.

Here again, it is possible to apply a linear magnetic

field gradient to encode linearly all spins along an axis at unique frequencies. Here the "frequency encoding axis" will be along one of the axes in the desired image, and therefore orthogonal to the slice-select direction.

It was also shown earlier that the induced EMF (voltage) in the detector results from the varying flux linkage between the precessing magnetization and the coil. The frequency of oscillation of the voltage is equal to the precessional frequency of the magnetization. Therefore, when the frequency encoding axis is applied, each spatial location along that axis is at a different frequency, thereby inducing a voltage in the detection coil at that frequency. All frequencies will appear simultaneously in the coil and simply add together. The amplitude of the voltage will be dependent on the amount of magnetization at each spatial location.[1]

Imagine a circular tube, as shown in Figure 1–8, and that we wish to image at position Za. A slice-select gradient is applied along the long axis of the tube, and an RF pulse of finite bandwidth is applied at the Lar-

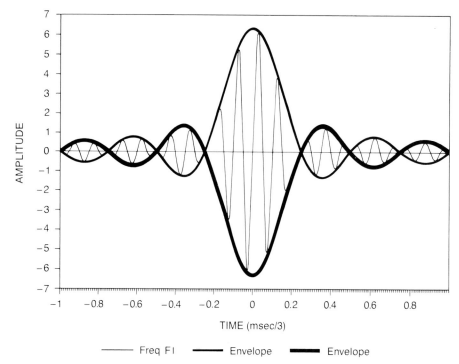

Figure 1–7. An RF envelope in the shape of a sine function has a uniform frequency distribution and a finite bandwidth, making it ideal for use in MR. Unfortunately, the pulse has an infinite time duration. Truncating the waveform in time preserves many of the advantages of the pulse, with only partial loss in edge profile. Better RF pulses are available, but this figure shows a typical envelope and the carrier frequency.

mor frequency of the spins at Za. The bandwidth of the pulse is related to the gradient strength in defining the slice thickness. The slice-select gradient is then turned off, and a frequency encoding linear magnetic field gradient is applied along the X-axis. The number of spins at each spatial location (and hence each frequency) along the axis is shown in Figure 1–8. Therefore, the signal in the coil is the sum of these frequencies, with the appropriate weighting to reflect the number of spins at each location. The signal in the coil is shown in Figure 1–8. The imager detects this signal, digitizes it (analog to digital conversion), and stores it in the computer. It would be desirable to examine the signal and determine both the frequency content (spatial location) and the amplitude (number of spins) of each frequency present. However, since all frequencies appear simultaneously, it is difficult to detect a single one. This is achieved by the Fourier transform (described more fully in the following section).

Up to this point, spatial localization along only one of the two image axes has been described as a frequency encoding. It is possible to show that each data point collected from the digitized coil signal can be related to a specific spatial frequency along that axis. Think of the image as a summation of a set of spatially varying waveforms, corresponding to different numbers of line pairs per millimeter (or centimeter). If we weight each of the waveforms appropriately and add them up, we can begin to produce an image, one-dimensional (Fig. 1–8) or two-dimensional (Fig. 1–8). It can be shown that each data point corresponds to a specific waveform (with some spatial variation in line pairs per millimeter), and the weighting is

determined from the amplitude of the detected signal. An alternative version of the units on the frequency domain data is cycles per centimeter. Immediately this should look familiar, as the standard Fourier transform is from time in seconds to frequency domain in cycles per second.[6, 12] Here, the spatial units are centimeters, and the frequency domain data are in cycles per centimeter. Note the similarity in the units. The important point is that the detected signal represents the spatial Fourier transform of the selected slice. To reconstruct the image in one dimension, an inverse Fourier transform must be performed. Now, each data point represents the contribution of a specific spatial frequency (line pairs per millimeter, if you will) to the resultant image. The Fourier conjugate variables are spatial frequency and position along the frequency encoding axis.[7, 14, 15]

Unfortunately, inverse Fourier transformation of the collected data only provides one-dimensional data of the object of interest. In order to create a two-dimensional image, spatial position along the second imaging axis must be obtained. Fortunately, this is easily accomplished by performing "phase encoding" along that axis. A short duration gradient is applied along the Y-axis prior to data collection. Therefore, each position along that axis has a different resonant frequency as determined by its spatial position and the gradient strength. The gradient is then shut off, so that the phase of each position along the axis is fixed before data collection. This is how the term "phase encoding" received its name. The experiment is repeated several times at different phase encoding gradient strengths.[14, 15]

Figure 1–9 shows a simplified MR pulse sequence,

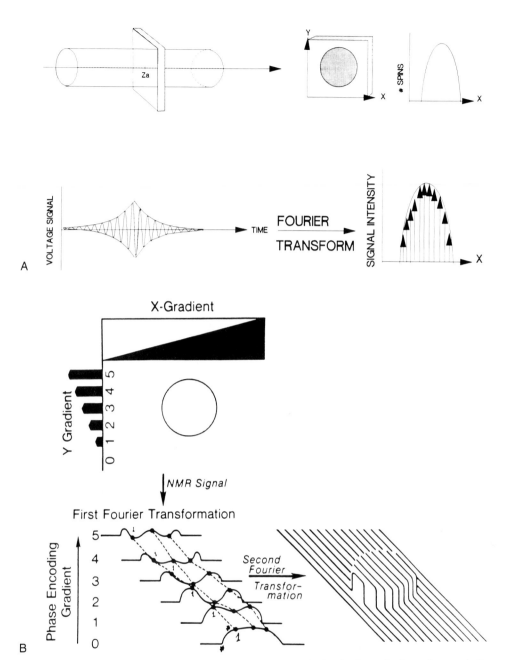

Figure 1-8. *A,* A slice along a tube at position Za is desired, and obtained using selective pulses and slice-select gradients. The projection of the tube onto the X-axis is shown. During data collection, all points along the X-axis are at different precessional frequencies. They induce voltages in the coil at that frequency and at an amplitude dependent on the number of spins at that frequency. The imaging experiment produces a signal in a detection coil like that shown, which is the sum of all signals from the various positions along the X-axis (different frequencies). The Fourier transform of the signal produces the projection of the signal onto the X-axis by taking the time domain signal and determining the various frequencies and their strength in the detected signal. *B,* Performing spatial encoding along two axes produces a set of data that contains information about spatial localization along both imaging axes. Fourier transformation of the various signals following unique "phase encodings" is shown. The final step in reconstructing the image is to perform the second Fourier transform. (From Harms SE, Morgan TJ, Yamanashi WS, et al. Principles of magnetic resonance. Radiographics 1984; 4:25–38.)

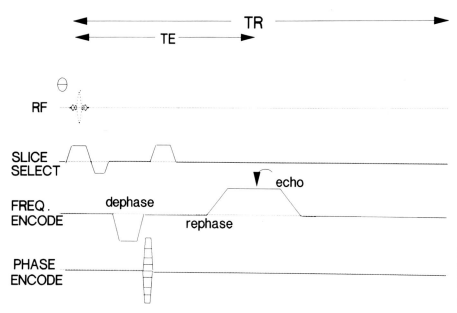

Figure 1–9. A typical gradient-echo pulse sequence is shown, with typical timings of the three imaging axes. The TR is actually much longer than that shown.

complete with slice selection and both frequency and phase encoding. It can be shown that the amount of phase encoding applied for a given experiment or "view" is given by:

amount of phase encoding is proportional to the duration of the phase encoding gradient wave form × gradient strength during phase encoding

Closer examination of the equation above shows that phase encoding is also in units of cycles per centimeter. Therefore, phase encoding performs the same task as data sampling of the induced voltage. The difference, however, is that phase encoding provides spatial frequency information about the subject along the imaging axis perpendicular to the frequency encoding direction. Therefore, by both phase encoding (probably more appropriately termed "spatial frequency encoding") and data sampling, the complete set of data obtained is the two-dimensional Fourier transform of the selected slice. In order to reconstruct the image, an inverse two-dimensional Fourier transform is required to take the data from the spatial frequency domain (the raw data, or digitized signals) to the spatial domain of the image.

The field of view along the phase encoding axis is proportional to:

$$\frac{1}{\text{phase encoding gradient step size} \times \text{duration of each gradient lobe}}$$

The resolution is equal to the field of view divided by the number of views (or data points) acquired. To increase the resolution, more phase encodings can be obtained for a given field of view, for example. To change the field of view, the strength and/or duration of the gradient lobe can be varied. A typical value of

the duration of each gradient lobe is about 3 to 5 msec, and the number of phase encodings, nenc, varies from typically 128 to 256.

Integration of Radiofrequency and Gradient Pulsing

At this point it is appropriate to describe a "generic" gradient-echo (sometimes called field-echo) pulse sequence (see Figure 1–9 again). The sequence begins by applying the slice-select gradient and RF pulse. This pulse is designed to have a finite bandwidth, as described previously, so that a finite slice thickness is obtained. The frequency offset of the pulse determines the spatial location of the selected plane. After completion of the RF pulse, the slice-select gradient often is applied negatively because the selective RF pulse can cause the excited spins from the front and back of the slice to be out of phase. The reversal of the gradient refocuses (or rephases) the spins so that they begin to precess as a coherent group.

Figure 1–9 shows that data collection does not begin immediately after the RF pulse. The RF transmitting coil often functions as the receiving coil as well. During transmission there may be several volts on the coil. During reception the induced signal in the coil may be microvolts, representing a 10^7 difference in the signal level associated with transmission and reception. Therefore, the coil's transmission voltage is allowed to die out before data collection. Further, some time is required to rephase the spins along the slice-select axis. It can be shown that the maximal signal in the X-Y plane would occur approximately halfway through the selective RF pulse. Therefore, since data collection cannot occur then, other techniques must be used to obtain a maximal signal in the detection plane.

Figure 1–9 also shows that the frequency encoding

gradient is applied negatively at first, then positively during data collection. The first gradient lobe (negative) acts to dephase the coherent group of spins in a controlled manner. Application of the gradient positively during data collection causes the spins to be rephased into forming an echo. This dephasing, followed by rephasing during data collection, allows data sampling to be performed away from the RF pulse, and also enables positive and negative spatial frequency information about the image to be obtained to simplify the two-dimensional Fourier transform reconstruction. The time that the spins rephase along the frequency encoding axis is called the echo time and is denoted by TE.[16] It should be apparent that, since each nucleus acts as a small source of magnetic field, and since the nuclei are moving randomly with respect to each other, the "time dependent" microscopic magnetic field of adjacent nuclei will cause the bulk magnetization to lose coherence and decay in magnitude. In addition to the microscopic magnetization, main field inhomogeneities cause the spins on a local level to be at slightly different field strengths, and therefore at slightly different precessional frequencies. This variation causes further loss of coherence. Together, the microscopic spin-spin interaction and the macroscopic field inhomogeneity cause the signal to decay at a rate given by $1/T2^*$. Therefore, following the RF pulse, the signal undergoes $T2^*$ relaxation. The amount that occurs is dependent on TE (the amount of time from excitation to detection). It should also be noticed that the interval between the dephase and rephase lobes of the frequency encoding axis determines the echo time, and therefore the amount of spin-spin relaxation that occurs from the start of the pulse sequence. The frequency encoding gradient strength, the data sampling interval, and the number of data points collected are adjusted to meet the desired field of view and resolution requirements in that direction.[14, 15]

Before data collection, however, the phase encoding gradient is applied to perform spatial frequency encoding along the other imaging axis. It is initiated and completed before data collection in most pulse sequences. Again, the phase encoding gradient strength, duration, and step size from one view to the next define the image spatial resolution and field of view along that axis in the image. Once data collection is finished, the remainder of the time is spent allowing the nutated magnetization to return toward equilibrium along the Z-axis. The entire sequence is reinitiated at a second phase encoding gradient value at a specific time later, called TR, the repetition time. The amount of spin-lattice relaxation that occurs from the initiation of one view to the next is dependent on TR and the T1 of the different tissues in the selected slice.[1, 2, 5] Typical values for the echo time range from about 8 to 120 msec, with corresponding TRs ranging from 50 to 3000 msec.

As shown in Figure 1–9, much time following data collection is spent with no gradient activity or data collection being performed. Therefore, to improve temporal efficiency, the pulse sequence is reinitiated at a different spatial location by simply changing the frequency offset of the RF pulse and repeating the gradient waveforms, once data collection is completed for one slice. This nesting of the data acquisition of multiple slices often allows information from all slices within the imaging volume to be obtained within one TR.

Each view of the pulse sequence may be repeated multiple times to exploit the fact that the MR signal adds linearly, with the noise adding as the square root of the number of repetitions. The ratio of the signal strength to the noise level increases with the square root of the number of repetitions of each view. Therefore, each view of the pulse sequence may be repeated several times to improve the amount of signal used in the reconstruction, relative to the amount of noise. This ratio of signal level to noise level is called the signal-to-noise ratio, and is discussed later.

There is a complex relationship between the signal intensity and the T1 and T2 relaxation times, the hydrogen concentration, the time to echo, and the pulse repetition time. The signal intensity (SI), and therefore the image intensity, at every spatial location is given by:

$$SI \propto \rho(x,y) \, (1 - e^{-TR/T1(x,y)}) \, e^{-TE/T2^*(x,y)}$$

if a 90-degree pulse is applied and TR $\gg$ T2*. T1(x,y), T2*(x,y), and $\rho(x,y)$ are the relaxation parameters and spin density of the tissue at any point in space x,y. TR and TE are acquisition parameters associated with the pulse sequence. SI is the signal intensity. This equation basically explains that the signal intensity in the generic sequence drawn earlier is dependent on the amount of magnetization available (spin density), the amount of recovery toward equilibrium between RF pulses (T1 term), and the amount of dephasing loss of signal following the RF pulse (T2 term).[1, 3, 5] Figure 1–10 shows a time-based history of the magnetization and signal in this pulse sequence. Other pulse sequences will be described later.

Advantage of the interleaved multislice acquisition:
1. Time efficiency.
Disadvantages of interleaved multislice acquisition:
1. The minimal slice thickness is limited by the maximal strength of the slice-select gradient.
2. The selective pulses do not lead to perfectly rectangular slice profiles. Therefore, RF pulses from adjacent slices interact, producing "cross-talk" between slices that further degrades slice profile and the amount of signal obtained in the images.

Three-Dimensional Data Acquisition

The spatial encoding along the frequency and phase encoding axes is independent since the axes themselves are orthogonal. Therefore, spatially encoding information along the slice-select axis can be performed in the same way as that of the phase encoding axis described earlier. That is, the slice-select and phase encoding axes can both be used for phase encoding. Here, a "slab" will be excited along the slice-select axis. This

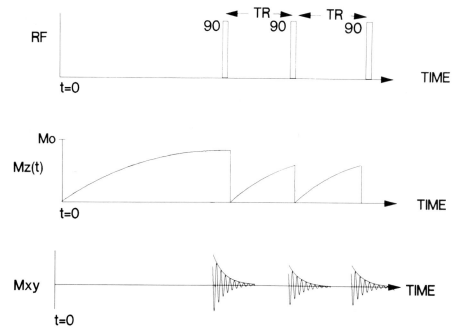

Figure 1–10. Over time, the initial equilibrium magnetization along Z develops. It is then nutated into the X-Y plane where it decays according to T2* and grows along Z via T1. The sequence is then repeated so that the same amount of magnetization is nutated into the X-Y plane following the second RF pulse.

slab represents a volume slightly greater than the previous multislice imaging volume, and is much greater than each of the individual slice thicknesses used before. After the RF pulse, rephasing is performed as before. However, phase encoding will be performed along both the phase encoding axis of the previous example and the slab-select axis. The resolution along the slab-select–phase encoding axis will be dependent on the parameters of the phase encoding used along that axis. Denote the number of phase encoding steps along the slab-select axis as $nenc_{ss}$, and the number along the primary phase encoding axis as nenc as before. The imaging time is now given by:

$$image\ acquisition\ time\ =\ TR * nenc * nenc_{ss} * reps$$

Advantages of three-dimensional image acquisition:
1. Problems associated with selective RF pulses for each slice are eliminated, since spatial position is defined along a phase encoding axis. Therefore, cross-talk and loss of signal due to imperfect RF profiles are eliminated (or at least reduced). Images obtained at the edges of the slab experience significant phase signal loss owing to the slab-selective RF pulse and are usually discarded.
2. Three-dimensional acquisition offers a technique for improved minimal slice thickness and improved signal, primarily as a result of avoiding selective pulses for defining spatial position.
3. It is possible to obtain nonsequential images from a specific imaging volume when short TRs are used. Specifically, if TR is so short that the various gradient, offset, and RF files cannot be reloaded into the computer for all the next spatial locations within TR, three-dimensional acquisitions will enable a multislice cover-

age of the imaging volume to be obtained. Often this is more time efficient than repeated two-dimensional single-slice scans to cover the same area.

Disadvantages of three-dimensional image acquisition:
1. For a given pulse sequence (specific TE, TR, FOV, and resolution), three-dimensional acquisition will take $nenc_{ss}$ times longer.
2. The reconstruction algorithm is more difficult, involves more data, and therefore takes longer.
3. Motion artifacts (discussed in a later chapter) can now appear along two phase encoding axes, instead of along one axis.

TIME TAKEN FOR PRODUCTION OF AN IMAGE

The time required to obtain all the data needed before image reconstruction depends on the repetition time, the number of views obtained (number of phase encoding steps), and the number of times each view is repeated. Therefore, the time required (T_{acq}) to perform a typical multislice imaging experiment is given by:

$$T_{acq}\ =\ TR * nenc * reps$$

where TR is the pulse repetition time, nenc is the number of phase encoding steps, and reps is the number of times each phase encoding gradient is repeated for a given slice. Interestingly, the number of slices does not affect imaging time as long as the total time spent in performing the acquisitions is less than the TR for one slice.

IMAGE RECONSTRUCTION: FOURIER TRANSFORMATION

The mathematical process of the Fourier transform performed on a time domain signal (the induced voltage) determines the frequencies present, their amplitude during detection, and their phase. Therefore, the Fourier transform (FT) can be applied to the detected voltage to determine the projection of the slice of the sample (tube of Figure 1–8) onto the frequency encoding axis, as shown earlier in Figure 1–8, since the amplitude of the frequencies present can be determined. The FT takes the time domain signal and converts it to frequency domain. Time and frequency are the Fourier conjugate variables for this one-dimensional example.

A few words about the FT are in order. First, because the signal has been digitized, a continuous function of the frequencies present in the signal cannot be obtained. Instead, discrete frequencies, corresponding to discrete locations, are produced. Fortunately, those frequencies between discrete values produced by the FT are "lumped" into the closest values.[12, 13] Therefore, although they are not obtained directly, all frequencies (corresponding to all spatial locations) are effectively accounted for. We can imagine that the frequency resolution of the FT is simply not sufficient to detect all frequencies discretely. However, frequency resolution of the FT is inversely related to the length of time spent collecting the data. Interestingly, since we have used frequency as a method of defining spatial location, the frequency resolution of the FT defines the spatial resolution in the image. Second, the digitization rate will be at least twice the highest frequency that can be determined without error (aliasing). Therefore, the digitization rate will define the highest frequency that should be allowed in the image, which will be from those at the edge of the field of view. Thus, the inverse of the digitization rate defines the highest frequency that can be present from the sample during data collection, and hence defines the gradient strength and size of the field of view. The number of data points collected multiplied by the resolution is equal to the field of view. These relationships in the imaging experiment are summarized in the three equations below:

1. $\Delta X = 1/(\text{npts } \gamma \Delta t_x G_x)$
2. field of view is proportional to time interval between digitizations^{-1} × gradient field strength^{-1}
3. bandwidth = field of view × gradient strength

where npts is the number of data points collected, t_x is the time interval between digitizations, G_x is the gradient strength (Gauss per centimeter), and γ is the gyromagnetic ratio (hertz per Gauss). Thus, the image bandwidth can be reduced by decreasing the frequency encoding gradient strength. To maintain the same resolution and field of view, the number of data points and/or the digitization interval must be increased.

Earlier it was mentioned that noise has a uniform distribution over all frequencies. Therefore, it appears desirable to limit the bandwidth in the imaging experiment to as low a level as possible, so that only a narrow band of frequencies is present in the detected signal. In this way, narrow band filters can be used in the detection of the signal, thereby reducing the total amount of noise in the image. Unfortunately, two factors prevent the widespread application of this technique. The first is that time limits involved in the imaging process prevent low-amplitude, long-duration data collections from occurring. This is described in more detail later. Second, chemical shift artifacts, associated with small resonant frequency differences between fat and water protons, increase with decreasing gradient strength (all other factors maintained to obtain the same FOV and resolution).

It is easy to understand why this occurs, and also why it occurs more prominently at high field strength. The resonant frequency of fat and water protons differs by about 3.5 ppm. At 0.5T, this corresponds to about 74 hertz difference. At 1.5T, it is about 220 hertz. The gradient strength times the field of view defines the bandwidth across the image. The number of unique points across the field of view defines the resolution, and hence the number of hertz per resolution element, or pixel. Now imagine fat and water at exactly the same spatial location. The imager will map them to the spatial location corresponding to the frequency they precess at. In this case, let us assume that we are at 1.5T, and that they resonate 220 hertz apart despite being at the same spatial location. If the image bandwidth is 14 KHz, and 256 data points are collected, the fat and water will be 4 pixels apart in the image, even though they are at the same location. If the image bandwidth is dropped to 7KHz by decreasing the gradient strength and increasing the duration of data collection and sampling interval, half the noise power will be in the image, yet the chemical shift between the fat and water will be 8 pixels, as opposed to 4 in the previous case. Therefore, image bandwidth, sampling interval, and the number of data points collected interact with the field of view in defining the amount of noise in the image, and the degree of chemical shift artifact.

T1, T2, AND SPIN-DENSITY CALCULATIONS AND IMAGES

The signal intensity in the images is theoretically a known function of imaging parameters such as TE, TR, and flip angle. Each pixel represents the manifestation of the T1, T2, and spin density of the tissue in the image signal intensity equation for the sequence used. Unfortunately, each pixel represents a single value of the mixture of T1, T2, and spin-density contributions to the image. Therefore, each pixel value is dependent on the three tissue characteristics. It is often desirable to obtain a second image dependent on two of the parameters identical to the first one, so that differences in signal intensity are a function of only the third parameter. Under these conditions it would be possible to calculate an estimate of the tissue parameter.

An example follows. Imagine obtaining a TE 20, TR 800 image over a specific field of view and slice thickness. The signal intensity at every spatial location is proportional to:

$$SI_1 \ \alpha \ (1 \ - \ e^{-800/T1(x,y)}) \ e^{-20/T2(x,y)}$$

A second image can then be obtained using a TE 20, TR 3000 pulse sequence. Here, the signal intensity is proportional to:

$$SI_2 \ \alpha \ (1 \ - \ e^{-3000/T1(x,y)}) \ e^{-20/T2(x,y)}$$

It is easily seen that the only difference in signal intensity between the two images is a result of differences in TR, and hence differences in spin lattice (T1) recovery. The ratio of the images gives:

$$SI_1/SI_2 \ = \ (1 \ - \ e^{-800/T1(x,y)})/(1 \ - \ e^{-3000/T1(x,y)})$$

so that estimates of T1 at each spatial position can be obtained by solving the above equation, often by creating a table of ratios of signal intensities as a function of T1, and then using the natural logarithm of the ratio of the images at the pixel value of interest. A similar technique can be used to obtain estimates of T2, by using different echo times and identical TRs in the two pulse sequences.

Unfortunately, every image, independent of the sequence used, is dependent on the spin density at that location. Other techniques must be used to obtain estimates of the spin density. It would be possible, for example, to solve for T1 and T2 as described above, substitute them into an equation for the signal intensity, and then find the relative differences in spin density at each spatial location.

Several attempts have been made in the past to determine accurate estimates of T1 and T2 using algorithms similar to these. Unfortunately, they have met with limited success for a variety of reasons. First, finite slice thicknesses have been used in order to obtain relatively noise-free images. Large slice thicknesses result in partial volume effects so that multiple tissues exist within each voxel, eliminating the possibility of assigning unique T1, T2, or spin densities to each location. Use of thin slices leads to significant noise levels, and therefore significant errors in the estimates. Use of multiple repetitions and thin slices leads to long imaging times, making the desired estimates impractical to obtain. Second, selective RF pulses lead to dephasing at the edges of the selected slice, and imperfect slice profiles that introduce additional errors into the estimation process. Three-dimensional techniques would eliminate these effects, but add to the scan time, as described earlier. Overall, T1, T2, and spin-density estimation techniques on whole-body MR imagers are of limited use in providing accurate estimates of these tissue parameters. Only qualitative differences should presently be inferred from results obtained from the various algorithms owing to the many unaccounted sources of error.

BASIC DESIGN OF AN MR MACHINE

The magnets and RF coils are arranged in layers on the surface of a large tube; the patient lies within this tube. The outermost structure is the large magnet, which produces a very strong uniform magnetic field. The strength of this magnet is kept constant during operation, except for time-dependent spatial variations resulting from the gradient system. The gradient fields are produced from three sets of coils, oriented orthogonally on the patient tube. Their strengths are changed repeatedly during scanning by varying the current flowing through them. Large amplifiers, similar to stereo amplifiers, are used to generate the high currents required for imaging. These are able to generate small gradient magnetic fields in any plane. Lying closer to the center of the circle are the RF coils. These transmit the RF energy required to nutate the spins from their orientation along the axis of the magnetic field, and receive the induced RF signal resulting from the precession of the spins in the X-Y plane.

The imager is also equipped with an RF amplifier used to take the RF transmission signal that is stored in the computer, amplify it, and send it to the RF transmit coil. This amplifier is similar to those used by radio stations for broadcasting their signal to their antenna, and thence through the atmosphere.

Once a signal is obtained from the patient, it must be amplified to a level that can be detected by current analog circuits. To simplify this task, a great deal of the electronics in the RF detection chain of the imager is dedicated to demodulating the RF signal from the megahertz range down to the kilohertz range. Since signal-to-noise ratio is an important determinant of image quality, it is important to design these circuits with as low a noise level as possible. Once the signal is converted to digital format (A/D conversion), it is stored in a computer. Often this same computer is responsible for storing and applying gradient waveforms, RF waveforms, controlling data sampling, and all other aspects of the imager's operation. After all data have been obtained, the computer reconstructs the image and displays it on a video monitor.

REFERENCES

1. Wolfe FL, Popp C. NMR. A primer for medical imaging. Thorofare, NJ: Slack, 1984.
2. Harms SE, Morgan TJ, Yamanashi WS, et al. Principles of nuclear magnetic resonance imaging. RadioGraphics 1984; 4:26–43.
3. General Electric. NMR: A perspective on imaging. Milwaukee, WI: General Electric Company, Medical Systems Operations.

4. Partain LC, Price RR, et al. The physical basis for NMR imaging. In: Partain CL, James AE, Rollo FD, Price RR, eds. Magnetic resonance imaging. Philadelphia: WB Saunders, 1983:73–93.

5. Wehrli FW, MacFall JR, Newton TH. Parameters determining the appearance of NMR images. In: Newton TH, Potts DG, eds. Advanced imaging techniques. Vol. 2. San Anselmo, CA: Clavadell Press, 1983.

6. Fukishima E, Roeder SB. Experimental pulse NMR: a nuts and bolts approach. Reading, MA: Addison Wesley, 1981.

7. Abragam A. Principles of nuclear magnetism. New York: Oxford University Press, 1978.

8. Slichter CP. Principles of magnetic resonance. New York: Springer-Verlag, 1980.

9. House WV. Theoretical basis for NMR imaging. In: Partain CL, James AE, Rollo FD, Price RR, eds. Magnetic resonance imaging. Philadelphia: WB Saunders, 1983:60–72.

10. Hinshaw WS, Lent AH. An introduction to NMR imaging: from the Bloch equations to the imaging equations. Proc IEEE 1983; 71(3):338–350.

11. Pykett IL. NMR imaging in medicine. Sci Am 1982; 246:5:78–88.

12. Brigham EO. The fast Fourier transform. Englewood Cliffs, NJ: Prentice-Hall, 1974.

13. Farrar TC, Becker ED. Pulse and Fourier transform NMR: introduction to theory and methods. New York: Academic Press, 1971.

14. King K, Moran PR. A unified description of NMR data collection strategies and reconstruction. Med Phys 1984; 11:1–14.

15. Kumar A, Welti D, Ernst RR. NMR Fourier zeugmatography. J Mag Res 1975; 18:69–83.

16. Hahn EL. Spin echoes. Phys Rev 1950; 80:580–584.

ADDITIONAL READINGS

Feinberg EA, Crooks LE, Sheldon P, et al. Inner volume MR imaging: technical concepts and their application. Radiology 1985; 156:743–747.

Holland GN. Systems engineering of a whole body proton magnetic resonance imaging system. In: Partain CL, James AE, Rollo FD, Price RR, eds. Magnetic resonance imaging. Philadelphia: WB Saunders, 1983:128–151.

Mansfield P. Echo planar MR imaging. NMR Images, May/June 1984:22–25.

Mansfield P, Morris PG. NMR imaging in biomedicine. Suppl 2, Advances in magnetic resonance. New York: Academic Press, 1982.

Moore WS. Basic physics and relaxation mechanisms. Br Med Bul 1984; 40(2):115–154.

Stark DD, Bradley WG. Magnetic resonance imaging. Washington, DC: CV Mosby, 1988:120–125.

Wehrli FW. Advanced MR imaging techniques. Milwaukee, WI: GE medical systems.

Basic Physics: Modifying and Interpreting the Magnetic Resonance Image

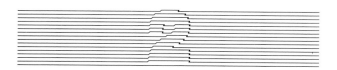

JEFFREY L. DUERK, Ph.D.

Many factors alter the MR image. MR imaging is a modality of tradeoffs, and alteration of any one factor often has both advantages and disadvantages. This chapter examines some of the factors affecting the image.

In conventional x-ray radiology the final image depends basically on *one* parameter, which is differential attenuation (absorption) of an x-ray beam by tissues. Different tissues attenuate the x-ray beam differently, thus enabling an image to be formed. On an x-ray, the order of the gray scale is fixed: bone appears white, soft tissue appears gray, fat appears a darker gray, and air appears black. The KV and mA determine the number and energy of x-ray photons, and the film sensitivity determines the gray scale. However, the principal parameter influencing the image is the attenuation of the x-ray.

Unlike x-ray imaging, MR imaging depends not on one but on at least *18* (and actually many more) separate parameters. These are:

1. The density of hydrogen atoms.
2. The T1 relaxation time.
3. The T2 relaxation time.
4. Blood flow.
5. Field of view.
6. Resolution.
7. Slice thickness.
8. TE.
9. TR.
10. RF profile, tip angle, and spatial uniformity.
11. Noise level (and bandwidth).
12. Gradient waveforms (including eddy currents).
13. Filtering schemes.
14. Transmit/receive coils.
15. Operating frequency field strength.
16. Nuclei of interest.
17. Data collection strategy (repetitions, echo planar, and so forth).
18. Other miscellaneous factors (such as temperature, artifacts).

19

FIELD STRENGTH AND MAGNET DESIGN

Advantages and Disadvantages of High Field Strength

Advantage of increasing field strength:
1. Increased signal intensity.
Disadvantages of increasing field strength:
1. Increased cost.
2. Increased artifacts—chemical shift motion sensitivity.
3. T1 relaxation time increases.
4. Increased risk of harm from magnetic foreign bodies within and without the patient.
5. Increased radiofrequency (RF) energy given to the patient. This may limit the number of slices obtainable.

Magnets

A magnetic field is required for MRI. There typically are three classes of magnets: permanent, resistive, and superconducting. Each has its own advantages and disadvantages.

Permanent Magnets

Permanent magnets are often made out of ceramic materials heated above their Curie temperature and cooled in the presence of a large magnetic field. As the ceramic cools, lattice forces exceed the magnetic forces on the molecules and atoms in the material. They are prevented from randomizing after the external magnetic field is removed, thereby remaining permanently magnetized. Large blocks of the ceramic materials can then be assembled into sheets to form a two-pole permanent magnet.

Advantages of permanent magnets:
1. Fringe magnetic fields, i.e., those outside the useful bore of the magnet, are limited in distance. This reduces the hazard of attracting stray objects into the magnet bore where the patient is located.
2. No external power supply is required to (a) get the magnet to field or (b) keep it at field.
3. The often vertical alignment of the field allows solenoidal coils to be used for detection of the MRI signal for most body parts.
Disadvantages of permanent magnets:
1. These magnets are relatively low in field strength (up to about 0.3T) unless additional supplemental resistive or superconducting windings are added.
2. They are heavy.
3. They cannot be turned off.

Resistive Magnets

Resistive magnets work on the basic principle that a current flowing through a wire produces a magnetic field. The wire is made into loops with the same current flowing through all loops. The magnetic field strength increases with the number of loops and with the amount of current flowing through them. Small-diameter wire is used so that a large number of loops of wire can be fitted into a small volume. Unfortunately, the resistance of the wire increases with length, and therefore with the number of loops. The resistance increases as the cross-sectional area of the wire decreases. Unfortunately, the power, and therefore the heat, dissipated in the magnet is proportional to the resistance of the magnet windings and to the amount of current squared. Thus, to reduce the amount of heat dissipated, low-resistance (yet finite) wire is used. The heat dissipation requires an external cooling system, like a radiator in an automobile, to keep the windings and magnet at a reasonable and constant temperature. The limitations of these magnets are primarily that they are limited to low field strength owing to tradeoffs in size for magnet windings, and heat dissipation. They also require a continuous supply of DC electrical current, and produce fringe fields extending beyond the magnet.

Superconducting Magnets

Superconducting magnets avoid the problems of heat by cooling special wire used for magnet windings below their superconducting temperature. Here, the wire has no resistance and therefore does not generate heat, regardless of diameter or current flow. Therefore, it is possible to generate a strong magnetic field using this type of magnet. The magnet windings are placed in a bath of liquid helium, which in turn is surrounded by a bath of liquid nitrogen. The liquid nitrogen insulates the helium from the external environment to reduce its conversion from liquid to gas. The magnet is designed to hold several hundred liters of both liquid gases, while maintaining magnet windings below their superconducting temperatures. Unfortunately, the insulation is not perfect, requiring periodic replenishment of the small fraction of lost liquid gases (perhaps weekly or biweekly). Alternatively, one can purchase a refrigeration unit to collect the boiled-off gases, automatically convert them back to liquid, and then resupply the magnet continuously.

If the magnet windings became nonsuperconducting, they would have a nonzero resistance, and would generate heat. This would boil off additional gases, limiting the magnet's ability to keep the remainder of the wire superconducting, thereby generating even more heat. The magnetic field collapses as current is converted to heat. This scenario is called a quench of the magnetic field. Despite what some may claim, this quench of the superconducting magnet is rare, and occurs spontaneously even more rarely.

Advantages of superconducting magnets:
1. High field strength without the need for external cooling systems or continuous supply of current.
2. Once the magnet becomes superconducting, and at field, no additional current is required.

Disadvantages of superconducting magnets:

1. They require periodic replenishment of liquid gases, or a refrigeration unit (which only reduces periodic replenishment of gases).

2. They can have significant fringe fields, thereby increasing the risk of attractive force–induced accidents.

3. They can (albeit rarely) quench, which requires significant reloading of liquid gases and possible damage to the magnet. Replacement of several hundred liters of liquid gas is a rather expensive proposition, considering that liquid nitrogen costs about as much as milk and liquid helium costs as much as 12-year-old scotch on a liter for liter comparison.

The advantages of high field strength, and hence higher signal levels, are considered by many to be a worthwhile tradeoff for the potential disadvantages.

Recently, magnet manufacturers have recognized the potential hazards of large fringe fields associated with high field superconducting magnets. Future magnets are anticipated to incorporate active or passive shielding of the fringe magnetic field. Active shielding incorporates a traditional superconducting winding magnet with a second magnet, placed outside the first, wound in the opposite direction and carrying the same current about fewer actual loops. In this way, the strength of the magnetic field inside the imager is the sum of the field produced by the traditional magnet minus the field from the additional windings in the opposite direction. The second set of windings, farther from the center bore of the magnet, produces a fringe field in the opposite direction of the main magnet's fringe field, leading to cancellation outside the magnet. The distance between the second set of windings and the traditional set determines the location of the cancellation of the fringe fields. This cancellation is achieved through more total magnet windings being required, and an overall significantly larger, heavier magnet. However, with fringe fields reduced, site design and building costs may be reduced to more than offset the additional cost of the magnet.

Magnetic Field Shielding

Construction costs for whole-body MR imagers often include steel plating to contain fringe fields within the magnet room. This method of reducing fringe fields in hallways, adjacent rooms, and rooms above or below the imager works by effectively "focusing" the magnetic field to travel through the metal as opposed to free space. To a certain extent, an analogy with current flowing through two possible paths can be used. Imagine that there are two current paths, one low resistance and one high resistance. The total current divides between the two paths, most of the current going through the path of least resistance. The magnetic field behaves somewhat similarly, by traveling through the path of highest permeability. That is, the magnetic field travels through the path that is "most permeable" to the magnetic field. The permeability of

pure iron and air is 4,000 and 1, respectively.[1] This mechanism for magnetic field containment is a form of shielding.

Imagine moving the steel in the walls closer and closer to the magnet, thereby gradually restricting the magnetic field to a smaller and smaller volume. A complete passive shielding, without the need for additional magnet windings (active shielding), could be obtained by placing a specific shape and a sufficient amount of the steel directly on the magnet proper. This would contain the field to approximately the volume enclosed by the combined magnet and steel shielding. To date, this mechanism has been used to perform both passive shielding and passive magnetic field shimming (field homogeneity optimization). Its primary advantage over active shimming lies in the slightly lower cost and slightly smaller magnets.

DETECTION COILS

Coil Design

The design of detector coils in MRI must balance several factors such as the size of the coil, its sensitivity, the resonant frequency, the bandwidth (or Q) of the coil, and the changes of the electrical circuit that occur by introducing a conducting medium (the patient) into it. A few basic rules govern the shape that the coil assumes. The first is Biot-Savart's law, which allows the spatial magnetic field resulting from passing a current through the coil to be determined.[1] The magnetic field produced by the coil at any point in space can be determined by summing the field components that arise from all infinitesimal sections along the length of the coil. The magnetic field at a fixed point in space resulting from a current flowing in the coil can be obtained by performing this summation while stepping along the entire length of the coil. By considering all points in space, or those within the region of interest of the coil, a magnetic field map from the coil can be determined.

The second rule applied is that of reciprocity. This rule states that a varying magnetic field at a fixed point in space will produce a current in the coil equal to the current that would be required to produce an alternating magnetic field of equal magnitude as the sample at that point in space. That is, we can use Biot-Savart's law to determine the magnetic field that would be produced by the coil and also the current that would be produced in the coil circuit from a varying magnetization at fixed points in space. We therefore have a mechanism to determine, a priori, the coil's spatial sensitivity. Similarly, we can determine the (spatial) uniformity of the coil's sensitivity. In order to vary these parameters, the shape of the coil must be changed.

While theoretically any coil can be used as a detector, we would prefer to maximize their response at the precessional frequency of the spins, and hence the frequency of the alternating magnetization in the X-Y plane (the Larmor frequency). To do this, a capacitor can be placed in parallel to the coil inductance to form a parallel resonant circuit.[2] This circuit produces a maximal voltage at a frequency given by:

$$\text{resonant coil frequency} = \frac{1}{2\pi\sqrt{\text{coil inductance} \times \text{parallel capacitance}}}$$

The shape of the coil, the type of wire used to form it, the number of turns, and many other factors influence the value of the inductance of the coil. Similarly, the net capacitance of the coil is dependent on the fixed capacitor used, on the type of wire used and its size, and to a smaller extent on the geometry of the wire. Therefore, the shape of the coil helps define the sensitivity, inhomogeneity, and inductance of the resonant circuit.

In MRI the potential subject population of interest and the anatomy of interest often impose constraints on the design of the detection coil, thereby limiting the number of degrees of freedom that are available in choosing its shape. However, once a shape has been determined, various sources of stray capacitance may force the inherent resonant frequency below that of the nuclei of interest. It is then necessary to insert additional circuitry or to redesign the coil to reduce the overall parallel capacitance.

A further problem is that of patient "loading" of the coil inductance. Here, the conductive medium of the body adds an additional source of magnetic permeability, altering the path of the flux linkage between the sample and the coil. Subsequently the inductance and also the stray capacitance within the coil are varied, thus changing the resonant frequency of the coil. Therefore, since each patient interacts with the coil differently, variable parallel or series capacitance can be added to the circuit so that the resonant frequency of the patient-coil system can be varied. Thus, capacitors can often be varied to allow the coil to be "tuned" to the resonant frequency of the nuclei of interest, to ensure that its performance is optimal for each patient.

An alternative approach to the loading problem often necessitating coil tuning is to design coils that eliminate or reduce patient electrical loading (capacitive) and account for approximately uniform magnetic (inductive) patient loading over the wide range of patients anticipated.[3] Here the coil would be designed to resonate initially above the Larmor frequency, so that the increased inductance of coil from the patient lowers the resulting desired resonant frequency of the coil to that of the nuclei of interest.

Another parameter is often used to characterize the response of a coil at frequencies about the Larmor frequency. This parameter is called the quality factor, or Q, of the resonant circuit and is a measure of the coil's frequency bandwidth.[2] That is, the Q of a detection circuit helps define the range of frequencies that

the coil is sensitive to and also the voltage gain in the resonant circuit above that of the coil alone. Ideally, a detection system (resonant circuit) should respond to a very narrow bandwidth, so that the amount of noise that enters the system is reduced. This would correspond to a high quality factor (high Q) corresponding to a narrow bandwidth, and a high voltage gain. Before a patient is placed on/in the coil, a typical Q might be 200 to 500. After loading, it is reduced to 20 to 100 or so. Therefore, the effect of the patient on the coil is to vary its inductance, shift the circuit's resonant frequency, and lower its Q, thereby increasing the coil's bandwidth and increasing the amount of noise in the images. It is therefore imperative to design coils with as high an unloaded and loaded Q as possible, or to design coils to eliminate or reduce patient loading.

Surface Coils

Advantages of surface coils:

1. They can be built to correspond to the shape of the body part to be imaged.

2. They are closer to the body and therefore detect a stronger signal.

Disadvantages of surface coils:

1. Detection of signal drops with distance from the coil; body parts closer to the coil produce a stronger signal.

Through the use of Biot-Savart's law and some basic electromagnetic theory, it is possible to explain why surface coils are widely used in MRI. Earlier, it was stated that Biot-Savart's law allows one to determine the sensitivity of a coil at any point in space through the concept of reciprocity. Analytically, Biot-Savart's law can be written as:

$$\vec{H} = \oint (I\, \vec{dL} \times \vec{a_R})/4\pi R^2$$

where H is the vector field, or sensitivity at any point in space, I is the current we assumed to move through the coil, dL describes the coil's shape through space, a_R is the direction between the coil and the point in space being evaluated, and R^2 is the distance from the coil to the point in space. Now, let us imagine that a 90-degree pulse has nutated the magnetization, from the spine, for example, into the X-Y plane. A whole-body coil will be several centimeters away, such that $1/R^2$ is a small number. On the other hand, a surface coil could be placed within millimeters of the spine, so that $1/R^2$ is much larger, resulting in higher sensitivity and thus increased signal from the spine if all other factors were the same.

A second advantage of surface coils is that they can be designed to have a sensitive volume limited to only the anatomic region of interest. The advantage of this is that patient noise, or thermal noise–induced variation in the coil voltage unrelated to the NMR signal from the patient, is often the dominant source of noise in MRI. Electronic noise is often secondary to patient noise. Therefore, any point in space that is both occupied by the patient and the coil will be a source of noise in the signal, regardless of whether that tissue is to be in the image. Again, imagine the body coil, and a surface coil, now in relation to noise. Body coils are often designed to have uniform sensitivity throughout an imaging volume that may be 50 cm^3 or more. The image we desire is again of the lumbar spine, as an example. The image will contain signal from the image plane that we selected with the RF pulses. The noise in the image will result from thermal noise from all points in the coil occupied by the subject. This may be a significant portion of the coil's sensitive volume. The surface coil image will be performed at the same spatial location, under the same pulse sequence conditions. However, it is designed to have a limited sensitive volume, so that the volume of the patient that contributes to the overall amount of patient noise is less. Therefore, the surface coil generally has increased sensitivity, corresponding to increased detected signal, and decreased noise through limitation of its sensitive volume.

The noise in MRI, although primarily attributed to patient sources, has some interesting characteristics that will be useful in describing a recent advance in transmission and/or detection coils, and also later when signal to noise and contrast to noise are discussed. The noise can be considered white noise, with equal strength at all frequencies. This implies that the noise signal superimposed on top of the MR signal is not correlated with the noise that occurs later. Because of this, adding N repetitions of the same signal gives rise to N times the signal, and an $N^{1/2}$ of the noise. Therefore, multiple repetitions on a sequence can give rise to an improvement in signal-to-noise ratio in NMR (or MRI). We can view this addition, or averaging, as being successful because there are multiple repetitions of the signal, with no repetition of the same noise signal.

Quadrature Coils

An alternative mechanism for producing independent noise signals is to design quadrature detection systems constructed of two separate coils. Each coil detects a different part of the magnetization in the X-Y plane: one detecting signal in the X and one detecting signal in the Y direction. Thus, the two coils give rise to two signals, each with their own noise content. By adding the signals a similar reduction in noise occurs, so that the effective signal-to-noise ratio in the quadrature coil becomes $\sqrt{2}$ times better than a similar nonquadrature (linear) coil.

Quadrature transmit coils offer two other advantages over linear (standard) transmit coils. The first is that they require half the transmitted power to achieve any degree pulse compared with linear coils. Basically, transmission in a linear coil involves the use of an oscillating RF pulse along one of the axes in the laboratory frame. This RF signal can be viewed as two separate signals, one rotating in the same direction as the precessing spins and one rotating in exactly the opposite direction.[4] Clearly, the component rotating at the same frequency as the precessing spins appears stationary in the rotating reference frame. The other component is viewed as precessing backward at twice the Larmor frequency and does not contribute significantly to the nutation of the spins from the Z-axis toward the X-Y plane. Thus, half the linearly transmitted RF pulse goes toward nutation, while the other half is of no use.

A quadrature coil is capable of producing the rotating RF field directly, thereby eliminating the production of the counterrotating (useless) component. Here, all the RF energy goes toward nutation of the spins. Figure 2–1 shows the effect of the rotating RF component (in the laboratory and rotating reference frame) nutating the magnetization from the Z-axis toward the X-Y plane. The second advantage of quadrature over linear coils lies in the fact that the induction of a B1-RF field for nutation in a coil is opposed, via Faraday's (or Lenz's) law, by an opposing field. In the linear transmission case, there are regions that the opposing field adds and subtracts from the applied field, thereby producing a nonuniform transmission (and reception) profile across a sample. Needless to say, the spatial distribution of this opposing field is dependent on the geometry of a sample, its conductivity, and the frequency of the applied field. A circular uniform phantom filled with a conducting fluid shows this effect well (Figs. 2–23A and 2–23C). Compared to a patient (Fig. 2–2A), the shading is more pronounced on the phantom images owing to longer uninterrupted eddy current paths and other geometric and conductivity effects.[5]

Quadrature coils, on the other hand, can be viewed as producing two similar distortion fields that are 90 degrees out of phase with one another. Here, the dark regions of one field can be superimposed on the bright bands from the component 90 degrees out of phase to produce an averaging effect. Similarly, this produces "bright on dark" averaging across other regions.[5] Therefore, the net effect is a more uniform transmission and reception field (Figs. 2–2B, and 2–23B and D). All images in Figures 2–2 and 2–23 were obtained on the same imager, same phantom, and same pulse sequence, or on the same volunteer under similar controlled conditions. Therefore, quadrature coils offer several significant advantages over linear coils for both transmission and detection.

SIGNAL INTENSITY

Summary of Tissue Factors Influencing Signal

A weak signal is obtained (on many pulse sequences) from tissues with:
1. Long T1 relaxation times.
2. Short T2 relaxation times.
3. Low concentration of hydrogen.

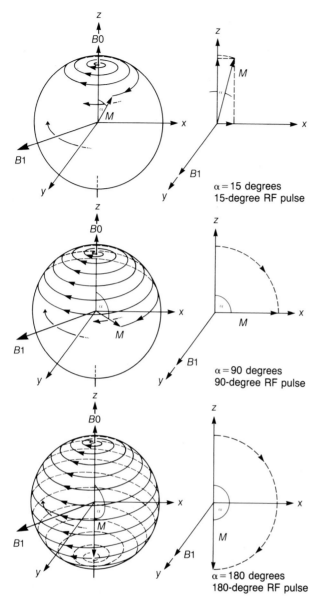

α = 15 degrees
15-degree RF pulse

α = 90 degrees
90-degree RF pulse

α = 180 degrees
180-degree RF pulse

Figure 2–1. Applying an RF pulse is shown in both the laboratory frame of reference and in the rotating reference frame. The tip angle is dependent on the strength of the B1 field and the amount of time it is applied. In the rotating frame the motion of the bulk magnetic moment is a simple precession about the B1 field that appears static. In the laboratory frame there is both precession and nutation about the oscillating B1 field. The description (mathematical) is much more complicated in the laboratory frame. However, the figure represents the nutation of Mz into the X-Y plane. (From Pykett IL. NMR imaging in medicine. Scientific American 1982; 246(5):78–88.)

4. Rapid flow.

A strong signal is obtained (on many pulse sequences) from tissues with:

1. Short T1 relaxation times.
2. Long T2 relaxation times.
3. High concentration of hydrogen.
4. Slow laminar flow.

We can generate images that depend primarily on T1

(T1 weighted), T2 (T2 weighted), or hydrogen concentration (spin density weighted).

The order of gray scale of tissues on MR images can be manipulated by utilizing different pulse sequences. Thus, for example, fluids can be made darker or whiter than muscle. The whiteness on an MR image is proportional to the strength of the signal received back from the body.

The reasons why T1 relaxation time, T2 relaxation time, and hydrogen concentration (or more appropriately, spin density) affect the signal strength and hence image whiteness are as follows:

1. The more hydrogen that is present in a defined area, the stronger is the overall signal received from that area.

2. T1 relaxation time. Tissues with a long T1 relaxation time yield a much weaker signal than tissues with short T1 relaxation times owing to incomplete recovery between RF pulses in many sequences. When the T1 relaxation time is short, hydrogen atoms that have been nutated away from equilibrium can quickly and fully recover and are then available to be flipped again by the next pulse sequence, causing more signal. Tissues with long T1 relaxation times cannot recover as quickly and are not available to be restimulated as rapidly. They therefore produce a weaker signal.

3. T2 relaxation time. Tissues with long T2 relaxation times often produce a strong signal and therefore appear white on images. T2 relaxation time is a parameter describing the time that the hydrogen atoms are rotating coherently in the transverse (X-Y) plane. The longer they keep rotating, the longer they keep yielding a signal, with the result that the overall signal from them is higher.

Simplified definitions of T1 and T2 relaxation times are:

T1. The longitudinal relaxation time. The parameter describing how the signal returns to equilibrium exponentially, characterized by a time constant, T1.

T2. The transverse relaxation time. After an RF flip into the X-Y plane, the net magnetic moment precesses about the transverse plane and generates a voltage in a receive coil (the MR signal). As the spins precess, they lose coherence, and the net magnetization decreases exponentially, owing to spin-spin interactions. T2 is the parameter that describes this exponential loss of magnetization.

Detailed Discussion

T1 Relaxation (Spin Lattice)

As we showed earlier, the energy of the MRI system is rather low in relation to thermal energies of the body (translation, rotation, and vibration of molecules) or the energies associated with common radiographic modalities such as x-ray.[6] The thermal agitation of the spin system in the weak earth's magnetic field prevents any significant net magnetic moment in the body from

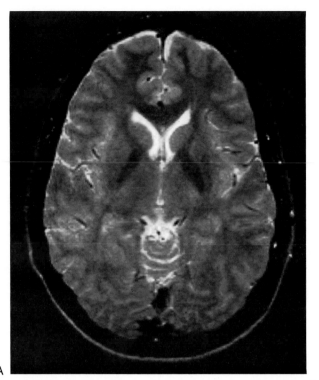
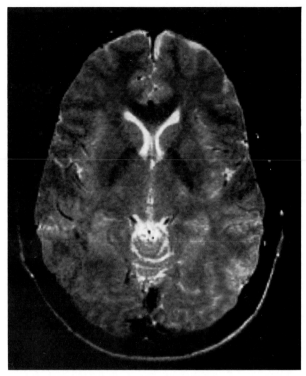

A   B

Figure 2–2. Quadrature coils offer a theoretical improvement of $(2)^{1/2}$ in signal to noise over linear coils. This figure shows two head images obtained using a linear coil (*A*) and a quadrature coil using the same pulse sequence. Note the improved SNR in (*B*).

being produced. However, once placed in a strong magnetic field, a net alignment of spins (hydrogen atoms) occurs as energy is given off by the protons to the surrounding lattice.[7,8] High energy spins opposed to the field give up a sufficient amount of energy to go through the transition from a high energy state to a low energy state (aligned with the field). However, the development of the net magnetic moment takes a finite amount of time since billions and billions of spins must give up their energy to the lattice. Further, the lattice accepts energy only until the energy associated with the net population difference is balanced by the thermal energy (or temperature) of the lattice.

We can use a basic analogy to this situation by thinking of a cup of hot water (the spin system) and the environment. When the water is taken off a hot stove, the mean temperature of the water molecules is significantly different from that of the environment, and a significant amount of energy is transferred from the water to the environment. The mean temperature of the water falls as the environment accepts the energy. However, the temperature of the environment does not change significantly since there is so much of it. As time goes on, the rate of energy transfer becomes less since the temperature difference between the two systems (water and environment) is so small. Eventually, the two are at the same temperature, called equilibrium, where the water transfers as much energy to the environment as the environment does to the water.

For our spin system and the lattice (the body), a similar situation develops. Here, high energy spins give up energy to the lattice, and a net population difference begins to develop rapidly. As time progresses, the system of spins and environment approaches a net magnetic moment corresponding to the equilibrium net alignment of spins. The rate of energy transfer becomes less as the system approaches equilibrium. This rate of development of net magnetic moment resulting from the transfer of energy from the spins to the lattice is characterized by a single parameter called T1, the spin-lattice relaxation rate. It can be shown that the net magnetization along the Z-axis (M_z), as a function of time (t), can be written as:

$$M_z(t) = M_o(1 - e^{-t/T1})$$

where M_o is the equilibrium magnetization, t is time, and T1 is the spin-lattice relaxation rate for the spins.[6–9] Therefore, the equilibrium magnetization is produced over time, at an exponential rate with a time constant given by T1. At higher field strengths, the energy difference between states is greater and the number of spins that will align is greater, both of which contribute to the known increase in T1 with increased field strength.[7,8]

Figure 2–3 shows a graph of the development of net magnetization along the Z-axis for two tissues with differing T1s and loss of signal in the X-Y plane, as

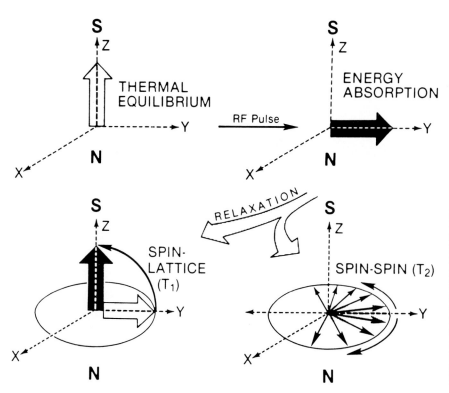

Figure 2–3. A sample placed in a magnetic field produces a net magnetic moment when in thermal equilibrium with the lattice. The moment is aligned with the magnetic field. An RF pulse is used to nutate the magnetization into the X-Y (detection) plane, where the spins begin to precess about the field, losing coherence and returning to equilibrium magnetization. The two processes are called spin-spin (T2) relaxation and spin-lattice (T1) relaxation, respectively. (From Harms SE, Morgan TJ, Yamanashi WS, et al. Principles of nuclear magnetic resonance imaging. RadioGraphics 1984; 4:26–43.)

described later in the discussion of T2. Figure 2–4 examines the difference of the development of magnetization along the Z-axis for tissues with different T1s.

The development of magnetization along the Z-axis is more difficult than described previously. For relaxation to occur, there must be some varying magnetic field in the X-Y plane to "stimulate" the spin to give up its energy. The probability of the spin undergoing spontaneous emission of the energy difference between the high and the low energy state varies inversely with the third power of the frequency, and is therefore an extremely remote possibility at the RF (megahertz) frequencies used in MRI.[10] Fortunately, the rotation, translation, and vibration of the lattice molecules provide this varying magnetic field on a local microscopic level. A concept, called the correlation time (τ_c), gives us a means of describing the motion of lattice molecules and hence variation of the magnetic fields near the spin.[7, 10] Imagine a large (or cold) and a small (or hot) molecule model for the lattice. The large molecule will tumble slowly, leading to rather low-frequency variation of the magnetic field associated with various portions of the molecule. The variation at the Larmor frequency of our spins will act to realign the spins along the Z-axis. Unfortunately, for the large molecules the variation is primarily low frequency, and provides little variation at the Larmor frequency. In this case, T1 would be long. If all the molecules were small, the range of frequencies would be high, yet the strength of the varying magnetic field at any specific frequency is low. This also produces little interaction at the Larmor

frequency, and a long T1 for the spin system. However, T1 is shortest when $1/\tau_c$ is approximately equal to the Larmor frequency of the nuclei of interest. Under these conditions, there are maximal strength frequency components at the Larmor frequency of the nuclei. Figures 2–5 and 2–6 provide examples of the frequency content of the variation of the magnetic field as a function of correlation time, and also the variation of T1 as the correlation time changes for a fixed nuclei in a fixed field.

The correlation time of the patient can be considered as a constant as the field strength is varied. After all, the molecules of the body are the same, and thus their motion is the same from one field strength to the next. What changes, however, is the Larmor frequency of the spins. This changes the frequency of varying magnetic fields in the X-Y plane required to obtain realignment of the spins along the Z-axis. Since the correlation time of the lattice is fixed, the frequency content of the varying magnetic fields is also fixed. Figure 5 shows that as the resonant frequency is increased, the strength of the frequency content of the varying magnetic fields at the new Larmor frequency is less.[8] This leads to reduced energy of interaction between the varying field and the spins, causing a slower relaxation toward equilibrium, and hence an increased T1. This is the source of increased T1 at higher magnetic fields. The frequency content of local magnetic fields is weaker at high frequencies than at lower resonant frequencies owing to the fixed correlation time of the lattice components.

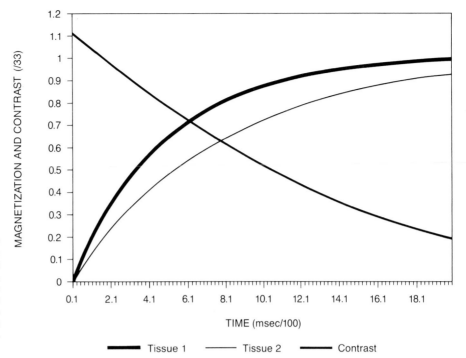

Figure 2–4. Once nutated into the X-Y plane, spin-lattice (T1) relaxation attempts to realign the spins along the axis of the magnetic field. To do this, spins must give up energy to the lattice. This figure shows the return to equilibrium of two tissues, with different T1s. The contrast curve details the relative difference in recovery between the two tissues over time.

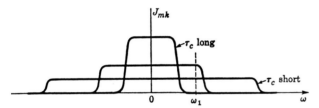

Figure 2–5. The correlation time of the lattice components provides a measure of the frequency content of the time-varying magnetic fields required to stimulate the spins into giving up the absorbed RF energy. Imagine a resonant frequency of the spin system being ω1. The long correlation time lattice provides little stimulation at ω1 since most of the frequency content is low frequency. On the other hand, the short correlation time lattice components have all frequencies present, yet little strength at ω1. Both of these conditions result in long T1s. There is, however, an ideal lattice that provides excellent stimulation at ω1 and a short T1. If the resonant frequency of the system is changed to a higher value (higher magnetic field strength), the lattices will have less energy at the higher frequency, and therefore a longer T1 will result. (From Slichter CP. Principles of magnetic resonance. New York: Springer-Verlag, 1980: 164–167.)

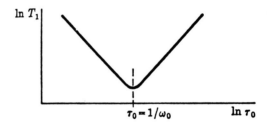

Figure 2–6. As the correlation time of a lattice increases or decreases, the T1 of the system at a fixed frequency also varies. Imagine increasing the correlation time of a lattice by heating it, and examining the T1. At some point the correlation time will provide optimal stimulation at the frequency of interest. Above or below that correlation time, T1 will lengthen. (From Slichter CP. Principles of magnetic resonance. New York: Springer-Verlag, 1980: 164–167.)

$$\omega_L(x, y) = \gamma B(x, y)$$
$$= \gamma(B_o + B\Delta(x, y))$$

where γ is the gyromagnetic ratio, B_o is the main static magnetic field, and $B(x,y)$ is the field inhomogeneity at every spatial location. Typical values of ΔB over the useful volume of a present 1.5T magnet are about 10 to 20 parts per million (ppm), which therefore represents a variation of the precessional frequencies of approximately 1,200 Hertz (at 64 MHz).

Immediately following the RF pulse, all the spins are oriented along one of the axes in the rotating reference frame (Fig. 2–7A). If all spins were at the same frequency, they would precess as a coherent group, all traveling together in their precession about the static magnetic field. However, since the field is inhomogeneous, some spins precess faster (positive ΔB) and

T2 Relaxation (Spin-Spin Decay)

Following the RF pulse, an oscillating voltage at the Larmor frequency is induced in a detection coil, since all protons are ideally at the same magnetic field strength. However, the main static magnetic field is not perfectly homogenous, which in turn sets up a variation of the precessional frequency of the protons in the magnetic field. The key concept to remember is that the precessional frequency of the spins in the XY plane ($\omega_L(x,y)$) is given by:

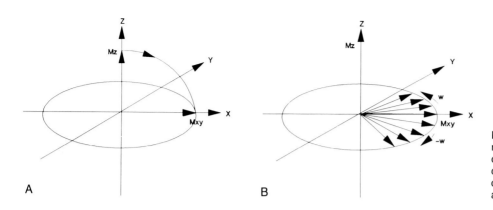

Figure 2–7. Once the spins are nutated into the X-Y plane, they dephase and lose coherence owing to (**A**) magnetic field inhomogeneities and (**B**) spin-spin interactions.

some precess slower (negative ΔB) than those at exactly the static magnetic field. Therefore, the spins lose coherence as the faster spins precess ahead and the slower spins fall behind (Fig. 2–7B).

This dephasing, or loss of coherence, causes the overall vector strength of the magnetic moment tipped into the X-Y plane to diminish over time. This loss of signal is called transverse relaxation and is characterized by a time constant, T2. It can be shown that the loss of signal follows an exponential relaxation curve, so that the magnetization in the X-Y plane (M_{xy}) following a 90-degree RF pulse is given by:

$$M_{xy}(t) = M_z\, e^{-t/T2^*}$$

where M_z is the amount of magnetization along the Z-axis prior to the RF pulse.

While the use of the inhomogeneity of the magnetic field is capable of describing a portion of the loss of signal in the X-Y plane, it is not complete. It provides only the loss of signal on a macroscopic level. To determine the additional causes of loss of coherence, the spin system on a microscopic (molecular) level must be examined. When this is done, the magnetic fields associated with portions of neighboring molecules contribute to a random source of dephasing as they rotate, translate, and vibrate. Similarly, the adjacent protons (or spins) contribute as they move about as well. Thus, transverse relaxation has the additional name of spin-spin relaxation owing to the interaction between neighboring magnetic moments causing a random loss of signal in the X-Y plane. Overall, the rate of loss of signal in the X-Y plane can be described as:

$$1/T2^* = 1/T2 + \gamma\Delta B$$

This expression states that the apparent rate of transverse relaxation (T2*) is determined from the true random spin-spin interaction (T2) plus a term due to the constant magnetic field inhomogeneity (ΔB) over the sample (or patient). Later it will be shown how to remove the constant inhomogeneity term so that the only source of loss of signal is due to T2 alone. Figure 2–8 shows the decay of the transverse magnetization due to T2.

Imagine a series of 90-degree RF pulses applied sequentially, TR apart in time, with TR much greater than T2, as described earlier. The amount of magnetization nutated into the X-Y plane is given by the amount of magnetization along the Z-axis prior to the RF pulse. That is:

$$M_z(t) = M_o(1 - e^{-TR/T1})$$

where different tissues may have different T1s. Thus, different tissues have different amounts of magnetization tipped into the X-Y plane. Once in the detection plane, the signals decay according to their T2*s. Thus, the signal strength in the X-Y plane for a simple repeated free induction decay sequence of 90-degree pulses is given by:

$$M_z(t) = M_o(1 - e^{-TR/T1})\, e^{-t/T2^*}$$

where different tissues may have differences in their T1s and T2s. Therefore, through analyses such as these, the contrast between tissues can be described for a variety of MR pulse sequences.

PULSE SEQUENCES

Summary of Practical Information

By the term pulse sequence, we mean the timing and nature of the RF exciting pulses that are beamed into the body and the gradient waveforms used for slice selection or spatial localization. Many different pulse sequences are available and each has definite advantages and disadvantages. A pulse sequence consists of a series of pulses of radiowaves (each of specific duration and strength), applied fairly rapidly in succession. The time interval between the start of one repetition of the pulse sequence and the start of the next is termed the pulse repetition time (TR). It is usually between 200 and 3,000 msec. In any pulse sequence the time between the excitation RF pulse (often a 90-degree pulse) and the moment at which the returned signal from the body is read is termed the time to echo (TE).

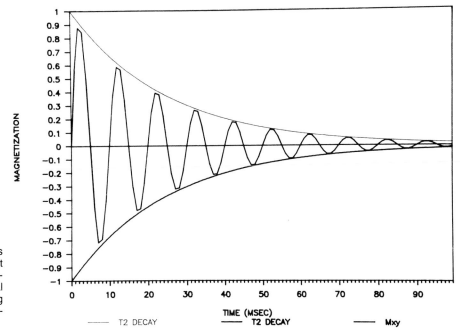

Figure 2-8. The loss of signal occurs as the magnetization precesses about the magnetic field at the Larmor frequency. This figure shows a typical free induction decay (FID) showing both the precession and the exponential decay.

Spin-Echo Pulse Sequences
Advantages:
1. Field inhomogeneity effects are eliminated.
2. Images can be obtained at different TEs (and the same TR) with a single repetition time; i.e., images can be obtained at multiple-echo times within a given TR.
Disadvantages:
1. TEs are routinely unavailable below about 10 msec.
2. Tissue heating effects (SAR) due to multiple RF pulses may limit the number of slices acquired for a given TR.
Effects:
1. Increasing TE: increases T2 weighting.
2. Increasing TR: increases signal strength.
    decreases T1 weighting of the image.
    increases the number of slices that can be obtained.
    increases scan time.
To obtain "T1 weighting" use:
 short TR and short TE
 TR less than approximately 600 msec
 TE as short as possible and less than approximately 40 msec
To obtain "T2 weighting" use:
 long TR and long TE
 TR: greater than approximately 1500 msec
 TE: greater than approximately 50 msec

Inversion Recovery Pulse Sequences
Advantages:
1. Can selectively depress signal from any tissue, e.g., fat (when used with a short time to inversion-STIR [short tau inversion recovery] sequence).

2. Can reduce or eliminate ghost motion artifacts from fat.
3. High contrast through strong T1 weighting.
4. Decrease chemical shift artifact (suppress fat).
5. Mixed T1, T2 contrast through use of varying TE on data collection.
Disadvantages:
1. Require a long imaging time.
2. Require a long reconstruction time if phase correction techniques are used.

Field (Gradient)-Echo Pulse Sequences
Advantages:
1. Can produce T2 weighted images with very short acquisition time.
2. Can be used with very short TEs and flip angles less than 90 degrees.
3. Can be performed rapidly.
Disadvantages:
1. Number of slices is limited (if short TR is utilized).
2. Contrast is sometimes decreased owing to field inhomogeneity.
3. Signal strength is decreased (worse signal-to-noise ratio).
4. Increased motion and flow artifacts.
5. Increased susceptibility to field inhomogeneity (worse at higher magnetic field strengths).
6. Flowing blood often appears white.
To obtain T1 weighted image use:
 short TE, 12 to 15 msec
 high flip angle, 45 to 90 degrees
To obtain T2 weighted image use:
 long TE, 50 to 90 msec, high flip angle

or

low flip angle, 5 to 20 degrees, short TE

To obtain spin density weighted image use:

short TE, 12 to 15 msec

high flip angle, long TR, 2,000 to 3,000 msec

Detailed Review

The following sections describe various pulse sequences currently available on many MR imagers, their contrast mechanism, and the impact of various changes in scan parameters on both signal to noise, and a parameter called contrast to noise. Terms such as "T1 weighted," "T2 weighted," and "spin density weighted" are used, but it should be recognized that these apply to the primary mode of contrast production between most tissues. This does not imply that the other parameters are not affecting contrast. All images are always a mix of contributions from their spin density, their T1, and their T2.[11]

Contrast-to-Noise Ratio

The contrast-to-noise ratio (CNR) is the percentage of signal intensity difference between tissues in the MR images. The basic contrast (C) between tissues is given by the expression below:

$$C = (SI_1 - SI_2)/SI_1 * 100\%$$

where SI_1 is the greater of the two signal intensities. This parameter is a measure of how different tissues appear in an image. Unfortunately, the presence of noise in the image adds some uncertainty to the signal intensities, thereby adding some uncertainty to the true contrast between tissue. The CNR between tissues is given by the ratio of the contrast to the peak-to-peak or root-mean-squared (RMS) noise in the image. CNR is a measure of how well the contrast between tissues is appreciated. Higher CNR indicates high contrast between tissues despite any noise in the image, and can result from moderate contrast and low noise, or exceptional contrast even with significant noise. A low CNR indicates that the contrast between tissues is not well appreciated, either because of lack of inherent contrast between them or because of uncertainty due to high noise levels.

Contrast-to-noise ratios and signal-to-noise ratios (SNR) both deal with aspects of image quality, yet are somewhat independent. Figure 2–9A is an image of the brain taken to intentionally have a high SNR and yet a low CNR. That is, the image is not grainy (high SNR), but there is not significant contrast between the different tissues in the brain (low CNR). Figure 2–9B shows the same anatomic location, but from a different pulse sequence. This image has a significantly degraded SNR and appears relatively "noisy" (low SNR). On the other hand, the contrast between tissues is quite good, indicative of a high CNR. The CNR and SNR change as pulse sequence timing parameters are varied.

Studies have reported that humans can detect signal intensity differences in the presence of noise if the CNR is approximately greater than 0.05, i.e., if the contrast in the absence of noise is greater than 5 percent. If the noise led to a 5 percent variation in the signal intensity in both tissues, it would be difficult, if not impossible, to differentiate between the two.

Gradient Echoes or Field Echoes

These represent one of the simplest MR imaging techniques available. The three parameters required to characterize the basic contrast mechanism are Θ (RF tip angle), TE (echo time), and TR (repetition time). The equation governing the contrast between tissue is given by:

$$SI \propto \sin\Theta\, \rho(x,y)\, (1 - e^{-TR/T1(x,y)})\, e^{-TE/T2^*(x,y)}/ (1 - \cos\Theta\, e^{-TR/T1(x,y)})$$

The first feature that stands out is that T2 contrast between tissue is dependent on T2*, and therefore on field homogeneity. Second, the contrast can be varied significantly as the RF tip angle is varied.

Assume that a 90-degree tip is used. Here the signal intensity for the various tissues becomes:

$$SI \propto \rho(x,y)\, (1 - e^{-TR/T1(x,y)})\, e^{-TE/T2^*(x,y)}$$

which indicates that TR and TE can both be used to alter signal intensity for that spin density. On the other hand, assume that a 5- to 10-degree RF pulse is used. Under these conditions the pixel value becomes proportional to:

$$SI \propto \sin\Theta\, \rho(x,y)\, e^{-TE/T2^*(x,y)}$$

That is, under these conditions, each tissue's signal intensity is primarily dependent on the T2* of the tissue (i.e., the T2 of the tissue and field inhomogeneity in that region). As we reach regions between 10 and 90 degrees, the repetition time, and hence T1, becomes more important.

Analyzing the contrast between tissues when 90 degrees is used is fairly simple if the equation is handled piece by piece. First, the signal intensity of any tissue in the body is dependent on the number of protons per unit volume (spin density) in that tissue. Second, the amount of magnetization nutated into the X-Y plane is dependent on the T1 of the material, and how long it has had to relax toward equilibrium since the last RF pulse. Finally, once that magnetization is in the X-Y plane, T2* decay occurs. Differences in T1, T2*, and spin density can all be exploited by appropriate selection of TR and TE.

T1 based contrast between tissues can be obtained by minimizing the contributions due to T2. To do this, short echo times of less than 20 msec are often used, so

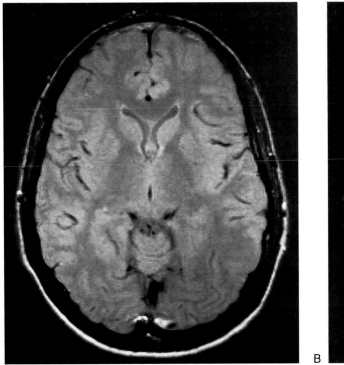
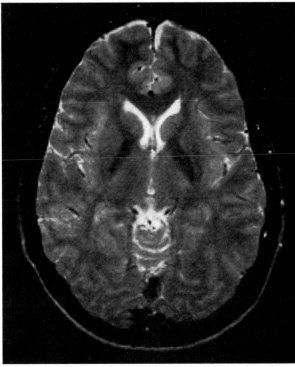

A   B

Figure 2–9. These images of the head are used to demonstrate differences in contrast to noise and signal to noise. **A** has high signal to noise yet low contrast between tissues; **B** has high contrast and low signal to noise. The only difference between the scans is the echo time.

that the T2 based exponential term is approximately equal to unity for all tissues (no T2* differences between them for normal tissue). This has the added benefit of providing data collection prior to any significant loss of signal due to T2* decay. Second, a short repetition time helps maximize contrast differences between tissues as a result of their T1. Unfortunately, short TRs indicate that only a short interval of time is available for spin lattice recovery. Therefore, although good T1 contrast would be obtained, the SNR would be rather poor. In the limit of decreasing TR there would be no contrast if no signal were obtained. (It is at this point that SNR and CNR become quite directly related.) Therefore, a short TE and a short TR (but not too short) are capable of exploiting T1 differences between tissues. As the TR is increased, greater amounts of signal are obtained from all tissues, yet the differences between them are reduced (percentage-wise) since they all tend toward their bulk magnetic moment associated with their spin density. Thus, increased signal would be obtained at the expense of reduced contrast (higher SNR, lower CNR).[4, 10–13]

On the other hand, it may be desirable to obtain images with contrast primarily due to spin density differences between tissues. Immediately, we know that short TEs are required to reduce T2* contrast. The portion of the contrast equation dealing with T1 differences must be made independent of T1. This can be done by using a repetition time much longer than the longest T1 in the selected slice. Thus, long TRs and short TEs are capable of producing spin density weighted contrast.

If T2* contrast is desired, either of the above two equations can be used. By using a partial tip angle, it is obtained immediately. Alternatively, the equation dealing with a 90-degree pulse would indicate that T2* contrast could be obtained at a long TR, typically 1,800 to 3,000 msec, to produce reduced T1 contrast. A long TE provides maximal T2* differentiation. Here again, however, we run into the problem of lack of signal, this time due to significant transverse relaxation prior to data collection. Therefore, the echo time must be adjusted to meet SNR and CNR tradeoffs. It should also be pointed out that the transverse relaxation in these examples deals with both T2, the spin-spin relaxation rate of the protons in that tissue, and with a term dealing with field inhomogeneity. Therefore, field echo imaging sequences generally use a short echo time, to reduce the amount of signal loss due to main field inhomogeneity dephasing. Second, since the sequence is sensitive to field inhomogeneity effects, artifacts are often produced in areas of high magnetic susceptibility differences. The amount of dephasing is worse at high field (for a given field difference in parts per million [ppm], as described shortly).

The most common technique for T2* based contrast

between tissue in the gradient-echo pulse sequences is through the partial tip angle techniques. The RF pulse tips the bulk magnetization away from the Z-axis, projecting a small component into the X-Y plane, and leaving most of the magnetization along the Z-axis. The signal in the X-Y plane decays according to T2*s of the tissues, while recovery along the Z-axis toward equilibrium is virtually complete, since very little was taken into the X-Y plane. A 10-degree tip, for example, projects a component into the X-Y plane that is 17.4 percent of the bulk magnetization value. A component 98.5 percent as strong as M_o is left along the Z-axis. Thus, once the RF pulse is completed, the magnetization is already 98.5 percent recovered to its bulk magnetic moment, and T1 differences are minimized, since they deal with recovery along the Z-axis.

The effect of field inhomogeneity on field-echo pulse sequences is field strength dependent. Field inhomogeneity is often measured in ppm, and can lead to some confusion related to the effect in field-echo scans. Imagine a 0.5T and a 1.5T magnet, both shimmed to give a mean field inhomogeneity of 10 ppm over the useful volume of the imager, with a mean inhomogeneity of 1 ppm per voxel. At 1.5T, the field variation (B) over one voxel is approximately:

$$\Delta B = 1 \times 10^{-6} * 1.5T$$
$$= 15 \text{ milli-Gauss}$$

At 0.5T, the same field inhomogeneity gives rise to a field variation of only 5.0 milli-Gauss. Therefore, the difference in the distribution of resonant frequencies over the voxel is three times higher at 1.5T than at 0.5T. This leads to a threefold increase in the amount of dephasing, for a given pulse sequence, at 1.5T compared with 0.5T despite the fields being at the same homogeneity. Therefore, the amount of loss of signal due to dephasing at 0.5T is less than at 1.5T. Similarly, the lower sensitivity to field variation at 0.5T leads to fewer (or less significant) magnetic field susceptibility difference artifacts than comparable images at 1.5T.

While gradient-echo techniques offer tremendous contrast flexibility, they suffer from being susceptible to significant losses of signal and artifact owing to main field inhomogeneities, or field distortions due to magnetic field susceptibility differences in the body that often occur near air-bone-tissue interfaces. However, they can often be used to produce T2-like weighted scans in a fraction of the time associated with other pulse sequences.

Spin-Echo Pulse Sequences

The most common type of MRI pulse sequence is the multislice spin-echo pulse sequence, or its variant the multiecho sequence. Figure 2–10 shows a typical example of a spin-echo pulse sequence. The principal difference between the spin-echo and gradient-echo sequences is the application of a 180-degree RF pulse halfway through the sequence, and a positive gradient

strength dephase lobe along the frequency encoding axis.

After application of the 90-degree pulse, the spins are rephased along the slice-select axis owing to induced phase shift across the slice thickness resulting from a selective RF pulse. They immediately begin to dephase owing to T2* resulting from random motion of nearby spins, and to constant magnetic field inhomogeneities. The frequency encoding axis (read axis) is applied positively to force the spins into a controlled dephasing. At this point, the net magnetization in the X-Y plane has dephased randomly from T2*, in a controlled manner from the application of the gradient, and in a contrast direction from the main field inhomogeneity. For the time being, the accumulated dephasing due to main field is signified by ψ. At a time (τ), a selective 180-degree pulse is applied at the same spatial location as the 90-degree pulse. This pulse effectively inverts, or reverses, the total accumulated dephasing. Therefore, following the 180-degree pulse, the dephasing due to the gradient pulse effectively appears as though the gradient had been applied negatively, while the accumulated phase due to the main field inhomogeneity is reversed as well, to a value of $-\psi$.

At this point, the spins continue to undergo dephasing owing to the main field. However, they start at an effective phase exactly opposite to that which they had accumulated in a time (τ) between the 90- and 180-degree pulses, i.e., $-\psi$. In the τ msec after the 180-degree pulse, they acquire the same amount of phase that they acquired in the milliseconds between the 90- and 180-degree pulses. Therefore, at τ msec after the 180-degree pulse, the total accumulated phase is $-\psi$ (90 to 180, then inverted by a 180-degree pulse) $+\psi$ (accumulated phase-in after the 180) = 0. That is, at 2τ after the 90-degree pulse the net dephasing is zero, and no loss of signal occurs owing to main field inhomogeneities. The recovery of the loss of signal associated with the main field has been termed the field echo, and should not be confused with the gradient echo. In this case, the field echo occurs at 2τ = TE.

During the interval following the 180-degree pulse, the frequency encoding gradient is applied positively as well, thereby effectively refocusing the controlled dephasing from its initial application. A gradient echo occurs when the amount of rephasing is exactly equal to the amount of dephasing induced prior to the 180-degree pulse. Typically, this is adjusted so that the gradient echo occurs at the same time as the field echo, and called the echo time, TE, as in the gradient-echo example.

The advantage of these sequences is that it is possible to eliminate the field inhomogeneity dependence from the T2* expression so that the only loss of signal in the X-Y plane is due to the random dephasing caused by spin-spin (T2) relaxation. Therefore, for a given echo time, the spin echo produces more signal by recovering signal lost due to main field dephasing that occurs in the gradient-echo sequence. The price that must be paid for the increased signal is the application of a second RF pulse, and a minimal echo time greater than that possible with gradient-echo sequence.

The same basic rules governing contrast in the gradient-echo sequence using a 90-degree pulse are applied to the spin-echo sequence also; the only difference is that $T2^*$ is replaced by T2. Figure 2–11 shows the difference in signal intensity nutated into the X-Y plane, and T1 contrast for two tissues as a function of TR. The point to note in this illustration is that T1

contrast is highest at low TR; however, the signal strength, and hence SNR, is lowest there. Nonetheless, as long TRs are used, less contrast is observed at the expense of improved SNR. Figure 2–12 shows the decay of magnetization in the X-Y plane for the two tissues, at an intermediate value of TR. The initial contrast in this illustration is due to differences in the amount of magnetization nutated into the X-Y plane.

As the echo time is increased, T2 mechanisms begin to dominate. Again, it should be apparent from the illustration that significant tradeoffs exist between con-

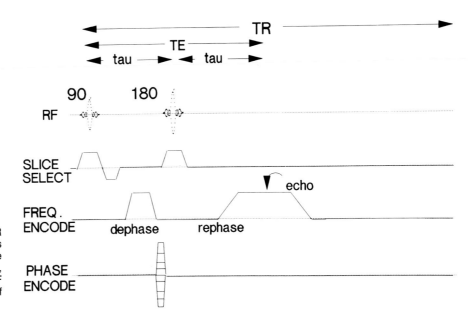

Figure 2–10. Typical spin-echo MR pulse sequence gradient waveforms are shown. Note that they are quite similar to those shown in Figure 1–9, with the exception of a 180-degree RF pulse required to obtain refocusing of magnetic field inhomogeneities.

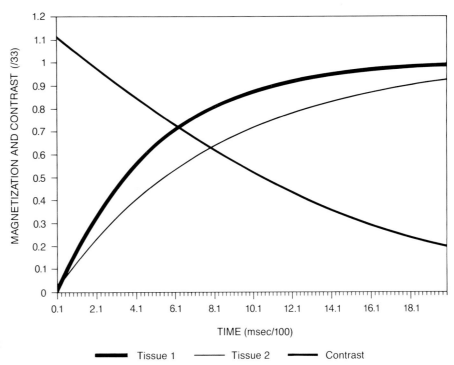

Figure 2–11. Differences in T1 between tissues can be used to generate contrast in resulting MR images. This figure shows the return toward equilibrium and the potential contrast between them as a result of T1 differences. Note that the highest contrast is obtained when the lowest signal levels are available. Similarly, the highest signal is when T1 contrast is lowest. Contrast between tissues and signal level (SNR) in the images must be balanced.

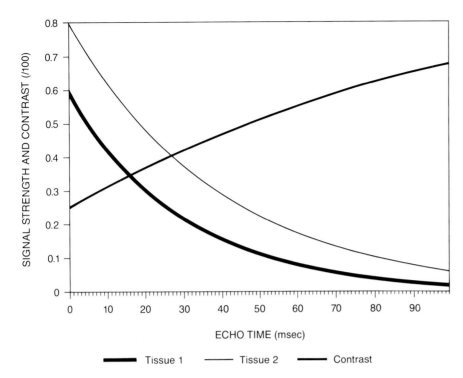

Figure 2–12. Similarly, T2 differences between tissues can be used as a mechanism of generating contrast in MR images. This figure shows the T2 decay of two tissues and the contrast between them. The initial contrast between them is due to differences in the amount of signal nutated into the X-Y plane. The highest contrast is again available when the signal level is least, and vice versa.

trast and signal strength. Table 2–1 shows the impact of changing various spin-echo parameters and the primary contrast mechanism between most tissues at 1.5T. Figure 2–13 shows how the spin-echo pulse sequence successfully rephases field inhomogeneity effects through the application of the 180-degree pulse. Field inhomogeneities continue to dephase the spins following the echo time. Similarly, the frequency encoding gradient adds a further controlled amount of dephasing, similar to that which occurs during the initial portion of the gradient-echo pulse sequence.[4, 11–13]

Figure 2–14*A* to *D* represents a duplication of the spin-echo phase effects presented in Figure 2–13. Figure 2–14*E* shows the spins continuing to dephase following the echo in the presence of field and gradient effects. It is possible to add a second 180-degree pulse to form a second echo. If data collection occurs about this point, it is possible to obtain a second image at the same spatial location, yet at a different echo time. Additional 180-degree pulses lead to additional echoes, and the potential for additional images. Therefore, multiple images can be obtained from the same spatial location following the selective 90-degree pulse through multiple applications of selective refocusing 180-degree RF pulses and subsequent data collection and frequency encoding.

This capability offers several potential advantages over conventional spin-echo techniques. First, data required to obtain multiple images from multiple slices can be collected from the same spatial location within one repetition time. While all images have the same repetition time, they have varied T2 contrast resulting

from differences in their echo times. This increases the time efficiency of the imaging pulse sequence (in number of images acquired per unit time) and also results in a wider variation of contrast between tissues. The price paid for the additional echoes is that a greater number of RF pulses must be applied.

The explanation for the effects of changing TE and TR is as follows. If the TR is very long, more hydrogen protons can recover between pulses and can be available for excitation by the next exciting pulse. As approximately 95 percent recovery occurs in a time of three times T1, the effect of increasing TR will almost cease once the TR is more than three times the T1 relaxation time. If the TR is long (much longer than the tissue with the longest T1), two adjacent tissues with different T1 relaxation times can both have complete T1 recovery of their hydrogen atoms during the repetition time. Their initial magnetization nutated into the X-Y plane will thus appear of similar intensity, with little T1 differentiation. With a shorter TR, more re-

Table 2–1. SCAN PARAMETERS AND CONTRAST

Typical TR	TE	Contrast mechanism
Long (>1,800 msec)	Long (>50 msec)	T2
Long	Short (<40 msec)	Spin density
Short (<600)	Short	T1
Poor		
Short	Long	T1, T2 (little signal)
Short (<100)	Short	T1 (little signal)
Long	Long (>150 msec)	T2 (little signal)

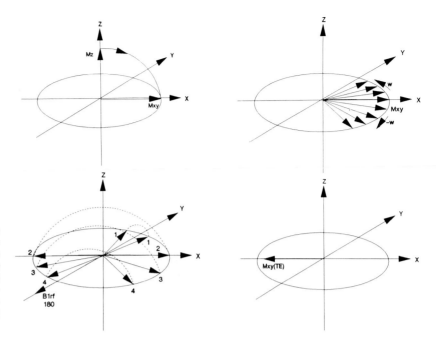

Figure 2–13. This figure demonstrates the time course of the magnetization in a spin-echo experiment, from the application of the 90 to the echo time. Once nutated into the X-Y plane, the spins dephase owing to the constant field inhomogeneities and the dephasing lobe of the read gradient. The 180-degree pulse flips the spins and causes an echo to form, as shown.

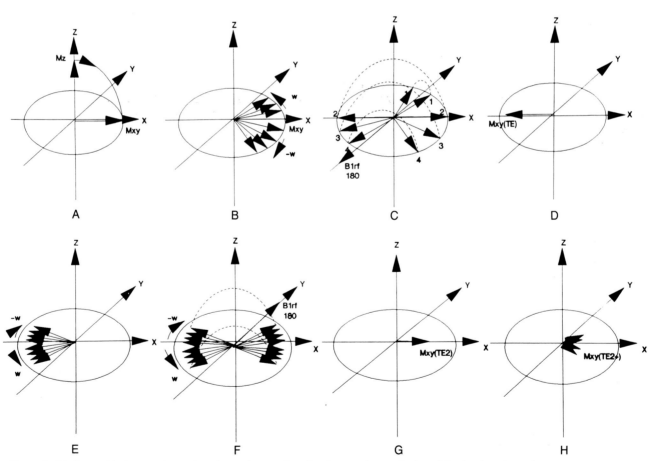

Figure 2–14. In a multiecho experiment the spins rephase at the echo, then continue to dephase following the echo, owing to both the gradient and the field inhomogeneities. It is possible to refocus the dephasing a second time by the application of another 180-degree pulse and another read gradient. Thus, once in the X-Y plane it is possible to generate multiple echoes, thereby forming images with variable T2 contrast and the same repetition time.

covery will occur in the tissue with the shorter T1 relaxation time. This tissue will have more spins (magnetization) available for reexcitation by the next exciting pulse and will therefore have more initial magnetization in the X-Y plane than the adjacent tissue with a longer T1 relaxation time.

Note that changing TE mainly affects T2 weighting, whereas changing TR mainly affects T1 weighting of the image. Problems associated with RF energy deposition are described in another chapter. However, it is important to realize that the human body absorbs RF energy required for nutation of the spins. There are both theoretical limits and FDA guidelines on the amount that can be deposited in a given amount of time, as described by the specific absorption rate (SAR). The human body's sensitivity to RF is not uniform over all frequencies of interest in MRI. Instead, it increases with frequency over those anticipated for potential use in MR. While SAR is typically not a problem below about 1.0T for proton imaging, it can impose severe limitations at 1.0T and above.

Common SAR limitations require modifications of TR, number of slices, or number of echoes acquired. Therefore, selection of multiecho sequences adds more RF pulses to a standard spin-echo scan, thereby increasing the amount of energy deposited. This can force tradeoffs between the desired contrast by necessitating the use of longer TRs to limit the amount of energy deposited per unit of time. Alternatively, fewer RF pulses can be applied, corresponding to fewer echoes or fewer slices. Therefore, tradeoffs with multislice multiecho sequences often revolve around the variations in the coverage of the desired imaging volume, or variations in the amount of contrast in the images.

Inversion Recovery Pulse Sequences

Beside the gradient-echo (with partial tip angles) and spin-echo pulse sequences, the next most common pulse sequence is the inversion recovery pulse sequence. This technique is also capable of providing some interesting tradeoffs in signal strength and contrast. Figure 2–15 shows the typical inversion recovery (IR) sequence. It is typically characterized by two parameters—TR, the pulse repetition time, and TI, the time between an initial 180-degree pulse and a second RF pulse to nutate the spins into the detection plane.

The sequence begins with a selective 180-degree pulse, applied at the location of the slice of interest. The bulk magnetization begins originally along the + Z-axis, and is inverted to alignment along the − Z-axis (Fig. 2–16*A*, *B*). The magnetization then attempts to return toward equilibrium via T1 relaxation. Since different tissues have different T1s, they relax at different rates. After some amount of recovery, a selective 90-degree pulse nutates the partially recovered magnetization of the tissues into the X-Y plane, exactly as done with the spin-echo pulse sequence. The only difference is that the amount of magnetization knocked into the X-Y plane depends on the interval of

time between the 180- and 90-degree pulses, and on the total repetition time. After all, even after the spins are nutated into the X-Y plane, they relax back toward the Z-axis.

Once in the X-Y plane, the remainder of the pulse sequence can be identical to the spin-echo sequence already described; i.e., the magnetization from the various tissues decays according to T2*. Application of a refocusing 180-degree pulse produces an echo at 2 = TE, thereby removing the field inhomogeneity loss of signal. However, it is not necessary to perform an inversion recovery with spin-echo data collection. Gradient-echo techniques for data collection are equally applicable. The basic equation governing signal intensity in the inversion recovery sequence is:

$$ SI \propto M_o(x,y) \, (1 \, - \, 2e^{-TI/T1(x,y)} \, + \, e^{-TR/T1(x,y)}) \, e^{-TE/T2(x,y)} $$

Here T2(x,y) is used to denote either T2 or T2*, depending on the pulse sequence.

The interesting feature of the inversion recovery sequences is that the dynamic range (range of possible pixel values) is twice that of the spin-echo sequence since negative values are now possible. Therefore the potential contrast between tissues is now twice as great. However, the primary contrast separation between tissues is a result of T1s since it is the longitudinal relaxation that gives rise to the factor of 2 increase in dynamic range. Therefore, inversion recovery scans are typically run with data collection techniques using an echo time as short (following the 90-degree pulse) as possible to reduce T2 effects. This also increases the amount of signal recovered since only small amounts of transverse relaxation are allowed to occur.

Inversion recovery sequences can also be run in a multislice mode. They are obtained by interleaving the pulse sequences for adjacent slices within the inversion time of the initial slice instead of concatenating pulse sequences following data collection. Typically, inversion times are on the order of 200 to 900 msec, which allows ample time for interleaving several slice data collections.

The second advantage of the IR scans is shown in Figure 2–17, which is the signal intensity for two different tissues as a function of variations in the inversion time. There is a unique TI for each tissue (for a given TR) at which it has no net magnetization. This occurs when the spins have recovered to the point at which half of their magnetization is along the − Z direction and half has recovered along + Z. If the magnetization is allowed to recover completely between repetitions, the zero point for each tissue is given as TI = 0.693*T1. However, the null point varies if changes in the repetition time lead to incomplete recovery between sequence repetitions. It is also possible to determine the zero crossing for incompletely recovered tissue. However, any change in TR or TI from that found to produce signal suppression leads to imaging away from the null point. The TR-TI pair uniquely defines the tissue T1 that will be completely suppressed from

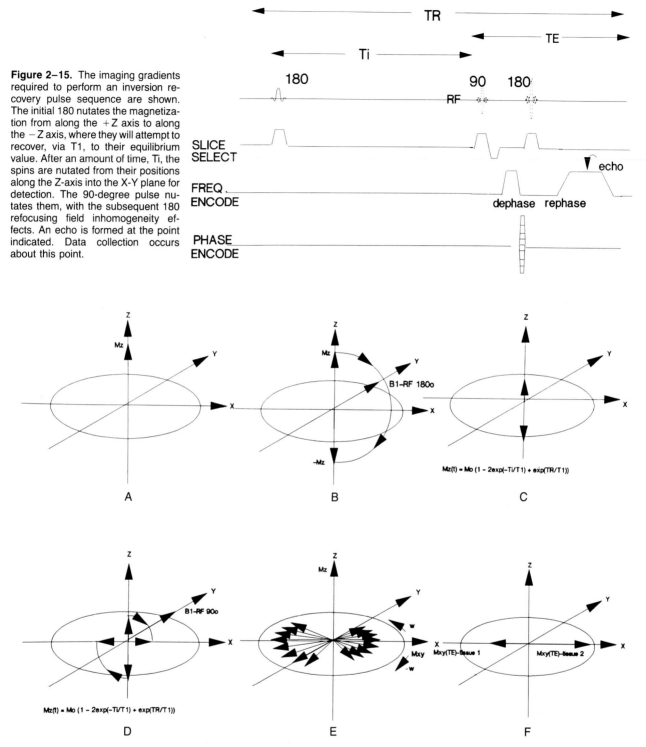

Figure 2–15. The imaging gradients required to perform an inversion recovery pulse sequence are shown. The initial 180 nutates the magnetization from along the +Z axis to along the −Z axis, where they will attempt to recover, via T1, to their equilibrium value. After an amount of time, Ti, the spins are nutated from their positions along the Z-axis into the X-Y plane for detection. The 90-degree pulse nutates them, with the subsequent 180 refocusing field inhomogeneity effects. An echo is formed at the point indicated. Data collection occurs about this point.

Figure 2–16. A graphic demonstration of the inversion recovery pulse sequence shows how the initial 180 flips the Mz (**A,B**). The magnetization recovers, as in (**C**). However, prior to complete recovery, the 90-degree pulse nutates the magnetization into the X-Y plane (**D**). There it dephases, as in the spin-echo sequence (**E,F**). The interesting part is that the amount knocked into the X-Y plane is strongly dependent on the T1 of the different tissues.

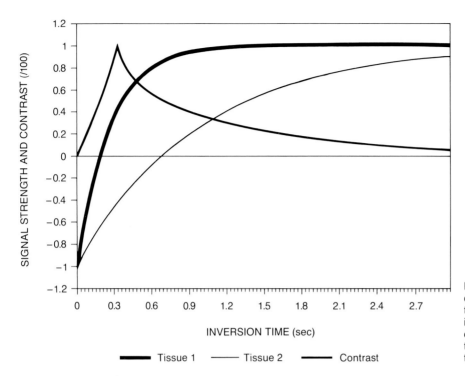

Figure 2–17. If the full dynamic range of the potential pixel values is used, contrast between tissues as a function of T1 is available as shown for variations in Ti of the pulse sequence. The magnetization nutated into the X-Y plane of the two tissues is also shown.

the image. Since different tissues generally have different T1s, they will have different null points as well.

STIR (short TI inversion recovery) pulse sequences have been used successfully to perform T1 weighted imaging, while suppressing the signal from fat. The advantage here revolves around the fact that the predominant contrast in motion artifact "ghosts" is between fat and the other tissues. By suppressing fat, the contrast within the ghosts is reduced, which also reduces their conspicuity. At 1.5T, fat has a T1 of between 200 and 300 msec, and can be suppressed with an inversion time of approximately 140 to 200 msec and a TR greater than 800. Unfortunately, most tissues have T1s longer than fat, forcing TRs to be significantly longer than 800 msec so that significant signal is obtained from them. Common STIR parameters for fat suppression at 1.5T form approximately a TI = 150–180 msec, TR = 2,000 msec, and TE = 30 msec pulse sequence.

The principal disadvantage of inversion recovery pulse sequences is that they generally require long imaging time, since the principal contrast advantage is obtained when all tissues have recovered completely. Typical repetition times for many inversion recovery scans are approximately 1,800 to 3,000 msec, which is almost as long as that required for spin-echo T2 weighted scans. Earlier, T1 weighted scans with spin-echo sequences were shown to use a short TR (200 to 800 msec), and therefore to require a relatively short imaging time. Although the T1 weighted spin-echo scans may offer less contrast than the inversion recovery sequences, they often offer enough to justify the reduced acquisition time.

The second disadvantage revolves around the mode of reconstruction of the acquired data. Ideally, the factor of 2 improvement in contrast to noise is easily obtained by performing a reconstruction and obtaining a "real" image. Typically, the Fourier transform provides a "real" and "imaginary" image. The phase between the two images can be related to various time delays, field inhomogeneities, and phase offsets in the pulse sequence. Both images usually have spatial variations corresponding to the phase effects. The good news is that these variations can be eliminated by taking the magnitude of the images. That is, the pixel value can be obtained without outphase variation. Typically, this is done for spin-echo sequences. The bad news is that this procedure makes all pixel values positive, and would reduce the dynamic range in an inversion recovery sequence by one-half and lead to a contrast versus TI relationship like that shown in Figure 2–18. Therefore, to exploit the complete dynamic range potential in inversion recovery sequences, a real reconstruction is desired without common spatial phase variation effects.

Methods centered around determining the spatial phase variation have been used to correct the alterations, while maintaining the complete dynamic range. However, the correction algorithms required to perform this modification may add significantly to the time required for image reconstruction.

Steady State Free Precession and Fast Scanning

One criticism of MRI is that the scan times are long relative to CT or other modalities. However, it should be remembered that in MRI, all spatial locations within the imaging volume are often acquired within one pulse sequence. In CT, each location is done se-

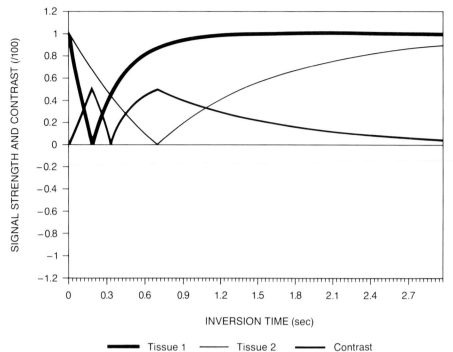

Figure 2–18. If a magnitude reconstruction is used, negative pixel values become positive, thereby reducing the dynamic range of the scan and altering the contrast between tissues. The initial contrast increases as before and begins to fall, as the one tissue goes through its zero crossing. At some point the contrast is zero as the magnetization of the two tissues becomes identical in magnitude. This occurs when one is positive and one is negative with respect to the Z-axis, but by the same amount. A similar contrast curve is then obtained as the second tissue approaches its zero crossing and beyond.

quentially. The total amount of time from the start of data collection to the end for each spatial location is less for a CT examination than for virtually all spin-echo, virtually all inversion recovery, and many gradient-echo sequences. Because of this, many MR examinations are subject to artifacts resulting from patient motion that may occur from the start to the end of the data collection process. In an attempt to reduce scan time, steady state free precession (SSFP) and fast scanning techniques have been developed for use in MRI. Some common names associated with these techniques are FAST, FLASH, FISP, GRASS, CE-FAST, and RARE, each with its own unique contrast properties.[14, 15]

SSFP is accomplished by applying a series of equal RF pulses to the sample, equal intervals apart in time. The pulses are applied very rapidly (TR < T1,T2), initially nutating magnetization into the X-Y plane with an arbitrary flip angle RF pulse. Assume that the detected signal following the first pulse would be relatively strong. In the X-Y plane, the signal is allowed to precess and begin to dephase according to T2*. A second RF pulse again tips magnetization from along the Z-axis toward the X-Y plane. However, if the time between pulses is less than T2*, the X-Y magnetization from the first RF pulse is tipped as well, so that some may remain in the X-Y plane and some return to the Z-axis (plus or minus direction, depending on the RF pulse sequence used). The signal strength would be less than that obtained with the first pulse, since the full amount of magnetization was not available along the Z-axis (some still in the X-Y plane). A third pulse is then applied, knocking new magnetization into the

X-Y plane, and some put back along the Z-axis from the second pulse. The spins that arrive in the X-Y plane for the second time now rephase and give a signal stronger than that produced from the last pulse, but less than the first pulse. Thus, the odd and even pulses produce alternately strong and weak pulses. However, as more and more pulses are applied, the difference between the odd and even signals is reduced. It can be shown that after a large number of pulses have been applied, the signals produced from odd and even pulses are equivalent, and all further pulses produce the same amount of signal. That is, a steady state has been achieved. The free precession refers to the fact that the signal is observed following the RF pulse, during the time when the spins are precessing about the static magnetic field.

The advantage is that an equilibrium (nonzero) amount of signal is obtained in a very short repetition time. Performing the MRI data collection using these sequences can therefore reduce imaging times, since TR is very short. Typical values for TR in SSFP sequences may be less than 50 msec, so that a 128^2 image can be obtained in about 6 seconds of true data collection. Performing multiple repetitions per view improves signal to noise, as shown earlier, and also leads to increases in scan time. However, it is possible to obtain MRI data collections in short intervals, so that breath holding can be used to eliminate respiratory motion artifacts, for example. Recent advances have reduced the total acquisition time to near 100 msec.

There are several reasons why these sequences have not gained widespread application. First, the difference in signal intensity between the tissues is dependent in a fairly complicated way on the T1, T2, RF flip angle, motion, and various parameters of the gradient portion of the pulse sequence. It is not a straightforward process to predict a priori how various tissues will appear in the images. The simple exponential relationships encountered with either spin-echo, inversion recovery, or gradient-echo sequences are conceptually easier to understand and "get a feel for." Second, the sequences are based around gradient echoes and are often subject to field inhomogeneity artifacts. Third, while they can often be obtained in one breath hold, they may have a very low SNR, and therefore may be limited diagnostically. Likewise, the sequences are often quite sensitive to view-to-view motion that may occur. Fourth, a tremendous body of information exists on more conventional sequences and the appearance of pathology in them. Unfortunately, the radiologic community does not have the same amount of information to draw on in using SSFP sequences, making the search for an appropriate screening sequence difficult. Fifth, the sequences are run in a single slice mode since the short repetition time does not allow interleaving to occur. Therefore, multiple slices can be obtained by either three-dimensional techniques or multiple replications of the same imaging sequence at sequential spatial locations. Often this sequential imaging of multiple slices can remove the time advantage that was gained from the reduced TR.

The principal advantage of the SSFP techniques is the wide range of potential contrast and the ability to obtain images similar to long TR, long TE (T2 weighted) spin-echo pulse sequences in a reduced examination time. Furthermore, sequential imaging at the same spatial location, yet at different times, allows serial images to be obtained for use in joint studies or dynamic studies after injection of contrast agents, and other orthopedic work. Although this provides interesting results, MRI may not be the examination of choice in these cases.

Several other reduced imaging time techniques have been proposed and developed over the years. One of the most ambitious and earliest of these was Mansfield's echo planar technique. The concept behind echo planar can be explained by imagining all data collection techniques as methods of covering a data space that is similar to a checkerboard. Conventional spin-echo imaging spans the checkerboard by selecting a row (corresponding to a specific phase encoding step), and then marching across the row (corresponding to collecting data during application of the read gradient). The next row is selected and covered one TR later, at the next phase encoding value. Echo planar imaging is accomplished by running up and down along the columns in a serpentine manner so that all blocks on the checkerboard are covered following one excitation. To achieve this result, the phase encoding gradient oscillates during data collection. Here, all data required for imaging are obtained after one data excitation. Complete data acquisition can be obtained in less than 50 msec.[16-18]

The limitation of these methods is that they require very strong, very rapidly switching phase encoding gradient systems. Many conventional imagers have not yet been designed to perform the rapid repeatable response required for successful implementation of these techniques. To simplify the technique, various methods were proposed to increase the number of phase encoding steps, applying oscillating gradients to cover a portion of data space. Repeating the sequence at different initial phase encoding values, followed by oscillating gradient application, maintains the resolution and field of view desired while reducing the number of phase encoding "steps" over conventional two-dimensional Fourier transform (2-DFT) MRI. Two, four, or possibly eight rows of the checkerboard could be covered following one RF pulse.

However, several problems associated with reconstruction, correction, and system calibration have limited the availability of these methods. Similar techniques, such as hybrid and snapshot imaging, are recent variations of the echo planar method.[19] Recent work has reduced the acquisition time to approximately 40 msec for a single slice, at an image matrix of 128^2.

Chemical Shift Imaging

Chemical shift imaging refers to techniques designed to produce images of fat or water separately, rather than together. One of the motivations for this imaging technique deals with the high signal intensity often associated with fat in conventional spin-echo or inversion recovery sequences. The short T1 of fat leads to it possessing a strong signal in many pulse sequences. Since motion artifact ghosts contain the same contrast as the tissue producing them, it is desirable to eliminate fat from the images. If this is accomplished, the conspicuity of ghosts is reduced. Similarly, the high signal intensity of fat reduces the contrast in the images by forcing the image gray scale to a narrow range in the tissues of interest, or alternatively reduces the dynamic range of the receiving system in the tissues of interest. On the other hand, fat images may be useful in areas not yet appreciated.

Two techniques have been advocated for performing chemical shift imaging. The first, the Dixon method, takes advantage of differences in the resonant frequency of the spins once in the X-Y plane.[20] The other technique deals with differences in resonant frequency during slice selection.[21]

The Dixon technique[20] has been popular for the last 3 or 4 years. The technique takes advantage of fat protons having a resonant frequency different from protons by approximately 3.5 ppm. At 1.5T, this is about 220 hertz difference. Following slice selection, spins from fat and water are nutated into the X-Y plane, where they immediately begin to dephase because of differences in their resonant frequency.

Imagine two groups of spins at the same spatial location. If they resonated at the same frequency, they would precess coherently in the X-Y plane. However, since they do not, the two travel as independent coherent groups (ignoring T2 effects). At some point in time, the two sets of spins will be exactly out of phase, leading to a cancellation of their signals. If imaging is performed at this point, the signal intensity on a pixel by pixel basis will be due to the difference in the signal strengths between the fat and the water. This has been termed the water-fat, or difference, image. At a later time, the two packets of spins will come together in the X-Y plane, as the fat spins "lap" the water spins. Imaging performed at this time produces the water + fat image.

To produce the difference and sum images, it is necessary to adjust the relative position of the gradient echo so that it occurs during the out-of-phase cancellation period, or during the in-phase addition period. At 1.5T, the spins come into phase approximately every 4.5 msec, requiring gradient-echo times at multiples of this. They are exactly out of phase every 2.2 msec plus $n*4.5$ seconds, where n is any integer. Therefore, the spins would be out of phase in the X-Y plane at approximately 6.7, 11, 15.5 (etc.) msec following the RF pulse. Data collection occurring so that the gradient echo peak occurs at the various in-phase or out-of-phase periods produces the corresponding sum or difference image.

The principal drawback of this technique is that it does not directly give fat or water images. Instead, they are the sum or difference images of the respective signal intensities of the constituent tissues on a pixel by pixel basis. Since fat has a short T1, it often gives rise to a stronger signal than that from an identical volume of water. Therefore, the difference image is not a direct measure of the percentage of fat or water in the voxel, but is instead a measure of their signal intensity difference. Second, even though the techniques have fat and water potentially out of phase, magnitude reconstruction loses the sign, and therefore does not identify one component as positive or negative. In order to get the fat or water image, the in-phase image must be obtained, so that each pixel represents the sum of signal intensities. The difference image (difference between signal intensities) can then be subtracted (added) from it to give water (fat) image alone. However, to generate these images correctly, it is often necessary to perform a correction owing to magnetic field inhomogeneities broadening the exact time that the tissues are in or out of phase.

Although this has been described as a gradient-echo sequence, it is possible to generate a spin-echo pulse sequence that accomplishes the same task by modifying the position of the 180-degree pulse so that the field echo and gradient echo occur at either the same time (in phase) or at a specific different time (difference image). The primary objection to the technique is that two sequences must be performed, along with image processing functions such as image subtraction and field correction, to obtain independent fat and water images.

The second type of chemical shift imaging selects a fat slice or a water slice as a result of differences in their resonant frequencies.[21] Imagine a selective RF pulse with a given bandwidth. A gradient along the slice-select axis leads to excitation of water protons at position B, with a slice thickness of δ. However, fat protons from a different position are excited by the RF pulse, since fat has a slightly different resonant frequency. Therefore, different positions are excited for the fat and water protons, as shown in Figure 2–19. This occurs in all MR imaging that uses selective pulses and a magnetic field gradient for slice selection. It is analogous to the chemical shift artifact seen along the frequency encoding axis. Application of the slice select gradient in the same direction for all pulses leads to fat and water protons from different spatial locations being obtained in the image. However, both sets of protons are tipped into the X-Y plane.

If the pulse sequence requires multiple RF pulses (as in a spin echo, or inversion recovery sequences), the magnetic field gradient used during application of the

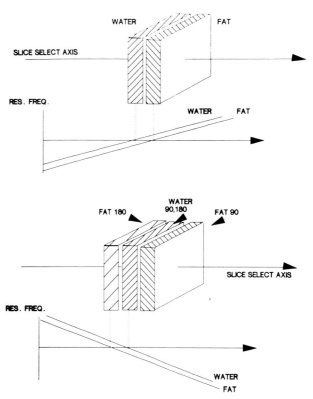

Figure 2–19. Application of the slice-select gradient sets up a magnetic field distribution along the axis. Fat and water slices at the same location, however, resonate at different frequencies owing to the magnetic field shielding effect of portions of the fat molecules. Therefore, despite the fact that the fat and water are at the same position, they resonate at different frequencies. In the presence of a linear field gradient, fat and water from different positions resonate at the same frequency. Therefore, application of a 90-degree pulse nutates slices of fat and water into the X-Y plane from different spatial locations. If the magnetic field gradient for the 180 is applied in the same direction as the 90, fat and water from different locations echo and appear in the image. Reversing the gradient for the 180 allows the fat slice excited by the 180 to be different from that excited with the 90. Therefore, it is possible to obtain a water slice alone.

second pulse can be reversed so that a fat slice on the opposite side of the water slice is affected. In the case of a spin-echo sequence, fat on the right side of the water slice could be excited by the 90-degree pulse, and a fat slice on the left by a 180-degree pulse. Since neither fat slice sees both the 90 and 180, they will not contribute signal to the image. Only the water spins become refocused as a result of seeing both the 90- and 180-degree pulses. Typically, the fat and water slices are separated by less than one slice thickness.

The bandwidth of the RF pulse and the gradient strength determine the width of the selected slices. The gradient strength determines how far apart in space the fat and water slices are located. To obtain a water image alone, the center of the fat slice must be at least at the edge of the water slice. If this occurs, the fat slice extends from the center of the water slice to one-half slice thickness outside the water slice. Reversing the slice-select gradient makes the excited fat slice for the second pulse extend from the center of the water slice to one-half slice thickness outside the water slice, yet in the opposite direction. In this way, the 90- and 180-degree fat slices do not overlap. Therefore, to accomplish this separation, knowledge of the bandwidth of the RF pulse, gradient strength, and chemical shift in hertz must be known. Since chemical shift is fixed, fat removal in conventional imaging can be performed by designing lower frequency RF pulses, so that the bandwidth of the pulse is at least twice the chemical shift at that frequency.

As an example, an RF pulse might have a bandwidth of 672 hertz, corresponding to the fat and water slices being one-third of the slice thickness apart. A lower frequency pulse could be obtained by time scaling the original by a factor of 1.5 (and reducing the amplitude by 66 percent), to obtain an RF bandwidth of approximately 448 hertz, or twice the chemical shift in hertz at 1.5T. The chemical shift frequency difference scales directly with field strength. However, the RF pulses used at different field strengths in MRI often have the same amplitude modulation and hence the same bandwidth as those used at 1.5T. Therefore, the spatial chemical shift between the excited fat and water slices is much less at lower frequencies.

The advantage of these sequences is that true fat or water images can be obtained. The only requirement is that the imager must be tuned to the resonant frequency of the desired component (fat or water) at the spatial location of interest. This is done during the setup stages of the pulse sequence.

The Appearance of Flowing Blood

The appearance of flowing blood is one of the most complicated phenomena to predict or interpret in MRI. Virtually every parameter of the MR pulse sequence has a direct effect on the appearance of flowing blood. The following section attempts to explain the effect of the flow velocity and of many of the pulse sequence parameters on the appearance of flowing blood.

The first parameter that should be discussed is the laminar flow velocity traveling through the selected slice. While steady laminar flow may not truly exist in the human body, it serves as a good approximation for many situations encountered. First, imagine that the flow velocity is zero, so that none of the blood within an excited slice "washes out" from one TR to the next. Here, the blood appears in the pulse sequence and produces a signal according to its spin density, T1, and T2.

However, in most situations, blood is moving. Imagine now that the flow velocity is small, so that only a small portion of the spins washes out of the selected slice during TR. They will be replaced by spins that are fully magnetized since they have never been in an imaging volume before. Therefore, the slice consists of partially magnetized spins that have a signal intensity given by their T1, T2, spin density, and the TE and TR of the pulse sequence. The rest of the spins are completely magnetized and give a signal strength dependent on the spin density and the TE of the sequence. Therefore, a greater signal level will be observed for the low velocity case than the no flow case since a portion of the partially saturated spins has been replaced by "fresh" full magnetized spins. This increase in flow signal level increases with flow velocity until the entire slice thickness of flowing spins is replaced by "fresh" spins within one TR. This occurs at all velocities greater than Z/TR. We have assumed that a negligible amount of signal has washed out of the slice from the time of the first RF pulse to the next during each view of the MRI pulse sequence.[22–26]

As the nonturbulent flow velocity increases, portions of the spins travel out of the selected slice from the first selective pulse to the second. In the case of the spin-echo sequence, spins travel out of the selected

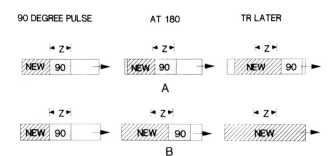

Figure 2–20. Slow and fast laminar flow can produce markedly different signals in a spin-echo (or any) pulse sequence. In the slow flow case (**A**), spins excited at the 90 do not move far prior to the 180, and give rise to a signal in the image. The strength of the signal is dependent on the inflow of fresh, fully magnetized spins into the slice. One TR later, the spins are fully magnetized, giving rise to an exceptionally strong signal from flowing blood. In the case of fast flow (**B**), most of the spins excited by the 90-degree pulse have gone downstream by the application of the 180. Therefore, while the slice consists of new spins, they have not seen the 90-degree pulse, and therefore do not contribute to the image. Therefore, a weak signal is obtained. At some velocity, dependent on the TE and slice thickness, all spins wash out in the (90–180) interval, producing no signal in the image.

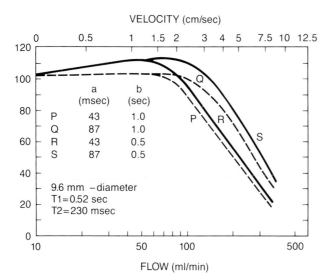

VELOCITY (cm/sec)

FLOW (ml/min)

	a (msec)	b (sec)
P	43	1.0
Q	87	1.0
R	43	0.5
S	87	0.5

9.6 mm – diameter
T1=0.52 sec
T2=230 msec

Figure 2–21. This figure shows the changes in signal intensity in four sequences of flowing fluid, doped to be similar in T1 to blood. The graph represents the increased signal associated with slow flow, a linear decrease in signal at intermediate velocity, and a loss of signal entirely at high flow rates. (From Bradley WG, Waluch V. Blood flow: magnetic resonance imaging. Radiology 1985: 154:443–450.)

slice in the interval of time between the 90- and 180-degree pulses. Therefore, during application of the 180-degree pulse, the slice consists of new protons that have seen no RF pulses, and those that were completely magnetized and have seen the 90-degree pulse. Following the 180, the spins in the slice of interest consist of protons seeing only the 180, and those that have seen both the 90 and 180. Only the second case of spins produces any detectable signal in the X-Y plane. However, the signal strength is less than the case when an insignificant number of spins is washed out of the selected slice. The signal strength continues to decrease until all spins wash out of the slice in the interval between the 90- and 180-degree pulses. This occurs at all velocities greater than or equal to Z/tau.[22, 23]

Figures 2–20 and 2–21 are diagrams of the various situations described and the signal intensity as a function of velocity for two TRs and two TEs. There are several points of interest to be obtained from the graph. First, the velocity of the peak signal for laminar through-plane flow situations is dependent on the slice thickness and TR of the pulse sequence. The velocity of zero signal in this case occurs at a velocity dependent on the slice thickness and echo times. Therefore, changes in slice thickness, echo time, or repetition time produce markedly different curves and different flow velocities for the peak and zero signal positions. The initial point on the graph also changes, since it is the signal strength of static blood in the pulse sequence.[23]

The second interesting feature of the graph is that a specific signal strength in the image can correspond to different velocities. This makes flow estimation from a single sequence impossible. Further, no matter what

sequence is employed, there will be a velocity limit at which all velocities greater than or equal to it produce no signal at all. In these cases it is possible only to state the lower limit of the velocity.

A second case of interest is laminar flow through the imaging plane of the selected slice. Imagine a vessel flowing diagonally across the selected slice. All spins in the slice that have seen both the 90- and 180-degree pulses appear in the final image. Imagine a proton at position A during application of the phase encoding gradient, as shown in Figure 2–22. It will obtain an effective position encoding at the spatial location that it occupies along the Y-axis at the time the gradient is applied, in this case Y_a. Later the read axis is applied to generate the echo, thereby encoding its position along the X-axis. The proton has moved from position A to B since the application of the phase encoding gradient. There is a time difference between the encoding of the position along each of the imaging axes during which the spin moves to a new position. The effective spatial position encoded for the moving in-plane proton is (X_b, Y_a). Therefore, laminar in-plane flow velocity will produce blood moving from within the vessel to adjacent to the lumen because of differences in time between spatial encoding along the axes. The shift away from the lumen depends on the direction of the fluid motion and on the time difference between phase encoding and the echo. The greater the velocity, the greater is the spatial discrepancy between the spin positions during phase encoding and echo time. Similarly, the discrepancy increases with increased time between phase encoding and the echo. If the motion is parallel to one axis or the other along its entire path, this artifact will not be produced.[27]

The previous discussions were based on the notion of single slice acquisitions. Unfortunately, most MRI sequences are run in a multislice mode, thereby complicating the appearance of the flowing blood even further. The concept of entrance slice effects must be examined. They will be defined as the effect of through-plane or in-plane flow as a function of the slice of interest within the imaging volume. Imagine for the time being that the slice of interest is the second one in the imaging volume. Here, blood will enter from the previous slice, therefore possibly having been nutated from one of the RF pulses. Thus, instead of entering the slice of interest fully magnetized, it can be completely magnetized, partially magnetized, or fully saturated, depending on the order (in time) that the slices are excited and on the flow velocity.[25, 26]

Imagine the flow velocity to be high enough to travel at least two slice thicknesses in one TR. Here, both the first and second slices will be filled with fresh spins. However, the velocity may lead to significant loss of signal due to washout within the echo time, or at lower velocities to high signal intensity in both slices. Alternatively, it is possible to have a velocity that only partially fills the latter slices, so that the intensity pattern within the vessels within the imaging volume is nonuniform as a function of position within the imaging

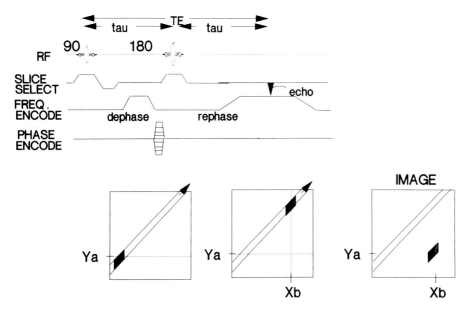

Figure 2–22. This figure demonstrates the source of the vascular misregistration problem encountered in MRI. Basically, the motion of the fluid at some angle to the imaging plane forces the spatial flow encoding of the coordinates of the spins to occur at two different times, thereby encoding the spatial position at the wrong location. Here, the Y coordinate of the indicated plug is as shown, well before the echo time. Once the Y coordinate has been encoded, the spins move to new X and Y coordinates as they move diagonally through the imaging plane. At the echo, the X-coordinate information is obtained. The net effect is to obtain an image with the fluid displaced from the lumen.

volume. Deep within the imaging volume, little full magnetization appears, owing to limitations in the flow velocity. Alternatively, deeper within the imaging volume, blood entering the slices has been excited at previous spatial locations, giving rise to a reduced signal intensity compared with the initial slice within the imaging volume. It is interesting to note that entrance slice effects occur at both ends of the imaging volume. In axial imaging sequences, for example, the upper slices have entrance slice effects from arterial blood, while the lower slices have it from venous blood returning to the heart. The overall appearance of the entrance slice effects is dependent on the flow velocity, the spatial location of the slice, the order in which the slices are acquired, and the parameters of the imaging sequence like TE and TR. Unfortunately, many flow rates and vessel diameters lead to nonsteady, even turbulent flow in various regions of the body. Therefore, the effect of turbulent flow must be considered. In the discussion of gradient moment nulling techniques, flow dephasing is discussed. It is shown there that many imaging gradients, primarily the read and slice-select axes, have sensitivity to flow velocity, acceleration, and higher order derivatives of motion, which can produce a net loss of signal.[28,29] For this to occur, there must be a velocity distribution within the voxel, as would occur in turbulent flow. Thus, the various spins inside the voxel are dephased differently, so that they no longer travel as a coherent group. It can be shown that the magnitude of the flow velocity distribution and the shape of the gradient waveform lead to the different amounts of dephasing. In-plane resolution and slice thickness influence these effects, since the amount of signal loss is dependent on spatial velocity distribution within the voxel. Often the dephasing exhibits itself as the "flow void" phenomenon. However, partial loss of signal can be obtained as well. Gradient moment nulling

acts to reduce this dephasing, independent of the flow velocity, acceleration, and all higher order derivatives of motion.

In addition to dephasing, the through-plane and in-plane effects described earlier continue to apply in turbulent flow. That is, the motion that occurs from one TR to the next and within the 90–180 interval influences the appearance of the flowing material as well. The only difference is that the amount of signal obtained from that entering the slice may be dephased, and therefore less than predicted if laminar or plug flow was assumed. One interesting example of a form of gradient moment nulling that is often incompletely appreciated is even echo rephasing (EER).[27,30,31] It can be shown that the amount of signal dephasing that accumulates from the start of a multiecho, spin-echo pulse sequence to the first echo leads to a net loss of signal. From the first echo, the protons continue to move through imaging gradients, and re-form another spin echo if an additional 180-degree pulse is applied. The net amount of dephasing that accumulates from the first to the second echo is seen to be exactly opposite that acquired from the start of the sequence to the first echo. That is, the net amount of dephasing from the start of the sequence to the second echo leads to a net increase of signal since the net dephasing of the constant velocity components is zero. All constant velocity spin dephasing is recovered and produces brighter signal in the second echo image than that obtained in the first.

Unfortunately, there are several factors of this phenomenon that are not commonly appreciated. First, the second echo time must often be exactly twice the first. Secondly, the gradient waveforms used must be symmetric for true EER to occur. In the discussion of gradient moment nulling, the gradient waveform was the "heart of the beast." This is also true in EER. That is, there are several requirements on the gradient waveforms for EER to occur. The original discussions of EER used gradient waveforms that met rephasing requirements at the second echo. However, this is not necessarily true for all even echo sequences. Further, EER may not be seen owing to washout effects that occur at high flow velocities. For example, the flow rate could be high enough that complete washout occurs within the time between the 90-degree pulse and the second 180-degree pulse, leading to no net signal in the image within the vessel lumen. Further, only constant velocity components of the flow are recovered. Since accelerative terms are still not recovered, significant dephasing can still occur.[32]

The bottom line of this is that the presence or absence of flow, as determined by the appearance of signal differences in the lumen between even echo images, is difficult to assess. Several parameters, including the gradient waveform, must be known, as well as the range of velocities expected. If EER does seem to occur, the presence of flowing material can be determined reasonably successfully. However, the magnitude of the velocity cannot be assured.

If EER does not appear to have occurred, often no statement about the presence or absence of flow can be determined because of dephased accelerative terms, incomplete refocusing of velocity terms due to the shape of the gradient waveforms used, or high velocity flow washout during the pulse sequence. Here again, additional factors that complicate this assessment are the gradient strengths used (i.e., motion sensitivity), slice thickness, TR, TE, RF pulses, resolution, and slice thickness.

SIGNAL INTENSITY: IMPROVING SIGNAL-TO-NOISE RATIO

How to Increase Signal

To increase SNR use:
1. Reduced resolution (large field of view).
2. Thick slices.
3. Long TR.
4. Short TE.
5. Increased magnetic field strength.
6. Decreased bandwidth across sample.
7. Increased number of repetitions.
8. Quadrature receiving coils.
9. Anti-aliasing techniques.

Disadvantages of the above factors:
1. Large field of view and thick slices reduce spatial resolution.
2. Decreasing bandwidth increases chemical shift artifact.
3. Long TR limits T1 weighting and short TE limits T2 weighting in the images.
4. Increasing repetitions increase total scan time.

Discussion of Signal-to-Noise Ratio

Much effort has been expended in describing the signal characteristics in an MR pulse sequence. Similarly, common sources of noise and noise characteristics have been described. It is now time to relate these two parameters in a more robust manner. The SNR can be defined as the ratio between the true NMR signal amplitude and the root-mean-square (RMS) noise value (or uncertainty) in the signal.[33] Since both signal and noise occur simultaneously during data acquisition, they cannot be separated independently. Therefore, to increase our confidence in the data (i.e., increase the SNR), we can attempt to increase the amount of signal present, or decrease the amount of noise.

In an image, the SNR is a measure of the "graininess" or "pixeliness" of the resultant image. It is not directly related to the ability to distinguish between tissues. The SNR in an image relates directly to the SNR in the acquired data. Therefore, a great deal of the design work in the construction of an MR imager relates to improving signal detection and noise immunity.

Techniques used to vary the amount of incoming noise in MRI, where patient thermal noise is often the dominant source of noise, are to increase the Q (decrease the bandwidth) of the detector coil, decrease the bandwidth of the MR pulse sequence, use quadrature detection, and perform and add multiple repetitions of each view. Other sources of noise that are not often dominant, yet still important, are the signal preamplifier noise figure (how noiseless is the initial amplification stage), the noise figure of the entire receive chain, and the digitization noise (digitization error).

Techniques used to increase the amount of signal detected often involve better design of receiver coils (including surface coils), improving RF pulses to provide more uniform slice profiles, or simply acquiring information over thicker slices, and with longer repetition times and shorter echo times. Unfortunately, some of these choices are not as desirable as others, as described below.

Figure 2–23 offers a comparison of the same pulse sequence applied on the same patient on the same day, using exactly the same scan parameters of field of view, slice thickness, resolution, RF pulses, and image bandwidth. The only difference between the two is the use of linear and quadrature receive coils. In this example, differences in signal to noise between the images are due to the quadrature coil having a 1.414 times improvement (theoretical) in signal to noise over the linear coil, since it effectively appears as two detectors. Since MR signal adds linearly (factor of 2) and noise adds as the square root of two, the net improvement in the SNR is $(2)^{1/2}$.

Before discussing pixel size and resolution, a semantic explanation of resolution terminology should be given. Resolution can be defined as the ability to detect

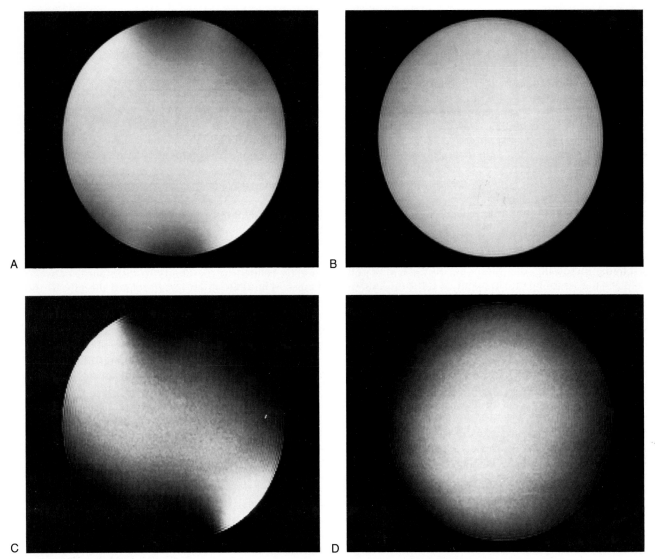

Figure 2–23. These images shows examples of the uniformity and signal-to-noise difference between linear and quadrature head coil images on a uniform phantom using the same pulse sequence in (**A**) and (**B**). Figures (**C**) and (**D**) show the same images under different window and level settings, demonstrating the variations in uniformity over the image.

adjacent tissues, or adjacent small objects. References to increased resolution imply that the resolving power, or ability to resolve objects as different, is increased. This is often achieved through decreased pixel size. Therefore, increased resolution is often associated with decreased pixel size.

On the other hand, references to decreased resolution imply that the ability to detect differences between adjacent tissues or small objects has diminished. This is often associated with increased pixel size. Thus, decreased resolution is often associated with increased pixel size.

The easiest way to examine the impact of various scan parameter selections on image SNR is to examine

two separate factors. The first is to examine how the scan parameter selections alter the amount of signal present in the voxel. Increasing the resolution decreases the pixel size, thereby reducing the amount of signal per voxel, leading to a reduced signal to noise (grainier image). Decreasing the resolution provides bigger voxels, therefore more spins per voxel, and a higher SNR. Similarly, increasing the slice thickness increases the amount of signal, while reductions lead to corresponding losses in the amount of signal present in each voxel. Unfortunately, partial volume effects become more severe and may limit the observed resolution to less than that predicted by the parameters of the pulse sequence (field of view, number of phase encodings or data points). Therefore, for a given pulse sequence, any scan parameter selection that increases the number of spins in a voxel increases the signal to noise if all other noise and bandwidth parameters are maintained. This includes providing for more T1 recovery through increased TR, or decreased spin-spin relaxation through shorter TEs.

The second way to examine the signal-to-noise question is to examine techniques for limiting the amount of noise. Adding multiple repetitions of each view leads to a net improvement in the signal to noise by N, where N is the number of repetitions. However, this increases scan time by N. It can be shown, as already described, that quadrature detection provides a similar mechanism for an improvement by 2 over the same pulse sequence run with a linear coil.

Alternatively, a narrower image bandwidth could be used by decreasing the frequency encoding gradient strength, increasing the sampling interval, and decreasing the sampling rate to maintain the same field of view and resolution. The bandwidth of frequencies across the subject is reduced. This lets in less noise, while maintaining signal strength, resolution, and field of view. However, as described earlier, the chemical shift artifact becomes greater by the same proportion as the reduction in the frequency encoding gradient. No increase in scan time is associated with this method, however.

Many manufacturers now offer anti-aliasing techniques along both the read and phase axes. They often require twice the number of data points and/or twice the number of phase encodings as a comparable scan in which aliasing is possible. The theory behind the technique is to acquire a scan with a field of view twice that desired in the final image. The resolution over the image is exactly as specified in the scan parameters. However, aliasing occurs about the edge of the acquired field of view that is twice that desired. Therefore, wraparound occurs outside the desired image. To accomplish this, the sampling rate is doubled while the gradient strength is decreased and the sampling interval halved. Along the phase encoding axis, the phase encoding step size is halved, and twice as many "views" are acquired. This effectively places a data point between those that would have been acquired in an "aliasable" scan on both the read and phase axes. Twice as many data are therefore obtained along both axes. Thus, a square root of 2 improvement is obtained along both axes, producing a net improvement by a factor of 2 in signal to noise over identical scans aliasing about the displayed field of view. This technique is comparable in signal to noise as a double repetition scan with half as many views. The scan time is identical to aliasing protection and the signal to noise is the same, yet aliasing has not occurred. Most manufacturers have allowed anti-aliasing along the read (frequency) encoding axis for some time since there is no time penalty associated with it. Anti-aliasing represents a technique for $(2)^{1/2}$ improvements in the SNR

due to acquiring a twofold difference between the acquired and displayed matrix. Likewise, since the gradient strength is reduced along the read axis, it is possible to reduce the image bandwidth, thereby acquiring less noise as well. The degree of oversampling along either axis is not limited to a factor of 2, and in fact can be any value provided appropriate changes are made in gradient strength, sampling, or phase encoding step size.

The description of image signal-to-noise presented here deals primarily with techniques that can be used once the basic pulse sequence has been chosen. SNR is a complicated function of many imaging parameters. As users of MR imagers, it is directly related to the size of the voxels as defined by the thickness of the slice and the resolution along the two image axes. It can be improved by performing multiple repetitions of the same view or by using anti-aliasing sequences or quadrature coils. Further, reductions in image bandwidth through reduced gradient strength and extending the data sampling can lead to improvements in the SNR as well. Unfortunately, other significant improvements that are continually being pursued by the manufacturer often require modifications to the imager, or redesign beyond the scope of this text. Refinements in selective RF pulses, eddy current compensation, detection coils, and state of the art electronics are examples of industry-based projects aimed at SNR improvements.

METHODS OF MOTION SUPPRESSION

Motion occurs from breathing, heart beat, vascular pulsation, body movement, peristalsis, and other forms of voluntary or involuntary motion. Many methods are available for reducing unwanted effects of motion, and many are explained in detail in relevant anatomic chapters. Gradient moment nulling techniques (such as MAST™, FLOW COMP, GRF) and spatial presaturation will be reviewed in detail in this section.[28,34] Methods of suppressing unwanted motion effects are:

1. Cardiac gating: RF pulse is triggered by the electrocardiogram (ECG) to coincide with heart beat.

2. Respiratory gating: data are collected during quiet phases of breathing.

3. Small field of view.

4. Short TE and TR pulse sequences.

5. STIR pulse sequence: reduces signal and therefore ghosting effects from fat.

6. Altering phase encoding axis: phase encoding occurs much more slowly than frequency encoding, so motion in any direction is displayed along the phase encoding axis.

7. Physical restraint.

8. Signal averaging: smooths the effects of motion.

9. Phase reordering, e.g., ROPE, COPE.

10. Gradient moment nulling, e.g., MAST.

11. Spatial presaturation.

Gradient Moment Nulling

The chapters dealing with Artifacts and both the Cardiovascular and Respiratory systems discuss the need for synchronizing the data collection of the pulse sequence with either the ECG or the chest wall movement. Gating to the source of motion has been shown to be an effective technique for reducing motion artifacts resulting from view-to-view variations in the spatial spin-density distribution. Recently, however, motion that occurs from the start of the pulse sequence to the center of data collection has been recognized as an important contributor to motion artifacts. These sources of motion artifacts, or loss of signal, are termed "in-view" or "within-view" artifacts. Gradient moment nulling is one technique for dealing with these sources of motion.[28, 35]

Typically, imaging gradients are designed to provide refocusing of static spins. In the initial discussion of the slice-select gradient, the rephasing gradient lobe after the RF pulse was shown to refocus static spins, from the front to the back of the slice. Similarly, the frequency encoding gradient was shown to refocus static spins at the echo time, TE. It has been assumed that all spins in the imaging volume were static during the application of the gradient pulses. Unfortunately, this frequently is not the case. The interaction of the motion of the spins and the imaging gradient leads to a net dephasing that is dependent on the magnitude of the various derivatives of motion (velocity, acceleration, jerk, and higher order derivatives of motion), and the gradient's sensitivity to those terms. The sensitivity of the gradient lobes can be described by time moment equations, as shown below for the case of a gradient's sensitivity to velocity.

$$S_v = \int \gamma G(t) \, t \, dt$$

This produces a net dephasing of the moving spins by the equation:

$$\Phi_v = e^{-j \, 2\pi \, S_v \, V}$$

Where V is the magnitude of the velocity along the gradient G(t).

As the velocity increases, so does the magnitude of the spin dephasing. Examples of this are numerous in cardiovascular imaging. Often, the lumen appears dark at spatial locations where the velocity of the moving blood is insufficient to wash out of the slice within the interval between the 90- and 180-degree pulses. The interaction between the motion and the imaging gradients produces significant dephasing and the common flow void phenomenon. Similar terms exist for acceleration and higher order derivative terms as well. These terms exist for motion along all gradient axes.

Gradient moment nulling is accomplished by designing gradient waveforms, primarily along the read and slice-select axes, whose S_v terms (and possibly higher terms) equal zero. That is, the gradients have no sensi-

tivity to velocity or higher orders of motion. Therefore, no spin dephasing occurs no matter how large or small the velocity. With no sensitivity, the gradients recover signal from moving spins independent of the magnitude of their velocity.

How is this accomplished? The read and slice-select gradients have lobes that must be applied for specific amounts of time, and at specific amplitudes. For example, the frequency encoding gradient's amplitude during data sampling is fixed, and the amount of time that it is on, in part, determines field of view, bandwidth, and resolution. Once these parameters are selected in the design of a read gradient, the only factor left to be determined is how long and how strong the dephasing portion of the gradient is applied. It can be shown that this is equivalent to finding a gradient that meets the following condition:

$$R = \int G(t) \, dt$$

Setting R = 0 at the echo time will determine the required area under the dephase lobe. Once the duration of this lobe is chosen, its amplitude is explicitly defined in order to meet the R = 0 requirement. Therefore, by defining the timing of a single lobe other than that required for data collection (dephase gradient), it is possible to determine the amplitude needed to form an echo and meet the imaging requirements.[36] If there is enough time available to define another gradient lobe, we can determine the amplitude of each that will allow us to meet imaging requirements (form an echo) and also refocus spins moving with a constant velocity. Adding more lobes allow us to refocus higher and higher orders of motion (acceleration, jerk, and so forth).

This technique permits additional terms to be refocused as long as time is available for the addition of more gradient lobes. For example, a TE40 read gradient has only has about 25 msec available for adding more lobes. The remainder is devoted to approximately 10 msec for application of RF pulses and 5 msec for the first part of data collection. More gradient lobes can be added until their total is 25 msec. Therefore, if velocity compensation is required, a minimum of two lobes other than the data collection lobe is needed. Compensation to acceleration would require three lobes to be placed within the 25 msec. Needless to say, the longer the echo time, the more time is available to add lobes, and hence compensate for various moments.

The techniques used to determine the required gradient lobe amplitudes are straightforward. However, fitting gradient lobes into time intervals is only half the battle. The algorithms define the gradient lobe amplitudes that allow the waveforms to meet the refocusing and imaging requirements. Often the imagers are simply incapable of producing the gradient strengths required for all lobes. Time and gradient strength are the two factors that often limit the number of moments compensated in a given pulse sequence. It is possible to specify gradient lobes' positions in time and their amplitudes (which can be produced by the imager), and still be unable to accomplish refocusing. The limitation would arise if the imager could not reach the specified gradient strength within the time intervals used in the analysis. Typical values for echo times and maximal number of moments that can be compensated with current imagers are given in Table 2–2.

Gradient moment nulling techniques (e.g., MAST™, GRF, Flow Comp) provide significant improvements in many imaging applications where gating is commonly not used. Improved resolution and reduced motion artifacts have been observed in neuroradiologic, orbit, and abdominal studies. Total signal variation is reduced by refocusing moving spins completely within each view. They offer no significant time penalty since multiple acquisitions or synchronization is not required. However, it is possible to use gradient moment nulling techniques in combination with gating to reduce both within-view and view-to-view sources of motion artifact.

There are a few potential drawbacks to these techniques. First, they often produce complete (or partial) refocusing of moving blood, thereby making the lumen appear bright. However, most radiologists are used to seeing the lumen as flow voids. The refocusing can be somewhat annoying until one becomes accustomed to it. In the case of cardiac imaging, these techniques are often undesirable, since the heart chambers can appear bright as the flowing blood is recovered. This is potentially a significant problem if differentiation of normal and infarcted myocardium is pursued, if tumor is suspected, or if valve regurgitation with cine field echo sequences is used. In the latter two cases, the flowing blood and abnormal tissue may both be high signal intensity, thereby reducing the contrast between them. In the former case, the regurgitant valve is often identified by the presence of turbulence and local flow voids. The gradient moment nulling techniques partially refocus the turbulence, reducing the ability to detect the dysfunction.

The other criticism of these techniques relates directly to the imager. First, they can be significantly louder than their nonrefocusing counterparts. Additional lobes and higher gradient strength both produce more noise. Second, the gradient waveform required for refocusing is explicitly defined. If the gradient waveform is distorted, owing to eddy currents, for example, the performance of the technique will be compromised, since the obtained gradient waveform differs from the theoretical solution. This results in imperfect refocusing.

Advantages and Disadvantages of Gradient Moment Nulling

Advantages:
1. Can be used routinely.
2. Decreases motion artifact.
3. Does not increase scan time.
4. Additional gating or other hardware not required.

Disadvantages:
1. Very small fields of view or thin slice thicknesses, owing to increased gradient demands (usually need field of view >30 cm) may not be routinely available.
2. Flowing blood appears white.
3. Difficult to obtain motion refocusing at short echo times.
4. Sensitive to eddy currents.
5. More noise than non-refocused scans.

Spatial Presaturation

A second source of motion artifacts has to do with variations in the signal intensity from view-to-view motion. While gating can often be used to eliminate the motion variation, it cannot, for example, adequately deal with signal intensity variations resulting from tissue moving into or within the slice differently from one view to the next. Again, the best example of this is cardiovascular imaging and the effect of blood flow. Even though cardiac images may be gated, blood flows into and out of the cardiac chambers differently from view to view. Therefore, the amount of signal lost in a spatially dependent manner is different for each view, despite successful cardiac gating. The goal of spatial presaturation techniques is to identify the regions outside of the volume of interest from where the blood is flowing, and saturate the signal from all tissues (including blood) in these regions. Here, the blood will enter the imaging volume completely saturated, as opposed to completely magnetized. Thus, the inherent amount of signal that can be observed from the blood is severely reduced, thereby reducing the motion artifact resulting from it.[34]

In a typical cardiac gated pulse sequence, for example, 12 1-cm thick axial slices can be obtained. Blood entering from the inferior vena cava will pass through the slices on its way to the right heart. As it travels from the lower body toward the imaging plane, it becomes completely magnetized to its equilibrium value of M_0. As it passes through the imaging volume, it becomes partially saturated as it encounters the selective excitation for each of the slices. As it enters the right heart, it probably is partially saturated and will therefore produce signal in the imaging plane following RF application. Blood entering from the superior vena cava, how-

Table 2–2. ECHO TIME AND COMMON MOMENT REFOCUSING

TE	Moments
<10 msec	0 (position only)
10–25	0,1 (position, velocity)
30–50	0–2 (position, velocity, acceleration)
>55	0–3 (position, velocity acceleration, jerk)

Variations in field of view, data sampling interval, gradient strength, slew rate, RF pulse durations, etc., affect these values. These are not theoretical limits, but those commonly observed.

ever, does not pass through the imaging volume, and will therefore enter the imaging volume completely magnetized. In the right heart, the two "forms" of blood will mix, giving some intermediate value of saturation. From one view to the next, the blood will flow into the imaging volume slightly differently, thereby giving signal intensity differences that will lead to flow motion artifacts.

Spatial presaturation acts to "kill" these artifacts through the application of successive, rapidly applied RF pulses to regions outside the imaging volume, to reduce the magnetization flowing into the region of interest to several orders of magnitude below the previous example. If we think of the imaging volume as a cube, spatial presaturation could theoretically be applied on all six sides.

It is also possible to use spatial presaturation to remove signal that (1) contributes to motion artifact, (2) is not in the area of the desired information, yet (3) would fall within the image plane. An example of this would be the abdominal wall in a sagittal or axial lumbar spine surface coil examination. In this example, the abdominal wall rarely contributes diagnostic information in the image, even though it can be a significant source of motion artifacts. Therefore, spatial presaturation could be used to suppress the signal from the abdominal wall, thereby reducing the extent of its motion artifact in the scan. Alternatively, spatial presaturation could be applied to regions outside that of interest to eliminate the possibility of aliasing.

Most presaturation techniques (such as BOSS, FLAK) require additional RF pulses to be applied to the subject. As mentioned earlier, however, the amount of RF energy applied to the body must be limited. Therefore, the degree of saturation, or the number of "sides" of the imaging volume saturated, may be limited. However, these techniques undoubtably add significant improvements in artifact reduction. Further, these techniques will be combined with gradient moment nulling and advanced gating techniques to remove in-view, view-to-view, and into-the-view sources of artifact even further than presently achieved.

IMAGE PROCESSING

Filtering and Anti-aliasing

The Fourier transform reconstruction (two- and three-dimensional) algorithms used in MRI produce discrete pixel values at each spatial location. Often a smoothing algorithm is applied to the final image to remove "pixeliness" resulting from producing discrete pixel values in the display of an image matrix size greater than that acquired. An example of this would be a 256 × 128 data matrix that would lead to a 256 × 128 image matrix. However, the resolution along one axis will be twice that along the other, necessitating the replication of pixels along one axis so that the displayed

image will be correctly sized. If the display is capable of 512 × 512, pixel values will be replicated along both axes, one by a factor of 2, and the other by a factor of 4 to use the entire display area. Unfortunately, this pixel replication makes the displayed images look "blocky." However, we know that tissue does not come in blocks, and often changes fairly gradually throughout the image plane. Therefore, it is possible to smooth the reconstructed matrix by weighting adjacent pixels and summing them. Each pixel then becomes a weighted average of its neighbors. This filtering smooths the image, removing the distinct edges of the reconstructed boxes. The range of adjacent pixels and their weighting determine how much smoothing or how much sharpness remains in the displayed images. Imagers often come with a wide range of filtering algorithms that can be used on the reconstructed images.

A second type of algorithm on most imagers is the ability to acquire a real image, at twice the field of view along one or both axes of the image plane. The resolution of the acquired matrix is equal to that desired. To accomplish this, twice as many views or twice as many data points are collected, at twice the field of view. The images are then reconstructed, and only the center part, corresponding to the area of interest, is displayed. For example, imagine that a 25-cm field of view is desired and that the in-plane resolution is to be 1 mm. This would require 256 data points to be collected per data sampling interval, and 256 phase encodings to be performed. The image generated under these conditions would have aliasing along the read and phase axes about the edges of the field of view. Performing the same sequence by acquiring twice the data points and twice the phase encodings (at half the step size for both) leads to a final image that is 512 × 512 at twice the field of view (50 cm). The center 256 × 256 part of the reconstructed image corresponds to a 25-cm field of view (FOV), with 1 mm resolution.

The advantage of the second method is that aliasing occurs about the edges of the acquired, not displayed, field of view. This is known as an anti-aliasing form of filtering. It is available by collecting a data matrix greater than the displayed matrix. It can also be obtained at any ratio of acquired to displayed field of view.

Zooming

A second technique for displaying a portion of the displayed, or acquired, field of view is to magnify or zoom the image. To perform this task, the original data points are used to generate additional pixels that fall between known acquired values. For example, imagine that the acquired display is 256 × 256 and that the acquired field of view is 25 cm, as in the previous example. The desired field of view may be approximately 20 cm, indicating that the displayed image should be the same displayed over the same number of pixels, yet over 80 percent of the original field of view.

Eighty percent of the original 256 × 256 data matrix corresponds to zooming the center 205 × 205 pixels to a 256 × 256 matrix. Zooming creates the pixel required to perform this remapping similarly to the smoothing process described earlier. The zooming process creates additional pixels in an intelligent fashion, by considering adjacent pixels, and assuming that transitions in pixel values occur with some reasonably gradual spatial variation. The advantages of zooming are that the displayed matrix can incorporate and expand on only the tissues of interest. Unfortunately, since pixels are created artificially, this technique cannot compare directly with the image that would be obtained by performing the pulse sequence at the spatial location of interest with the field of view obtained by zooming. It is often impossible to obtain the image under the desired conditions, necessitating the use of zooming to obtain an approximation to the resolution and signal to noise desired.

Surface Coil Correction

The variations in signal intensity resulting from spatial differences in the sensitivity of the receiving coil are often fairly gradual. Surface coil correction algorithms attempt to normalize the intensity across the image plane. In this way, the variation in intensity resulting from the coil can be made less conspicuous. Figure 2–24 shows the one-dimensional variation of a coil across a field of view. Surface coil correction would scale the intensity at each spatial location by line B in the figure. The product of A and B at all locations is approximately 1.0 and removes the spatial variation associated with the coil.

Unfortunately, an accurate knowledge of the coil's sensitivity pattern for each patient over all fields of view would be required to perform the simple scaling described. A more robust pattern of correction is desired that automatically accounts for these differences. Fortunately, the spatial variation is low frequency, occurring gradually over space within the image plane. Therefore, a subset of the acquired data set, corresponding to the low-frequency variations in the image, can be used as a model to the variation in signal intensity resulting from the coil. A 256 × 256 data set could be used to reconstruct the whole image, complete with spatial variation resulting from the coil. The central 32 × 32 would provide information about the low-frequency variation in signal intensity over the field of view. This 32 × 32 matrix can be interpolated up to a 256 × 256 matrix, and smoothed so that a reasonably accurate and smooth signal intensity variation resulting from the coil can be obtained. The reconstructed image is then divided by the surface coil image obtained from the central part of the data. This division is done on a pixel by pixel basis, to normalize over the image plane.

The advantage of this technique for surface coil image reprocessing is that the correction map is determined from the image itself. There is no need to maintain a set of correction maps for the various coils over the ranges of field of view, and positioned over different regions of the image plane. Further, the 32 × 32 reconstruction takes rather less time than does the interpolation.

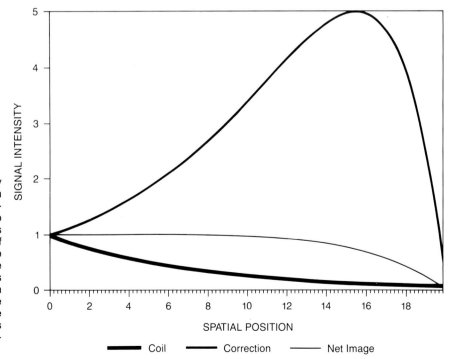

Figure 2–24. The surface coil intensity falloff is often fairly gradual as shown in a one-dimensional example of a coil applied on a uniform object. It is possible to examine the variation of the signal as obtained from the low-frequency part of the image to generate a correction map that normalizes the intensity over the field of view. The correction applied is also shown. The net result in a uniform object is presented to show that some falloff cannot be corrected. However, the normalization of the uniform object is fairly accurate and may offer advantages over no correction.

The actual rescaling of the image does take an additional amount of time. However, the correction does not add a tremendous burden to the reconstruction and is often worth the extra time required to obtain a more uniform signal. Depending on the techniques available on the imager, it is often possible to perform the correction on the images during periods of low demand on the imager.

SPECTROSCOPY

Recently, spectroscopic information has been obtained from various nuclei on slightly modified MR imagers. The two nuclei of interest in NMR spectroscopy for human applications are primarily 1H and 31P. The 1H work has been portrayed as an addition to a conventional scan, since the resonant frequency of the compounds of interest is approximately equal to the Larmor frequency of the remainder of the protons in the body. The 31P work is of interest owing to phosphorus being a major "player" in cell energetics through ATP, ADP, inorganic phosphate, phosphocreatine, and so forth.

Different metabolic or neurotransmitter compounds of interest have protons or phosphorus nuclei with slightly different resonant frequencies owing to electron cloud portions of the molecule shielding some of the nuclei from part of the main static magnetic field. The amount of shielding depends on the shape and constituents of the molecule. Thus, the different molecules of interest often have slightly different resonant frequencies because of differences in structure and composition.[10, 37] Generally, the shift in resonant frequencies is less than 10 ppm, or less than 640 hertz for protons at 64 MHz. Once nutated into the X-Y plane, the nuclei precess at their resonant frequency and induce a voltage in the coil at that frequency.

Unfortunately, the concentration of the nuclei in the compounds of interest is a factor of at least 1,000 less than the concentration of the water in the body. Therefore, since so few of the compounds are available, the signal level from the compounds will be small as well. Thus, in order to obtain adequate signal-to-noise levels in many spectroscopic examinations, it is necessary to increase the size of the voxel from 1 mm × 1 mm × 5 mm to about 2 cm × 2 cm × 2 cm. Further, the dynamic range of the system must be adjusted so that detectable levels of the compound of interest can be detected in the presence of water for 1H work. Thus, techniques must be available for suppressing the water resonant signal, while simultaneously detecting the compounds of interest. Fortunately, these techniques have been developed.

The spins from the nuclei of interest must then be nutated into the detection plane, while the unwanted resonances are suppressed. This often entails performing selective excitation along all three imaging axes so that only the voxel of interest produces signal in the X-Y plane. Once the proposed spectroscopic voxel has been nutated into the X-Y plane, a signal is observed that is the sum of varying sinusoids, whose strength is proportional to the concentration of the compound at that frequency in the voxel of interest. A one-dimensional Fourier transform is then applied to the signal to separate the individual frequencies and their concentrations. The compounds are then identified according to their known shift in resonant frequency, in parts per million. Often, multiple repetitions are performed to increase the signal to noise of the resulting spectrum. A variety of techniques have been developed to perform the spatial localization and water suppression.

31P spectroscopy requires a different resonant frequency owing to differences in 1H and 31P gyromagnetic ratios. Therefore, 31P spectroscopy on an imager requires both separate coils tuned to the resonant frequency of 31P at the field strength used, and an imager that can be adjusted to the alternate resonant frequency with little if any loss in performance (other than the amount of time required to make the conversion).

Figure 2–25 shows an example of 1H and 31P spectra obtained on a muscle before and after occlusion.[37] A great deal of effort has been put forth for NMR spectroscopy on clinical MR imagers, but its clinical usefulness and relevance have not yet been conclusively established.

SUMMARY AND CONCLUSIONS

The goal of this chapter has been to refamiliarize those already working in the field of MRI with many of the physical principles of NMR. Further, it is hoped that this chapter has given some insight to those just beginning, or contemplating further work in MRI. The myriad of potential variables has been partially explored, leaving almost an infinite number still to be covered. To a certain extent, MRI may offer yet unknown potential or may suffer unforeseen pitfalls as these variables are explored in the future. However, at this point, its future seems promising.

The basic physics involved in the production of longitudinal magnetization were presented, as were the methods required for nutating it into a plane adequate for detection. The signal used for RF transmission and the resultant induced voltage in a coil were described. Relaxation toward equilibrium and relaxation in plane were also discussed.

Two of the most important concepts presented in this chapter were the SNR in an image and the CNR. Signal to noise was discussed as the "graininess" of the image, with high signal level relative to patient and electronic noise offering the clearest, least mottled images. Attempts to improve the SNR can be seen to be centered around two predominant methods. The first deals with getting more spins (protons) in each voxel, by increases in slice thickness, or decreasing the in-plane resolution. The price paid for this is poorer resolution and increased partial volume effects that may reduce the observed resolution below that predicted by parame-

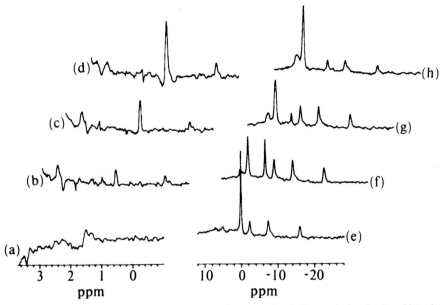

Figure 2–25. The 1H and 31P spectra obtained from a rat leg before and after ligation. Note the changes in the relative strength of the various peaks in both the 1H (a–d) and 31P (e–h) spectra with time. The primary compound in the 1H is lactate. Note the change in lactate production from before occlusion (a) to approximately 1 hour later. Signal peak assignments in the 31P spectra (e–h) spectra from right to left have been identified as alpha, beta, and gamma phosphates in ATP, phosphocreatine (0 ppm), inorganic phosphate, and phosphomonoesters. Figure (e) was obtained before ligation, and f–h 13, 26, and 52 minutes later. Note the difference in pH over time, as obtained from the shift position difference between inorganic phosphate and phosphocreatine. Note also the changes in peak strengths over time. (From Williams SB, Gadian DG, Proctor E, et al. Proton NMR studies of muscle metabolites in vivo. J Magn Res 1985; 63:407–412.)

ters of the data collection. Parameters, such as field of view, only lead to differences in signal to noise if the physical size of the voxel (resolution) changes as well. Therefore, the basic techniques for improving signal to noise deal with increasing the size of the voxel.

The second method for altering the image signal-to-noise dealt with changing the amount of signal detected in the X-Y plane, through variations in TE, TR, or TI, or by using alternate pulse sequences. Examples were presented that showed how signal-to-noise improvements obtained through these techniques force compromises to be made with the image contrast. Variations in these parameters often lead to variations in image contrast that alternately improve the image signal to noise and reduce the differentiation between tissues.

Alternative techniques for reducing the image noise through reductions in the image bandwidth were presented. The method was described as extending the data collection interval while simultaneously reducing the frequency encoding gradient. In this way, the bandwidth across the image and across each voxel is reduced, so that narrower bandwidth filters can be used in the receive chain of the imager. Here, the tradeoff in the image is between signal to noise and chemical shift artifact. In the head and some areas of the body, the advantages to be gained are worth the increased shift in position of the fat signal. A second method for increasing the image signal to noise, while not affecting con-

trast, is through multiple repetitions of each view. Here, the tradeoff is between signal to noise and imaging time. Imaging time increases directly with the number of repetitions per view, signal to noise increasing as the square root of the number of repetitions.

Techniques were presented that described methods for slice localization. Predominantly 2-D and 3-D techniques were described. The advantage of 3-D acquisition is that improvements in the slice profile can be obtained that improve the amount of detected signal in the X-Y plane, since selective RF pulses are not used to define individual slices. 3-D techniques take at least N times longer (N is the number of slices) than a conventional 2-D multislice scan for many pulse sequences, but some of the fast techniques cannot be obtained in 2-D multislice mode, which necessitates 2-D sequential or 3-D data collection strategies. The basic problem with 2-D techniques is that the selective pulses used to define slice position lead to cross-talk between images (presently quite slight) and spin dephasing at the edges of the slice profile, which leads to incomplete signal recovery during detection.

Some of the more interesting recent pulse sequences were also described. Most were centered around two areas: reducing scan time and reducing the effects of motion. All have applications and benefits that were described. However, only the gradient moment nulling techniques have presently gained widespread application and use. The use of chemical shift imaging will undoubtably open new horizons in imaging as well. The role of spectroscopy in the future is undoubtably further off, yet still an important topic.

It would be nice if MRI were a simple, easy to understand imaging modality, but it is not. However, it is the number of variables that affect image quality and contrast that makes MRI such a powerful tool, with only partially realized potential. The bottom line on imaging, however, is that any parameter that is changed, whether it be field of view, slice thickness, tip angle, number of views, or TR, will lead to changes in the appearance of the resultant images, with widespread ramifications throughout. MRI is not a tool that has cookbook recipes for finding lesions optimally. Therefore, one must explore the impact of the many variables, balancing contrast, signal to noise, resolution, imaging time, and end image interpretability until appropriate selections and understanding are obtained. Often the final selections chosen will be similar to those of others, with minor differences as required to balance individual specific tradeoffs and needs.

REFERENCES

1. Hayt WH. Engineering electromagnetics. 3rd ed. New York: McGraw-Hill, 1974.
2. Hayt WH, Kemmerly JE. Engineering circuit analysis. 3rd ed. New York: McGraw-Hill, 1978.
3. American Radio Relay League. Radio engineers handbook.
4. Hinshaw WS, Lent AH. An introduction to NMR imaging: from the Bloch equations to the imaging equations. Proceedings of the IEEE 1983; 71(3):338–350.
5. Patrick J. Picker International, personal communication, April 10, 1989.
6. House WV. Theoretical basis for NMR imaging. In: Partain CL, James AE, Rollo FD, Price RR, eds. Magnetic resonance imaging. Philadelphia: WB Saunders, 1983:60–72.
7. Slichter CP. Principles of magnetic resonance. New York: Springer-Verlag, 1980.
8. Abragam A. Principles of nuclear magnetism. New York: Oxford University Press, 1978.
9. Partain RC, Price RR, et al. The physical basis for NMR imaging. In: Partain CL, James AE, Rollo FD, Price RR, eds. Magnetic resonance imaging. Philadelphia: WB Saunders, 1983: 73–93.
10. Fukishima E, Roeder SB. Experimental pulse NMR: a nuts and bolts approach. Reading, MA: Addison Wesley, 1981.
11. Wehrli FW, MacFall JR, Newton TH. Parameters determining the appearance of NMR images. In: Newton TH, Potts DG, eds. Advanced imaging techniques. Vol 2. San Anselmo, CA: Clavadell Press, 1983.
12. Wolfe FL, Popp C. NMR: a primer for medical imaging. Thorofare, NJ: Slack, 1984.
13. General Electric. NMR: a perspective on imaging. Milwaukee, WI: General Electric Company, Medical Systems Operations.
14. Gyngell ML, Palmer ND, Eastwood LM. The application of SSFP in 2D-FT MR imaging. SMRM, Fifth Annual Meeting, August 19–22, 1986, Montreal. 3:666–667.
15. Sebok DA, Yeung HN. Gradient reversal echo, equilibrium driving—a new method of rapid imaging. SMRM, Fifth Annual Meeting, August 19–22, 1986, Montreal. 3:936–937.
16. Mansfield P, Morris PG. NMR imaging in biomedicine. Suppl 2. Advances in magnetic resonance. New York: Academic Press, 1982.
17. Mansfield P. Echo planar MR imaging. NMR Images, May–June 1984:22–25.
18. Ordidge RJ, Mansfield P, Doyle M. Real time movie images by NMR. Br J Radiol 1982; 55:729–733.
19. Haacke EM, Clayton JR, Linga NR, Bearden FH. Demonstration of a flexible fast scan technique. Radiology 1984; 153:244.
20. Dixon WT, Faul DD, Gado MH, et al. Using the chemical shift difference between water and lipid in proton imaging. Radiology 1984; 153:65.
21. Park HW, Kim DJ, Cho ZH. Gradient reversal and its applications to chemical-shift-related NMR imaging. Mag Res Med 1987; 4:526–536.
22. Axel L. Blood flow effects in magnetic resonance imaging. Am J Roent 1984; 143:1157–1166.
23. Bradley WG, Waluch V, Lai KS, et al. The appearance of rapidly flowing blood in magnetic resonance images. Am J Roent 1984; 143:1167–1174.
24. Bradley WG, Waluch V. Blood flow: magnetic resonance imaging. Radiology 1985; 154:443–450.
25. George CR, Jacobs G, MacIntyre WJ, Lorig RJ, et al. Magnetic resonance intensity patterns obtained from continuous and pulsatile flow models. Radiology 1984; 151:421–428.
26. Grant JP, Back C. NMR rheotomography: feasibility and clinical potential. Med Phys 1983; 42(3):938–940.
27. Ehman RL, Felmlee J, Julsrud PR, Gray JE, et al. Vascular misregistration: a helpful sign in clinical MR imaging characterizing blood flow within the plane of selection. Radiology 1985; 157:121.
28. Duerk JL, Pattany PM. Analysis of imaging axes' significance in motion artifact reduction technique: MRI of turbulent flow and motion. Mag Res Imag 1989; 7:251–263.
29. Constantinesco A, Mallet J, Bonmartin A, Lallot C, Briguet A. Spatial flow velocity phase encoding gradients in NMR imaging. Mag Res Imag 1983; 2:335–340.
30. Crooks LE, Mills C, Davis PL, Brandt-Zawadzki M, et al. Visualization of cerebral abnormalities by NMR imaging: The effects of imaging parameters on contrast. Radiology 1982; 144:843–852.
31. Waluch V, Bradley WG. NMR even echo rephasing in slow laminar flow. JCAT 1984; 8(4):594–598.
32. Katz J, Peshock RM, McNamee P, et al. Analysis of spin-echo rephasing with pulsatile flow in 2DFT magnetic resonance imaging. Mag Res Med 1987; 4:307–322.
33. Henkelman RM. Measurement of signal intensities in the presence of noise in MR images. Med Phys 1985; 12(2):232–233.
34. Ehman RL, Felmlee JP, Julsrud PR, et al. Technique for eliminating flow artifacts and for improving the depiction of vascular anatomy in MRI—description and clinical application. Mag Res Imag (Suppl 1) 1987; 5:33.
35. Pattany PM, Phillips J, Chiu LC, et al. Motion artifact suppression technique (MAST) for magnetic resonance imaging. JCAT 1987; 11:3.
36. Duerk JL. A magnetic resonance imaging gradient modulation technique for motion artifact reduction and flow quantification. Case Western Reserve University, Biomedical Engineering Department, Cleveland, Ohio, November 1986.
37. Williams SB, Gadian DG, Proctor E, et al. Proton NMR studies of muscle metabolites in vivo. J Mag Res 1985; 63(2):407–412.
38. Farrar TC, Becker ED. Pulse and Fourier transform NMR: introduction to theory and methods. New York: Academic Press, 1971.

ADDITIONAL READINGS

Feinberg EA, Crooks LE, Sheldon P, et al. Inner volume MR imaging: technical concepts and their application. Radiology 1985; 156:743–747.

Hahn EL. Spin echoes. Phys Rev 1950; 80:580–584.

Hanly P. Magnets for medical applications of NMR. Br Med Bull 1984; 40(2):125–131.

Harms SE, Morgan TJ, Yamanashi WS, et al. Principles of nuclear magnetic resonance imaging. RadioGraphics 1984; 4:26–43.

Holland GN. Systems engineering of a whole body proton magnetic resonance imaging system. In: Partain CL, James AE, Rollo FD, Price RR, eds. Philadelphia: WB Saunders, 1983:128–151.

Hoult DI. NMR imaging techniques. Br Med Bull 1984; 40(2):132–138.

King K, Moran PR. A unified description of NMR data collection strategies and reconstruction. Med Phys 1984; 11:1–14.

Kumar A, Welti D, Ernst RR. NMR Fourier zeugmatography. J Mag Res 1975; 18:69–83.

Moore WS. Basic physics and relaxation mechanisms. Br Med Bull 1984; 40(2):120–124.

Moran PR. A flow zeugmatographic interlace for NMR imaging in humans. Mag Res Imag 1982; 1:197–203.

Pykett IL. NMR imaging in medicine. Sci Am 1982; 246(5):78–88.

Rabi II, Ramsey NF, Schwingerm J. Use of rotating coordinates in magnetic resonance problems. Rev Mod Phys 1954; 26(2):167–171.

Stark DD, Bradley WG. Magnetic resonance imaging. Washington, DC: CV Mosby, 1988.

Wehrli FW. Advanced MR imaging techniques. Milwaukee, WI: GE Medical Systems.

Young IR. Considerations affecting signal and contrast in NMR imaging. Br Med Bull 1984; 40(2):139–147.

Artifacts

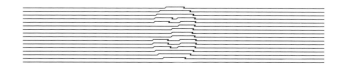

PETER ROTHSCHILD, M.D.
MURRAY SOLOMON, M.D.
JOSEPH CARLSON, Ph.D.

A knowledge of artifacts is more important in MRI than in almost any other imaging procedure in radiology. There are many causes of artifacts on MR images. Artifacts can obscure pathology, degrade overall image quality, and lead to false-positive or false-negative diagnoses. Although it is the job of the MR system engineer to minimize the potential for artifacts, some will inevitably occur. The radiologist reading MR scans should be able to understand the basic physics and origin of these artifacts. This knowledge will assist an analysis of areas of abnormal signal intensity seen on an MR image and help avoid misinterpreting an artifact for a pathologic condition. Furthermore, throughput can be increased when precautions are taken to eliminate common artifacts, especially those that are patient induced.

Artifacts can be divided into two simple categories. The most frequently encountered group are patient induced. These include patient motion (external or internal), metallic implants, braces, dental work, metal in clothes, eye makeup, residual Pantopaque, hair clips, iron fillings, and other metallic objects. This category of artifact is the most frequent cause of poor-quality MR studies and repeat examinations. The other major category of artifacts stems from the MRI equipment and includes system failures, inherent artifacts in data collection and reconstruction, and environmental factors. Murphy's law ("Whatever can go wrong will go wrong") definitely applies to this group of artifacts.

PATIENT-INDUCED ARTIFACTS

Motion

Motion artifact is probably the most frequently encountered and most disturbing artifact in MRI (Fig. 3–1). The cause can be divided into gross body motion and physiologic motion[1] (i.e., bowel peristalsis, cerebrospinal fluid [CSF] pulsation, cardiac pulsation, and respiratory motion). Motion in any direction in a two-dimensional Fourier transformation (2D-FT) results in artifacts that are displayed in the phase encoding direction. This motion artifact is present in the image as spatial misregistration of the data or ghosts. As little as 2 mm of motion can seriously degrade edge detection.[2,3] Generally less apparent in an MR image is motion perpendicular to the imaging plane. This motion does not introduce any obvious ghosts in 2D-FT MRI, but rather a loss of resolution in the slice direction as data from different projections are acquired from different sections. Motion artifacts are more apparent at higher field strengths. The explanation for this is not completely understood but may be related to the higher absolute field inhomogeneity. This is shown in the example of a sagittal knee scan performed at 0.064T that shows no phase encoding artifacts from the pulsating popliteal artery (Fig. 3–2) and the same knee performed on a 0.35T system showing pulsation artifacts from the popliteal artery (Fig. 3–3). The

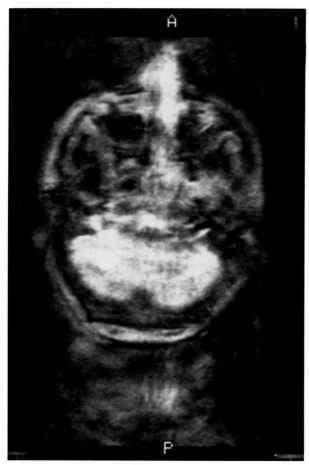

Figure 3–1. *Diagnosis: Motion artifact. Axial head scan.* This was a very uncooperative patient and motion artifact is seen throughout the image. Sedation is often the best way to eliminate this type of motion artifact.

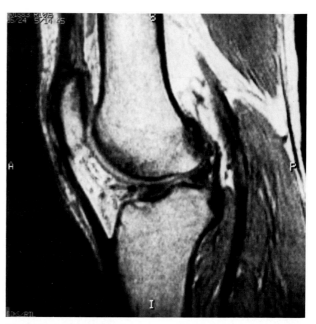

Figure 3–2. *Diagnosis: Lack of pulsation artifact.* Sagittal knee scan at 0.064T obtained in the plane of the popliteal artery without the use of presaturation or flow compensation. Note the lack of pulsation artifact that is seen at higher field strength magnets, as in Figure 3–3.

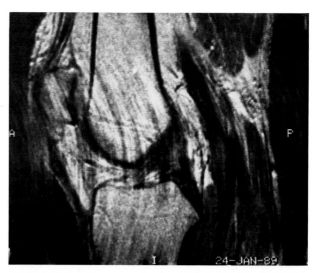

Figure 3–3. *Diagnosis: Pulsation artifacts.* Sagittal 0.35T knee scan. Phase encoding pulsation artifacts are seen throughout the knee. The contour of the artifact corresponds to the vessel of origin. These artifacts can mimic meniscal or ligamentous tears. Presaturation, flow compensation, and reordered phase encoding are ways to decrease these artifacts in the area of interest.

perplexing problem of motion in MRI has led to many interesting solutions. Only the most useful methods are discussed here (see also the chapters on the physics of MRI and the gastrointestinal [GI] system).

Sedation

The obvious solution for gross patient motion is sedation. Noise from the gradients and claustrophobia from lying in a confined space contribute to patients' anxiety and diminish their ability to lie still. The recent development of a quiet and open MR system operating at 0.064T alleviates many of these difficulties. Many children can be imaged in this system without sedation, since it is quiet and less imposing than other MR systems. The child's parents are always encouraged to be in the MR suite with the child (Fig. 3–4).

Gating

Sedation does not help physiologic motion (Fig. 3–5). Pulsation artifact can be decreased by synchronizing the MR sequence with the r wave of the

cardiac cycle (Fig. 3–6).[4] Electrocardiographic (ECG) gating decreases flexibility in selecting TR (must be equal to a multiple of the R-R interval) and assumes a regular heart rate, since most MR systems today cannot eliminate data acquired during ectopic beats. Another disadvantage is the time it takes to

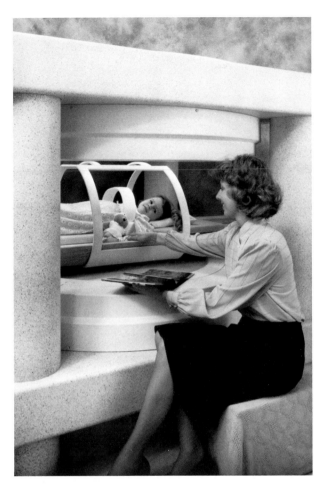

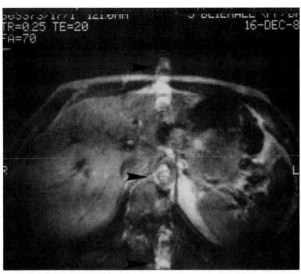

Figure 3–5. *Diagnosis: Pulsation artifact.* Breath-hold abdominal MR scan. Pulsation artifact from the aorta is seen in the phase encoding direction. This artifact could easily be mistaken for a lesion in the left lobe of the liver. The use of reordered phase and frequency encoding can help resolve a difficult case. Also, the use of cardiac gating for non–breath-hold sequences or presaturation pulses can help eliminate this artifact.

Figure 3–4. *Diagnosis: Low field MRI.* 0.064T system manufactured by Diasonics. The open design of this magnet has excellent patient acceptance and easier patient monitoring during the examination. Furthermore, the low field eliminates the danger from flying projectiles, and the much weaker gradients are almost inaudible.

connect the ECG leads and the technical setup of the gating mechanism.

Presaturation

Another very successful method of decreasing motion is presaturation,[5] the object of which is to minimize signal from whatever is moving. Therefore, when the computer misplaces this signal along the phase encoding axis, it will not be distracting. Presaturation uses repeated radiofrequency (RF) pulses applied to the area responsible for the motion and outside the area of interest in the slice. An example of presaturation for a lumbar spine study is seen in Figure 3–7. The abdomen anterior to the lumbar spine has been presaturated with repeated RF pulses to eliminate most of the signal from this portion of the abdomen. Also, tissue outside the slices can be presaturated with multiple 90-degree RF pulses, so that when the blood enters the area being imaged it will have low signal intensity. This has proved very helpful in decreasing the vascular ghost, especially at high field. Presaturation technique allows any TR to be used and does not increase the scan time, but it does increase the RF power deposited in the patient. At higher field strengths with certain pulse sequences, this may exceed FDA guidelines.

Breath Hold

For cooperative patients, respiratory motion may be eliminated by obtaining breath-hold scans (see Fig. 3–5) lasting approximately 30 seconds. This is more difficult to achieve in children than in adults. Generally, these scans do not have the resolution or signal-to-noise ratios of the longer scans, but they significantly decrease motion artifact, making them useful in abdominal imaging. Repeated sets of breath-hold scans can be averaged to improve signal-to-noise ratios.

Reordered Phasing and Frequency Encoding

Reordered phasing and frequency encoding is a simple method to alter motion artifacts (Fig. 3–8).[6] Since ghost artifacts are displayed in the phase encoding axis, by swapping the latter with the frequency encoding axis, motion artifact can be moved to a different part of the image away from important structures. This is most frequently performed in the spine, especially the thoracic spine. Instead of having the phase encoding artifacts from the pulsating heart and major blood vessels projected over the spine, these can be moved so that the spine is not obscured by motion artifact. There is no penalty for this method, but care must be taken when using it not to choose a matrix that is smaller than the field of view in the phase encoding axis, or wraparound can be a major problem (Fig. 3–9). Altering the phase encoding axis does not reduce motion arti-

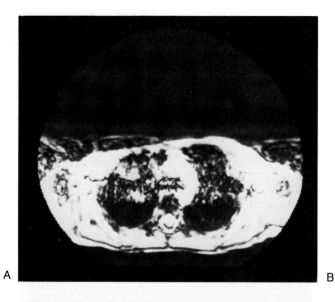

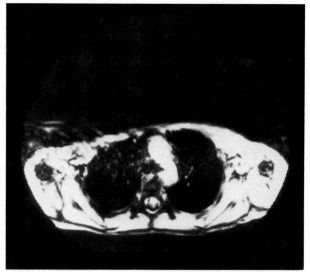

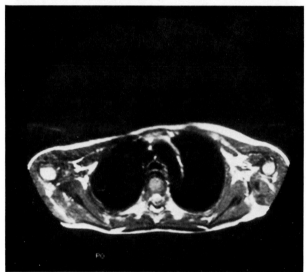

Figure 3–6. *Diagnosis: Effect of image acquisition technique on aortic pulsation artifact. All images are transverse thoracic images at the level of the aortic arch.* **A,** Field echo (550/12) without cardiac gating. Marked pulsation artifact is seen throughout the image. **B,** Field echo (800/12) with cardiac gating. There is significant reduction of the pulsation artifact. **C,** Spin echo (670/26) with cardiac gating. There is further reduction in the pulsation artifact.

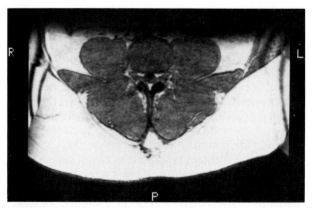

Figure 3–7. *Diagnosis: Presaturated pulse sequence.* Axial lumbar spine. The anterior portion of the abdomen has been presaturated and hence is of low signal intensity. Notice the lack of motion artifact over the area of interest in the spine.

fact, but merely moves it to a different part of the image. In some cases it can be an effective and simple technique to decrease motion artifact in the area of interest. Imaging techniques also affect the appearance of motion artifacts. For example, field-echo (gradient-echo) pulse sequences are far more sensitive to motion than the more current conventional spin-echo techniques (Fig. 3–10) and should therefore not be used for areas of the body where motion is a problem.

Image Averaging

One of the simplest ways to reduce motion artifact is image averaging, which has proved most helpful for respiratory motion. It does not require extra equipment but can significantly increase the time of the examination, which can lead to increased patient fatigue and motion.

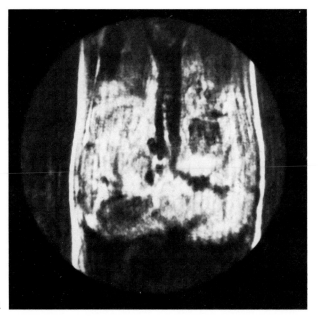 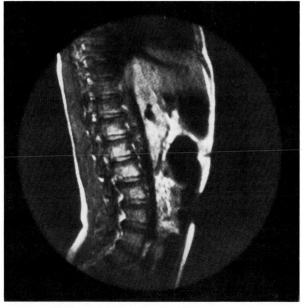

A   B

Figure 3–8. *Diagnosis: Effect of changing imaging plane on motion artifact. Alteration of the imaging plane can sometimes result in a reduction of motion artifact.* ***A,*** *Coronal T1 spin-echo image (700/30). There is marked motion artifact due to aspiration. Phase encoding is from side to side.* ***B,*** *Sagittal T1 weighted image (700/30). Alteration of the acquisition plane and phase encoding has resulted in a significant reduction of the respiratory motion artifact. Phase encoding is from front to back of the patient.*

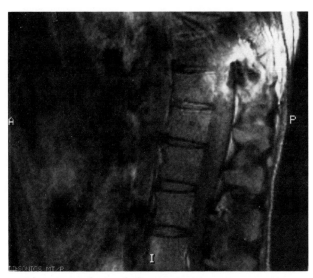

Figure 3–9. *Diagnosis: Wraparound artifact. Sagittal spine.* An unusual-looking area of increased signal with a loss of the superior lumbar vertebra is identified. This lesion is an artifact from wraparound of the sacrum and air in the rectum in a patient with a normal lumbar spine.

Flow Compensation

Flow compensation (gradient moment nulling) is a new and promising method of decreasing physiologic motion (see the chapters on the physics of MRI).[7] It involves the use of gradient manipulation to refocus out-of-phase signal from motion of arteries, veins, the GI system, and CSF. Flow compensation can compensate for higher orders of motion such as acceleration and pulsatility. The disadvantages are the increased time the gradient must be on per imaging sequence, limitation on the minimal TE value that can be utilized, and the decreased number of slices obtained for a given TR. Flow compensation is an excellent way to decrease motion artifact and will be used more often in the future, especially for techniques making CSF appear white, such as a partial flip sequence (Fig. 3–11).

Magnetic Field Inhomogeneity

Implanted Metal and Metallic Objects

After motion, the next most troublesome artifact routinely encountered is focal field inhomogeneity. The quality of images in MRI is highly dependent on the extreme uniformity (parts per million) of the static magnetic field. Metal appliances such as vena caval filters,[8,9] joint prostheses (Fig. 3–12), dental work (Fig. 3–13),[10] metal fragments (Figs. 3–14, 3–15), surgical clips,[11] mascara and eye makeup (Fig. 3–16), jewelry, hairpins (Fig. 3–17), metal in clothing (Fig. 3–18), and dentures (Fig. 3–19) all can cause a warping of the main magnetic field at a specific location. Magnetic metals warp the local magnetic field because of their own intrinsic magnetic field. Nonmagnetic metals have currents induced in them by the gradients.

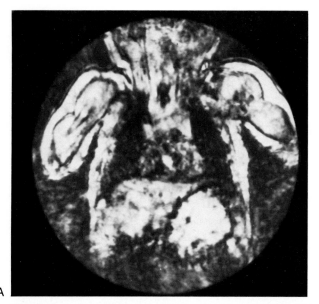
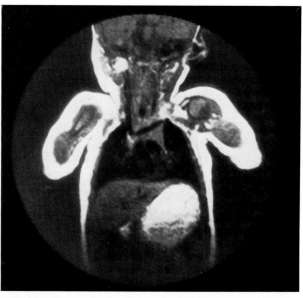

A   B

Figure 3–10. *Diagnosis: Demonstration of the increased sensitivity of field-echo imaging techniques to motion. Both images are coronal images through the thorax, acquired with cardiac gating.* **A,** Field-echo image (560/12). There is severe artifact due to motion. **B,** Spin-echo image (460/20). The spin-echo images are much less sensitive to motion than field-echo images. There is much less artifact due to motion on this image.

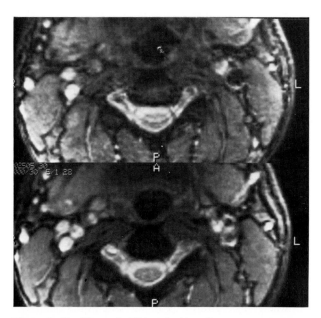

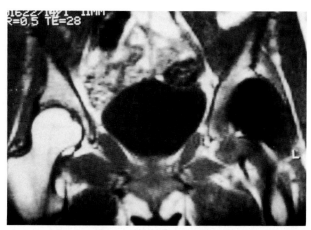

Figure 3–12. *Diagnosis: Artifact from a prosthetic hip.* Coronal T1 WI MR pelvic scan. In the region of the left hip is an area of signal void, which is secondary to artifact from the prosthetic hip. Artifact from a prosthetic hip is often worse on CT than on MRI.

Figure 3–11. *Diagnosis: With and without flow compensation.* A partial flip axial of a normal cervical spine with and without flow compensation: top image without, bottom image with flow compensation. Note how the lower image does not have the artifact overlying the cord, which could mask a lesion.

These electric currents create a local magnetic field that distorts the main magnetic field. Magnetic metals cause a much greater artifact than nonmagnetic metals. It is the electromagnetic field associated with these metallic devices that interferes with and distorts

(warps) the main magnetic field, causing gross spatial mismapping of anatomic detail. This is secondary to the fact that the linear relationship between spatial location, phase angle, and frequency is no longer valid. MR images derive their spatial information from the deliberate alteration of magnetic fields, which are assumed by the MR computer to be perfectly homogeneous. If this main magnetic field is disturbed by metal artifact, spatial misregistration occurs. Furthermore, these metallic objects can cause large variations in the

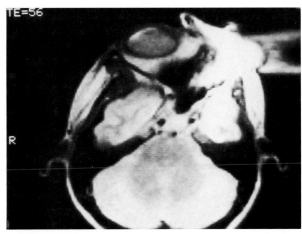

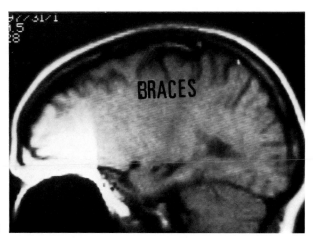

Figure 3–13. *Diagnosis: Artifact from orthodontic braces.* **A, B,** Axial and sagittal head scans. Distortion and high signal intensity are identified in the left facial, orbital, and temporal areas. This is an artifact commonly seen in patients with orthodontic braces. One must be very careful not to misinterpret the high signal in the temporal lobes of these patients as a pathologic condition. It may be helpful to have the technologist record whether patients have metal anywhere in their bodies that is not removed before the MR scan, especially dentures or braces.

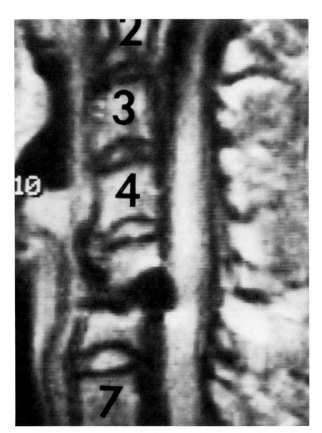

Figure 3–14. *Diagnosis: Ferromagnetic material artifact.* Sagittal cervical spine. The patient is postoperative at the C5–C6 level, at which there is an area of signal loss with a small band of high-intensity signal superiorly and inferiorly. This artifact is due to distortion of the main magnetic field by ferromagnetic material. In this case the artifact is from small (probably microscopic) metallic fragments left behind from previous surgery. These fragments often cannot be seen on CT or plain films but can have a profound effect on the MR images.

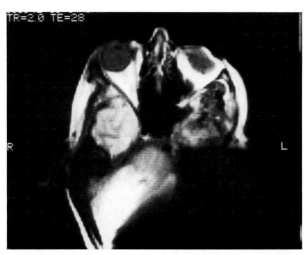

Figure 3–15. *Diagnosis: Artifact from a metal plate.* Axial head MR scan. Profound loss of signal in the posterior left aspect of the head is identified, secondary to an artifact from a metal plate in the occipital area.

local fields, which in turn cause rapid dephasing of nearby protons, leading to loss of signal. Cosmetics tend to be a frequent offender and one that is easy to correct by simply asking patients to remove all makeup before an MR examination. Certain pigments in makeup contain ferrous material that causes the dropout of signal and distortion of the main magnetic field.[12] Another substance not often thought of as an artifact is Pantopaque, which is frequently left behind in the subarachnoid space and can easily be misinterpreted on T1 and T2 WI image as blood (Fig. 3–20).

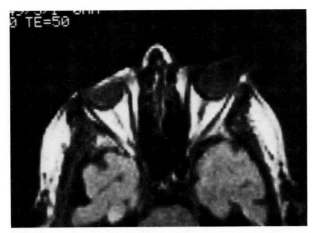

Figure 3–16. *Diagnosis: Artifact from makeup.* Axial head scan. There is distortion of the anterior portions of both globes and orbital rims. Notice the linear area of high signal intensity anterior to the right eye and the severe lateral distortion of the left eye. This is artifact from makeup, which can be easily eliminated by having the patient wash off all makeup.

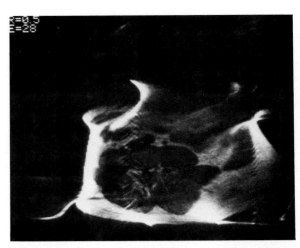

Figure 3–18. *Diagnosis: Artifacts from metal studs in the jeans.* Axial lumbosacral spine scan. Artifacts are seen in the anterior portion of the abdomen. This patient wore her blue jeans into the magnet, and the metal studs in the jeans were responsible for this profound artifact. It is important to have patients remove their street clothes, especially metal-containing clothing such as bras, and change into hospital gowns.

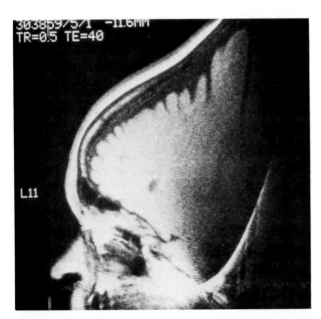

Figure 3–17. *Diagnosis: Artifact from hairpins.* Sagittal head scan. Elongation and distortion of the posterior skull is secondary to hairpins worn into the magnet by the patient (the conehead effect). Careful patient preparation should eliminate this problem.

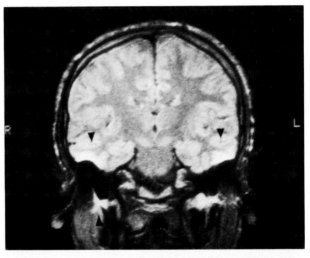

Figure 3–19. *Diagnosis: Artifacts from dentures. Coronal head MR scan.* There is an area of increased signal in the inferior temporal lobe bilaterally (*upper arrow*). The lower arrowhead points to increased signal intensity from the patient's dentures, which are responsible for the increased signal in both temporal lobes. If only an axial scan had been obtained, this artifact could have been misinterpreted as a pathologic condition.

Tissue Magnetic Susceptibility

A related but unavoidable artifact is seen in the inhomogeneities introduced in the magnetic field by the variations in magnetic susceptibility of different tissues in the patient. Because tissue has a different susceptibility from that of air, small distortions of the field are evident at tissue-air interfaces. This is most noticeable in the regions of the sinuses as a bright interface on one side and a signal void on the other. For both ferrous and susceptibility artifacts, gradient reversal sequences are much more susceptible to image artifacts than spin echo.

EQUIPMENT ARTIFACTS

The other large group of artifacts in MR are those due to the equipment used to obtain an MR image. They range from inherent artifacts in the data collec-

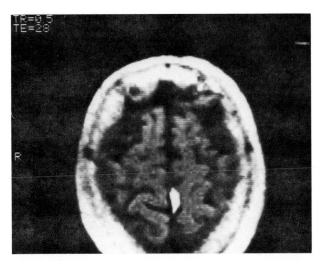

Figure 3–20. *Diagnosis: Pantopaque in the subarachnoid space.* Axial T1 WI head scan. A high-intensity lesion to the left of the falx is seen. This lesion was also bright on the T2 weighted image. The differential diagnosis is blood, fat, or paramagnetic substance. Plain films or CT scans of the head can be very helpful to differentiate this high signal from other pathology.

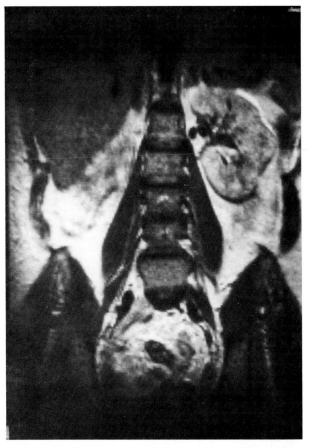

Figure 3–21. *Diagnosis: Chemical shift artifact.* Coronal abdomen scan. There is a band of increased signal from the superior border and a band of decreased signal from the inferior border of the left kidney. The frequency axis is from superior to inferior and the high-frequency side is superior. Chemical shift occurs because fat protons experience a smaller magnetic field than water protons at the same location; therefore, the fat signal is shifted to the low-frequency side.

tion and reconstruction algorithms to a failure in any part of the electronics or computer system.

Chemical Shift Artifact

The artifact most frequently discussed in this group is chemical shift (see also the chapters on the physics of MRI).[13] This shift is caused by the MR computer placing a signal coming from a voxel in the patient being imaged into an incorrect pixel on the CRT screen. The error occurs in the frequency encoding axis. This signal placement is done by measuring the frequency of the signal returning from a voxel in the patient and placing that signal intensity in the corresponding pixel location on the CRT screen. Fat has a large cloud of electrons that shield its hydrogen protons from the main magnetic field: i.e., fat protons see a weaker main magnetic field than water protons at the same location. Since the frequency of signal returning from the hydrogen protons is proportional to the strength of the magnetic field felt, fat protons have a lower frequency than water protons at the same voxel location. The computer then places the fat signal toward the low-frequency side and the water toward the high-frequency side. Chemical shift artifact is most noticeable at fat-water interfaces. A linear or crescent signal void toward the high frequency end of the frequency encoding axis is observed (Fig. 3–21). This should not be misinterpreted as a pathologic process; it can be verified as a chemical shift artifact by simply swapping the frequency and phase encoding axes. Since the amount of shift is proportional to the field strength, chemical shift tends to be more of a problem at high field strength such as 1.5 or 2T than at middle and low magnetic strengths.[13]

Aliasing

The other major artifact secondary to image reconstruction is aliasing.[6, 14] This is seen when the dimension of a body part in the plane of an MR image exceeds the field of view. The area outside the field of view is replicated and superimposed (folded over) onto the opposite side of the image (see Fig. 3–9). Aliasing can occur in the phase and frequency encoding axes but is not often seen in the frequency encoding axis, since filters are used in this axis to eliminate wraparound. Aliasing or phase wrap occurs because of undersampling of the data points and can be eliminated by increasing the sampling rate. This is done by increasing the phase encoding steps or pixel size so that the field of view matches or is larger than the body part to be imaged.

Of all artifacts presented in this chapter, aliasing is the one most often misinterpreted as a pathologic lesion by beginners in MR imaging (Fig. 3–22). When extremities are being imaged, the use of RF shields

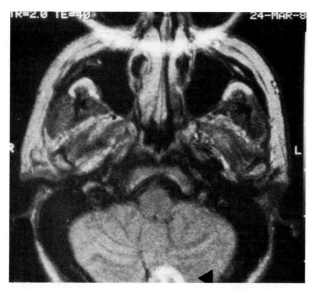

Figure 3–22. *Diagnosis: Wraparound artifact.* Axial head scan. The area of high signal intensity anteriorly overlying the anterior maxillary sinus and nasal cavity is wraparound from the scalp fat from the back of the head. The more confusing area of increased signal overlying the posterior cerebellum is not a pathologic lesion such as a posterior fossa hematoma, but the patient's nose. This artifact is not exactly midline because the patient's head was slightly rotated. Aliasing occurs when the diameter of the field of view is smaller than the body part to be imaged. This is most frequently seen in the phase encoding axis, since this wraparound can be filtered out in the frequency encoding axis.

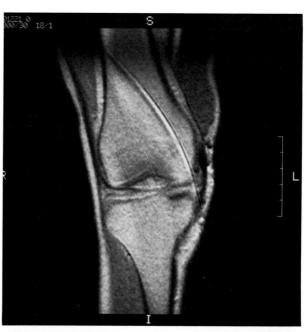

Figure 3–23. *Diagnosis: Wraparound artifact.* Coronal knee scan. There is a linear area of increased signal laterally, extending superiorly to the joint, which is wraparound from the subcutaneous fat of the patient's other leg. The use of RF shields on the nonimaged leg will eliminate this artifact.

wrapped around the arm or leg that is not being imaged can be helpful. This prevents the nonimaged extremity from returning a signal and eliminates phase wrap from that extremity (Fig. 3–23).

Gibbs Phenomenon

A less frequently observed artifact but one often present is the Gibbs phenomenon (edge effect, truncation error).[15, 16] This is most frequently observed at the interface between low and high signal intensity, i.e., the brain and calvarium (Fig. 3–24).[17] Truncation error presents as alternating linear bands of bright and dark signal parallel to the interface that dampen out quickly with distance from the interface. The artifact can be decreased by decreasing pixel size (e.g., by decreasing the field of view or increasing the matrix size). It is important that this artifact be differentiated from gross patient motion. If the artifact interfering with the study is a truncation error and not patient motion, the examination does not need to be repeated with sedation, but the field service representative should be called. Gibbs ringing is easily removed, but at the cost of some blurring in the image. This is done with a moderate amount of electronic filtering of the image.

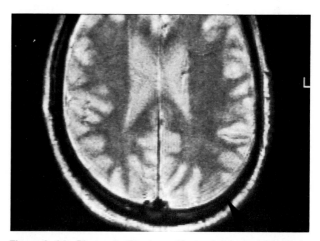

Figure 3–24. *Diagnosis: Ringing artifact.* Axial scan of the brain shows multiple dark and light bands at the interface of the brain and skull. This ringing artifact does not extend through the image as motion artifact would; it is important to differentiate these two.

Hardware Failures

The final class of artifacts consists of those due to failures in the hardware of the MR imaging system. Gradient power supply failure causes partial or complete loss of the gradients, which leads to distortion of the image in the plane of the gradient that failed (Figs. 3–25, 3–26). Another source of artifact is RF noise

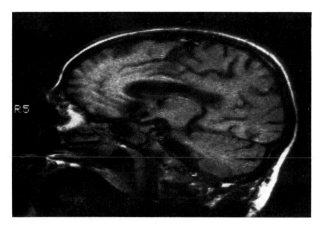

Figure 3–25. *Diagnosis: Partial failure in the Z-gradient power supply.* Sagittal brain scan. The head is foreshortened from top to bottom.

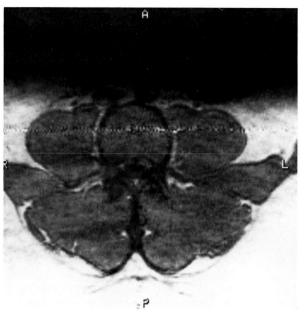

Figure 3–27. *Diagnosis: Free induction decay (FID) leak.* Axial lumbar spine with presaturation. There is a linear area of abnormal signal consistent with an FID leak.

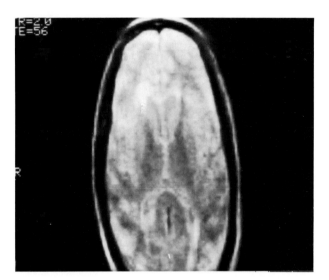

Figure 3–26. *Diagnosis: Partial failure in the X-gradient power supply.* Axial brain scan. The head is foreshortened from left to right.

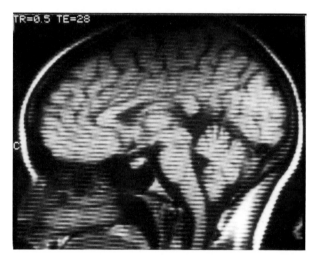

Figure 3–28. *Diagnosis: Herringbone artifact.* Sagittal head scan shows a herringbone pattern secondary to a bad light bulb releasing RF energy. This occurs with alternating current and can be very transient. A herringbone artifact can also occur with a failure in the amplifiers or other parts of the MR system.

from outside the MR scanner, which can easily exceed the inherently weak NMR signal. An example is an FM RF leak into the MR room, which has a characteristic appearance of a line of signal along the phase encoding direction in the image (Fig. 3–27). Old light bulbs that blink emit a spectrum of RF energy and lead to a herringbone appearance on the MR image (Fig. 3–28). Improper adjustment of the RF transmitter power can lead to nonuniformity across an image. This is generally caused by an excessive amount of RF energy: instead of a 90-degree–180-degree spin echo, the system performs a 270-degree–540-degree flip sequence. Generally this makes the nonuniformity in the RF field much more apparent and may show up as a dropout in the center of the image (Fig. 3–29).

Use of Surface Coils

The use of surface coils also causes an artifact with decreasing signal intensity from tissues farthest from the coil (Fig. 3–30). Intensity variations pose the greatest difficulty in viewing an image with a fixed window since nearby and more distant tissue cannot be viewed simultaneously. Recently, software corrections

among the more common, and most can be eliminated through careful evaluation of the patient and the basic MR system. For a practicing radiologist, the ultimate goal is to provide a reliable diagnosis and increase throughput by an understanding of artifacts in MR imaging.

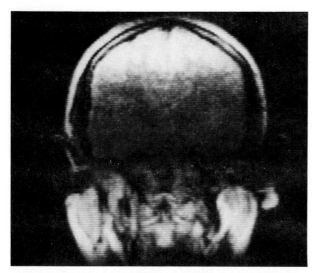

Figure 3–29. *Diagnosis: Artifact seen with too much RF power.* This coronal head scan was performed with the same RF energy used for body MR. The alternating band of increased and decreased signal is characteristic of the artifact seen with too much RF power. Instead of a 90-degree flip, a 180-degree flip is obtained. A similar artifact occurs when too little RF energy is used for the 90-degree flip.

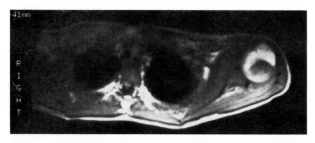

Figure 3–30. *Diagnosis: Signal loss due to use of a surface coil.* T1 weighted transverse image through the upper thorax with a surface coil behind the left scapula. The lower signal of the muscle on the right side of the chest, compared with the left side, is not due to pathology, but to a signal dropoff artifact from use of surface coils.

that compensate for signal dropoff have been introduced into several systems.

This summary of artifacts is not meant to be comprehensive. However, the MR artifacts presented are

REFERENCES

1. Ehman RL, McNamara MT, Brasch RC, et al. Influence of physiologic motion on the appearance of tissue in MR images. Radiology 1986; 159:777–782.
2. Lewis CE, Prato FS, Drost DJ, Nicholson RL. Comparison of respiratory triggering and gating techniques for the removal of respiratory artifact in MR imaging. Radiology 1986; 160:803–810.
3. Clark JA, Kelly WM. Common artifacts encountered in magnetic resonance imaging. Radiol Clin North Am 1988; 26:893–920.
4. Lanzer P, Botvinick EH, Schiller NB, et al. Cardiac imaging using gated magnetic resonance. Radiology 1984; 150:121–127.
5. Felmlee JP, Ehman RL. Spatial presaturation: a method for suppressing flow artifacts and improving depiction of vascular anatomy in MR imaging. Radiology 1987; 164:559–564.
6. Kelly B. Image artifacts and technical limitations. In: Brant-Zawadzki M, Norman D, eds. Magnetic resonance imaging of the central nervous system. New York: Raven Press, 1987.
7. Haacke EM, Lenz GW. Improving MR image quality in the presence of motion by using rephasing gradients. AJR 1987; 148:1251–1258.
8. Teitelbaum GP, Bradley WG, Klein BD. MR imaging artifacts, ferromagnetism, and magnetic torque of intravascular filters, stents, and coils. Radiology 1988; 166:657–664.
9. Liebman CE, Messersmith RN, Levin DN, Lu CT. MR imaging of inferior vena caval filters: safety and artifacts. AJR 1988; 150:1174–1176.
10. Hinshaw DB, Holshouser BA, Engstrom HIM, et al. Dental material artifacts on MR images. Radiology 1988; 166:777–779.
11. Laakman RW, Kaufman B, Han JS, et al. MR imaging in patients with metallic implants. Radiology 1985; 157:711–714.
12. Sacco DC, Steiger DA, Bellon EM, et al. Artifacts caused by cosmetics in MR imaging of the head. AJR 1987; 148:1001–1004.
13. Weinreb JF, Brateman L, Babcock EE, et al. Chemical shift artifact in clinical magnetic resonance images at 0.35T. AJR 1985; 145:183–185.
14. Bellon EM, Haacke EM, Coleman PE, et al. MR artifacts: a review. AJR 1986; 147:1271–1281.
15. Czervionke LF, Czervionke JM, Daniels DL, Haughton VM. Characteristic features of MR truncation artifacts. AJR 1988; 151:1219–1228.
16. Lufkin RB, Pusey E, Stark DD, et al. Boundary artifact due to truncation errors in MR imaging. AJR 1986; 147:1283–1287.
17. Wood ML, Henkelman RM. Truncation artifacts in magnetic resonance imaging. J Mag Res Med 1985; 2:517–526.

Safety and Biologic Effects

MICHAEL A. KUHARIK, M.D.
RICHARD R. SMITH, M.D.

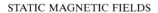

Magnetic resonance continues to be a rapidly advancing imaging technology. Although not all questions regarding its biologic effects are completely answered, it is clear that MR, as currently employed in clinical imaging, is a safe procedure with no known direct detrimental effects. There is, however, a potential hazard from the magnetic forces on metallic implants and foreign bodies. Additionally, further research is necessary because of the growing interest in MR field strengths beyond 2T as well as the use of newer, more powerful radiofrequency (RF) pulses designed to shorten examination time.

There is a vast literature on the effects of magnetic fields and RF deposition on biologic systems, ranging from humans to bacteria to biologic molecules. Many of these experiments are contradictory, poorly controlled, anecdotal, or inapplicable to human clinical MR imaging.[1] This chapter reviews the important physiologic effects and potential hazards to patients exposed to the MR environment. This information should provide a basis for a rational approach to the screening of patients referred for this procedure. The potential health hazards of MR imaging can be divided into three causative categories:

1. The static magnetic field.
2. The time-varying magnetic fields (TVMF) of the gradient coils.
3. The pulsed RF electromagnetic field.

STATIC MAGNETIC FIELDS

Clinical MR imaging uses magnets with a field strength of less than 2T; most high field systems operate at 1.5T. The intensity of the magnetic field de-creases rapidly with increasing distance from magnet bore (distance^{-3}). For a 1.5T magnet, the fringe field is reduced to 5 gauss (0.00005T) at a distance of approximately 40 feet from the magnet center (Fig. 4–1). This 5-gauss line becomes important in relation to patient and visitor safety. Magnetic shielding can also be used to reduce the distance of the 5-gauss line and the fringe field to an area within the scanning room.

Hazards from Implanted Metallic Objects

Ferromagnetic materials are metals such as iron, cobalt, nickel, and stainless steel (type 400 series) that have the inherent ability to concentrate magnetic lines and interact with the magnetic field.[2] Silver, tantalum, and the type 300 series stainless steel with a high concentration of chromium or nickel are not magnetic and are in widespread use in orthopedic devices, surgical clips, and suture material.[2] A patient with an implanted ferromagnetic or metallic object exposed to the MR environment is subject to potential harm. The interaction of the object with the magnetic fields may result in torque or movement, induction of electric currents, heating, and MR image distortion.

The force of attraction between a ferromagnetic object (bioimplant) and the magnet depends on the magnetic field gradient and not on the total magnetic field strength. In other words, the force of attraction depends on how rapidly the magnetic field changes with distance. Once the patient (and bioimplant) are within the bore of the scanner, there is no magnetic gradient, and therefore no force of attraction is experienced. However, the ferromagnetic object will attempt to align its long axis with the long axis of the static mag-

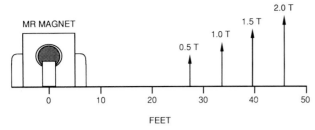

Figure 4–1. *The 5-gauss fringe field lines for MR unshielded magnets measured in feet parallel to the magnet bore.* The fringe field is less at points perpendicular to the magnet bore. At 1.5T, the 5-gauss line is approximately 40 feet.

netic field. This torque force can be potentially dangerous, depending largely on the location, field strength, and degree of ferromagnetism. Many of the older intracranial aneurysm clips are ferromagnetic, and clip motion possibly leads to vessel damage and resultant hemorrhage, ischemia, or death.[3] A number of nonferromagnetic aneurysm clips are currently available. However, an MR examination is still contraindicated unless the exact type of clip is known.[4]

Most prosthetic heart valves manufactured after 1964 are not ferromagnetic and pose no problems during MR imaging.[6] Most cochlear implants are not magnetic; however, MR imaging can result in damage to the prosthesis or pain to the patient from induced signals or heating during MR examination.[5] Most stainless steel orthopedic implants, including prosthetic joints, pins, and rods, are not ferromagnetic and are not affected by MR. These nonmagnetic metals, however, "bend" the magnetic flux lines and preferentially absorb RF radiation, resulting in MR image distortion and artifacts adjacent to these metallic objects. fected by MR. These nonmagnetic metals, however, "bend" the magnetic flux lines and preferentially absorb RF radiation, resulting in MR image distortion and artifacts adjacent to these metallic objects.

Cardiac pacemakers can be affected by induced currents caused by the changing field gradients or by the patient moving into the static magnetic field. Magnetization of its electronic components may result in damage or malfunction. Activation of the read switch on a demand pacemaker can occur in field strengths greater than 100 gauss, resulting in an asynchronous mode of operation.[7] Although this usually has no adverse effects on the patient, areas with magnetic fields of 5 gauss or greater must be labeled with warning signs and controlled.

Hazards from Nonimplanted Metallic Objects

The force of attraction between a ferromagnetic object and the magnet is related to the size and shape of the object, the degree of ferromagnetism, the strength of the magnetic field, and (most important) the distance between the two. Because the intensity of the magnetic field increases to the third power as a ferromagnetic object approaches the magnet, both large and small objects are potentially dangerous. At a distance of 3 to 4 feet from the bore of a 1.5T magnet, a ferromagnetic object will experience a force of approximately ten times its weight.[5] Probably the most serious hazard of the MR environment is injury from the small metallic projectiles that are accidentally brought into the magnet field. Objects such as pens, hairclips, earrings, and scissors can be drawn into the magnet at high velocity and, because of their small weight, at a relatively great distance from the bore of the magnet. For this reason, all patients must be thoroughly screened for metallic objects, and MR staff must always be aware of these hazards.

Biologic Effects

It is emphasized that there are no known adverse effects on human subjects from static magnetic fields up to a field strength of 2T.[1,5,7] There are, however, a number of known bioeffects that potentially can cause physiologic changes at field strengths higher than 2T.

The flow of an electrically conductive fluid such as blood within the static magnetic field produces a current in a direction that opposes the magnetic field in which it resides.[5] In theory, these currents could oppose the flow of blood through the vasculature, leading to a decrease in blood flow velocity. Although animal experiments show no observable change in the blood flow characteristics at 1.5T,[8] an estimated reduction in blood flow rate for humans in a 5T field is approximately 70 percent.[5] Another effect of these induced voltages is seen in T-wave alterations that appear on the electrocardiogram (ECG). These occur without any physiologic change in the intrinsic electrical activity of the heart.[9]

Molecular and cellular anisotrophy is the alignment of these structures with the flux lines of the magnetic field. Studies have been performed on retinal rods, DNA, and deoxygenated sickled erythrocytes that temporarily align with the magnetic field. There are no known deleterious effects on health.[5,7]

Current Guidelines for Patient Exposure to Static Magnetic Fields

The national Center for Devices and Radiological Health through the Food and Drug Administration (FDA) has suggested that no significant risk exists for static magnetic fields of 2T or less.[5,11] It should be noted that these values are only guidelines (Table 4–1) and not absolute restrictions. Research, both animal and human, is presently being conducted at field strengths of up to 4T.

TIME-VARYING MAGNETIC FIELDS

Rapidly applied magnetic field gradients are used to spatially encode the RF signal emitted by the irradiated tissues for MR imaging. Although these gradient fields are of small absolute strength (10 to 100 gauss per meter), it is the rapid change over time that leads to its potential bioeffects. These time-varying magnetic fields (TVMF) generate internal electric currents in a conducting medium such as nerves, muscles, and blood vessels. The effects of the TVMF depend on the pulse duration and strength, the wave shape, the pulse rate, and the distribution of the induced current within the body.

Biologic Effects

It is difficult to calculate the exact magnitude of the induced current from a given applied gradient field because of the many variables. In general, there are no known adverse effects associated with the TVMF of clinical MR imaging.[5, 10]

Flickering illuminations induced in the visual field, magnetophosphenes, can occur as a result of exposure to TVMF.[7] This phenomenon is probably due to the slight torquing of the cone cells leading to electric stimulation. It is completely reversible and has no known long-term effects.[5] Magnetophosphenes have been experimentally produced at TVMF that are within the range of clinical MR equipment.[1, 7]

Ventricular fibrillation and nerve conduction interference can be potentially induced by TVMF. However, these effects require induced current densities approximately 10,000 times greater than those induced with current MR clinical parameters.[1]

Current Guidelines for Patient Exposure to TVMF

New MR strategies and pulsing parameters are continually being developed in an effort to shorten examination time. Many of these techniques result in increasing TVMF strengths. For this reason, continual investigation in this area is required before a comprehensive safety range is established. The FDA indicates that exposures of up to 3T per second are safe, but does not provide a time duration guideline (Table 4–1).

RADIOFREQUENCY FIELDS

Radiofrequency coils are used to irradiate the nuclei selected for imaging. Usually a circumferential body coil that surrounds the patient is utilized to transmit this RF field, and the entire volume of tissue within the coil is irradiated. Then, either the same body coil or a surface coil adjacent to the area of interest can be used to receive the transmitted signal. This surface coil, however, must be unreceptive during the transmission of the RF from the body coil. This prevents heating of the surface coil, which may burn the patient's skin if the coil is in direct contact with it.

Biologic Effects

The most important consequence of RF exposure used in clinical MR is the generation of heat in the irradiated tissues. The heat comes from the oscillating magnetic fields and RF energy. Electric currents are produced within the body tissues, secondary to the applied rapidly oscillating magnetic field from the RF coils. These currents tend to produce heat within the resistive body fluids.[1, 7] RF energy is partly transferred to body tissues in the form of heat. The amount of RF absorption into a system is measured as a unit called the specific absorption rate (SAR), expressed as watts per kilogram. It relates to the rate with which the energy is deposited per unit of tissue.[13] RF absorption (SAR) is dependent on the pulse duration and repetition rate, RF frequency (related to field strength, approximately 64 MHz at 1.5T), tissue conductivity, object size, and coupling between the RF coil and the subject.[12]

After the deposition of RF energy into the body, the heating of the tissues results in a conduction of the heat to the superficial surfaces of the body for heat loss by radiation and evaporative mechanisms. For most patients using present MR equipment and imaging parameters, there is no significant change in core body or skin temperature during MR imaging.[5, 14] However, patients suspected of having compromised or underdeveloped thermoregulatory systems, such as premature infants or febrile individuals, may be candidates for core body temperature monitoring (with a rectal temperature probe).

Large metallic implants may result in local heating secondary to RF absorption. The amount of temperature elevation is minimal and of no clinical consequence.[15]

Table 4–1. CURRENT FDA GUIDELINES FOR MAXIMAL STATIC MAGNETIC FIELD, TIME-VARYING MAGNETIC FIELDS, AND RF EXPOSURE

MR Component	Recommended Limits
Static field	2.0T
TVMF	3.0T/sec
RF SAR	0.4 watts/kg (whole body)
	2.0 watts/kg (in any gram)

TVMF, Time-varying magnetic field; SAR, specific absorption rate.

Current Guidelines for Patient Exposure to RF Energy

The FDA report indicates that no significant risk exists when the SAR is less than 0.4 watts per kilogram as averaged over the entire body or 2.0 watts per kilogram in any gram of tissue (Table 4–1).[11] To put these values into perspective, the basal metabolic rate of an adult is approximately 1.3 watts per kilogram, and 18 watts per kilogram for strenuous exercise.[5] High-field MR devices, particularly when certain RF pulsing strategies are utilized to obtain multisection-multiecho sequences, have the tendency to generate SARs that exceed the advised SAR limit.[14] Patients experimentally exposed to SARs up to three times the recommended limit experienced no significant temperature, pulse, or blood pressure elevation.[14] However, when approximately six times the routine imaging RF power was deposited experimentally into dogs in a clinical MR unit, significant elevation in deep and superficial tissue temperatures was found.[16] Further research is therefore warranted, and continued caution in the operation of present high-field MR imaging is advised. In addition, if the SARs exceed the limit advised by the FDA, care should be taken not to wrap patients tightly with blankets. The imaging room should be maintained at a relatively low temperature and humidity, along with good airflow through the bore of the magnet to enhance the patient's heat-losing mechanisms.[16]

GENERAL PATIENT AND PUBLIC SAFETY

The MR imager is usually contained within a restricted area, access to which is normally through a supervised entry. A 5-gauss field line is posted with warning signs adjacent to the restricted area, as required by the FDA. This is primarily to exclude patients with pacemakers from this area. Magnetized credit cards and tapes, analog watches, and other instruments can also be damaged within the 5-gauss line.

The room should be securely locked when not in use or when trained personnel are not present. In-service training sessions for the custodial and patient transportation services are also important to avoid needless accidents.

The patient and any other support personnel (nurses or parents of a young child) entering the MR scanning room should be thoroughly screened and questioned about the presence of any metallic material on or within them. Such free objects if undetected may result in hazardous projectiles.

Although pregnancy is not usually applicable to a pediatric population, it should be noted that the FDA guidelines do not specifically address the risks from MRI. In general, MRI is not believed to be hazardous to the fetus.[5, 15]

Finally, as more and more acutely ill and less stable patients are being evaluated with MRI, situations requiring emergency cardiopulmonary resuscitation (CPR) and direct medical intervention may arise during this procedure. The MR technologists, physicians, and other personnel monitoring the patient must act quickly to initiate CPR and remove the patient from the MR environment. Much of the resuscitation equipment is ferromagnetic and might be dangerous if taken into the scanning room. Also, the magnetic field may interfere with the function of this equipment.

SUMMARY

The MR environment can be divided into three categories corresponding to the static magnetic field, the TVMF from the gradient coils, and the pulsed RF electromagnetic fields. Although each has known biologic effects, there are no known deleterious or long-term health effects from current clinical MR imaging. The major concern with regard to the safety of the patient and operator is the presence of internal or external metallic objects that can be influenced by the MR environment. A few medical devices, such as cardiac pacemakers and certain cerebral aneurysm clips, are incompatible with an MR examination. For these reasons, the safety of MR imaging to a large degree depends on the awareness of its potential risks to the patient and an effective screening of patients to exclude those at risk of injury. Constant caution and continuing research are required as MR field strengths increase and new RF pulsing parameters are developed.

REFERENCES

1. Budinger TF, Cullander C. Health effects of in vivo magnetic resonance. In: James TL, Margulis AR, eds. Biomedical magnetic resonance. San Francisco: Radiology Research and Education Foundation, 1984:421–441.
2. Barrafato D, Henkelman RM. Magnetic resonance imaging and surgical clips. Can J Surg 1984; 27:509–512.
3. New PF, Rosen BR, Brady TJ, et al. Potential hazards and artifacts of ferromagnetic and nonferromagnetic surgical and dental materials and devices in nuclear magnetic resonance imaging. Radiology 1983; 147:139–148.
4. Shellock FG. MR imaging of metallic implants and materials: a compilation of the literature. AJR 1988; 151:811–814.
5. Pavlicek W. Safety considerations. In: Stark DD, Bradley WG, eds. Magnetic resonance imaging. St. Louis: CV Mosby, 1988:244–257.
6. Soulen RL, Budinger TF, Higgins CB. Magnetic resonance imaging of prosthetic heart valves. Radiology 1985; 154:705–707.
7. Budinger TF. Biological and environmental hazards. In: Higgins CB, Hricak H, eds. Magnetic resonance imaging of the body. New York: Raven Press, 1987:539–545.
8. Smith H. Revised guidance on acceptable limits of exposure during nuclear magnetic resonance clinical imaging. The National Radiological Protection Board ad hoc advisory group on nuclear magnetic resonance clinical imaging. Br J Radiol 1983; 56:947–977.
9. Budinger TF. Nuclear magnetic resonance in vivo studies: known thresholds for health effects. J Comput Assist Tomogr 1981; 5:800–811.

10. Tenforde TS. Interaction of time-varying ELF magnetic fields with living matter. In: Polk C, Postow E, eds. Biological effects of electromagnetic fields. Boca Raton: CRC Press, 1986.

11. Guidelines for evaluating electromagnetic exposure risk for trials of clinical NMR systems. Washington, DC: Center for Devices and Radiological Health, Food and Drug Administration, 1982.

12. Bottomley PA, Andrew ER. RF magnetic field penetration, phase shift and power dissipation in biological tissue: implications for NMR imaging. Phys Med Biol 1978; 23:630.

13. Bushong SC. Biologic effects of MRI. In: Bushong SC, ed. Magnetic resonance imaging—physical and biological principles. St. Louis: CV Mosby, 1988:326–335.

14. Shellock FG, Crues JV. Temperature, heart rate, and blood pressure changes associated with clinical MR imaging at 1.5T. Radiology 1987; 163:259–262.

15. Shellock FG, Crues JV. Safety considerations in magnetic resonance imaging. MRI Decisions 1988; Jan:25–30.

16. Shuman WP, Haynor DR, Guy AW, et al. Superficial- and deep-tissue temperature increases in anesthetized dogs during exposure to high specific absorption rates in a 1.5T MR imager. Radiology 1988; 167:551–554.

Sedation, Anesthesia, and Patient Monitoring

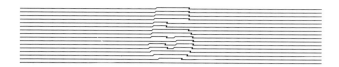

MICHAEL A. KUHARIK, M.D.

The elimination of patient motion is fundamental to optimal imaging of any kind. In conventional radiography, motion problems are eliminated by the use of very short radiographic exposure times of $1/100$ of a second or less. Motion problems are most troublesome with computer-generated sectional imaging because these techniques require long imaging times. This problem was first encountered in computed tomography (CT). In the early days of CT, single slice scan times were as long as 15 seconds. Although scan times have now been reduced to 2 seconds or less, motion is still a problem in some patients, and a small percentage of patients require sedation. Motion causes significant problems in MR imaging because of the long data acquisition time, which can exceed 15 minutes for a single imaging pulse sequence. The spontaneous movement of infants and children constitutes the single greatest impediment to the acquisition of high-quality MR images in the pediatric population. Sedation therefore assumes an important role in pediatric MR imaging.

SEDATION FOR MRI

The pediatric patient has a number of unique needs that require attention for successful MR imaging. These include control of the environment within the MR scanner, careful patient monitoring, an understanding and discussion of parental concerns, and (most important) safe sedation. Neonates and young infants should be wrapped in blankets or plastic wrap to help preserve body heat in the relatively cold MR imaging suite.

Levels of Sedation

The section on anesthesiology of the American Academy of Pediatrics published an excellent review of pediatric sedation in 1985, defining three levels of sedation:

1. Conscious (light) sedation. This is the level to be utilized by nonanesthesiologists and is the level of sedation that radiologists use in the MR or CT environment. It represents a minimal depressed level of consciousness that retains the patient's ability to maintain a patent airway independently, respond to physical stimulation and commands, and retain protective reflexes.

2. Deep sedation. This is a controlled state of depressed consciousness from which the patient is not easily aroused and in which there is some loss of protective airway reflexes.

3. General anesthesia. A state of unconsciousness with loss of protective reflexes and ability to respond to physical stimulation.[1]

Selection of Patients for Sedation

In general, all patients under 5 years of age and older uncooperative patients require sedation. Most patients over the age of 5 cooperate and remain still if the study is explained to them. From some patients, particularly those with mental retardation, it may not be possible to obtain cooperation even if they are over the age of 5. Fortunately, claustrophobia is not as common in children as in adults, but when present it may also be an indication for sedation. In the adult population, claus-

75

trophobia during MR examinations has been reported in approximately 4 to 7 percent of studies.[2,3] In infants, it may sometimes be possible to avoid sedation by merely feeding them and then wrapping them warmly and securely in a blanket. Once it has been decided that a patient will require sedation, it must be determined whether to utilize light sedation administered by the radiologist, or deep sedation or general anesthesia administered by an anesthesiologist. A few centers use general anesthesia for all patients requiring sedation. We do not believe that this is practical, first because of the time involved in performing general anesthesia, second because of the increased cost, and third because light sedation can safely be administered without the need for an anesthesiologist. A select group of patients, however, always require general anesthesia. These include individuals with severe systemic disorders, particularly those involving the cardiovascular, respiratory, or central nervous system. Other patients to be included in this group are children with suspected CNS depression, chronic obstructive lung disease, sleep apnea, impaired gag or swallowing reflexes, or impaired liver function. Each institution must define its own criteria for the use of deep sedation or general anesthesia, but if there is doubt it is probably safer to err on the side of general anesthesia. Fortunately, most pediatric patients requiring sedation for the MR examination are from the outpatient population and none of the above indications for general anesthesia are relevant. This means that light sedation can be administered in most cases.

Requirements for a Successful and Safe Sedation Program

Sedation involves much more than merely administering a sedative agent. To be run safely, a sedation program must incorporate all of the following features.

Facility

The MR facility should have an emergency cart or kit readily accessible. This should include all the necessary drugs and equipment for resuscitation. In addition, the room must be equipped with an oxygen delivery system and a suction apparatus. Staff should be familiar with the use of this equipment.

Parental Involvement

There must be an effective mechanism for giving the parents presedation instructions for their child. There should be a minimal period of starvation of 4 to 8 hours depending on the patient's age. Informed consent from the parents or guardians may be obtained prior to sedation and they must be given a careful explanation of the MR imaging procedure.

Presedation Evaluation

Before light sedation is administered, the criteria for the use of general anesthesia should again be reviewed and one should ensure that no indications for general

anesthesia are present. The patient should be examined for acute illness such as respiratory infection, for which one would consider postponing the MR study. The patient's weight must be recorded. Medications the patient is receiving, particularly sedatives, must be documented. Baseline recording of vital signs must also be obtained.

Monitoring During MR Scanning

All the noninvasive physiologic monitoring data obtained during the MR examination should also be recorded periodically during the study. This is particularly important because direct visualization of the patient in the MR unit is suboptimal. Data to be monitored and recorded include blood pressure, temperature, heart rate, respiratory rate, blood oxygen saturation, and end tidal CO_2. The dosage and route of administration of the sedative agent should also be recorded. Any intravenous line placed for the delivery of a sedating agent should be maintained during the scan.

Patient Discharge

The patient must be evaluated before discharge. Specific discharge criteria must be defined and met, and documented as such. The patient is ready for discharge when he or she can obey commands, talk, and walk if old enough, and when the vital signs are stable and close to the presedation level. The parents must be given specific written instructions regarding restriction of activity and eating during the recovery phase. They should also receive a written statement of the type and dosage of sedative utilized.

Pediatric Sedation Techniques and Regimens

In selecting a sedative, the safety of the patient must at all times be the primary consideration. Numerous sedation regimens have been used in the pediatric population for CT and invasive procedures such as angiography or myelography. These procedures require both a sedative and an analgesic agent. For MRI no analgesic agent is required. The ideal sedation agent should be safe, predictable, and efficient with a controllable duration of action and no adverse side effects. Although no such agent exists, one should seek a regimen that is safe and dependable for use on a daily basis. It is helpful if all patients can be relatively sleep deprived, but this usually is not practical.

Chloral Hydrate

This oral agent has long been used to successfully sedate infants undergoing electroencephalography (EEG) and CT. It probably remains the most widely used sedation agent for outpatient imaging studies (both CT and MRI). The recommended dosage of chloral hydrate varies in the literature, but most reports recommend approximately 75 to 80 mg per kilogram to a maximal total dose of 100 mg per kilogram.[3,4] The total dosage should not exceed 2,000 mg.

This drug has a wide margin of safety, is easy to administer, and has a record of many years of safe experience with its use. A disadvantage of chloral hydrate is that it is ineffective in sedating approximately 15 percent of patients who receive it; this is especially true in children over the age of 2 years.[4] Also, because the agent is given orally, the induction time is unpredictable and can be prolonged. Strain and colleagues noted an induction time range of 30 to 105 minutes; 16 percent of patients needed a second dose.[5] The duration of the sedation can also be long, another serious drawback.[6]

Pentobarbital (Nembutal)

This short-acting barbiturate, used intravenously (IV), is rapidly gaining popularity for pediatric sedation during imaging. Because the drug is used IV, there is a rapid onset of activity (less than 60 seconds), which allows reliable titration of the dose to the patient's response.[5] This is the most attractive feature, which is not shared by the relatively unpredictable absorption of drugs administered orally, rectally, or intramuscularly (IM). Both the induction and recovery times are significantly shortened compared with those of chloral hydrate.[5] The usual dosage is 5 mg per kilogram. One-half of the dose (2.5 mg per kilogram) is administered first over a period of 30 seconds, and the patient's response is monitored for 1 minute.[7] If required, the second half of the dose is then slowly given, the amount given again being titrated with the patient's response. An additional dose of 1 mg per kilogram can be given if needed to a total dosage of 6 mg per kilogram.[7] The sedation failure rate is extremely low (approximately 1 percent), and centers using this drug have demonstrated its safety.[5,7] The degree of respiratory depression is said to be less than that from narcotic analgesics and even less than that from chloral hydrate.[8] The IV route may be the preferred one since it offers an effective means of drug titration, with the average dosage administered less than the calculated maximum for most patients. It is also more comfortable than IM injections, and maintains vascular access if additional sedation, resuscitation, or IV contrast material is required.

Intramuscular Nembutal has also been used to premedicate infants and children for CT scanning.[9] A dose of 5 to 6 mg per kilogram is given 30 minutes before the examination.[5] The disadvantages of this method include inconsistent absorption with delayed induction, more patient discomfort than with IV administration, and lack of IV access for repeat sedation if needed.

AMPS (Atropine, Meperidine, Promethazine, and Secobarbital)

This intramuscular "cocktail" has also been used for children undergoing CT examinations.[4,9] Thompson and colleagues[4] described a sedation failure rate of 12 percent, compared with the oral chloral hydrate failure rate of 15 percent. However, since this difference is insignificant and since chloral hydrate can be given orally, it would appear that the latter is preferable. Other disadvantages of AMPS are the potential car-

diopulmonary depression caused by the meperidine, the increased risks of multiple drugs, and the necessity of two IM injections because secobarbital is incompatible with the other drugs.[10] Thompson and colleagues listed the dosages and methods of administration of this relatively complicated regimen.[4]

"Cardiac Cocktail"

Meperidine, 25 mg per milliliter; chlorpromazine, 6 mg per milliliter; and promethazine, 6 mg per milliliter make up this well-known IM regimen used extensively for pediatric cardiac catheterization. The dosage is 0.1 ml per kilogram with a maximum of 2 ml.[9] All the drugs are compatible and can be given as a single injection 10 to 20 minutes before the scan. The major disadvantage of this cocktail is the relatively high dose of meperidine (2.5 mg per kilogram). This dosage is probably appropriate for relatively painful procedures such as angiography in which the narcotic analgesic effect is necessary. However, the risk of medullary depression in an inherently painless imaging procedure is probably not appropriate. In addition, both meperidine and chlorpromazine can cause hypotension.[11]

Ketamine (Ketalar)

Ketamine hydrochloride, although used by the anesthesiologists, is thought to be unacceptable for routine outpatient use because of the risks of increased intracranial pressure in hydrocephalic children, its prolonged action, and its hallucinogenic effects during recovery.[4,12]

Diazepam (Valium)

Intravenous diazepam is useful to calm anxious adults during a somewhat intimidating MR examination. It is, however, often ineffective in the sedation of children and is not safe in the higher doses required to immobilize them properly.[4]

In general, the type of pediatric sedation regimen chosen by an MR facility is usually the same protocol used in the institution's CT scanning service. Here they have usually accumulated experience with a particular sedation agent. At the Indiana University Medical Center MRI Facility we have chosen oral chloral hydrate in patients under the age of 18 months and IV Nembutal for those over 18 months. This was decided after a retrospective review of our experience in both CT and MRI in which either chloral hydrate or Nembutal was used during the past few years. Whichever sedation regimen is chosen, it is important to use it consistently and comfortably, and to evaluate its performance periodically.

ANESTHESIA AND MECHANICAL VENTILATION DURING MRI

In the early years of MRI, patients requiring general anesthesia or mechanical ventilation were not able to undergo MRI because ventilators could not be used in the MR imaging room. Most ventilators are electronically controlled and contain moving ferromagnetic materials. This causes interference with the normal function of the ventilator and degrades MR image quality. With increasing involvement of interested anesthesiologists in the management of patients requiring anesthesia or ventilatory support during MRI, many of these problems have been solved.

General anesthesia during an MR procedure should be reserved for the critically ill and the small group of patients in whom light sedation is judged unsafe or has previously failed. In general, the induction of anesthesia is performed outside the scanning suite, and the patient is then transferred to the MR imaging couch in the anesthetized state. Because of the patient's enclosed environment when inside the magnet bore, almost all patients are intubated for airway control when under general or deep anesthesia. If inhalation anesthesia is used within the MR imaging suite, the anesthetic machine must be placed far from the magnet, with a long breathing system to deliver fresh gas to the patient.[2] A totally intravenous anesthesia technique is probably easier to use while within the MR suite, with a member of the anesthesia team monitoring the depth of anesthesia during the procedure.[13] The unique MR environment also creates a number of problems related to the physiologic monitoring of these patients. Monitoring during an MR procedure is discussed in the next section.

The choice between spontaneous, manual, or mechanically controlled ventilation is made by the individual anesthesiologist for each patient, but it is important to consider the choice of breathing system or ventilator used during MRI. All anesthetized patients, including those breathing spontaneously, are intubated and attached to an oxygen delivery system.[13] Neonates and infants are usually ventilated by hand with a breathing circuit devoid of ferromagnetic material.[14]

For patients requiring controlled mechanical ventilation, two approaches are possible. The first is to place a standard ventilator far from the bore of the magnet with long extension tubes connected to the patient. This approach creates the problem of compensating for the compression volume and the increased flow resistance of the extended circuit, which can range up to 50 feet (depending on magnetic field strength).[2,15] The second approach is to place a ventilator adjacent to or within the bore of the magnet. Such a ventilator should have no ferromagnetic components and its function should not be influenced by the MR environment. Ventilators specifically designed to be used during MRI have recently become commercially available. These devices are pneumatically powered (using compressed oxygen) and contain no electric or ferromagnetic components.[15,16] They are usually encased in aluminum, do not interfere with MR image acquisition, and do not cause imaging artifacts. Manufacturers of MRI-compatible ventilators are listed in the Appendix at the end of the chapter.

MONITORING DURING MRI

The monitoring of most adults and nonsedated older children during MRI requires little more than closed circuit television and a two-way intercommunication system. Seriously ill or combative patients, as well as infants and young children, require sedation or general anesthesia. Effective monitoring of vital signs and well-being during MRI is mandatory. MRI as a diagnostic imaging modality is being used more commonly in this group of patients, but monitoring is made difficult because of the unique environment in an MR imaging suite.

Problems Associated with Monitoring

After adequate sedation, the patient is placed on the MR couch and moved into the bore of the magnet. The general physical construction of an MR imager is such that the patient is almost completely concealed from visual observation and is inaccessible to direct physical contact. Manual control of the airway and vital sign monitoring become difficult. This is particularly true in infants and children in whom the center of the cylindric magnet is farther from the bore opening relative to body size. In addition, the incompatibility of various medical monitors with the strong magnetic field and radiofrequency (RF) interaction creates new problems for effective patient monitoring and MR image acquisition.

The selection of monitoring devices to be used within the MR imaging suite requires consideration of a number of factors. The effect of the MR imager on these devices depends on the strength of the magnetic field, the proximity to the imager, the number of ferromagnetic elements within the monitor, and the design of its electronic circuitry. In general, the stronger the magnetic field, the closer the monitoring device to the magnet, and the more ferromagnetic material used in the device, the greater is the danger of pulling the device into the magnet bore, with resultant patient injury or damage to the imager and monitor. The magnetic field can distort the display of a cathode ray tube and potentially affect the monitor's internal magnetic or mechanical switches.[17] Rapidly changing gradient fields and RF pulses, for example, can induce a current within the circuitry of an electrocardiographic (ECG) display.[18]

Additional problems arise from influences that the monitors have on RF excitation pulses, MR signal detection, and magnetic field homogeneity. These interactions generally result in image degradation, artifacts, and a decrease in the image signal-to-noise ratio (SNR). Monitoring or ECG wires and leads attached to the patient can act as antennae for the emitted RF signals, thus decreasing the total signal received by the imager's coils.[19] Direct electric connections between monitoring devices within the MR suite and the adjacent control room can introduce RF interference, and should be avoided.[2] The monitor may also emit its own RF signal, induced by the rapidly changing magnetic gradients upon loops of wire within the monitor or produced as a part of the normal function of the monitor.[19] If this spurious RF signal is near the operating frequency range of the MR imager (approximately 64 MHz at 1.5T), an artifactual signal will be received by the imager's coils and will contribute to the image.[19] This can appear as a single linear artifact perpendicular to the frequency encoding axis, representing a single stray RF signal, or can result in generalized streaky artifacts that render the images uninterpretable. It should be noted that the presence of these artifacts on one imaging system may not occur on other systems operating at different field strengths. The larger and more ferrous the monitor, as well as the closer to the imager, the greater is the disturbance of the magnetic field homogeneity and subsequent image distortion.

The overall result of these interactions between the monitor and the MR imager is a decrease in the SNR and an increase in image degradation. Monitoring devices must therefore be carefully selected and each separately evaluated with respect to its disruptive interaction upon image acquisition. Conversely, the monitor's ability to function accurately within the hostile MR environment must be confirmed before its clinical use.

Methods of Monitoring

Most conventional physiologic monitoring devices are not designed or easily adapted for use in the MR environment. However, solutions have been found to some of the problems described above in dealing with MR imaging monitoring incompatibilities. Some commercial manufacturers have modified various noninvasive monitors, which can now be used in the harsh MR environment (see the Appendix).

In general, monitoring devices should be placed as far away from the magnet bore as possible to prevent the malfunction of these instruments as a result of attraction by the magnetic field. Increased distance also lessens the effects of magnetic field inhomogeneity and a reduction in the SNR of the image. Extension cables or tubing can be used to accomplish this, with nylon or plastic connectors replacing the metallic fittings. Fiberoptic cables can be substituted for wires to transmit electric signals, and a fiberoptic pressure transducer can be used to obtain physiologic pressure monitoring.[20] A number of methods and devices are available to monitor sedated or anesthetized patients noninvasively. A brief outline of these is given below.

Blood Pressure Monitoring

Blood pressure is periodically measured by means of the oscillometric technique with a pressure transducer connected to a pressure cuff via a pneumatically filled hose.[21] The addition of an extension hose with nonmetallic connectors will allow the pressure monitor to be positioned away from the magnet to avoid undesirable interactions. It has been reported, however, that the cuff inflation can disturb lightly sedated pediatric patients, leading to patient motion artifacts.[21]

Heart Rate–ECG Monitoring

Conventional ECG methods with patient electrode wires leaving the scanner usually create both image and monitor readout artifacts. Telemetric ECG with a remote receiver has been used successfully during MR imaging.[22,23] Fiberoptic transmission of the ECG signals to a distant monitor, usually within the control room, is a common method of cardiac gating MR images as well as ECG monitoring. However, some MR systems require the study to be cardiac gated if this type of ECG monitor is to function properly.

Heart rate monitoring can be obtained by a number of methods, usually in association with another measurement such as blood pressure, ECG, or capillary blood flow. Ultrasonic Doppler flow detectors and plethysmographic measurement of the arterial pulse of the finger have also been used to monitor heart rate during MR procedures.[21,22]

Cutaneous Blood Flow Monitoring

A laser-Doppler velocimetry system with fiberoptic signal transmission has been used during MRI to monitor blood flow and heart rate noninvasively. This technique detects the Doppler broadened scattered light from the moving red blood cells within the cutaneous capillary bed.[24]

Body Temperature Monitoring

Rectal temperature can be monitored during MRI by a temperature probe. This is usually appropriate only in premature neonates whose body temperature homeostasis is underdeveloped.

Respiratory Monitoring

Respiratory movements can be monitored by chest wall bellows attached to a pressure transducer. This technique, however, is capable only of determining respiratory effort and cannot detect apneic episodes associated with upper airway obstruction.[21] This problem has been overcome with the development of pulmonary gas exchange monitors, which evaluate exhaled nasal cannula carbon dioxide by optical infrared absorption technique, and display respiratory rate with preset apnea alarms. They can also display expired air end-tidal carbon dioxide concentrations.

Arterial Oxygen Saturation Monitoring (Pulse Oximeter)

Spectrophotometric assessment of arterial hemoglobin oxygen content by measuring the amount of light transmitted through the capillary bed can be obtained by use of a pulse oximeter.[25] These monitors usually display blood oxygen saturation and pulse rate, each with preset alarms.

A few noninvasive monitors are directly MR compatible, and most require certain modifications such as tubing or cable extensions in order to place the unit as far away from the magnet as possible (at least 8 to 10 feet). These monitors require a prepurchase trial period with the MR imager with which it is proposed to be used. This trial should include use with both infants and adults; head, body, and surface utility coils; and the commonly employed pulse sequence protocols. Both the proper operation of the monitor and the diagnostic quality of the images in sedated or otherwise compromised patients should be carefully assessed before these devices are purchased.

APPENDIX: EQUIPMENT SUPPLIERS

The following is a list of physiologic monitoring devices that are compatible with MRI. Most require minimal modifications such as extension tubing or cables.

HEART RATE/BLOOD PRESSURE MONITOR

Omni-Trak 3100 MRI Unit
Omega 1400
Invivo Research, Inc.
3061 West Albany
Broken Arrow, OK 74012
(800) 331-3220   (918) 250-0566

CUTANEOUS BLOOD FLOW/HEART RATE MONITOR

Medpacific LD 5000
Laser-Doppler Capillary Perfusion Monitor
Medpacific Corporation
6701 6th Avenue South
Seattle, WA 98108
(206) 763-9177

BPM 403A Perfusion Monitor
TSI, Inc.
500 Cardigan Rd.
P.O. Box 64394
St. Paul, MN 55164
(612) 483-0900

Model 811 Ultrasonic Doppler Flow Detector
Parks Medical Electronics, Inc.
P.O. Box 5669
Aloha, OR 97006
(800) 547-6427   (503) 649-7007

PULSE OXIMETRY MONITOR

1040 Pulse Oximeter
Biochem International, Inc.
W 238 N 1650 Rockwood Dr.
Waukesha, WI 53188
(800) 558-2345   (414) 542-3100

3700 Oximeter
Ohmeda Instruments
P.O. Box 7550
Madison, WI 53707
(800) 345-2700   (608) 221-1551

RESPIRATORY RATE/APNEA MONITOR

515 Respiration Monitor
Biochem International, Inc.
W 238 N 1650 Rockwood Dr.
Waukesha, WI 53188
(800) 558-2345   (414) 542-3100

TEMPERATURE MONITOR

Luxtron Fluoroptic Thermometry System
1060 Terra Bella Avenue
Mountain View, CA 94043
(415) 962-8110

MRI COMPATIBLE VENTILATOR

Omni-Vent Series D/MRI
CMS Medical, Inc.
702 Jayhawk Tower
700 Jackson
Topeka, KS 66603
(913) 234-8199

Monaghan 225 SIMV Ventilator
Monaghan Medical Corporation
P.O. Box 978
Plattsburgh, NY 12901
(518) 561-7330   (800) 833-9653

REFERENCES

1. Committee on Drugs, Section on Anesthesiology. Guidelines for the elective use of conscious sedation, deep sedation, and general anesthesia in pediatric patients. Pediatrics 1985; 76:317–321.
2. Nixon C, Hirsch NP, Ormerod IE, Johnson G. Nuclear magnetic resonance—its implications for the anaesthetist. Anaesthesia 1986; 41:131–137.
3. Bydder GM. Clinical nuclear magnetic resonance imaging. Br J Hosp Med 1983; 29:348–356.
4. Thompson JR, Schneider S, Ashwal S, et al. The choice of sedation for computed tomography in children—a prospective evaluation. Radiology 1982; 143:475–479.
5. Strain JD, Harvey LA, Foley LC, Campbell JB. Intravenously administered pentobarbital sodium for sedation in pediatric CT. Radiology 1986; 161:105–108.
6. Burchart GJ, White TJ III, Stegle RL, et al. Rectal thiopental versus an intramuscular cocktail for sedating children before computed tomography. Am J Hosp Pharm 1980; 37:222–224.
7. Strain JD, Campbell JB, Harvey LA, Foley LC. IV Nembutal: safe sedation for children undergoing CT. AJNR 1988; 9:955–959.
8. Kurosu Y, Keats AS. Comparative respiratory effects of commonly used hypnotic and analgesic drugs in the young and aged. Anesthesiology 1959; 20:131.
9. Heinz ER. Techniques in imaging of the brain. Part II: Premedication and sedation. In: Rosenberg RN, ed. The clinical neurosciences: IV neuroradiology. New York: Churchill Livingstone, 1984:204–207.
10. Mitchell AA, Louik C, Lacouture P, et al. Risks to children from CT scan premedication. JAMA 1982; 247:2385–2388.
11. Anderson RE, Osborn AG. Efficacy of simple sedation for pediatric computed tomography. Radiology 1977; 124:739–740.
12. Crumrine RS, Nulsen FE, Weiss MH. Alterations in ventricular fluid pressure during ketamine anesthesia in hydrocephalic children. Anesthesiology 1975; 42:758–761.
13. Boutros A, Pavlicek W. Anesthesia for magnetic resonance imaging. Anesth Analg 1987; 66:367.
14. McArdle CB, Richardson CJ, Nicholas DA, et al. Developmental features of the neonatal brain: MR imaging. Radiology 1987; 162:223–229.
15. Smith DS, Askey P, Young ML, Kressel HY. Anesthetic management of acutely ill patients during magnetic resonance imaging. Anesthesiology 1986; 65:710–711.
16. Dunn V, Coffman CE, McGowan JE, Ehrhardt JC. Mechanical ventilation during magnetic resonance imaging. Mag Reson Imag 1985; 3:169–172.
17. Higgins CB, Lanzer P, Stark D, et al. Imaging by nuclear magnetic resonance in patients with chronic ischemic heart disease. Circulation 1984; 64:523–531.
18. McArdle CB. MRI helps detect injury in neonatal infant brain. Diag Imag 1987; Nov:272–276.
19. McArdle CB, Nicholas DA, Richardson CJ, Amparo EC. Monitoring of the neonate undergoing MR imaging: technical considerations. Radiology 1986; 159:223–226.
20. Roos CF, Carroll FE Jr. Fiber-optic pressure transducer for use near MR magnetic fields. Radiology 1985; 156:548.
21. Shellock FG. Monitoring during MRI. Medical Electronics 1986; Sept:93–97.
22. Rothe JL, Nugent M, Gray JE, et al. Patient monitoring during magnetic resonance imaging. Anesthesiology 1985; 62:80–83.
23. Lieberman JM, Alfidi RJ, Nelson AD. Gated magnetic resonance imaging of the normal and diseased heart. Radiology 1984; 152:465–470.
24. Stern MD, Lappe DL, Bowen PD, Chimosky JE. Continuous measurement of tissue blood flow by laser-Doppler spectroscopy. Am J Physiol 1977; 232:441–448.
25. Wukitsch MW, Petterson MT, Tobler DR, Pologe JA. Pulse oximetry: analysis of theory, technology, and practice. J Clin Monit 1988; 4:290–301.

SECTION

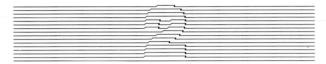

2

HEAD AND SPINE IMAGING

Normal Anatomy and Development of the Brain

STEVEN J. FAGAN, D.O.
SHARON E. BYRD, M.D.

PROTOCOLS
  Posterior Fossa
  Sella–Juxtasellar Region
  Cerebral Hemispheres
MYELINATION

GRAY–WHITE MATTER SIGNAL INTENSITY
RELATIONSHIPS
IRON DEPOSITION
GADOLINIUM–DTPA

Magnetic resonance imaging of the pediatric brain provides excellent anatomic detail and tissue characterization. To the neuroradiologist, the ability to image the brain in multiple planes is an especially valuable asset when attempting to display the complex anatomy of the intracranial structures. Obtaining the multiplane images without using ionizing radiation, and without having to disturb or reposition the sedated child, gives MR a unique and important role in pediatric neuroradiology.

The MR evaluation of the normal pediatric brain, unlike adult studies, must take into consideration the continuing, rapid development that normally occurs during the first 2 years of life. The pediatric brain undergoes certain fundamental changes that dramatically affect the MR images during early childhood. These changes are related to the normal process of white matter myelination, the changing water content of the gray and white matter, and early iron deposition.[1-7]

Although the brain continues to grow, develop, and mature into early adulthood, for practical purposes the brain of a 2-year-old child can be used as the norm for the pediatric brain. In this chapter the normal anatomy of the brain along with its variations is discussed and illustrated, using MR images in the sagittal, axial, and coronal planes. Various pulse sequences are used depending on the anatomic features being illustrated and the age of the patient. Our routine pulse sequences and parameters are listed in Table 6–1.

Our material was obtained with a General Electric 1.5T Signa MR scanner. References are provided for extensive reviews of the embryology, functions, and neuroanatomy of the brain, which are beyond the scope of this chapter.[8-13]

PROTOCOLS

At our institution a routine examination consists of T1 and T2 weighted axial images. An initial localizer sequence provides T1 weighted sagittal images. Coronal images are added as necessary to further evaluate anatomy and pathology. Intravenous gadolinium–DTPA (0.1 mmol per kilogram) is employed when searching for, or evaluating, a lesion known to disrupt the normal blood-brain barrier.

Posterior Fossa

Axial images at the level of the medulla oblongata show the normal surface contour (Fig. 6–1). The ventral median sulcus separates the corticospinal tracts (pyramids) from the more lateral olives. Prominent dorsolateral lobulations represent spinocerebellar tracts forming the inferior cerebellar peduncles. The inferior extent of the fourth ventricle separates the medulla from the inferior vermis and tonsils. The vallecula and cisterna magna are well seen on axial images at the level of the medulla. The vallecula is a cerebrospinal fluid (CSF) canal extending from the midline outlet of the fourth ventricle (Magendie) to the cisterna magna. The cerebellar tonsils form the lateral walls of the vallecula. Normally, the vallecula should not be greater than 2 mm in diameter. The vallecula leads to the cisterna magna, which can vary considerably in size in children. A large cisterna magna is considered normal in children as long as there is not any associated mass effect on the cerebellum. The flow void of the basilar or vertebral arteries is normally seen ventral to the medulla within the medullary cistern.

Table 6–1. MR PROTOCOLS FOR ROUTINE EVALUATION OF THE PEDIATRIC BRAIN: PULSE SEQUENCES AND IMAGING PLANES

Routine Brain		
T1 sagittal "localizer" (head coil)		
T1 axial		
T2 axial		
	Under 2 yr	**Over 2 yr**
Field of view	Less than 24 cm	24 cm
Slice thickness	3 or 5 mm	5 mm
Slice gap	0.5 or 1 mm	1 mm
Excitations	2 or 4	2
Matrix	192 or 256 × 256	128, 192, or 256 × 256

Routine Sella	
	Under or Over 2 yr
T1 sagittal "localizer" (head coil)	
T1 and T2, axial and coronal, as required by clinical information	
Field of view	8–16 cm
Slice of thickness	3 mm
Slice gap	0.5 mm
Excitations	4
Matrix	192 or 256 × 256

[a] T1 parameters: Spin echo TR 500–700/TE 20–30
[b] T2 parameters: TR 2,000/TE 30, 90
[c] In a patient under 2 yr of age, it may be advantageous to increase TR above 2,000 to 3,000–3,500 and TE above 90 to 120 to 160 msec when the degree of myelination is being evaluated
[d] Motion Compensation:
   T1: Arterial flow compensation may be required; cardiac gating may be necessary for small field of view, high-resolution images
   T2: Cardiac gating and venous/CSF flow compensation required

At a slightly higher level the pons expands the ventral aspect of the brain stem. From the pons, the middle cerebellar peduncles (brachium pontis) course dorsolaterally into the cerebellar hemispheres. The fourth ventricle is now more prominent between the tegmentum and the cerebellar vermis. Within the cerebellopontine angle, cranial nerves VII and VIII can be seen coursing from the pontomedullary junction to the internal auditory canals. More superiorly, cranial nerve V exits the ventral lateral surface of the pons and travels anteriorly through the routine cistern to become the gasserian ganglion within Meckel's cave.

At the higher level of the mesencephalon, or midbrain, corticospinal tracts are forming ventrolateral masses—the cerebral peduncles. The substantia nigra is deep to these tracts. Dorsal to these extrapyramidal nuclei, the decussation of the superior cerebellar peduncles arches across the posterior aspect of the midbrain. In the most dorsal region of the midbrain, a midline CSF flow void marks the location of the cerebral aqueduct. The CSF flow void is the result of propagation of the systemic arterial pulse wave.[14] The inferior and superior colliculi flank the cerebral aqueduct and make up the quadrigeminal plate or tectum. Axial images through the superior colliculus may also demonstrate paired red nuclei dorsomedial to the substantia nigra. At this level the superior cerebellar vermis is imaged in the midline, posterior to the mesencephalon. This axial level also includes the circle of Willis, and it is normal to see flow voids surrounding the mesencephalon as the posterior cerebral arteries bend around the midbrain, coursing posteriorly. Occasionally one may see focal high signal or signal void representing the anterior pontomesencephalic vein, or the lateral mesencephalic vein, closely applied to the ventral or lateral surfaces, respectively, of the pons and mesencephalon.

Sagittal images of the brain illustrate the unique ability of MR to image accurately in multiple planes. The sagittal view provides the radiologist with an opportunity to evaluate the configuration and relationships of midline structures (Fig. 6–2). In the posterior fossa the brain stem and cerebellum surface anatomy is clearly depicted at short repetition and echo times (TR-TE). The foramen magnum is limited by the occipital bone (opisthion) posteriorly, and fat between the dens and clivus (basion) anteriorly. Thus, the normally capacious foramen magnum can be evaluated with respect to the position of the cerebellar tonsils. The tonsils normally do not extend below the level of the foramen magnum, but may extend 2 to 3 mm below an imaginary line drawn between the inferior margins of the opisthion and basion.[15] The position of this line must be estimated owing to the lack of signal in cortical bone. The midsagittal short TR-TE image of the posterior fossa includes the brain stem (medulla, pons, and mesencephalon), fourth ventricle, and cerebellum. The decussation of the superior cerebellar peduncles appears as a region of low signal immediately above the pons, while the medial lemniscus curves behind the pons. Flow voids may indicate the location of the cerebral aqueduct, internal cerebral veins, vein of Galen, straight sinus, and basilar artery. Each lobule of the cerebellum can be identified. The quadrigeminal plate can be seen protruding dorsally into its own cistern above the superior cerebellar vermis.[8–10, 16–19]

Sella–Juxtasellar Region

The cavernous sinuses are paired, symmetric venous channels that lie on either side of the pituitary fossa (Fig. 6–3). The medial walls are formed by the sphenoid bone, while the normally straight or concave lateral walls are made up of dura. The two trabeculated sinuses communicate with each other via anterior and posterior intercavernous sinuses beneath the dura of the diaphragma sellae. An additional communication, the occipital transverse sinus, is located more posteriorly. At the posteroinferior aspect of each cavernous sinus is an oval space, Meckel's cave, which contains the gasserian ganglion and rootlets of cranial nerve V. Cranial nerves III, IV, V-1, VI, and V-2 travel through the cavernous sinus, each within its own fibrous sheath derived from the lateral walls of the sinus. The most prominent structure coursing through the cavernous

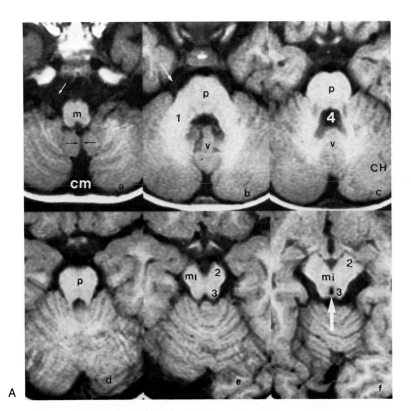

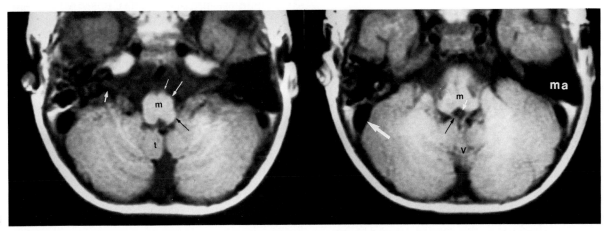

Figure 6–1. *Normal posterior fossa in a 2-year-old child (600/20).* **A,** Axial images from inferior to superior (*a* to *f*). *a,* Medulla (m), vallecula (*small black arrows*), cisterna magna (cm), cranial nerves IX to XI complex (*small white arrow*). *b,c,d,* Pons (p), cranial nerve V (*long white arrow*), fourth ventricle (4), middle cerebellar peduncle (1), vermis (v), cerebellar hemisphere (CH). *e,f,* Midbrain (mi) with cerebral peduncles (2) anteriorly and colliculi (3) posteriorly, aqueduct (*white arrow*). **B,** Normal posterior fossa in a 2-year-old child (600/20). Axial images from inferior to superior. *A,* Medulla (m) with demonstration of pyramid (*thin white arrow*), olive (*long white arrow*) and inferior cerebellar peduncle (*black arrow*), cranial nerves VII and VIII (*short white arrow*), cerebellar tonsils (t). *B,* Medulla (m), fourth ventricle (*small white arrow*), inferior medullary velum (*black arrow*), vermis (v), mastoid air cells (ma), sigmoid sinus (*large white arrow*).

sinus is the intercavernous segment of the internal carotid artery (ICA), which creates a conspicuous flow void on MR images.

In coronal sections these cranial nerves have a constant relationship to the ICA. Cranial nerve III is superolateral, the diminutive cranial nerve IV is lateral, and cranial nerves V-1 and VI are inferolateral to the ICA. A prominent venous space separates the ICA

from cranial nerve V-2, which is located at the most inferior aspect of the cavernous sinus. The signal intensities of the cranial nerves are approximately those of the corpus callosum. The nerves, and their spatial relationships to each other, are imaged to best advantage in the coronal plane, but individual nerves may be difficult to identify in neonates and young children. Meckel's cave has a low signal intensity (only slightly

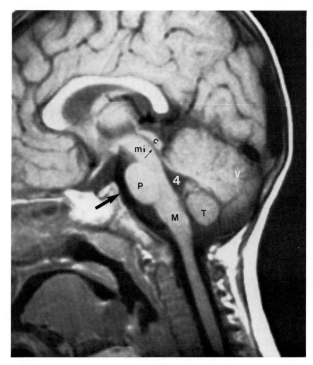

Figure 6–2. *Normal posterior fossa in a 2-year-old child (600/20).* Sagittal image of brain stem. Medulla (m), pons (p), midbrain (mi) with signal void of the basilar artery (*large black arrow*) anterior to the pons, cerebellar tonsil (t), fourth ventricle (4), vermis (v), aqueduct (*small black arrow*) just beneath the collicular plate (c).

greater than CSF) on short TR-TE images and a high signal intensity on long TR-TE images.[8–10, 20–24]

The pituitary gland within the sella turcica results from the embryologic combination of tissue derived from Rathke's pouch and the hypothalamus. At birth the pituitary gland is approximately one-fifth the size of an adult gland and exhibits considerable protein synthetic activity. This increased activity is thought by some investigators to account for the "bright" appearance of the pituitary gland on short TR-TE images of neonates. In children and young adults the pituitary gland has signal intensity similar to white matter on short TR-TE and long TR-TE images. In both neonates and children the posterior lobe has higher signal intensity than the anterior lobe, although this difference in signal intensities may not be apparent in the bright neonatal pituitary gland (Fig. 6–4). The higher signal intensity within the posterior lobe may be due to lipid in the pituicytes of the pars nervosa. The pituitary gland should be distinguished from any adjacent high-signal-intensity marrow within the sphenoid bone.

The coronal plane is especially useful in evaluating the size and shape of the pituitary gland. The superior surface is flat or concave, and symmetry is an important normal finding. An exception to this may be noted in teenage girls at menarche or beyond, when the pitui-

tary gland may normally reach 1 cm in diameter with a convex superior surface. The diaphragma sellae appears as a thin band of negligible signal intensity above the pituitary gland. The coronal plane is very useful in evaluating both the cavernous sinus and pituitary gland, but the axial plane best demonstrates the optic chiasm and the anterolateral course of the optic nerves. The chiasm and the intracranial portions of the optic nerves are outlined by the low signal intensity of the surrounding CSF on short TR-TE images. The signal intensity of the nerves is similar to that of white matter.[8–10, 25–28]

Cerebral Hemispheres

A midsagittal image and a series of axial and coronal images are used to identify structures within the cerebral hemispheres, including the basal ganglia, thalamus, and deep white matter structures. For a detailed review of the functional neuroanatomy of the brain, the reader is referred to several excellent articles and texts.[8–12] The ease with which the brain is imaged in multiple planes with MR obligates the neuroradiologist to have a three-dimensional concept of neuroanatomy.

The short TR-TE midsagittal plane shows midline structures in excellent detail (Fig. 6–5). As in other planes, the structures are identified more easily by their characteristic shape and location than by a particular signal intensity during any given pulse sequence. The limits and recesses of the third ventricle can be identified. They are the infundibular recess leading to the infundibulum, supraoptic recess, lamina terminalis, anterior commissure, fornix, suprapineal recess, habenula, pineal recess, posterior commissure, mesencephalon, and mamillary body. The corpus callosum is the largest commissure between the hemispheres and forms the roof of the lateral ventricles. At birth the neonatal corpus callosum has a uniform thin appearance with a signal intensity similar to or slightly greater than the centrum semiovale. During the ensuing 6 to 8 months the corpus callosum grows into its adult configuration. The genu becomes more prominent and the splenium acquires its rounded, bulbous appearance (Fig. 6–6). The body of the corpus callosum enlarges more slowly and focal thinning is considered a normal variant.[29–31]

The pineal gland lies between the quadrigeminal plate and the splenium of the corpus callosum on midsagittal sections. It has a signal intensity of intermediate strength. Pineal calcification is common in adults but is rare in children under 10 years of age, and its presence suggest neoplasm. Because calcification, like cortical bone, lacks mobile protons, a signal loss is observed on MR images. Gradient-echo acquisition using a partial flip angle appears to be more sensitive than routine spin-echo sequences for the detection of

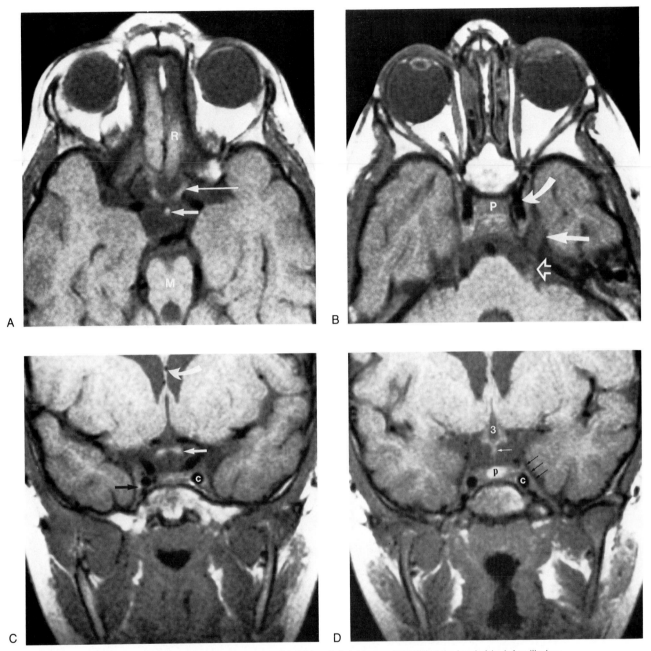

Figure 6–3. *Normal cavernous sinus region in a 2-year-old child.* **A,** Axial image (600/20) at the level of the infundibulum (*short white arrow*). The optic nerve (*long white arrow*) is seen coursing toward the orbit. Midbrain (M); gyrus rectus (R). **B,** Axial image at the level of the inferior aspect of the pituitary gland (P). The cavernous carotid artery (*curved arrow*) creates a conspicuous flow void. Cranial nerve V (*open arrow*) is barely visible as it courses anteriorly toward Meckel's cave (*arrow*). **C,** Coronal image through the optic chiasm (*white arrow*). Carotid artery (C) within the cavernous sinus; septal vein (*curved white arrow*) within the septum pellucidum. Note the small punctate region of high signal intensity inferolateral to the cavernous carotid artery, representing cranial nerves VI and V-1 (*black arrow*). **D,** Coronal image through the pituitary gland (P). The infundibular recess of the third ventricle (3) is directly superior to the infundibulum (*white arrow*). C, Carotid artery within the cavernous sinus; *black arrows,* lateral wall of the cavernous sinus.

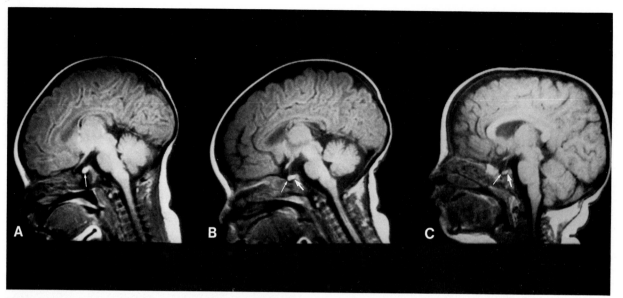

Figure 6–4. *Normal pituitary glands. Midsagittal short TR/TE images.* ***A,*** A "bright" pituitary (*arrow*) is seen in this 9-day-old infant. The anterior and posterior lobes cannot be distinguished. ***B,*** In this 1-month-old infant the pituitary is still bright, but the anterior lobe (*small arrow*) has slightly less SI than the posterior lobe (*large arrow*) and the difference is difficult to appreciate. ***C,*** The anterior and posterior lobes of the pituitary are distinguishable in this 10-month-old child. The SI of the posterior lobe (*large arrow*) remains high, while the anterior lobe (*small arrow*) is now isointense to gray matter.

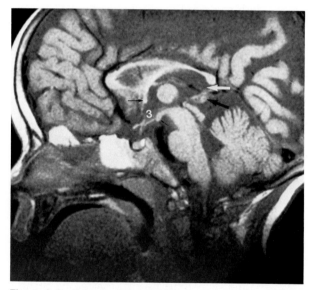

Figure 6–5. *Normal midline anatomy in a 2-year-old child with severe atrophy.* Sagittal view (600/20) demonstrating the mamillary body (*small black arrow*) of the hypothalamus, anterior recesses of the third ventricle (3), anterior commissure (*medium black arrow*), suprapineal recess (*white arrow*) with the pineal gland (*large black arrow*) posteriorly.

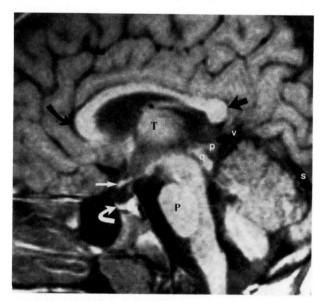

Figure 6–6. *Normal midline anatomy, midsagittal view (600/20).* In this 8-year-old child the corpus callosum has changed from its early uniform thickness to its adult configuration. Note the normal prominent genu (*curved black arrow*) and bulbous splenium (*black arrow*). T, Thalamus; p, pineal gland; q, quadrigeminal plate; s, straight sinus; v, vein of Galen; P, pons. *White arrow* indicates the optic chiasm. *Curved white arrow* indicates the anterior lobe of the pituitary gland. (Note normal high signal intensity of the posterior lobe.)

intracranial calcifications, but may not be sensitive enough to detect subtle punctate calcifications within the pineal gland. MR also lacks specificity when imaging calcification.[9, 32–35]

The sectional anatomy of the brain has been described in detail with use of axial and coronal planes.[8, 10–12] The cortical surface of the cerebral hemispheres and the deep cerebral structures are easily imaged by MR. Representative axial sections will be described, followed by coronal sections. Axial images are obtained in a plane parallel to the canthomeatal line.

The first section is at the level of the centrum semiovale, above the lateral ventricles (Fig. 6–7A). In this section the interhemispheric fissure is uninterrupted, dividing the hemispheres. The convoluted cortex is seen covering both the lateral and medial aspects of each hemisphere. Deep to each ribbon of cortex, interdigitating white matter converges to form the centrum semiovale within each hemisphere.

At the lateral aspect of each hemisphere a prominent central fissure or sulcus divides the hemisphere into roughly equal anterior and posterior halves—the frontal and parietal lobes. The precentral gyrus is immediately anterior to the central sulcus and is the primary motor region of the brain. The postcentral gyrus, representing the primary sensory region of the brain, lies immediately posterior to the central sulcus. Both of these major gyri and the central sulcus extend from the level of the sylvian fissure over the convexities onto the medial surfaces of each hemisphere. Therefore, at this axial level the precentral and postcentral gyri are seen on both the lateral and medial surfaces of the hemisphere. A flow void representing the superior sagittal sinus may be seen at the anterior and posterior extent of the interhemispheric fissure.

The next axial section is at the high ventricular level (Fig. 6–7B). Here the interhemispheric fissure is not continuous from anterior to posterior, but rather is interrupted in the midline of the body of the corpus callosum. The depth of the interhemispheric fissure reaches the cingulate gyrus anteriorly and posteriorly, since this gyrus curves around the corpus callosum deep within the medial surface of each hemisphere. The bodies of the lateral ventricles have a lateral concave configuration. The anterolateral extent forms the frontal horns, while posterolaterally they enlarge slightly to form the atria. Portions of the choroid plexus within the lateral ventricles may be seen. The head of the caudate nucleus may be sectioned on this or lower levels bulging into the frontal horn, forming its lateral wall. The remainder of the hemispheres consist of gyral convolutions and interdigitating white matter tracts.

The low ventricular axial section reveals a more complex array of deep gray and white matter structures (Fig. 6–7C). The thalamus forms the lateral wall of the thin midline third ventricle. At the anterior aspect

of the third ventricle, CSF continuity can often be seen between the third ventricle and the lateral ventricles, via the Y-shaped foramina of Monro. Numerous quantitative methods have been described to evaluate the size of the ventricles, especially the lateral ventricles, and thereby determine whether ventriculomegaly exists. In daily practice, however, ventricular size is estimated by visual inspection of the axial MR images. In children under 2 years of age, and especially during the first 6 months of life, mild enlargement of the ventricles and subarachnoid spaces is a frequent finding and is considered normal. Minimal asymmetry of the brain, including the ventricles, is also a normal finding. In addition, long TR-TE images may reveal differences in signal intensities between the intraventricular and extraventricular CSF spaces, reflecting the subtle increase in protein concentration in the latter.[36–40]

The septum pellucidum is seen as a thin midline structure separating the lateral ventricles posterior to the genu of the corpus callosum. The septum pellucidum is created during the embryologic fusion of the cerebral hemispheres. Before complete fusion there is a cavity. The portion of the cavity anterior to the columns of the fornix is called the cavum septum pellucidum; the cavity posterior to the columns is the cavum vergae. Fusion begins posteriorly and progresses anteriorly. Thus, the cavum vergae is the first space to be obliterated. Fusion is usually complete during the first months of life, but 15 percent of children aged 6 months to 16 years have a persistent cavum septum pellucidum (Fig. 6–8). If a cavum is defined as a space 1 mm or greater between the leaves of the septum pellucidum, virtually all neonates have a cavum septum pellucidum, although this may not be apparent on MR images.[41]

The anterior and posterior limbs of the internal capsule meet at an obtuse angle or genu. Anteromedial to the anterior limb is the head of the caudate nucleus. Posteromedial to the posterior limb is the thalamus. Lateral to each internal capsule is the wedge-shaped lentiform nucleus, composed of a medial globus pallidus and a lateral putamen. The external capsule defines the lateral extent of the putamen. A barely visible claustrum and an extreme capsule complete the outward progression to the cortical gray matter of the insula. The signal intensities of these deep gray matter structures (thalamus, caudate nucleus, globus pallidus, putamen, and claustrum) parallel that of the cortical gray matter. The internal capsule's signal intensity varies with the extent of myelination, eventually becoming similar to that of cortical white matter.

Anterior to the frontal horns of the lateral ventricles, the genu of the corpus callosum limits the depth of the anterior aspect of the interhemispheric fissure. Posterior to the thalamus, the splenium of the corpus callosum similarly limits the depth of the posterior aspect of the interhemispheric fissure. Posterior to the splenium in the midline, the flow void of the vein of Galen

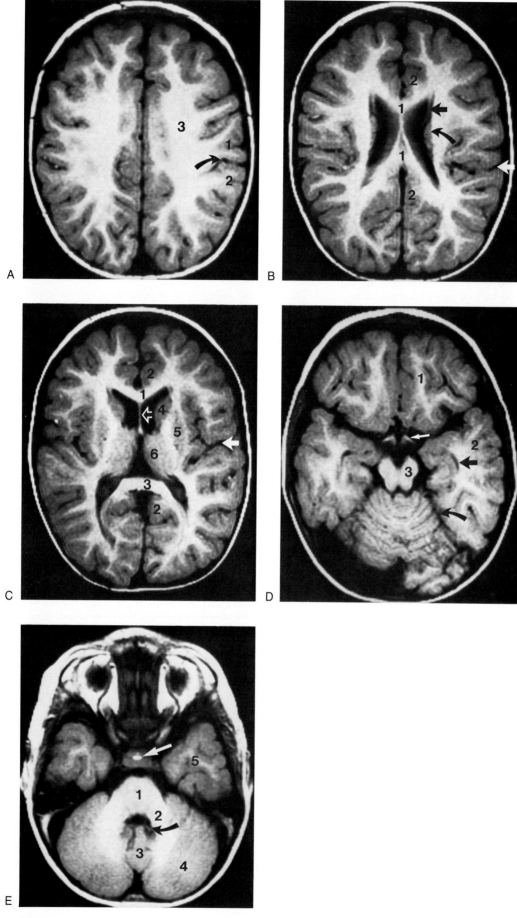

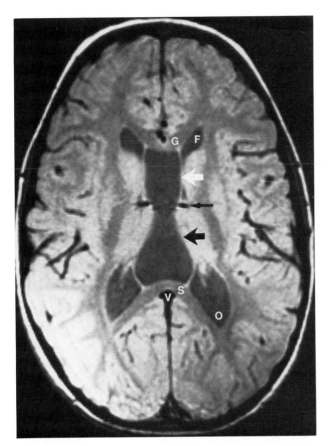

Figure 6–8. *Normal cavum.* Axial image (SE 200/20) shows a prominent cavum septum pellucidum (*large white arrow*) and vergae (*large black arrow*) in a 6-year-old child. G, Genu of the corpus callosum; S, splenium of the corpus callosum; F, frontal horn of the lateral ventricle; O, occipital horn of the lateral ventricle; V, vein of Galen. *Black arrow* indicates flow void created by the thalamostriate vein as it courses toward its junction with the internal cerebral vein.

is imaged, and it is not unusual to see the midline linear flow voids created by the internal cerebral veins within the cistern of the velum interpositum.

At this axial level the lateral ventricles consist of frontal horns anteriorly, and the atria and occipital horns posteriorly. The deep extent of the sylvian fissure is the prominent feature of the lateral cortical surface. The infolded cortical tissue is the frontal, parietal, and temporal opercula. The frontal lobe and a

small portion of the parietal lobe lie anterior to the sylvian fissure in this plane, while the temporal and occipital lobes are posterior.

Anterior to the genu of the corpus callosum, along the medial surface of the cortex, the cingulate and superior frontal gyri are seen. Posterior to the splenium of the corpus callosum, the medial surface of the cortex is more extensive. Once again the posterior extent of the cingulate gyrus is seen. A prominent landmark, the parieto-occipital sulcus, is seen in cross section separating the parietal lobe from the more posterior occipital lobe.

Axial images at the infraventricular level section the inferior aspects of each frontal and temporal lobe (Fig. 6–7*D*). Anteriorly, the interhemispheric fissure separates the gyrus recti and is contiguous posteriorly with the stellate-appearing suprasellar cistern. The sylvian cistern extends laterally between the frontal and temporal lobes.

The temporal horns of the lateral ventricles are seen as curvilinear CSF structures in the medial aspects of each temporal lobe. The mamillary bodies and optic tract may be seen in the suprasellar cistern, anterior to the midbrain. At this level the tentorium is also sectioned. Because of its configuration, structures lateral to the cut surfaces of the tentorium are supratentorial, while those structures medial to cut surfaces are infratentorial. Thus, the superior vermis of the cerebellum is seen posteriorly in the midline at this axial level.

MYELINATION

The MR appearance of the pediatric brain changes considerably during the first 2 years of life. The MR appearance of the brain in children under 2 years of age is due to two factors: (1) the changing water content of the gray and white matter and (2) the myelination process of the white matter. In the developing brain, myelination of the white matter progresses in an orderly fashion, beginning in intrauterine life around the eighth month of fetal gestation and nearing completion at about 2 years of age (although myelination continues until early adulthood). At birth, myelination can be seen in portions of the brain stem, cerebellum, posterior limb of the internal capsule, optic radiations, centrum semiovale, and parietal subcortical white matter (Figs. 6–9, 6–10).[42–47]

◄ **Figure 6–7.** *Normal cerebral hemisphere, axial images in a 17-month-old child (600/20).* **A,** Supraventricular level. *Curved arrow,* central fissure separating the frontal and parietal lobes; 1, precentral gyrus (primary motor region); 2, postcentral gyrus (primary sensory region); 3, centrum semiovale. **B,** High ventricular level. The interhemispheric fissure is now interrupted by the corpus callosum (1). *Black arrow,* lateral ventricle; *curved black arrow,* caudate nucleus; *white arrow,* central fissure; 2, cingulate gyrus. **C,** Low ventricular level. 1, Genu of corpus callosum; 2, cingulate gyrus; 3, splenium of the corpus callosum; 4, head of the caudate nucleus; 5, lentiform nucleus; 6, thalamus; *white arrow,* sylvian fissure; *open white arrow,* septum pellucidum. **D,** Infraventricular level. The tip of the temporal horn of the lateral ventricle (*black arrow*) is visible within the medial aspect of the temporal lobe (2). Optic tracts (*white arrow*) within the suprasellar cistern converge to form the optic chiasm. 1, Frontal lobe; 3, midbrain; *curved black arrow,* flow void created by the tentorium. Structures medial to the tentorium are infratentorial; lateral structures are supratentorial. **E,** Level of the pituitary gland and pons. *White arrow,* pituitary gland; *curved black arrow,* fourth ventricle; 1, pons; 2, brachium pontis; 3, cerebellar vermis; 4, cerebellar hemisphere.

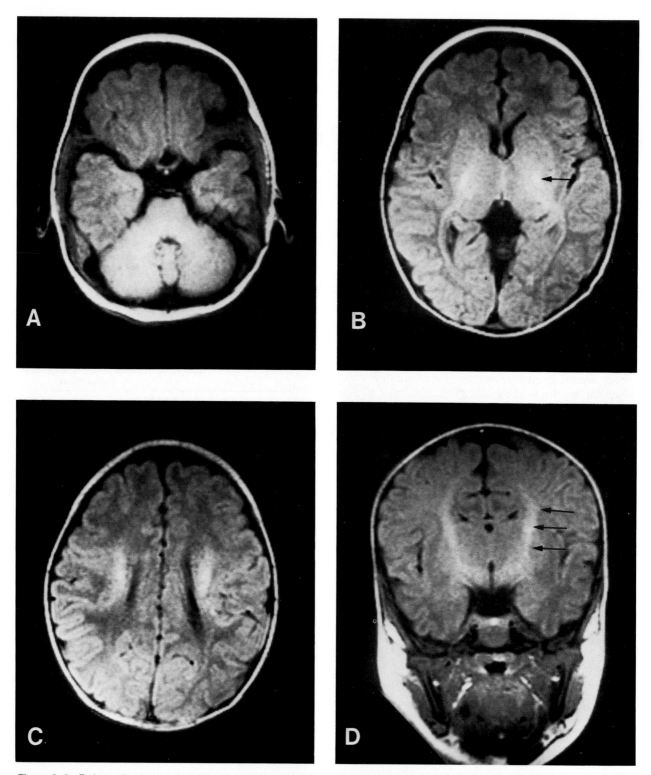

Figure 6–9. *Early myelination in a 1-month-old child.* Short TR/TE. Axial images show high SI within the brain stem and the middle cerebellar peduncles (***A***), indicating myelination. Note the similar high SI of the subcutaneous fat. In ***B*** the high SI extends superiorly through the posterior limb of the internal capsule (*arrow*) and reaches the midportion of the centrum semiovale (***C***). Note how the subcortical white matter is of lower SI than the cortical gray matter on these short TR/TE images. In these unmyelinated portions of the white matter tracts, the SI does not parallel that of the subcutaneous fat. The coronal image (***D***) clearly illustrates the increased SI of the myelinated tracts (*arrows*) extending up through the internal capsule into the centrum semiovale region.

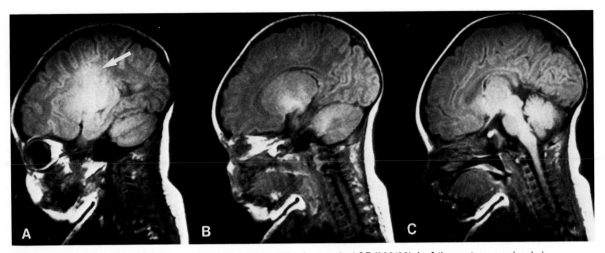

Figure 6–10. *Normal early myelination pattern in a 9-day-old infant sagittal SE (900/20).* In **A** the centrum semiovale is only sparsely myelinated above the internal capsule. Note the patchy increased SI within the central portion of the centrum semiovale (*arrow*). The myelinated, high SI internal capsule extends inferiorly and medially (**B**) to join the myelinated white matter tracts of the brain stem (**C**).

Myelination progresses rapidly during the first 2 years of life and Table 6–2 can be used as a guide to when myelin begins in certain brain structures and when the myelin in these structures is at least 50 percent mature. Myelin is a lipid, and the signal intensity on T1 images is greater than, and on T2 images less than, gray and nonmyelinated white matter. Since MR is very sensitive to the amount of water in a given tissue, the signal intensity of myelinated and nonmyelinated white matter tissue can be compared and used as an indicator of brain maturity.

GRAY-WHITE MATTER SIGNAL INTENSITY RELATIONSHIPS

During the first year of life, the MR appearance of the infant brain is due primarily to the changing water content of the gray and white matter. Water is being rapidly lost from the white matter and less rapidly from the gray matter at this time. After 1 year of age, the process of myelination gains more prominence in influencing the MR appearance of the pediatric brain.

In the neonatal brain, because of the minimal degree of myelination and the increased amount of water in the white matter relative to the gray matter, the signal intensity of the white matter on T1 is less than, and on T2 greater than, adjacent gray matter. The nonmyelinated white matter demonstrates hypointensity on T1 and hyperintensity on T2. This MR appearance continues until about 6 months of age (Fig. 6–11).

The MR appearance of the pediatric brain at 6 to 12 months of age demonstrates an isointensity of gray and nonmyelinated white matter. The water content of these two tissues is such that the relaxation times are similar and the brain demonstrates the isointense (gray) appearance on T1 and T2 images. The myelinated white matter structures continue to demonstrate their characteristic signal changes (Fig. 6–11).

Table 6–2. TIMETABLE FOR MYELINATION OF SPECIFIC BRAIN STRUCTURE

Structure	Myelination
Posterior Fossa	
Brain stem (corticospinal tract of tegmentum)	Present at birth; mature by 6 mo
Cerebellar peduncles	Present at birth; mature by 6 mo
Cerebellar hemisphere	Small amount of myelin present laterally at birth; mature by 6 mo to 1 yr
Diencephalon	
Dorsal thalamus (stria medullaris thalami)	Present at birth; mature by 6 mo to 1 yr
Telencephalon	
Optic radiations	Preset dorsally at birth; mature by 6 mo
Internal capsule	Posterior limb myelinated at birth; begin to see myelin in anterior limb by 4 mo; at 8 mo equal myelination in posterior and anterior limbs; myelin mature in internal capsule by 1 yr
Cingulum	Begins at 2 mo; mature by 6–12 mo
Corpus callosum	Begins in splenium by 4–6 mo and continues anteriorly into body, genu, and rostrum; mature throughout corpus callosum by 1 yr
Postcentral gyrus (subcortical white matter)	Present at birth
Precentral gyrus (subcortical white matter)	Begins at 2–3 wk
Lobes of Brain (Subcortical White Matter)	
Calcarine cortex	
Heschl's gyrus	
Precentral gyrus	
Posterior frontal	Mature by 6.5–15 mo
Posterior parietal	
Occipital pole	
Subcortical white matter association fibers of: temporal lobe	
temporal pole	Mature by 21–26.5 mo
frontal pole	

Adapted from refs. 44, 45, 47.

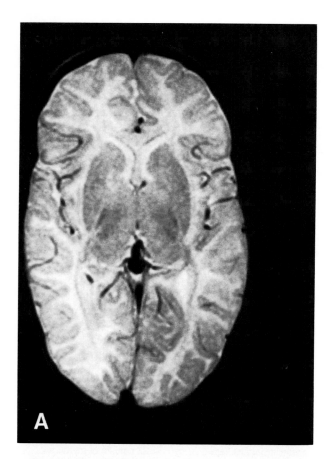

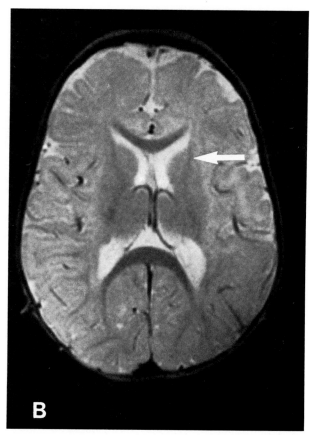

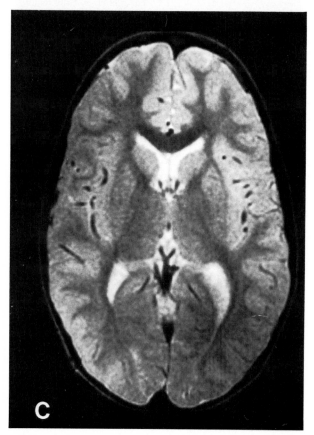

Figure 6–11. *Normal myelination. Long TR/TE axial images.* **A,** A 3-month-old infant. The white matter is of higher SI than the gray matter, indicating a lack of myelination. The exception is the posterior limb of the internal capsule (*arrow*), which is becoming myelinated and has a decreased SI. **B,** A 13-month-old infant. At this time myelination has progressed to the point that the white matter SI is similar to that of adjacent cortical gray matter. The SI of the corpus callosum is significantly decreased, indicating more advanced myelination. Note how the anterior limb of the internal capsule has become myelinated (*arrow*). **C,** A 6-year-old child. The whit matter tracts are now completely myelinated and the SI is significantly lower than that of the gray matter. White matter now has MR properties similar to lipid, and its SI will parallel that of subcutaneous fat.

After 1 year of age, the myelination process has progressed to the level at which it has begun to have a dramatic effect on the MR appearance of the pediatric brain. By this time, there is a noticeable reversal of the MR appearance from the neonatal picture. The infant brain begins to resemble more the adult brain. By 2 years of age (when 90 percent of the white matter tracts are myelinated), the pediatric brain for practical purposes resembles the adult brain; the signal intensity of white matter on T1 is greater than, and on T2 less than, gray matter (the white matter is bright on T1 and dark on T2 images). The use of a TR greater than 2,000 msec (2,500 to 3,500) and a TE of greater than 90 msec (100 to 160) further contrasts the signal intensities of gray and white matter and can be extremely useful in the evaluation of the myelination process, especially in children under 2 years of age (Fig. 6–11).

IRON DEPOSITION

Beginning at approximately 6 months of age, certain sites within the brain begin to preferentially accumulate ferric iron. Histologic staining demonstrates in-volvement of the globus pallidus (6 months), substantia nigra (9 to 12 months), red nucleus (18 to 24 months), and dentate nucleus (3 to 7 years). Iron accumulation plateaus in the late teens or twenties, low concentrations of iron eventually being found throughout the gray and white matter of the cerebrum and cerebellum. The areas of high iron concentration exhibit a decrease in T2 relaxation time, resulting in decreased signal intensity on long TR-TE images obtained with a high field strength magnet (Fig. 6–12).[48]

GADOLINIUM–DTPA

The increased signal intensity or "enhancement" of intracranial structures after intravenous administration of 0.1 mmol per kilogram of gadolinium–DTPA parallels that of contrast enhancement with CT (Fig. 6–13). Structures that have an incomplete or absent blood-brain barrier demonstrate increased signal intensity on short TR-TE images owing to shortening of the T1 relaxation time. Rapidly flowing blood and normal cerebral tissue with an intact blood-brain barrier do not enhance. Structures that normally enhance

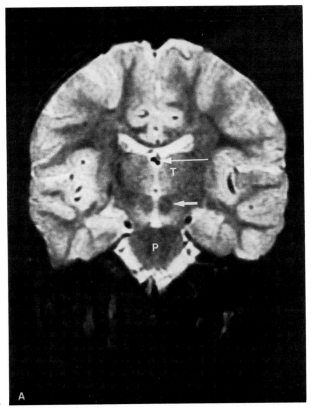
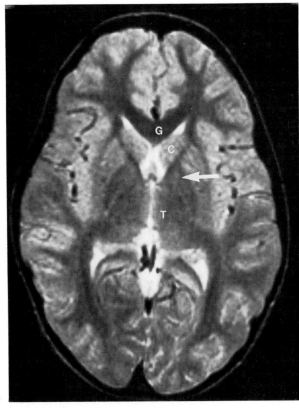

Figure 6–12. *Normal iron deposition.* **A,** Coronal view (2100/80) shows decreased SI in the red nucleus (*short arrow*) secondary to iron deposition in an 8-year-old child. **B,** Axial view (2500/80) shows decreased SI in the globus pallidus (*arrow*) secondary to iron deposition in a 6-year-old child. T, Thalamus; P, pons; G, genu of the corpus callosum; C, head of the caudate nucleus. In **A,** *long arrow* indicates flow voids created by the paired internal cerebral veins within the cistern of the velum interpositum.

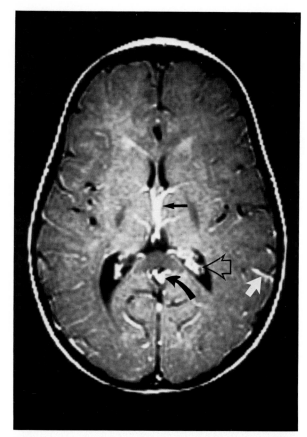

Figure 6–13. *Normal axial postgadolinium image in a 2-year-old child (750/20). Black arrow,* internal cerebral veins; *open arrow,* choroid plexus; *curved black arrow,* vein of Galen; *white arrow,* cortical vein.

with gadolinium–DTPA include the pituitary gland, infundibulum, pineal gland, dural reflections such as the falx cerebri, tentorium and walls of the cavernous sinus, paranasal sinus and nasal mucosa, choroid plexus, retinal choroid, and small blood vessels.[10, 49, 50]

MR is the best imaging modality to date for evaluating the pediatric brain. It provides excellent delineation of normal anatomic structures as well as demonstrating the early development and maturation of the pediatric brain. A fundamental understanding of the normal appearance of the pediatric brain aids in accurate interpretation of MR images and serves as the foundation for the evaluation of true abnormalities.

REFERENCES

1. Dietrich RB, Bradley WG, Zaragoza EJ, et al. MR evaluation of early myelination patterns in normal and developmentally delayed infants. AJNR 1988; 9:69–76, AJR 1988; 150:889–896.
2. Baierl P, Forster C, Fendel H, et al. Magnetic resonance imaging of normal and pathological white matter maturation. Pediatr Radiol 1988; 18:183–189.
3. McArdle CB, Richardson CJ, Nicholas DA, et al. Developmental features of the neonatal brain: MR imaging. Part I. Gray-white matter differentiation and myelination. Radiology 1987; 162:223–229.
4. Nowell MA, Grossman RI, Hackney DB, et al. MR imaging of white matter disease in children. AJNR 1988; 9:503–509, AJR 151:359–365.
5. Johnson MA, Pennock JM, Bydder GM, et al. Clinical NMR imaging of the brain in children: normal and neurologic disease. AJNR 1983; 4:1013–1026, AJR 1983; 141:1005–1018.
6. Barkovich AJ, Kjos BO, Jackson DE, Norman D. Normal maturation of the neonatal and infant brain: MR imaging at 1.5T. Radiology 1988; 166:173–180.
7. Brant-Zawadzki M. MR imaging of the brain. Radiology 1988; 166:1–10.
8. Daniels DL, Haughton VM, Naidich TP. Cranial and spinal magnetic resonance imaging: an atlas and guide. New York: Raven Press, 1987.
9. Newton TH, Ports DG, eds. Radiology of the skull and brain. St Louis: CV Mosby, 1977.
10. Starke DD, Bradley WG. Magnetic resonance imaging. St Louis: CV Mosby, 1988.
11. Gado M, Hanaway J, Frank R. Functional anatomy of the cerebral cortex by computed tomography. JCAT 1979; 3:1–19.
12. Naidich TP, Daniels DL, Haughton VM, et al. Hippocampal formation and related structures of the limbic lobe: anatomic MR correlation. Part I. Surface features and coronal sections. Radiology 1987; 162:747–754.
13. DeGroot J. Functional neuroanatomy by magnetic resonance imaging. In: Brant-Zawadzki M, Norman D, eds. Magnetic resonance imaging. New York: Raven Press, 1987.
14. Citrin CM, Sherman JL, Gangarosa RE, Scanlon D. Physiology of the CSF flow-void sign: modification by cardiac gating. AJNR 1986; 7:1021–1024, AJR 1987; 148:205–208.
15. Barkovich AJ, Wippold FJ, Sherman JL, Citrin CM. Significance of cerebellar tonsillar position on MR. AJNR 1986; 7:795–799.
16. Han JS, Bonstelle CT, Kaufman B, et al. Magnetic resonance imaging in the evaluation of the brainstem. Radiology 1984; 150:705–712.
17. Flannigan BD, Bradley WG, Mazziotta JC, et al. Magnetic resonance imaging of the brainstem: normal structure and basic functional anatomy. Radiology 1985; 154:375–383.
18. Daniels DL, Williams AL, Haughton VM. Computed tomography of the medulla. Radiology 1982; 145:63–69.
19. Press GA, Hesselink JR. MR imaging of cerebellopontine angle and internal auditory canal lessions at 1.5T. AJNR 1988; 9:241–252, AJR 1988; 150:1371–1381.
20. Daniels DL, Pech P, Mark L, et al. Magnetic resonance imaging of the cavernous sinus. AJNR 1985; 6:187–192, AJR 1985; 144:1009–1014.
21. Harris FS, Rhoton AL. Anatomy of the cavernous sinus: a microsurgical study. J Neurosurg 1976; 45:169–180.
22. Braffman BH, Zimmerman RA, Rabischong P. Cranial nerves III, IV, and VI: a clinical approach to the evaluation of their dysfunction. Semin Ultrasound, CT and MR 1987; 8:185–213.
23. Kapila A, Chakeres DW, Blanco E. The Meckel cave: computed tomographic study. Part I. Normal anatomy. Radiology 1984; 152:425–433.
24. Daniels DL, Pech P, Pojunas KW, et al. Trigeminal nerve: anatomic correlation with MR imaging. Radiology 1986; 159:577–583.
25. Daniels DL, Pojunas KW, Kilgore DP, et al. MR of the diaphragma sellae. AJNR 1986; 7:765–769.
26. Sze G, Pardo F, Kucharczyk W, et al. The posterior pituitary gland: MR correlation with anatomy and function. Presented at the annual meeting of the ASNR, New York, NY, May 1987.
27. Wolpert SM, Osborne M, Anderson M, Runge VM. The bright pituitary gland—a normal MR appearance in infancy. AJNR 1988; 9:1–3.
28. Daniels DL, Herfkins R, Gager WE, et al. Magnetic resonance imaging of optic nerves and chiasm. Radiology 1984; 152:79–83.
29. Reinarz SJ, Coffman CE, Smoker WRK, Godersky JC. MR imaging of the corpus callosum: normal and pathologic findings

and correlation with CT. AJNR 1988; 9:649–656, AJR 1988; 151:791–798.

30. Barkovich AJ, Kjos BO. Normal postnatal development of the corpus callosum as demonstrated by MR imaging. AJNR 1988; 9:487–491.

31. Curnes JT, Laster DW, Koubek TD, et al. MRI of corpus callosal syndromes. AJNR 1986; 7:617–622.

32. Alas SW, Grossman RI, Gomori JM, et al. Calcified intracranial lesions: detection with gradient-echo-acquisition rapid MR imaging. AJNR 1988; 9:253–260, AJR 1988; 150:1383–1389.

33. Kilgore DP, Strother CM, Starshak RJ, Haughton VM. Pineal germinoma: MR imaging. Radiology 1986; 158:435–438.

34. Ganti SR, Hilal SK, Stein BM, et al. CT of pineal region tumors. AJNR 1986; 7:97–104, AJR 1986; 146:451–458.

35. Grant EG, Williams AL, Schellinger D, Slovis TL. Intracranial calcification in the infant and neonate: evaluation by sonography and CT. Radiology 1985; 157:63–68.

36. Harwood-Nash DC, Fitz CR. Pneumoencephalography. In: Harwood-Nash DC, Fitz CR, eds. Neuroradiology in infants and children. St Louis: CV Mosby, 1976.

37. Kleinman PK, Zito JL, Davidson RI, Raptopoulos V. The subarachnoid spaces in children: normal variation in size. Radiology 1983; 147:455–457.

38. McArdle CB, Richardson CJ, Nicholas DA, et al. Developmental features of the neonatal brain: MR imaging. Part II. Ventricular size and extracerebral space. Radiology 1987; 162:230–234.

39. Shapiro R, Galloway SJ, Shapiro MD. Minimal asymmetry of the brain: a normal variant. AJR 1986; 147:753–756.

40. Brant-Zawadzki M, Kelly W, Kjos B, et al. Magnetic resonance imaging and characterization of normal and abnormal intracranial cerebrospinal fluid (CSF) spaces: initial observations. Neuroradiology 1985; 27:3–8.

41. Shaw CM, Alvord EC. Cava septi pellucidi et vergae: their normal and pathological states. Brain 1969; 92:213–224.

42. Norton WT. Formation, structure, and biochemistry of myelin. In: Siegel GJ, Albers RW, Agranoff BW, Katzman R, eds. Basic neurochemistry. Boston: Little, Brown, 1981:63–69.

43. Yakovelev PI, Lecours AR. The myelogenetic cycles of regional maturation of the brain. In: Minkowski A, ed. Regional development of the brain in early life. Oxford: Blackwell Scientific Publications, 1967:3–79.

44. Brody BA, Kinney HC, Kloman AS, Gilles FH. Sequence of central nervous system myelination in human infancy. I. An autopsy study of myelination. J Neuropathol Exp Neurol 1987; 46:283–301.

45. Homes GL. Morphological and physiological maturation of the brain in the neonate and young child. J Clin Neurophysiol 1986; 3:209–238.

46. Kinney HC, Brody BA, Kloman AS, Gilles FH. Sequence of central nervous system myelination in human infancy. II. Patterns of myelination in autopsied infants. J Neuropathol Exp Neurol 1988; 47:217–234.

47. Quencer RM. Maturation of normal primate white matter: computed tomographic correlation. AJR 1982; 139:561–568.

48. Drayer B, Burger P, Darwin R, et al. Magnetic resonance imaging of brain iron. AJNR 1986; 7:373–380, AJR 1986; 147:103–110.

49. Berry I, Brant-Zawadzki M, Osaki L, et al. Gd–DTPA in clinical MR of the brain: extraaxial lesions and normal structures AJNR 1986; 7:789–793, AJR 1986; 147:1231–1235.

50. Kilgore DP, Breger RK, Daniels DL, et al. Cranial tissues: normal MR appearance after intravenous injection of Gd-DTPA. Radiology 1986; 160:757.

Congenital Malformations of the Brain

H. SYLVESTER CHUANG, M.D.
MARY K. EDWARDS, M.D.
A. JAMES BARKOVICH, M.D.

The most common congenital malformations in man occur in the brain and skull. About 60 to 80 percent of all stillbirths and about 40 percent of all infant deaths are attributed to malformations of the central nervous system (CNS).[1] However, the incidence of congenital cranial malformations is higher than the statistics of infant mortality suggest, because many malformations are compatible with life and some may not be detected until adulthood.

The improvement provided by magnetic resonance imaging (MRI) in our ability to diagnose and understand congenital malformations of the brain is more than an academic exercise. Many malformations, although not curable, may be treatable. For example, temporal lobectomy is now an accepted treatment for refractory focal seizures, a common problem in congenital brain malformations. A better understanding of the complex cerebral malformations also affords the clinician a better foundation for counseling parents about the prognostic and genetic implications of their child's malformation.

Although pneumoencephalography, angiography, and later computed tomography (CT) and neurosonography provided fairly accurate methods of studying congenital malformations, MRI is far better at evaluating these complex disorders.[2-4] Because of the improved tissue contrast, the ability to acquire multiplanar images, and the improved vascular contrast enhancement of MRI, it surpasses all other imaging modalities in the accurate diagnosis of brain malformations. Admittedly, CT remains more accurate in demonstrating calcification and disorders of bone, angiography may better define the vascular anatomic defects, and ultrasonography may have an advantage in demonstrating cystic collections. For the investigation of simple congenital lesions, CT may suffice. Nevertheless, MRI provides the best method of evaluating the complex cerebral malformations, possibly directing further investigation depending on the MR findings.

All congenital cerebral malformations involve a deviation in form and structure from normal that occurs during intrauterine development. To a large extent the stage of development during which the insult occurs, rather than the specific etiologic event, controls the appearance of the eventual malformation.[3] Many factors may result in congenital brain malformations, including genetic, infectious, vascular, traumatic, toxic, and idiopathic etiologies; idiopathic causes, unfortunately, remain the most common.[5]

The classification of congenital disorders of the brain by DeMyer is summarized in Table 7–1.[6] In its simplest form, the classification divides malformations into two major categories: those that cause major anatomic defects, the organogenetic disorders, and those that cause focal tissue defects, the histogenetic disorders.

Table 7–1. CEREBRAL MALFORMATIONS

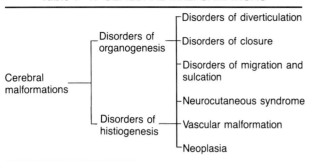

The classification may be further subdivided by separating the organogenetic disorders into different stages of development resulting in diverticulation disorders, closure disorders, and migrational or sulcation disorders. Each of these occurs at a predictable stage of brain development. This classification does not include hydrocephalus and destructive lesions of the brain. Hydrocephalus and destructive lesions such as porencephalic cysts are best understood as isolated disorders resulting from specific insults or events. They may be found alone or superimposed on the disorders of histogenesis and organogenesis.

DISORDERS OF DIVERTICULATION

Defects in the division of the cerebral hemispheres and in the formation of ventricles, termed disorders in diverticulation, are the earliest congenital malformations. Vesiculation of the primitive prosencephalon, occurring between the fourth and eighth weeks of fetal development, results in the formation of the telencephalon (cerebral hemispheres) and diencephalon (thalamus).[5] An insult to the embryo at this stage may result in the prosencephalon failing to cleave to form two separate hemispheres. The diverticulation disorders therefore consist of the various forms of holoprosencephaly and septo-optic dysplasia. Some authors regard septo-optic dysplasia as the mildest form of holoprosencephaly.[5]

Holoprosencephaly

The term holoprosencephaly, replacing the older name arrhinencephaly, is the preferred term for incomplete separation of the two cerebral hemispheres.[7] The subdivisions of holoprosencephaly (lobar, semilobar, and alobar) are based on the degree of separation of the holosphere. It is important to realize that the transition from one form of holoprosencephaly to another is not distinct and the various forms are sometimes difficult to differentiate.

In all forms of holoprosencephaly the olfactory bulbs and tracts are missing.[8] Hypotelorism is seen in all forms but is more severe in the more severe forms of holoprosencephaly. The extreme form of hypotelorism is the cyclops, in which all children also have alobar holoprosencephaly.[8] The presence of hypotelorism helps to differentiate the dorsal cyst of agenesis of the corpus callosum from holoprosencephaly. Midline facial defects are common in holoprosencephaly, ranging from midline cleft to absent philtrum.[8] Most patients with holoprosencephaly have associated lissencephaly, the most severe migrational anomaly. Other forms of migrational anomalies may also be found. Migrational anomalies are to be expected, since diverticulation occurs before sulcation and migration. Arrest in diverticulation would therefore affect the sulcation and migration that come later.

Alobar holoprosencephaly is the most severe form in which all or most of the two cerebral hemispheres and thalami are fused.[7] The third ventricle is incorporated into the fused lateral ventricles. The holoventricle appears as an inverted "U" on coronal views. The sylvian fissures are not formed and the falx cerebri is completely absent. In 20 percent of cases a dorsal arachnoid cyst is present (Fig. 7–1).[8]

In semilobar holoprosencephaly, with intermediate severity of fusion of the hemispheres, there is more division between the two cerebral hemispheres, but the thalami are almost completely fused (Fig. 7–2).[7] The temporal horns show some degree of development and the sylvian fissure is formed. The third ventricle is

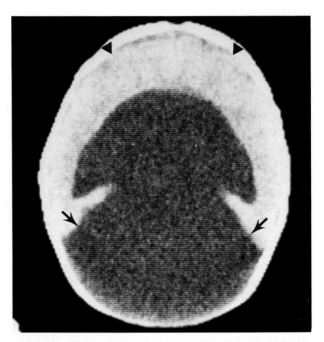

Figure 7–1. *Alobar holoprosencephaly.* CT scan shows an associated dorsal cyst (*arrows*). Note the absence of sulcation in the fused frontal lobe (*arrowheads*).

partially incorporated into the lateral ventricles (Fig. 7–3), however, and there is almost complete absence of the falx cerebri.

The mildest type of holoprosencephaly is the lobar form. The diagnosis may be difficult to make from CT scans, especially if gray and white differentiation is not good and if coronal views are not performed. MRI, with improved definition of gray and white matter, defines well the extent of the holoprosencephalic defect (Fig. 7–4). On axial MR scans, the frontal horns of the lateral ventricles are small and poorly defined. The trigone and the occipital horns are mildly dilated.[9] The white matter in the frontal lobe is seen to cross the midline to join the white matter of the opposite hemisphere.[9]

Septo-optic Dysplasia

Septo-optic dysplasia, also known as DeMorsier's syndrome, was first described in 1956.[10] DeMorsier identified the triad of absence of the septum pellucidum, hypoplasia of the optic nerves, and hypoplasia of the infundibulum.[10] The corpus callosum is usually thinned but present, and the anterior third ventricle is bulbous. The falx cerebri is always present and is not deficient. The absence of the septum pellucidum results in square-shaped, fused frontal horns of the lateral ventricles with a flat roof and rounded lateral angles.[11, 12] The coronal projection best defines

the anomaly (Fig. 7–5). Occasionally, septo-optic dysplasia is found in association with agenesis of the corpus callosum. In this case, the MR and CT appearance of the brain are indistinguishable from agenesis of the corpus callosum alone. Scans such as STIR, which define the optic nerve (described in the chapter on the Orbit), are helpful in demonstrating optic nerve atrophy, and therefore in diagnosing septo-optic dysplasia that complicates agenesis of the corpus callosum.

DISORDERS OF CLOSURE

The four most common malformations resulting from disorders of closure are meningoencephalocele (including Chiari malformation, meningocele, and anencephaly), agenesis of the corpus callosum, and Dandy-Walker syndrome.[3] It should be understood that the disorders of organogenesis may overlap. When multiple cranial anomalies occur, there is often an anomaly of closure of diverticulation associated with a migrational anomaly, such as heterotopia.[5]

Meningoencephalocele or Encephalocele

Meningoencephalocele is the herniation of brain and meninges through a defect in the skull and dura mater. The term meningocele is reserved for the herniation of a sac containing only meninges and cerebrospinal fluid

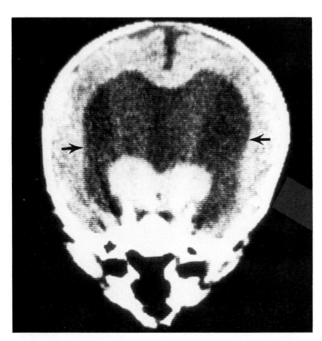

Figure 7–2. *Semilobar holoprosencephaly.* CT scan in the coronal projection demonstrates the typical shape of the fused lateral ventricles and an inverted "U" configuration (*arrows*).

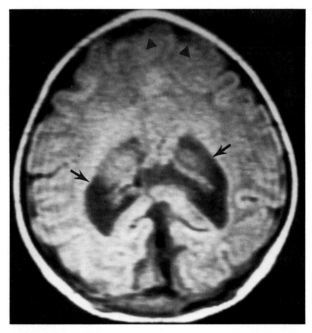

Figure 7–3. *Semilobar holoprosencephaly.* Axial T1 weighted MR images demonstrate the fused lateral ventricles (*arrows*) and frontal lobes. Note the sulcation anomaly in the frontal lobes (*arrowheads*).

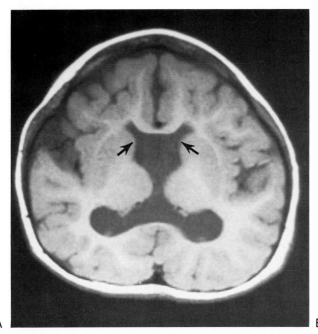

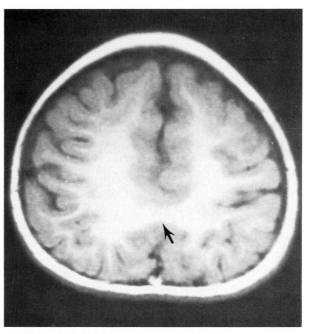

A   B

Figure 7–4. *Lobar holoprosencephaly.* ***A,*** Axial T1 weighted image shows the typical appearance of squared lateral ventricles (*arrows*) and the absence of the septum pellucidum. ***B,*** Axial T1 weighted image at a higher level shows fusion of the white matter between the two hemispheres (*arrow*).

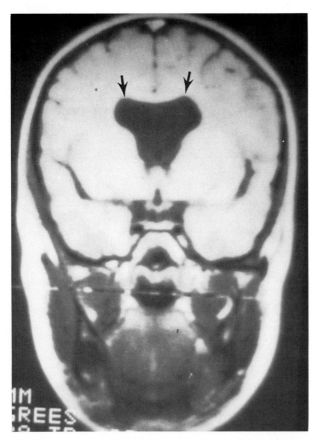

Figure 7–5. *Septo-optic dysplasia.* Coronal T1 weighted MR image shows the typical appearance of squared frontal horns of the lateral ventricles (*arrows*) and absence of the septum pellucidum.

(CSF).[10] A skull defect without herniation of brain or meninges is called cranium bifidum occultum. Other cerebral anomalies are often associated with encephaloceles, which occur in 0.3 to 4 percent of live births.[5, 8] The defects in closure at the cephalic end of the neural tube causing encephaloceles are less common than those at the caudal end. Meningoencephaloceles occur between 6 and 16 times less frequently than spina bifida.[1]

The etiology of meningoencephaloceles is unclear but is probably multifactorial. A genetic influence is often apparent, there being an increased incidence in families with other CNS malformations. Radiation and toxic chemicals have been used to induce meningoencephaloceles experimentally.

Most encephaloceles occur in the midline, although a rare case of lateral encephalocele is occasionally demonstrated. In America and Europe the most common site for meningocele is posteriorly, in the parieto-occipital location; in Russia and Southeast Asia a frontal location is more common.[13, 14]

Posterior encephaloceles may occur above or below the tentorium, or may split the tentorium and herniate contents of both the supra- and infratentorial compartments. When the tentorium is split, there is an absence of the straight sinus, which is replaced by the paramedian veins draining that region (Fig. 7–6).[13] The ability of MRI to demonstrate the malformation in the sagittal plane has been of utmost value in understanding the components of the encephalocele and in planning the surgical repair. MRI shows the location of the encephalocele and the contents of the herniated sac. Herniated

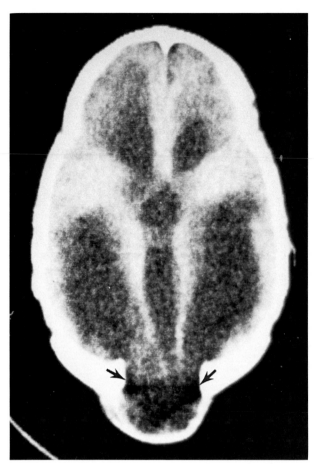

Figure 7–6. *Parietal occipital encephalocele.* Axial CT scan demonstrates a midline parietal occipital encephalocele (*arrows*).

brain and CSF have normal signal characteristics on T1 weighted sequences. A CSF tract may be demonstrated extending from the quadrigeminal plate cistern into the encephalocele.

The second most common site of meningoencephalocele is the frontal nasal region, where it is known as a frontal ethmoidal encephalocele (Fig. 7–7). The defect is in the base of the anterior cranial fossa in the ethmoid region. The herniated cerebral tissue is mostly dystrophic.[15, 16] Agenesis of the corpus callosum is a common associated anomaly.[17] All patients with frontal encephalocele have hypertelorism.

Encephaloceles occur at the craniovertebral junction with a frequency almost as common as that of frontal encephaloceles (Fig. 7–8). This is associated with a Chiari III malformation. Chiari described three variations of hindbrain malformations.

CHIARI I MALFORMATION. This consists of herniation of the cerebellar tonsils through the foramen magnum into the cervical canal. It has also been termed tonsillar ectopia.[5, 18] Chiari I malformation is frequently asymptomatic until adulthood or may be found as an incidental finding on MRI.[19] Hydrocephalus is a common associated finding and fre-

quently is the source of the presenting symptoms.[19] Syringomyelia has been found in up to 50 percent of patients with Chiari I malformations.

MRI has been of value in demonstrating both the low tonsils and the associated syrinx. On MR images the sagittal and coronal views are best for demonstrating the findings of Chiari I. The tonsils are usually seen as triangular structures with the base at the cephalad, protruding out of the foramen magnum (Fig. 7–9). Generally the tonsils must be measured more than 3 mm below the foramen magnum before the diagnosis of Chiari I is given.[20]

CHIARI II MALFORMATION. Also known as Arnold-Chiari malformation, this includes herniation of the cerebellar tonsils, vermis, and medulla into the cervical canal with associated elongation and displacement of the fourth ventricle as well. Spinal dysraphism, often with myelomeningocele, always accompanies this malformation. There are many associated intracranial findings in Chiari II malformation. Hydrocephalus is common, often resulting from aqueductal stenosis, probably related to the frequent finding of beaking of the tectum of the midbrain. Fenestration of the falx is a common finding, with interdigitation of the two cerebral hemispheres across the interhemispheric fissure. A small posterior fossa is present, an enlarged tentorial hiatus permits upward herniation of the cerebellum, and an enlarged foramen magnum allows downward herniation of the inferior cerebellum and brain stem.

Several theories have been proposed to explain this anomaly. A complete discussion of the embryogenesis of neural tube closure and myelomeningocele can be found in the chapter on Spinal Dysraphism. Russell proposed that Chiari II malformation is a primary developmental dysplasia occurring at the third week of fetal life.[21] Barry and colleagues suggested that an overgrowth of the hindbrain at the fourth week of gestation is the predominant factor.[22] A third theory by Gardner and colleagues is that in utero hydrocephalus causes the neural tube to remain open.[23] The hydrocephalus associated with Chiari II malformation does seem to be more of a problem after the myelomeningocele defect is repaired.

MRI has been found to demonstrate the multiple cranial findings of the Chiari II malformation better.[24–27] Sagittal images reveal to great advantage the extent of cerebellar herniation and fourth ventricle elongation. The inferior position of the cervicomedullary junction and inferior displacement of the brain stem can be well seen (Fig. 7–10). The advantage of MRI in defining the anatomy of the cervicomedullary region may be of utmost significance in the planning of posterior fossa decompression and upper cervical laminectomy for patients with symptoms of brain stem and cord compression.

MRI defines well the tectal beaking (Fig. 7–11) and upward herniation of the superior vermis (Fig. 7–12) through an enlarged tentorial hiatus. The shape of the

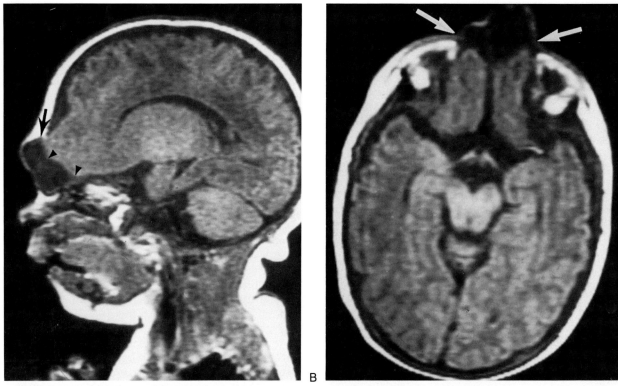

A   B

Figure 7–7. *Frontal ethmoid encephalocele.* **A,** Sagittal T1 weighted MR image shows a bony defect in the frontal ethmoid region with the meningocele sac (*arrow*) and herniated brain tissue (*arrowheads*) protruding through the bony defect. **B,** Axial T1 weighted image confirms the bony skull defect with a herniated meningocele sac containing CSF (*arrows*).

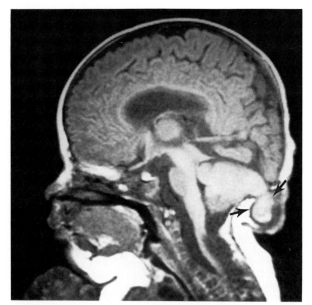

Figure 7–8. *Occipital encephalocele at the cervicovertebral junction.* Sagittal T1 weighted MR image demonstrates the encephalocele with herniated cerebellar tissue (*arrows*). This configuration is consistent with a Chiari III malformation.

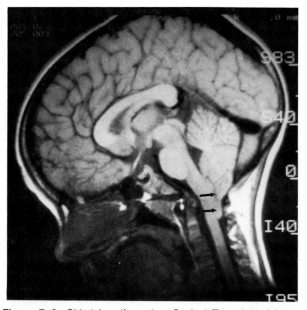

Figure 7–9. *Chiari I malformation.* Sagittal T1 weighted image demonstrates clearly tonsillar herniation through the foramen magnum (*arrows*).

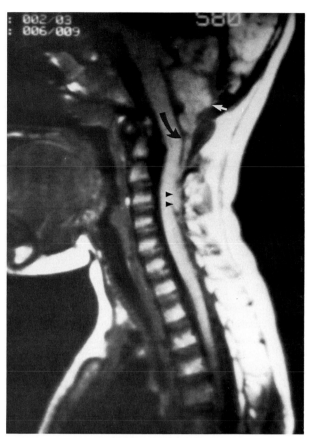

Figure 7–10. *Chiari II malformation.* Sagittal T1 weighted MR image shows herniated tonsils (*arrowheads*) and vermis (*arrow*). The fourth ventricle is elongated, with the cervicomedullary junction located within the cervical region (*curved arrow*).

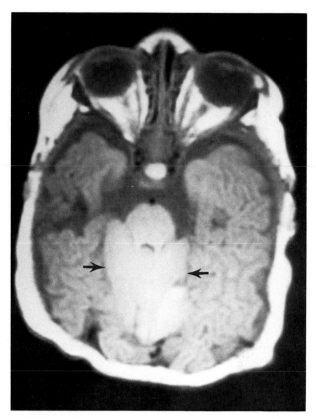

Figure 7–12. *Chiari II malformation.* Axial T1 weighted image at the level of the tentorial hiatus shows a psuedomass (*arrows*) consisting of cerebellar tissue herniating upward through the tentorium.

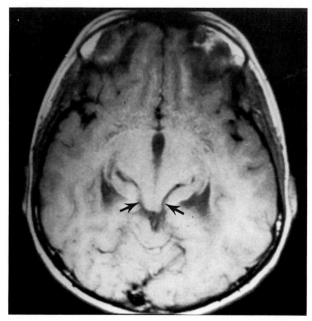

Figure 7–11. *Chiari II malformation.* Axial T1 weighted image at the level of the midbrain shows beaking of the tectum (*arrows*).

lateral ventricles is best demonstrated on axial images (Fig. 7–13). Enlargement of the occipital horns and atria results from deficiency of the white matter in the forceps major, creating the appearance of fetal colpocephaly. Squaring or beaking of the frontal horns is caused by large caudate nuclei that impress upon the infralateral frontal horns, and by a deficiency of the forceps minor. MRI may also demonstrate callosal hypoplasia or absence and deficiency of the falx cerebri, with interdigitation of the cerebral hemispheres (Fig. 7–14).

CHIARI III MALFORMATION. A variant of the occipital encephalocele, this is characterized by herniation of the hindbrain into a meningeal lined sac located at the foramen magnum. The entire contents of the posterior fossa are usually included in the encephalocele, with variable buckling of the brain stem into the encephalocele defect. MRI has improved the ability of the radiologist to define the extent of brain stem herniation into the encephalocele, a matter of extreme importance to the neurosurgeon. The contents of the encephalocele are usually dysplastic and of no functional value except for the brain stem, which must be preserved for respiration. The remaining intracranial findings of Chiari III malformation are similar to those of Chiari II.

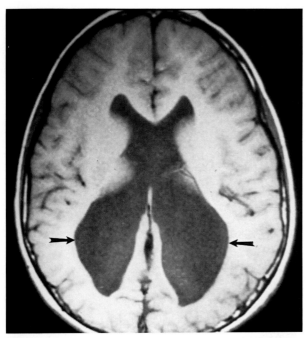

Figure 7–13. *Colpocephaly.* Axial T1 weighted image shows expansion of the atria of the lateral ventricles (*arrows*) with normal frontal horns. This configuration is seen in both Chiari II and Chiari III malformations.

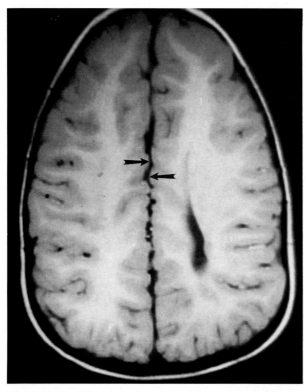

Figure 7–14. *Chiari II malformation.* Axial T1 weighted images show irregular intrahemispheric fissure (*arrows*), due to a deficient falx and interdigitation of the gyri.

Agenesis of the Corpus Callosum

Absence of the corpus callosum may be caused either by a failure of formation or by later destruction of the callosal fibers.[27–29] The corpus callosum forms at the third month of embryonic development. In complete agenesis it is believed that the disconnected fibers of the corpus callosum become the lateral Probst bundles.[30]

The anterior horns of the lateral ventricles are widely spread in agenesis of the corpus callosum and are not dilated.[31, 32] The bodies and especially the occipital horns are dilated, presumably owing to the absence of a forceps major. This results in a colpocephalic configuration of the lateral ventricles on axial images (Fig. 7–15).[33–35] The sagittal and coronal MR images are the best from which to make the diagnosis of absence of the corpus callosum (Fig. 7–16).

The corpus callosum may be completely or partially absent. It forms from anterior to posterior; an insult to the fetal brain during callosal development that causes partial agenesis therefore always results in absence of the posterior portion of the corpus callosum (Fig. 7–17). In rare cases a small focal vascular insult occurring after callosal development is complete causes partial destruction or absence of a portion of the corpus callosum, with sparing of the splenium and posterior portions. This form of callosal injury is better termed

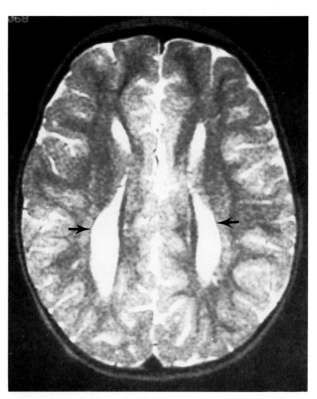

Figure 7–15. *Agenesis of the corpus callosum.* T2 weighted axial MR images show parallel lateral ventricles with a teardrop shape of the atria (*arrows*) consistent with colpocephaly.

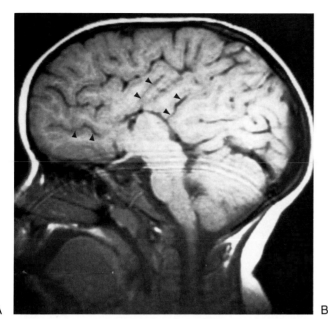

A

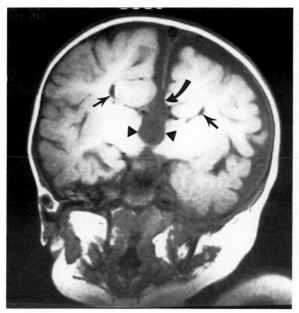

B

Figure 7–16. *Agenesis of the corpus callosum.* ***A,*** Sagittal T1 weighted image best defines the absence of the corpus callosum, with sulci radiating from the brain stem in a radial distribution (*arrowheads*). ***B,*** Coronal T1 weighted image demonstrates separated lateral ventricles (*arrows*) with upward displacement of the third ventricle (*arrowheads*) and absence of the callosal fibers. The interhemispheric fissure (*curved arrow*) appears to connect with the third ventricle.

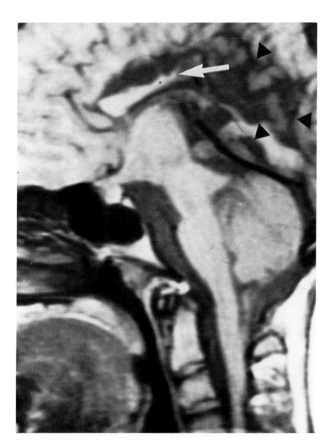

Figure 7–17. *Partial agenesis of the corpus callosum.* Sagittal T1 weighted image demonstrates the genu and anterior body of the corpus callosum terminating (*arrow*) at the level of the midbody. Associated encephalomalacia is present in the parietal lobes (*arrowheads*).

partial absence, rather than partial agenesis, of the corpus callosum (Fig. 7–18).

Partial agenesis of the corpus callosum is often associated with other congenital cerebral malformations, most commonly ectopic gray matter[33] and to a much lesser extent polymicrogyria.[36] Another associated anomaly is lipoma of the corpus callosum (Fig. 7–19).[37] Only a fraction of the cases of agenesis of the corpus callosum have associated lipomas, but the converse is not true. In approximately 50 percent of cases of lipoma of the corpus callosum, there is at least partial agenesis.[38] An interhemispheric arachnoid cyst, often in connection with the high-positioned third ventricle, is present in approximately 15 to 20 percent of cases.[39] Porencephalic cysts may be found in association with destruction of the corpus callosum.[28]

Dandy-Walker Syndrome

The Dandy-Walker syndrome is characterized by complete or partial absence of the vermis, hypoplasia of the cerebellum, and cystic dilatation of the fourth ventricle, probably due to atresia of the foramina of Luschka and Magendie.[40–42] Gardner proposed the hypothesis that the Dandy-Walker syndrome is closely allied to the Chiari malformations and therefore belongs to the broad category of disorders of closure of the neural tube. The Dandy-Walker syndrome results from intrauterine insult occurring between the fourth and sixth weeks of gestation, the time of development of the vermis and cerebellum.[41] The cystic dilatation of the fourth ventricle is usually due to obstruction of the

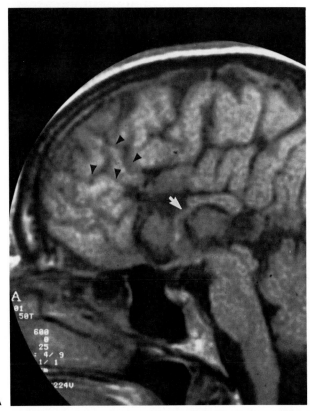

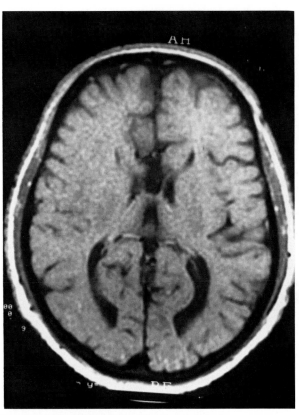

A

B

Figure 7–18. *Partial destruction of the corpus callosum.* **A,** Sagittal T1 weighted image shows irregular destruction of the genu and anterior body of the corpus callosum (*arrow*) with associated radial anomaly of the midline sulci (*arrowheads*). **B,** Axial T1 weighted image confirms the destruction of the anterior portion of the corpus callosum.

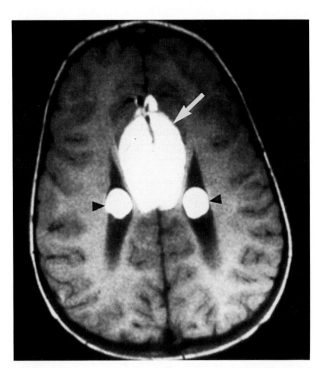

Figure 7–19. *Lipoma of the corpus callosum.* T1 weighted axial image shows a huge midline corpus callosum lipoma (*arrow*) with extension into the lateral ventricles (*arrowheads*) associated with agenesis of the corpus callosum.

outlet foramina, although it is not usual to have obstuction of the cerebral aqueduct as well.

"Dandy-Walker variant" is a term used to describe cases of only partial absence of the vermis, normal cerebellar hemispheres, and absence of hydrocephalus. The distinctions between Dandy-Walker syndrome and Dandy-Walker variant are often unclear, and many cases described as variant in the past may now be considered to be a mild form of the Dandy-Walker syndrome.

Sagittal MR images define clearly the extent of the vermian dysplasia, although the degree of cerebellar hemispheric hypoplasia is better seen on axial MR views (Fig. 7–20).[32, 43] MRI also provides excellent definition of other associated anomalies, posterior fossa encephalocele, agenesis of the corpus callosum, and heterotopia (Fig. 7–21).[43]

DISORDERS OF MIGRATION AND SULCATION

The cells from the germinal matrix migrate to the cortex between 8 and 16 weeks of intrauterine life to form the six layers of cerebral cortex. Any interruption of the migrating neuroblasts at the third to fifth months of gestation results in a migration disorder.[44] Lissen-

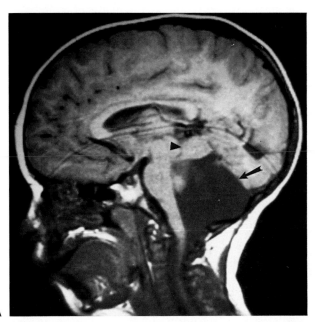

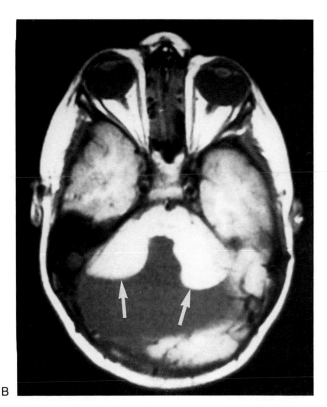

A

B

Figure 7–20. *Dandy-Walker cyst.* **A,** Sagittal T1 weighted image shows a large cyst (*arrow*) in the posterior fossa and dysplastic vermis (*arrowhead*). **B,** Axial T1 weighted image shows hypoplastic cerebellar hemispheres (*arrows*).

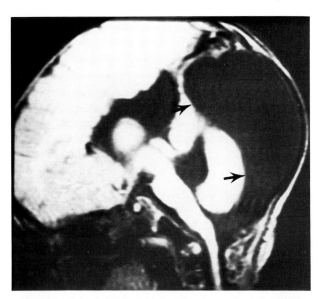

Figure 7–21. *Dandy-Walker cyst with agenesis of the corpus callosum.* Sagittal T1 weighted image shows a huge Dandy-Walker cyst (*arrows*) and agenesis of the corpus callosum.

cephaly, polymicrogyria, schizencephaly, and heterotopia are migrational disorders that can be suggested by MRI. Megalencephaly has many features similar to lissencephaly on the cellular level and should also be included in the migrational disorders.[44]

Migrational disorders include abnormalities in sulcation such as lissencephaly and polymicrogyria, and focal disruption of normal gray and white matter patterns such as heterotopia and schizencephaly. There are many variations of the sulcation anomalies that are apparent on gross inspection, but appear similar on MR or CT scanning. These include pachygyria (large shallow sulci), ulegyria (scarred brain with shallow sulci), and polymicrogyria (many small shallow sulci).

These anomalies may occur independently, but not uncommonly in association with other malformations of closure, diverticulation, or other migrational anomalies. It is typical for an agyric brain to contain many areas of heterotopia. Pachygyria, ulegyria, and polymicrogyria may all be present in the same brain as well. Megalencephaly, both unilateral and bilateral, is characterized by severe sulcation anomaly, commonly agyria, but areas of pachygyria and polymicrogyria may also be present. MRI provides the best diagnostic tool for the detection and characterization of migrational anomalies.

Lissencephaly

In lissencephaly, the sulcation pattern may be that of agyria or pachygyria,[44] depending on the age of the fetus when the intrauterine insult occurred. In both, the cerebral cortex is thicker than normal and has an abnormal four-layered structure, instead of the normal six layers.[45–47] The white matter is reduced and the ventricles are enlarged. Clinical signs vary, depending on the severity of the malformation. Complete agyria

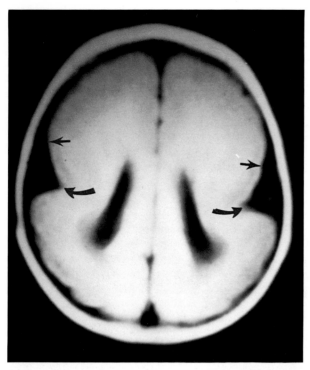

Figure 7–22. *Lissencephaly with agyria.* Axial T1 weighted image demonstrates a smooth brain (*straight arrows*) indicating agyria. Incomplete formation of the sylvian fissure (*curved arrows*) is typical of lissencephaly.

results in a lack of psychomotor development, microcephaly, axial hypotonia, pyramidal signs, and seizures.[44] Less severe cases, with pachygyria, may show only slow mental development and seizures.

The MR appearance of agyria is absence of sulcation except for the primary fissure that forms the sylvian fissure. No gyri are seen. The white matter does not show any branching into the gray matter. The lateral ventricles are abnormally dilated but no obstruction is present (Fig. 7–22). The MR appearance of pachygyria is not as severe as that of agyria, although the patterns are similar. The white matter is abnormal, with only rudimentary branching of white matter into the gray matter. Agyria and pachygyria may also be focal in the occipital or temporal lobes, where the abnormal sulcal pattern may serve as a seizure focus (Fig. 7–23).

Polymicrogyria

On gross examination, polymicrogyria is characterized by multiple small, shallow gyri. Although polymicrogyria differs from pachygyria histologically, the various forms of sulcation anomaly are similar in function.[44] Areas of polymicrogyria may serve as a focus for seizures but do not appear to have functioning cortex.[45] Ectopic gray matter, or heterotopia, is frequently found in association with polymicrogyria. MRI is able

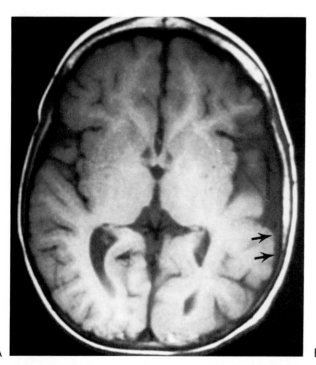

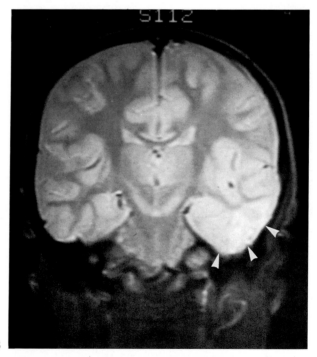

A B

Figure 7–23. *Pachygyria.* **A,** Axial T1 weighted image shows large gyri and abnormal sulcation (*arrows*) in the left parietal region. **B,** Coronal T2 weighted sequence shows lack of extension of the white matter (*arrowheads*) into the thickened gray matter in the region of pachygyria.

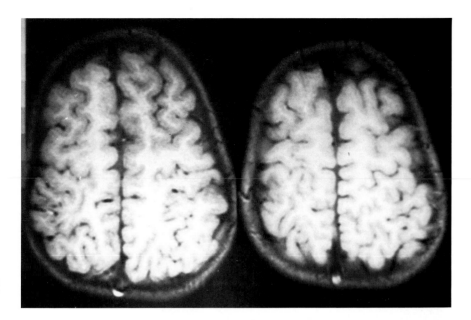

Figure 7–24. *Polymicrogyria.* Axial T1 weighted image of small, poorly formed gyri near the vertex.

to demonstrate the anomaly as many small gyri with a smooth outline (Fig. 7–24).

Megalencephaly

Megalencephaly consists of abnormal enlargement of one or both cerebral hemispheres.[44] In this condition, it is true that more is not better. When the condition is bilateral, the infant is profoundly retarded, with epilepsy. Unilateral megalencephaly is one of the conditions predisposing children to refractory seizures.[48] If diagnosed early, hemispherectomy may permit the child to live a fairly normal life, with only mild paresis. The infant brain is described as plastic, in that each hemisphere is capable of performing the functions of the other hemisphere. When the abnormal unilateral megalencephalic hemisphere is removed in the perinatal period, the opposite hemisphere retains the ability to control both halves of the body, and to perform other higher cortical functions. In this condition it is vital to establish the diagnosis early.

In megalencephaly there is dysplastic enlargement of the lateral ventricles on the affected side and thickening of the cortical gray matter. The white matter has an abnormal branching pattern and is not myelinated. There is a lack of sulcation, and microscopically it resembles lissencephaly.[44, 48–50] MRI provides an excellent method of evaluating the abnormal white matter and sulcation pattern to establish the diagnosis early (Fig. 7–25).[49]

Schizencephaly

Schizencephaly, literally cleft brain, was first characterized by Yakovlev and Wadsworth in 1946 as a congenital malformation of the brain separate from en-

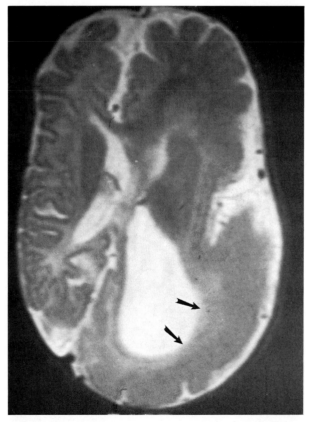

Figure 7–25. *Unilateral megalencephaly.* Axial T2 weighted image shows enlargement of the left hemisphere and ventricle with increased cortical thickness (*arrows*) and poor myelination of the ipsilateral white matter.

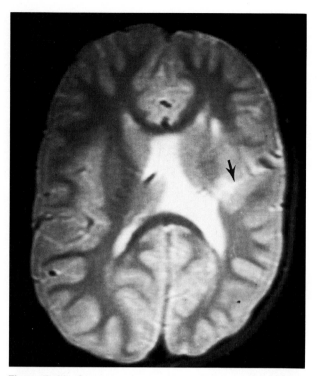

Figure 7–26. *Open-lip schizencephaly, mild.* Axial T2 weighted image shows a CSF-containing cleft (*arrow*) on the left with extension from the lateral ventricle to the subarachnoid space. The cleft is lined by gray matter.

cephaloclastic porencephaly secondary to a vascular insult.[51] The cleft may be unilateral, although it is usually bilateral. It commonly occurs in the region of the primary fissure. The cleft, lined by ependyma and gray matter, is quite different from porencephaly, which is simply a cystic destruction within normally formed cortex.

Schizencephaly is divided into open-lip and closed-lip types.[52] In open-lip schizencephaly the cleft communicates from the subarachnoid space to the lateral ventricle (Fig. 7–26). The cleft may be large and there may be expansion of the extracerebral space (Fig. 7–27). In the closed-lip type, communication does not occur at the ventricular level, but there is gray matter abutting the ventricular wall. In two-thirds of patients with schizencephaly, there is associated septo-optic dysplasia, again suggesting a developmental rather than an ischemic origin. MRI provides an excellent way to establish the diagnosis by demonstrating the gray matter lining the cleft (Fig. 7–28).[53]

Heterotopia

Heterotopia, or ectopic gray matter, results from an arrest or disturbance in the radial migration of neuroblasts originating at the germinal matrix.[44] Heterotopias occur as isolated anomalies but are frequently

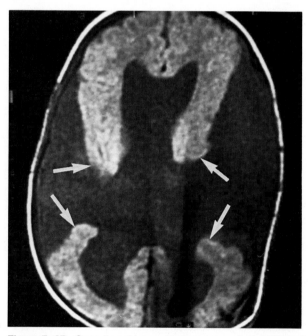

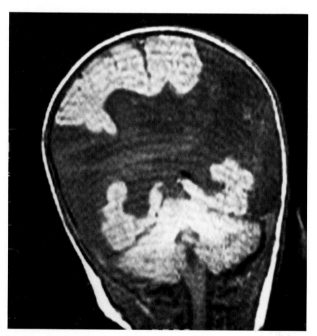

Figure 7–27. *Open-lip schizencephaly, severe.* **A,** Axial T1 weighted image demonstrates a severe form of bilateral schizencephaly with gaping holes (*arrows*) allowing communication between the ventricles and enlarged arachnoid spaces. **B,** Coronal T1 weighted image confirms the massive communication between the ventricles and subarachnoid space.

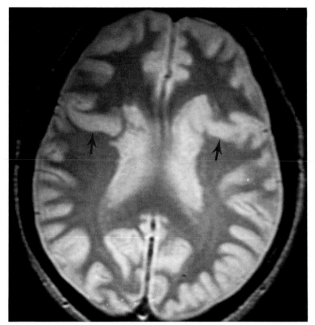

Figure 7–28. *Closed-lip schizencephaly.* Axial T2 weighted sequence shows bilateral clefts lined by gray matter (*arrows*) extending to the frontal horns of the lateral ventricles.

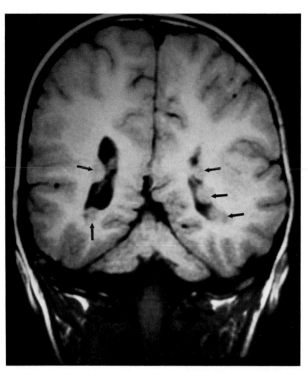

Figure 7–29. *Ectopic gray matter.* Coronal T1 weighted sequences show extensive heterotopia (*arrows*) lining the lateral ventricles.

found in association with other malformations. On MR images heterotopias appear as lumps of gray matter protruding into the lateral ventricles (Fig. 7–29).[54] In children with extensive heterotopias the appearance may be that of a double layer of gray and white matter in the cerebral hemispheres (Fig. 7–30).[55]

NEUROCUTANEOUS SYNDROMES

Neurocutaneous syndromes and phakomatoses are synonymous terms, referring to a group of inherited diseases with both neurologic and cutaneous features. Although the neurologic and cutaneous manifestations may appear in isolation, they more commonly are found in conjunction with a variety of ophthalmic, visceral, endocrine, and bony lesions. These syndromes include neurofibromatosis, tuberous sclerosis, Sturge-Weber syndrome, and von Hippel-Lindau syndrome. Intracranial tumors may develop in most of these syndromes, but rarely cause the presenting symptoms. The most common use of neuroimaging in these syndromes is to monitor a patient with a known syndrome for the development of CNS neoplasms. Occasionally, though, as in tuberous sclerosis, the cutaneous and neurologic manifestations of the disease may not be pathognomonic for the disease at an early stage, and MRI may establish the diagnosis. MRI is also useful in defining non-neoplastic manifestations of these diseases. Ultimately, the role of MRI is to help establish the diagnosis and monitor CNS manifestations in order to plan therapy and help primary physi-

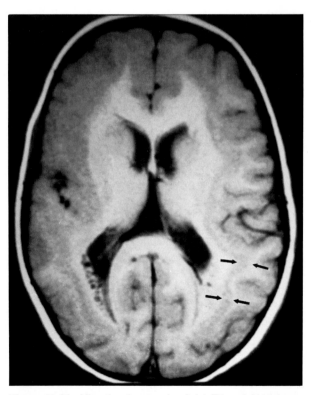

Figure 7–30. *Migrational anomaly.* Axial T1 weighted image shows double rows of gray and white matter (*arrows*).

cians provide families with informed prognostic and genetic counseling.

Neurofibromatosis

Neurofibromatosis, or von Recklinghausen's disease, is the most common of the neurocutaneous syndromes, occurring in 0.04 percent of the population.[56] Neurofibromatosis is inherited by autosomal dominant transmission, with high penetrance and variable expression.[57] Approximately one-third of cases are new mutations.[58] The diagnosis is usually made when there is a positive family history, and café au lait spots are observed on the skin. Two distinct forms of the disease have been defined, with distinct differences in clinical manifestations and chromosomal defects on different genes.[59, 60] The criteria for the diagnosis of types I and II neurofibromatosis, established by the NIH Consensus Conference on Neurofibromatosis in 1987, are summarized in Table 7–2.[61] Type I neurofibromatosis occurs approximately 17 times as frequently as type II. Both types are autosomal dominant. Patients with bilateral acoustic neuromas are classified as having type II neurofibromatosis.

The most common cranial and spinal MR findings in children with neurofibromatosis are optic gliomas, heterotopias, parenchymal gliomas, cranial nerve neuromas, meningiomas, hydrocephalus, osseous dysplasia, and neurofibromas of the spine and orbit.[62, 63] The tumors and dysplasias of the orbit, brain, and spine are described in more detail in the chapters devoted to these regions.

MRI has been of great value in defining the number and extent of the many CNS manifestations of neurofibromatosis. Optic chiasmal gliomas are commonly

Table 7–2. CRITERIA FOR THE DIAGNOSIS OF NEUROFIBROMATOSIS

Neurofibromatosis Type I

Any two of the following criteria:
1. Six or more café au lait spots larger than 5 mm in children and 15 mm in teenagers and adults
2. At least two neurofibromas or one plexiform neurofibroma
3. Axillary or inguinal freckling
4. Optic nerve glioma
5. Two or more iris nodules
6. Characteristic bony lesion, such as sphenoid wing dysplasia or thinning of the long bone cortex, with or without pseudarthrosis
7. A parent, sibling, or child with definite NF-I.

Neurofibromatosis Type II

The diagnosis is established by the presence of:
Bilateral acoustic neuromas
or
A first-degree relative with NF-II
and
Unilateral acoustic neuromas or two of the following: neurofibromas of skin, plexiform neurofibroma, schwannoma, glioma, meningioma, or presenile posterior cataract

associated with separate areas of abnormal signal in the basal ganglia and optic tracts on T2 weighted sequences, termed heterotopias (Fig. 7–31).[64] These heterotopias, seen only on MRI, may be the only intracranial findings, and the significance of these lesions is not clear. It has been suggested that they are abnormal hamartomatous collections of glial cells with the potential of developing into neoplasms.[64] Benign gliomas are common in neurofibromatosis, but as many as 3.5 percent of children with neurofibromatosis have malignant tumors.[57] The exquisite contrast enhancement seen on T1 weighted sequences with gadolinium-DTPA administration makes MRI the procedure of choice for diagnosing neuromas and meningiomas (Fig. 7–32). Hydrocephalus associated with neurofibromatosis, uncommon in children under 8 years of age, is usually the result of aqueductal stenosis (Fig. 7–33).[57]

Tuberous Sclerosis

Tuberous sclerosis, or Bourneville's disease, is characterized by the clinical triad of mental retardation, epilepsy, and adenoma sebaceum. Of this triad, mental retardation is the most variable finding, adenoma sebaceum usually does not appear before the age of 6 years, and epilepsy of unknown cause is frequently the presenting clinical problem. MRI or CT may be of utmost importance in establishing the diagnosis and in monitoring the intracranial manifestations of the disease.[65, 66] The mode of inheritance is autosomal dominant, with incomplete penetrance and variable expressivity. At least one-half of the cases represent new mutations, often with a more severe clinical course.[57] Tuberous sclerosis involves multiple organ systems, with hamartomatous lesions common in the skin, brain, orbit, heart, kidney, and bones.

Intracranial manifestations are found early in life. Subependymal nodules are the most constant finding.[65] They are located in the lateral ventricles, usually at the caudothalamic junction. They are commonly small (2 to 3 mm), round, multiple, calcified, and nonenhancing on CT or MRI (Fig. 7–33). Calcification of the subependymal nodules, making them highly apparent on CT, is progressive with age. MRI may demonstrate subependymal nodules, but not as conspicuously as CT.[65, 66] Cortical hamartomas, or nodules, are larger, measuring 1 to 3 cm, and are much more apparent on MRI than on CT (Fig. 7–34).[65] These cortical lesions, thought to be the epileptic foci, do not enhance on either CT or MRI and do not appear to have any malignant potential. They appear as bright areas on T2 weighted MR sequences. Giant cell astrocytomas may develop, almost always at the foramen of Monro, commonly causing obstructive hydrocephalus (Fig. 7–35). Contrast enhancement is common but does not imply malignancy.[66] The giant cell astrocytomas are usually observed, and are resected only if

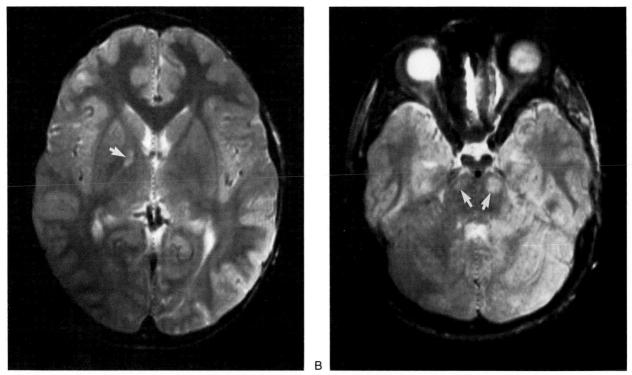

Figure 7–31. *Neurofibromatosis with heterotopias.*   ***A,*** Axial T2 weighted sequence at the level of the internal capsule shows a focal increased signal (*arrow*) consistent with heterotopia. ***B,*** Axial T2 weighted sequence at the level of the pons in the same patient shows two areas of abnormal signal (*arrows*).

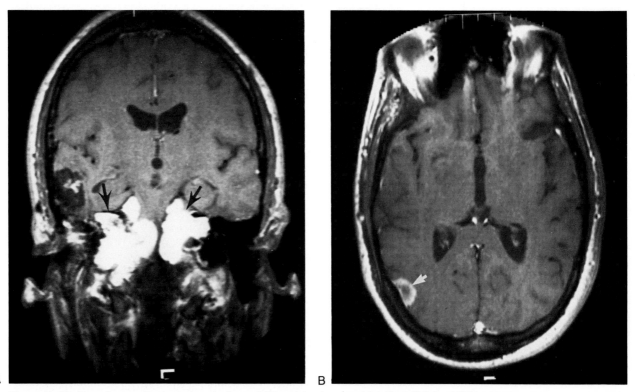

Figure 7–32. *Type II neurofibromatosis.*   ***A,*** Coronal T1 weighted sequence with gadolinium-DTPA enhancement shows bilateral acoustic neuromas (*arrows*). ***B,*** Axial T1 weighted sequence with gadolinium-DTPA enhancement in the same patient shows a small meningioma (*arrow*).

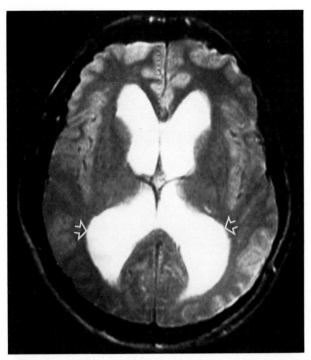

Figure 7–33. *Neurofibromatosis with hydrocephalus.* Axial T2 weighted sequence shows moderate hydrocephalus involving the lateral ventricles (*arrows*) in a patient with neurofibromatosis.

complications develop, such as hemorrhage, refractory hydrocephalus, or malignant degeneration with tumor invasion.

Sturge-Weber Syndrome

Sturge-Weber, a noninherited syndrome, has neurocutaneous manifestations confined to the face and brain. These include a port-wine nevus of the forehead, ipsilateral piadural vascular malformation, epilepsy, focal neurologic deficits, and mental retardation. The skin angioma and the intracranial vascular malformation arise from a common embryologic origin, and an abnormal development of the primordial capillary system has been proposed as a mechanism.[57]

CT scanning has revealed characteristic unilateral, gyriform calcifications in the ipsilateral cerebral hemisphere, with opacification of the angiomatous territory and adjacent cerebral tissue. There is ipsilateral atrophy, with enlargement of the ventricle and sulci. MRI demonstrates the same findings as CT, but the gyriform calcifications appear as areas of signal void. Areas of increased signal appear in the adjacent white matter on T2 weighted sequences, possibly related to the steal phenomenon (Fig. 7–36). Enlargement of the

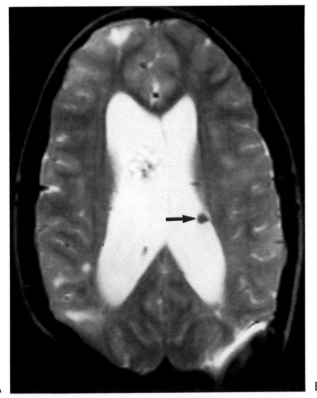

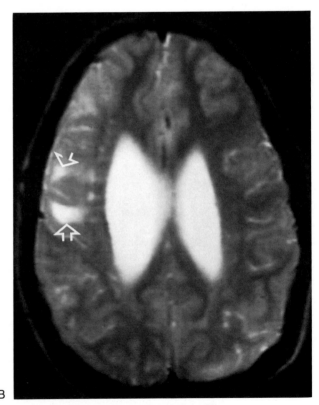

A   B

Figure 7–34. *Tuberous sclerosis.*   ***A,*** Axial T1 weighted sequence shows a small subependymal nodule creating a filling defect within the lateral ventricle (*arrow*). ***B,*** Axial T2 weighted sequence shows a bright signal within the cortex consistent with cortical hamartomas (*arrows*).

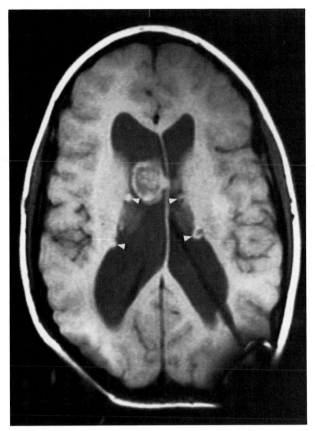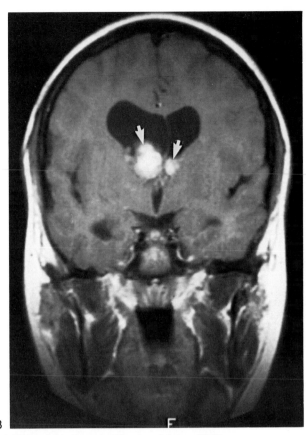

A B

Figure 7–35. *Tuberous sclerosis with giant cell astrocytoma.* **A,** Axial T1 weighted image without gadolinium-DTPA enhancement shows subependymal nodules (*arrowheads*) and a large filling defect in the right lateral ventricle due to a giant cell astrocytoma. **B,** Coronal T1 weighted image with gadolinium-DTPA enhancement shows bilateral enhancing giant cell astrocytomas at the level of the foramina of Monro (*arrows*).

choroid plexus[67] and accelerated myelination in infants with Sturge-Weber disease have been reported.[68] Either CT or MRI may be of value in the early detection of the Sturge-Weber syndrome in children with a port-wine nevus of the face, before the onset of seizures.

HYDROCEPHALUS

Enlarged ventricles are a common finding in children, both as an isolated finding and in association with other disorders. The term hydrocephalus is reserved for cases in which the enlargement of the ventricles is due to obstruction of either the ventricular system, the subarachnoid spaces, or the arachnoid granulations. When the ventricles are enlarged because of decreased surrounding parenchyma, the term cerebral atrophy is usually applied.

In neonates and infants it may be difficult on both MRI and CT to differentiate between atrophy and a communicating form of hydrocephalus, in which the ventricles and subarachnoid spaces are both dilated.[69] Correlation with head size usually helps; there is enlargement of the head in communicating hydrocephalus and a small head size with atrophy.

Although most cases of hydrocephalus remain well studied by CT, MRI has certain advantages in the evaluation of enlarged ventricles. MRI defines better the extent of subependymal reabsorption of CSF, with bright signal appearing boldly in the periventricular white matter.[69] Tectal plate gliomas, an uncommon but serious cause of hydrocephalus, may be subtle on CT scans, but are seen as characteristic bright lesions on T2 weighted MR scans. Sagittal MR scanning is of great value in defining the point of obstruction within the cerebral aqueduct (Fig. 7–37).[70] Gradient-echo imaging may be helpful in demonstrating absent flow in aqueductal stenosis.[71]

ARACHNOID CYST

Arachnoid cysts are collections of CSF between two layers of arachnoid. They are commonly found in the base of the middle cranial fossa, cerebellopontine angle cistern, and suprasellar cisterns, but they may occur

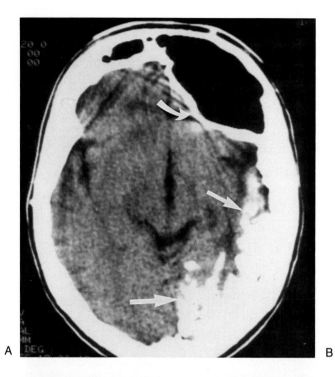

A

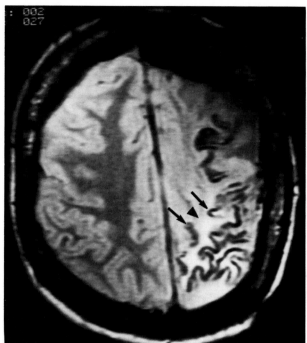

B

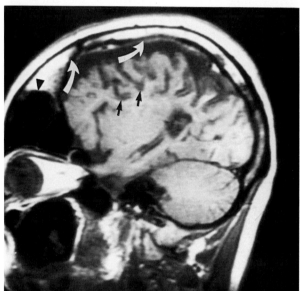

C

Figure 7–36. *Sturge-Weber syndrome.* ***A,*** Axial nonenhanced CT scan shows extensive calcification in the atrophic left cerebral hemisphere (*arrows*). Note the expansion of the frontal sinus consistent with cerebral hemiatrophy (*curved arrow*). ***B,*** Axial T2 weighted sequence shows signal void within the areas of calcification (*arrows*) and a bright signal in the adjacent cerebral cortex due to the steal phenomenon (*arrowhead*). ***C,*** Sagittal T1 weighted sequence shows signal void in a gyriform configuration due to cortical calcification (*straight arrows*). Cerebral hemiatrophy is apparent, with enlargement of the frontal sinus (*arrowhead*) and a thickened calvarium (*curved arrows*).

anywhere there is arachnoid. When the cysts occur in the region of the third ventricle, quadrigeminal cistern, or cisterna magna, hydrocephalus may result. Arachnoid cysts probably arise in utero from the progressive trapping of CSF in a potential space formed from a duplication of arachnoid. The cysts continue to enlarge, eventually expanding the overlying bone and compressing or displacing the adjacent brain parenchyma. MRI offers little advantage over CT in the evaluation of arachnoid cysts. Cysts appear as uncomplicated CSF collections on either CT or MRI, with the CSF of cysts appearing isointense to the ventricles. In

one case, MRI showed a hygroma in a child with acute headache and papilledema related to recent subdural rupture of an arachnoid cyst (Fig. 7–38).

CEREBELLAR DYSGENESIS

Cerebellar atrophy may be an isolated malformation or may accompany other cerebral malformations, such as the Chiari malformations and the Dandy-Walker syndrome.[72] Cerebellar atrophy also is often the result of chronic phenytoin therapy. Olivopontocerebellar

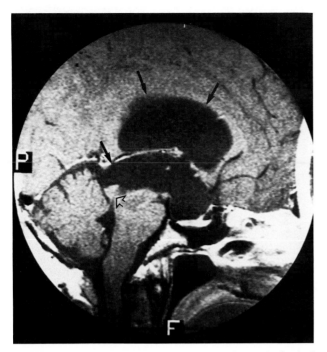

Figure 7–37. *Hydrocephalus due to aqueductal stenosis.* Sagittal T1 weighted image shows severe hydrocephalus involving the third and lateral ventricles (*arrows*) due to aqueductal stenosis (*open arrow*).

degeneration and Friedrich's ataxia are two of the common causes of primary cerebellar atrophy. Some reports suggest that focal atrophy of the inferior posterior vermian lobules is associated with autism.[73] In each of these conditions, MRI provides the best method of evaluating the extent of cerebellar atrophy or dysgenesis. The sagittal image defines the vermian involvement best, and the axial or coronal images provide the best views of the hemispheric atrophy (Fig. 7–39).[72]

PORENCEPHALY

Focal destructive lesions of the fetal brain occur in response to vascular, infectious, or toxic insults (Fig. 7–40). The appearance of focal destructive lesions is strongly related to the age of the fetus when the insult occurred.[6,8] These lesions may present with findings similar to neonatal injury when they occur late in gestation (Fig. 7–41). An early insult is often associated with disorders of migration or sulcation. Intrauterine infection, or TORCH (toxoplasmosis, rubella, CMV, herpes, and now AIDS) is described in the chapter on Infection of the Spine. The increase in HIV infection and drug use in mothers is reflected in the number of

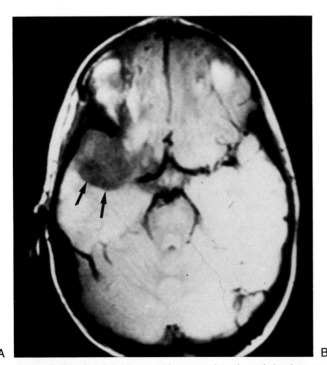

A

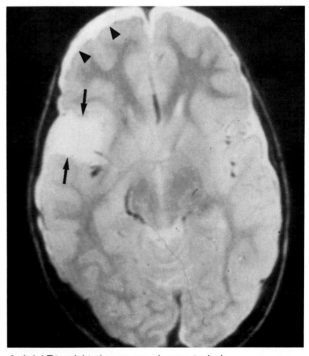

B

Figure 7–38. *Arachnoid cyst with rupture into the subdural space.* **A,** Axial T1 weighted sequence shows a typical middle cranial fossa arachnoid cyst (*arrows*). **B,** Axial T2 weighted sequence at a higher level shows an arachnoid cyst (*arrows*) and associated expansion of the subdural space (*arrowheads*).

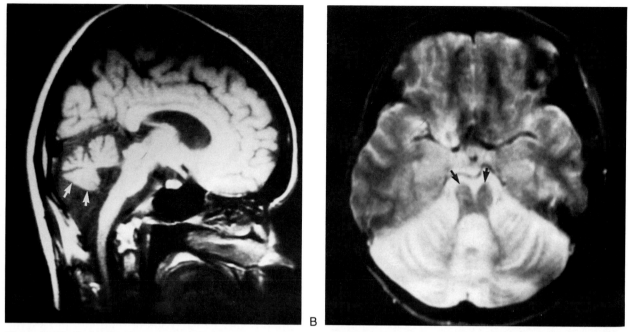

A

B

Figure 7–39. *Cerebellar degeneration.* **A,** Sagittal T1 weighted sequence shows marked atrophy of the cerebellar vermis (*arrows*). **B,** Axial T2 weighted sequence shows associated atrophy of the cerebellar hemisphere and a small brain stem (*arrows*).

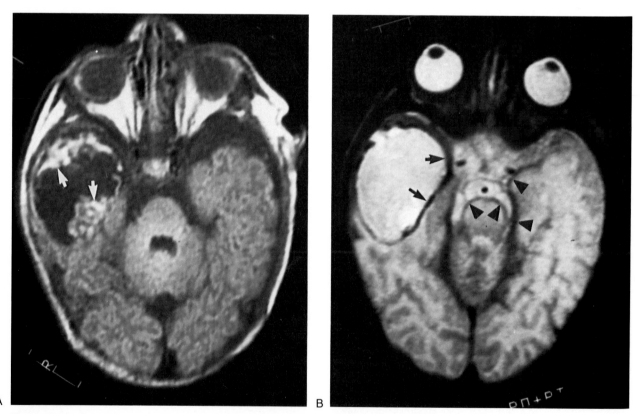

A

B

Figure 7–40. *Congenital porencephalic cyst due to intrauterine parenchymal hemorrhage.* **A,** Axial T1 weighted sequence shows hemorrhagic products within a right temporal porencephalic cyst (*arrows*). **B,** Axial T2 weighted sequence shows hemosiderin lining the porencephalic cyst (*arrows*) and subarachnoid space (*arrowheads*).

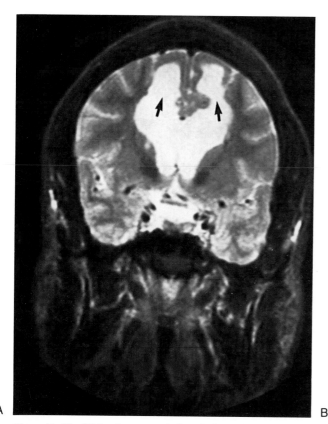
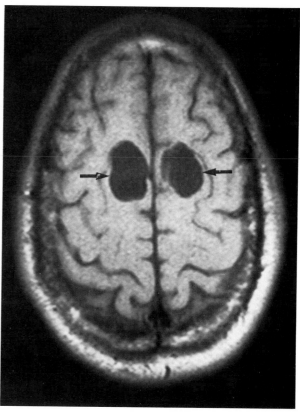

Figure 7–41. *Bilateral porencephaly.* ***A,*** Coronal T2 weighted sequence shows bilateral porencephalic cavities (*arrows*) in communication with the lateral ventricles. ***B,*** Axial T1 weighted sequence shows symmetric CSF-containing cysts (*arrows*).

congenital malformations in this population (Fig. 7–42). MRI may provide additional information to the CT examination if porencephaly accompanies a more extensive malformation or involves posterior fossa structures.

Hydranencephaly, intrauterine bilateral infarcts in the internal carotid distribution, is easily diagnosed with CT and does not require MR examination to define or treat the malformation.

MESIAL SCLEROSIS

MRI is being used with greater frequency to diagnose the source of seizures. Coronal T2 weighted images appear to be most helpful in detecting subtle lesions in the temporal lobe, which are the most common source of focal epilepsy.[74] One of the elusive causes of temporal lobe seizures is mesial sclerosis, or scarring of the medial temporal lobe.[75] It appears pathologically as small areas of focal, usually unilateral, scarring, with atrophy and focal enlargement of the temporal horn of the lateral ventricle. There have been several reports of the use of MRI in the diagnosis of mesial sclerosis (Fig. 7–43).[75] Because the lesion is small and subtle, even on MRI, there has been

some skepticism about the role of MRI in the diagnosis of mesial sclerosis. If the diagnosis can be made, it is clear that thin scans are necessary and that the same levels in the temporal lobe must be compared.

CONCLUSION

The ability of MRI to demonstrate congenital malformations with clarity in all projections is both an opportunity and a challenge. Because gray and white matter differences are more apparent on MRI than on CT, lesions involving migrational disturbances can be diagnosed with greater certainty. Sagittal MR scans demonstrate callosal, brain stem, and foramen magnum lesions with exquisite detail that was not previously available. The contrast sensitivity of MRI makes it possible to diagnose subtle lesions such as mesial sclerosis. However, there are still many unexplored possibilities. The challenge remains to use MRI to further an understanding of the pathogenesis of these malformations. New pulse sequences need to be explored to maximize the diagnostic yield of MRI. With improved anatomic definition on MRI, the radiologist is also challenged to learn and understand more detailed cerebral anatomy and embryology.

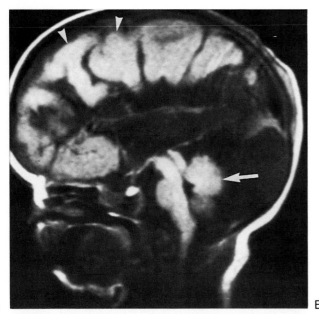

A

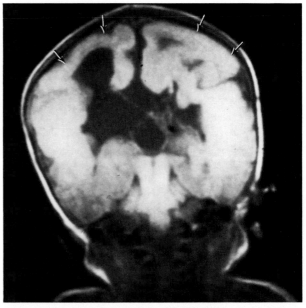

B

Figure 7–42. *Porencephaly with associated migrational and developmental anomalies in an infant born of a mother with a history of cocaine abuse.* **A,** Sagittal T1 weighted sequence shows agenesis of the corpus callosum, an atrophic cerebellum (*arrow*), and large, poorly formed gyri (*arrowheads*). **B,** Coronal images confirm extensive malformations with large, poorly formed gyri (*arrows*).

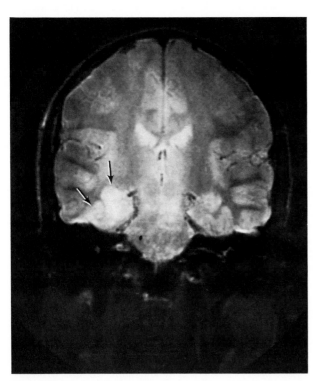

Figure 7–43. *Mesial sclerosis.* Coronal T2 weighted sequence shows abnormal signal in the right hippocampal region (*arrows*) in a patient with refractory seizures.

REFERENCES

1. Record RG, McKeown T. Congenital malformations of the central nervous system. A survey of 230 cases. Br J Soc Med 1949; 4:183–219.
2. Zimmerman RA, Bilaniuk LT, Johnson MH, et al. MRI of central nervous system: early clinical results. AJNR 1986; 7:587–594.
3. Van Der Knaap MS, Valk J. Classification of congenital abnormalities of the CNS. AJNR 1988; 9:315–326.
4. Han JS, Benson JE, Kaufman B, et al. MR imaging of pediatric cerebral abnormalities. J Comput Assist Tomogr 1984; 8: 103–114.
5. Harwood-Nash DC, Fitz CR. Congenital malformations of the brain. In: Neuroradiology in infants and children. Vol 3. St Louis: CV Mosby, 1976:998–1053.
6. DeMyer W. Classification of cerebral malformations. Birth Defects: Original Article Series VII 1971; 1:78–93.
7. Yakovlev PL. Pathoarchitectonic studies of cerebral malformations. III. Arrhinencephalies (holotelencephalies). J Neuropathol Exp Neurol 1959; 18:22.
8. Muller J. Congenital malformations of the brain. In: Rosenberg RN, ed. The clinical neurosciences. Vol 3. Neuropathology. New York: Churchill Livingstone, 1983:1–33.
9. Byrd SE, Naidich TP. Common congenital brain abnormalities. Radiol Clin North Am 1988; 26:755–772.
10. Barkovich AJ, Fram EK, Norman D. Septo-optic dysplasia: MR imaging. Radiology 1989; 171:189–192.
11. Storm RL, DeBenito R. Bilateral optic nerve aplasia associated with hydranencephaly. Ann Ophthalmol 1984; 16:988–992.
12. Manelfe C, Rochiccioli P. CT of septo-optic dysplasia. AJR 1979; 133:1157–1160.
13. Suwanwela C, Suwanwela N. A morphological classification of sincipital encephalomeningoceles. J Neurosurg 1972; 36: 201–211.
14. Barrow N, Sumpson DA. Cranium bifidum. Investigation, prognosis, management. Aust Paediatr J 1966; 2:20–26.
15. Lister J. Nasal glioma. J Laryngosc 1963; 77:34–42.

16. Pensler JM, Bauer BS, Naidich TP. Craniofacial dermoids. Plast Reconstr Surg 1988; 82:953–958.
17. Naidich TP, Osborn RE, Bauer B, Naidich MJ. Median cleft face syndrome: MR and CT data from 11 children. J Comput Assist Tomogr 1988; 12:57–64.
18. Barkovich AJ, Wippold FJ, Sherman JL, Citrin CM. Significance of cerebellar tonsillar position on MR. AJNR 1986; 7: 795–799.
19. DeLaPas RL, Brady TJ, Buonanno FS, et al. Nuclear magnetic resonance (NMR) imaging of Arnold-Chiari type I malformation with hydromyelia. J Comput Assist Tomogr 1983; 7:126–129.
20. Aboulezz AO, Sartor K, Geyer CA, et al. Position of the cerebellar tonsils in patients with Chiari malformation. J Comput Assist Tomogr 1985; 9:1033–1036.
21. Russell DS. Observations on the pathology of hydrocephalus. Med Res Counc Resp No. 265, 1949.
22. Barry A, Patten BM, Stewart BH. Possible factors in the development of the Arnold-Chiari malformation. J Neurosurg 1957; 14:285–301.
23. Gardner SJ, Smith JL, Padget DH. The relationship of Arnold-Chiari and Dandy-Walker malformations. J Neurosurg 1972; 36:481–486.
24. Naidich TP, Pudlowski RM, Naidich JB. Computed tomographic signs of Chiari II malformation. Part II. Midbrain and cerebellum. Radiology 1988; 134:391–398.
25. Wolpert SM, Anderson M, Scott RM, et al. Chiari II malformation: MR imaging evaluation. AJNR 1987; 8:783–792.
26. El Gammal T, Mark EK, Brooks BS. MR imaging of Chiari II malformation. AJNR 1987; 8:1037–1044.
27. Atlas SW, Zimmerman RA, Bilaniuk LT, et al. Corpus callosum and limbic system: neuroanatomic MR evaluation of developmental anomalies. Radiology 1986; 160:355–362.
28. Barkovich AJ, Kjos BO. Normal postnatal development of the corpus callosum as demonstrated by MR imaging. AJNR 1988; 9:487–491.
29. Marburg O. So-called agenesis of the corpus callosum (callosal defect): anterior cerebral dysraphism. Arch Neurol Psychiatry 1949; 61:297.
30. Probst FP. Congenital defects of the corpus callosum: morphology and encephalographic appearances. Acta Radiol (Diagn) 1973; 331(Suppl):1.
31. Curnes JT, Laster DW, Koubeck TD, et al. MRI of corpus callosal syndromes. AJNR 1986; 7:617–622.
32. Davidson HD, Abraham R, Steiner RE. Agenesis of the corpus callosum: magnetic resonance imaging. Radiology 1985; 155:371–373.
33. Barkovich AJ, Norman D. Anomalies of the corpus callosum: correlation with further anomalies of the brain. AJNR 1988; 9:493–501.
34. Atlas SW, Shkolnik A, Naidich P. Sonographic recognition of agenesis of the corpus callosum. AJR 1985; 145:353–361.
35. Byrd SE, Harwood-Nash DC, Fitz CR. Absence of the corpus callosum: computed tomographic evaluation in infants and children. J Canad Assoc Radiol 1978; 29:108–112.
36. Norman RM. Malformations of the nervous system, birth injury and diseases of early life. In: Blackwood W, McMenemey WH, Myer A, et al., eds. Greenfield's neuropathology. 2nd ed. London: Edward Arnold Publishing, 1963.
37. Friedman RB, Segal R, Latchaw RE. Computerized tomographic and magnetic resonance imaging of intracranial lipoma. J Neurosurg 1986; 65:407–410.
38. Sutton D. Radiological diagnosis of lipoma of corpus callosum. Br J Radiol 1949; 22:534.
39. Zingesser L, Schechter M, Gonatas N, et al. Agenesis of the corpus callosum associated with an interhemispheric arachnoid cyst. Br J Radiol 1964; 37:905.
40. Raimondi AJ, Samuelson G, Yarzagaray L, Norton T. Atresia of the foramina of Luschka and Magendie: the Dandy-Walker cyst. J Neurosurg 1969; 31:202.
41. Hart MN, Malamund N, Ellis WG. The Dandy-Walker syndrome: clinicopathological study based on 28 cases. Neurology 1972; 22:771.
42. Dandy WE, Blackfan KD. Internal hydrocephalus: an experimental clinical and pathological study. Am J Dis Child 1914; 8:406.
43. Hanigan WC, Wright R, Wright S. Magnetic resonance of the Dandy-Walker malformation. Pediatr Neurosci 1985–86; 12:151–156.
44. Barkovich AJ, Chuang SH, Norman D. MR of neuronal migration anomalies. AJNR 1987; 8:1009–1017.
45. Byrd SE, Osborn RE, Bohan TP, Naidich TP. The CT and MR evaluation of migrational disorders of the brain. Part I. Lissencephaly and pachygyria. Pediatr Radiol 1989; 19:151–156.
46. Byrd SE, Osborn RE, Bohan TP, Naidich TP. The CT and MR evaluation of migrational disorders of the brain. Part II. Schizencephaly, heterotopia and polymicrogyria. Pediatr Radiol 1989; 19:219–222.
47. Osborn RE, Byrd SE, Naidich TP, et al. MR imaging of neuronal migrational disorders. AJNR 1988; 9:1101–1106.
48. Fitz CR, Harwood-Nash DC, Boldt DW. The radiographic features of unilateral megalencephaly. Neuroradiology 1978; 15:145–148.
49. Kalifa GL, Chiron C, Sellier N, et al. Hemimegalencephaly: MR imaging in five children. Radiology 1987; 165:29–33.
50. Towsend JJ, Nielson SL, Malamud N. Unilateral megalencephaly, hamartoma or neoplasm? Neuroradiology 1975; 25:448–453.
51. Yakovlev PI, Wadsworth BC. Schizencephalies: study of the congenital clefts in the cerebral mantle. Part I. Clefts with fused lips. Part II. Clefts with hydrocephalus and lips separated. J Neuropathol Exp Neurol 1946; 5:116–130.
52. Bird RC, Gilles GH. Type I schizencephaly: CT and neuropathologic findings. AJNR 1987; 8:451–454.
53. Barkovich AJ, Norman D. MR imaging of schizencephaly. AJNR 1988; 9:297–302.
54. Hayden SA, Davis KA, Stears JC, Cole M. MR imaging of heterotopic gray matter. J Comput Assist Tomogr 1987; 11: 878–879.
55. Barkovich AJ, Jackson DE Jr, Boyer RS. Band heterotopias: a newly recognized neuronal migration anomaly. Radiology 1989; 171:455–458.
56. Riccardi VM. Von Recklinghausen neurofibromatosis. N Engl J Med 1981; 305:1617–1628.
57. Diebler C, Dulac O. Neurocutaneous syndromes. In: Pediatric neurology and neuroradiology. Berlin: Springer-Verlag, 1987.
58. Holt JF. Neurofibromatosis in children. AJR 1978; 130: 615–639.
59. Barker D, Wright E, Nguyen K, et al. Gene for von Recklinghausen neurofibromatosis is in the pericentromeric region of chromosome 17. Science 1987; 136:1100–1102.
60. Rouleau GA, Wertelecki W, Haines JL, et al. Genetic linkage of bilateral acoustic neurofibromatosis to a DNA marker on chromosome 22. Nature 1987; 329:246–248.
61. Dunn DW, Roos KL. Neurofibromatosis; an update. Indiana Med 1988; 81:207–215.
62. Zimmerman RA, Bilaniuk LT, Metzger RA, et al. Computed tomography of orbital-facial neurofibromatosis. Radiology 1984; 146:113–116.
63. Crawford AH. Neurofibromatosis in children. Acta Orthop Scand 1986; 57:1–60.
64. Bognanno JR, Edwards MK, Lee TA, et al. Cranial MR imaging in neurofibromatosis. AJNR 1988; 9:461–467.
65. Roach ES, Williams DP, Laster DW. Magnetic resonance imaging in tuberous sclerosis. Arch Neurol 1987; 44:301–303.
66. McMurdo SK Jr, Moore SG, Brant-Zawadzki M, et al. MR imaging of intracranial tuberous sclerosis. AJR 1987; 148: 791–796.
67. Stimac GK, Solomon MA, Newton TA. CT and MR on angiomatous malformations of the choroid plexus in patients with Sturge-Weber disease. AJNR 1986; 7:623–627.
68. Jacoby CG, Yuh WTC, Afifi AK, et al. Accelerated myelination in early Sturge-Weber syndrome demonstrated by MR imaging. J Comput Assist Tomogr 1987; 11:226–231.
69. Britton J, Marsh H, Kendall B, et al. MRI and hydrocephalus in childhood. Neuroradiology 1988; 30:310.

70. Novetsky GJ, Berlin L. Aqueductal stenosis: demonstration by MR imaging. J Comput Assist Tomogr 1984; 8:1170–1171.

71. Atlas SW, Mark AS, Fram EK. Aqueductal stenosis: evaluation with gradient echo rapid MR imaging. Radiology 1988; 169:449.

72. Yuh WTC, Segal HD, Senac MO, et al. MR imaging of Chiari II malformation associated with dysgenesis of cerebellum and brain stem. J Comput Assist Tomogr 1987; 11:188–191.

73. Courcheane E, Hesselink JR, Jernigan TL, et al. Abnormal neuroanatomy in a nonretarded person with autism: unusual findings with magnetic resonance imaging. Arch Neurol 1987; 44:335–341.

74. Triulzi F, Franceschi M, Fazio F, et al. Nonrefractory temporal lobe epilepsy: 1.5T MR imaging. Radiology 1988; 166:181–185.

75. Maertens PM, Machen BC, Williams JP, et al. Magnetic resonance imaging of mesial temporal sclerosis: case reports. CT 1987; 11:136.

Trauma and Mechanical Disorders of the Brain

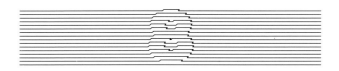

JAMES R. BOGNANNO, M.D.

Head trauma is a major cause of childhood morbidity, with at least one in ten individuals sustaining significant head injury during childhood. Most of these head injuries are mild; only about 10 percent are defined as serious.[1] These serious injuries carry high morbidity and mortality rates.[2] Reports in the literature suggest that up to one-half of children who survive a moderate or severe head injury have some degree of learning impairment after returning to school.[3] Even children who retain normal learning abilities may show persistent neuropsychological dysfunction.[4,5] Head injuries therefore are important, because the long-term sequelae may affect a child's learning and language functions and lead to future academic, psychological, or behavioral disturbances.[6]

Computed tomography (CT) has played a crucial role in the evaluation of the child with acute head injury.[7,8] Its greatest impact has been in the detection of surgically treatable intracranial hematomas. Despite this important contribution, CT has been found relatively insensitive compared with neuropathologic studies, for the detection and characterization of other types of brain injury.[9–11] Some recent reports indicate that cranial MRI is superior to CT for the detection and characterization of certain types of traumatic brain injury.[12–15] The implication of these reported findings is that MRI in conjunction with other clinical factors allows a more accurate prediction of the eventual neurologic recovery after craniocerebral injury.

INITIAL EVALUATION OF THE HEAD INJURED PATIENT

MR imaging in the acute traumatic setting is hindered by problems of possible malfunction of life support and monitoring equipment within strong magnetic fields, significantly longer scan times of MRI compared with CT, and the marked sensitivity of MRI to patient motion, with subsequent image degradation. In addition, because of site considerations, MR units are frequently distant from emergency care areas and radiology departments. Another potential drawback of MRI is that acute hemorrhagic conditions, with oxyhemoglobin still present, may be isointense to brain tissue on spin-echo images,[16] and acute hematomas containing deoxyhemoglobin may not be visible at low and intermediate magnetic field strengths with spin-echo techniques.[16–18] Acute subarachnoid blood is also difficult to identify with MRI.[19] CT, on the other hand, has the advantages of sensitivity for detecting acute intracranial hemorrhagic mass lesions, relatively rapid scan times, and ready availability.

In summary, although MRI has many advantages in craniocerebral imaging, the ready availability and quickness of CT and its adequate sensitivity for the detection of surgically treatable hemorrhagic mass lesions leave CT the imaging tool of choice in the initial neuroradiologic evaluation of the patient with acute head trauma.

MECHANISMS OF HEAD INJURY

Pediatric head injuries can be classified into several age-related groups. Neonates most commonly sustain injury from the normal forces of labor or from obstetric instrumentation. In noninstrumented deliveries, slow, steady pressure of the baby's head against the maternal pelvic side wall can occasionally cause "ping pong ball" fractures of the skull, subarachnoid or subdural hematomas, and soft tissue scalp injury. Misapplication of obstetric forceps may result in soft tissue lacerations, depressed or linear skull fractures, and/or extracerebral or parenchymal hemorrhages. Rarely, stretch injury of the spinal cord and the cervicomedullary junction may be seen after a traumatic delivery.

In infants and toddlers, short falls occasionally cause uncomplicated skull fractures that usually have few serious consequences. Various reports indicate that up to 95 percent of serious head injuries in this age group are the result of child abuse.[20, 21] Shaking or whiplash injury appears to be the most common mechanism resulting in the characteristic interhemispheric subdural hematomas.[22, 23] A skull fracture with an epidural hematoma or underlying brain contusion is usually the result of a direct blow to the head or a fall down stairs.

From 2 years of age through the first decade, most severe head injuries are due to motor vehicle accidents. These take two forms: a child pedestrian may be directly hit by a car, or an unrestrained child in a car may suffer cervicocranial trauma due to rapid acceleration and deceleration forces.

After the first decade, direct impact trauma accounts for most head injuries. These frequently result from sports injuries or accidents on bicycles or motorbikes that cause focal cerebral injury.

MAGNETIC RESONANCE APPEARANCE OF HEMORRHAGE

A brief review of the MR appearance of hemorrhage is appropriate, since most severe cranial injuries involve some degree of hemorrhage. The appearance of blood on the MR image is dependent on the oxidation state of the hemoglobin and its environment. Both of these vary with time in a relatively predictable fashion, creating characteristic changes in the signal of the blood collection. These factors allow a rough approximation of the age of the hemorrhage. The appearance of hemorrhage is also dependent on the magnetic field strength, with preferential T2 proton relaxation enhancement more pronounced at higher field strengths. Table 8–1 provides a summary of the molecular forms and oxidation states of hemoglobin and its breakdown products and their respective MR signal characteristics observed on spin-echo imaging.

The oxidation state of hemoglobin directly influences the relaxation rates of surrounding protons. The tertiary molecular structure of the heme-protein moiety affects the accessibility of these surrounding protons to the iron center, thus modifying the relaxation enhancement potential of this paramagnetic substance. The paramagnetism of the various forms of oxidized hemoglobin with its available unpaired electrons is the major influencing factor on the MR appearance of hemorrhage. Circulating oxyhemoglobin has been shown to be diamagnetic, one of the heme irons' four unpaired electrons being shared with the oxygen molecule, resulting in a low-spin ferrous (Fe^{2+}) form with a single unpaired electron in the outer shell.[24, 25] In the absence of oxygen the heme iron retains its four unpaired electrons and exists in the paramagnetic or high-spin state of deoxyhemoglobin.[25] While static susceptibility experiments have shown deoxyhemoglobin to be paramagnetic,[24] aqueous solutions of this compound do not enhance proton relaxation and therefore show little or no effect on T1 or T2 relaxation times of the solution. This occurs primarily because of stearic hindrance to the access of water molecules to the paramagnetic heme iron, and also because deoxyhemoglobin has an inefficient exchange of energy between unpaired electrons and surrounding water protons.[26] Since the interaction of the dipole of the electron and that of the local hydrogen nucleus falls off as the sixth power of the distance between them, the hydrogen nuclei must be able to approach within several angstroms of the paramagnetic center for relaxation enhancement to occur.[27] The effective distance for the interaction to occur is approximately 3 angstroms.[28] This close approach is prevented by the tertiary configuration of the protein moiety of deoxyhemoglobin, thereby limiting any paramagnetic effects on surrounding water protons.

Table 8–1. SUMMARY OF PHYSICAL AND MR IMAGING CHARACTERISTICS OF HEMOGLOBIN AND ITS BREAKDOWN PRODUCTS

	Oxyhemoglobin	Intracellular Deoxyhemoglobin	Extracellular Deoxyhemoglobin	Intracellular Methemoglobin	Extracellular Methemoglobin	Intralysosomal Hemosiderin
Oxidation state of iron	Fe^{2+}	Fe^{2+}	Fe^{2+}	Fe^{3+}	Fe^{3+}	Fe^{3+}
No. of unpaired electrons	0	4	4	5	5	5
Paramagnetic	No	Yes	Yes	Yes	Yes	Yes
Proton relaxation enhancement mechanism T1 WI/T2 WI	None/None	None/PT2	None/None	PEDD/PT2	PEDD/None	None/PT2
Signal intensity on T1 weighted images	No change	Slightly ↓ or no change	No change	↑	↑ ↑	Slightly ↓ or no change
Signal intensity on T2 weighted images	No change	↓ ↓	No change	↓ ↓	No change or ↑	↓ ↓

PT2 = preferential T2; PEDD = Proton electron dipole-dipole.

Within intact red blood cells the paramagnetic effects of deoxyhemoglobin induce a strong magnetic field gradient across the red cell membrane. Free diffusion of water molecules across the membrane allows the molecules to experience local magnetic nonuniformity between the intra- and extracellular space, promoting irreversible spin-spin dephasing. This effect is increased as the square of the applied magnetic field and as the square of local gradient induced by the paramagnetic deoxyhemoglobin.[29, 30] This accounts for the more pronounced T2 shortening effect seen with higher magnetic field strength magnets. The effect of intracellular deoxyhemoglobin is therefore a preferential T2 shortening, which accounts for the lack of signal from hemorrhage seen on long TR, long TE images, with more pronounced effect seen with increased echo times. Relatively little effect is seen on short TR, short TE images and long TR, short TE images, with blood relatively iso- to slightly hypointense to brain with these pulse sequences.

Once hemoglobin is removed from the circulation, a lack of oxygen results in failure of aerobic metabolism. Eventually a lack of glucose results in anaerobic metabolism failure. Absence of these energy-producing metabolic pathways results in subsequent failure of the methemoglobin reductase systems required to keep the heme iron in its reduced ferrous (Fe^{2+}) form.[31] The result is oxidative conversion to ferric (Fe^{3+}) methemoglobin. In methemoglobin the sixth coordination site, which held the molecular oxygen in oxyhemoglobin, is occupied by a water or hydroxyl molecule ligand, depending on the pH. Access of the water molecule to the heme iron occurs because of an alteration of the tertiary structure of the globin chain. Exchange of water molecules between the aqueous solvent and the water ligand promotes proton relaxation enhancement, known as inner sphere effects.[32] Increased accessibility of the solvent protons to the heme iron allows a shorter distance of closest approach by nearby water protons, and enables proton relaxation enhancement of these solvent water protons to occur. Methemoglobin has a more efficient exchange of energy than deoxyhemoglobin and therefore a shorter relaxation time. These last two effects are known as outer sphere effects.[33] The result of the inner and outer sphere of influence effects is significant T1 shortening in aqueous solution.[33]

These combined effects have been termed proton electron dipole-dipole proton relaxation enhancement (PEDD PRE).[16] The appearance on short TR, short TE images is therefore that of high signal from the aqueous methemoglobin. On long TR images, aqueous methemoglobin has high signal due to its long T2 relaxation rate from the aqueous and protein components. There is some T2 shortening effect from the PEDD PRE interactions, although this is small compared with the effect on the T1 relaxation rate.[34] This results in minimal, if any, discernible changes on long TR, long TE images. Within intact red blood cells the effect of methemoglobin on short TR, short TE sequences is similar to that of aqueous solutions owing to the PEDD PRE effects. The effect seen on long TR, long TE images is similar to, or more pronounced than, that seen with deoxyhemoglobin, i.e., marked hypointensity due to heterogeneity of the magnetic field induced by the methemoglobin contained within the intact red cell membranes causing T2 shortening by PTZ PRE effects.[30]

Further oxidative degradation of hemoglobin results in the formation of hemichromes, globin compounds with the iron in the ferric state (Fe^{3+}) and the sixth coordination site occupied by a ligand from the globin molecule itself.[25] Physiologic response mechanisms to intraparenchymal hematomas include phagocytosis of free hemoglobin products by macrophages. Within the lysosomes of these macrophages, the hemoglobin products are converted to the insoluble macromolecule, hemosiderin. These hemosiderin-laden macrophages are not removed from the site of the hemorrhage and persist there indefinitely. The electrons of hemosiderin are shielded from contact with water hydrogens and thus have no significant T1 shortening effects, although they do induce inhomogeneity of the local magnetic field gradient, and therefore cause T2 shortening.[30] The effect on imaging is therefore to produce marked signal loss in the area of deposition of these hemosiderin-laden macrophages on long TR, long TE pulse sequences. No significant effects are generally seen on short TR, short TE images.

SKULL FRACTURES

Patients sustaining craniocerebral trauma severe enough to cause a skull fracture are usually studied initially with head CT and plain films of the skull. The MR evaluation of a skull fracture is not usually of primary importance in the initial evaluation and treatment of such patients. CT has been found to be more sensitive for the detection of skull fractures than MRI, and even when a fracture is detected by MRI, its extent is usually underestimated.[35] Work by Zimmerman and colleagues[36] on the subject of skull fracture has elaborated several unique characteristics of skull fractures on MRI as well as some shortcomings of MRI compared with CT. Fractures can be missed on MR images. Since cortical bone lacks mobile protons, it causes no signal on MRI. If there is no fluid or blood traversing a fracture crevice, the fracture will not be evident, since no interruption of the bone's normal hypointense signal will be seen. Also, since air has few mobile protons, a fracture traversing an adjacent air cell may be missed. Another pitfall is that air may provide a false-positive appearance of a fracture fragment by simulating a free fragment of bone within soft tissues or blood, particularly in the temporal bone region.

When fractures are identified with MRI they usually possess one or more of the following features: (1) absence or disruption of the normal black line of cortical bone; (2) displacement of the black line of cortical bone into adjacent tissue, with or without outlining of this by clot or fluid; (3) blood or fluid traversing the black line of cortical bone in a nondisplaced fracture; and (4) herniation or displacement of orbital fat into an adjacent paranasal sinus through a fracture of the bony orbit.[37] These findings should be sought in areas adjacent to associated injuries such as cortical contusion, parenchymal hemorrhage, and epidural and/or subcutaneous hematoma (Fig. 8–1). Zimmerman and colleagues found that six of eight temporal bone fractures with the above characteristics were identifiable by MRI.[36]

EXTRACEREBRAL FLUID COLLECTIONS

MRI can provide exquisite detail in delineating extracerebral fluid collections, owing in part to its multiplanar imaging ability. It also provides excellent representation of blood products and other fluids, differentiating abnormal fluid collections from adjacent normal structures. Bony streak artifacts and partial volume problems encountered with CT do not occur on MR images.

Subarachnoid Hemorrhage

CT is more sensitive than MRI in detecting acute subarachnoid hemorrhage.[17, 19] Several factors contribute to the relative lack of sensitivity of MRI to subarachnoid blood: (1) oxyhemoglobin may take longer to desaturate in the cerebrospinal fluid (CSF), because of its relatively high oxygen content, and the conversion of hemoglobin to methemoglobin is probably required to cause signal alteration in the CSF on T1 weighted images;[26, 38] (2) the long T2 relaxation times of CSF may somewhat counterbalance the paramagnetic effects of intracellular deoxyhemoglobin; (3) red cell lysis may occur, and extracellular deoxyhemoglobin causes no paramagnetic effect; and (4) pulsatile flow of CSF may also contribute to signal loss on spin-echo images.[39] In the subacute setting, 1 week or more after injury, the sensitivity of MRI may be greater than that of CT because the blood products will have been almost completely converted to methemoglobin with its full effect of T1 shortening, and because the sensitivity of CT to subarachnoid blood decreases with time.[40, 41]

Subarachnoid bleeding after trauma is usually the result of cerebral contusion with injury to the leptomeninges and surface blood vessels. For this reason, subarachnoid hemorrhage is usually found adjacent to cerebral contusions and in the interhemispheric fissure.[42] The spread of trauma-induced subarachnoid blood throughout the CSF cisterns is uncommon unless there has been intraventricular bleeding and diffusion of blood through the outlets of the fourth ventricle.[43] On long-term follow-up, focal areas of superficial hemosiderosis, appearing as linear areas of low signal intensity, may occasionally be identified in the area of a previous subarachnoid hemorrhage (Fig. 8–2).[44]

Subdural Fluid Collections

Childhood subdural hematomas have a peak incidence during the first 6 months of life, and of these, approximately 80 percent are bilateral.[45] Subdural hematomas may be classified as acute or chronic. Pathologically there is disruption of the cortical veins as they bridge the subdural space before draining into the dural sinuses. The high incidence of subdural hemorrhage in infancy is thought to be due to the relatively large subarachnoid space at this age, allowing increased mobility of the brain within the cranium. Most subdural bleeds are probably due to a shaking injury from child abuse. The MR appearance of subdural hematoma is that of the characteristic crescentic extracerebral fluid collection, which does not extend into the sulci. Signal characteristics vary, depending on the stage of evolution of the blood products.

Acute Subdural Hematoma

Children with acute subdural hematomas present with seizures, elevated intracranial pressure, disturbances of consciousness, and only occasionally focal neurologic deficits. In neonates or infants, hypovolemic shock may be a presenting finding. When identified by CT scanning, approximately two-thirds of acute subdural hematomas are located along the inner table of the calvarium, and one-third in the interhemispheric fissure.[46] Associated underlying parenchymal injury is common and may account for mass effect out of proportion to the size of the hematoma. Posterior fossa subdural hematomas are relatively uncommon, and are found primarily in newborns after difficult or breech delivery.[47] As subdural hematomas progress from the acute to the chronic stage, they tend to enlarge. The increasing size is due to oozing from the surrounding highly vascular membranes that develop with time, and possibly to the osmotic effects of the protein-rich fluid within the hematoma.

On MR images obtained at high magnetic field strength (1.5T), acute subdural hematomas (when deoxyhemoglobin is the predominant form of hemoglobin) show signal hypointensity to brain on long TR, long TE images and isointensity to brain on short TR, short TE images. This may lead to poor visualization of thin subdural hematomas, which may be difficult to differentiate from the normal hypointensity of the adjacent inner table of the skull and intermediate signal of adjacent brain on spin-echo imaging.[12] Evolution of blood products results in formation of methemoglobin within approximately 1 week (Fig. 8–3). The paramagnetic effect of the methemoglobin shortens T1 relaxation, which results in a high signal from the hematoma on short TR, short TE images. This markedly increases the conspicuity of even very small subdural

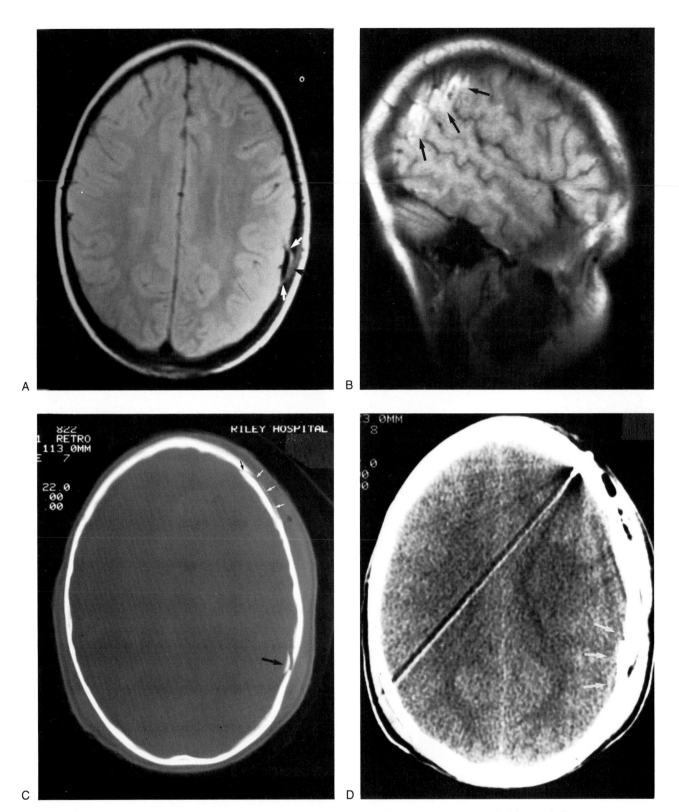

Figure 8–1. *Skull fracture following blunt head trauma.* ***A,*** Proton density MR image reveals a small skull fracture in the left parietal bone with hyperintense fluid between the small fragment and calvarium (*arrows*). ***B,*** T1 weighted MR image reveals subjacent hemorrhagic cortical contusion with hyperintense signal from methemoglobin (*arrows*). ***C,*** Bone window from CT scan approximately 1 week before MRI shows the small left parietal skull fracture identified on the latter (*large arrow*). A second anterior left frontal skull fracture (*small arrows*) was not identified on the MRI. ***D,*** Brain window from the same CT scan exemplifies the relative lack of CT sensitivity to identification of small amounts of cortical hemorrhagic contusion (*arrows*). An intracranial pressure monitor is present in the left frontal lobe.

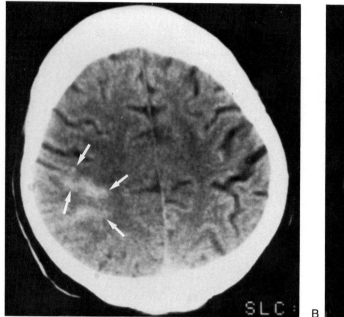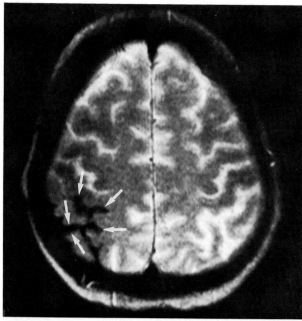

Figure 8–2. *Superficial siderosis after post-traumatic subarachnoid bleeding.* ***A,*** CT scan after closed head injury reveals subarachnoid hemorrhage within the sulci of the right parietal lobe (*arrows*). ***B,*** Long TR, long TE MR image 2 months after the CT scan seen in ***A.*** Marked signal hypointensity is present in the same region as the subarachnoid hemorrhage seen on the CT scan (*arrows*). This is secondary to staining of the brain surface by hemosiderin.

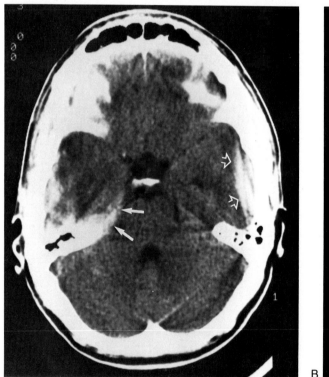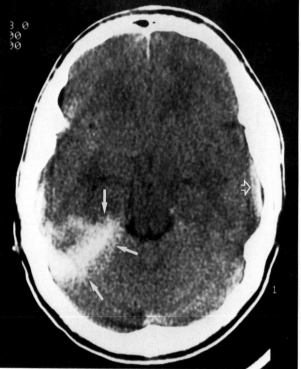

Figure 8–3. *A 15-year-old hemophiliac boy after a fall from a bicycle. Subdural and epidural hematomas.* ***A, B,*** CT scan upon admission reveals subdural hematoma layering along the tentorium on the right (*arrows*). There is a probable left middle cranial fossa epidural hematoma on the left (*open arrows*). Streak artifact frequently degrades CT image quality in the middle cranial fossa and in the base of the anterior cranial fossa. ***C, D,*** Short TR, short TE axial MR images reveal the relatively thin right-sided subdural hematoma (*arrows*), which is much more extensive than that anticipated by the CT scan. There is a lentiform epidural hematoma in the left middle cranial fossa (*open arrows*). Mass effect from the right-sided subdural hematoma is manifested by effacement of the right lateral ventricle. ***E, F,*** Coronal long TR, long TE images reveal the subdural hematoma layering along the tentorium and right temporal area (*short arrows*). The left middle cranial fossa epidural hematoma with its biconvex configuration is well defined (*open arrows*). Hyperintense signal on both the short TR and long TR images of the subdural hematomas is consistent with extracellular methemoglobin. Hyperintense and isointense signal on the short TR image and hyperintense and hypointense signal on the long TR image from the epidural hematoma are consistent with the presence of both extra- and intracellular methemoglobin, as well as intracellular deoxyhemoglobin.

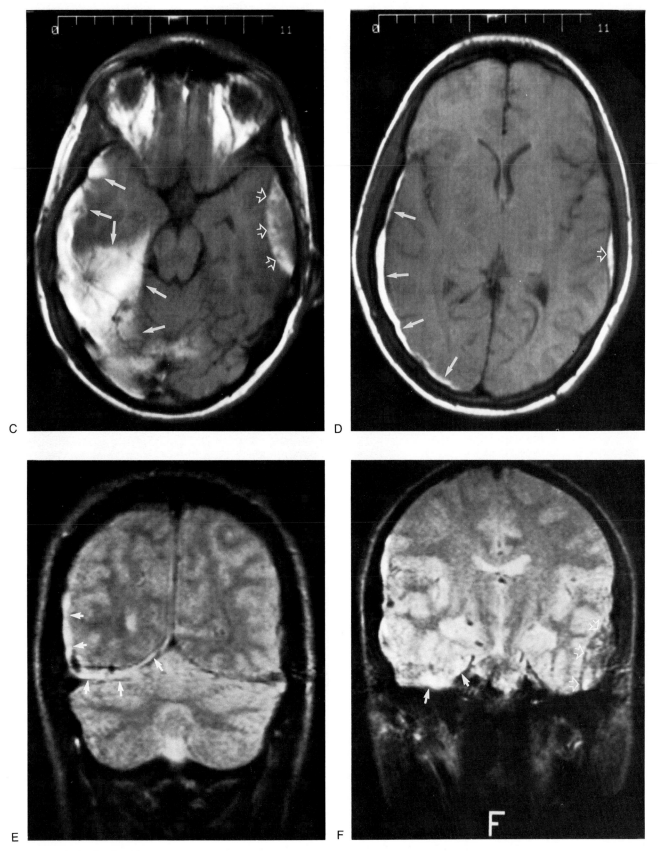

Figure 8–3. *Continued.*

collections. The persistence of methemoglobin for weeks to months allows ready identification of the hematomas on MRI. During this time, subdural hematomas are frequently isodense on CT.[48]

Chronic Subdural Fluid Collections

Chronic subdural fluid collections may contain CSF, proteinaceous fluid, chronic blood products, or mixed subacute and chronic blood products. In our experience, most chronic subdural fluid collections contain fluid with high signal on long TR, long TE images and slightly increased signal intensity from that of normal CSF on short TR, short TE images. Small amounts of methemoglobin layering in the collection are occasionally seen, and presumably arise from small amounts of repeat hemorrhage from the friable vascular membranes that develop around chronic subdural fluid collections. The MR appearance is therefore somewhat variable, ranging from signal characteristics similar to that of CSF to high signal intensity on all spin-echo sequences, such as that seen in subacute hemorrhage with dilute methemoglobin.[31]

Chronic subdural fluid collections in the pediatric population can be divided into three categories: (1) infantile chronic subdural hematomas, (2) childhood chronic subdural hematomas, and (3) subdural hygromas. Infantile chronic subdural hematomas are characteristically discovered on physical examination of infants between the ages of 2 and 6 months. Enlargement of the head with a bulging fontanelle and retinal hemorrhages are common physical findings. The etiology of this entity is child abuse in most cases, usually secondary to shaking injury (Fig. 8–4). The location is characteristically posterior in the interhemispheric fissure.

Childhood chronic subdural hematomas are relatively rare.[49] When they do occur, there is usually a history of previous injury. Symptoms and signs such as headache, diminished mental status, and papilledema are usually present and are similar to those found in

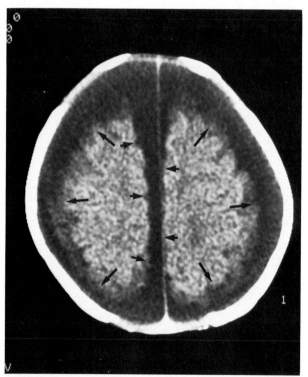 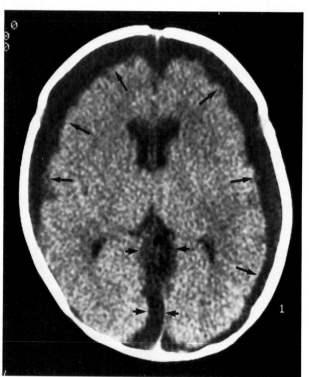

A   B

Figure 8–4. *Child abuse in an infant: the shaken baby syndrome.* **A, B,** CT scans of this 14-month-old chronically abused child reveal characteristic low-density chronic subdural fluid collections at the convexities bilaterally (*arrows*) and in the interhemispheric fissure (*short arrows*). **C,** Short TR, short TE coronal image during the same hospitalization shows high signal from subdural fluid collections consistent with protein and/or small amounts of dilute methemoglobin. Some layering along the outer arachnoid membrane of higher signal fibrinous material is present (*small arrows*). A septation through the right-sided subdural fluid collection is present (*arrowheads*). **D, E,** Long TR, long TE axial and parasagittal images reveal high signal from the subdural fluid collections (*arrows*), greater than that seen from the cerebrospinal fluid (*arrowheads*). The septation within the subdural fluid is nicely visualized on the parasagittal image. **F,** Short TR, short TE image obtained 3 months after the MR study shown in **C, D,** and **E.** There is persistent high signal from the chronic subdural fluid collections, suggesting continued bleeding (*arrows*). A subdural drain has been placed (*small arrows*).

Figure continues on following page.

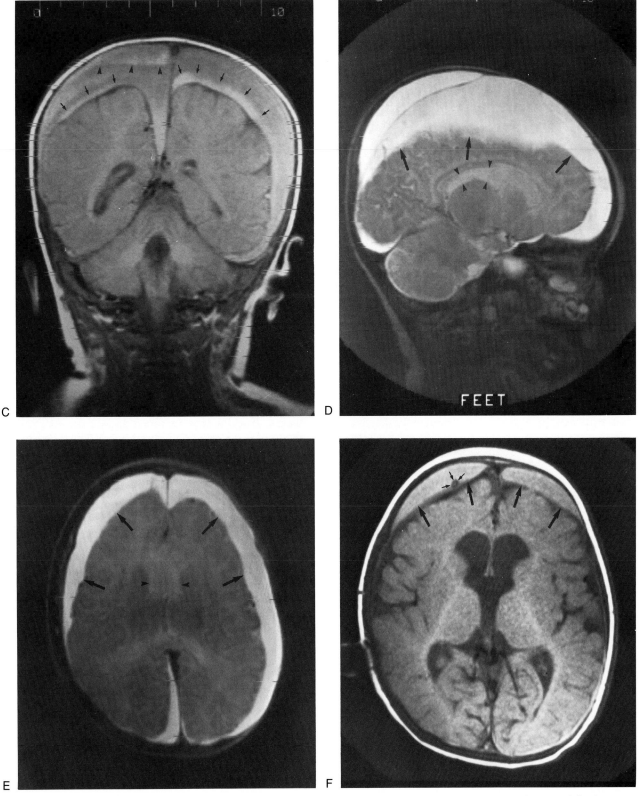

Figure continues on following page.

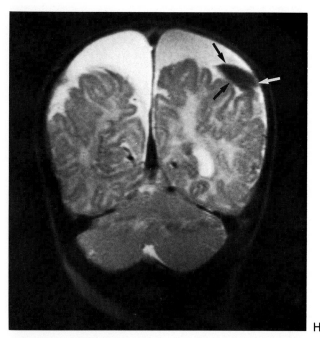

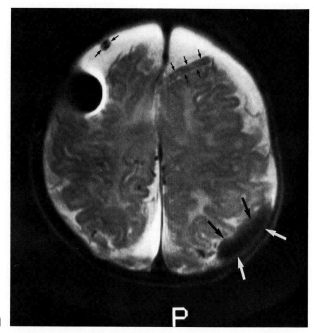

Figure 8–4. *Continued.*
G, H, Long TR, long TE coronal and axial images reveal a small amount of deoxyhemoglobin present within a locule in the left subdural hematoma (*arrows*). Subdural drains are present bilaterally (*small arrows*). Metal artifact is from the shunt reservoir.

adult chronic subdural hematomas. As in adults, children with atrophy or enlarged subarachnoid spaces are more prone to chronic subdural hematomas because of excessive mobility of the cerebrum within the cranial vault.

Subdural hygroma, a subdural collection of CSF, probably results from trauma causing a small tear in the arachnoid, and subsequent leakage and dissection of CSF into the subdural space. This may cause headaches and occasionally papilledema. The fluid within the collection has the low protein content of CSF, as opposed to the high protein content of chronic subdural hematomas (Fig. 8–5). The signal characteristics of subdural hygromas on MRI should exactly parallel those of other CSF spaces, whereas the signal from chronic subdural hematomas usually reflects the presence of blood products, with subtle T1 shortening relative to CSF (brighter signal on short TR, short TE images).

Epidural Hematomas

Epidural hematomas, relatively rare in infants and children, are nevertheless a serious and treatable complication of craniocerebral trauma. Acute epidural hematomas are usually first detected by CT scanning and managed by surgical evacuation. The source of bleeding is frequently venous in children, unlike adults, in whom a laceration of a branch of the middle meningeal artery is the most common cause. Venous bleeding probably occurs as a result of a stripping action exerted

on the dura by sudden inward bending of the relatively plastic calvarium from a direct blow.[43] In 30 to 40 percent of children with epidural hematomas, no skull fracture can be detected.[50] The clinical presentation in infants may be acute owing to hypovolemic shock, or delayed because patent sutures expand to accommodate the hematoma, thus preventing a rise in intracranial pressure.

The evolution of blood products in epidural hematomas is similar to that of subdural hematomas. The characteristic appearance is that of a biconvex mass separate from the brain. In the deoxyhemoglobin stage, clot retraction may produce extrusion of serum around the periphery of the clot. On T2 weighted sequences, this serum appears bright, contrasting with the dark line of the elevated dura, separating clot from bright CSF in the subarachnoid space (Fig. 8–6). With progression to the methemoglobin stage, high signal intensity will be seen throughout the epidural hematoma on both T1 and T2 weighted spin-echo images. Precise localization of epidural hematomas in multiple planes, definition of their relationship to the dural sinuses, and absence of significant partial voluming or beam-hardening artifacts make MRI a superb modality for imaging in the subacute period.

PARENCHYMAL INJURY

The pathophysiologic processes that occur within the brain parenchyma at the time of injury are complex.[51] The goal of imaging is to characterize these

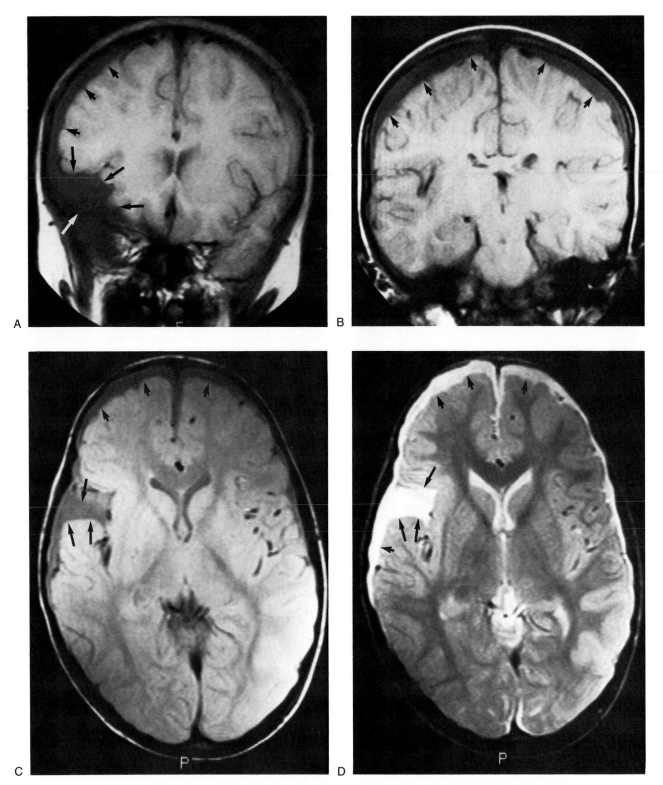

Figure 8–5. *Subdural hygroma. A 12-year-old boy who presented with headache and papilledema 1 month after minor head trauma from a bicycle accident.   **A, B,** Short TR, short TE images in coronal projection show a right-sided middle cranial fossa arachnoid cyst (large arrows) Bilateral subdural hygromas are present over the convexities (short arrows).* Signal characteristics of these fluid collections parallel the T1 relaxation characteristics of cerebrospinal fluid (CSF). **C, D,** Multiecho axial sequence with long TR and short and long echo times. Signal characteristics of the arachnoid cyst (*arrows*) in the middle cranial fossa on the right as well as the subdural hygromas (*short arrows*) parallel that of the CSF.

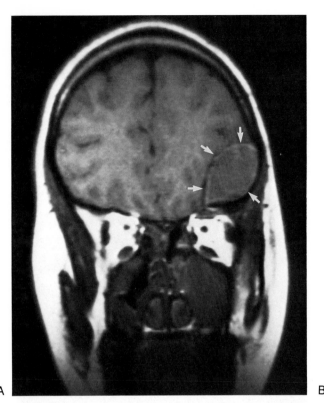
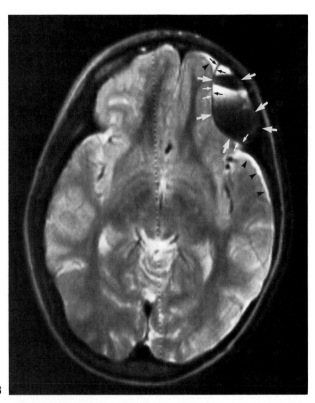

A   B

Figure 8–6. *Epidural hematoma. A 6-year-old girl after closed head injury from an automobile accident.* ***A,*** Short TR, short TE coronal image reveals a biconvex epidural hematoma in the left anterior cranial fossa (*arrows*). Signal characteristics are relatively isointense to brain. A small amount of high signal from within the fluid collection suggests some oxidative conversion to methemoglobin. ***B,*** Axial long TR, long TE image showing hypointense signal from deoxyhemoglobin within the epidural hematoma (*arrows*). Some extrusion of serum and the presence of methemoglobin are seen as layers of high signal within the hematoma. The dark line of dura (*small arrows*) contrasts with the high signal fluid within the epidural hematoma and a small adjacent subdural hematoma (*arrowheads*).

processes, assess their severity, determine whether they are progressive, and evaluate any permanent sequelae. Various specific types of cerebral injury have been identified by CT scanning and correlated with pathogenetic mechanisms.[8, 52, 53] Several reports have indicated the usefulness of MRI in the evaluation of these patients.[12, 14, 54] This section offers a brief review of the MR characteristics and pathogenetic mechanisms of the various types of parenchymal brain injury. These are discussed separately but it is important to remember that they are rarely identified as isolated findings, and that multiple foci of injury are usually found as well as multiple types of injury in the same patient.

Contusion

Contusions are superficial sites of brain injury where mechanically induced tissue and cellular disruption occur. These are frequently associated with some degree of bleeding, ranging from cortical petechiae (Fig. 8–7) to gross hemorrhage (Fig. 8–8). The degree of the injury may vary, depending on the force, from superficial bruising to cortical necrosis extending into the underlying white matter. Hemorrhagic contusions are the most common hemorrhagic parenchymal lesion seen on CT scanning[8] and are twice as common in children as in adults.[43] These typically result from impact injury: either direct contact of the inner table of the skull with the brain surface, or contact of the brain surface with the skull during rapid rotational acceleration-deceleration movements.[55] The most common sites of contusion are the base of the frontal lobes and temporal lobes, resulting from contact with the adjacent rough edges of the inner table of the skull along the floor of the anterior cranial fossa, sphenoid wings, and petrous ridges.[56, 57] Contusion also frequently accompanies skull fractures, depressed or nondepressed. The degree of contusion is typically greatest at the apices of the involved gyri, with relative sparing of cortex within adjacent sulci. MRI is more sensitive than CT in detecting hemorrhage in cortical contusions. The latter are hemorrhagic on MR examination in approximately 50 to 60 percent of cases, as opposed to CT, in which hemorrhage is found in only approximately 20 to 25 percent of contusions.[13, 57, 58] The lack of sensitivity of CT in the anterior and middle cranial fossae is due to streak artifacts and volume averaging with adjacent bone.

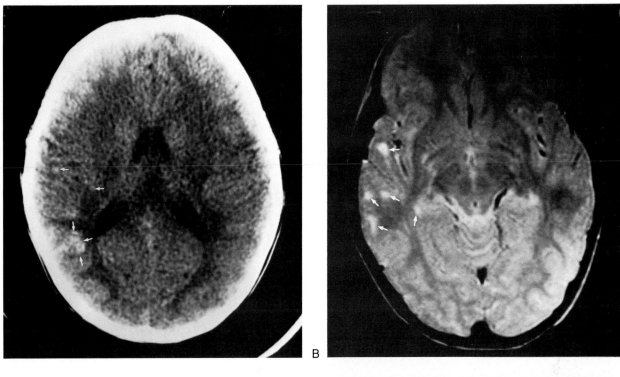

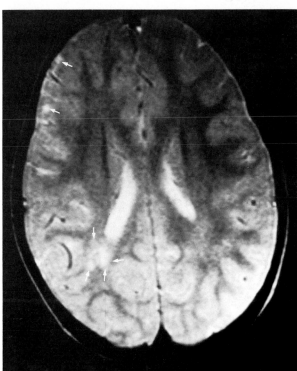

Figure 8–7. *Petechial hemorrhages following closed head injury.* ***A,*** CT scan reveals numerous focal high-density lesions in the right hemisphere (*arrows*). ***B, C,*** Long TR, long TE images reveal many more focal hemorrhages than those seen on CT. These are identified as high signal foci (*arrows*) scattered about the right cerebral hemisphere.

Acute contusion appears on MRI as high signal from edema in the cerebral cortex and subjacent white matter on long TR, long TE images. Slight hypointensity on the short TR, short TE images may be present. If there are hemorrhagic components, deoxyhemoglobin will cause marked hypointensity on the long TR, long TE images; this is usually surrounded by a zone of hyperintense signal from the vasogenic edema.[35] The hemorrhagic areas are iso- to hypointense on short TR, short TE images until conversion of the deoxyhemoglobin to intracellular methemoglobin occurs (usually after 3 to 6 days), when high signal will be encoun-

Text continues on page 143.

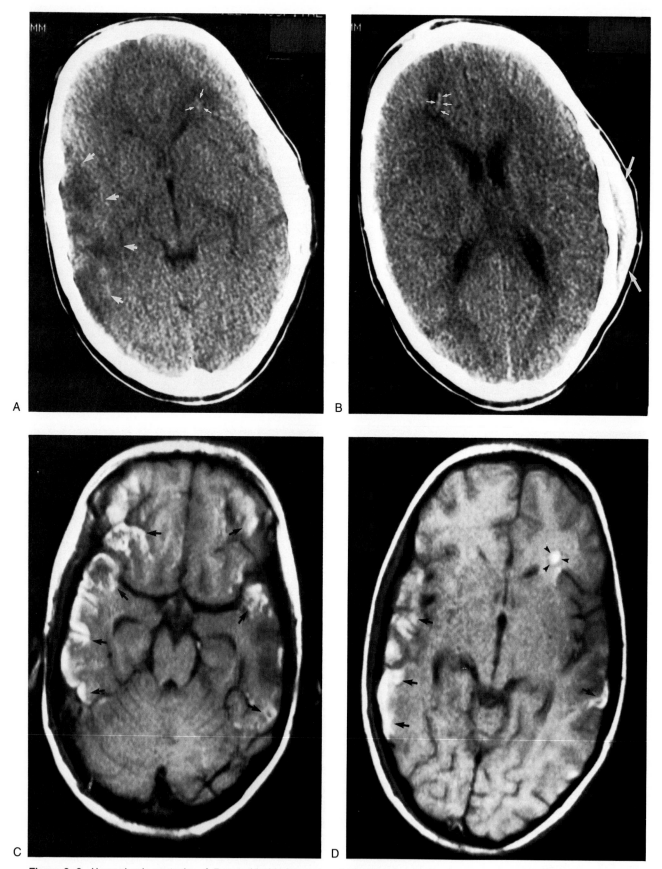

Figure 8–8. *Hemorrhagic contusion. A 7-year-old girl after a closed left-sided head injury from an automobile acci-dent.* **A, B,** CT scan at the time of trauma reveals evidence of injury in the left parietal scalp (*arrows*). Contrecoup hemorrhagic cortical contusion and edema is identified in the right temporal lobe (*short arrows*). Also, scattered hemor-rhagic shearing injuries are seen in the frontal lobes bilaterally (*small arrows*). **C** to **E,** Short TR, short TE axial images 1 week after the CT scan. Extensive hemorrhagic cortical contusion is identified in the temporal lobes bilaterally, as well as in

Figure continues on following page.

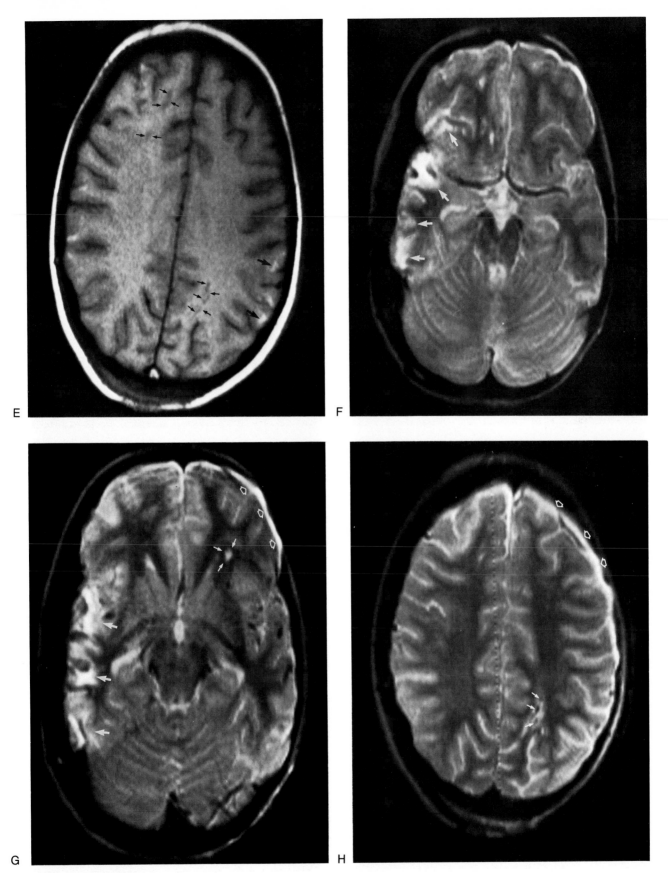

Figure 8–8. *Continued.*
the base of the frontal lobes and in the left temporal and parietal areas (*short arrows*). There is hemorrhagic shear injury in the left frontal lobe (*arrowheads*). Other nonhemorrhagic shearing injuries are identified in the right frontal lobe and in the left parietal occipital white matter (*small arrows*). *F* to *H,* Long TR, long TE images reveal edema subjacent to the areas of cortical contusion (*short arrows*). Some early hemosiderin deposition around the periphery of the hemorrhagic shear injury in the left frontal lobe is noted, as well as a small amount of hemosiderin or deoxyhemoglobin in the left parietal occipital shearing injury (*small arrows*). A small left subdural hematoma is present (*open arrows*).

Figure continues on following page.

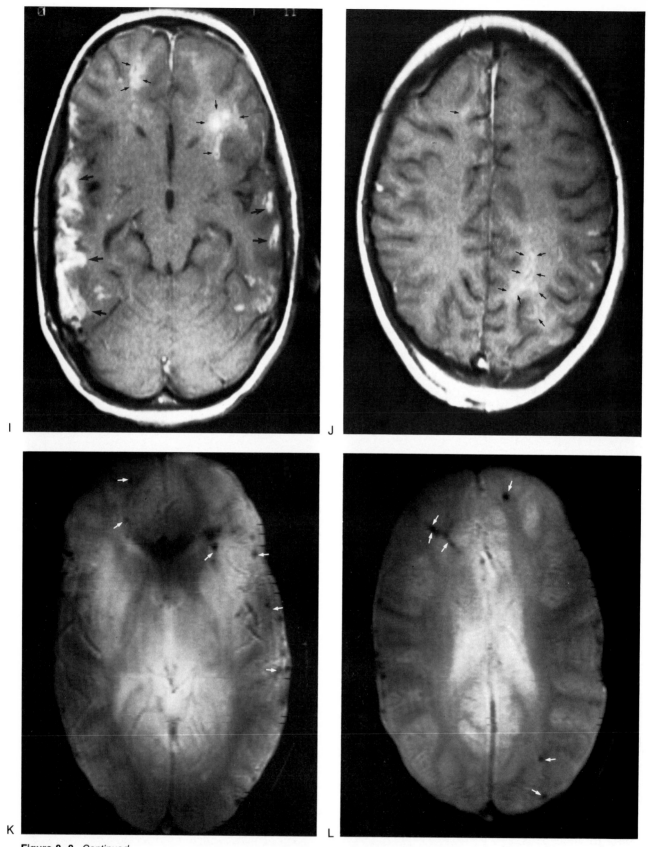

Figure 8–8. *Continued.*
I, J, Gadolinium-enhanced images reveal some enhancement of the cortical contusion and subjacent white matter (*short arrows*). There is also rather marked enhancement of the numerous foci of shearing injury (*small arrows*). *K, L,* Short flip angle gradient-recalled echo images obtained on a follow-up MR scan 6 months after the initial injury. There are numerous foci of hemosiderin deposition throughout the white matter consistent with extensive small hemorrhagic shear injuries throughout the cerebrum (*small arrows*).

tered on short TR, short TE images and hypointense signal on long TR, long TE images. With cell lysis, high signal is encountered on both long TR, long TE and short TR, short TE images. At this point, differentiation of the hemorrhagic components on long TR, long TE images may be difficult. In chronic stages hemosiderin deposition, with hypointense signal on long TR, long TE images, may be encountered in areas of hemorrhagic contusion.[57] Encephalomalacia is also identified, with widening of the subarachnoid spaces and irregularity and thinning of the surface of the involved portion of the brain on short TR, short TE images. On long TR, long TE images, residual high signal intensity at the involved site is present consistent with loss of normal cellularity, gliosis, and scarring.

Intraparenchymal Hematoma

Intraparenchymal hematoma is relatively unusual in children as opposed to adults with comparable head trauma. This is presumably related to the increased plasticity of the calvarium in children. Parenchymal hematomas are usually caused by closed head injury. Severe overlying contusion is common. The hematoma is generally in the frontal or temporal lobe. The center of the hematoma is usually deep within the white matter, or in the contused cortex. Temporal lobe hematoma in the neonate is due to birth trauma, usually associated with obstetric instrumentation, the overlying temporal area being compressed by the blades of the forceps. Hematomas arise as a result of disruption of penetrating blood vessels entering the white matter, or because of extensive bleeding within a hemorrhagic contusion dissecting into subjacent white matter (Fig. 8–9). A small percentage present as delayed hematomas, appearing 1 to 7 days after injury (Fig. 8–10). These are a readily identifiable and treatable cause of sudden deterioration after head injury, and their diagnosis frequently follows surgical drainage of an extra-axial hematoma, which may have been acting to tamponade the intraparenchymal bleeding. The overall incidence of parenchymal hematomas following trauma is approximately 5 percent, relatively low compared with that of contusion.[8, 59] The incidence in children is approximately one-third that of adults.[53]

The evolution of intraparenchymal hematomas has been well characterized by Gomori and colleagues.[16, 30] The signal characteristics of the different stages of hemoglobin oxidation do not vary from those seen in other hemorrhagic conditions. The distribution of the different oxidation products within the hematoma does follow a characteristic pattern, however. Fresh clot, with oxyhemoglobin and plasma present, is hypointense to brain on short TR, short TE images and hyperintense on long TR, long TE images. Reactive edema is identified by increased signal surrounding the hematoma. This is observed within the first 24 hours, in the hyperacute stage. After 24 hours, resorption of plasma and conversion of oxyhemoglobin to deoxyhemoglobin occurs, causing the characteristic hypointense signal on long TR, long TE images. This acute stage persists for approximately 3 to 7 days and is also associated with surrounding vasogenic edema. After this, the subacute stage ensues, with conversion of the deoxyhemoglobin to methemoglobin, initially around the periphery, then migrating to the central core of the hematoma. This is generally complete within about 2 weeks. The chronic phase is heralded by the appearance of macrophages around the periphery of the hematoma cavity and the conversion of hemoglobin to hemosiderin. Phagocytosed hemosiderin is deposited within the macrophage lysosomes. The methemoglobin within the center of the hematoma may persist for weeks or years. Eventually, the center of the hematoma is left with non–iron-containing heme pigments known as hematoidins, which are not paramagnetic and have signal characteristics of simple protein solutions, hypointense on short TR, short TE images and hyperintense on long TR, long TE images. The hemosiderin-laden macrophages do not migrate from the brain and persist around the periphery of the previous hematoma for years, leaving characteristic telltale evidence of the previous hemorrhagic event as low-intensity hemosiderin staining (Fig. 8–11).

Shearing Injury

MRI is much more sensitive than CT in displaying the nonhemorrhagic consequences of trauma and is often able to demonstrate the cause of unexplained neurologic deficits.[12] Shearing injury is a major cause of unexplained deep coma or a persistent vegetative state in patients showing no CT evidence of a significant focal mass lesion.[9] Holbourn[55] followed by Lindenberg and colleagues[60] postulated that shearing injuries result from unbalanced mechanical forces acting on the brain during rapid rotational or nonlinear acceleration-deceleration motions of the calvarium and brain. The brain, with very little rigidity and extreme incompressibility, is subject to shear strains in areas of different consistencies, such as gray-white matter junctions. Rotational accelerations produce shearing strains across axon tracts within the hemispheres. These forces appear to be most commonly induced by high-speed motor vehicle accidents with rapid deceleration.[9, 61] This results in disruption of groups of axons and occasionally their accompanying blood vessels. Typical distribution of these injuries is at the corticomedullary junctions and parasagittal white matter structures of the corpus callosum, internal capsule, and midbrain as well as the basal ganglia and thalamus.[9, 61, 62] As might be expected, shearing injury is frequently associated with other forms of injury. In our experience, cortical contusion is the most common form of associated injury (Figs. 8–8, 8–12).

The sensitivity of MRI in detecting hemorrhagic and

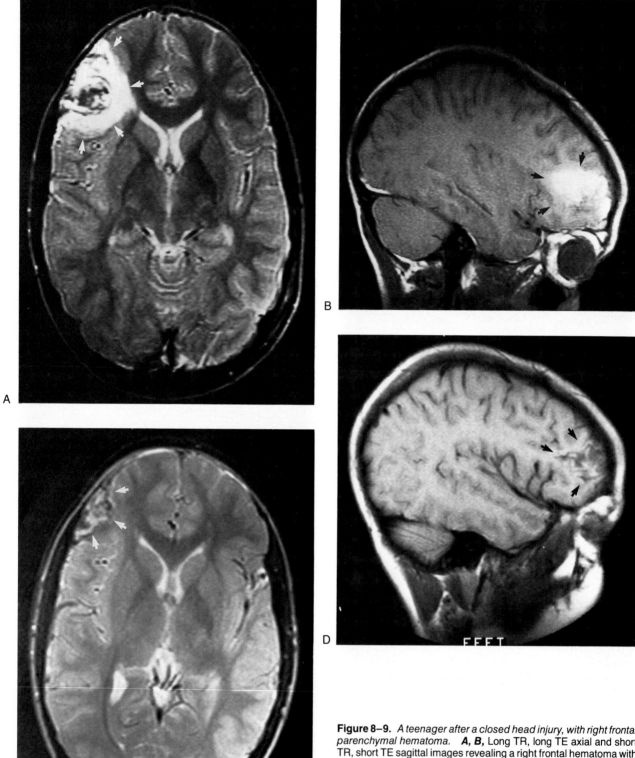

Figure 8–9. *A teenager after a closed head injury, with right frontal parenchymal hematoma.* ***A, B,*** Long TR, long TE axial and short TR, short TE sagittal images revealing a right frontal hematoma with surrounding edema (*arrows*). There is low signal deoxyhemoglobin centrally on the long TR image. Peripheral high signal met-hemoglobin is best seen on the short TR image. ***C, D,*** Follow-up MR scan 2 months later. Long TR, long TE axial and short TR, short TE sagittal images reveal resolution of the edema and hematoma. Residual encephalomalacia with some hemosiderin staining is noted on the axial image (*arrows*).

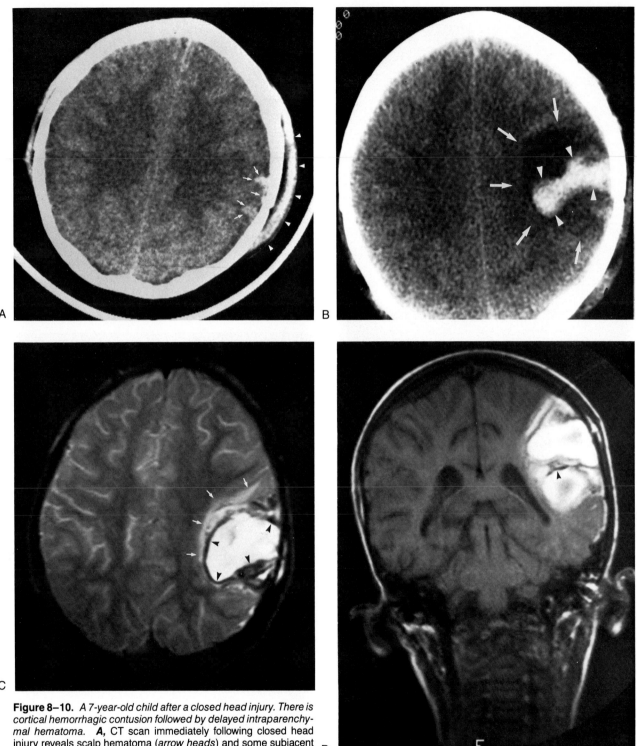

Figure 8–10. *A 7-year-old child after a closed head injury. There is cortical hemorrhagic contusion followed by delayed intraparenchymal hematoma.* **A,** CT scan immediately following closed head injury reveals scalp hematoma (*arrow heads*) and some subjacent cortical contusion and subarachnoid bleeding (*arrows*). **B,** Follow-up CT scan 4 days later after an acute deterioration in mental status and neurologic examination. A delayed intraparenchymal bleed has occurred with high-density blood in the hematoma (*arrowheads*) and surrounding edema (*arrows*). **C, D,** Long TR, long TE axial and short TR, short TE coronal MRI obtained one week after the CT scan, showing delayed hematoma formation. A small amount of residual edema persists around the hematoma (*arrows*). A rim of hypointense hemosiderin staining about the periphery of the hematoma is present (*arrowheads*). The central portion of the hematoma has converted to high signal methemoglobin.

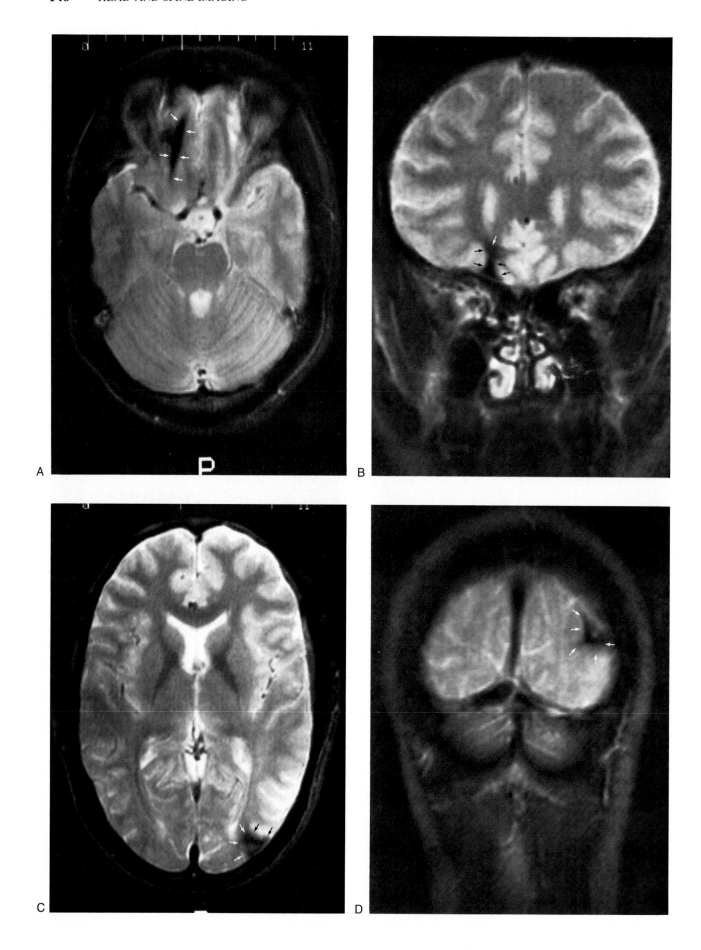

A

B

C

D

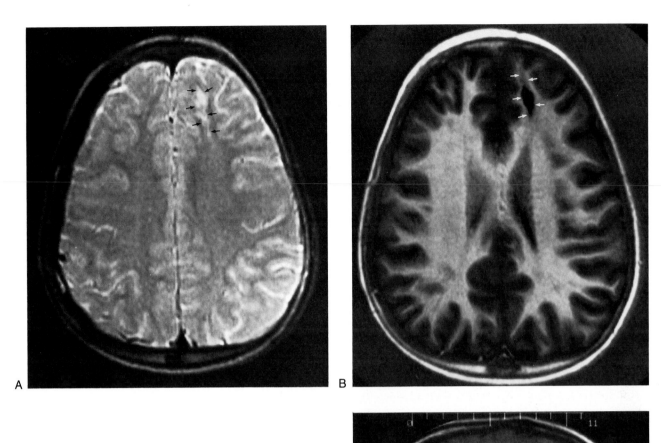

Figure 8–12. *Shearing injury and contusion. Closed head injury after a motor vehicle accident.* **A,** Long TR, long TE axial image reveals a focal area of high signal in the left frontal lobe consistent with a white matter shearing injury (*arrows*). **B,** Inversion recovery (TI = 600 msec) scan reveals the white matter shearing with low signal within the cleft (*arrows*). **C,** Short TR, short TE parasagittal image reveals an area of hypointense signal corresponding to the left frontal shearing injury (*arrows*). Some hemorrhagic cortical contusion along the base of the frontal lobe is also present (*arrowheads*).

◀ **Figure 8–11.** *Hemosiderin staining from old hemorrhage. A 33-year-old man status post head trauma as a teenager, now with an intractable seizure disorder. A CT scan in the same period as the MRI was unremarkable.* **A, B,** Axial and coronal long TR, long TE images reveal hemosiderin staining along the base of the right frontal lobe (*arrows*). **C, D,** Same studies, different levels. Hemosiderin staining is also present in the left parietal occipital cortex (*arrows*). These areas presumably represent coup and contrecoup hemorrhagic lesions that have left telltale evidence of hemosiderin staining.

nonhemorrhagic shear injuries is superior to that of CT scanning.[12,57] Areas of acute nonhemorrhagic shear injury on MRI appear as high signal foci on long TR, long TE images. Occasionally, clefts within the white matter are identified on short TR, short TE images or inversion recovery images, which maximize gray-white matter differentiation (Figs. 8–12, 8–13). After resolution of edema the focal areas of axonal disruption may or may not be apparent on the short TR, short TE images, but persist as focal areas of encephalomalacia identifiable on long TR, long TE images. On long-term follow-up a pattern of generalized atrophy may be identified, presumably relating to parenchymal loss from wallerian degeneration. Hemorrhagic shearing injuries follow the same temporal signal characteristics as other parenchymal hemorrhages. Owing to the small size of shearing injuries, the usual pattern of concentric formation of methemoglobin from the periphery inward may not be as readily discernible as in large hematomas (Fig. 8–14). Follow-up examination of these patients may reveal numerous small foci of hemosiderin deposition at areas of previous shearing injury. This is particularly conspicuous on pulse sequences sensitive to areas of magnetic susceptibility effects such as short flip angle gradient-recalled echo images, which produce T2* weighted images (see Fig. 10–8).

Malignant Edema

Twenty to 50 percent of children in post-traumatic coma within the first 24 hours show a pattern on head CT of diffuse bilateral cerebral edema.[53,63] Sixty percent of these show elevation of intracranial pressure within the first 72 hours.[53] Malignant cerebral edema apparently is unique to the pediatric age group. The mean age of patients with malignant edema is 6 years.[53] Whether this is a form of injury or a phenomenon occurring in response to injury is uncertain. This entity does not appear to be entirely due to cerebral edema but it is probably due in part to loss of cerebral autoregulation with hyperemia.[64] Inciting events are thought to include trauma, hypotension, and hypercarbia.[64] The CT appearance of diffuse cerebral edema has been well documented and correlated with intracranial pressures.[53] The findings on CT include sulcal effacement, ventricular compression, and obliteration of the perimesencephalic cisterns. Currently, no reports of the MR appearance of malignant edema have appeared. This is probably due to the severe nature of the underlying injuries and the complications of managing malignant edema. These patients usually require extensive monitoring and life support equipment, which in most cases makes MRI difficult. Aggressive management of these patients has resulted in relatively

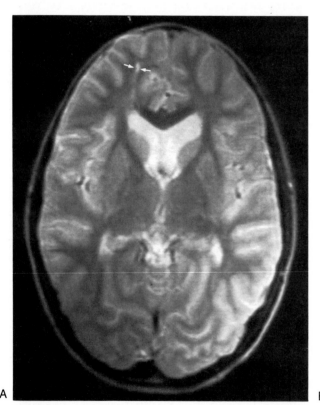
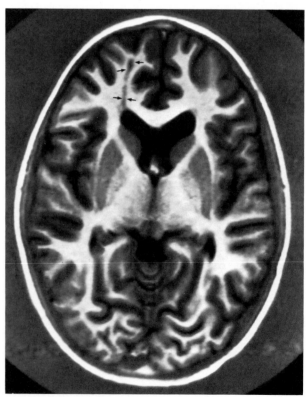

A   B

Figure 8–13. *The same patient as in Figure 9–1.* **A,** Long TR, long TE axial image reveals edema around a focal shearing injury of the right frontal lobe white matter. **B,** Inversion recovery technique (TI = 600 msec). Hypointense signal from the white matter shearing injury in the right frontal lobe is well defined on this pulse sequence (*arrows*), which maximizes gray and white matter differentiation.

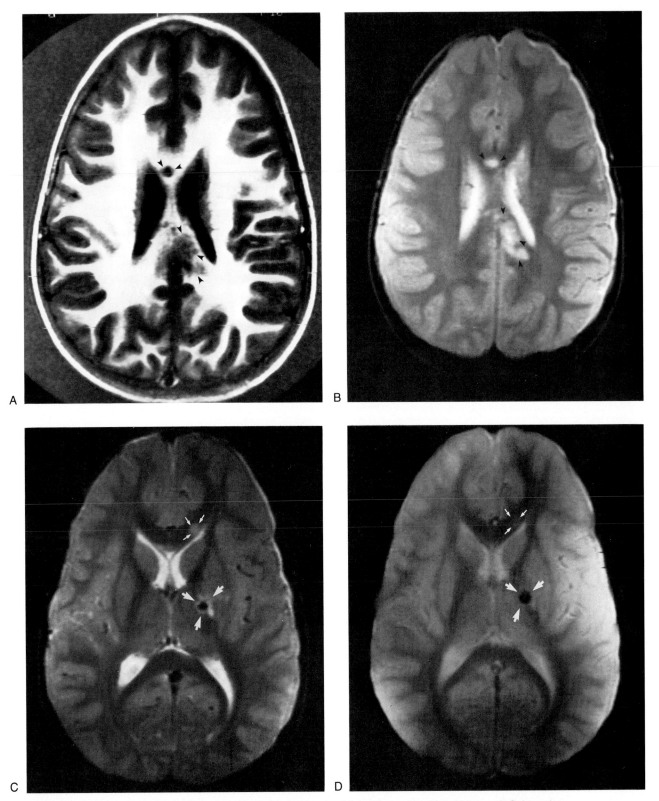

Figure 8–14. *Extensive hemorrhagic and nonhemorrhagic shearing injury after a closed head injury.* **A, B,** Inversion recovery (TI = 600 msec) axial and long TR, long TE axial images at similar levels. Nonhemorrhagic shearing injury is identified in the genu of the corpus callosum as well as in the splenium of the corpus callosum (*arrowheads*). **C, D,** Long TR, long TE axial and short flip angle gradient-recalled echo axial images at similar levels. The nonhemorrhagic shearing injury in the left limb of the genu of the corpus callosum is less apparent on the gradient-recalled echo image (*small arrows*). Surrounding edema around the hemorrhagic shearing injury in the posterior limb of the internal capsule on the left is less apparent (*short arrows*). The hypointense signal from the deoxyhemoglobin is slightly more pronounced on the gradient-recalled echo image.

Figure continues on following page.

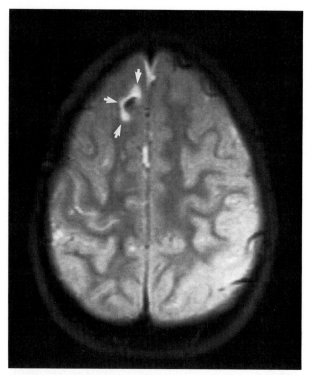

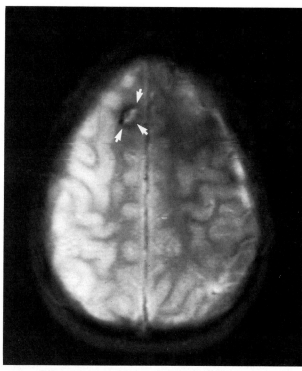

E

F

Figure 8–14. *Continued.*
E, F, Axial long TR, long TE and axial short flip angle gradient-recalled echo images through similar levels reveal a gray-white matter junction hemorrhagic shearing injury in the right frontal lobe (*arrows*). Signal hypointensity due to the presence of paramagnetic substances is somewhat more conspicuous on the gradient-recalled echo image.

low morbidity and mortality rates; in approximately 75 percent of patients there is a satisfactory outcome and normalization of CT findings.[63, 65]

CHILD ABUSE

Intracranial injury is the leading cause of death in cases of child abuse and is a major factor leading to the sequelae of mental retardation and neurologic impairment.[22, 66, 67] Most abused children are under 2 years of age.[68] The two major mechanisms in the production of cerebral injury are shaking and beating of the head with direct blows.[53] CT has represented a major advance in the evaluation of the abused child, documenting the characteristic occipitoparietal and interhemispheric subdural hematomas found in the shaken baby syndrome[23] as well as parenchymal brain and calvarial injuries from impact trauma. In a series of abused children with head injury, Zimmerman and colleagues reported a mortality rate of one-third and a morbidity rate of one-third (defined as permanent neurologic sequelae).[68] This same report also indicated a mortality rate of 5 percent from shaking injury but a 53 percent incidence of permanent neurologic deficit.[68]

CT has the advantage of being able to demonstrate bony abnormalities and acute subarachnoid blood, but has been shown to be relatively insensitive compared with MRI in detecting small subdural hematomas and posterior fossa hemorrhage.[69] MRI has the advantage that the absence of bone artifact makes small subdural fluid collections more apparent. MRI also provides superb delineation of the various types of parenchymal injury discussed earlier in this chapter. The characteristic temporal changes in hemorrhage identified with MRI may also have legal implications in terms of documenting and approximating the age of previous hemorrhagic injury, and determining whether the patient has sustained recurrent injury. The initial evaluation of the abused child should probably include head CT in view of its ready availability and rapidity. However, for follow-up and further evaluation, MRI is the method of choice for detection and characterization of intracranial injury, particularly in patients whose CT results are normal.

SEQUELAE OF TRAUMA

MRI provides exquisite detail in the depiction of hemorrhagic products, but it is its great sensitivity to other changes within the brain after trauma that sets it apart from CT. MRI may have a role in predicting the prognostic outcome of various types of injury, although further study correlating MRI with follow-up neuropsychological testing is necessary. After trauma, generalized atrophic changes of the brain are seen in up to 30 percent of survivors of severe head trauma.[70] The morphologic characteristics of post-traumatic atrophy are generalized sulcal enlargement along with ventriculomegaly. This should not be confused with post-traumatic communicating hydrocephalus, in which there is enlargement of the frontal and temporal horns together with enlargement of the third and fourth ventricles. Communicating hydrocephalus has less sulcal enlargement and is also distinguished by the presence of periventricular transependymal CSF re-

sorption. The time course also differs in that post-traumatic hydrocephalus develops in most patients by the end of the second post-traumatic week.[70] Generalized ventricular enlargement from atrophy is typically seen 2 or more months after injury.[43]

Focal atrophic changes following head trauma correspond to the location of the acute injury, usually in areas of previous contusion. In children sustaining injury in the first 2 years of life, multicystic encephalomalacia may be a sequela of focal brain injury (Fig. 8–15). MRI is better at defining the location of these

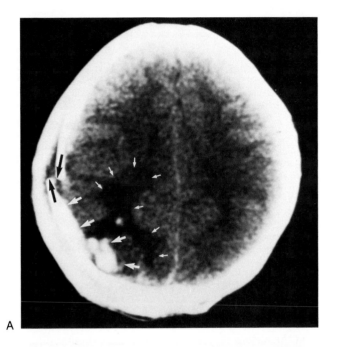

A

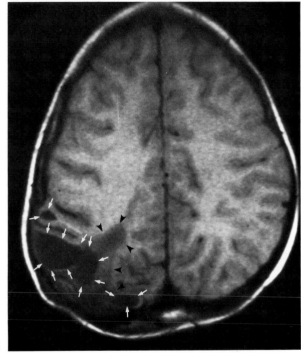

B

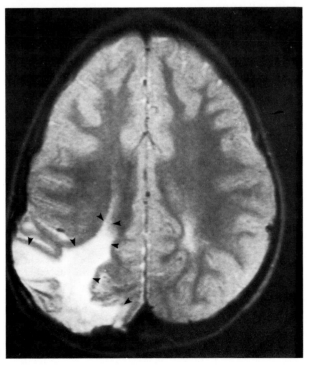

C

Figure 8–15. *Encephalomalacia after trauma. A 4-year-old patient who sustained an impact injury to the right parietal occipital area at age 2 years.* **A,** *CT scan at the time of injury reveals skull fracture (*black arrows*), underlying parenchymal hematoma (*short arrows*), and edema and/or infarction (*small arrows*). **B, C,** MR scan 2 years after the initial injury was performed to evaluate chronic swelling at the traumatic site. Axial short TR, short TE and long TR, long TE images through similar levels reveal encephalomalacia (*arrowheads*) with cystic expansile changes (*arrows*).*

encephalomalacic changes with multiplanar imaging and lack of artifact from adjacent bone. MRI will undoubtedly prove invaluable in correlating the structural image with the functional abnormalities determined by neuropsychological testing.

REFERENCES

1. Bruce DA, Schut L, Sutton LN. Pediatric head injury. In: Wilkins RH, Rengachary SS, eds. Neurosurgery. New York: McGraw-Hill, 1985: 1600–1604.
2. Bruce DA, Schut L, Bruno LA, et al. Outcome following severe head injuries in children. J Neurosurg 1978; 48:679–688.
3. Heiskanen O, Kaste M. Late prognosis of severe brain injury in children. Dev Med Child Neurol 1974; 16:11–14.
4. Bowden HN, Knights RM, Winogram HW. Speeded performance following head injury in children. J Clin Exp Neuropsych 1985; 7:39–54.
5. Gulbrandson GB. Neuropsychological sequelae of light head injury in older children six months after trauma. J Clin Neuropsychol 1984; 6:257–268.
6. Luerssen TG, Hesselink JR, Ruff RM, et al. Magnetic resonance imaging of craniocerebral injury: clinical and research considerations. Conc Pediatr Neurosurg 1987; 7:190–208.
7. Dublin AB, French BN, Rennick JM. Computed tomography in head trauma. Radiology 1977; 122:365–369.
8. Zimmerman RA, Bilaniuk LT, Genneralli T, et al. Cranial computed tomography in diagnosis and management of acute head trauma. AJR 1978; 131:27–34.
9. Zimmerman RA, Bilaniuk LT, Gennarelli T. Computed tomography of shearing injuries of the cerebral white matter. Radiology 1978; 127:393–396.
10. French BN, Dublin AB. The value of computerized tomography in the management of 1000 consecutive head injuries. Surg Neurol 1977; 7:171–183.
11. Gentry LR, Godersky JC, Thompson B. MR imaging of head trauma: review of the distribution and radiopathologic features of traumatic lesions. AJR 1988; 150:663–672.
12. Zimmerman RA, Bilaniuk LT, Hackney DB, et al. Head injury: early results of comparing CT and high-field MR. AJR 1986; 147:1215–1222.
13. Gentry LR, Godersky JC, Thompson B, Dunn VD. Prospective comparative study of intermediate-field MR and CT in the evaluation of closed head trauma. AJR 1988; 150:673–682.
14. Han JS, Kaufman B, Alfidi RJ, et al. Head trauma evaluated by magnetic resonance and computed tomography: a comparison. Radiology 1984; 150:71–77.
15. Snow RB, Zimmerman RD, Gandy SE, et al. Comparison of magnetic resonance imaging and computed tomography in the evaluation of head injury. Neurosurgery 1986; 18:45–52.
16. Gomori JM, Grossman RI, Goldberg HI, et al. Intracranial hematomas: imaging by high field MR. Radiology 1985; 157:87–93.
17. De La Paz RL, New PFJ, Buonanno FS, et al. NMR imaging of intracranial hemorrhage. J Comput Assist Tomogr 1984; 8:599–607.
18. Zimmerman RA, Bilaniuk LT, Grossman RI, et al. Resistive NMR of intracranial hematomas. Neuroradiology 1985; 27:16–20.
19. Bradley WG, Schmidt PG. Effect of methemoglobin formation on the MR appearance of subarachnoid hemorrhage. Radiology 1985; 156:99–103.
20. McClelland CQ, Rekate H, Kaufman B, Persse L. Cerebral injury in child abuse: a changing profile. Childs Brain 1980; 7:225–235.
21. Billmire ME, Myers PA. Serious head injury in infants: accident or abuse? Pediatrics 1985; 75:340–342.
22. Caffey J. The whiplash-shaken infant syndrome: manual shaking by the extremities with whiplash-induced intracranial and intraocular bleedings, linked with residual permanent brain damage and mental retardation. Pediatrics 1974; 54:396–402.
23. Zimmerman RA, Bilaniuk LT, Bruce D, et al. Interhemispheric acute subdural hematoma: computed tomographic manifestation of child abuse by shaking. Neuroradiology 1978; 16:39–40.
24. Pauling L, Coryell C. The magnetic properties and structure of the hemochromogens and related substances. Proc Natl Acad Sci USA 1936; 22:159–163.
25. Wintrobe MM, Lee GR, Boggs DR, et al. Clinical hematology. Philadelphia: Lea & Febiger, 1981.
26. Singer JR, Crooks LE. Some magnetic studies of normal and leukemic blood. J Clin Engin 1978; 3:237–243.
27. Drayer B, Burger P, Darwin R, et al. Magnetic resonance imaging of brain iron. AJNR 1986; 7:373–380.
28. Gomori JM, Grossman RI, Hackney DB, et al. Variable appearances of subacute intracranial hematomas on high-field spin-echo MR. AJNR 1987; 8:1019–1026.
29. Edelman RR, Johnson K, Buxton R, et al. MR of hemorrhage: a new approach. AJNR 1986; 7:751–756.
30. Gomori JM, Grossman RI. Head and neck hemorrhage. In: Kressel HY, ed. Magnetic resonance annual. New York: Raven Press, 1987:71–112.
31. Rappaport SI. Introduction to hematology. New York, Harper & Row, 1971.
32. Hecht-Leavitt C, Gomori JM, Grossman RI, et al. High-field MR imaging of hemorrhagic cortical infarction. AJNR 1986; 7:587–594.
33. Koenig SH, Brown RD, Lindstrom TR. Interactions of solvent with the heme region of methemoglobin and fluoromethemoglobin. Biophys J 1981; 34:397–408.
34. Bradley WG. MRI of hemorrhage and iron in the brain. In: Stark DD, Bradley WG, eds. Magnetic resonance imaging. St. Louis: CV Mosby, 1988: 359–374.
35. Zimmerman RA. Magnetic resonance of head injury. In: Taveras H, Ferrucci J, eds. Radiology: diagnosis/imaging/intervention. Philadelphia: JB Lippincott, 1988; 37A:1–12.
36. Zimmerman RA, Bilaniuk LT, Hackney DB, et al. Magnetic resonance imaging in temporal bone fracture. Neuroradiology 1987; 29:246–251.
37. Zimmerman RA, Bilaniuk LT, Hackney DB, et al. Magnetic resonance imaging of paranasal sinus hemorrhage. Radiology 1987; 162:111–114.
38. Bloembergen N, Purcell E, Pound RV. Relaxation effects in nuclear magnetic resonance absorption. Phys Rev 1948; 73:679–712.
39. Brant-Zwadzki M. MR imaging of the brain. Radiology 1988; 166:1–10.
40. Van Gijn J, Van Dongen KJ. The time course of aneurysmal hemorrhage on computed tomograms. Neuroradiology 1982; 23:153–156.
41. Adams JP, Kassell NF. CT and clinical correlations in recent aneurysmal subarachnoid hemorrhage: a preliminary report of the cooperative aneurysm study. Neurology 1983; 33:981–988.
42. Dolinskas C, Zimmerman RA, Bilaniuk LT. A sign of subarachnoid bleeding on cranial computed tomography of pediatric head trauma patients. Radiology 1978; 126:409–411.
43. Zimmerman RA. Evaluation of head injury: supratentorial. In: Taveras H, Ferrucci H, eds. Radiology: diagnosis/imaging/intervention. Philadelphia: JB Lippincott, 1988; 37:1–18.
44. Gomori JM, Grossman RI, Bilaniuk LT, et al. High-field MR imaging of superficial siderosis of the central nervous system. J Comput Assist Tomogr 1985; 9:972–975.
45. Milhorat TH. Pediatric neurosurgery. In: Contemporary neurology series, Vol 16. Philadelphia: FA Davis, 1978.
46. Diebler C, Dulac O. Cranial trauma. In: Diebler C, Dulac O, eds. Pediatric neurology and neuroradiology. Heidelberg: Springer-Verlag, 1987:343–355.
47. Hernansanz J, Munoz F, Rodriguez D, et al. Subdural hematomas of the posterior fossa in normal weight newborns. J Neurosurg 1984; 61:872–974.
48. Moon KL Jr, Brant-Zawadzki M, Pitts LH, et al. Nuclear magnetic resonance imaging of CT-isodense hematomas. AJNR 1984; 5:319–322.
49. Rahme ES, Green C. Chronic subdural hematoma in childhood and adolescence. JAMA 1961; 176:424–426.

50. Hammock MK, Milhorat TH. Trauma. In: Hammock MK, Milhorat TH, eds. Cranial computed tomography in infancy and childhood. Baltimore: Williams & Wilkins, 1981:97–129.

51. Jennett B, Teasdale G. Management of injuries. In: Contemporary neurology series, Vol 20. Philadelphia: FA Davis, 1981.

52. Zimmerman RA, Bilaniuk LT, Bruce D, et al. Computed tomography of pediatric head trauma: acute general cerebral swelling. Radiology 1978; 126;403.

53. Zimmerman RA, Bilaniuk LT. Computed tomography in pediatric head trauma. J Neuroradiology 1981; 8:257.

54. Gandy WE, Snow RB, Zimmerman RD, et al. Cranial nuclear magnetic resonance imaging in head trauma. Ann Neurol 1984; 16;254–257.

55. Holbourn AHS. The mechanics of brain injuries. Br Med Bull 1945; 3:147–149.

56. Hadley DM, Teasdale GM, Jenkins A, et al. Magnetic resonance imaging in acute head injury. Clin Radiol 1988; 39:131–139.

57. Hesselink JR, Dowd CF, Gealy ME, et al. MR imaging of brain contusions: a comparative study with CT. AJR 1988; 150:1133–1142.

58. Zimmerman RA, Bilaniuk LT, Dolinskas C, et al. Computed tomography of acute intracerebral hemorrhagic contusion. Comput Tomogr 1977; 1:271.

59. Koo AH, LaRoque RL. Evaluation of head trauma by computed tomography. Radiology 1977; 123:345.

60. Lindenberg R, Fisher RS, Kurlacher SH, et al. Lesions of the corpus callosum following blunt mechanical trauma to the head. Am J Pathol 1955; 31:297–317.

61. Strich SJ. Shearing of nerve fibres as a cause of brain damage due to head injury. A pathological study of twenty cases. Lancet 1961; 2:443–448.

62. Peerless SJ, Rewcastle NB. Shear injuries of the brain. Can Med Assoc J 1966; 96:163–185.

63. Bruce DS, Alavi A, Bilaniuk LT, et al. Diffuse cerebral swelling following head injuries in children: the syndrome of "malignant brain edema." J Neurosurg 1981; 54:170–178.

64. Zimmerman RA. Radiology of brain failure. In: Grevnick A, Safar P, eds. Clinics in critical care medicine. Vol 2, Brain failure and resuscitation. New York: Churchill Livingstone, 1981.

65. Berger MS, Pitts CH, Lovely M, et al. Outcome from severe head injury in children and adolescents. J Neurosurg 1985; 62:194–199.

66. Caffey J. On the theory and practice of shaking infants. Its potential residual effects of permanent brain damage and mental retardation. Am J Dis Child 1972; 124:161–169.

67. Greg GS, Elmer E. Infant injuries: accident or abuse? Pediatrics 1969; 44:434–439.

68. Zimmerman RA, Bilaniuk LT, Bruce D, et al. Computed tomography of craniocerebral injury in the abused child. Radiology 1979; 130:687–690.

69. Alexander RC, Schor DP, Smith WL. Magnetic resonance imaging of intracranial injuries from child abuse. J Pediatr 1986; 109:975–979.

70. Gudemen SK, Kishore RRS, Becker DP, et al. Computerized tomography in the evaluation of incidence and significance of post-traumatic hydrocephalus. Radiology 1981; 141:597–602.

Tumors of the Brain

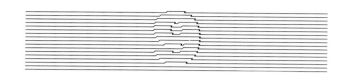

PATRICIA C. DAVIS, M.D.

Brain tumors represent the second most common neoplasia arising in the pediatric population, and thus represent a significant source of morbidity and mortality in children. Fortunately, these lesions are relatively infrequent, with an estimated incidence of 2.4 per 100,000 children in the United States.[1] Advances in management of these lesions have been relatively slow for many reasons.[1] The relatively small numbers of children evaluated at any given medical center create difficulties in obtaining a large enough population for controlled studies of specific therapies. Large lesions or those in critical areas may not be amenable to complete or extensive resection. Small children with an immature nervous system are more susceptible to the adverse effects of radiation therapy than are older children and adults. The blood-brain barrier is a formidable obstacle to the penetration of effective chemotherapeutic agents, although extensive research continues into new agents and improved systems for their delivery.

A variety of brain neoplasms encountered in the pediatric population are described below, grouped by pathologic type.[2] Typical findings at presentation, general gross and microscopic pathologic features, therapeutic approaches, and imaging findings are discussed sequentially for each neoplasm. Magnetic resonance (MR) findings are stressed, particularly those performed after administration of gadolinium–DTPA enhancement. The dosage administered in children is 0.1 mmol per kilogram, given slowly intravenously over 1 to 2 minutes.

GLIOMA

Glial origin tumors account for 70 to 85 percent of primary intracranial neoplasms in the pediatric population, and astrocytomas account for 21 to 45 percent of this group.[1] Histologic grading systems for astrocytoma correlate reasonably well with survival and biologic behavior, although survival also varies with the location of the primary tumor.[2]

A variety of grading systems are in use that generally separate the lower-grade tumors with a relatively favorable prognosis from their more aggressive counterparts, the malignant astrocytoma and glioblastoma multiforme. Kernohan and colleagues suggested a grading system using grades 1 to 4 in increasing order of histologic malignancy.[3] Controversy continues over inclusion of glioblastoma multiforme in the astrocytoma category, since this disorder may arise as a de novo malignancy rather than as a progression of a preexisting, more differentiated form of astrocytoma.[2] Other divisions based on cell morphology and growth pattern are termed protoplasmic, pilocytic, fibrillary, gemistocytic, and so forth.[2] The simplest grading system includes three categories: low grade, anaplastic, and glioblastoma multiforme. All grading systems suffer from some ambiguity in defining the limits of each category and from sampling error in these histologically variable tumors.

The following discussion focuses on astrocytoma on the basis of the anatomic location of the tumor, since the prognosis, therapeutic approach, and associated clinical findings depend on the site of the primary neoplasm.

Cerebellar Astrocytoma

Cerebellar astrocytoma accounts for about 11 percent of primary central nervous system (CNS) tumors in children and carries an excellent prognosis after surgical resection of up to 94 percent at 10 years.[1,2] Approximately one-third of childhood posterior fossa tumors are cerebellar astrocytomas, with no definite sex predilection.[4] These tumors commonly occur in the first two decades, with a peak late in the first decade and early in the second decade. Cerebellar astrocytomas commonly harbor cysts, are well circumscribed, and are relatively surgically resectable.

Cerebellar astrocytoma may occur in the cerebellar vermis or hemispheres in children, older patients tending to have eccentric hemispheric lesions. Extension into or origin within the vermis is common, although cerebellar astrocytoma infrequently presents within the fourth ventricle. Cerebellar astrocytoma is well defined grossly, and up to 80 percent are frankly cystic,[5,6] with hemispheric tumor more commonly cystic than its vermian counterpart. A solitary cyst peripheral to a neoplastic mural nodule, or a diffuse multicystic form surrounded by tumor matrix, is typical. The solitary cyst wall of tumors with a mural nodule tends to be composed of gliotic tissue from degenerated glial cells, although biopsy is required to exclude active tumor. The cysts contain highly proteinaceous yellow or brown fluid. Infrequently a predominantly solid tumor is identified. Cystic or solid forms may diffusely infiltrate adjacent tissues or leptomeninges on microscopic appearance.[2,7]

Although marked variation occurs histologically within these tumors, the most common or "juvenile" type is a mixed tumor with compact areas of fibrillary cells and spongy areas with microcysts and stellate astrocytes.[2] These characteristics closely resemble those of juvenile pilocytic astrocytoma of the third ventricular region. A less common form, occurring in approximately 15 percent of cerebellar astrocytomas[2] and particularly in adolescence, is the diffuse astrocytoma with fibrillary stellate or piloid cells and few microcysts. These diffusely infiltrating astrocytomas are the ones most commonly implicated in anaplastic change and have a less favorable prognosis than the more common juvenile cerebellar astrocytoma.[2] Clinically and histologically malignant cerebellar astrocytomas are uncommon, although rare malignancy and secondary neoplastic seeding of the subarachnoid space have been described.[2,8,9] An association has been described

between malignant cerebellar astrocytoma and neurofibromatosis.[2] Histologic abnormalities such as multinucleated giant cells, nuclear hyperchromasia, and endothelial proliferation are common and do not correlate with a poor prognosis.[7] Hemorrhage occasionally occurs spontaneously into the cystic tumors with a mural nodule, but otherwise is distinctly unusual. Calcospherites occur in about 25 percent of cases.[2] Leptomeningeal invasion is noted in about 15 percent but does not connote malignant change or adversely affect survival.

Common presenting complaints with cerebellar astrocytoma include a long course of morning vomiting and headache, followed by clumsiness or frank ataxia. The insidious onset of hydrocephalus may be inapparent until significant secondary visual loss has occurred. Episodic unconsciousness, also called cerebellar fits, is noted in about 10 percent of cases.[5,6] Physical examination may reveal lateralizing signs of cerebellar dysfunction suggesting eccentricity of the tumor, or truncal ataxia in midline tumors. Papilledema or macrocephaly may be encountered, although children with large tumors may have remarkably few recognizable deficits.[4]

The treatment of choice for cerebellar astrocytomas is as complete a surgical resection as possible, since a complete removal is generally curative without further therapy. Recurrence is likely after partial removal, so that repeat surgery may be needed. Incomplete removal of the mural nodule in cystic masses is associated with recurrence, although the gliotic wall may be left in place if surgical biopsies confirm the absence of active tumor. Tumor recurrences tend to appear locally and may be very delayed (e.g., after more than 10 years). The common mixed form carries a 25-year survival rate of 94 percent, compared with 38 percent for the diffuse type, which is more difficult to resect completely.[10] Radiation therapy to the tumor bed is controversial in patients with incomplete resections owing to the relative radioresistance of this tumor, but may significantly prolong the interval before recurrence.[11] Spinal and subarachnoid seeding are sufficiently uncommon that craniospinal radiation therapy is not routinely performed unless a frankly malignant cerebellar tumor is encountered.[8,9] Experience with medical therapy is limited, chemotherapy being considered only in patients with inoperable recurrences that are refractory to radiation therapy.

MRI of cerebellar astrocytoma reveals an eccentric mass in the cerebellar hemisphere or vermis, which usually displaces without invading or expanding the fourth ventricle (Fig. 9–1). The mass and its cystic components are commonly iso- to hypointense in comparison with adjacent normal cerebellum with T1 weighting, and hyperintense to normal tissues with proton density and T2 weighting.[12–16] Cysts have intermediate signal intensities depending on the protein content of the fluid within, and hemorrhagic cysts are atypical in these low-grade tumors.[12] In spite of the mass effect, the location of the fourth ventricle is usu-

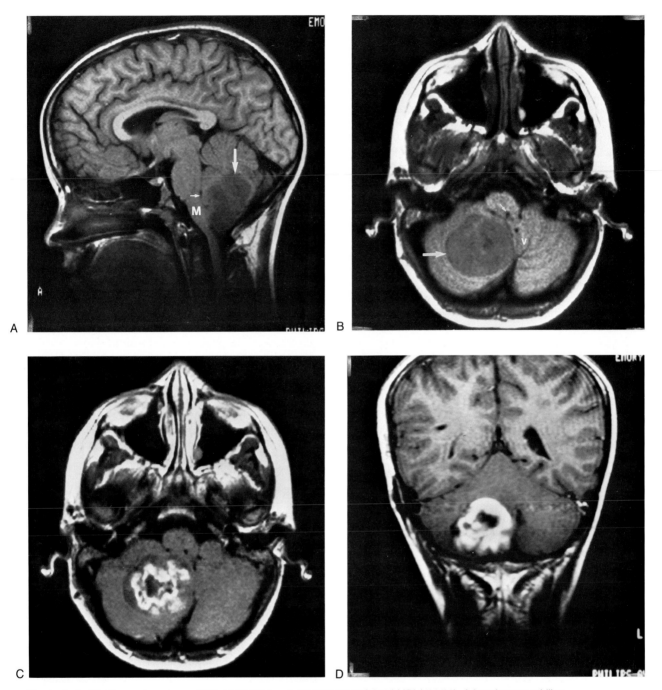

Figure 9–1. *Fibrillary astrocytoma of the cerebellum.*   *A,* Sagittal T1 weighted MRI (500/20). A hypointense midline mass (*large arrow*) expands and infiltrates the inferior cerebellum with secondary compression of the medulla (M) and fourth ventricle (*small arrow*). *B,* Axial T1 weighted MR (700/20). A hypointense intraaxial mass (*large arrow*) of the right cerebellar hemisphere displaces the inferior vermis (V) and compresses the inferior fourth ventricle (*small arrow*). The cystic nature of this mass is inapparent on this sequence. *C,* Axial T1 weighted MR (700/20) after gadolinium–DTPA. The diffuse multicystic configuration of the tumor with irregular enhancing circumferential tumor is demonstrated. *D,* Coronal T1 weighted MRI (700/20) after gadolinium–DTPA. Multiplanar images are useful in demonstrating this lesion anatomically for surgical planning.

ally apparent on MRI even when obscured on computed tomography (CT). Multiplanar MRI allows differentiation between intra- and extra-axial components with greater clarity than with CT.[16] The tumor margins are relatively well defined, although cyst, tumor, and edema may be indistinguishable on T2 weighted noncontrast MRI (Fig. 9–1). The associated mass effect upward at the tentorial notch, or downward with displacement of the inferior vermis and tonsils, is readily apparent on T1 weighted sagittal and coronal scans. The absence of beam-hardening artifacts on multiplanar imaging is particularly advantageous for anatomic localization of this lesion, although rather dense calcifications on CT may be undetected by MRI.[17] The remarkable sensitivity of MRI compared with CT for detection of parenchymal pathology permits identification and localization of masses that may be undetected by CT.[16]

Enhancement with gadolinium–DTPA results in superior differentiation of tumor margins from associated edema, although microscopic tumor may extend beyond the limits of recognizable blood-brain barrier disruption on both contrasted CT and MRI (Fig. 9–1). Enhancement aids the recognition of cystic components that may mimic solid neoplasia on noncontrast studies, and allows localization of the mural nodule in tumors composed primarily of a solitary cyst. Very low-grade astrocytomas may have no enhancement after gadolinium. Pre- and post-gadolinium–DTPA MR studies are important for evaluation of these patients after surgical resection, since postoperative gliosis and encephalomalacia may be difficult to differentiate from residual tumor on noncontrast MRI. Enhancement with associated mass effect suggests neoplasia, particularly if postsurgical complications such as hematoma and abscess are clinically unlikely. Recent surgical margins may enhance on both CT and MRI, at times rendering differentiation of residual tumor and scar difficult. In this situation, baseline and follow-up scans are important for demonstrating a gradual decline in postsurgical enhancement with time, while that associated with residual or recurrent tumor remains stable or progresses.[18]

About one-half of cerebellar astrocytomas have a typical eccentric hemispheric location. Others arising in the midline, involving both the vermis and hemispheres or directly invading the fourth ventricle, mimic more aggressive tumors such as medulloblastoma or ependymoma. Cystic masses with a mural tumor nodule are typical of cerebellar astrocytoma; however, in older pediatric patients, hemangioblastoma may have a similar appearance. Diffuse astrocytoma without recognizable cysts may mimic other masses such as medulloblastoma and ependymoma.

CT scans of cerebellar astrocytoma classically reveal a cystic eccentric and enhancing mass of the cerebellar hemisphere or vermis.[19,20] The fourth ventricle is displaced rather than invaded, and secondary obstructive hydrocephalus is common. Calcifications may be rec-

ognizable in 10 to 25 percent of tumors; otherwise these masses are hypodense to adjacent brain on noncontrast CT.[19] Other common CT appearances include a solitary large cyst with an associated enhancing mural nodule, or a solid tumor with multiple intrinsic cysts of varying sizes. Less frequently the tumor may be diffuse, ill defined, and entirely solid in radiographic appearance. Enhancement is variable, some tumors demonstrating little or no recognizable enhancement on CT. The margins of the tumor and its relationship to the fourth ventricle may be difficult to define anatomically on CT owing to limited enhancement and associated beam-hardening artifacts. Angiography, although not generally necessary, demonstrates an avascular lateral or posterior compartment mass.

Brain Stem Glioma

Brain stem gliomas are primarily pediatric lesions, accounting for 10 to 15 percent of CNS tumors in children. Most are either astrocytoma or glioblastoma multiforme. The peak age of presentation is 5 to 14 years,[1] although these have been described in children under 1 year of age and in late adulthood.[2] A slight male sex predominance has been noted.[4]

Presenting complaints in children with brain stem tumors are related to infiltration of the parenchyma itself, with hydrocephalus and increased intracranial pressure late findings in approximately two-thirds of patients.[4] Only those with tumors arising near the aqueduct present early with hydrocephalus. Cranial nerve palsies; hemiparesis or quadriparesis; pyramidal syndrome unilaterally or bilaterally; and behavioral problems including somnolence, hyperactivity, emotional lability, and even coma may occur. Additional signs include disorders of eye movement with nystagmus. Ataxia reflects damage to cerebellar crossing fibers in the pons or direct invasion of the cerebellum. Bulbar deficits with difficulty in swallowing, absent gag reflex, and tongue atrophy suggest involvement of the medulla.[4]

Most brain stem neoplasms are of astrocytic origin, and fibrillary or pilocytic types are common. The cells themselves are fibrillated, with the pilocytic pattern of growth imposed by insinuation within preexisting pontine tracts. These tumors may infiltrate normal tracts of the brain stem and cerebellar white matter extensively before secondary deficits occur.[4] Up to 40 percent are frankly malignant, as in glioblastoma multiforme. Brain stem gliomas may be eccentric or may involve virtually the entire brain stem diffusely. Those involving the pons and medulla tend to be more aggressive than those of the midbrain. Extension into the adjacent thalamus from midbrain tumors is common, while those of the pons and medulla eccentrically infiltrate into the cerebellum. Cyst formation occurs in either benign or malignant forms, but hemorrhagic or necrotic cysts are characteristically associated with glioblastoma multiforme. Exophytic growth into the posterior fossa cisterns, particularly the cerebellopontine angle (CPA) and lateral recesses of the fourth ventricle, is present in a minority of cases. A small subset (20 percent) of very benign pilocytic brain stem gliomas have been described that show no mitotic activity or anaplasia and carry an associated prolonged favorable course.[2]

Intrinsic brain stem gliomas generally are not surgically resectable owing to their location and the risk of further damage to the brain stem, although preliminary evidence suggests that the uncommon small, well-localized pilocytic tumors at the cervicomedullary junction may be aggressively resected.[21] Occasionally, exophytic components or a tumor in accessible locations may be decompressed or debulked surgically, but diffuse or malignant tumors benefit little from aggressive resection.[22] Stereotactic biopsy of lesions of the brain stem may be performed with a low risk of complications in experienced hands,[23] providing a histologic confirmation of neoplasia and its type. Although tumor grading from the small sample obtained is difficult, a biopsy confirms neoplasia and prevents a misdiagnosis in patients with disorders such as encephalitis, ischemia, and demyelinating disease. A record of the histologic tumor type and grade is also useful for prognostic purposes. Cysts with mass effect may be decompressed or shunted palliatively, using open or stereotactic techniques. More aggressive forms including glioblastoma multiforme occasionally metastasize via the cerebrospinal fluid (CSF) to the cisterns, ventricles, and spinal canal. Radiation therapy is the mainstay of treatment for brain stem glioma; it has a significant palliative effect and provides longer survival in patients with lower-grade astrocytomas receiving at least 5,000 rads.[24, 25] Radiation therapy is less effective in patients with glioblastoma multiforme.[26] Chemotherapy is an area of active investigation but as yet has been disappointing in both single- and multi-agent trials.[27] In spite of the relatively benign histologic appearance of some brain stem tumors, relentless progression locally is the rule, with increasing neurologic deficits until death.[28] The 5-year survival rate is 20 to 30 percent.[2, 4]

MRI is exquisitely sensitive in detecting brain stem pathology, and allows recognition and characterization of lesions that may be totally inapparent on CT.[29–31] This is particularly true for brain stem tumors that have little associated mass effect or fail to enhance after contrast medium administration (Fig. 9–2). MRI is markedly sensitive for intraparenchymal pathology, eliminates artifact from bone, and can be performed in any plane.[29–31] The cranial and caudal margins of the lesion, extension into adjacent tissues such as the thalamus, and associated cyst formation are readily demonstrated (Fig. 9–3). Lesions of the aqueductal region may be inapparent or may mimic aqueductal stenosis on CT, but on MRI are readily recognizable on the basis of signal intensities and distortion of adja-

cent structures. Downward extension into or adjacent to the cervical spinal cord is readily demonstrated on MRI; thus, high cervical cord and brain stem tumors are better differentiated by MRI than by other imaging modalities. MRI provides direct visualization of the fourth ventricle, which typically is displaced but not invaded by tumor, and of extension laterally into the cerebellum. The superior anatomic definition provided by MRI permits differentiation of normal tissues displaced by exophytic tumor from those directly invaded by neoplasm. Untreated brain stem gliomas rarely hemorrhage spontaneously; thus, the MR demonstration of breakdown products of blood suggests another diagnosis such as hemangioma or arteriovenous malformation rather than tumor.[32]

Gadolinium−DTPA enhancement is useful for defining tumor margins apart from edema analogous to iodinated contrast and CT.[33] On gadolinium MRI as on contrast-enhanced CT, brain stem gliomas may demonstrate no associated enhancement or may infiltrate well beyond the enhancing margins revealed on either examination. Gadolinium is also necessary for MR detection of CSF seeding, which may occur with glioblastoma multiforme and malignant astrocytoma.

On CT, brain stem gliomas characteristically enlarge the normal outline of the brain stem, with secondary displacement of the fourth ventricle and effacement of the adjacent cisterns (Fig. 9–2).[34] On CT without contrast, gliomas are variably hypo-, iso-, or hyperdense compared with normal brain. In the series by Kingsley and Kendall, calcifications and cysts recognizable on CT occurred in 12 percent of brain stem tumors.[20] Those that result in no detectable enhancement may be difficult to recognize on CT, particularly in the lower brain stem where beam-hardening artifacts from adjacent dense bone are prominent. Distortions of the adjacent CSF spaces and ventricular system may point to the tumor location. Before the availability of MRI, CT cisternography was commonly required to confirm the presence and extent of isodense nonenhancing tumors. Approximately half demonstrate mild to moderate enhancement after administration of intravenous contrast material in an inhomogeneous manner.[20] Enhancement may be diffuse, nodular, ring-like, or patchy, thus mimicking non-neoplastic diseases such as vascular malformations and inflammatory processes (Fig. 9–3). There are no consistent CT features that allow differentiation among brain stem gliomas of varying grades, or between brain stem tumors and other disorders such as abscess, demyelination, radionecrosis, arteriovenous malformation (AVM), other kinds of tumor, and infarction.[23]

Deep Basal Ganglia, Thalamic, and Callosal Glioma

Primary tumors of the deep structures of the brain excluding the relatively benign hypothalamic-chiasmal group are uncommon, accounting for approximately 6

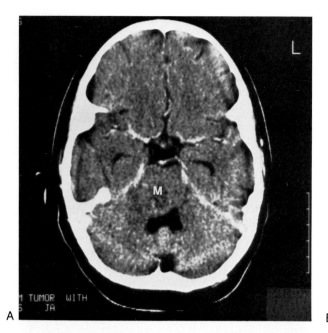

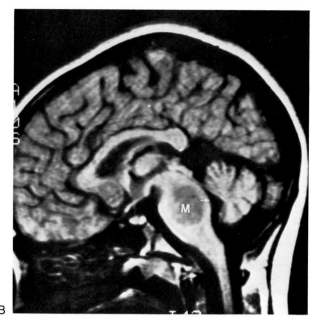

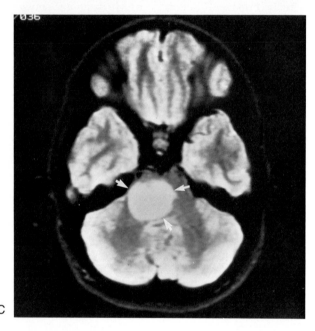

Figure 9–2. *Brain stem astrocytoma.* **A,** Contrast-enhanced CT. An ill-defined inhomogeneous mass is demonstrated in the pons and right middle cerebellar peduncle. **B,** T1 weighted MRI (800/25). The intraaxial pontine mass (M) is hypointense to normal brain and expands the pons with effacement of the fourth ventricle (*arrow*). **C,** T2 weighted MRI (2000/70). The lesion (*arrow*) is homogeneously hyperintense on T2 weighting and is well differentiated from normal parenchyma. With this sequence, tumor and edema are indistinguishable.

percent of primary brain tumors in children.[4] The biologic behavior and patient survival rates vary with the degree of malignancy, although these generally are more aggressive than their midline counterparts arising in the hypothalamus and optic chiasm.

Deep gray and white matter tumors present with headaches and nonspecific symptoms of increased intracranial pressure due to secondary hydrocephalus. Other symptoms and signs are variable and nonspecific, including behavioral changes, emotional lability, memory loss, and speech difficulties. Movement disorders including choreiform movements, tremor, ataxia, and dysmetria may be present owing to inter-

ference with the cerebellorubrothalamic tracts, subthalamus, and basal ganglia.[4, 35] Visual symptoms include field cuts from involvement of the optic pathways or pressure on the midbrain, and visual loss related to hydrocephalus. Unilateral motor weakness suggests involvement of the adjacent internal capsule.

The full range of astrocytic tumors occurs in the deep structures, with approximately an equal distribution between benign pilocytic and malignant astrocytoma–glioblastoma multiforme.[4] Both benign and malignant forms extend by direct infiltration along white matter pathways, especially in the subependymal location, or remotely in the CSF.

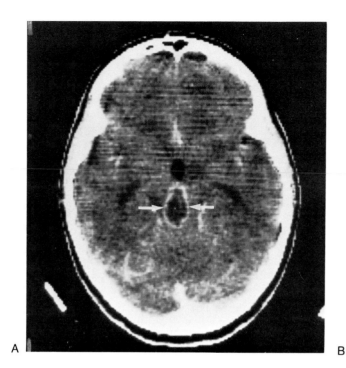

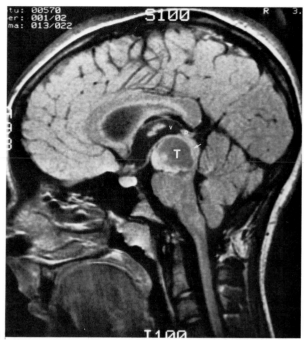

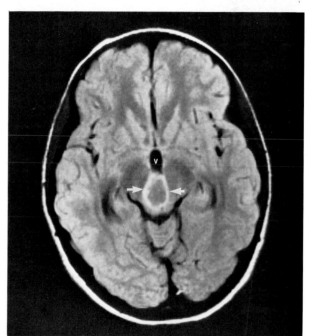

Figure 9–3. *Astrocytoma of the midbrain.* **A,** Contrast-enhanced CT. A ring-enhancing lesion (*arrows*) of the midbrain is partially obscured by artifacts from a stereotactic head holder during CT-guided biopsy. **B,** Sagittal proton density image (1500/20). The relationship of the tumor (T) to the cerebral aqueduct (*arrow*), pineal gland (p), and third ventricle (v) is better demonstrated on MRI. **C,** Axial proton density image (2000/20). A hyperintense midbrain lesion (*arrows*) results in effacement of the posterior third ventricle (v) and hydrocephalus.

Primary treatment of these tumors is radiation therapy after a confirmatory biopsy. A tissue diagnosis is important in order to exclude non-neoplastic lesions such as infarction, demyelinating disease, and encephalitis, which may have an identical presentation and imaging appearance. These infiltrative tumors are not usually resectable owing to their location, with some evidence suggesting that extensive resection provides no significant prolongation of survival.[36] A variety of chemotherapeutic agents have been employed with little documented success, although investigations seeking better combinations and methods of administration of chemotherapy continue. The overall prognosis for survival approaches 50 percent at 5 years for patients with histologically benign tumors; there are very few 5-year survivors with malignant tumors.[36]

Thalamic and basal ganglia tumors are readily recognizable as hyperintense, homogeneous deep masses distorting normally recognizable gray matter nuclei of this region on T2 weighted MRI. Multiplanar T1 weighted images may better define anatomic contrast between the tumor and adjacent CSF of the third ventricle and cisterns (Fig. 9–4). These tumors are iso- to mildly hypointense with T1 weighting; cystic regions and spontaneous hemorrhage are uncommon. Corpus callosal lesions expand and distort the corpus callosum and extend variably bilaterally into the hemispheres (Fig. 9–5). Gadolinium–DTPA is a useful adjunct for tumors that actively disrupt the blood-brain barrier; however, CT studies reveal that approximately half of the low-grade and malignant thalamic astrocytomas have no associated enhancement.[33, 36] Subependymal, cisternal, and spinal seeding into the CSF, which may develop with these malignant conditions, enhances with gadolinium (Fig. 9–5).

The MR appearance of this group of astrocytic tumors is not specific. Other glial and primitive neuroectodermal tumors (PNET) may be encountered in this area, and non-neoplastic disorders including encephalitis, infarction, and demyelinating disease may have an identical MR appearance (Fig. 9–6). For this reason, MRI has not eliminated the need for a tissue diagnosis via open or stereotactic biopsy.

On CT, thalamic and basal ganglia tumors are typically ill-defined hypo- or isodense masses that are primarily recognizable by distortion of the adjacent parenchyma or CSF spaces. Some benign or malignant tumors demonstrate contrast enhancement, but those with less associated blood-brain barrier disruption are difficult to localize and quantitate on CT. Before the

development of MRI, CT cisternography was commonly required to define the extent of these lesions.

Hypothalamic–Optic Chiasmal Glioma

Hypothalamic and optic chiasmal origin tumors are usually low-grade midline tumors that carry a better prognosis than other supratentorial astrocytomas. These are grouped together since they may be indistinguishable clinically, radiographically, and pathologically.[2] The optic chiasm and hypothalamus are in close anatomic proximity, and neoplasms of this area readily extend along normal neural tracts between these tissues. Gliomas originating in the optic pathways represent 3 to 5 percent of intracranial tumors in children. Approximately half the children with optic glioma have neurofibromatosis, while about 3 to 10 percent of children with neurofibromatosis have optic pathway glioma.[4, 37, 38] The peak incidence is between ages 2 and 6 years, and 75 percent occur within the first decade of life.[39] The association of these tumors with neurofibromatosis may be underestimated because of the difficulty in confirming this diagnosis in very small children.

These tumors usually are juvenile pilocytic astrocytomas and rarely are histologically malignant in children, although malignancy has been described in adults.[40, 41] They are composed of mature astrocytes without anaplasia. Pilocytic forms develop when fibril-

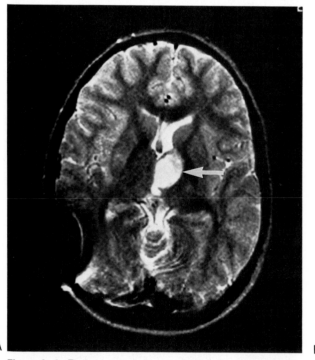
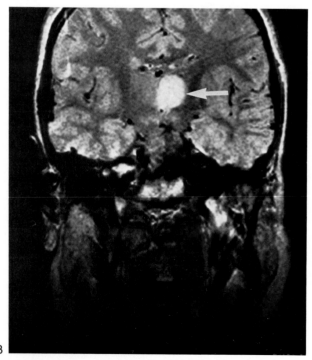

A   B

Figure 9–4. *Thalamic astrocytoma.* **A, B,** Axial (1900/90) and coronal (1800/30) images. A focal lesion (*arrow*) of the thalamus results in a mass effect on the third ventricle, with secondary hydrocephalus requiring shunting.

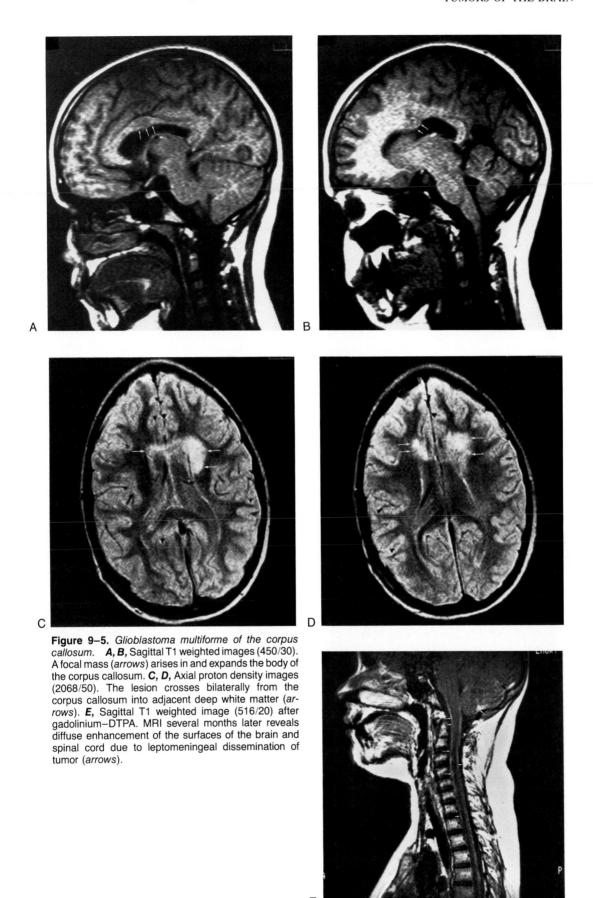

Figure 9–5. *Glioblastoma multiforme of the corpus callosum.* **A, B,** Sagittal T1 weighted images (450/30). A focal mass (*arrows*) arises in and expands the body of the corpus callosum. **C, D,** Axial proton density images (2068/50). The lesion crosses bilaterally from the corpus callosum into adjacent deep white matter (*arrows*). **E,** Sagittal T1 weighted image (516/20) after gadolinium–DTPA. MRI several months later reveals diffuse enhancement of the surfaces of the brain and spinal cord due to leptomeningeal dissemination of tumor (*arrows*).

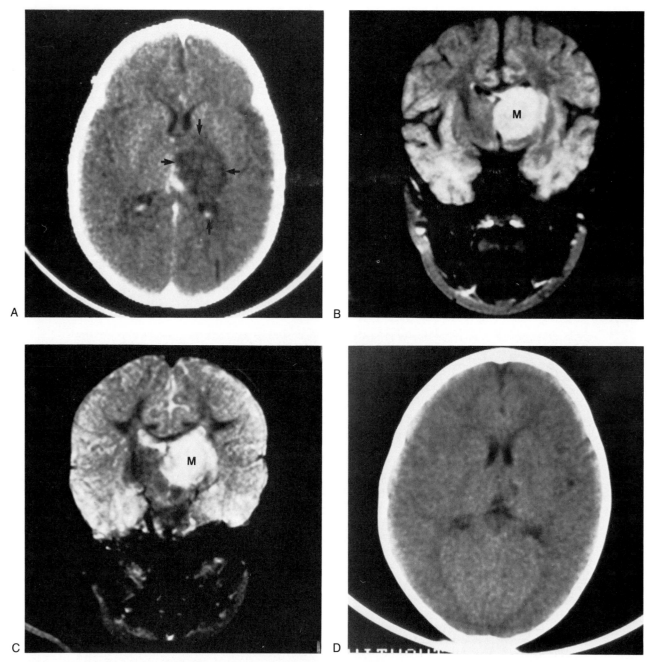

Figure 9–6. *Presumed encephalitis mimicking neoplasia. A 2-year-old girl with subacute onset of nausea, vomiting, and right hemiparesis.* **A,** Contrast-enhanced CT. A hypodense nonenhancing lesion (*arrows*) is present in the left thalamus that is suggestive of glioma. **B, C,** Coronal proton density and T2 weighted images (2000/50, 2000/100). The thalamic mass (M) is uniformly hyperintense to adjacent normal brain. **D,** Noncontrast CT. A follow-up CT 4 weeks later demonstrates spontaneous near-resolution of the mass without intervening therapy; thus, this mass is not neoplastic in etiology.

lary astrocytomas are forced into elongated parallel forms owing to constraints by the surrounding tissues, such as white matter tracts.[2] Piloid or pilocytic tumors are those growing along tracts of nerve processes with secondary long parallel alignment of the astrocytic cell processes. Microcysts are common, although grossly apparent cysts and spontaneous hemorrhage are infrequently noted without histologic evidence of malig-

nancy. Although grossly these tumors are well defined, direct infiltration into adjacent deep gray matter and infiltration of the meninges are common pathologically.

Hypothalamic infiltration by astrocytoma results in a spectrum of clinical abnormalities primarily of an endocrinologic nature. These include diabetes insipidus, growth failure, hypoglycemia, obesity, lethargy, precocious or delayed puberty, and accelerated long bone growth. Occasionally these children present with the diencephalic syndrome, a sign-symptom complex referring to a euphoric but emaciated child, typically less than 3 years old, with a voracious appetite due to a hypothalamic tumor.[42, 43]

Visual signs and symptoms predominate in tumors of the optic pathways, although involvement of both optic pathways and hypothalamus frequently results in a combination of visual and hypothalamic symptoms.[44, 45] Small children may have abnormal eye movements without overt visual deficits. Nystagmus is common with chiasmal involvement. Tumors confined to the optic nerve generally occur with neurofibromatosis and result in proptosis, unilateral visual loss, and optic atrophy. Infiltration of the optic pathways is associated with variable patterns of visual loss; thus, children with sizable chiasmal masses may have significant preservation of vision. Large tumors of this region result in secondary obstructive hydrocephalus.

An ongoing controversy continues over the natural history of these tumors in patients with neurofibromatosis. Some investigators suggest that the biologic behavior of this tumor in neurofibromatosis is more akin to that of a hamartoma than to a true neoplasia; accordingly, therapy should be limited or omitted.[37, 38, 44] A summary of the literature by Cohen and Duffner, however, suggests that approximately half will follow a prolonged benign course and that no clear predictors allow differentiation of this group from those with a more aggressive course.[4] Very young children with large chiasmal-hypothalamic tumors at presentation may have a poorer prognosis than older children in whom such tumors are smaller at presentation.[45] Tenny and colleagues report a 5-year survival rate of 50 percent for patients with lesions of the chiasm and posterior optic pathways, although long-term survivors with anterior or posterior pathway tumors are well known.[46]

Management of children with hypothalamic-chiasmal tumors is controversial because of the unpredictable course of these tumors.[37] Some authors advocate an approach of observation without treatment, while others point to evidence of stabilization of progression after radiation therapy.[47] Surgical approaches also vary; large tumors that infiltrate deeply may be biopsied or debulked to a limited degree. Those confined to the optic nerve with significant secondary visual loss and sparing of the chiasm may be completely resected.[46]

MR examination of children with hypothalamic or optic pathway gliomas reveals frank enlargement of the involved structures on coronal T1 weighted images, with a signal intensity often iso- or slightly hypointense compared with normal brain (Fig. 9–7).[48–52] Deep extension of these lesions into the thalami, basal ganglia, and optic radiations is best demonstrated with multiplanar T2 weighted sequences (Figs. 9–8, 9–9). MRI may also reveal previously unsuspected paren-

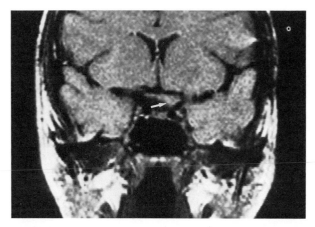

Figure 9–7. *Optic chiasmal glioma.* Coronal T1 weighted MRI (600/50). The optic chiasm is focally enlarged (*arrow*) owing to a small chiasmal glioma.

chymal neoplasia, gliomatosis, or hamartomas in children with neurofibromatosis (Figs. 9–9, 9–10).[48] MRI noninvasively provides the anatomic detail of the suprasellar cistern necessary to localize these lesions for surgical or therapeutic planning. MR examinations of lesions involving the chiasm should include the orbits, since optic chiasmal lesions commonly involve the intraorbital optic nerves (Fig. 9–11).

Enhancement after gadolinium is variable: some masses enhance intensely and others minimally (Figs. 9–10, 9–12). Even those with intense enhancement are histologically low-grade tumors, so that the degree of enhancement has little correlation with the degree of malignancy.

The differential diagnosis for homogeneous, solid infiltrating masses that enlarge and infiltrate the optic pathways and hypothalamus is limited, with deep midline astrocytoma by far the most likely diagnosis. Ependymoma arising from the third ventricle can mimic these lesions, but rarely infiltrates and enlarges the hypothalamus and optic chiasm. Hypothalamic hamartoma, an uncommon lesion presenting with precocious puberty, requires biopsy for differentiation from astrocytoma. An example has been reported of a large childhood meningioma of the chiasm with no apparent dural origin that mimicked chiasmal glioma.[53] Craniopharyngioma is usually cystic and displaces, rather than infiltrates, the optic chiasm. Suprasellar germinoma is uncommon but may appear solid and infiltrating and may enhance in a manner similar to that of a hypothalamic glioma. Masses arising within the third ventricle or within the sella present little diagnostic difficulty owing to the superb anatomic information depicted by MRI.

On CT, chiasmal and hypothalamic masses result in a full appearance of the suprasellar cistern with variable enhancement. Orbital extension is readily identified, but contrast CT provides only a limited evaluation of intracranial disease.[54–56] Direct coronal scans are

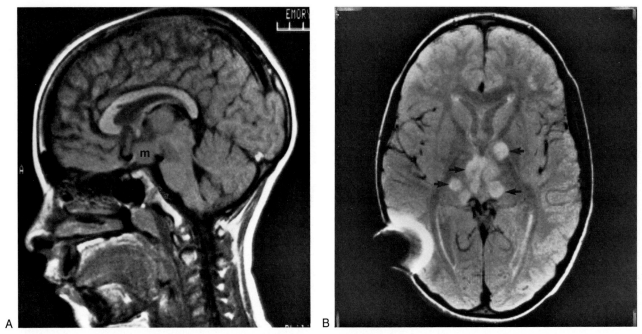

Figure 9–8. *Hypothalamic-chiasmal glioma.* **A,** Sagittal T1 weighted image (500/30). A focal mass (M) enlarges and obscures definition of the chiasm and hypothalamus. On this image the suprasellar mass is readily distinguishable from the pituitary gland and sellar structures below. **B,** Axial proton density image (2000/30). The parenchymal extension of this lesion (*arrow*) into the thalamus bilaterally was not appreciated with T1 weighting.

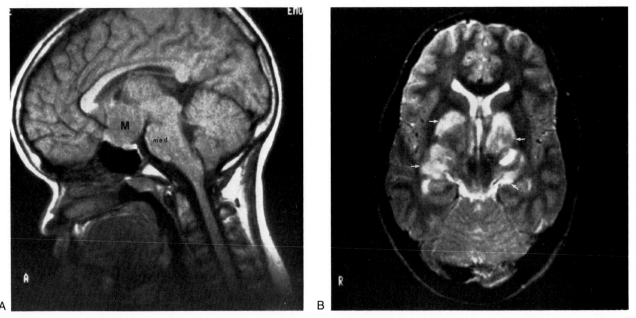

Figure 9–9. *Neurofibromatosis 1 and hypothalamic-chiasmal glioma.* **A,** Sagittal T1 weighted image (499/29). A clinically suspected extensive hypothalamic and chiasmal mass (M) is demonstrated. The focal enlargement of the medulla (med) was clinically silent and may represent hamartoma-gliosis or an asymptomatic glioma. **B,** Axial T2 weighted image (2015/90). Extensive infiltration (*arrows*) of deep gray matter posteriorly to the level of the optic tracts and adjacent to the tumor is best evaluated with T2 weighted images.

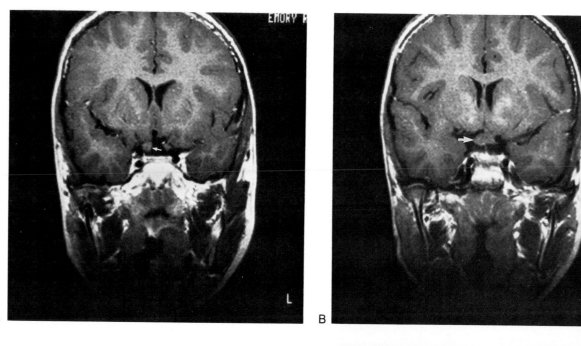

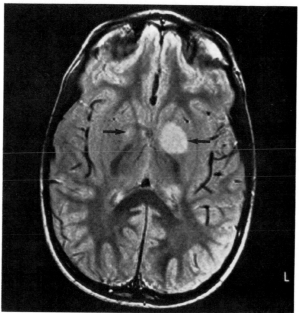

Figure 9–10. *Extensive optic pathway glioma and neurofibromatosis 1.* ***A, B,*** *Coronal T1 weighted images with gadolinium–DTPA (700/20). Focal enlargement of the right intracranial optic nerve (*small arrow*) and of the chiasm (*large arrow*) is demonstrated. Note the absence of enhancement of this low-grade neoplasm after gadolinium administration.* ***C,*** *Axial proton density weighted image (1900/20). Additional lesions (*arrows*) of the striate nuclei bilaterally were inapparent on T1 weighted imaging.*

required to differentiate these suprasellar masses from third ventricular or sellar masses; before the development of MRI detailed CT cisternography was necessary for surgical planning. On CT, hypothalamic-chiasmal masses are more difficult to differentiate from craniopharyngioma than on MRI, and the suprasellar cisternal anatomy is not as well demonstrated. Angiography, infrequently required for evaluation of these patients, reveals a hypovascular to avascular mass with secondary displacement of the vessels around the circle of Willis. A moyamoya appearance with stenosis or occlusion of the supraclinoid internal carotid arteries and associated parenchymal infarcts has been described with or without previous radiation therapy.[45,57,58]

Hemispheric Supratentorial Astrocytoma

Supratentorial tumors of the pediatric population account for up to 55 percent of CNS primary tumors, and most of these are astrocytoma.[2,4] Deep midline

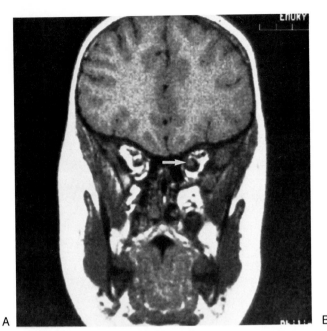

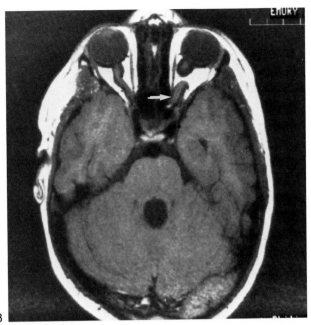

Figure 9–11. *Optic nerve glioma.* **A, B,** Coronal and axial T1 weighted images (566/20). Diffuse enlargement of the left optic nerve (*arrow*) is revealed in this 12-year-old boy. The anatomic extent of the glioma is mapped on MRI; thus, more invasive techniques such as CT cisternography are avoided.

tumors have a slightly better prognosis than hemispheric tumors. Prognosis varies with the location and degree of malignancy of these neoplasms.

Gross examination of hemispheric astrocytoma reveals a diffusely infiltrating, ill-defined tumor of white

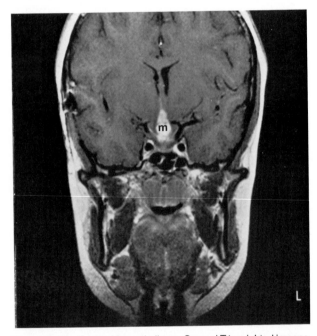

Figure 9–12. *Optic chiasmal glioma.* Coronal T1 weighted images after gadolinium–DTPA (516/20). An intensely enhancing chiasmal mass (m) is seen in the suprasellar cistern. An old craniotomy site is present on the right.

and gray matter, or a discrete mass, perhaps with one or more cysts. A particularly well-defined cystic benign astrocytoma with a mural tumor nodule carries an excellent prognosis after resection, analogous to its counterpart in the cerebellum. Hemispheric astrocytomas may occur anywhere in the supratentorial region, although relatively few involve the occipital lobes.[2] These lesions may infiltrate deep gray matter nuclei or cross the midline in the corpus callosum and septum pellucidum. Necrosis and hemorrhage occur in proportion to foci of anaplasia within the tumor.[2]

Lower-grade tumors are usually fibrillary in nature, although focal areas of pilocytic or gemistocytic astrocytoma are common. Microscopically, most astrocytomas are inhomogeneous, often including nonastrocytic elements such as oligodendroglia. Protoplasmic astrocytes are generally restricted to gray matter, especially of the cerebral cortex. Astrocytes that have a swollen cytoplasm with short, thick processes are referred to as gemistocytic and generally connote a more aggressive tumor. Piloid or pilocytic tumors are typical of deep midline astrocytomas rather than hemispheric lesions. Protoplasmic astrocytoma is uncommon in relatively pure form, with the exception of superficial temporal lobe masses; it commonly contains foci of cystic degeneration. Fibrillary astrocytomas are more commonly hemispheric in adults than in children.[2] These tumors form glial fibrils, resulting in a firm texture with occasional cyst formation, and usually push adjacent neural structures without destroying them. Foci of anaplasia are common microscopic findings within an otherwise low-grade astrocytoma, and may evolve over time. Associated with anaplasia are necrosis, spontaneous hemorrhage, nuclear pleomorphism, frequent mitotic figures, and increased cellularity.

Presenting complaints in children with astrocytoma include headache, evidence of increased intracranial pressure, seizures, and neurologic deficits related to the tumor location.[4] Seizure activity is greatest with tumors located in the temporal lobes or sensorimotor cortex, and is more problematic in benign than in malignant tumors.[4, 59] Headaches, increased intracranial pressure, neurologic deficits, focality of seizure disorders, or a change in seizure frequency suggests a structural lesion such as astrocytoma as the cause.[60, 61] The most complete surgical resection possible is the initial treatment of choice for most astrocytomas, followed by radiation therapy to the tumor bed. A possible exception is the malignant astrocytoma–glioblastoma multiforme, which has a very poor prognosis in spite of surgical resection. An incomplete surgical resection of this lesion results in palliation at best; thus, in this case, a limited biopsy followed by radiation therapy is an option.[62, 63] Low-grade hemispheric astrocytomas, excluding deep midline tumors, have about a 30 to 40 percent 5-year survival, compared with a survival of less than 20 percent for higher-grade tumors.[2, 64] Notably, most of the survivors in this group have grade III astrocytomas, with a maximum of 5 to 10 percent 5-year survival in grade IV astrocytoma and glioblastoma multiforme. Trials with a variety of chemotherapeutic agents are ongoing, but to date little objective palliation has been achieved. Astrocytoma typically recurs at the site of the primary tumor, although malignant astrocytoma may seed to the sub-arachnoid space or rarely may metastasize extraneurally. Extraneural metastases to lung and lymph nodes have been described, less commonly to bone and liver.[4] Accessible recurrences may be palliatively treated with repeat surgery, although dedifferentiation into higher-grade tumors is common. CSF seeding is common with glioblastoma multiforme but is often overshadowed clinically by progression of the primary tumor.[2]

MRI is very sensitive for detection of hemispheric tumors of all grades and may demonstrate lesions that are undetectable on CT.[65–68] These lesions are homogeneous or inhomogeneous, and hypointense to isointense to normal brain on T1 weighted images (Figs. 9–13, 9–14). T2 weighting reveals a hyperintense mass with borders that are inseparable from surrounding edema. Calcifications are underestimated or inapparent on MRI,[17] but MRI is very sensitive for detection of subacute or chronic hemorrhage in more aggressive tumors that may not be apparent on CT. Multiplanar MRI with thin slices and flow compensatory sequences provides the unique ability to detect subtle lesions such as temporal lobe masses.[65, 68] Although MRI is very sensitive for lesion detection and localization, tissue confirmation remains necessary, since many neoplastic and non-neoplastic lesions have a similar MR appearance.

Gadolinium enhancement should be included in the MR evaluation of these tumors to better define tumor margins, to assess CSF seeding in malignancy, and to better differentiate tumor from edema or sequelae of therapy.[69–71] Low-grade astrocytoma may result in no

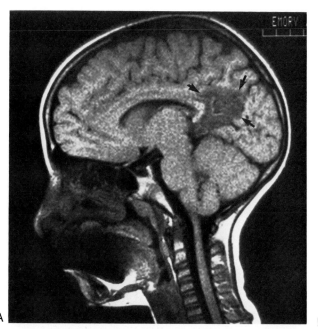

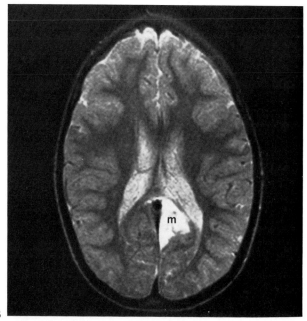

A   B

Figure 9–13. *Low-grade hemispheric astrocytoma.* **A,** Sagittal T1 weighted image (575/20). A focal, well-circumscribed hypointense mass (*arrows*) is defined in the medial occipital lobe. **B,** Axial T2 weighted image (2068/100). The mass (M) is hyperintense, well circumscribed, and relatively homogeneous with little associated edema or displacement of normal structures.

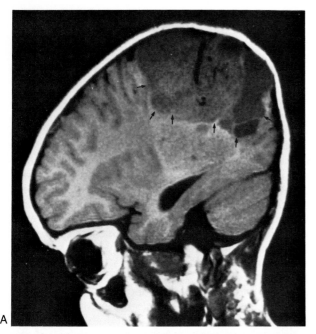
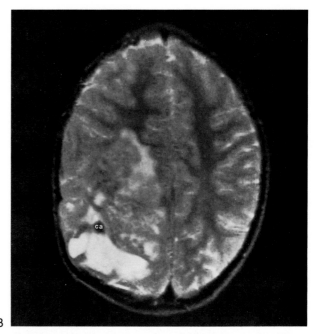

A B

Figure 9–14. *Glioblastoma multiforme.* **A,** Sagittal T1 weighted image (500/20). A large, inhomogeneous, cystic, and calcified hemispheric mass (*arrows*) has involved and expanded the adjacent calvarium. **B,** Axial T2 weighted image (2000/90). The inhomogeneous hyperintense mass contains a focal hypointense region area of calcification (Ca).

recognizable enhancement with gadolinium–DTPA, presumably owing to minimal or absent disruption of the blood-brain barrier (Fig. 9–15).

Before the development of MRI, CT was the imaging modality of choice to evaluate hemispheric astrocytoma. The sensitivity of CT is limited in small lesions, superficial lesions that may be masked by adjacent bone artifacts, and nonenhancing lesions with little mass effect. In addition, CT is performed in axial or coronal planes only. The advantages of CT include more rapid scanning and increased sensitivity to acute hemorrhage and calcification. Hemispheric astrocytomas enhance variably and calcifications are common, particularly in lower-grade tumors.

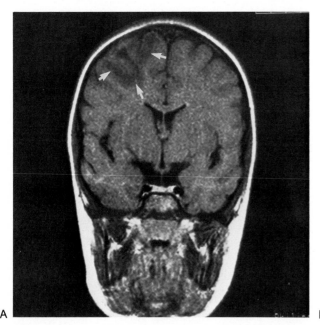
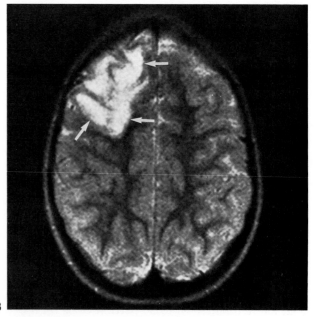

A B

Figure 9–15. *Low-grade hemispheric astrocytoma.* **A,** Coronal T1 weighted image after gadolinium enhancement (680/30). A well-defined, hypointense, hemispheric mass (*arrows*) has no recognizable enhancement. **B,** T2 weighted image (2208/100). The extent of this intra-axial mass (*arrows*) is better demonstrated.

MEDULLOBLASTOMA

Medulloblastoma is predominantly a tumor of childhood and represents approximately 25 percent of pediatric intracranial tumors. Approximately half occur in the first decade, with a second peak at ages 20 to 24 years.[2] A male predominance of up to 4:3 has been described, with a mean age at presentation of 6.5 years.[64,72] Medulloblastoma occurring in adulthood may have a more benign course and a better prognosis. Medulloblastoma occurs only in the posterior fossa, but medulloblastoma and other histologically similar tumors occurring elsewhere have been grouped in the general category of primitive neuroectodermal tumors.[73,74] Although medulloblastoma typically occurs sporadically without a genetic or familial association, it has occasionally been described in families. Other associations include nevoid basal cell carcinoma syndrome (Gorlin's syndrome), Turcot's syndrome (glioma-polyposis), ataxia-telangiectasia, xeroderma pigmentosum, and blue rubber-bleb nevus syndrome.[2] No conclusive data link medulloblastoma to neurofibromatosis, viral exposure, or occupational-environmental exposures,[75] although a seasonal predilection has been described.[76]

Medulloblastoma commonly produces symptoms related to increased intracranial pressure from hydrocephalus such as morning vomiting with or without nausea.[2,77] Visual loss from increased intracranial pressure tends to be unreported or unnoticed until quite advanced. Cerebellar or pyramidal syndromes from extension outside the fourth ventricle may be prominent. An abnormal head position may be noted, as may neuropathies of the sixth and seventh cranial nerves. Occasionally a fulminant course develops with frank coma or intratumoral hemorrhage. Additional neurologic deficits may be present at diagnosis owing to the propensity of this tumor to spread along CSF pathways of the brain and spinal cord.

Therapy is directed at as complete a surgical resection as possible, since a complete resection is associated with a better prognosis. After resection, craniospinal radiation is performed, with a higher dose to the posterior fossa.[78] Chemotherapy should be considered in order to delay radiation therapy in very young children, or for recurrences. Tumor staging does not necessarily correlate with prognosis.[79,80] Overall 5-year survival with surgical resection followed by radiation therapy ranges from 40 to 80 percent; late recurrences result in a reduced 10-year survival of about 40 to 50 percent.[2] The quality of life of surviving children, particularly young children, may be adversely affected by the neoplasm itself or by sequelae of therapy.[81] The prognosis is generally poorer for children in whom the condition is diagnosed in the first 2 years of life.[76] Recurrences occur locally at sites of incomplete resection, and ultimately 10 to 50 percent of patients develop spinal metastases.[2] These remote deposits may directly invade parenchyma, or cross into the subdural space by direct extension or by growth along perivascular sheaths of blood vessels. Medulloblastoma may seed via a ventricular shunt to the pleura or peritoneum. Other extraneural metastases are uncommon (5 percent), but reported sites include bone, bone marrow, lymph nodes, and occasionally liver and lungs.[2]

Medulloblastoma is a soft, friable, predominantly midline neoplasm of the vermis and adjacent cisterna magna that commonly occupies and obscures the fourth ventricle. It often arises in the inferior vermis. Rarely, cysts, calcifications, and necrosis are noted before therapy. Spontaneous hemorrhage occasionally occurs at presentation. Medulloblastoma may extend eccentrically into the cerebellar hemispheres, the cerebellopontine angle (CPA), or the brain stem. Although medulloblastoma appears well circumscribed on gross examination, the adjacent tissues are diffusely invaded on microscopic views.[82] Histologically, medulloblastoma appears as an extremely cellular tumor of predominantly hyperchromatic small cells with frequent mitoses and leptomeningeal invasion. Occasional neuronal differentiation accounts for its histologic similarity to neuroblastoma. The cell of origin of this tumor is generally thought to be a germinal cell of the medullary epithelium, although the fetal granular layer of Obersteiner or rests of primitive cells in the posterior medullary velum have been implicated.[2] More mature differentiated tumors are termed ganglioneuroma (gangliocytoma) and ganglioglioma.[2]

A desmoplastic variant of medulloblastoma with a substantial component of fibrous connective tissue tends to be eccentric and more commonly occurs in older patients. This variant has been said to carry a slightly better prognosis than the more common variety of early childhood, although recent series, including that of Packer and colleagues, discount this.[83,84] Other studies suggesting that the degree of differentiation of the medulloblastoma correlates with prognosis have not been confirmed.[84] Desmoplastic medulloblastoma extends laterally from the fourth ventricle or arises primarily in the cerebellar hemisphere more often than the classic childhood form of medulloblastoma.[82]

Other variants of medulloblastoma recognized by the World Health Organization classification include medullomyoblastoma, which contains muscle fibers, and medulloepithelioma, with large undifferentiated cells resembling primitive neural or medullary epithelium.[82] An uncommon melanotic variant of medulloblastoma has been described.[2] A distinct cerebellar tumor that is indistinguishable from supratentorial neuroblastoma is generally considered a subgroup of medulloblastoma. These rare variants are clinically similar in behavior to typical medulloblastoma.

MR imaging of medulloblastoma demonstrates a midline posterior fossa mass arising in or adjacent to the fourth ventricle with variable eccentricity (Fig. 9–16). On T1 weighted images, medulloblastoma re-

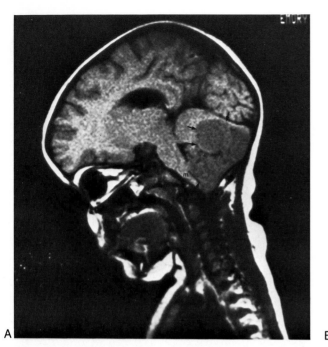
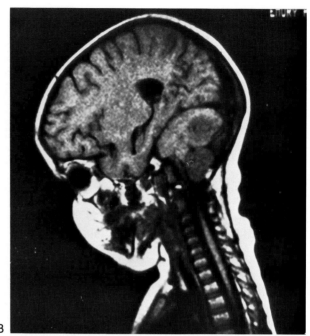

A   B

Figure 9–16. *Medulloblastoma.* ***A, B,*** Adjacent sagittal T1 weighted images (700/30). A hypointense mass (*arrows*) involves the inferior medullary velum of the fourth ventricle and extends into the cerebellar vermis and hemisphere. The medulla (m) is displaced anteriorly. An ependymoma might have an identical appearance on MRI.

sults in a well-defined mass that is iso- or hypointense compared with normal parenchyma. Multiplanar T1 weighted images provide excellent contrast between soft tissues and CSF, and thus anatomic distortions of posterior fossa structures and tumor growth within the fourth ventricle are well seen. The signal intensities of both tumor and associated parenchymal edema are increased on proton density and T2 weighted images in comparison with normal brain, so that tumor margins and edema are often difficult to differentiate. Uncommonly, spontaneous intratumoral hemorrhage at presentation results in an increased signal from methemoglobin on T1 and T2 weighted images with associated variable areas of signal loss attributable to deoxyhemoglobin (most evident on T2 weighted images) or hemosiderin in the subacute phase (Fig. 9–17). Obstructive hydrocephalus is frequent. Atypical features of medulloblastoma are common, rendering confident differentiation of this tumor from other posterior fossa masses difficult (Fig. 9–18).[85]

Subarachnoid and subependymal dissemination of tumor may be present initially or upon follow-up of these patients. Occasionally CSF metastases are nodular and masslike or alter CSF intensities sufficiently for recognition on T1 weighted images (Fig. 9–19).[86, 87] Leptomeningeal metastases are often inapparent on T2 weighted images owing to masking of high-intensity lesions by CSF. Less extensive seeding with diffuse coating of the brain and dura or small nodules lacking mass effect may be underestimated or entirely inapparent on noncontrast MRI (see CNS metastases below). Subependymal spread of tumor may blend with

periventricular signal abnormalities due to hydrocephalus and/or radiation therapy and similarly be overlooked on noncontrast MRI.

MR studies of patients with medulloblastoma both at presentation and at follow-up should be performed with intravascular contrast enhancement. Medulloblastoma enhances moderately to markedly on T1 weighted images after administration of gadolinium–DTPA owing to enhancement of areas of blood-brain barrier disruption.[33] This enhancement permits gross definition of tumor margins apart from secondary parenchymal edema, which is problematic on noncontrast MR studies. Gadolinium–DTPA enhancement is also helpful for differentiation of tumor from postoperative changes based on the morphology of the enhancing lesions and the progression of enhancement on sequential studies. Early in the postoperative period, differentiation between residual tumor, postoperative enhancement, and surgical complications such as infection or hematoma may be difficult, requiring follow-up examination or occasionally surgical exploration.[18] Leptomeningeal seeding that may be entirely hidden on noncontrast studies enhances with gadolinium–DTPA and is readily recognizable (Fig. 9–20).

CT scans performed without contrast material reveal medulloblastoma as a slightly hyperdense midline posterior fossa solid mass with marked enhancement, either homogeneously or inhomogeneously. It may grow exophytically into the CPA and cisterna magna, or may fill the fourth ventricle. Subarachnoid and subependymal spread in the CSF at diagnosis or upon follow-up

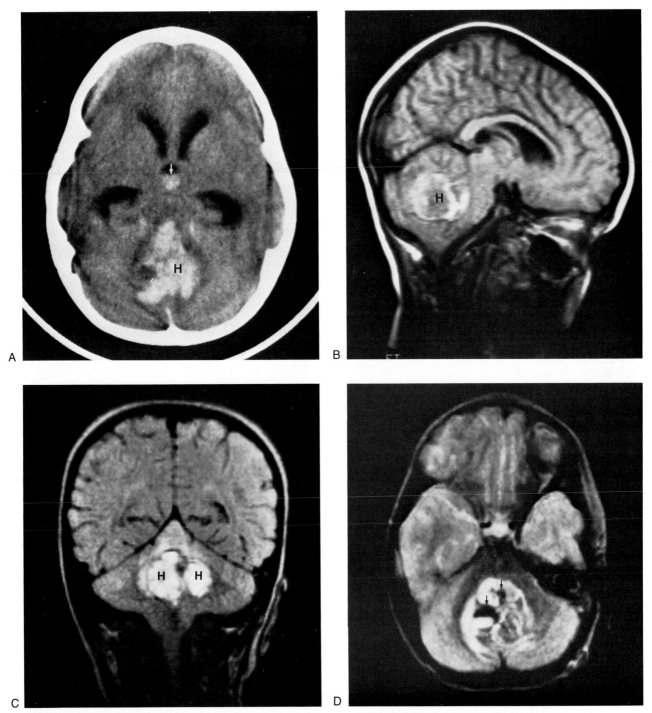

Figure 9–17. *Medulloblastoma. Spontaneous intratumoral and intraventricular hemorrhage at presentation in a 5-year-old boy. Angiography revealed mass effect with no evidence of vascular malformation, and the primary tumor was discovered during surgical exploration for decompression of the hematoma.* **A,** *Noncontrast CT. An extensive midline posterior fossa hemorrhage (H) with reflux into the third ventricle (small arrow) and secondary hydrocephalus is demonstrated. The tumor was obscured by hemorrhage.* **B, C,** *Sagittal and coronal T1 weighted images (900/26). An inhomogeneously hyperintense hematoma (H) expands the fourth ventricle and extends bilaterally into the cerebellum. The slightly hypointense areas centrally and absence of a hypointense peripheral border suggest that this hemorrhage is subacute. The primary tumor is obscured by the hemorrhage.* **D,** *Axial T2 weighted image (2200/100). Central areas of hypointensity (arrow) are present within the mass, suggestive of deoxyhemoglobin related to a subacute hemorrhage.*

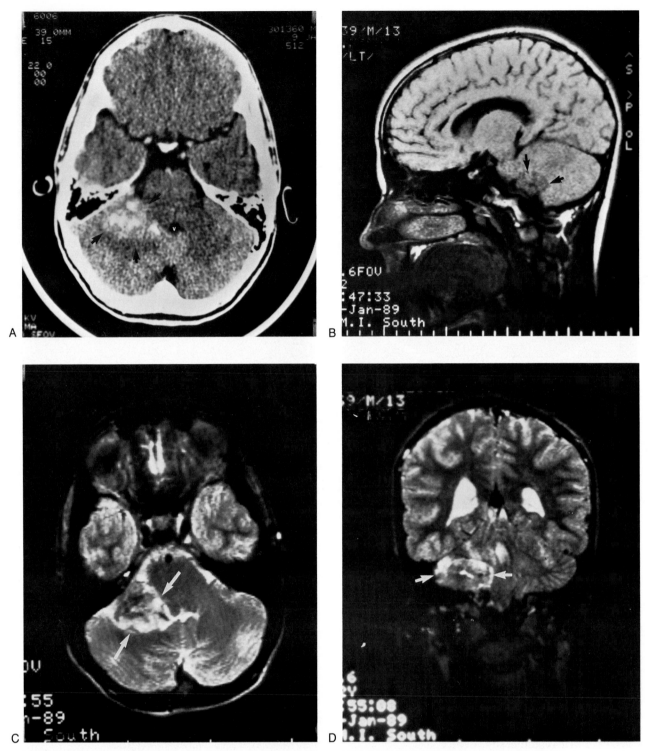

Figure 9–18. *Desmoplastic medulloblastoma.* ***A,*** Contrast-enhanced CT. A calcified and enhancing eccentric mass (*arrows*) has its medial margin adjacent to the fourth ventricle (v). ***B,*** Parasagittal T1 weighted image (517/33). A slightly hypointense mass (*arrows*) is seen eccentrically in the region of the middle cerebellar peduncle. ***C, D,*** Axial (2000/96) and coronal (2278/120) T2 weighted images. Multiplanar MRI provides additional anatomic localization of this inhomogeneous lesion (*arrows*).

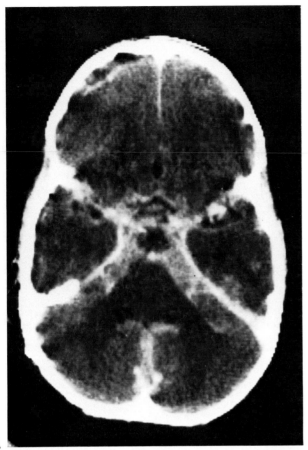
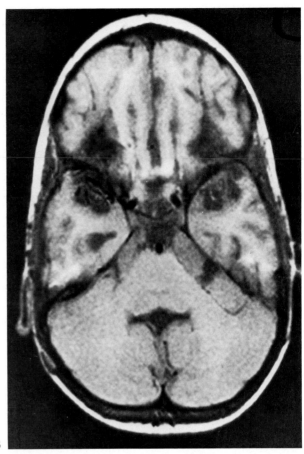

A   B

Figure 9–19. *Disseminated medulloblastoma. A 4-year-old child presented with meningismus and low-grade fever that mimicked an infectious process. Diffuse leptomeningeal dissemination of medulloblastoma had occurred at presentation, and a very tiny primary tumor was identified only on microscopic postmortem examination.* **A,** Contrast-enhanced CT. Marked diffuse enhancement of all cisterns and of the fourth ventricular margins compatible with leptomeningeal metastasis or diffuse basilar meningitis. **B,** T1 weighted axial image (600/30). The cisterns and subarachnoid spaces have a diffuse, abnormally increased intensity.

results in a diffuse or nodular enhancement of meningeal-ependymal surfaces, although superficial meningeal enhancement on CT may be obscured by the overlying dense calvarium.[88, 89] Hydrocephalus is typical at presentation.

Although the above description applies to typical medulloblastoma, one or more atypical features occur often enough for medulloblastoma to be indistinguishable from other posterior fossa neoplasms. Atypical characteristics on CT examination include cyst formation, necrosis, spontaneous hemorrhage, calcifications, eccentricity, direct supratentorial extension, and a lack of recognizable contrast enhancement.[85] These atypical features have been described in up to 47 percent of previously untreated medulloblastoma.

Advantages of multiplanar MRI compared with CT include elimination of beam-hardening artifact from the skull base, resulting in superior visualization of tumor around the inferior fourth ventricle, foramen magnum, and upper cervical spine. The relationship of

the fourth ventricle and the tumor mass are better evaluated on MRI.

The differential diagnosis of medulloblastoma primarily includes ependymoma and cerebellar astrocytoma. Ependymoma most closely mimics medulloblastoma on MRI both in intensity patterns and in location. Intratumoral calcifications favoring ependymoma may not be apparent on MRI, making preoperative differentiation of these lesions difficult. This may have little clinical relevance, however, since surgical resection is the treatment of choice for both tumors. The desmoplastic variant of medulloblastoma in particular mimics other lesions owing to its eccentricity, occasional calcification at presentation, and epicenter remote from the fourth ventricle. Direct invasion of the fourth ventricle favors medulloblastoma over astrocytoma. Occasionally the primary tumor is so small that it may be unrecognizable, and symptoms related to leptomeningeal metastases are the presenting findings (Fig. 9–19).

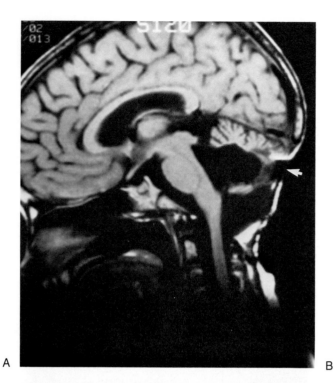

A

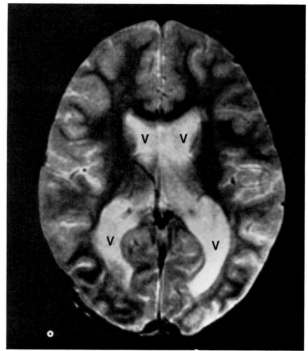

B

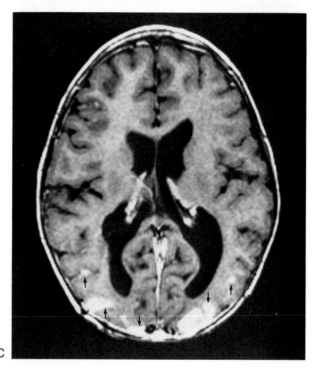

C

Figure 9–20. *Medulloblastoma. A follow-up examination in a 10-year-old girl who had undergone previous surgical resection of medulloblastoma.* **A,** *T1 weighted sagittal image (800/20). The posterior fossa craniotomy (arrow) and site of resection are demonstrated, with no evidence of recurrence.* **B,** *T2 weighted axial image (2000/70). The child has mild ventriculomegaly (V) without definable masses or evidence of recurrence.* **C,** *T1 weighted image (600/20) after gadolinium-DTPA. Multiple focal sulcal enhancing masses (arrows) are now apparent, suggestive of leptomeningeal dissemination. On the last follow-up, the child continued to do well without clinical or CSF evidence of recurrent disease. (Courtesy of the Medical College of Georgia, Department of Radiology, Section of Neuroradiology.)*

EPENDYMOMA AND EPENDYMOBLASTOMA

Ependymoma accounts for approximately 5 to 10 percent of all intracranial tumors and approximately 6 percent of all gliomas.[2,4] It arises from differentiated ependymal cells of any ependymal cell–lined surface.

Choroid plexus lesions, considered by some authors as a subset of ependymoma, are discussed elsewhere. Rests of ependymal cells in the lateral recesses of the fourth ventricle, at other points of sharp angulation of the ventricular surfaces, and at variable distances from the ventricles in the adjacent white matter may account for the common occurrences of ependymoma in the fourth ventricle and in the supratentorial periventricu-lar white matter.[2] About 40 percent arise in the supra-tentorial space and 60 percent in relation to the fourth ventricle.[2] The mean age of incidence is 5 to 7 years, with a peak in the first 2 years of life. Ependymomas occur in both sexes, but a male predominance of 1.7 to 1 has been described for ependymoblastoma.[89] Epen-dymoblastoma is considered a subset of PNET and is an embryonal, aggressive, highly cellular tumor of young children.[90]

Presenting signs and symptoms of posterior fossa ependymomas include those of increased intracranial pressure from hydrocephalus, cerebellar ataxia, and cranial nerve palsies. Pyramidal signs such as hemi-plegia, quadriplegia, and nystagmus are common.[4] Su-pratentorial lesions result in deficits related to their location and malignancy, with secondary seizure disor-ders common. Benign or malignant ependymoma and ependymoblastoma may spread into the CSF, with resultant cord compression or other neurologic defi-cits.

Surgical resection or debulking with shunting as needed for hydrocephalus is routine; the use of subse-quent local or craniospinal radiation depends on the histologic appearance of the tumor and its proximity to the spinal canal. Complete surgical removal of poste-rior fossa ependymomas generally is not possible owing to infiltration of the fourth ventricular floor. Chemotherapy, although under investigation, has thus far been of limited value. It is generally reserved for ependymoblastoma, tumors that seem to be malignant either clinically or histologically, or recurrences after radiation. Histologic malignancy correlates poorly with the clinical course.[2] Overall, intracranial epen-dymoma results in a 5-year survival of 20 to 30 per-cent,[4] with frequent local and CSF recurrences. Spinal seeding develops in approximately 10 percent, with rare extraneural metastases to lymph nodes, lungs, liver, bone marrow, scalp, and diaphragm.[91,92] Median postoperative survival in ependymoblastoma is 12 to 20 months, with very few 3-year survivors.[93]

Ependymoma may occur in association with any ependymal surface, although the roof or floor of the fourth ventricle is a common site of origin.[2] It com-monly infiltrates or fills the fourth ventricle and may extend laterally into the lateral recesses or cerebello-pontine angle, superiorly along the aqueduct, or inferi-orly to the cervical spine. Intraventricular forms may be papillary on gross examination and resemble cho-roid plexus papilloma. Malignant ependymoma of the posterior fossa occasionally presents in infancy.[2] Su-pratentorial ependymoma is histologically malignant more commonly than its posterior fossa counterpart; some series suggest an incidence of malignancy ap-proaching 50 percent.[94] Supratentorial ependymoma may be intraventricular, both intra- and extraventricu-lar, or entirely extraventricular with only a small exten-sion to the ventricular margin. Ependymoblastoma predominantly occurs supratentorially, and aggres-

sively infiltrates adjacent tissues and the leptomen-inges. Subependymoma, possibly of reactive or hamar-tomatous origin, is a subset noted typically in older adults characterized by intraventricular location, mul-tiplicity, lobulated appearance, and benign growth pat-tern.[2] Myxopapillary ependymoma is virtually re-stricted to conus lesions.

Intracranial ependymomas are categorized histo-logically as epithelial, papillary, and cellular, all with a similar prognosis. On microscopic examination, epen-dymomas typically contain ependymal epithelium, ependymal rosettes, and perivascular pseudorosettes. Ependymoma may be extensively cystic, with calcifica-tion present in 44 percent.[91] Histologically noted ma-lignancy such as anaplasia, pleomorphism, and high mitotic rates are uncommon, accounting for approx-imately 5 percent of intracranial ependymomas. More mature malignant forms are termed malignant epen-dymoma, although the histologic appearance does not reliably correlate with survival.[95] Anaplastic or malig-nant ependymoma shows histologic evidence of epen-dymal differentiation and is not synonymous with the embryonal or undifferentiated form of ependymoblas-toma. The term ependymoblastoma is reserved for the largely undifferentiated embryonal form with occa-sional obvious rosettes, a subset of the PNET cate-gory.[90]

To date, there has been no reported large series of MR findings of ependymoma or ependymoblastoma, but limited observations suggest that ependymoma and ependymoblastoma have MR intensity patterns similar to those of other tumors. Variable hypointen-sity on T1 and hyperintensity on T2 are typical. Multi-planar MR images demonstrate those arising in the posterior fossa either within or directly involving the fourth ventricle, with variable lateral and craniocaudal extension. Those arising low in the fourth ventricle, adjacent to the medulla, or extending into the upper cervical spine are better defined on MRI than on CT (Fig. 9–21). Calcifications, although common on CT, are infrequently recognizable on MRI, resulting in difficulty in differentiation of medulloblastoma from ependymoma.

Supratentorial ependymoma has signal characteris-tics similar to its posterior fossa counterpart, with a greater tendency toward associated cyst formation (Fig. 9–22). Calcifications, although common, are of-ten inapparent on MRI. This MR limitation is rela-tively minor, since calcifications are common in other supratentorial neoplasms and are not specific for this tumor. Multiplanar MRI is superior to CT for delinea-tion of the relationship of the neoplasm to the ventricu-lar system, and for surgical and radiation planning. An aggressive, infiltrating, supratentorial tumor with ill-defined borders and associated edema favors the diag-nosis of a more aggressive malignant ependymoma or ependymoblastoma, but on MRI these may be indis-tinguishable from each other and from more benign forms of ependymoma (Fig. 9–23). Gadolinium con-

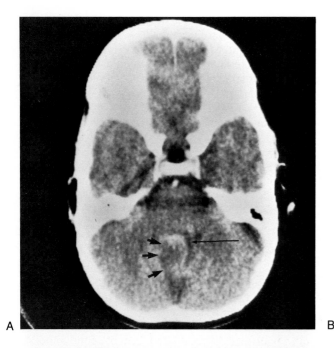

A

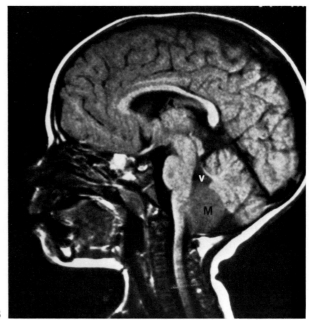

B

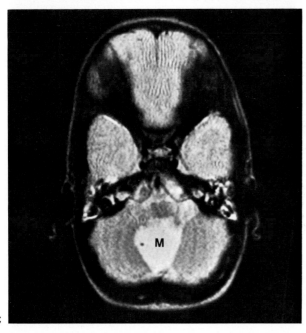

C

Figure 9–21. *Ependymoblastoma. A 1-year-old girl with persistent nausea and vomiting.* ***A,*** Contrast-enhanced CT. Minimal enhancement of a mass in the inferior vermis (*short arrows*) is noted associated with distortion of the adjacent fourth ventricle (*long arrow*). ***B,*** Sagittal T1 weighted image (500/30). A hypointense inferior vermian mass (M) is better shown with invagination of the fourth ventricle (V). ***C,*** Axial T2 weighted image (2500/60). The mass (M) is uniformly hyperintense relative to normal brain.

trast enhancement should be routinely included in the MR evaluation of these tumors because it permits better differentiation of tumor margins from associated edema and from postradiation and postoperative abnormalities.[34] In addition, gadolinium markedly improves the sensitivity of MRI both intracranially and in the spinal canal for detection of metastases to the leptomeninges, a relatively common occurrence in both ependymoma and ependymoblastoma.[96]

The morphologic and intensity patterns of ependymoma on MRI are not specific to this tumor; thus, the differential diagnosis includes medulloblastoma and cerebellar astrocytoma. Supratentorial masses having a similar appearance include other glial series tumors, PNET (especially neuroblastoma), choroid plexus papilloma and carcinoma, or (remotely) intraventricular meningioma.

On noncontrast CT, posterior fossa ependymoma typically is predominantly isodense to brain with focal calcifications. After intravenous contrast enhancement, most of these tumors enhance homogeneously or inhomogeneously, although occasionally no recognizable enhancement occurs.[97] Posterior fossa tumors may be midline within or around the fourth ventricle

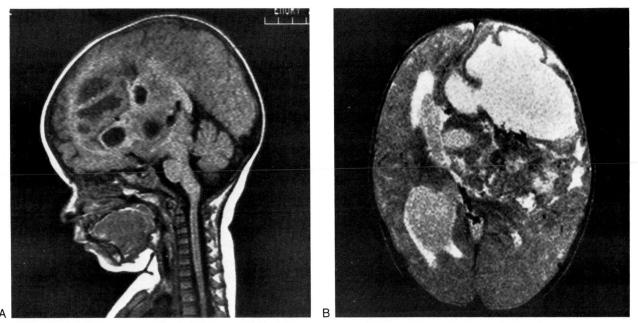

Figure 9–22. *Ependymoma. An 11-month-old girl with extensive, proven supratentorial ependymoma.* **A,** Sagittal T1 weighted image (469/30). An extensive inhomogeneous left frontal lobe mass contains cystic components. **B,** Axial T2 weighted image (2538/100). An extensive inhomogeneous and ill-defined frontal lobe mass has resulted in midline shift and secondary dilatation of the contralateral ventricle.

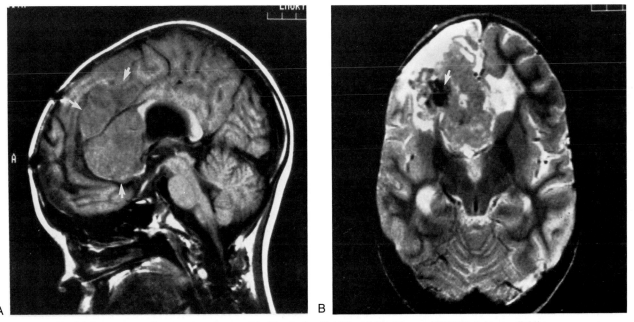

Figure 9–23. *Malignant ependymoma in a 9-year-old girl.* **A,** Sagittal T1 weighted image (566/20). A large, slightly hypointense mass (*arrows*) expands the corpus callosum and displaces the ventricular system posteriorly and inferiorly. **B,** Axial T2 weighted image (2180/80). The mass extends from the corpus callosum eccentrically into the right frontal lobe. Focal hypointense areas (*arrow*) may reflect calcification or sequelae of previous hemorrhage.

or may expand the fourth ventricle; there are rare reports of spontaneous hemorrhage. Eccentricity is not uncommon, and lesions may extend or originate laterally in the cerebellar hemisphere, lateral recesses, or CPA. The extent of these lesions may be difficult to define on CT owing to interference from dense bone artifacts of the skull base. Supratentorial ependymoma more commonly contains recognizable cysts, and approximately half have associated edema and hydrocephalus.[98] Ependymoblastoma is not usually calcified. It enhances moderately to markedly and may be frankly invasive, with ill-defined margins.[98] CT is limited by imaging planes and by beam-hardening artifacts around the skull base, so that MRI may be required as a supplemental examination for anatomic definition of these neoplasms and for therapeutic planning. CSF metastases are commonly hidden on CT, but are well demonstrated by gadolinium-enhanced MRI. Before the availability of the latter, reliable localization of spinal metastases required myelography.

NEUROBLASTOMA AND PRIMITIVE NEUROECTODERMAL TUMORS

First classified in 1973 by Hart and Earle,[74] primitive neuroectodermal tumors (PNET) include several tumors common in children and young adults that have a malignant histologic appearance and a poor prognosis. Most occur within the first decade, approximately one-fourth in infants under 2 years of age.[99] No sex predominance has been noted. PNET may occur anywhere in the neuraxis, including the spinal cord.[99–104]

The PNET categorization is controversial since it includes a variety of histologically distinct tumors in one category;[2] some authors therefore suggest that this terminology be dropped. Primitive tumors without foci of differentiation are termed primary CNS neuroblastoma or medulloblastoma, depending on the tumor location. In particular, Horten and Rubinstein[103] suggest that these purely undifferentiated forms warrant a separate terminology and should not be considered under the broad category of PNET. Medulloblastoma, ependymoblastoma, medulloepithelioma, and pineoblastoma are discussed elsewhere.

Gross examination of neuroblastoma reveals a sharply defined mass that is often lobulated, cystic, or necrotic and not infrequently hemorrhagic.[2, 100] Favored locations include the parietal and occipital lobes.[101] Histologically the tumor appears hypercellular, with at least 90 percent of the tumor composed of small undifferentiated cells having little cytoplasm.[74, 102] Mitoses are numerous, as are foci of necrosis and endothelial hyperplasia. Although the tumor is predominantly undifferentiated, small foci of differentiation into glial or neuronal cell types may be present. Electron microscopy is generally necessary to differentiate neuroblastoma from other primitive neuroectodermal tumors. These aggressive tumors may invade locally, spread within the CSF with neoplastic deposits, or rarely metastasize extraneurally to lung, lymph nodes, liver, diaphragm, and pericardium.[4]

Children with neuroblastoma or other PNET generally show signs and symptoms of increased intracranial pressure related to the large size of these lesions at presentation or related to secondary hydrocephalus. They may be surprisingly free of symptoms and deficits relative to the size of the tumor.[4] The average survival ranges from 5 to 36 months,[2, 74, 99] with a 30 percent survival for neuroblastoma at 5 years.[2, 100] Treatment consists of surgical resection to the extent possible, followed by radiation therapy.[104] A better prognosis has been suggested for cystic than for solid tumors. Limited prolongation of survival has been described following aggressive radiation therapy and multiagent chemotherapy,[4, 100] but experience to date is limited.[99] These tumors tend to spread in the CSF, so that craniospinal radiation therapy or chemotherapy may be indicated. Extraneural metastases to bone, lymph nodes, and liver have been reported.[2]

Few reports describe the MR appearance of these lesions. A series limited to study of primary neuroblastoma found that these lesions occur in equal proportion as large parenchymal lesions or as intraventricular and periventricular masses (Fig. 9–24).[105] The MR appearance is nonspecific, with inhomogeneous increased signal on T2 weighted images and mild to moderate hypointensity on T1 weighted images. Spontaneous hemorrhage, a relatively frequent event in neuroblastoma, results in characteristic MR signal abnormalities from hematoma (Figs. 9–25, 9–26). Spontaneous subacute to chronic intratumoral hemorrhages are evident on MRI as foci of increased signal intensity on T1 weighted images. There are no characteristic features that permit ready preoperative differentiation from more common tumors such as astrocytoma or ependymoma, or among different subsets of PNET. Intraventricular neuroblastoma is radiographically indistinguishable from meningioma, papilloma, and ependymoma. Cysts are common in parenchymal lesions, calcifications being more apparent on CT than on MRI. Multiplanar MRI is helpful for anatomic localization of these lesions relative to the adjacent ventricular system. Noncontrast MRI is inferior to CT for recognition of tumor seeding or tumor recurrence around cysts and at operative sites; accordingly, gadolinium–DTPA should be used for initial and follow-up examinations of these patients.

The CT appearance of PNET is more widely reported[106–110] but is nonspecific. Neuroblastoma commonly appears as a large cystic and calcified parenchymal mass on noncontrast CT, and enhances inhomogeneously after administration of iodinated contrast material. CT is limited to axial and coronal planes of imaging. CT is insensitive for demonstration of subacute or chronic hemorrhage, a relatively common finding in PNET. Subarachnoid or ependymal seeding is common, resulting in focal or diffuse enhancement of intracranial meningeal and ventricular surfaces with contrast CT. Both CT and MRI reveal these tumors to be indistinguishable from more common entities such as astrocytoma and ependymoma.

GANGLIOGLIOMA AND GANGLIOCYTOMA

Gangliocytoma, also termed ganglioneuroma, is a rare tumor containing exclusively mature ganglion cells in a stroma of spindle cells with calcospherites.

Masses of histologically similar appearance that contain a mixture of mature ganglial and astrocytic cells are termed ganglioglioma. These tumors account for approximately 4 percent of primary CNS tumors in children. Eighty percent of cases of ganglioglioma and gangliocytoma occur in patients under age 30,[2] although these have been encountered in middle-aged and older adults. Up to 10 percent are identified in infants, suggesting both a neoplastic and a developmental process beginning in utero.[2] These have also been called desmoplastic cerebral neuroblastoma of infancy. Ganglioglioma is much more common than

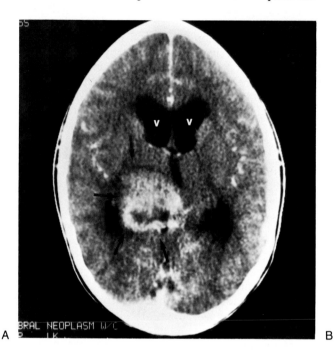

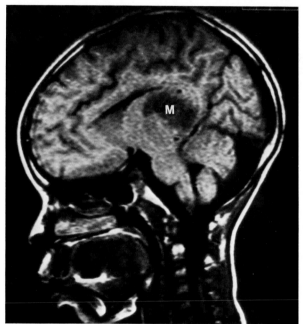

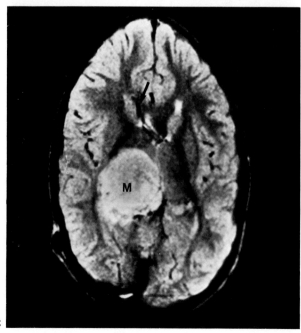

Figure 9–24. *Malignant small cell tumor of the thalamus (PNET).* **A,** Contrast-enhanced CT. An enhancing mass (*arrows*) involves the right thalamus with associated hydrocephalus. Lateral ventricle (V). **B,** Sagittal T1 weighted image (500/30). The thalamic mass (M) is ill defined and hypointense compared with normal parenchyma. The ventricles are decompressed after shunting. **C,** Proton density image (2000/50). The hyperintense right thalamic mass (M) distorts the third ventricle and pineal region. A ventricular shunt catheter (*arrow*) is seen in the right frontal horn.

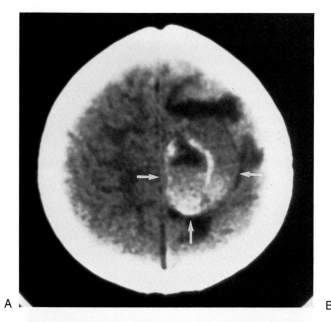

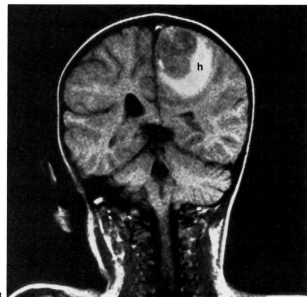

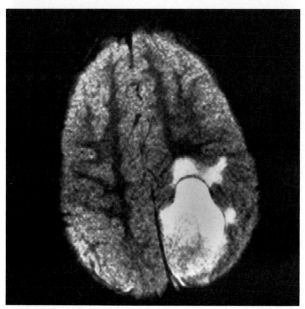

Figure 9–25. *Neuroblastoma. A 4-year-old child with spontaneous hemorrhage of a proven convexity neuroblastoma at presentation.* **A,** Noncontrast CT. The convexity mass (*arrows*) is hyperdense, compatible with intratumoral hemorrhage. **B,** Coronal T1 weighted image (620/30). A mixed-intensity intra-axial mass (*arrows*) is seen in the left parietal lobe with a hyperintense periphery secondary to subacute hemorrhage (h). **C,** Axial proton density image (2000/30). The mass has a nonspecific high intensity relative to brain on this sequence.

gangliocytoma. Frequent locations include the temporal lobe and floor of the third ventricle, although examples have been described in virtually all locations.

Ganglioglioma and gangliocytoma are similar in behavior clinically and are firm, well-defined, often cystic masses on gross examination. Ganglioneuroma and gangliocytoma tumors contain cells of neuronal origin, with Nissl substance and neurofibrils on a scanty background of supporting tissue. Microscopic evidence of Nissl substance and neurofibrils is necessary for identification of a ganglion origin cell, and engulfment of ganglial cells by another tumor type must be excluded.[2] The cells generally are well differentiated, and mitoses are notably absent. Gangliogliomas also contain neoplastic astrocytic elements along with neuronal cells in

variable proportions.[2] Scattered small neuroblastic cells are encountered in both types, and calcospherites are common. A controversy exists concerning whether these tumors of mature cell types are truly neoplastic or are dysplastic and hamartomatous. Associated congenital or developmental abnormalities are encountered in 5 percent of patients.[2] Malignant forms and metastases are exceedingly uncommon, although the glial elements of ganglioglioma may differentiate into more typical and more aggressive glial tumors.

A distinct form encountered in the cerebellum, which may be diffuse or focal, has variously been termed dysplastic gangliocytoma of the cerebellum, Purkinjeoma, gangliocytoma dysplasticum, or Lhermitte-Duclos.[111–113] This varied terminology reflects the con-

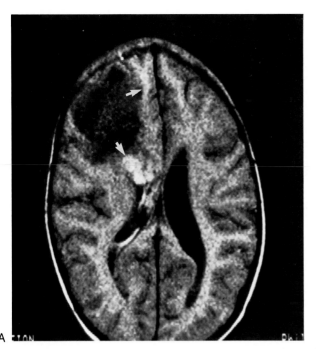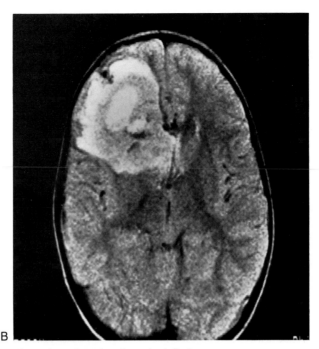

A   B

Figure 9–26. *Neuroblastoma. Spontaneous intraventricular hemorrhage from a large frontal cystic and calcified, proven neuroblastoma.* ***A,*** Axial T1 weighted image (500/30). The large right frontal mass is inhomogeneously hypointense with the exception of hyperintense medial foci of hemorrhage (*arrows*) in and adjacent to the right lateral ventricle. ***B,*** Axial proton density image (2000/30). The mass is nonspecifically hyperintense to normal brain.

troversy over the neoplastic versus the hamartomatous native of this lesion. Characteristically a thickening of the folia and loss of normal cerebellar architecture occurs over a limited area, with a reduction in the normal adjacent white matter. Microscopically, the component axons of the superficial molecular layer of the cerebellar folia appear thickened, and the granular cell layer underneath it is replaced by large neuronal elements.[114] The normal folia of the cerebellum are enlarged and appear thickened in this disease.

Surgical biopsy or resection of these masses is generally indicated to confirm the diagnosis and for symptomatic relief from mass effect.[115–117] The benign nature and slow course of these lesions generally do not warrant aggressive radiation or chemotherapy, with the rare exception of those that show malignant degeneration. A prolonged course with nonspecific symptoms is common before these very low-grade lesions are diagnosed.

The marked sensitivity of MRI to processes that distort or disrupt normal parenchyma is particularly useful for definition of these lesions, because their benign nature is associated with little secondary edema and little disruption of the blood-brain barrier (Figs. 9–27, 9–28).[113, 118] T1 weighted images depict secondary anatomic distortion of normal structures (Fig. 9–28). The intensities on T1 weighted images are variable, revealing hypo-, iso-, and slightly hyperintense masses (Fig. 9–29).[118] Cysts are mildly hypointense and not typically fatty or hemorrhagic (Fig.

9–30). Dense calcifications may be apparent as focal regions of decreased signal on both T1 and T2 weighted images. Although the intensity of these lesions on T2 weighted images is variable, these sequences are useful for evaluation of the extent of intraparenchymal involvement (Fig. 9–29). In some cases the intensities on T2 weighted images are so similar to those of normal parenchyma that lesions are recognized only by distortion of normal parenchymal anatomy.[118] Castillo and colleagues reported one surgically and histologically proven ganglioglioma that was undetected by MRI on either T1 or T2 weighted sequences.[118] Although little experience with gadolinium–DTPA and these lesions has been reported, variable enhancement is to be expected on the basis of CT studies.

On CT these tumors tend to be intraparenchymal masses that are isodense to normal brain, with recognizable cysts or calcifications.[119, 120] Secondary edema is not a prominent associated finding. Enhancement may occur after administration of iodinated contrast material, although this finding is variable. No specific CT characteristics provide confident differentiation of this lesion from other neoplastic processes.

The differential diagnosis includes other more common intraparenchymal or intraventricular masses such as astrocytoma, ependymoma, neuroblastoma, and oligodendroglioma. The cerebellar lesions have a rather specific appearance, since few other masses thicken the cortex without frank invasion of the white matter.

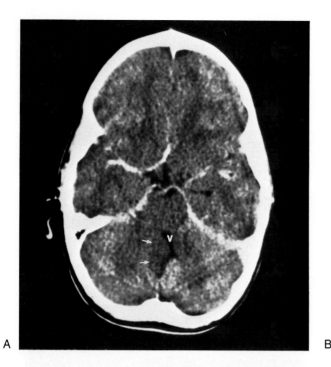

A

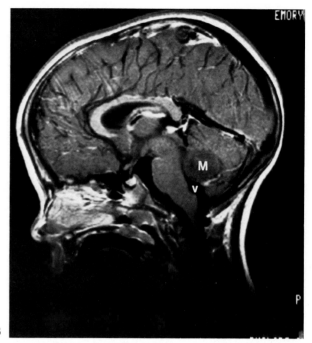

B

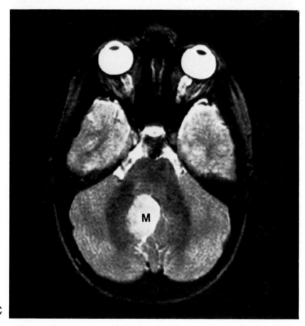

C

Figure 9–27. *Gangliocytoma. A young girl with an atypical seizure disorder and surgically proven gangliocytoma.* **A,** Contrast-enhanced CT. The vermis (*arrows*) and fourth ventricle (V) are distorted, but no discrete or enhancing mass is recognizable. **B,** Sagittal T1 weighted image (650/20) after gadolinium–DTPA. The focal nonenhancing mas (M) expands the vermis and distorts the fourth ventricle (V). **C,** Axial T2 weighted image (2000/90). The hyperintense vermian mass (M) displaces the fourth ventricle and has little associated edema.

OLIGODENDROGLIOMA

Oligodendroglioma is an uncommon glial neoplasm of the cerebral hemispheres that occurs at all ages, but accounts for less than 1 percent of CNS tumors in children.[4] An adolescent and male predominance has been noted in pediatric examples of this supratentorial tumor.[121]

Oligodendrogliomas are histologically mixed gliomas with a predominance of oligodendroglial ele-

ments. Greater recognition of this heterogeneity by electron microscopy in recent years has resulted in an increased reported frequency of tumors designated as mixed oligodendroglioma and astrocytoma. They may grossly be firm in appearance or have necrotic, cystic, friable, or frankly calcified components. Calcifications occasionally are inapparent radiographically, but are virtually always noted on histologic examination. A mucoid or gelatinous texture is not uncommon, with inconspicuous cysts and necrosis. Spontaneous hemor-

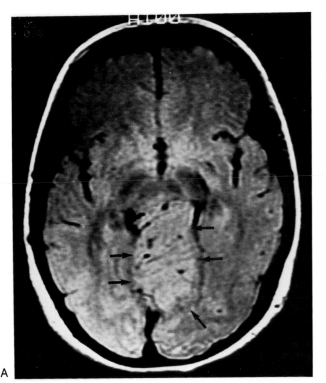 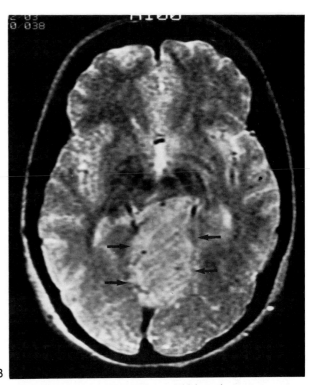

A   B

Figure 9–28. *Ganglioglioma.* ***A,*** Proton density image (2000/30) and ***B,*** T2 weighted image (2000/90) reveal thickened superior vermian folia and mass effect in this recurrent proven ganglioglioma (*arrows*).

rhage may have catastrophic consequences. Common sites include frontal and temporal lobes, with rare cerebellar and spinal origins.[2]

Microscopically these tumors appear as compact masses containing swollen oligodendroglia with a sparse supporting matrix. Calcifications are generally located in proximity to the blood vessels, and may progress to frank bone formation with a lamellar organization.[2] A general lack of correlation exists between histologic evidence of aggression and the clinical be-

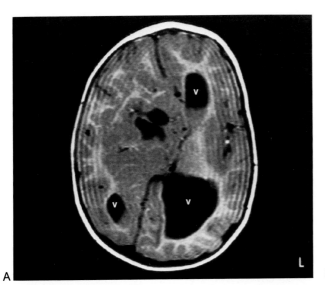 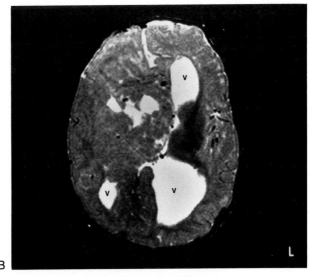

A   B

Figure 9–29. *Ganglioglioma. An infant with a right cerebral hemisphere, proven ganglioglioma. Note the difficulty in differentiation of this lesion from a dysplastic or hamartomatous malformation.* ***A,*** *T1 weighted image (500/30). A dysplastic right deep hemispheric mass is associated with right-to-left midline shift and contralateral ventriculomegaly. V, Ventricle.* ***B,*** *T2 weighted image (2000/90). The signal intensities of the solid portions of the mass are similar to normal brain, and cystic components resemble CSF on both sequences. V, Ventricle.*

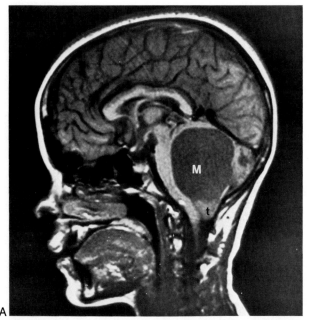
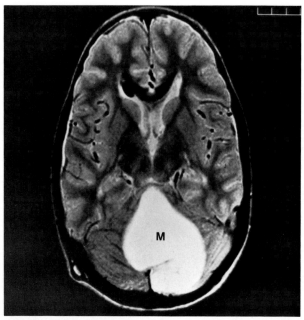

A   B

Figure 9–30. *Cystic ganglioglioma.* **A,** Sagittal T1 weighted image (500/20). The large hypointense mass (M) markedly compresses the fourth ventricle and displaces the cerebellar tonsils (T) downward. **B,** Axial T2 weighted image (2440/50). The mass (M) is homogeneously hyperintense, with poor demonstration of an associated enhancing mural mass identified on contrast-enhanced CT. Gadolinium–DTPA was unavailable at the time of this examination. This lesion is radiographically indistinguishable from cystic cerebellar astrocytoma.

havior of the tumor. Part of this difficulty stems from the reporting of malignant oligodendroglioma as glioblastoma multiforme.[122] These tumors may remain stable in a benign fashion for many years, but late degeneration into a clinically malignant form is not uncommon.[123–125] There are no distinct histologic characteristics denoting the transition between benign and malignant progression of tumor, and thus the outlook for survival is unpredictable.[2] Leptomeningeal seeding may be extensive and progressive or longstanding and fibrotic, with rare extraneural metastases.

Clinical symptoms and signs relate to the location of these tumors and to increased intracranial pressure. Seizure disorders and headache are common, as are long survivals.[122] Dohrmann and colleagues reported a 70 percent 5-year and a 58 percent 10-year survival in a small series of children with oligodendroglioma, although other series described widely variable survival rates due to the unpredictable progression of this tumor to sarcoma or glioblastoma multiforme.[2, 121, 125]

Surgical resection is the primary treatment of choice, with radiation therapy either after resection or at the time of recurrence.[126] Aggressive recurrences and those with spinal seeding may warrant a combined approach with radiation therapy and chemotherapy, although the efficacy of this approach has not been conclusively demonstrated.

Few reports describe the MR appearance of oligodendroglioma. Lee and Van Tassel describe oligodendroglioma as typically hypointense on T1 weighted

and hyperintense on T2 weighted images, with calcifications generally inapparent.[122] The major role of MRI is to define lesions relative to adjacent tissues for surgical and radiation planning (Fig. 9–31).[126] A small percentage have foci of hyperintensity on T1 weighted images, perhaps related to previous hemorrhage. On the basis of CT patterns of enhancement, oligodendrogliomas should enhance variably after gadolinium administration. However, confirmation of this awaits further experience with MR contrast agents.

Noncontrast CT generally reveals an iso- or slightly hypodense mass with foci of calcification.[127, 128] Mild or ill-defined enhancement is seen in approximately 50 percent, and up to 30 percent demonstrate associated edema.[122] Calcifications may be nodular, shell-like, or ringlike in appearance.[128]

The differential diagnosis includes other glial masses, most commonly astrocytoma and ganglioglioma or gangliocytoma. Neuroblastoma and other PNET may be calcified and enhancing, although these may be more aggressive in radiographic appearance than oligodendroglioma.

CHOROID PLEXUS PAPILLOMA AND CARCINOMA

Choroid plexus papilloma and carcinoma are uncommon neoplasms, accounting for less than 1 percent of all CNS primary tumors. They occur in both children

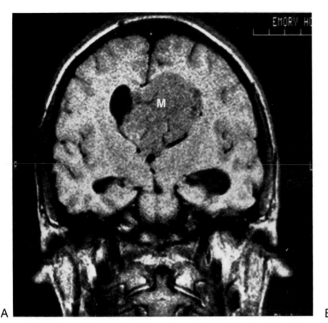

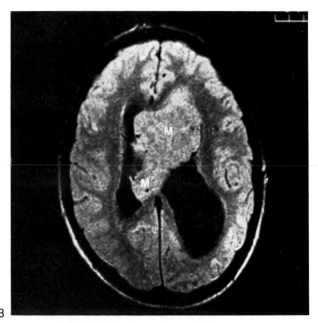

A   B

Figure 9–31. *Oligodendroglioma. A mass arising in the left frontal lobe projects primarily into the ventricular system in a 20-year-old patient with a long history of headaches.* **A,** Coronal T1 weighted image (500/30). A mildlly hypointense mass (M) arises from the left deep frontal white matter and extends bilaterally into the frontal horns. Calcifications are subtle areas of focal hypointensity on this image and are easily overlooked. **B,** Axial image (2000/30). The mass (M) extends posteriorly within the ventricular system and has resulted in an obstructive hydrocephalus.

and adults; approximately 40 to 50 percent present during the first decade. About 20 percent are identified in children under 1 year of age, and occasional congenital examples are recognized during the neonatal period.[2, 89, 129] A male predominance has been reported.[2]

In Herren's series,[130] 32 percent arise from the lateral ventricle, 60 percent from the fourth, and 8 percent from the third. In children, most arise from the choroid plexus of the lateral ventricles (particularly the left), while in adults a fourth ventricular or cerebellopontine angle origin is more common. Uncommonly these tumors are bilateral or extend through the choroidal fissure into the quadrigeminal plate cistern. Malignant forms are uncommon (10 to 20 percent),[131] tending to occur in younger pediatric patients.

Choroid plexus papillomas arise from and are attached to choroid plexus epithelium, and thus have a pink or reddish-gray globular or cauliflower-like appearance on gross examination.[2] Approximately one-fourth have focal areas of ependymal differentiation, occasionally making it difficult to distinguish these tumors pathologically from ependymoma. Dense calcification is not unusual. Benign forms are slow-growing masses that characteristically expand the adjacent ventricular walls without invasion of the adjacent parenchyma.

Microscopically, papillomas are characterized by arborizing frondlike papillae with collagen in their stroma, lined by single-layered or pseudostratified cuboidal to columnar epithelium.[2, 132] Occasional mitotic

figures, atypia, microscopic infiltration, and ependymal differentiation are present in benign papillomas, which may not adversely affect the prognosis.[132] About 10 percent of choroid plexus papillomas are malignant. These invade adjacent parenchyma and histologically show a loss of regular papillary architecture, variability in cell size and shape, conspicuous mitoses, and occasional giant nuclei.

Presenting symptoms typically are those of increased intracranial pressure with papilledema or vomiting.[89] This results from mass effect with secondary ventricular obstruction, from overproduction of CSF with secondary hydrocephalus, or from repeated small hemorrhages with a secondary communicating hydrocephalus. Subarachnoid hemorrhage or focal signs such as hemiparesis are uncommon.

Complete surgical resection is generally curative in benign papilloma and may result in resolution of associated hydrocephalus.[132] Malignant choroid plexus papilloma or carcinoma carries a poor prognosis in spite of surgery, radiation, and chemotherapy. Radiation therapy is not routine for papilloma, but is reserved for recurrences, anaplastic tumors, and (in selected examples) for incompletely excised tumors. Leptomeningeal spread is common in malignant and exceptional in benign choroid plexus tumors, and extraneural spread is unusual.

Few reports describe MR findings in choroid plexus papilloma or carcinoma. Radkowski and colleagues[129] described a neonatal papilloma as a large lobulated tumor of mixed intensity. Tumor intensities in the absence of hemorrhage should be similar to those of other neoplasms on MRI, i.e., hypo- to isointensity on T1 weighted and hyperintensity on T2 weighted images. Choroid plexus papilloma and carcinoma not uncommonly hemorrhage spontaneously, resulting in foci of hyperintensity on T1 weighted images and variable hypointensity on T2 weighted images peripherally (hemosiderin) or centrally (deoxyhemoglobin) (Fig. 9–32).[133] Associated intraventricular or subarachnoid hemorrhage may not be seen on MRI. Multiplanar imaging with MRI provides detailed localization of these intraventricular masses relative to the choroid plexus and periventricular tissues, and aids recognition of solely intraventricular masses apart from those with an extraventricular component. Malignant choroid plexus papillomas may mimic other aggressive intra- and periventricular masses,[134] but multiplanar MR imaging facilitates a correct diagnosis by demonstrating an epicenter within the choroid plexus. Large or dense calcifications are recognizable on MRI, although small calcifications are more apparent with CT.

Gadolinium enhancement assists definition of the mass itself, differential diagnosis, and recognition of CSF seeding; it thus should be routinely included in the MR examination of these patients (Fig. 9–32). Gadolinium–DTPA enhancement is helpful postoperatively for evaluation of recurrent or residual tumor apart from surgical abnormalities.[18]

On CT, choroid plexus papillomas are iso- to hyperdense intraventricular masses before contrast administration, which arise from sites of normal choroid plexus, i.e., atria of lateral ventricles, the roof of the third ventricle, or centrally or eccentrically in the foramina of Luschka of the fourth ventricle. The choroid plexus typically appears engulfed rather than displaced by papilloma, whereas other masses tend to displace the choroid plexus.[134] Hydrocephalus is a common sequela. Marked contrast enhancement of a mass with well-defined margins is characteristic, and masses are occasionally bilateral. Tumor extension outside the ventricular system into adjacent parenchyma suggests malignancy, while spread along CSF pathways either intraventricularly or in the subarachnoid space occurs with malignant or occasionally with benign disease.

Supplemental angiography may be required preoperatively in addition to CT or MRI to define the major arterial supply of these lesions and to exclude a vascular malformation. Angiographic findings are those of a hypervascular intraventricular mass with associated enlargement of the choroid plexus arterial supply. Additionally, venous aneurysms and an intense tumor stain are typical.

A variety of masses should be considered in the differential diagnosis of an intraventricular mass in a child.[135] A papillary or cauliflower-like mass is typical of choroid plexus papilloma and may be recognizable on imaging studies. Many intraventricular lesions enhance with intravascular contrast agents, but a generally avascular mass on angiography favors a diagnosis of astrocytoma, ependymoma, medulloblastoma, craniopharyngioma, or inflammatory cyst (i.e., cysticercosis) rather than choroid plexus papilloma or car-

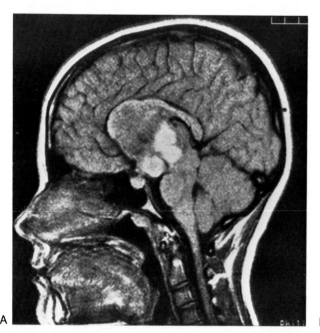
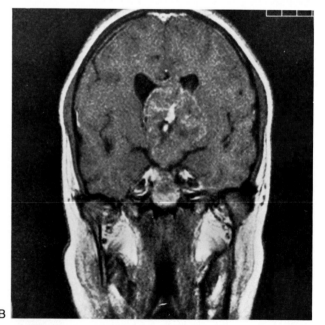

A   B

Figure 9–32. *Benign choroid plexus papilloma of the third ventricle.* **A,** Sagittal T1 weighted image (575/30). A mixed-intensity mass with foci of hyperintensity, presumably representing intratumoral hemorrhage, expands the third ventricle and extends upward into the frontal horns of the lateral ventricles. **B,** Coronal T1 weighted image (575/30) after gadolinium–DTPA. The intraparenchymal extent into the adjacent thalamus is better defined after contrast administration, but evidence of previous hemorrhage is obscured by the enhancement of the lesion.

cinoma. Enhancing masses that may be hypervascular on angiography include meningioma (usually with neurofibromatosis and a prolonged tumor stain), arteriovenous malformations (rapid arteriovenous shunting without tumor stain), choroid plexus papilloma and carcinoma, and other uncommon malignant or aggressive tumors. Intraventricular masses associated with the choroid plexus that enhance poorly or not at all include xanthogranuloma, ependymal or arachnoid cysts, and rarely dermoid or epidermoid.

PINEAL REGION MASSES

Pineal region masses are conveniently grouped into several major categories (adapted from Russell and Rubinstein):[2]

1. Germ cell tumors, including germinoma, benign teratoma, malignant teratoma, embryonal carcinoma, choriocarcinoma, endodermal sinus tumors, and chorioepithelioma.

2. Pineocytoma (formerly called "pinealoma").

3. Pineoblastoma.

4. Glial tumors such as astrocytoma and glioblastoma multiforme.

5. Others: hamartoma, lipoma, meningioma arising from the tentorium or velum interpositum, and nonneoplastic cysts.

Pineal region masses account for 2 to 8 percent of intracranial masses in pediatric patients. Of these, about half are germ cell tumors, glial tumors in this region being quite uncommon. The normal pineal gland is not greater than 1 cm in length,[136-138] and thus any pineal region calcification or mass exceeding this size requires careful evaluation. Although benign cysts of the pineal gland are common incidental findings in adults on MRI and at autopsy,[139,140] the incidence and significance of these benign cysts in the pediatric population are not generally known. Pineal calcifications are uncommon in small children,[136] and early or prominent pineal calcification in a child warrants careful evaluation. About 25 percent of pineal region masses are benign and encapsulated.

Owing to the radiosensitivity of certain pineal region masses (e.g., germinoma) and the risks of open surgical biopsy, a trial of radiation therapy without biopsy has been a common diagnostic and therapeutic approach in children with a pineal region mass.[141-144] With the advent of safer microsurgical and stereotactic biopsy techniques, a tissue diagnosis is generally obtainable and warranted.[145]

Symptoms common to all pineal region masses include those of increased intracranial pressure with hydrocephalus, and visual disturbances such as Parinaud's syndrome (failure of upward gaze associated with loss of convergence and accommodation). Precocious puberty is uncommon, although an increased frequency has been described in patients with teratoma.[142,146]

Germ Cell Tumors

Germ cell tumors arise from primordial germ cells that persist as isolated rests in a variety of locations. Germinoma, also called atypical teratoma and dysgerminoma, accounts for more than half of tumors in the germ cell category. Others include teratoma, embryonal carcinoma, endodermal sinus tumors (yolk sac carcinoma), choriocarcinomas, and mixed tumors.[2,147-149]

In the CNS, germ cell tumors occur in decreasing frequency in the pineal region, suprasellar cistern, and region of the fourth ventricle; germinoma is more commonly suprasellar.[150] A strong male predominance (90 percent) has been described for germ cell tumors of the pineal region,[2] and a variable sex predominance, for suprasellar germinoma. These are predominantly tumors of children and young adults, with a peak at puberty. Suprasellar germinomas are associated with disturbed growth or diabetes insipidus from interference with pituitary stalk or gland function, and may coexist with a pineal germinoma.[150] Pineal region germ cell tumors commonly are diagnosed in patients between 10 and 21 years of age and have been described with Klinefelter's syndrome.[150]

Teratoma of the pineal region is rare, is more commonly malignant than benign, and is encountered almost exclusively in males in their second and third decades. Teratomas may occur elsewhere in the CNS, including the suprasellar region, the spinal meninges, the cerebral hemispheres, or occasionally in the posterior fossa.[89] These tumors rarely present as massive lesions in infancy, replacing normal parenchyma and extending into the orbit or neck.[2] These are heterogeneous masses with variable foci of hair, cartilage, bone, calcification, fat, teeth, and cysts of a dermoid or epidermoid nature containing cholesterol-laden fluid or "crankcase" fluid from previous hemorrhage. Pure epidermoid or dermoid cysts of this region are extremely rare.[2] Immature forms are more prone to hemorrhage and necrosis,[2] and carry a less favorable prognosis than more differentiated mature teratoma. Mixed tumors with teratoma, carcinoma, and germinoma elements are common and carry a variable prognosis.

Presenting findings include those described above for pineal masses in general. Germ cell tumors also may result in precocious puberty,[151] and both germinoma and infrequently teratocarcinoma may produce suprasellar masses with secondary diabetes insipidus and decreased stature.[145] Abnormal levels of human chorionic gonadotropin or luteinizing hormone may be present with either germinoma or malignant teratoma and have been associated with a higher rate of dissemination or a poor prognosis. Elevated CSF alpha-fetoprotein generally occurs only in malignant teratoma and other germ cell tumors harboring elements of yolk sac origin.[146]

Germinomas are highly malignant tumors with a

propensity to spread in the CSF (7 to 57 percent)[2] and to infiltrate adjacent tissues, particularly the hypothalamus, third ventricle, and spinal cord.[146] Rarely metastases to lung and bone, or to abdomen and pelvis in association with ventriculoperitoneal shunting, have been described (3 percent).[146] Longer survivals are associated more with germinoma than other germ cell tumors, although invasion of adjacent structures and spinal seeding connote an unfavorable prognosis. Accurate staging of the extent of disease and histologic confirmation of tumor type are useful in order to determine those patients who should receive full craniospinal radiation or chemotherapy. Embryonal carcinoma and endodermal sinus tumors are highly malignant and less responsive in general to therapeutic measures than germinoma.[2] Choriocarcinoma is very rare, tending to be well demarcated and hemorrhagic. Recent studies suggest a beneficial response of these tumors to chemotherapy.[2]

Pathologically, germinomas may engulf or displace the normal pineal gland, with normal pineal calcifications remaining. An association between the pineal gland and neuroendocrine function is likely based on the locations of these tumors, common association of endocrinologic disturbances, strong male sex predominance, and peak presentation at puberty.[147–149] Germinomas are densely cellular malignant tumors with occasional teratoid elements. Teratomas are quite variable in maturity and in cell type, with differentiation variably into fat, cartilage, bone, and calcification. Additionally, epidermoid or dermoid cysts may be the predominant component of a pineal region teratoma, pure dermoid or epidermoid cysts of this region being extremely uncommon.[2] Endodermal sinus tumors examined by electron microscopy form glandlike spaces, with endodermal cells having prominent microvilli.[2] Choriocarcinoma is composed of syncytiotrophoblastic and cytotrophoblastic cells on histologic examination.

Pineal Parenchymal Tumors

The category of pineal parenchymal tumors includes pineocytoma, pineoblastoma, and transitional tumors between these categories. These account for approximately 20 percent of all pineal region masses. The peak age of incidence of these tumors is in the first decade. Pineocytoma tends to occur in older children or adults and has a relatively benign course; the aggressive form of pineoblastoma occurs in young male children. The symptoms are as those described above for pineal region masses in general, although children with pineoblastoma may have additional deficits related to invasion of adjacent neural structures. Trilateral retinoblastoma refers to a rare but well-documented association between bilateral retinoblastoma and coexistent pineoblastoma, which is usually hereditary.[2]

Pineocytoma is a calcified, well-defined tumor that occasionally contains cysts, but rarely undergoes necrosis. It may replace or displace the normal pineal gland and may contain microscopic foci of hemorrhage.[2] Focal infiltration of adjacent normal tissues is uncommon. Pineocytoma may differentiate into mature glial or neuronal cells, resulting in astrocytoma or ganglioglioma of the pineal gland. In contrast, pineoblastoma is an embryonal, highly malignant tumor, which has been included in the PNET category. It commonly has infiltrating, ill-defined margins; associated edema; and uncommon calcifications. The histologic appearance of pineoblastoma is similar to that of medulloblastoma, being composed of dense small cells with occasional spontaneous hemorrhage and necrosis.[2] Leptomeningeal and ventricular metastases are common sequelae of pineoblastoma, but may occur with any pineal parenchymal tumor. Transitional forms between pineoblastoma and pineocytoma are occasionally described.[2]

Pineocytomas without neuronal differentiation carry a guarded prognosis, with few long-term survivors.[2, 152] Those tumors with differentiation have an associated long survival rate and carry a much more favorable prognosis. The outlook in pineoblastoma is extremely guarded in spite of surgery, radiation therapy, and chemotherapy.

Miscellaneous Pineal Region Masses

A variety of other masses have been described in the peripineal region, including glioma, meningioma, hemangiopericytoma, arachnoid cyst, vein of Galen aneurysm, chemodectoma, and benign cyst. Glioma, meningioma, and benign cysts occur with sufficient frequency to warrant further discussion.

A variety of glial origin tumors may present in the pineal region, originating from adjacent structures such as the thalamus, diencephalon, and splenium of the corpus callosum. These most commonly are of astrocytic origin, although ependymoma, glioblastoma multiforme, choroid plexus papilloma, and others have been described.[2] Symptoms reflect those of pineal region masses in general and those of the adjacent neural tissues involved. Meningioma presenting in the peripineal region usually arises from the adjacent tentorium or from the velum interpositum,[2] and is an uncommon tumor of childhood in the absence of neurofibromatosis.

Non-neoplastic pineal cysts containing clear watery or proteinaceous fluid are noted in as many as 40 percent of autopsies as incidental findings.[139, 140] These may be formed by the neuroglial elements of the gland or be part of a degenerative process, and may become quite large.[2]

Imaging of Pineal Region Masses

The role of MRI in imaging pineal masses thus far has been to provide excellent anatomic definition of the mass itself and its adjacent tissues for surgical planning and follow-up examinations (Fig. 9–33). Although calcification is poorly depicted, the anatomic detail afforded by MRI largely offsets this limitation (Fig. 9–34). In children with hydrocephalus, MRI may demonstrate small tumors that are not detected by CT (Fig. 9–35).[153]

Experience with MRI and histologically proven pineal masses to date is insufficient to describe tumor-specific MR intensity patterns or characteristics. A small series suggests that germinoma without embryonal elements tends to be isointense to normal brain on

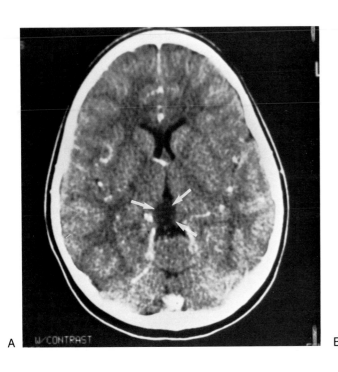

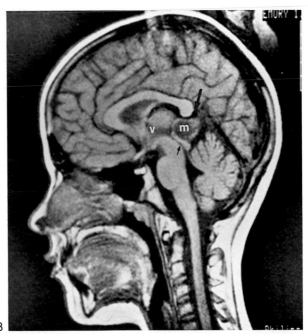

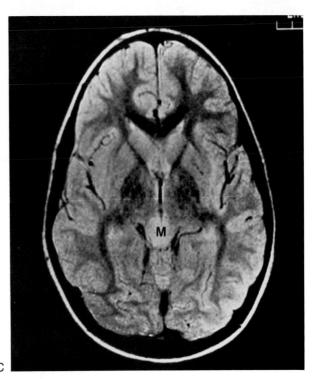

Figure 9–33. *Pineal epidermoid cyst.* ***A,*** Contrast-enhanced CT. The pineal region mass (*arrows*) is ill defined and nonenhancing. ***B,*** Sagittal T1 weighted image (500/30). The relationship of the pineal mass (m) to the midbrain (mb), aqueduct (*small arrow*), vein of Galen (*large arrow*), and third ventricle (v) is readily determined. ***C,*** Axial proton density image (2000/50). The mass (M) is mildly hyperintense to normal brain, and distorts the midbrain and posterior third ventricle.

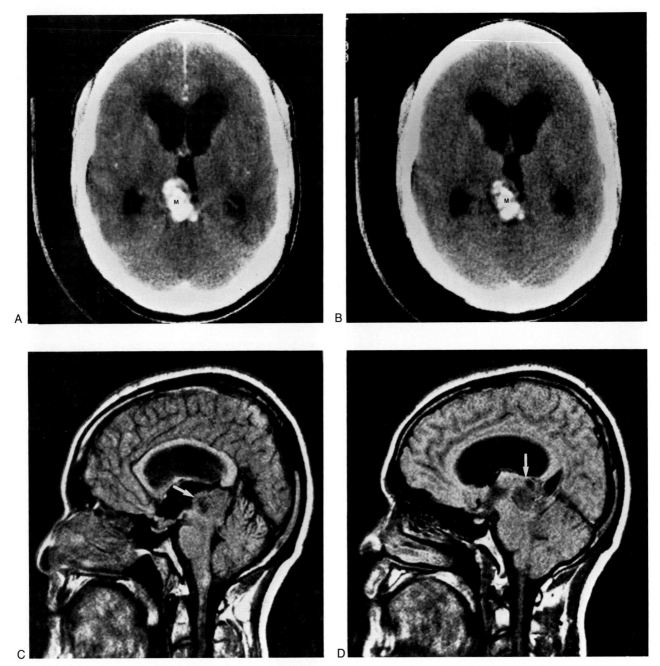

Figure 9–34. *Pineocytoma (unproven).* ***A, B,*** Pre- and postcontrast CT. The markedly calcified mass (M) enhances slightly after intravenous contrast administration. ***C, D,*** The mass (*arrow*) is homogeneously hypointense on T1 weighted sagittal images (500/30); however, the degree of calcification present could easily be underestimated from this study.

all pulse sequences.[154] Multiplanar T1 weighted images provide contrast between CSF, pineal region masses, the vein of Galen, and normal parenchyma. With T1 weighting, thalamic, aqueductal, or vascular lesions that displace the pineal gland are readily identified and differentiated from those arising from the gland itself. In general, pineal masses are homogeneously or inhomogeneously isointense to hypointense relative to normal parenchyma on T1 weighted sequences (Fig.

9–36). Infrequently, focal areas of increased signal suggest fatty elements or previous hemorrhage (Fig. 9–35). On T2 weighted studies, pineal lesions are variable in intensity (Fig. 9–37). Heavily calcified masses may be mildly hypointense, although most pineal masses are hyperintense compared with brain. Smaller calcifications are inapparent on MRI. Ill-defined tumor margins and associated secondary edema suggest aggressive or malignant tumor, but both be-

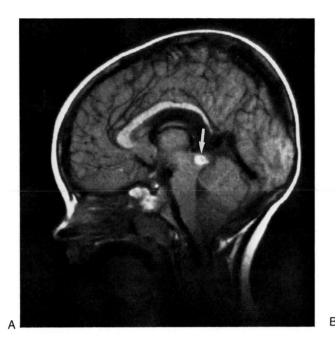

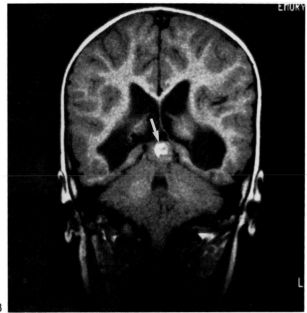

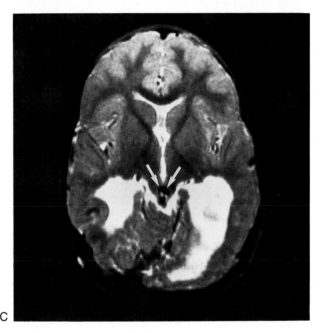

Figure 9–35. *Pineal teratoma in an infant with secondary obstructive hydrocephalus.* ***A, B,*** Sagittal and coronal T1 weighted images (499/29). The pineal region mass (*arrow*) is markedly hyperintense to normal parenchyma, suggesting either a fatty or a hemorrhagic mass. ***C,*** Axial T2 weighted image (2200/90). The mass (*arrows*) is markedly hypointense to normal brain on this sequence. This suggests a paramagnetic shortening of T2 relaxation, perhaps related to previous hemorrhage. Note the persistent ventriculomegaly.

nign and malignant masses may be well circumscribed on MRI (Figs. 9–38, 9–39).

Recent MR descriptions of benign cysts of the pineal gland in adults raise questions concerning the incidence of benign cysts seen on MRI in children.[140] Until further MR experience is available, a cautious course is reasonable when a small cystic pineal mass is encountered in an asymptomatic child, perhaps including CSF evaluation, detailed neurologic and visual evaluation, and follow-up MR examinations.

Gadolinium administration should be included for initial study of a pineal mass to define the primary lesion, distinguish between cystic and solid masses, exclude an associated suprasellar lesion (e.g., germinoma), and assess leptomeningeal seeding. Follow-up examinations after surgery or radiation of malignant lesions and of those with a propensity to metastasize to the leptomeninges should also include gadolinium enhancement.

On CT, germinomas generally result in a well-defined iso- or slightly hyperdense mass with uniform definite enhancement.[136, 146, 155–158] The normal pineal calcifications may be engulfed by tumor, or the pineal gland may be adjacent to and displaced by the mass. Calcifications are generally those that are normal for the age of the patient,[136] calcification in the tumor itself

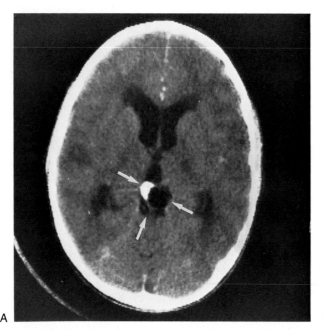

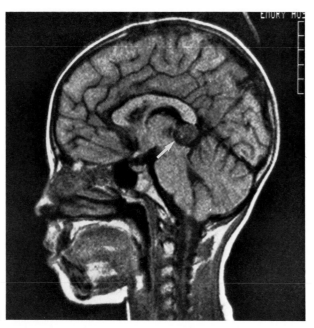

A   B

Figure 9–36. *Pineal teratoma.* ***A,*** Axial CT scan after contrast enhancement. The mass (*arrows*) is eccentrically calcified and contains a cystic region. ***B,*** On sagittal T1 weighted image (500/30), the mass (*arrow*) is mildly, nonspecifically hypointense to normal brain. Note the differing MR intensities of this lesion compared with the teratoma seen in Figure 9–35.

being uncommon. Germinomas may infiltrate adjacent tissues or result in enhancing ependymal or subarachnoid seeding at presentation.

Teratomas are inhomogeneous, with a wide range of densities on CT. A pineal region mass with prominent calcifications or even teeth and very low attenuation regions (fat) is suggestive of teratoma; however, teratomas vary widely in their component densities. Although frank invasion, edema, and ill-defined margins suggest malignant teratoma, the latter commonly is well defined and radiographically indistinguishable from a benign teratoma.[146] Both forms may enhance after contrast administration. Uncommon CT descriptions of rarer types of malignant germ cell tumors suggest variable patterns of calcification, homogeneity, and enhancement such that a firm histologic diagnosis based on CT alone is unreliable.[145]

Pineocytoma radiographically presents as a well-defined calcified mass with variable to no enhancement after intravenous contrast administration. Pineoblastoma, on the other hand, is more aggressive in appearance, with frequent enhancement, rare calcification, and invasion of adjacent structures such as the superior vermis. Enhanced ependymal and subarachnoid surfaces suggest associated leptomeningeal dissemination of tumor. A lucent or necrotic center favors pineoblastoma over pineocytoma radiographically.[156]

Miscellaneous masses of the pineal region are variable in CT appearance and enhancement characteristics. A hyperdense or calcified mass with homogeneous enhancement and a broad-based tentorial

margin suggests peripineal meningioma. Pineal cysts are infrequently detectable by CT in the absence of hemorrhage or frank mass effect. Before the advent of MRI, anatomic evaluation of the pattern of distortion of the pineal region cisterns and brain stem often required direct coronal imaging, reformatting, or CT cisternography.

CONGENITAL INCLUSION MASSES

Congenital inclusion masses include a variety of lesions attributed to developmental inclusion of tissues of variable types in aberrant locations. These include teratoma, dermoid, epidermoid, lipoma, and other rare masses such as melanotic tumor of infancy.

CNS teratoma is rare, accounting for less than 2 percent of pediatric CNS neoplasms. Teratomas occur in the pineal region in male children and contain elements of endoderm, mesoderm, and ectoderm (see pineal region tumors). Other favored locations include the suprasellar cistern and posterior fossa.[2] A variety of other locations have been described, infants under 6 months of age being particularly prone to large lesions in unusual sites. An increased frequency has been described in the Japanese population.[159] These tumors are variable in behavior, with malignant forms not infrequent. Teratomas are inhomogeneous pathologically, often containing cysts related to desquamation of lining cells or occasionally bone or teeth.

Dermoids and epidermoids are inclusion masses of ectodermal origin thought to arise from aberrant inclu-

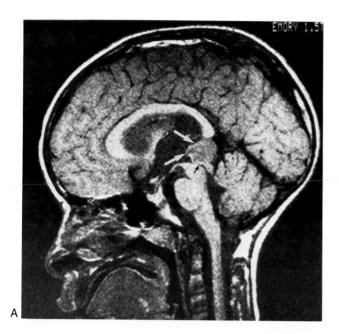

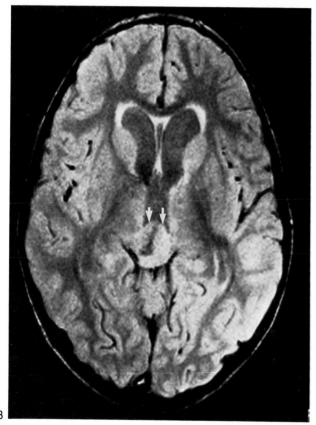

Figure 9–37. *Pineal germinoma.* ***A,*** Sagittal T1 weighted image (500/30). The mass (*large arrows*) is nonspecifically hypointense on this sequence, with compression of the aqueduct (*small arrow*). ***B,*** Axial proton density image (2000/50). The mass (*arrows*) is eccentrically inhomogeneous, but the signal intensities offer no tissue specificity as to the tumor type present.

sions at the time of neural groove closure in the third to fifth fetal week. Dermoids are uncommon midline masses that may be associated with a tract through the calvarium and skin. Skin appendages and hair are present in dermoid and notably absent in epidermoid. Dermoids represent earlier inclusions than epidermoids and thus tend to lie closer to the midline than the more laterally placed epidermoids.[2] Dermoids occur in the posterior fossa, at the base of the brain, or at the anterior fontanelle. Isolated pure dermoid is distinctly uncommon in the pineal region, although dermoid cysts have been described in association with other germ cell tumors of this region. The dermoid contains sebaceous glands and fatty material with inclusion hairs, or may be mucinous in content. Occasional calcifications are present in the cyst wall.[2] An associated dermal sinus may provide a tract for infection by traversing the occipital bone to the overlying skin. Complete excision is curative, and malignant degeneration is very rare. Spillage of cyst contents into the subarachnoid space results in a severe granulomatous meningitis. Dermoids tend to present in adulthood, although pediatric examples are not exceptional.

Epidermoids and mixed tumors, including epidermoid and dermoid elements, are more common than dermoids. Epidermoids, also called cholesteatoma, are usually encountered in adults, perhaps because of their slower growth, although they have been described in infants and children. Epidermoids may arise later embryologically, resulting in more lateral locations intracranially, in the cranium, pericranial tissues, and rarely within the cerebral parenchyma.[2] Common locations include the cerebellopontine angles, suprasellar cistern, and calvarium. A tract to the skin surface has been described, particularly with epidermoids of the posterior fossa. Epidermoids may also arise within the petrous bone as an inclusion mass, not to be confused with the acquired cholesteatoma associated with chronic infection of the middle ear. The cyst contents may include cholesterol-rich debris from the epithelial cyst wall, although the cyst fluid may also be brown-gray and viscid. Desquamation from the cyst wall results in gradual expansion of these lesions. Complete surgical excision is curative and these tumors have little potential for malignant degeneration.[106]

Lipomas of the CNS are inclusion masses of developmental origin. Larger CNS masses may provoke symptoms of mass effect on adjacent structures or seizures. They are often associated with other developmental abnormalities, particularly partial or complete agenesis of the corpus callosum.[161, 162] In the absence of other anomalies, lipomas tend to be incidental findings at autopsy or during imaging for other abnormalities. The most common site is that surrounding the corpus callosum, followed by the quadrigeminal plate cistern and suprasellar cistern. Microscopically, lipomas are seen to contain adipose cells with a variable collagen background matrix and capsule.[2] Occasional intermingling of other cell types, including neural elements,

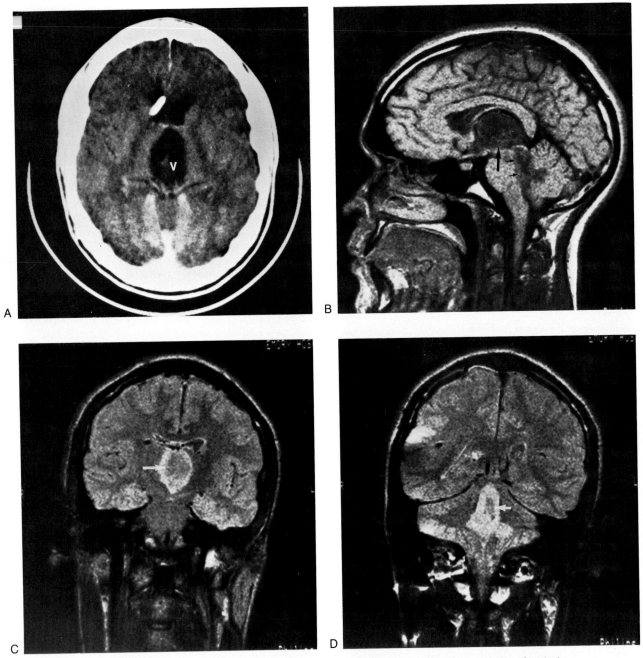

Figure 9–38. *Pineoblastoma in a teen-aged boy with hydrocephalus that failed to respond to shunting. Surgical exploration confirmed intraventricular extension from pineoblastoma.* **A,** Axial contrast-enhanced CT. The third ventricle (V) is markedly expanded, and failed to decompress after shunting. **B,** Sagittal T1 weighted image (700/30). The third (*large arrow*) and fourth (*small arrow*) ventricles are filled with tissue that is slightly hyperintense compared with normal CSF, and the normal tissues of the posterior third ventricle and pineal are obscured. **C, D,** Coronal proton density images (2100/50) confirm that the third and fourth ventricles are filled with abnormal tissue (*arrows*) rather than CSF.

supports the theory of a developmental origin for these lesions.

Another rare inclusion or ectopic tumor is the melanotic neuroectodermal tumor of infancy.[2, 163] This inclusion mass occurs in the mandible or adjacent to the anterior fontanelle in infancy and is thought to arise from neuroblastic cells, perhaps of neural crest origin.

These are pigmented masses containing melanin that are curable with complete excision. They can recur rapidly and disseminate if incompletely resected.

Complete surgical resection is the preferred treatment for all the lesions described above, with the exception of lipoma. Malignant teratoma requires radiation therapy and perhaps chemotherapy; the others are

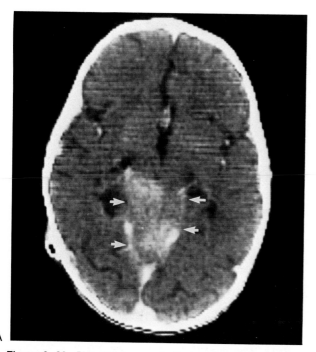

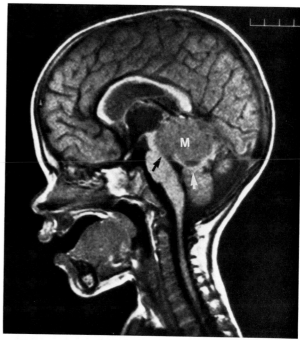

A   B

Figure 9–39. *Pineoblastoma.* **A,** Contrast-enhanced CT. The mass (*arrows*) enhances markedly and has poorly defined borders. **B,** Sagittal T1 weighted image (500/20). The mass (M) is mildly hypointense to normal brain and has invaded the brain stem (*black arrow*) and superior cerebellum (*white arrow*).

not generally radiation sensitive. Recurrences of these benign tumors may require repeated surgical resection.

MRI has proved superior to CT for localization and characterization of these lesions.[164, 165] Multiplanar images aid surgical planning, particularly for the soft epidermoid, which tends to extend along cisternal pathways with little mass effect relative to the tumor size. Epidermoids may contain cholesterol-laden cysts that are specifically recognizable on MRI based on an increased signal intensity on T1 weighted images without the foci of T2 shortening seen in hemorrhagic lesions. Others have variable cyst contents resulting in iso- to hypointense signals on T1 weighted images, and iso- to hyperintensity on T2 weighted images (Fig. 9–40). Dermoids are much less common than epidermoids. They characteristically have very fatty or cholesterol-laden cysts with resultant high signal on T1 weighted images (Fig. 9–41). Teratomas are highly variable in intensity on MRI and inhomogeneous on both T1 and T2 weighted images (Fig. 9–42). Lipomas are bright on T1 weighted images and have a gradual loss of intensity with T2 weighting (Fig. 9–43). Multiplanar MRI is advantageous for demonstration of associated midline abnormalities such as agenesis of the corpus callosum. Melanotic neuroectodermal tumor of infancy presents on MRI as a mass in proximity to the anterior fontanelle with a bright signal on T1 weighted images due to melanin within the tumor itself (Fig. 9–44).[163]

Little is known of enhancement characteristics with

gadolinium in these lesions, but from CT data it is expected that teratomas, particularly those harboring malignancy, would enhance.[166–168] Dermoids and epidermoids should not typically demonstrate enhancement.

Teratoma on CT is an inhomogeneous mass with associated enhancement. Fat or calcifications may be detectable, and malignant teratoma generally enhances after intravenous contrast administration. Direct coronal CT is helpful to improve localization of lesions of the pineal region. Dermoids and epidermoids are generally hypodense to adjacent brain and nonenhancing. Although a density in the fatty range may be recognizable, they are often closer to water in density and thus difficult to distinguish from arachnoid cysts.[166–168] Lipomas are hypodense to CSF on CT, although associated calcifications are common. Melanotic tumor of infancy is an extra-axial mass localized around the anterior fontanelle with variable intracranial and extracranial extension, and enhancement after contrast administration.

CRANIOPHARYNGIOMA

Craniopharyngioma is the most common sellar region mass of childhood, accounting for approximately 50 percent of masses in this location, and 6 to 10 percent of intracranial tumors in children.[4] Craniopharyngioma arises from epithelial remnants of Rathke's pouch, an embryonic tract between the phar-

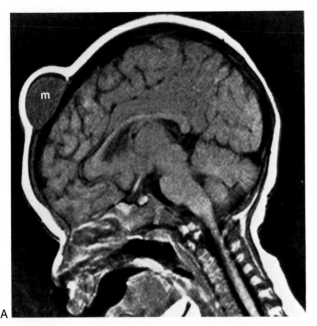
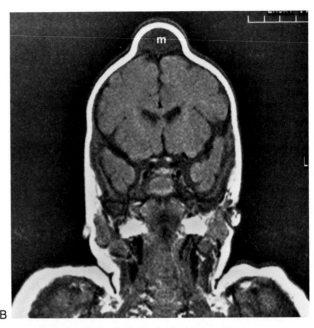

A   B

Figure 9–40. *Epidermoid. A mass is apparent at the anterior fontanelle in a 4-month-old girl.* **A, B,** Sagittal and coronal images with T1 weighting demonstrate a well-defined extra-axial mass (m) that is hypointense to brain and expands the outer table of the calvarium.

ynx and pituitary gland. It is customarily separated from other inclusion masses described above, although it has histologic similarities.[2] Craniopharyngioma occurs with a bimodal peak in childhood from approximately 6 to 12 years and in adults of the fourth to fifth decade.[1,2] It commonly is suprasellar in location, with variable extension into the adjacent third ventricle; cisterns of the anterior, middle, or posterior cranial fossa; or sella turcica. Occasionally (5 percent), this tumor is found strictly within the sella, or third ventricle, and very rarely ectopically in the sphenoid bone, nasopharynx, cerebellopontine angle, or pineal gland.[169]

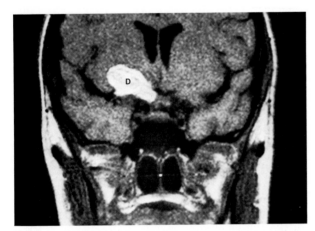

Figure 9–41. *Dermoid.* Coronal T1 weighted image (700/30). Proven intracranial dermoid (D) of the suprasellar cistern in a young girl is hyperintense to brain, suggesting its fatty or cholesterol content.

Presenting signs and symptoms from craniopharyngioma include headaches, visual loss with field cuts, short stature, diabetes insipidus, and hypothyroidism from interference with the hypothalamic-pituitary axis.[89] Additional signs and symptoms of increased intracranial pressure may be prominent in patients with hydrocephalus. Meticulous microsurgical techniques permit resection, although tumor adherence to adjacent structures such as the hypothalamus and cavernous sinus limit complete excision.[170,171] Approximately 50 percent of patients treated with surgical resection eventually have local recurrence of tumor, so that radiation therapy may be necessary. The 5-year survival rate in patients with craniopharyngioma is as high as 80 percent.[2,7]

Pathologically, craniopharyngioma is a benign, slow-growing neoplasm characterized by cords or rests of stratified squamous or columnar epithelium in a loose fibrous stroma.[2] It has an adamantinomatous pattern resembling the architecture of the enamel portions of teeth. Cyst formation is very common, present in 84 percent of a series of craniopharyngiomas studied at the Armed Forces Institute of Pathology.[7] Up to 60 percent may be almost entirely cystic.[172] Reasons for cyst formation in craniopharyngioma include central degenerative changes in cellular rests, stromal degenerative changes, or accumulation of debris related to maturation and desquamation of squamous epithelial cells.[172] Calcification occurs in at least 75 percent of cases. A continuum has been described pathologically in sellar region inclusion masses, the most benign form being a simple inclusion or epidermoid cyst, progressing to Rathke's pouch cyst (see discussion to follow),

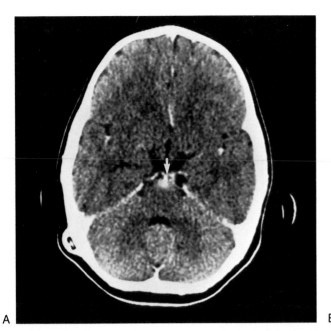
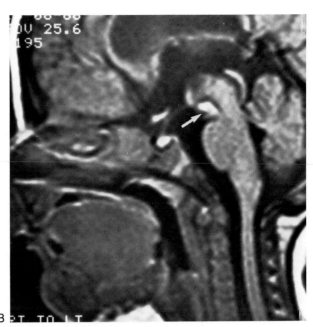

A   B

Figure 9–42. *Teratoma. A mass is present in the interpeduncular cistern in a newborn after shunting for coexisting aqueductal stenosis.* **A,** Contrast-enhanced CT. The mass (*arrow*) is ill defined in relation to the brain stem and major vessels. **B,** Sagittal T1 weighted image. The fatty component of the lesion (*arrow*) and its relationship to the midbrain and interpeduncular cistern are better demonstrated.

benign cystic craniopharyngioma, and craniopharyngioma.[2]

Craniopharyngioma has a variable MR appearance depending on the constituent solid, cystic, and cholesterol-laden components of the mass.[17,33,172–177] Thin (3-mm) coronal and sagittal images depict the anatomic extent of this lesion (Figs. 9–45, 9–46). Pre-

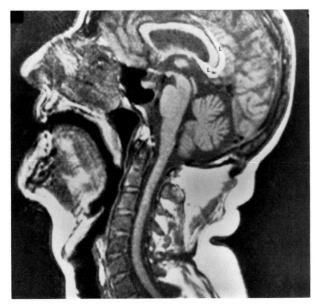

Figure 9–43. *Lipoma.* Sagittal T1 weighted image (500/20). Incidental lipoma (L) surrounding the corpus callosum in an adult. Note the high signal intensity characteristic of fat. In this example, the corpus callosum is structurally intact.

and post-gadolinium T1 weighted studies help to differentiate the solid and cystic components of this lesion. Craniopharyngioma enlarges or obliterates the infundibulum, displaces the chiasm, and often extends upward to distort or invade the floor of the third ventricle (Fig. 9–45). It may extend laterally, anteriorly, or posteriorly into the parasellar cisterns, with secondary displacement of the adjacent brain parenchyma. The normal infundibulum is isointense to brain on noncontrast MRI and is not larger in diameter than the adjacent basilar artery.[178] Craniopharyngiomas are usually hyperintense to brain on T2 weighted images, although Pusey and colleagues describe one example in which a cystic tumor with a high keratin content and bony trabeculae was hypointense on all sequences.[175] Intensities on T1 weighted sequences vary from hypo- to hyperintense, particularly in cystic areas. Hyperintense cysts on T1 weighted images may result from high cholesterol concentration within the cyst, or methemoglobin related to previous spontaneous hemorrhage or surgical exploration. Cystic portions of these tumors may also be hypo-, iso- or mildly hyperintense relative to brain, attributed to the variable keratin and protein content of these cysts, and to volume averaging of tumor with areas of calcification. Larger dense calcifications may result in a recognizable area of signal loss on all pulse sequences, but smaller calcifications are not apparent on MRI owing to volume averaging with adjacent tissues.

With MR imaging, a distinct plane is virtually always detectable between suprasellar and sellar structures; thus, classic craniopharyngioma is depicted as a mass of the suprasellar cistern distinct from the pituitary

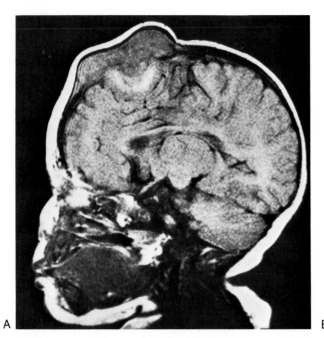

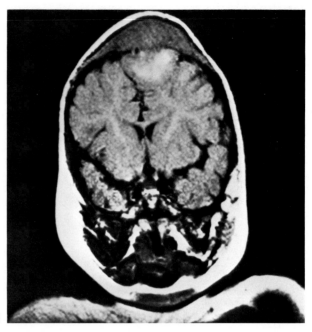

Figure 9–44. *Melanotic neuroectodermal tumor of infancy.* Sagittal (**A**) and coronal (**B**) T1 weighted images (500/30). An infant with a rapidly expanding mass involving the anterior fontanelle. The foci of hyperintensity within the mass are attributed to T1 shortening from melanin.

gland. The normal pituitary gland is recognized on MRI on the basis of its morphologic appearance and intensities similar to those of normal brain parenchyma. It may be obscured or destroyed by extensive intrasellar extension of craniopharyngioma, or by craniopharyngioma arising in the sella.

On CT, craniopharyngioma tends to be heterogeneous before contrast administration, with inhomogeneous enhancement of a well-defined suprasellar mass after such administration.[179, 180] Craniopharyngioma typically obscures visualization of the optic chiasm and infundibulum. Direct coronal scans aid local-

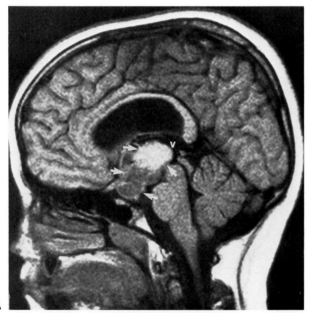

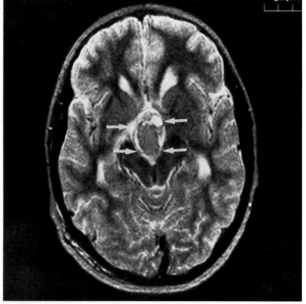

Figure 9–45. *Craniopharyngioma.* **A,** Sagittal T1 weighted image (575/30). The suprasellar mass (*arrows*) is inhomogeneous with focal areas of increased intensity and extension into the third ventricle (V). **B,** T2 weighted image (2489/100). The mass (*arrows*) has multiple component intensities. The area of hyperintensity in **A** has particularly lost signal, suggesting lipid or cholesterol content.

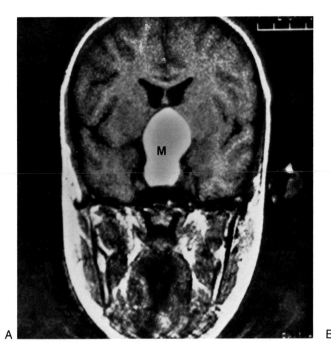

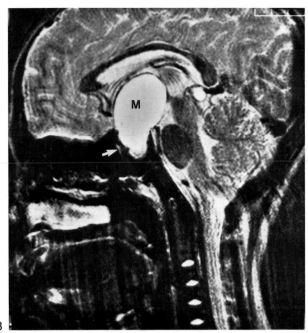

Figure 9–46. *Craniopharyngioma.* **A,** Coronal noncontrast T1 weighted image (500/30). The mass (M) has a homogeneous high intensity and extends upward from the sella. **B,** Sagittal T2 weighted image (2000/90). The mass (M) is uniformly hyperintense on T2 weighting, with displacement inferiorly of the pituitary gland (*arrow*) and expansion of the sella turcica.

ization of the mass relative to the sella, although beam-hardening artifacts from the skull base are often problematic. Before the development of MRI, CT cisternography was required to define these masses relative to the sellar contents, infundibulum, and chiasm. Recognizable hypodense cysts and calcifications are characteristic, although rarely the proteinaceous contents of cysts render them iso- to hyperdense to brain and thus indistinguishable from solid neoplastic masses.[179] Careful comparison of pre- and postcontrast studies demonstrating absence of central enhancement in the areas in question aids in making this distinction. Calcifications are typical in pediatric patients with craniopharyngioma, but less common in adults with this disorder (30 to 50 percent).[180] Plain skull films reveal erosion of the sella turcica downward and calcifications in the suprasellar cistern. Additional findings secondary to long-standing hydrocephalus include prominent convolutional markings and demineralization of the skull base in older children, or spread sutures and macrocephaly in younger children.

Compared with CT, coronal and sagittal MRI better demonstrate the extent of the tumor and its relationship to adjacent structures. In particular, the relationship of tumor to the third ventricle, optic chiasm, hypothalamus, and pituitary gland is better seen with MRI than with CT. For newly diagnosed or recurrent lesions, the superior demonstration of the extent of tumor by MRI is helpful for planning the surgical approach and in demonstrating the relationship of tumor to adjacent key structures. MRI avoids the awkward

positioning required for coronal CT and its associated bone-related artifacts. Metallic artifacts related to previous surgery are in some cases less troublesome on MRI than on CT. Nonenhancing components of craniopharyngioma may be difficult to localize confidently on CT but are readily identified on MRI. Gadolinium administration with MRI helps to demonstrate cystic regions in a manner similar to that of CT. Small calcifications and bone detail such as the sellar floor are better demonstrated with CT, but demonstration of the mixed cystic and solid components of the tumor by gadolinium-enhanced MRI makes visualization of calcification less essential in suggesting the correct diagnosis.

The differential diagnosis of craniopharyngioma in children includes a variety of suprasellar masses including optic-hypothalamic glioma, adenoma, teratoma, germinoma, and other glial tumors. Demonstration of tumoral cysts is the key to the diagnosis of craniopharyngioma, since other suprasellar masses are infrequently cystic in the absence of previous radiation therapy. Rathke's pouch cyst and benign cystic craniopharyngioma are within the histologic spectrum of craniopharyngioma (see below) and require tissue examination for exclusion. With gadolinium-enhanced MRI, demonstration of enhancing solid components within the mass strongly favors craniopharyngioma and excludes Rathke's pouch cyst. The rare suprasellar epidermoid, dermoid, or teratoma may have calcification and a complex multicystic appearance. These may also contain fatty or cholesterol-laden cysts that mimic those of craniopharyngioma. Arachnoid cysts occur in the suprasellar region, but the uncomplicated cyst matches CSF in intensity on all pulse sequences. Optic-hypothalamic and other glial tumors are infrequently cystic or hemorrhagic and engulf neural tissues such as the chiasm in a characteristic fashion. Pituitary macroadenoma originates in the sella, is uncommon in children, and is infrequently cystic or hemorrhagic. Aneurysm is uncommon in children and has a characteristic relationship to major vessels, with evidence of flow and concentric layers of high and low signal intensity on T1 weighted images, representing organizing clot within the aneurysm wall.

RATHKE'S CLEFT CYSTS

Rathke's cleft cysts are benign epithelial cysts of the sella or suprasellar cistern. Although some confusion in terminology exists in the literature, cuboidal, columnar, or squamous lined benign cysts in the sellar and suprasellar region are included within this category.[2, 172] These cysts are thought to arise from remnants of Rathke's cleft, an embryologic upward growth of oral stomodeum toward the neurohypophysis that contributes to the formation of the pituitary gland. Rathke's cleft cysts are grouped histologically in the spectrum of craniopharyngioma but are not considered neoplastic. These small epithelial cysts are common incidental asymptomatic findings at autopsy but may enlarge sufficiently to produce mass effect on the adjacent pituitary gland, infundibulum, and hypothalamus.

The clinical presentation includes visual disturbances related to chiasmal compression, headache, diabetes insipidus, and endocrinologic disorders such as hyperprolactinemia, hypopituitarism, and growth disturbance. These cysts typically are discovered in the third to fifth decades, but may occur in the pediatric population. Surgical exploration with biopsy, cyst drainage, and resection of the cyst wall is considered curative, and radical resection or radiation therapy is unnecessary.[181]

Pathologically, Rathke's cleft cysts are believed to arise as expansions of Rathke's cleft remnants within the sella.[2] The simplest cysts are lined by a single cell layer of epithelial origin, often with ciliated or goblet cells. More complex cysts have a fibrotic wall with occasional calcification. The cyst contents vary from serous to mucous to keratinizing with accumulated desquamated debris. Cysts containing little debris, protein, and cholesterol are similar to CSF in content. A transitional form that histologically falls between Rathke's cleft cyst and craniopharyngioma has been called benign cystic craniopharyngioma.[182]

The signal intensity of Rathke's cyst on MR is variable (Figs. 9–47, 9–48). It may mimic normal CSF on all sequences,[183] resulting in difficulty in differentiating it from an arachnoid cyst of the sella or suprasellar cistern. Others are iso- or hyperintense on T1 weighted sequences, reflecting variable protein and cholesterol content of the cyst fluid.[184] With T2 weighting the cyst intensity often is increased, although those with prominent keratinization or high cholesterol may be hypointense, analogous to intensities described in craniopharyngioma. Infrequently, Rathke's cleft cysts enhance after gadolinium–DTPA or contain calcium, with resultant difficulty in differentiation from craniopharyngioma (Fig. 9–48).[2] These masses may be intrasellar, suprasellar, or both.

On CT, Rathke's cleft cysts are homogeneous or heterogeneous intra-, supra-, or both intra- and suprasellar masses with little or no contrast enhancement. Cysts may be hypodense, although iso- or hyperdense cysts relative to brain mimic solid masses.[183] Calcification is infrequently demonstrated within the cyst wall.

Simple Rathke's cleft cysts do not enhance after administration of intravenous iodinated contrast material or gadolinium. Enhancement has been described on CT in transitional forms, e.g., benign cystic craniopharyngioma,[183] and in Rathke's cleft cysts with evidence of septic or aseptic inflammation.[183, 185]

HAMARTOMA

Ectopic foci of gray matter or hamartomas are encountered scattered throughout the major white matter tracts as incidental findings at autopsy, possibly related to seizure foci. They may be masslike or exophytic, particularly in those arising from the floor of the third ventricle involving the mamillary bodies or tuber cinereum.[2] Hamartomas may be isolated or associated with other congenital anomalies. They have been associated with precocious puberty, partial complex seizures, intellectual and behavioral difficulties, and acromegaly.[186, 187] Other anomalies may be present such as the Hall-Pallister syndrome (dysplastic olfactory bulbs; absent pituitary gland; hypoplastic thyroid and adrenal glands; cryptorchidism; cardiac, renal, and anal anomalies; syndactyly).[188]

Gross examination of the hypothalamic hamartoma reveals a lobular mass of gray matter that on histologic appearance is made up of normal neurons and glial tissues. Fibers may extend from these masses into the adjacent normal tracts of the hypothalamic region. A histologic progression has been noted between hamartoma and gangliocytoma (ganglioneuroma), suggesting an intermediate lesion between hamartoma and true neoplasia.[2] Ectopic hamartomas may occur extracranially, particularly involving the soft palate or nasal bridge.

Hamartomas are benign lesions that generally require no surgical resection or radiation therapy. Resection or biopsy may be required to exclude low-grade neoplasia, which may have an identical presentation and radiographic appearance. There are insufficient data to assess the therapeutic role of surgical excision in

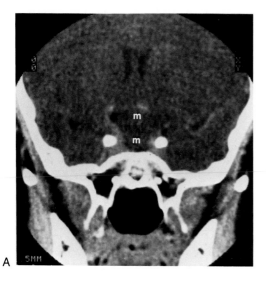

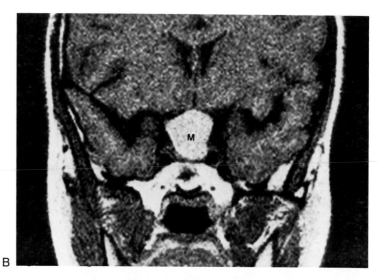

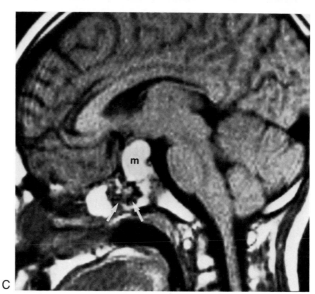

Figure 9–47. *Rathke's cleft cyst, recurrent.* **A,** Coronal contrast-enhanced CT. The intra- and suprasellar mass (m) is poorly defined owing to lack of contrast enhancement and low density. **B,** Coronal T1 weighted image (500/30). The intra- and suprasellar cyst (M) is hyperintense compared with brain and CSF, and thus is much better defined in MRI. On noncontrast MRI, this mass is indistinguishable from a craniopharyngioma. **C,** Sagittal T1 weighted image (500/30). The extent of the mass (m) upward into the suprasellar cistern and displacement of normal structures are again depicted. Note the mixed intensities within the sphenoid sinus (*arrows*) from previous trans-sphenoidal surgery.

hamartomas arising from the hypothalamus for control of endocrinologic disturbances.[2]

On MRI, hamartomas distort adjacent anatomic structures on T1 weighted images and have a hyperintense signal on T2 weighted images (Fig. 9–49).[189] Those of the hypothalamic region are indistinguishable without biopsy from astrocytoma. In other locations, they result in focal masses with intensities mimicking normal gray matter in abnormal locations. Although experience with gadolinium enhancement of these lesions is limited, variable enhancement is expected on the basis of CT data.

Hamartomas are isodense to normal gray matter on CT. Enhancement is variable, with some demonstrating no detectable enhancement after intravenous contrast administration. These may be difficult to recognize on CT; CT cisternography was required for localization of these lesions before the advent of MRI.

INTRASELLAR MASSES

Most sellar region masses in children are suprasellar, intrasellar neoplasms in pediatric patients being uncommon. The differential diagnosis in children includes intrasellar craniopharyngioma; Rathke's cleft, benign, and epidermoid cysts; adenoma; histiocytosis X; and rare germ cell tumors (Fig. 9–50). Infrequently the sellar region is invaded by direct extension from an adjacent nasopharyngeal or skull base primary neoplasm, or is a site of metastatic disease.

Pituitary adenoma is a benign proliferation of a normal anterior pituitary gland cell with associated disruption of the acinar pattern of the gland. Adenomas in pediatric patients account for approximately 10 percent of all adenomas and are very rare before age 10 years.[2] Adenomas in children are generally secretory or hormonally active adenomas and may be of any size

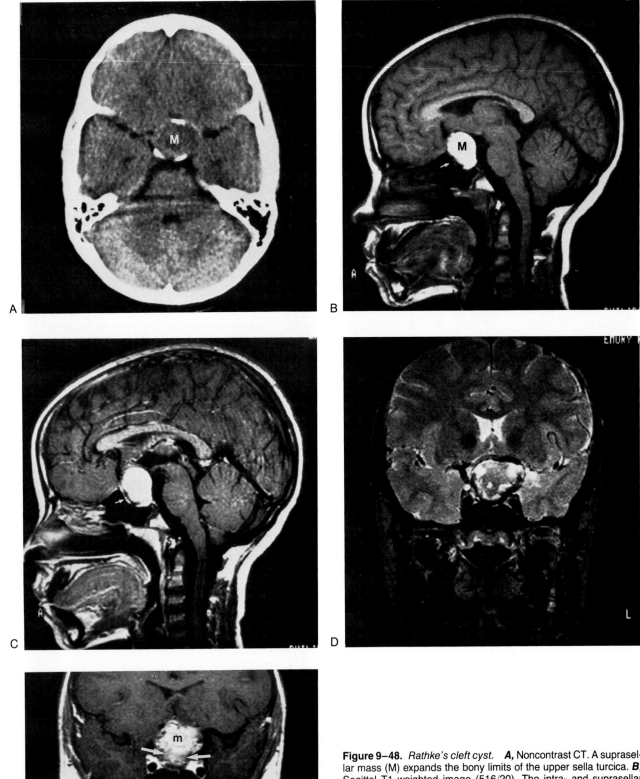

Figure 9–48. *Rathke's cleft cyst.* **A,** Noncontrast CT. A suprasellar mass (M) expands the bony limits of the upper sella turcica. **B,** Sagittal T1 weighted image (516/20). The intra- and suprasellar mass (M) is uniformly hyperintense compared with normal brain. The pituitary gland (*arrow*) is displaced anteroinferiorly. **C,** Sagittal T1 weighted image (616/20) after gadolinium–DTPA. The pituitary gland (*arrow*) enhances inhomogeneously but little enhancement has occurred of the mass itself. **D,** Coronal T2 weighted image (1980/90). The mass is inhomogeneous, with multiple areas of signal loss reflecting its cholesterol content. **E,** Coronal T1 weighted image (516/20) after gadolinium–DTPA. Contrast enhancement of the normal pituitary gland renders the border between the gland (*arrows*) and the mass (m) less apparent.

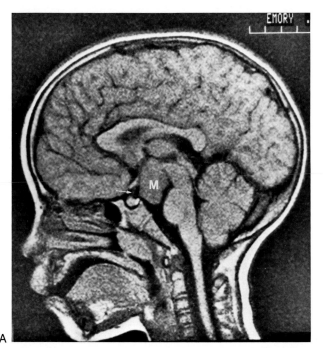
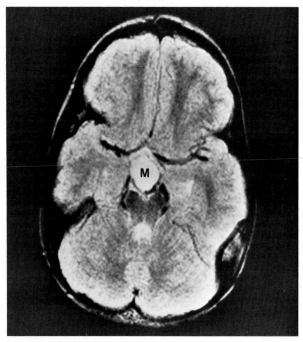

A B

Figure 9–49. *Hypothalamic hamartoma.* **A,** Sagittal T1 weighted image (523/30). The hypothalamic mass (M) extends exophytically inferiorly from the mamillary bodies with displacement anteriorly of the infundibulum (*arrow*). **B,** Axial T2 weighted image (2000/100). The mass (M) is uniformly hyperintense to normal brain on this sequence. On MR this lesion is indistinguishable from a hypothalamic glioma, although its posterior location and exophytic growth are typical of hamartoma.

at presentation. Those occurring during puberty may be more invasive, particularly prolactin-secreting tumors with prolactin levels of more than 500 ng/per milliliter, although other studies dispute this finding.[190,191]

Signs and symptoms are related to endocrinologic abnormalities of hypersecretion, interference with the normal hypothalamic-pituitary axis, or mass effect on the chiasm. As for adult adenomas, prolactin-secreting lesions are the most common type encountered; nonfunctioning adenomas are very uncommon in children. Treatment for ACTH- and GH-secreting tumors is surgical, i.e., trans-sphenoidal resection. Medical therapy (e.g., bromocriptine), surgery, or both may be required for prolactin-secreting lesions. Radiation therapy is reserved for symptomatic recurrence after resection that fails to respond to medical therapy. Malignancy is uncommon and is diagnosed on the basis of proven metastases, since benign and malignant adenomas are histologically similar.

Pathologically, adenomas are made up of proliferations of normal cells of the anterior pituitary gland.[2] Their secretory products reflect the cell type involved, with occasional reports of plurihormonal secretion from a single cell type. Hemorrhage and necrosis occur in larger tumors, but calcifications are uncommon.

On MRI, sagittal localizer images are followed by thin coronal T1 weighted images in patients suspected of harboring an adenoma (Fig. 9–51). Using these

sequences, enlargement of the gland and extension superiorly into the suprasellar cistern, or inferior erosion into the sphenoid sinus, are apparent.[192–194] Frank extension into the cavernous sinus results in asymmetry of the cavernous sinuses due to infiltration with tumor that is similar in intensity to that of the intrasellar lesion.[193–195] Macroadenomas most commonly have intensities similar to those of normal brain on MRI, with the exception of those containing necrotic cysts (hypointense on T1, hyperintense on T2 weighted images) or previous hemorrhage (hyperintense on T1 with hypointense foci on T2 weighted images attributable to deoxyhemoglobin or hemosiderin). Microadenomas may be hypointense to normal gland on thin high-resolution T1 weighted images, but proven microadenomas may result in no MR abnormalities. In this setting, T1 weighted MR studies performed immediately after gadolinium administration may permit detection of a microadenoma as a filling defect in the otherwise enhanced normal pituitary gland (Fig. 9–52).[196–198] Surgically proven microadenomas have been described with no abnormalities on noncontrast MRI or on MRI with gadolinium–DTPA; thus the diagnosis of microadenoma remains a joint effort, taking into account clinical, radiographic, and endocrinologic factors. The normal gland may be physiologically enlarged both at puberty and with pregnancy, so that evidence of gland enlargement alone is not sufficient for a diagnosis of adenoma. MR

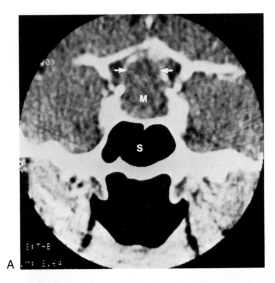

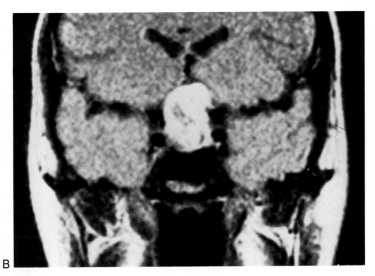

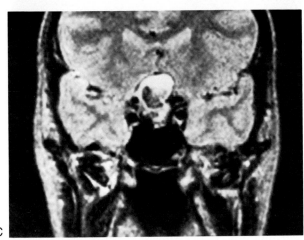

Figure 9–50. *Epidermoid. Intrasellar mass in a young girl with symptoms of chiasmal compression. Preoperative diagnosis was pituitary apoplexy, but at surgery a hemorrhagic intrasellar epidermoid was identified.* ***A,*** *Contrast-enhanced CT. The intrasellar mass (M) with suprasellar extension (*arrows*) is hypodense to brain, with only peripheral enhancement. Sphenoid sinus (S).* ***B,*** *Coronal T1 weighted image (620/30). The mass is hyperintense, with ill-defined foci of hypointensity, and arises from the sella.* ***C,*** *Coronal T2 weighted image (2000/100). The mass is less homogeneous in intensity, with foci of marked T2 shortening around the periphery and within the mass, suggesting subacute hemorrhage, which was not suspected on the basis of CT findings.*

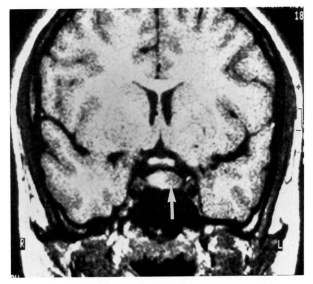

Figure 9–51. *Microadenoma.* T1 weighted image (516/29). A 15-year-old girl with hyperprolactinemia and a focal left-sided hypo-intense intrasellar mass (*arrow*) compatible with microadenoma.

findings must be correlated with endocrinologic and clinical findings in all cases.

Contrast-enhanced CT has been the imaging modality of choice for demonstration of large or small adenomas, and only recently has largely been replaced by MRI.[199,200] Approximately 50 to 60 percent of microadenomas are recognizable on CT as hypodense filling defects in contrast to the normally enhancing gland on scans immediately after contrast administration.[200] Additional findings include intrasellar mass effect such as focal elevation of the diaphragma sellae, displacement contralaterally of the infundibulum, overall gland enlargement, and focal sellar floor erosion. Microadenomas, particularly in Cushing's disease, may result in few or no abnormalities on direct coronal high-resolution CT. Thus, surgical exploration may be indicated based on clinical, endocrinologic, and petrosal venous sampling without demonstration of a focal lesion.[199,200] Macroadenomas (larger than 10 mm) result in an abnormally increased gland height with or without inhomogeneity or necrosis. The nor-

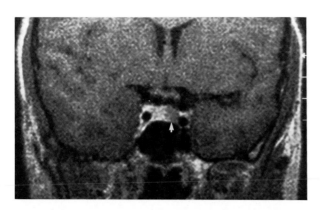

Figure 9–52. *Microadenoma.* T1 weighted image (516/20). A 16-year-old girl with hyperprolactinemia has a left-sided intrasellar hypointense mass (*arrow*), identified only after gadolinium enhancement, compatible with a microadenoma. The normal pituitary gland, the infundibulum, and the cavernous sinus normally enhance with gadolinium–DTPA.

mal gland is typically indistinguishable from macroadenoma or from isodense microadenoma on contrast-enhanced CT.

MENINGIOMA

Meningioma is an uncommon childhood tumor, accounting for no more than 3 to 4 percent of intracranial tumors in children.[2] Approximately one-fourth of meningiomas occur in association with neurofibromatosis. These patients may have multiple meningiomas or meningioma and other CNS tumors. Meningioma may also be induced by radiation therapy, but infrequently is identified in the pediatric population because of the long period of latency from time of radiation to tumor development.[201–203] Although a relationship between meningioma and trauma has been suggested, a causal relationship has not been confirmed.[204, 205] In children, these tumors tend to be discovered in the second decade, although symptoms may have been present for many years.[206]

Meningiomas arise from arachnoid cells in any location, but the calvarium adjacent to the sagittal sinus is the most common site, probably owing to the concentration of arachnoid villi in this location. Other sites include the tentorium, skull base, and infrequently the orbit, optic canal, and extracranially with extension from the calvarium or skull base into the scalp and face. Meningiomas may arise from the tela choroidea or choroid plexus, especially of the left lateral ventricle. Meningioma in childhood is more commonly cystic, devoid of a dural margin (i.e., intraventricular), and located in the posterior fossa than its adult counterpart.[4] In a series summarizing 75 reported pediatric patients with meningioma, Numaguchi and colleagues noted an incidence of 20 percent infratentorially and 13

percent intraventricularly.[206] Cyst formation has been attributed to tumor degenerative changes, loculations of adjacent CSF space, or reactive gliosis.[206–208]

Meningiomas are typically broad-based tumors with a dural attachment, although they may be globular or even dumbbell in shape, especially when arising from the falx. They displace but rarely invade the adjacent brain. Spread along the dura is common, and those adjacent to major venous sinuses may encroach upon or occlude the sinus. Remote metastases are uncommon. The cut surface may be gritty, especially in psammomatous forms due to calcification, and frank bone formation may be present. The adjacent calvarium may be hyperostotic from osteogenic invasion or in reaction to the meningioma. In other, perhaps faster growing tumors, the adjacent bone may be eroded or destroyed.

A number of different histologic types of meningioma have been described, as listed by Russell and Rubinstein:[2] (1) syncytial, (2) transitional, (3) fibroblastic, (4) angioblastic, and (5) malignant meningioma and sarcoma. Of these, the biologic behavior of the first three groups is benign and similar, so that the clinical significance of distinguishing among these is limited. The angioblastic meningioma, also called hemangiopericytoma, is more vascular and more aggressive than the previous categories. Malignant meningioma and primary meningeal sarcoma are rare, but preferentially arise in children.[2]

Presenting signs and symptoms in children reflect ventricular obstruction with hydrocephalus in those tumors arising within the ventricular system or in the posterior fossa. Other neurologic symptoms reflect mass effect on the adjacent brain or cranial nerves along the skull base.[4, 89] Treatment consists of surgical resection; a complete resection carries approximately a 20 percent recurrence rate at the site of previous surgery. Recurrences are more frequent in masses incompletely resected. Repeated surgical resection may be required for these radiation-resistant masses.

Meningioma has a variable intensity pattern on MRI, most commonly being hypo- or isointense to brain on T1 weighted images and hyperintense on T2 weighted images compared with cerebral white matter (Figs. 9–53, 9–54).[209–211] Compared with cortex, meningiomas may be isointense on all sequences, with resultant difficulty in visualization of these lesions on noncontrast MRI and at low field strengths. High-resolution techniques may reveal a well-defined hypointense interface between the tumor and adjacent brain attributed to a venous capsule, CSF fluid cleft, or dural margin, which improves lesion localization (Fig. 9–54). Additional helpful signs include mass effect with buckling of the junction between gray and white matter, and a heterogenous intensity pattern within the tumor itself.[209–211] Dense tumor calcifications may be recognized on MRI as areas of signal hypointensity resulting from averaging with adjacent tissues, but smaller calcifications are not apparent.[212] Associated

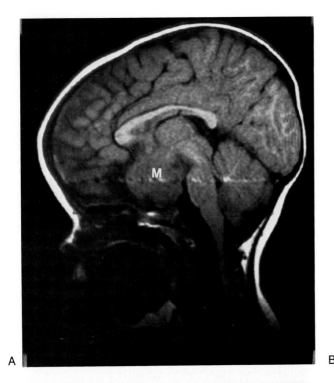

A

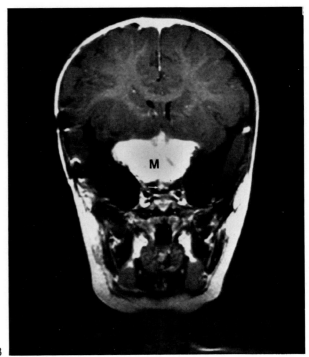

B

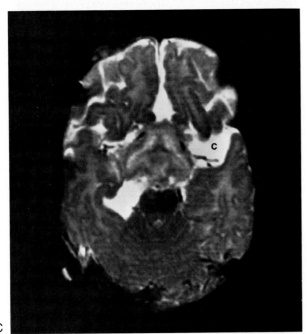

C

Figure 9–53. *Meningioma. A meningioma arising from the chiasm with erosion of the sella turcica in a young girl.* **A,** Sagittal T1 weighted image (500/30). An extensive mass (M) that is isointense to normal brain expands and obliterates definition of the optic chiasm and hypothalamus. **B,** Coronal T1 weighted image after gadolinium–DTPA enhancement (500/30). The mass (M) enhances markedly and spares the pituitary gland (*arrow*). Cysts extending into the sylvian fissures are difficult to distinguish from CSF on this sequence. **C,** Axial T2 weighted image (2000/90). The mass engulfs the optic chiasm, and associated cysts (c) enlarge the adjacent sylvian fissures bilaterally.

calvarial hyperostosis and bone destruction are better recognized on CT. MRI eliminates associated beam hardening or Hounsfield CT artifacts from bone; thus, lesions of the skull base are better evaluated. According to Elster and colleagues,[211] in 75 percent of cases the signal intensity on MRI correlates with the histologic type of meningioma present. In that series, angioblastic and syncytial meningiomas resulted in

marked hyperintensity on T2 weighted images, while those that were predominantly fibroblastic or transitional were hypointense to cortex on T2 weighted images.

Although larger lesions may be adequately defined on noncontrast studies, contrast-enhanced MRI provides superior lesion definition. With gadolinium enhancement, even small lesions are well defined. The

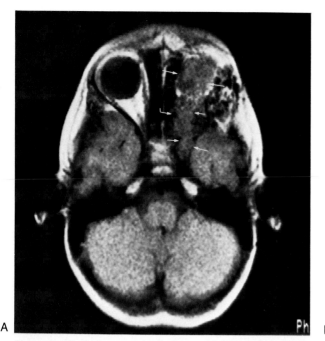
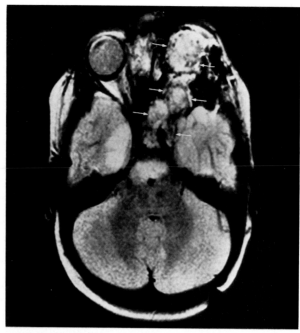

Figure 9–54. *Optic nerve meningioma with intracranial extension. A left intraorbital optic nerve meningioma extends posteriorly to involve the superior orbital fissure and cavernous sinus and invade the frontal lobe.* **A,** Axial T1 weighted image (500/30). The extensive orbital mass (*arrows*) contrasts with orbital fat, but the intracranial component in the cavernous sinus is isointense to brain parenchyma. **B,** Axial proton density (2000/50) image demonstrates extensive tumor (*arrows*) in the suprasellar and prepontine cisterns, medial right middle cranial fossa, and right frontal lobe.

optimal sequences on MRI for meningioma evaluation include multiplanar pre- and postcontrast T1 weighted images of the lesion, with T2 weighted images useful for demonstration of edema within the adjacent brain (Fig. 9–53).[213, 214] Slice thickness varies with lesion size, 5- to 6-mm images being reasonable for screening examinations; small lesions require thinner slices for greater detail. For example, lesions of the cavernous sinus, orbit, and internal auditory canal require 2- to 3-mm slices. Flow-sensitive techniques such as gradient-echo or phase sequences timed to demonstrate signal changes of flowing blood in relation to the cardiac cycle are useful to confirm the patency of major venous sinuses adjacent to the meningioma. Multiplanar gadolinium–DTPA MR studies are generally sufficient for preoperative tumor localization, and demonstrate the typical enhancement pattern and location of these extraaxial lesions. Angiography is occasionally used preoperatively to define the arterial blood supply, localize major draining veins, and assess the patency of major venous sinuses. In intraventricular lesions, a dense tumor stain lasting well into the venous phase suggests meningioma and aids differentiation from the hypervascular choroid plexus papilloma.

Meningioma is usually hyperdense to brain on noncontrast CT, with moderate to marked enhancement. Recognizable calcifications are common. Using wide CT windows, hyperostosis or osteolytic changes may be noted in the underlying bone, as well as enlarged vascular grooves. Macrocephaly or calvarial asym-

metry may result in small children. Meningioma typically has a broad interface with the calvarium and displaces the adjacent brain. Its margins are well defined, although these tumors may be associated with vasogenic edema in the underlying compressed brain. Uncommonly, aggressive forms may invade the brain parenchyma and blur the definition of tumor margins. Cysts within or adjacent to the tumor are better defined after contrast enhancement.[206–208] Lesions of the posterior fossa and foramen magnum may be obscured on CT by artifact from adjacent dense bone. Intraventricular forms are difficult to differentiate from other enhancing choroid plexus masses on CT. Meningioma arising orbitally from the optic nerve sheath results in a focal mass or diffuse enlargement of the optic nerve. Coronal imaging is helpful for differentiation of optic nerve from the enhancing meningioma surrounding it, compared with the diffuse enhancement and enlargement of the nerve itself in glioma.[215]

The differential diagnosis of meningioma in children includes meningeal sarcoma, malignant meningioma, dural metastasis, lymphoma, leukemia, or very rare lesions such as malignant fibrous histiocytoma, primary melanotic neuroectodermal tumor of infancy, or primary melanoma. Dural lesions of the cerebellopontine angle include meningioma and acoustic neuroma. Parasellar meningioma may resemble neuroma or glioma, but associated bone abnormalities and displacement, rather than enlargement of normal neural tissues, are helpful differential features.

HEMANGIOBLASTOMA

Hemangioblastoma is typically a cerebellar tumor of young male adults, but may be identified in the older pediatric population or rarely in infancy.[216] Occasional supratentorial examples have been documented.[2] Pediatric cases generally occur at or after puberty in association with von Hippel-Lindau disease (VHL), although the marked variability of this phakomatosis with many incomplete or atypical presentations is perhaps better termed hemangioblastomatosis.[217] Estimates suggest that approximately 20 percent of cerebellar capillary hemangioblastomas are associated with VHL.[2] In association with VHL, multiple lesions may be identified as well as retinal angiomatosis, cysts of the pancreas or kidney, adenomas of adrenal gland or liver, pheochromocytoma, epididymal tumors, liver carcinoma, and hypernephroma with an autosomal dominant inheritance.[4, 89, 218]

Presenting complaints from cerebellar hemangioblastoma include focal cerebellar deficits with ataxia and balance difficulties or hydrocephalus with increased intracranial pressure.[4] Asymptomatic lesions may be encountered in screening evaluations of affected kindreds.

Hemangioblastoma arises singly or multiply in the cerebellum or spinal cord. Syringomyelia is common with spinal lesions, and recurs until associated tumors are removed. Cerebellar lesions are often cystic (60 to 75 percent),[218–220] arising anywhere in the cerebellum and occasionally in the area postrema of the medulla. They may extend into the fourth ventricle or present as a mass within the medulla. Rarely, supratentorial hemangioblastoma has been described.[2] Secondary polycythemia is attributed to erythropoietin production by these tumors.

Gross examination reveals a well-defined mass with cysts containing xanthochromic or hemorrhagic fluid.[2] A predominant cyst with a tumor nodule is frequent. The neoplasia itself is vascular and firm, and spontaneous intratumoral hemorrhage is not uncommon. Lipid may be visible grossly on the tumor surface, as may vascular cavernous lesions. Microscopic evaluation reveals a mesh of capillary and cavernous blood spaces without mitoses.

Surgical resection is the treatment of choice and is curative if the mass is completely resected.[221] Local recurrences develop at sites of incomplete resection. Malignancy associated with these lesions is exceedingly uncommon, although several cases of intraspinal dissemination have been reported.[222] Multiple lesions or a positive family history warrant screening of family members in order to detect early lesions of VHL.

MRI reveals one or more cerebellar masses, often with associated cysts (Fig. 9–55).[223] The cysts and tumor may be hypointense on T1 weighted images, although those with previous hemorrhage are hyperintense relative to adjacent brain. T2 weighting reveals a hyperintense mass not readily separable from secondary edema. These are indistinguishable on MRI from cerebellar astrocytoma, but tend to affect an older patient population. Gadolinium–DTPA MRI markedly enhances these vascular tumors, and should be routinely included in the evaluation of these tumors and in screening evaluations of affected kindreds. Without gadolinium–DTPA, tumor nodules may go unrecognized owing to masking by the adjacent cysts (Fig. 9–55). Additional screening of the spinal cord after gadolinium–DTPA is warranted to exclude additional tumors and syringomyelia.

Contrast-enhanced CT of hemangioblastoma reveals a well-defined posterior fossa mass that is either cystic with a tumor nodule or solid with marked enhancement.[224, 225] CT is limited in sensitivity for detection of small lesions, tumor nodules, lesions close to the foramen magnum, and lesions within the medulla. Before MRI, angiography or myelography was required to diagnose small lesions of the posterior fossa and spine.[224]

Differential diagnoses in children include cystic cerebellar astrocytoma and uncommon cystic medulloblastoma and ependymoma. Occurrence in an older pediatric population, multiplicity, a positive family history or other stigmata of VHL, and marked enhancement after contrast administration are suggestive of this diagnosis.

NEUROFIBROMATOSIS

Neurofibromatosis is an inherited disorder of mesodermal and ectodermal tissues transmitted as an autosomal dominant trait with variable penetrance and frequent spontaneous mutations.[2, 226–228] Older terminology described a central and a peripheral form with differing distributions of neoplasia. More recent investigations suggest a categorization based on chromosomal abnormalities and designated as neurofibromatosis 1 and 2.[2, 229]

Neurofibromatosis 1 is the common form, being inherited as an autosomal dominant or sporadic mutation of chromosome 17. It results in a variety of lesions, including café au lait spots, intertriginous freckling, iris hamartomas, skin neurofibromas, optic glioma, and spinal and peripheral neurofibromata.[2, 227–230] Specific lesions encountered in neurofibromatosis 1 include optic pathway glioma, third ventricular–hypothalamic glioma, cerebellar astrocytoma, varied supratentorial gliomas and glioblastoma, spinal cord astrocytoma, cord ependymoma, and rarely retinal astrocytomas.[2] Diffuse gliosis and gliomatosis may be indistinguishable, resulting in infiltrating masses of the supra- or infratentorial parenchyma and spinal cord. In strict usage, von Recklinghausen's disease applies only to neurofibromatosis 1.

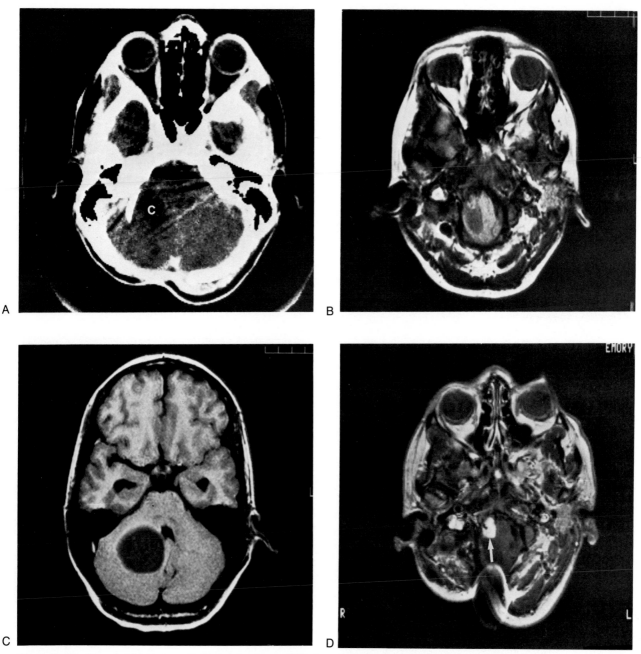

Figure 9–55. *Hemangioblastoma.* ***A,*** Contrast-enhanced CT. A cystic (C) right cerebellar mass containing "typical tumor fluid" was surgically explored, but no distinct tumor nodule was identified on CT or at surgery. A shunt was placed within the cyst. ***B, C,*** Axial T1 weighted images (500/30). A convincing tumor nodule was not recognizable. ***D,*** Axial T1 weighted images (500/30) after gadolinium–DTPA. A discrete enhancing tumor nodule (*arrow*) was recognized immediately adjacent to the medulla, which on reexploration was proved to represent hemangioblastoma.

Neurofibromatosis 2 is rare, is associated with lesions of chromosome 22, and typically includes bilateral acoustic neuroma or unilateral acoustic neuroma with other tumors (schwannoma, meningioma, or glial tumors) or familial evidence of neurofibromatosis.[229] Meningiomas in this category tend particularly to involve the choroid plexus of the lateral ventricle. The above-described neoplasms are discussed individually elsewhere in this chapter.

Controversies exist regarding the management of masses associated with neurofibromatosis. Some argue that the gliomas of neurofibromatosis, particularly of the optic pathways, are more akin to hamartomas than to true neoplasia.[230] For this reason, a plan of careful

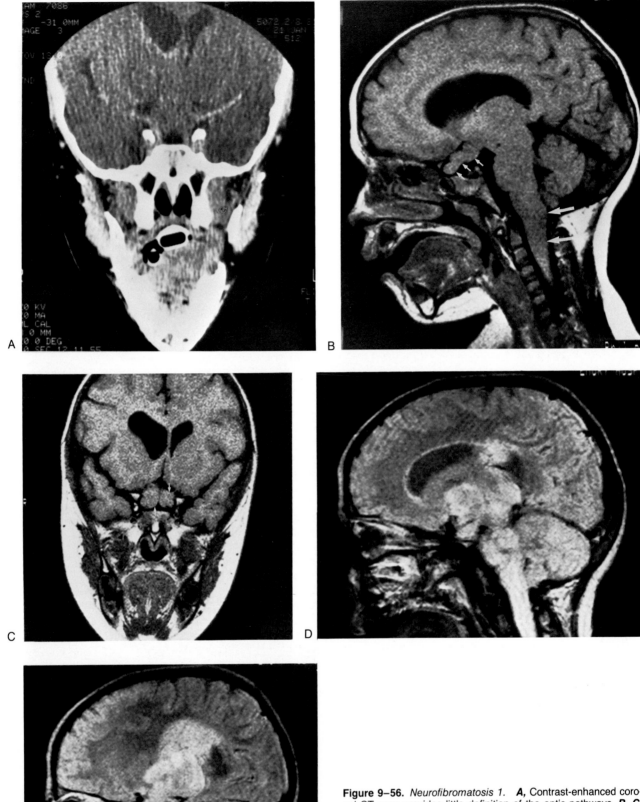

Figure 9–56. *Neurofibromatosis 1.* ***A,*** Contrast-enhanced coronal CT scan provides little definition of the optic pathways. ***B, C,*** Sagittal and coronal T1 weighted images (500/30). The optic chiasm, tracts, and intracranial optic nerves are expanded by glioma (*small arrows*) that is isointense to normal parenchyma. In addition, note the asymptomatic enlargement of the medulla and upper cervical spinal cord (*large arrows*). ***D, E,*** Proton density sagittal images (2000/50). Extensive asymptomatic intra-axial lesions are identified throughout the brain stem and deep gray matter. They may represent either asymptomatic neoplasia or hamartoma-gliomatosis.

212

medical observation without surgery or radiation therapy may be considered. In other cases, however, a clear pattern of tumor progression with sequelae necessitates intervention.

MRI has proved preferable to CT for diagnosis and follow-up of CNS manifestations of both forms of neurofibromatosis.[231–234] On MRI, T1 weighted images demonstrate distortions of normal anatomy due to intra-axial or larger extra-axial masses (Fig. 9–56). CNS lesions that infiltrate the brain parenchyma are better evaluated by T2 weighting. Extra-axial lesions enhance markedly after gadolinium administration, thus facilitating recognition and localization of these lesions. Bilateral acoustic neuromas are readily demonstrated on MRI. Larger acoustic neuromas present as masses originating at the porus acusticus with extension into the cerebellopontine angles (Fig. 9–57). Smaller intracanalicular lesions are best detected after gadolinium administration. Gadolinium is also useful for differentiation of intra-axial tumor margins apart from associated edema, and for differentiation of postsurgical abnormalities from residual or recurrent neoplasia.

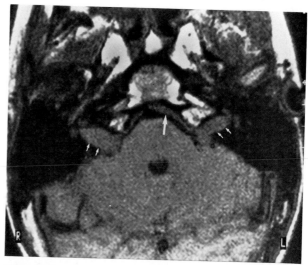

Figure 9–57. *Neurofibromatosis 2.* A young boy who presented with intraventricular meningioma, and on prolonged follow-up developed two separated spinal meningiomas and bilateral acoustic neuromas. Axial T1 weighted image (616/20). Bilateral acoustic neuromas (*small arrows*) expand the internal auditory canals and extend into the CPA cisterns. Thickened extra-axial tissue (*large arrow*) against the clivus is presumed to represent en plaque meningioma extending cranially from a lesion at C2.

CENTRAL NERVOUS SYSTEM METASTATIC DISEASE

Metastases within the CNS may develop from hematogenous dissemination of a non–CNS primary tumor, or by seeding from systemic or CNS diseases within the CSF. Hematogenous metastases to brain parenchyma are uncommon in the pediatric population, most commonly resulting from hematopoietic malignancies. Skull metastases to the bone or adjacent dura arise in neuroblastoma, lymphoma, and leukemia. Uncommon skull primary tumors and tumors arising adjacent to the skull base (orbit, nasopharynx, middle ear) may invade the CNS, as in chondrosarcoma, osteosarcoma, rhabdomyosarcoma, and nasopharyngeal malignancy. Leptomeningeal seeding in the intracranial space or spinal canal results from systemic disorders generally of the hematopoietic system, e.g., leukemia and lymphoma, or from CNS primary tumors.[2] The more common CNS primary tumors associated with metastasis in the subarachnoid space include medulloblastoma, pineal germ cell tumors, pineoblastoma, ependymoma, PNET (particularly primary CNS neuroblastoma), and malignant astrocytoma (Fig. 9–58). The frequency of dissemination in the subarachnoid space justifies craniospinal radiation at the time of diagnosis in medulloblastoma and leukemia; this decision in other tumors depends on the proximity of the primary tumor to CSF spaces, the histologic appearance, and CSF evidence of dissemination.

Leptomeningeal dissemination historically connotes a poor prognosis, although palliation and prolongation of survival are now being obtained by use of aggressive radiation and multiagent chemotherapy. Hematogenous metastases to brain parenchyma from an extraneural primary tumor generally carry a poor prognosis in spite of aggressive therapy.

Hematogenous metastases to brain parenchyma are identified as multiple lesions of variable size that disrupt the blood-brain barrier, with or without associated vasogenic edema and mass effect. Their multiplicity, enhancement, and tendency to cluster at the gray-white junction and in the middle cerebral artery territory suggest this diagnosis, although inflammatory and demyelinating diseases may have a similar appearance. In immunocompromised patients such as those with congenital or acquired immunodeficiency, transplants, and AIDS, multiple diseases may coexist in the same patient. Immunocompromised children may also develop second primary lesions such as meningioma, meningeal sarcoma, glioblastoma multiforme, and radiation necrosis (Fig. 9–59). For this reason, careful monitoring of response to therapy and stereotactic biopsy should be considered. In selected patients, positron emission tomography may be a useful adjunct to differentiate radiation necrosis from tumor recurrence.[235,236]

Although hematogenous metastases may be recognized on T2 weighted MRI, recent experience has shown that this technique is neither sufficiently sensitive nor specific for confirmation of metastases. Prob-

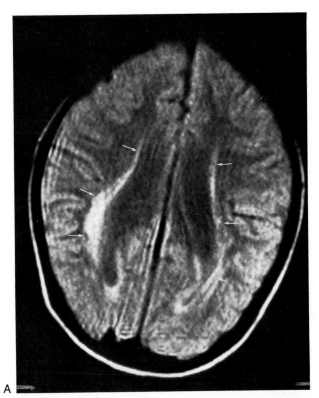

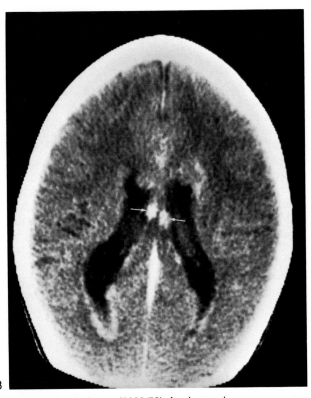

A

B

Figure 9–58. *Leptomeningeal dissemination from brain stem glioma.* **A,** Proton density image (2000/50). An abnormal high signal (*arrows*) around the lateral ventricles is compatible with leukoencephalopathy from radiation or chemotherapy, transependymal absorption of CSF related to hydrocephalus, or subependymal spread of tumor. This study was performed before the availability of gadolinium–DTPA. **B,** Contrast-enhanced CT. The enhancement around the ventricles and the nodules (*arrows*) on the septum pellucidum proved to be ependymal spread of malignant astrocytoma. With the availability of gadolinium–DTPA, similar information could be obtained from contrast-enhanced MRI.

lems with noncontrast MRI include failure to depict small lesions with little mass effect, those adjacent to CSF interfaces, and those adjacent to other metastatic or nonmetastatic abnormalities.[237,238] Noncontrast MRI is not sufficiently sensitive for detection of leptomeningeal metastases.[86] Although frank nodular masses are recognizable, smaller nodules and diffuse neoplastic coating of meningeal or ependymal surfaces may be inapparent. For this reason, gadolinium enhancement with T1 weighted MRI is essential for evaluation of patients in whom hematogenous or leptomeningeal metastases are suspected.[238] Gadolinium–DTPA markedly improves the sensitivity of MRI for detection of seeding of the brain and spinal canal, although postsurgical or inflammatory meningeal enhancement may have a similar appearance.[87,96] A precontrast T1 weighted image is useful in order to differentiate hemorrhagic or fatty masses with a short T1 from those enhancing with gadolinium.

Before the advent of MRI, contrast-enhanced CT was the imaging modality of choice in patients suspected of hematogenous or leptomeningeal CNS metastases.[239] CT, particularly with high-contrast dose techniques and delayed scanning, detects multiple enhancing masses with or without associated vasogenic edema. CT is limited, however, for detection of lesions adjacent to dense bone owing to interference from Hounsfield artifact. CT of leptomeningeal dissemination of tumor may reveal a diffuse coating of enhancing neoplasia on brain or dural surfaces, frank nodular masses with or without displacement of normal tissues, or communicating hydrocephalus. Meningeal carcinomatosis commonly is not apparent on CT, requiring CSF chemical and cytologic testing for diagnosis.[240] Subependymal spread of tumor similarly results in a diffuse coating of the ventricular surfaces, or in nodular masses on ventricular surfaces. Obstructive hydrocephalus may rarely occur when these lesions are located at the foramen of Monro or the aqueduct of Sylvius.

Acknowledgment: The author gratefully acknowledges the expert assistance of Francine Hollowell for editing and of Roz Vecchio for photography.

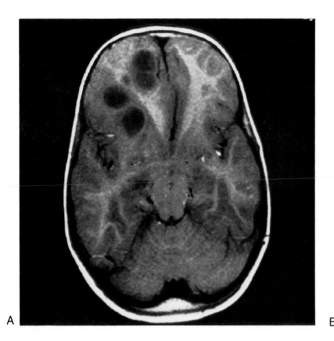

A

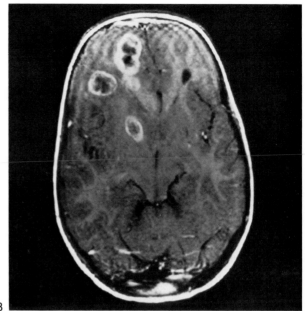

B

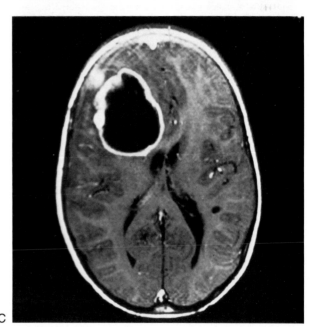

C

Figure 9–59. *Glioblastoma multiforme (GBM). A teen-aged boy who was considered cured of leukemia after extensive therapy and bone marrow transplant developed multiple masses within the right frontal lobe. These were biopsied and proved to represent multifocal GBM.* ***A,*** *Axial T1 weighted image (500/20). Multiple ringlike hypointense lesions and mass effect are apparent in the right frontal lobe.* ***B, C,*** *Axial T1 weighted images (500/20) after gadolinium–DTPA. Multiple masses with necrotic-cystic centers and enhancing margins are apparent.*

REFERENCES

1. Duffner PK, Cohen ME, Freeman AI. Pediatric brain tumors: an overview. CA 1985; 35:287–301.
2. Russell DS, Rubinstein LJ. Pathology of tumors of the nervous system. 5th ed. Baltimore: Williams & Wilkins, 1989.
3. Kernohan JW, Mabon RF, Svien HJ, Adson AW. Symposium on a new and simplified concept of gliomas (a simplified classification of gliomas). Proc Mayo Clin 1949; 24:71.
4. Cohen ME, Duffner PK. Brain tumors in children. Principles of diagnosis and treatment. New York: Raven Press, 1984.
5. Gol A, McKissock W. The cerebellar astrocytomas. A report on 98 verified cases. J Neurosurg 1959; 16:287–296.
6. Gol A. Cerebellar astrocytomas in children. Am J Dis Child 1963; 106:21–24.
7. Rubinstein LJ. Tumors of the central nervous system. Firminger HI, Washington, DC: Armed Forces Institute of Pathology, 1972:32–34.
8. Shapiro K, Shulman K. Spinal cord seeding from cerebellar astrocytomas. Childs Brain 1976; 2:177–186.
9. Bernell WR, Kepes JJ, Seitz EP. Late malignant recurrence of childhood cerebellar astrocytoma. Report of two cases. J Neurosurg 1972; 37:470–474.

10. Gjerris F, Klinken L. Long-term prognosis in children with benign cerebellar astrocytoma. J Neurosurg 1978; 49:179–184.

11. Griffin TW, Beaufait D, Blasko JC. Cystic cerebellar astrocytomas in childhood. Cancer 1979; 44:276–280.

12. Kjos BO, Brant-Zawadzki M, Kucharczyk W, et al. Cystic intracranial lesions: magnetic resonance imaging. Radiology 1985; 155:363–369.

13. Randell CP, Collins AG, Young IR, et al. Nuclear magnetic resonance imaging of posterior fossa tumors. AJNR 1983; 4:1027–1034.

14. Sze G. Pediatric posterior fossa tumors. MRI Decisions Nov-Dec. 1988:17–26.

15. Kucharczyk W, Brant-Zawadzki M, Sobel D, et al. Central nervous system tumors in children: detection by magnetic resonance imaging. Radiology 1985; 155:131–136.

16. Lee BCP, Kneeland JB, Deck MDF, Cahill PT. Posterior fossa lesions: magnetic resonance imaging. Radiology 1984; 153:137–143.

17. Oot RF, New PFJ, Pile-Spellman J, et al. The detection of intracranial calcifications by MR. AJNR 1986; 7:801–809.

18. Bird CR, Drayer BP, Medina M, et al. Gd-DTPA-enhanced MR imaging in pediatric patients after brain tumor resection. Radiology 1988; 169:123–126.

19. Zimmerman RA, Bilaniuk LT, Bruno L, Rosenstock J. Computed tomography of cerebellar astrocytoma. AJR 1978; 130:929–933.

20. Kingsley DPE, Kendall BE. The CT scanner in posterior fossa tumours of childhood. Br J Radiol 1979; 52:769–776.

21. Epstein F, McCleary EL. Intrinsic brain-stem tumors of childhood: surgical indications. J Neurosurg 1986; 64:11–15.

22. Hoffman JH, Becker L, Craven MA. A clinically and pathologically distinct group of benign brain stem gliomas. Neurosurgery 1980; 7:243–248.

23. Abernathey CD, Camacho A, Kelly PJ. Stereotaxic suboccipital transcerebellar biopsy of pontine mass lesions. J Neurosurg 1989; 70:195–200.

24. Kim TH, Chin HW, Pollan S, et al. Radiotherapy of primary brain stem tumors. Int J Radiat Oncol Biol Phys 1980; 6:51–57.

25. Stroink AR, Hoffman HJ, Hendrick EB, Humphreys RP. Diagnosis and management of pediatric brain-stem gliomas. J Neurosurg 1986; 65:745–750.

26. Golden GS, Ghatak NR, Hirano A, French JH. Malignant glioma of the brainstem. A clinicopathological analysis of 13 cases. J Neurol Neurosurg Psychiatry 1972; 35:732–738.

27. Fulton DS, Levin VA, Wara WM, et al. Chemotherapy of pediatric brain-stem tumors. J Neurosurg 1981; 54:721–725.

28. Albright AL, Price RA, Guthkelch AN. Brain stem gliomas of children. A clinicopathological study. Cancer 1983; 52:2313–2319.

29. Han JS, Bonstelle CT, Kaufman B, et al. Magnetic resonance imaging in the evaluation of the brainstem. Radiology 1984; 150:705–712.

30. Flannigan BD, Bradley WG, Mazziotta JC, et al. Magnetic resonance imaging of the brainstem: normal structure and basic functional anatomy. Radiology 1985; 154:375–383.

31. Johnson MA, Pennock JM, Bydder GM, et al. Clinical NMR imaging of the brain in children: normal and neurologic disease. AJR 1983; 141:1005–1018.

32. Lemme-Plaghos L, Kucharczyk W, Brant-Zawadzki M, et al. MR of angiographically occult vascular malformations. AJNR 1986; 7:217–222.

33. Powers TA, Partain CL, Dessler RM, et al. Central nervous system lesions in pediatric patients: Gd-DTPA-enhanced MR imaging. Radiology 1988; 169:723–726.

34. Bilaniuk LT, Zimmerman RA, Littman P, et al. Computed tomography of brain stem gliomas in children. Radiology 1980; 134:89–95.

35. Bendheim PI, Berg MO. Ataxic hemiparesis from a midbrain mass. Ann Neurol 1981; 9:405–407.

36. Bernstein M, Hoffman HJ, Halliday WC, et al. Thalamic tumors in children. J Neurosurg 1984; 61:649–656.

37. Hoyt WR, Baghdassarian SA. Optic glioma of childhood: natural history and rationale for conservative management. Br J Ophthalmol 1969; 53:793–798.

38. Stern J, DiGiacinto GV, Housepian EM. Neurofibromatosis and optic gliomas: clinical and morphologic correlations. Neurosurgery 1980; 4:524–528.

39. Chutorian AM, Schwartz JF, Evans RA, Carter S. Optic gliomas in children. Neurology 1964; 14:83–95.

40. Wilson WB, Feinsod M, Hoyt WF, Nielsen SL. Malignant evolution of childhood chiasmal pilocytic astrocytoma. Neurology 1976; 26:322–325.

41. Hoyt WF, Meshel LG, Lessell S, et al. Malignant optic glioma of adulthood. Brain 1973; 96:121–132.

42. Burr IM, Slovin AC, Danish RK, et al. Diencephalic syndrome revisited. J Pediatr 1976; 88:439–444.

43. Russell A. A diencephalic syndrome of emaciation in infancy and childhood. Arch Dis Child 1951; 26:274.

44. Stern J, Jakobiec FA, Housepian EM. The architecture of optic nerve gliomas with and without neurofibromatosis. Arch Ophthalmol 1980; 98:505–511.

45. Davis PC, Hoffman JC, Weidenheim KM. Large hypothalamic and optic chiasm gliomas in infants: difficulties in distinction. AJNR 1984; 5:579–585.

46. Tenny RT, Laws ER, Younge BR, Rush JA. The neurosurgical management of optic glioma. Results in 104 patients. J Neurosurg 1982; 57:452–458.

47. Danoff BF, Kramer S, Thompson N. The radiotherapeutic management of optic nerve gliomas in children. Radiat Oncol Biol Phys 1980; 6:45–50.

48. Brown EW, Riccardi VM, Mawad M, et al. MR imaging of optic pathways in patients with neurofibromatosis. AJNR 1987; 8:1031–1036.

49. Pomeranz SJ, Shelton JJ, Tobias J, et al. MR of visual pathways in patients with neurofibromatosis. AJNR 1987; 8:831–836.

50. Linder B, Campos M, Schafer M. CT and MRI of orbital abnormalities in neurofibromatosis and selected craniofacial anomalies. Radiol Clin North Am 1987; 25:787–802.

51. Daniels DL, Yu S, Pech P, Haughton VM. Computed tomography and magnetic resonance imaging of the orbital apex. Radiol Clin North Am 1987; 25:803–818.

52. Naheedy MH, Haag JR, Azar-Kia B, et al. MRI and CT of sellar and parasellar disorders. Radiol Clin North Am 1987; 225:819–848.

53. Castillo M, Davis PC, Ross W, Hoffman JC. Primary meningioma of the chiasm and the optic nerves in a child: CT and MR appearance. JCAT 1989; 13:679–681.

54. Byrd SE, Harwood-Nash DC, Fitz CR, et al. Computed tomography of intraorbital optic nerve gliomas in children. Radiology 1978; 129:73–78.

55. Fletcher WA, Imes RK. Chiasmal gliomas: appearance and long-term changes demonstrated by computerized tomography. J Neurosurg 1986; 154:159.

56. Savoiardo M, Harwood-Nash DC, Tadmor R, et al. Gliomas of the intracranial anterior optic pathways in children. Radiology 1981; 138:601–610.

57. Kurokawa T, Tomita S, Ueda K, et al. Prognosis of occlusive disease of the circle of Willis (moyamoya disease) in children. Pediatr Neurol 1985; 1:274–277.

58. Hilal SK, Solomon GE, Gold AP, Carter S. Primary cerebral arterial occlusive disease in children. Part I: Acute acquired hemiplegia. Part II: Neurocutaneous syndromes. Radiology 1971; 99:71–94.

59. Backus RE, Millichap JG. The seizure as manifestation of intracranial tumor in childhood. Pediatrics 1962; 29:978–984.

60. Livingston S. The diagnosis and treatment of convulsive disorders in children. Springfield, IL: Charles C Thomas, 1954:24.

61. Page LK, Lombroso CT, Matson DD. Childhood epilepsy with late detection of cerebral glioma. J Neurosurg 1969; 31:253–261.

62. Salcmon M. Supratentorial gliomas: clinical features and surgical therapy. In: Wilkins RH, Rengachary SS, eds. Neurosurgery. New York: McGraw-Hill, 1985:579–590.

63. Frankel SA, German WJ. Glioblastoma multiforme. Review of 219 cases with regard to natural history, pathology, diagnostic methods, and treatment. J Neurosurg 1958; 15:489–503.
64. Farwell JR, Dohrmann GH, Flannery JT. Central nervous system tumors in children. Cancer 1977; 40:3123–3132.
65. Aaron J, New PFJ, Strand R, et al. NMR imaging in temporal lobe epilepsy due to gliomas. JCAT 1984; 8:608–613.
66. Earnest F, Kelly PJ, Scheithaure BW, et al. Cerebral astrocytomas: histopathologic correlation of MR and CT contrast enhancement with stereotactic biopsy. Radiology 1988; 166:823–827.
67. Latack JT, Abou-Khalil BW, Siegel GJ, et al. Patients with partial seizures: evaluation by MR, CT, and PET imaging. Radiology 1986; 159:159–163.
68. Ormson MJ, Kispert DB, Sharborough FW, et al. Cryptic structural lesions in refractory partial epilepsy: MR imaging and CT studies. Radiology 1986; 160:215–219.
69. Graif M, Bydder GM, Steiner RE, et al. Contrast-enhanced MR imaging of malignant brain tumors. AJNR 1985; 6:855–862.
70. Brant-Zawadzki M, Berry I, Osaki L, et al. Gd-DTPA in clinical MR of the brain: 1. Intraaxial lesions. AJNR 1986; 7:781–788.
71. Claussen C, Laniado M, Schorner W, et al. Gadolinium-DTPA in MR imaging of glioblastomas and intracranial metastases. AJNR 1985; 6:669–674.
72. Farwell JR, Dohrmann GJ, Flannery JT. Medulloblastoma in childhood: an epidemiological study. J Neurosurg 1984; 61:657–664.
73. Rorke LB. Origin and histogenesis of medulloblastoma. In: Zeltzer RM, Pochedly C, eds. Medulloblastomas in children. New concepts in tumor biology, diagnosis, and treatment. New York: Praeger, 1986:14–21.
74. Hart MN, Earle RM. Primitive neuroectodermal tumors of the brain in children. Cancer 1973; 32:890–897.
75. Finlay JL. Natural history and epidemiology of medulloblastoma. In: Vinken PJ, Bruyn GW, eds. Tumors of the brain and skull. Part 3. New York: Elsevier, 1975:167–194.
76. McFarland DR, Horwitz H, Saenger EL, Bahr GK. Medulloblastoma—a review of prognosis and survival. Br J Radiol 1969; 42:198–214.
77. Milstein JM. Medulloblastoma: historical, diagnostic, and prognostic factors. In: Zeltzer PM, Pochedly C, eds. Medulloblastomas in children. New concepts in tumor biology, diagnosis, and treatment. New York: Praeger, 1986:76–86.
78. Tomita T, McLone DG. Medulloblastoma in childhood: results of radical resection and low-dose neuraxial radiation therapy. J Neurosurg 1986; 64:238–242.
79. Silverman CL, Simpson JR. Cerebellar medulloblastoma: the importance of posterior fossa dose to survival and patterns of failure. Int J Radiat Oncol Biol Phys 1982; 8:1869–1876.
80. Berry MR, Jenkin RDT, Keen CW, et al. Radiation treatment for medulloblastoma. A 21-year review. J Neurosurg 1981; 55:43–51.
81. Hirsch JF, Reiner D, Czernichow P, et al. Medulloblastoma in childhood. Survival and functional results. Acta Neurochir 1979; 48:1–15.
82. Zulch KJ. Medulloblastoma. In: Zulch KJ, ed. Brain tumors. Their biology and pathology. 3rd ed. Berlin: Springer-Verlag, 1986:324–340.
83. Chatty EM, Earle KM. Medulloblastoma. A report of 201 cases with emphasis on the relationship of histologic variants to survival. Cancer 1971; 28:977–983.
84. Packer RJ, Sutton LN, Rorke LB, et al. Prognostic importance of cellular differentiation in medulloblastoma of childhood. J Neurosurg 1984; 61:296–301.
85. Zee CS, Segall HD, Miller C, et al. Less common CT features of medulloblastoma. Radiology 1982; 144:97–102.
86. Davis PC, Friedman NC, Fry SM, et al. Leptomeningeal metastasis: MR imaging. Radiology 1987; 163:449–454.
87. Krol G, Sze G, Malkin M, et al. MR of cranial and spinal meningeal carcinomatosis: comparison with CT and myelography. AJNR 1988; 9:709–714.
88. Enzmann DR, Norman D, Levin V, et al. Computed tomography in the follow-up of medulloblastomas and ependymomas. Radiology 1978; 128:57–63.
89. Diebler C, Dulac O. Pediatric neurology and neuroradiology. Cerebral and cranial diseases. Berlin: Springer-Verlag, 1987.
90. Rubinstein LJ. The definition of the ependymoblastoma. Arch Pathol 1970; 90:35–45.
91. Liu HM, McLone DG, Clark S. Ependymomas of childhood. II. Electron microscopic study. Childs Brain 1977; 3:281–296.
92. Glasauer FE, Yuan RHP. Intracranial tumors with extracranial metastases. Case report and review of the literature. J Neurosurg 1963; 20:474–493.
93. Dohrmann GJ, Farwell JR, Flannery JT. Ependymomas and ependymoblastomas in children. J Neurosurg 1976; 45:273–283.
94. Centeno RS, Lee AA, Winter J, Barba D. Supratentorial ependymomas. J Neurosurg 1986; 64:209–215.
95. Ross GW, Rubinstein LJ. Lack of histopathological correlation of malignant ependymomas with postoperative survival. J Neurosurg 1989; 70:31–36.
96. Sze G, Abramson A, Krol G, et al. Gadolinium-DTPA in the evaluation of intradural extramedullary spinal disease. AJNR 1988; 9:153–164.
97. Swartz JD, Zimmerman RA, Bilaniuk LT. Computed tomography of intracranial ependymomas. Radiology 1982; 143:97–101.
98. Armington WG, Osborn AG, Cubberley DA, et al. Supratentorial ependymoma: CT appearance. Radiology 1985; 157:367–372.
99. Bennett JP, Rubinstein LJ. The biological behavior of primary cerebral neuroblastoma: a reappraisal of the clinical course in a series of 70 cases. Ann Neurol 1984; 16:21–27.
100. Duffner PK, Cohen ME, Heffner RR, Freeman AI. Primitive neuroectodermal tumors of childhood. An approach to therapy. J Neurosurg 1981; 55:376–381.
101. Berger MS, Edwards MSB, Wara WM, et al. Primary cerebral neuroblastoma. J Neurosurg 1983; 59:418–423.
102. Rubinstein LJ. Cytogenesis and differentiation of primitive central neuroepithelial tumors. J Neuropathol Exp Neurol 1972; 31:7–26.
103. Horten BC, Rubinstein LJ. Primary cerebral neuroblastoma. A clinicopathological study of 35 cases. Brain 1976; 99:735–756.
104. Kosnik EJ, Boesel CP, Bay J, Sayers M. Primitive neuroectodermal tumors of the central nervous system in children. J Neurosurg 1978; 48:741–746.
105. Davis PC, Wichman RD, Takei Y, Hoffman JC. CT and MR of primary cerebral neuroblastoma. AJNR 1990; 11:115–120.
106. Zimmerman RA, Bilaniuk LT. CT of primary and secondary craniocerebral neuroblastoma. AJNR 1980; 1:431–434.
107. Chambers EF, Turski PA, Sobel D, et al. Radiologic characteristics of primary cerebral neuroblastoma. Radiology 1981; 139:101–104.
108. Latchaw RE, L'Heureux PR, Young G, Priest JR. Neuroblastoma presenting as central nervous system disease. AJNR 1982; 3:623–630.
109. Kingsley DPE, Harwood-Nash DCF. Radiological features of the neuroectodermal tumors of childhood. Neuroradiology 1984; 26:463–467.
110. Pearl GS, Takei Y, Bakay RAE, Davis PC. Intraventricular primary cerebral neuroblastoma in adults: report of three cases. Neurosurgery 1985; 16:847–849.
111. Lhermitte J, Duclos P. Sur un ganglioneuroma diffus du cortex du cervelet. Bull Assoc Franc Etude Can 1920; 9:99–107.
112. Ambler M, Pogacar S, Sidman R. Lhermitte-Duclos disease (granule cell hypertrophy of the cerebellum). Pathological analysis of the first familial cases. J Neuropathol Exp Neurol 1969; 28:622–647.
113. Smith RR, Grossman RI, Goldberg HI, et al. MR imaging of

Lhermitte-Duclos disease: a case report. AJNR 1989; 10:187–189.

114. Carter JE, Merren MD, Swann KW. Preoperative diagnosis of Lhermitte-Duclos disease by magnetic resonance imaging. J Neurosurg 1989; 70:135–137.

115. Sutton LN, Packer RJ, Rorke LB, et al. Cerebral gangliogliomas during childhood. Neurosurgery 1983; 13:124–128.

116. Demierre B, Stinchnoth FA, Hori A, Spoerri O. Intracerebral gangliogliomas. J Neurosurg 1986; 65:177–182.

117. Mizuno J, Nishio S, Barrow DL, et al. Ganglioglioma of the cerebellum: case report. Neurosurgery 1987; 21:584–588.

118. Castillo M, Davis PC, Takei Y, Hoffman JC. Intracranial ganglioglioma: MR and CT findings in 18 patients. AJNR 1990; 11:109–114.

119. Zimmerman RA, Bilaniuk LT. Computed tomography of intracerebral gangliogliomas. J Comput Tomogr 1979; 3:24–30.

120. Dorne HL, O'Gorman AM, Melanson D. Computed tomography of intracranial gangliogliomas. AJNR 1986; 7:281–285.

121. Dohrmann GJ, Farwell JR, Flannery JT. Oligodendrogliomas in children. Surg Neurol 1978; 10:21–25.

122. Lee YY, Van Tassel P. Intracranial oligodendrogliomas: imaging findings in 35 untreated cases. AJNR 1989; 10:119–127.

123. Chin HW, Hazel JJ, Kim TH, Webster JH. Oligodendrogliomas. I. A clinical study of cerebral oligodendrogliomas. Cancer 1980; 45:1458–1466.

124. Earnest F, Kernohan JW, Craig WM. Oligodendrogliomas. A review of 200 cases. AMA Arch Neurol Psych 1950; 63:964–976.

125. Barnard RO. The development of malignancy in oligodendrogliomas. J Pathol Bacteriol 1968; 96:113–123.

126. Shuman WP, Griffin BR, Haynor DR, et al. The utility of MR in planning the radiation therapy of oligodendroglioma. AJNR 1987; 8:93–98.

127. Dolinkas CA, Simeone FA. CT characteristics of intraventricular oligodendrogliomas. AJNR 1987; 8:1077–1082.

128. Vonofakos D, Marcu H, Hacker H. Oligodendrogliomas: CT patterns with emphasis on features indicating malignancy. JCAT 1979; 3:783–788.

129. Radkowski MR, Naidich TP, Tomita T, et al. Neonatal brain tumors: CT and MR findings. JCAT 1988; 12:10–20.

130. Herren RY. Papilloma of the choroid plexus. Arch Surg 1941; 42:758–774.

131. Carpenter DB, Michelsen WJ, Hays AP. Carcinoma of the choroid plexus. Case report. J Neurosurg 1982; 56:722–727.

132. McGirr SJ, Ebersold MJ, Scheithauer BW, et al. Choroid plexus papillomas: long-term follow-up results in a surgically treated series. J Neurosurg 1988; 69:843–849.

133. Gomori JM, Grossman RI, Hackney DB, et al. Variable appearances of subacute intracranial hematomas on high-field spin-echo MR. AJR 1988; 150:171–178.

134. Silver AJ, Ganti SR, Hilal SK. Computed tomography of tumors involving the atria of the lateral ventricles. Radiology 1982; 145:71–78.

135. Morrison G, Sobel DF, Kelley WM, Norman D. Intraventricular mass lesions. Radiology 1984; 153:435–442.

136. Zimmerman RA, Bilaniuk LT, Wood JH, et al. Computed tomography of pineal, parapineal, and histologically related tumors. Radiology 1980; 137:669–677.

137. Harwood-Nash DC, Fitz CR. Neuroradiology in infants and children. Vol 2. St Louis: CV Mosby, 1976:484–486.

138. Erlich SS, Apuzzo MLJ. Review article: the pineal gland: anatomy, physiology, and clinical significance. J Neurosurg 1985; 63:321–341.

139. Megyeri L. Cystic changes in the pineal body. Frankfurt Z Pathol 1960; 70:699–704.

140. Lee DH, Norman D, Newton TH. MR imaging of pineal cysts. JCAT 1987; 11:586–590.

141. Brady LW. The role of radiation therapy. In: Schmidek HH, ed. Pineal tumors. New York: Masson, 1977:127–132.

142. Abay EO, Laws ER, Grado GL, et al. Pineal tumors in children and adolescents. Treatment by CSF shunting and radiotherapy. J Neurosurg 1981; 55:889–895.

143. Wara WM, Jenkin RDT, Evans A, et al. Tumors of the pineal and suprasellar region: Children's Cancer Study Group treatment results 1960–1975. Cancer 1979; 43:698–701.

144. Hitchon PW, Abu-Yousef MM, Graf CJ, et al. Management and outcome of pineal region tumors. Neurosurgery 1983; 13:248–253.

145. Futrell NN, Osborn AG, Cheson BD. Pineal region tumors: computed tomographic–pathologic spectrum. AJNR 1981; 2:415–420.

146. Jooma R, Kendall BE. Diagnosis and management of pineal tumors. J Neurosurg 1983; 58:654–665.

147. Sculte FJ, Herrmann HD, Muller D, et al. Pineal region tumours of childhood. Eur J Pediatr 1987; 146:233–245.

148. Herrick MK. Pathology of pineal tumors. In: Neuwelt EA, ed. Diagnosis and treatment of pineal region tumors. Baltimore: Williams & Wilkins, 1984:55–56.

149. Tapp E, Huxley M. The histologic appearance of the human pineal gland from puberty to old age. J Pathol 1972; 108:137–144.

150. Jennings MR, Gelman R, Hochberg F. Intracranial germ-cell tumors: natural history and pathogenesis. J Neurosurg 1985; 63:155–167.

151. Kitay JI. Pineal lesions and precocious puberty: a review. J Clin Endocrinol Metab 1954; 14:622–625.

152. D'Andrea AD, Packer RJ, Rorke L, et al. Pineocytomas of childhood. A reappraisal of natural history and response to therapy. Cancer 1987; 59:1353–1357.

153. Edwards MSB, Hudgins RJ, Wilson CB, et al. Pineal region tumors in children. J Neurosurg 1988; 68:689–697.

154. Kilgore DP, Strother CM, Starshak RJ, Haughton VM. Pineal germinoma: MR imaging. Radiology 1986; 158:435–438.

155. Wood JH, Zimmerman RA, Bruce DA, et al. Assessment and management of pineal-region and related tumors. Surg Neurol 1981; 16:192–210.

156. Ganti SR, Hilal SK, Stein BM, et al. CT of pineal region tumors. AJNR 1986; 7:97–104.

157. Hildenbrand PG, Gabrielsen TO, Dorovini-Zis K, et al. Radiology of primary intracranial yolk-sac (endodermal sinus) tumors. AJNR 1983; 4:991–993.

158. Naidich T, Cacayorin ED, Stewart WA, et al. Germinal-cell tumor of the pineal gland. AJR 1986; 146:1246–1252.

159. Ito T. Pathology of brain tumors. Acta Pathol Jap 1958; 8:415.

160. Bannerjee T, Krigman MR. Intracranial epidermoid tumor: discussion of four cases. South Med J 1977; 70:726–727.

161. Zettner A, Netsky MG. Lipoma of the corpus callosum. J Neuropathol Exp Neurol 1960; 19:305–319.

162. Gerber SS, Plotkin R. Lipoma of the corpus callosum. J Neurosurg 1982; 57:281–285.

163. Atkinson G, Davis PC, Patrick LE, et al. Melanotic neuroectodermal tumor of infancy: MR findings and a review of the literature. Accepted for publication, Pediatr Radiol 1989; 20:20–22.

164. Olson JJ, Beck DW, Crawford SC, Menezes AH. Comparative evaluation of intracranial epidermoid tumors with computed tomography and magnetic resonance imaging. Neurosurgery 1987; 21:357–360.

165. Kjos BO, Brant-Zawadzki M, Kucharczyk W, et al. Cystic intracranial lesions: magnetic resonance imaging. Radiology 1985; 155:363–369.

166. Banna M. Intracranial cholesteatoma. Clin Radiol 1977; 28:161–164.

167. Davis KR, Roberson GH, Taveras JM, et al. Diagnosis of epidermoid tumor by computed tomography. Radiology 1976; 119:347–353.

168. Zimmerman RA, Bilaniuk LT, Dolinskas CA. Cranial computed tomography of epidermoid and congenital fatty tumors of maldevelopmental origin. J Comput Tomogr 1979; 3:40–50.

169. Benitez WI, Sartor KJ, Angtuaco EJC. Case report: craniopharyngioma presenting as a nasopharyngeal mass: CT and MR findings. JCAT 1988; 12:1068–1072.

170. Hoffman HJ, Hendrick EB, Humphreys RP, et al. Management of craniopharyngioma in children. J Neurosurg 1977; 47:218–227.

171. Fischer ED, Welch K, Belli JA, et al. Treatment of cranio-pharyngiomas in children: 1972–1981. J Neurosurg 1985; 62:496–501.

172. Petito CK, DeGirolami U, Earle KM. Craniopharyngiomas: a clinical and pathological review. Cancer 1976; 37:1944–1952.

173. Karnaze MG, Sartor K, Winthrop JD, et al. Suprasellar lesions: evaluation with MR imaging. Radiology 1986; 161:77–82.

174. Freeman MP, Kessler RM, Allen JH, Price A. Craniopharyngioma: CT and MR imaging in nine cases. JCAT 1987; 11:810–814.

175. Pusey E, Kortman KE, Flannigan BD, et al. MR of craniopharyngiomas: tumor delineation and characterization. AJR 1987; 149:383–388.

176. Hillman TH, Peyster RG, Hoover ED, et al. Case report: infrasellar craniopharyngioma: CT and MR studies. JCAT 1988; 12:702–704.

177. Holland BA, Kucharcyzk W, Brant-Zawadzki M, et al. MR imaging of calcified intracranial lesions. Radiology 1985; 157:353–356.

178. Seidel FG, Towbin R, Kaufman RA. Normal pituitary stalk size in children: CT study. AJR 1985; 145:1297–1302.

179. Braun IF, Pinto RS, Epstein F. Dense cystic craniopharyngiomas. AJNR 1982; 3:139–141.

180. Fitz CR, Wortzman G, Harwood-Nash DC, et al. Computed tomography in craniopharyngiomas. Radiology 1978; 327:687–691.

181. Boggan JE, Davis RL, Zorman G, Wilson CB. Intrasellar epidermoid cyst. J Neurosurg 1983; 58:411–415.

182. Eisenberg HM, Weiner RL. Benign pituitary cysts. In: Wilkins RH, Rengachary SS, eds. Neurosurgery. Hightstown, NJ: McGraw-Hill, 1985:932–934.

183. Kucharczyk W, Peck WW, Kelly WM, et al. Rathke cleft cysts: CT, MR imaging, and pathologic features. Radiology 1987; 165:491–495.

184. Maggio WW, Cail WS, Brookeman JR, et al. Rathke's cleft cyst: computed tomographic and magnetic resonance imaging appearances. Neurosurgery 1987; 21:60–62.

185. Okamoto S, Handa H, Yamashita J, et al. Computed tomography in intra- and suprasellar epithelial cysts (symptomatic Rathke's cleft cysts). AJNR 1985; 6:515–519.

186. Diebler C, Ponsot G. Hamartomas of the tuber cinereum. Neuroradiology 1983; 25:93–101.

187. Asa SL, Scheithauer BW, Bilbao JM, et al. A case for hypothalamic acromegaly: a clinicopathological study of six patients with hypothalamic gangliocytomas producing growth hormone–releasing factor. J Clin Endocrinol Metab 1984; 58:796–803.

188. Nurbhai MA, Tomlinson BE, Lorigan-Forsythe B. Infantile hypothalamic hamartoma with multiple congenital abnormalities. Neuropathol Appl Neurobiol 1985; 11:61–70.

189. Nishio S, Fujiwara S, Aiko Y, et al. Hypothalamic hamartoma. Report of two cases. J Neurosurg 1989; 70:640–645.

190. Kanter SL, Mickle JP, Hunter SB, Rhoton AL. Pituitary adenomas in pediatric patients: are they more invasive? Pediatr Neurosci 1986; 12:202–204.

191. Richmond I, Wilson C. Pituitary adenomas in childhood and adolescence. J Neurosurg 1978; 49:163–168.

192. Lee BCP, Deck MDF. Sellar and juxtasellar lesion detection with MR. Radiology 1985; 157:143–147.

193. Davis PC, Hoffman JC, Spencer T, et al. MRI of pituitary adenoma: CT, clinical and surgical correlation. AJNR 1987; 8:107–112, AJR 1987; 148:797–802.

194. Bilaniuk LT, Zimmerman RA, Wehrli FW, et al. Magnetic resonance imaging of pituitary lesions using 1.0 to 1.5 T field strength. Radiology 1984; 153:415–418.

195. Daniels DL, Pech P, Mark L, et al. Magnetic resonance imaging of the cavernous sinus. AJNR 1985; 6:187–192.

196. Davis PC, Hoffman JC, Malko JA, et al. Gadolinium-DTPA and MR imaging of pituitary adenoma: a preliminary report. AJNR 1987; 8:817–823.

197. Dwyer AJ, Frank JA, Doppman JL, et al. Pituitary adenomas in patients with Cushing disease: initial experience with gadolinium-DTPA-enhanced MR imaging. Radiology 1987; 163:421–426.

198. Doppman JL, Frank JA, Dwyer AJ, et al. Gadolinium-DTPA enhanced MR imaging of ACTH-secreting microadenomas of the pituitary gland. JCAT 1988; 12:728–735.

199. Syvertsen A, Haughton VM, Williams AL, Cusick JF. The computed tomographic appearances of the normal pituitary gland and pituitary microadenoma. Radiology 1979; 133:385–391.

200. Davis PC, Hoffman JC, Tindall GT, Braun IF. CT-surgical correlation in pituitary adenomas: evaluation in 113 patients. AJNR 1985; 6:711–716.

201. Moss SD, Rockswold GL, Chou SN, et al. Radiation-induced meningiomas in pediatric patients. Neurosurgery 1988; 22:758–761.

202. Soffer D, Pittaluga S, Feiner M, Beller AJ. Intracranial meningiomas following low-dose irradiation to the head. J Neurosurg 1983; 59:1048–1053.

203. Rubenstein AB, Shalit MN, Cohen ML, et al. Radiation-induced cerebral meningioma: a recognizable entity. J Neurosurg 1984; 61:966–971.

204. Cushing H, Eisenhardt L. Meningiomas, their classification, regional behavior, life history, and surgical end results. Springfield, IL: Charles C Thomas, 1938:69–73.

205. Annegers JF, Laws ER, Kurland LT, Grabow JD. Head trauma and subsequent brain tumors. Neurosurgery 1979; 4:203–206.

206. Numaguchi Y, Hoffman JC, O'Brien MS, et al. Meningiomas in childhood and adolescence. Neurol Med Chin 1978; 18:119–127.

207. Parisi G, Tropea R, Giuffrida S, et al. Cystic meningiomas. Report of seven cases. J Neurosurg 1986; 64:35–38.

208. Dell S, Ganti SR, Steinberger A, McMurtry J. Cystic meningiomas: a clinicoradiological study. J Neurosurg 1982; 57:8–13.

209. Spagnoli MV, Goldberg HI, Grossman RI, et al. Intracranial meningiomas: high-field MR imaging. Radiology 1986; 161:369–375.

210. Zimmerman RD, Fleming CA, Saint-Louis LA, et al. Magnetic resonance imaging of meningiomas. AJNR 1985: 6:149–157.

211. Elster AK, Challa VR, Gilbert TH, et al. Meningiomas: MR and histopathologic features. Radiology 1989; 170:857–862.

212. Holland BA, Kucharcyzk W, Brant-Zawadzki M, et al. MR imaging of calcified intracranial lesions. Radiology 1985; 157:353–356.

213. Zimmerman RD, Fleming CA, Saint-Louis LA, et al. Benign extraaxial tumors: contrast enhancement with Gd-DTPA. Radiology 1987; 163:427–429.

214. Berry I, Brant-Zawadzki M, Osaki L, et al. Gd-DTPA in clinical MR of the brain: 2. Extraaxial lesions and normal structures. AJNR 1986; 7:789–793.

215. Daniels DL, Williams AL, Syvertsen A, et al. CT recognition of optic nerve sheath meningioma: abnormal sheath visualization. AJNR 1982; 3:181–183.

216. Neumann HP, Eggert HR, Weigel K, et al. Hemangioblastomas of the central nervous system. A 10-year study with special reference to von Hippel-Lindau syndrome. J Neurosurg 1989; 70:24–30.

217. Escourolle R, Poirier J. Manual of basic neuropathology. 2nd ed. Philadelphia: WB Saunders, 1978.

218. Cohen ME, Duffner PK. Von-Hippel Lindau disease. In: Hoffman HJ, Epstein F, eds. Disorders of the developing nervous system: diagnosis and treatment. Boston: Blackwell Scientific Publications, 1986:625–634.

219. Olivecrona H. The cerebellar angioreticulomas. J Neurosurg 1952; 9:317–330.

220. Jeffreys R. Clinical and surgical aspects of posterior fossa hemangioblastomas. J Neurol Neurosurg Psychiatr 1975; 38:105–111.

221. Sanford RA, Smith RA. Hemangioblastoma of the cervicomedullary junction. Report of three cases. J Neurosurg 1986; 64:317–321.

222. Mohan J, Brownell B, Oppenheimer DR. Malignant spread of hemangioblastoma: report of two cases. J Neurol Neurosurg Psychiatry 1976; 39:515–525.

223. Sato Y, Waziri M, Smith W, et al. Hippel-Lindau disease: MR imaging. Radiology 1988; 166:241–246.

224. Seeger JF, Burke DP, Knake JE, Gabrielsen TO. Computed tomographic and angiographic evaluation of hemangioblastomas. Radiology 1981; 138:65–73.

225. Fill WL, Lamiell JM, Polk NO. The radiographic manifestations of von Hippel-Lindau disease. Radiology 1979; 133:289–295.

226. Riccardi VM. Von Recklinghausen neurofibromatosis. N Engl J Med 1981; 305:1617–1626.

227. Rubenstein LJ. The malformative central nervous system lesions in the central and peripheral forms of neurofibromatosis. A neuropathological study of 2 cases. Ann NY Acad Sci 1986; 486:14–29.

228. Riccardi VM, Eichner JE. Neurofibromatosis. Phenotype, natural history, and pathogenesis. Baltimore: Johns Hopkins University Press, 1986.

229. Martuza RL, Eldridge R. Neurofibromatosis 2 (bilateral acoustic neurofibromatosis). N Engl J Med 1988; 318:684–688.

230. Holt JF. Neurofibromatosis in children. AJR 1978; 130:615–639.

231. Zimmerman RA, Bilaniuk LT, Metzger RA, et al. Computed tomography of orbital-facial neurofibromatosis. Radiology 1983; 146:113–116.

232. Mikhael MA, Ciric IS, Wolff AP. MR diagnosis of acoustic neuromas. JCAT 1987; 11:232–235.

233. Hurst RW, Newman SA, Cail WS. Multifocal intracranial MR abnormalities in neurofibromatosis. AJNR 1988; 9:292–296.

234. Mayer JS, Kulkarni MV, Yeakley JW. Craniocervical manifestations of neurofibromatosis: MR versus CT studies. JCAT 1987; 11:839–844.

235. Curnes JT, Laster DW, Ball MR, et al. Magnetic resonance imaging of radiation injury to the brain. AJNR 1986; 7:389–394.

236. DiChiro G, Oldfield E, Wright DC, et al. Cerebral necrosis after radiotherapy and/or intraarterial chemotherapy for brain tumors: PET and neuropathologic studies. AJNR 1987; 8:1083–1091.

237. Claussen C, Laniado M, Schorner W, et al. Gadolinium-DTPA in MR imaging of glioblastomas and intracranial metastases. AJNR 1985; 6:669–674.

238. Russell EJ, Geremia GK, Johnson CE, et al. Multiple cerebral metastases: detectability with Gd-DTPA-enhanced MR imaging. Radiology 1987; 165:609–618.

239. Shalen PR, Hayman LA, Wallace S, Handel SF. Protocol for delayed contrast enhancement in computed tomography of cerebral neoplasia. Radiology 1981; 139:397–402.

240. Ascherl GF, Hilal SK, Brisman R. Computed tomography of disseminated meningeal and ependymal malignant neoplasms. Neurology 1981; 31:567–574.

Inflammation and Infection of the Brain

RICHARD R. SMITH, M.D.
MICHAEL A. KUHARIK, M.D.

In addition to the increased sensitivity that MRI has demonstrated in the evaluation of intracranial tumors, this modality has shown a superb ability to detect intracranial infection.[1] Computed tomography (CT) can be useful in larger, relatively well established parenchymal infections, but MRI has shown utility in diagnosing early, small, focal infectious processes.[2] MRI has been particularly useful in evaluating areas difficult to visualize on CT, including the inferior frontal lobes, the temporal lobes, and the contents of the posterior fossa. The introduction of postgadolinium MRI has markedly improved the detection of meningeal abnormalities.[3] Complications related to intracranial infection appear better evaluated with MRI than with CT.[4]

As well as the increased sensitivity to the presence of intracranial lesions, MRI may give greater specificity by allowing differentiation of some infectious disease states from noninfectious disorders. This may include the ability to distinguish cystic neoplasm from abscess and infected from noninfected extra-axial fluid collections.[5,6]

However, MRI may not be as useful in the evaluation of congenital infections such as toxoplasmosis and cytomegalic virus, whose only manifestation may be parenchymal calcification. The development of gradient-echo imaging and its ability to detect calcification may in the future lead to MRI being the imaging modality of choice for the evaluation of patients with these diseases.[7]

MENINGITIS AND ITS COMPLICATIONS

Meningeal infection can be divided into bacterial and aseptic types. The aseptic group includes viral, chemical, and miscellaneous categories. These miscellaneous causes include tuberculosis, fungus, and syphilis as well as granulomatous meningeal involvement such as that seen in sarcoidosis or Whipple's disease. In children the bacterial and viral forms are most common. Tubercular and fungal meningitis are discussed under those specific disease processes. This chapter does not deal with meningeal infiltration secondary to sarcoidosis and other miscellaneous forms of meningeal inflammation.

Meningitis is an inflammatory involvement of the pia-arachnoid. The etiology of acute bacterial meningitis can be correlated with the patient's age. Schochet divided the pediatric etiologic bacterial agents into four categories, depending on the patient's age:[8]

Neonates:
  Escherichia coli.
  Group B streptococci.
  Listeria monocytogenes.
Two to Three Months:
  Group B streptococci.
  Streptococcus pneumoniae.
  Haemophilus influenzae.
Three Months to Three Years:
  Haemophilus influenzae.
  Streptococcus pneumoniae.

Neisseria meningitidis.
Over Three Years:
   Streptococcus pneumoniae.
   Neisseria meningitidis.

Although most cases of meningitis arise secondary to hematogenous dissemination from a distant focus of suppuration or colonization, direct extension from a focus of infection such as the middle ear cavity or paranasal sinuses is more commonly seen in children. Research suggests that after septicemia the bacteria enter the cerebrospinal fluid (CSF) through the choroid plexus and are distributed by normal CSF flow.[9–11] Bacteria are then able to invade the meninges. With further infection the meningeal vessels become congested and thrombosed, and an exudate forms, which is generally most prominent in the basal cisterns.[8] Exudate does cover the cerebral hemispheres but is most evident in the sulci. Bacterial meningitis exudate is generally yellow or greenish. The exudate initially has a predominance of polymorphonuclear leukocytes, but with chronicity other inflammatory cells are seen. The exudate may extend into the neural parenchyma along Virchow-Robin spaces, the so-called perivascular spaces that are filled with CSF.[8]

Viral meningitis may also be spread by hematogenous dissemination.[12] In most cases the specific viral etiology is unknown, but in 50 percent of proved cases the pathologic agent is enterovirus, including coxsackievirus and echovirus.[12] Almost any virus is capable of causing meningitis. Most viral meningitides in children occur in patients under 1 year of age.

Some clinical features relating to specific organisms may be helpful in diagnosis, but most cases of meningitis are radiographically indistinguishable from one another. *E. coli* meningitis is generally acquired from the mother. Predisposing factors have included prematurity, prolonged labor, and complicated delivery.[8] Congenital defects such as myelomeningoceles have also been associated with this entity. Group B streptococcus meningitis is more common than *E. coli* meningitis but appears to have similar predisposing factors.[8] Intrapartum streptococcal infection is generally a more fulminant systemic disease than is streptococcal infection acquired later. *H. influenzae* is the most common cause of meningitis in children beyond the neonatal age but under 3 years.[13] Most infections are due to the type B organism. Direct cerebral parenchymal involvement is more common with *H. influenzae* meningitis. *N. meningitidis* affects older children and is generally acquired from asymptomatic carriers who harbor the organism in the nasopharynx.[8] *S. pneumoniae* generally has very excessive exudate present, particularly over the convexities of the cerebral hemispheres.[14] It has been postulated that this represents early initial involvement of arachnoidal villae.

The clinical symptoms, which are well recognized in adults, are often absent in infants. The clinical features of bacterial meningitis may be more systemic in infants than in adults and there may be a relative lack of signs suggesting meningeal irritation.[12] Fever, vomiting, irritability, and anorexia may be the only clinical features. Altered states of consciousness and seizures as well as a bulging fontanelle may occur later when the infection is more well established. In older children, as in adults, fever, headache, vomiting, photophobia, stiff neck, and a positive Kernig's sign are present.[12] An altered mental status is common.

Viral meningitis usually presents over a longer time course. The patient may have "flu-like" symptoms for several hours or days before the onset of generally mild meningeal symptoms.[12]

The diagnosis of meningitis still rests on CSF examination following lumbar puncture. Care should be taken, however, to rule out an intracranial mass lesion, such as abscess, before performing the puncture.[12] The presence of papilledema or focal neurologic signs should suggest such a lesion.[15]

CSF examination includes evaluation of cell count and differential, protein, glucose, lactic acid, Gram stain, latex agglutination, and culture and sensitivity. Blood cultures should also be obtained.

The results of CSF studies, described below, are subject to a significant amount of variability, but the "classic" findings of meningitis will be discussed. In general, bacterial meningitis has greater than 1,200 white blood cell (WBC) count per cubic millimeter, with a predominance of neutrophils.[12] High protein and lactic acid and low glucose levels are also suggestive of a bacterial etiology. The latex agglutination study rapidly tests for several specific bacterial agents. Gram stain usually identifies the bacteria. Culture and sensitivity studies remain very useful. Viral meningitis usually shows a CSF cell count of 10 to 500 WBC per cubic millimeter with a lymphocytic predominance.[12] CSF glucose and lactic acid are normal, with only minimal elevation of protein. Gram stains are negative. In most cases the virus is not isolated. CSF studies in neonatal bacterial meningitis are often more similar to the "classic" viral findings.[12]

Treatment of meningitis must be undertaken rapidly and should be instituted within minutes of blood and CSF collection. Neonates generally receive ampicillin and gentamicin. Young children are usually started on ampicillin and chloramphenicol, while older children are given penicillin alone.[12] The initial regimen will of course be altered by Gram stain, latex agglutination, and culture and sensitivity results as they are received. Treatment of viral meningitis is usually symptomatic.

Even with appropriate treatment, a near-30 percent mortality rate persists for acute bacterial meningitis. Associated neurologic sequelae in survivors are also common. Most cases of viral meningitis resolve without significant mortality and morbidity.

The complications of meningitis, discussed later, include the following:

1. Communicating or obstructive hydrocephalus.
2. Infarction.
3. Venous or dural sinus thrombosis.

4. Ventriculitis.

Although extra-axial collections, cerebritis, and abscess are also potential complications of meningitis, they will be discussed separately.

Before the introduction of MRI, CT was generally used to rule out an increase in intracranial pressure that might preclude early lumbar puncture, or to evaluate the presence of any complications related to meningeal infection. CT was generally poor in demonstrating meningitis. Although some cases of meningeal enhancement, generally in the basal cisterns, could be seen within several days of the clinical onset of meningitis, most study results were normal.[16] Furthermore, the presence of contrast enhancement in early cases did not turn out to be of prognostic significance. The findings on CT examination of acute meningitis, as described above, include enhancement of the menin-

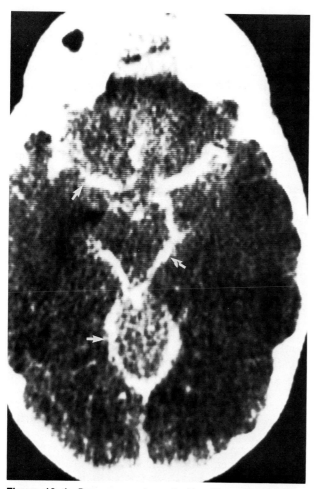

Figure 10–1. *Pneumococcal meningitis.* The axial CT scan taken after intravenous contrast material administration demonstrates marked enhancement of the basal meninges (*arrows*). The perimesencephalic cisterns, the sylvian fissures, and the margins of the tentorium show marked increased attenuation. The decreased attenuation in the supratentorial structures was secondary to diffuse infarction.

ges (Fig. 10–1).[17, 18] In the basal cisterns this is generally associated with a slight increased density of the subarachnoid space on unenhanced studies. Convexity meningeal enhancement is difficult to appreciate because of the "averaging" of the bright calvarial bone with the convexity meningeal enhancement. Another finding that may be evident on CT examination is the presence of communicating hydrocephalus, indicative of an inability of CSF to pass through the arachnoid granulations into the superior sagittal sinus.[19] Presumably these granulations are occluded by infectious debris. Communicating hydrocephalus presents with enlargement of the lateral ventricles, often including the temporal horns, as well as some prominence of the convexity and basal subarachnoid spaces.

Nonenhanced MRI was not particularly useful in the direct evaluation of meningitis. Abnormal increased signal in the basal cisterns, representative of replacement of normal CSF by inflammatory debris, could occasionally be seen on T1 weighted images, but this was uncommon.[20] Communicating hydrocephalus has a similar appearance on both MRI and CT. With the introduction of gadolinium-DTPA into clinical imaging, the ability of MRI to image meningeal inflammation directly has been dramatically enhanced. A recent report by Mathews and colleagues described the appearance of meningeal inflammation.[3] These authors found that a thin and relatively uniform enhancement of large sections of the meninges was present in documented cases of meningitis (Figs. 10–2, 10–3). The abnormalities were more prevalent in bacterial cases. The degree of enhancement in patients whose condition had bacterial or viral etiologies was similar, however. Not all cases with pyogenic meningitis enhanced. In addition, this type of enhancement was nonspecific for infection. It was also seen after the placement of a ventriculoperitoneal shunt.

Lumbar puncture and culture should remain the primary method for the diagnosis of meningitis. However, MRI may be useful in cases with increased intracranial pressure that preclude lumbar puncture, and cases in which CSF results are not clear-cut and further evidence of meningeal inflammation is sought.

Hydrocephalus

A variety of complications may arise secondary to meningitis. As described previously, communicating hydrocephalus or even obstructive hydrocephalus may be present, if debris lodges in the cerebral aqueduct or obstructs outflow of the fourth ventricle. On both CT and MRI in communicating hydrocephalus, there is prominence of the lateral ventricles and cortical sulci (Fig. 10–4). Obstructive hydrocephalus can also be imaged by CT and MRI. Symptoms referable to hydrocephalus are generally present, and ventricular decompression may be necessary in some cases.

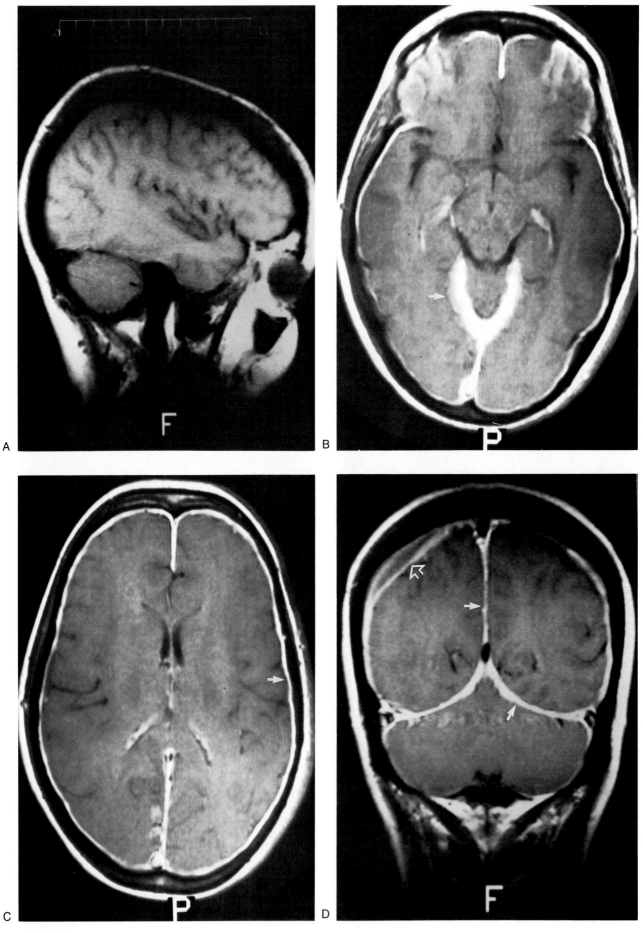

A

B

C

D

224

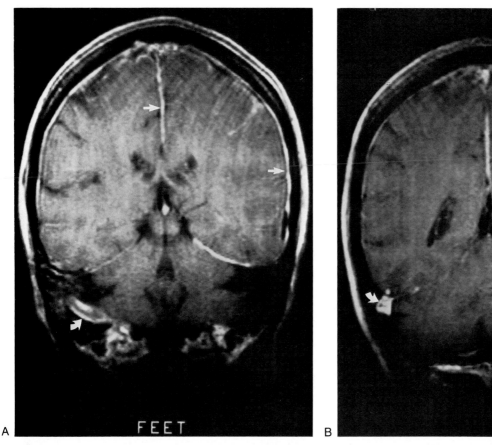

Figure 10–3. *Pneumococcal meningitis.* **A, B,** Postgadolinium coronal T1 weighted images (600/26) demonstrate linear and relatively diffuse meningeal enhancement (*arrows*). **B** shows an associated subarachnoid collection of pus (*open arrow*), which was proved at autopsy. Adjacent cortical enhancement is identified. A second associated finding in this case was thrombosis of the right transverse and sigmoid sinus (*curved arrow*).

Infarction

Meningitis-related cerebral infarction is not uncommon. The inflammatory exudate that is present in the basal cisterns bathes the large arterial branches as well as the smaller penetrating arterial branches.[12] Arterial spasm, compression from prominent exudate, or direct thrombosis of the vessels may occur. Large branch occlusion will result in cortical infarction; this may be localized or generalized, and if severe can result in complete supratentorial necrosis, also called multicystic encephalomalacia.[21] Occlusion of small penetrating vessels may result in well-defined lacuna-type infarcts in the basal ganglia. CT demonstrates the marked low density and mass effect seen in acute infarcts. Subacute infarction may enhance with intravenous iodinated contrast material (Fig. 10–5A). On MR examination the infarct may be seen as a focal or diffuse area of decreased signal on T1 weighted images, and marked increased signal on T2 weighted images (Fig. 10–5A,C). Subacutely, these infarcts, as well as any meningeal component of inflammation, may enhance following gadolinium-DTPA administration.

Venous and Dural Thrombosis

Venous thrombosis may occur secondary to meningitis and may involve either cortical branches or the dural sinuses. With cortical venous thrombosis and infarction, associated parenchymal hemorrhage often occurs. Dural sinus thrombosis may be present as a result of the meningeal inflammation, or may be secondary to the primary focus of suppuration, such as otitis media or a periorbital infection.

CT examination demonstrates a venous infarct as a focal area of decreased attenuation, perhaps with associated high-density hemorrhage (Fig. 10–6A), in a

◄ **Figure 10–2.** *Haemophilus influenzae meningitis.* **A,** Sagittal nonenhanced MRI (600/26) demonstrates no meningeal abnormality. **B** to **D,** Axial and coronal T1 weighted (600/26) images obtained after intravenous gadolinium-DTPA administration demonstrate profound meningeal enhancement (*arrows*). The diffuse enhancement is smooth and linear. The coronal view (**D**) demonstrates an associated subdural effusion (*open arrow*). The outer and inner margins of the effusion show enhancement. No underlying cortical enhancement is appreciated.

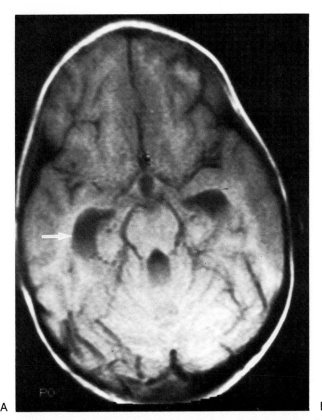
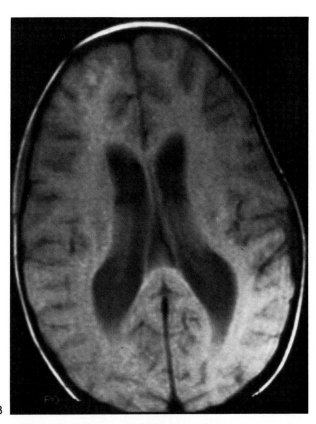

A   B

Figure 10–4. *Communicating hydrocephalus.* **A, B,** Axial nonenhanced T1 weighted images (600/26) demonstrate lateral ventricular enlargement including the temporal horns (*arrow*). This child with *H. influenzae* meningitis developed communicating hydrocephalus during the course of his illness that ultimately required ventricular decompression.

nonvascular distribution.[22] Dural sinus thrombosis may be seen as an area of increased density on the noncontrasted CT examination,[23] secondary to the increased density of the intraluminal clot. With intravenous contrast, the so-called empty triangle or delta sign may be present.[24] The dural leaflets enhance more than the intraluminal thrombus, resulting in a filling defect within the involved sinus.

MRI shows an area of venous infarction as a focal low-signal and high-signal zone on T1 and T2 weighted images, respectively (Fig. 10–6*B*). Acute hemorrhagic products are generally evident by marked decreased signal intensity on the T2 weighted images consistent with deoxyhemoglobin. Before the introduction of MRI, angiography was often necessary to confirm the CT findings of dural sinus thrombosis. The latter may be diagnosed on MRI by the absence of the usual flow void (Fig. 10–7).[26] This requires both T1 and T2 weighted images and generally necessitates multiple imaging planes. If only T2 weighted images are taken, the low intensity of acute clot, deoxyhemoglobin, may mimic a flow void. T1 weighted images, however, demonstrate signal within the involved sinus that is similar to gray matter in these acute thromboses. Conversely, high signal on a T1 weighted image in the dural sinus may be a manifestation of thrombosis with methemoglobin or only flow-related enhancement. An alternate

imaging plane or the presence of a flow void on T2 weighted images will be helpful in excluding sinus thrombosis. Recently, a septic dural thrombosis that had signal isointense to brain on T1 weighted images and hyperintense to brain on T2 weighted images was reported.[27] Presumably this represents the septic nature of this dural thrombosis, and the septic products present may alter the usual blood breakdown schema or appearance. This report also showed that the open triangle or delta sign can be demonstrated on gadolinium-enhanced MRI.

Ventriculitis

Ventriculitis may occur from the extension of leptomeningeal infection but can also be seen after extension or rupture of a parenchymal abscess into the ventricles. Ventriculitis may also be noted following ventricular shunt placement. There is generally a diffuse ventricular dilatation, perhaps secondary to obstruction at the outlet of either the third or fourth ventricles from the inflammatory debris. Intraventricular septations may also be noted. CT scanning demonstrates the dilated ventricles and may show a thin rim of enhancement along the infected ependymal surface (Fig. 10–8*A*).[19] On MRI, focal abnormal in-

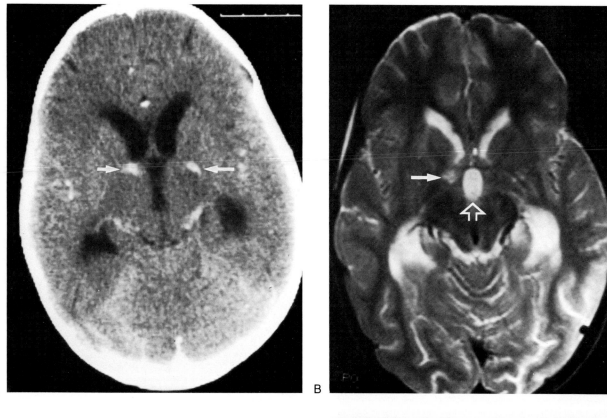

A

B

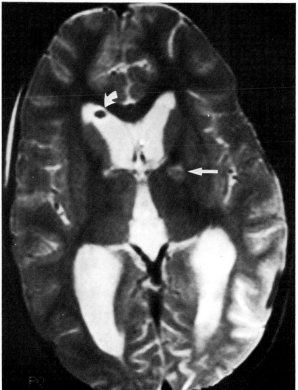

Figure 10–5. *Meningitis-associated infarction.* **A,** Axial CT scan after intravenous contrast administration demonstrates bilateral foci of enhancement in the distribution of the lenticulostriate arteries consistent with infarction (*arrows*). Basal meningeal enhancement was also identified on lower images. **B, C,** Axial T2 weighted images (2500/80) show abnormal increased signal in the left lenticulostriate distribution (*arrows*). Enlargement of the lateral and third ventricles (*open arrow*) consistent with early hydrocephalus is also identified. A ventricular catheter is identified in the frontal horn (*curved arrow*).   C

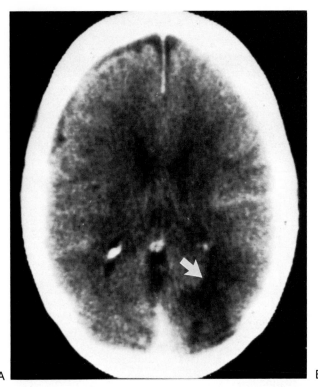
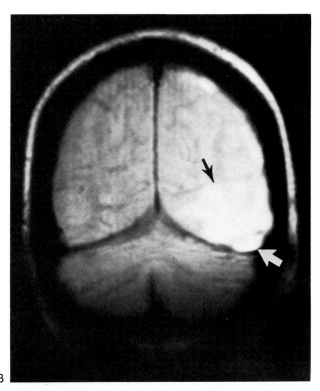

A   B

Figure 10–6. *Venous infarct.* ***A,*** Enhanced axial CT scan demonstrates a focal area of decreased attenuation in the left parietal occipital region (*arrow*). This is in a nonvascular distribution. No hemorrhage could be identified. ***B,*** Coronal proton density image (2000/20) shows abnormal increased signal intensity in the inferior left temporo-occipital lobe (*black arrow*). No hemorrhage was identified on MRI. An associated left transverse sinus thrombosis is evident (*white arrow*). This patient had *H. influenzae* meningitis.

creased signal in the periventricular region is usually evident on long TR images. After intravenous gadolinium-DTPA administration, T1 weighted images demonstrate the fine ependymal enhancement that may be seen on CT (Fig. 10–8).

Subdural and Extradural Collections

These collections may be sterile or infected. Epidural abscess and subdural empyema are the terms used for purulent collections in the epidural and subdural spaces, respectively. Subdural effusion represents a sterile extra-axial fluid accumulation.

Subdural collections in children are speculated to arise secondary to dural reaction, owing to irritation of the dura by the infected subarachnoid fluid in meningitis.[28] Infection of the collection is presumed to arise from rupture of an arachnoid villa, rupture of a vein into the subdural space with spillage of infected material, or primary infection of the dura through the bloodstream. Subdural empyema may also occur after trauma or by direct extension of infection from the paranasal sinuses of middle ear cavities. Epidural empyemas are more likely to arise following trauma or operation, or secondary to sinusitis or mastoiditis. In

children, epidural abscess is frequently found adjacent to otitic infections.

Symptomatology of the infected extra-axial collections may include fever, lethargy, meningeal symptoms, seizures, or coma.[29, 30] In addition, symptoms related to the mass effect of the extra-axial collection may be present.

CT examination of epidural abscess reveals a lens-shaped extra-axial collection that is slightly denser than CSF. With intravenous contrast an enhancing rim, the displaced dura, is often identified (Fig. 10–9A). Epidural abscess can cross the midline, whereas subdural empyema cannot. CT in subdural empyema shows a crescenteric low-density collection over the convexities, within the interhemispheric fissure, or both. The density is slightly greater than that of CSF. The rim may enhance after intravenous contrast administration. This enhancing rim is dependent on the development of granulation tissue. If there is underlying cortical irritation, gyriform enhancement and effacement of the cortical sulci may also be noted. Both the epidural and subdural infections also demonstrate mass effect. The noninfected subdural effusions are also of low density and in the same areas as the infected collections. No marginal enhancement or underlying gyriform enhancement will be evident. Mass effect will be

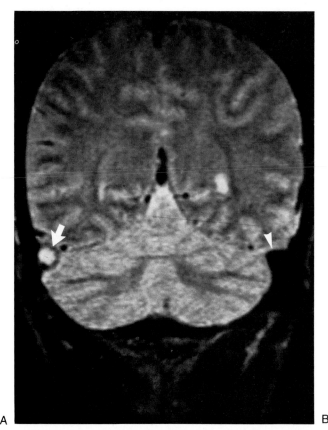
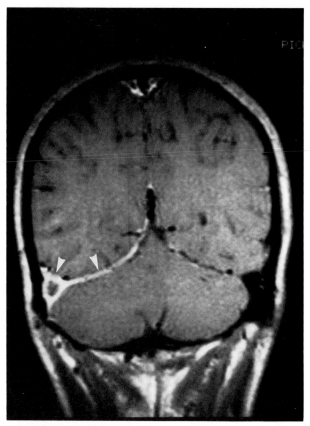

A   B

Figure 10–7. *Dural sinus thrombosis.* ***A,*** Unenhanced T2 weighted image (2000/80) demonstrates abnormal signal within the right transverse sinus (*arrow*). The left transverse sinus is patent, as shown by the presence of the flow void (*arrowhead*). ***B,*** T1 weighted image (600/26) following gadolinium-DTPA administration demonstrates abnormal enhancement of the margins of the right transverse sinus as well as the right tentorium (*arrowheads*). Abnormal signal consistent with thrombosis is identified in the right transverse sinus; its signal characteristics are similar to that of brain. The combination of the enhancement and sinus thrombosis produces a "delta sign," as described previously on CT. This thrombosis was associated with otitis-related meningitis. (From Harris TM, Smith RR, Koch KJ. Gadolinium-DTPA enhanced MR imaging of septic dural sinus thrombosis. J Comput Assist Tomogr 1989; 13:682–684.)

noted. Small extra-axial collections or collections in areas known to be difficult to image by CT, such as the middle cranial fossa, may be missed.

MRI is a superb modality for detection of extra-axial fluid collections. Recent reports describing extra-axial collections continue to demonstrate the superiority of MRI over CT in revealing these collections, particularly when they are small.[6] The MR examination of epidural abscess demonstrates a fluid collection over the convexity that is relatively biconvex (Fig. 10–9B,C). The signal intensity of the abscess is greater than that of CSF on T1 weighted images, and is greater than or equal to the intensity of CSF on T2 weighted images. A well-defined dural margin representing the medial aspect of the abscess appears as a well-demarcated, focal area of decreased signal on both T1 and T2 weighted images. Associated mass effect will be seen. In a recent report, no underlying parenchymal abnormalities were appreciated with epidural abscesses.[6] Presumably, gadolinium-DTPA injection would demonstrate enhancement of the dural margin, which rep-

resents the medial border of the abscess. Subdural empyema is manifest on MRI as a fluid collection over the convexity, in the interhemispheric fissure, or both. The signal intensity of the fluid is greater than CSF on T1 weighted images and may be greater than or equal to CSF signal on T2 weighted images (Fig. 10–10). The sharp low-signal area representing the dura, which is seen along the medial aspect of an epidural abscess, is not identified with subdural empyema. The collection generally has an abrupt interface with the brain parenchyma. Abnormal increased signal on T2 weighted images is commonly seen in the underlying cortex, presumably related to edema, ischemia, or infection. Mass effect is also noted. The collections are generally linear or crescenteric in shape. The lateral and medial margins of the subdural empyema may enhance after gadolinium-DTPA injection, and enhancement of the adjacent cortex may also be noted. Sterile subdural collections have demonstrated signal characteristics similar to those of the infected collections (Fig. 10–11). Underlying signal abnormality in the cortex, however,

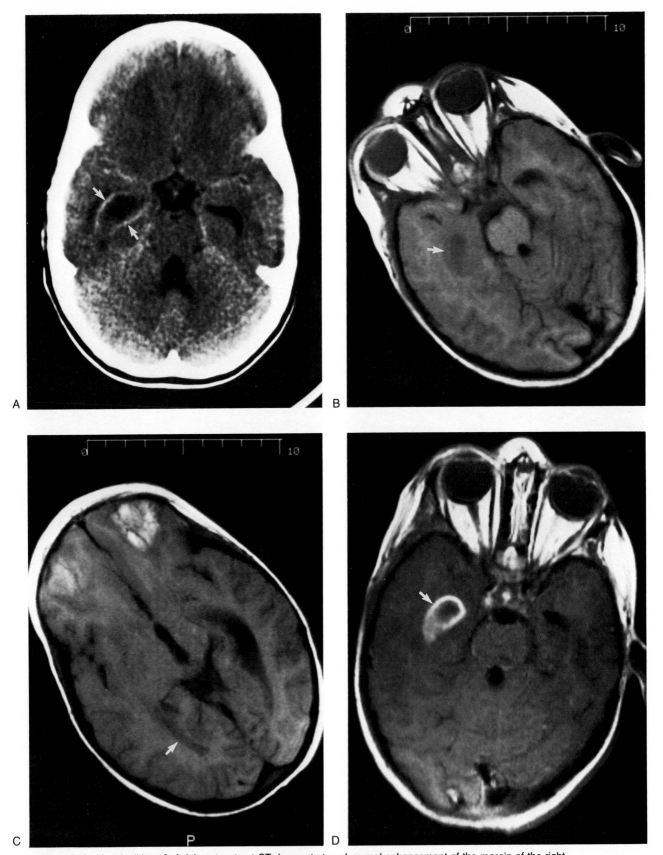

Figure 10–8. *Ventriculitis.* ***A,*** Axial postcontrast CT demonstrates abnormal enhancement of the margin of the right temporal horn (*arrows*). There also is associated ventricular dilatation. ***B, C,*** Axial unenhanced T1 weighted images (600/26) show abnormal signal intensity within the right lateral ventricle. The margins of the right lateral ventricle are also irregular and not well defined (*arrows*). ***D, E,*** Axial T1 weighted images (600/26) after gadolinium-DTPA administration demonstrate marked enhancement of the margins of the right lateral ventricle (*arrows*). The choroid plexus of the left lateral ventricle (*arrowhead*) has normal enhancement. ***F,*** Axial T2 weighted image (2500/80) shows abnormal signal surrounding the right temporal horn. The signal intensity within the right temporal horn (*arrow*) is also greater than that of CSF seen in either the left temporal horn or the suprasellar cistern.

Figure continues on following page.

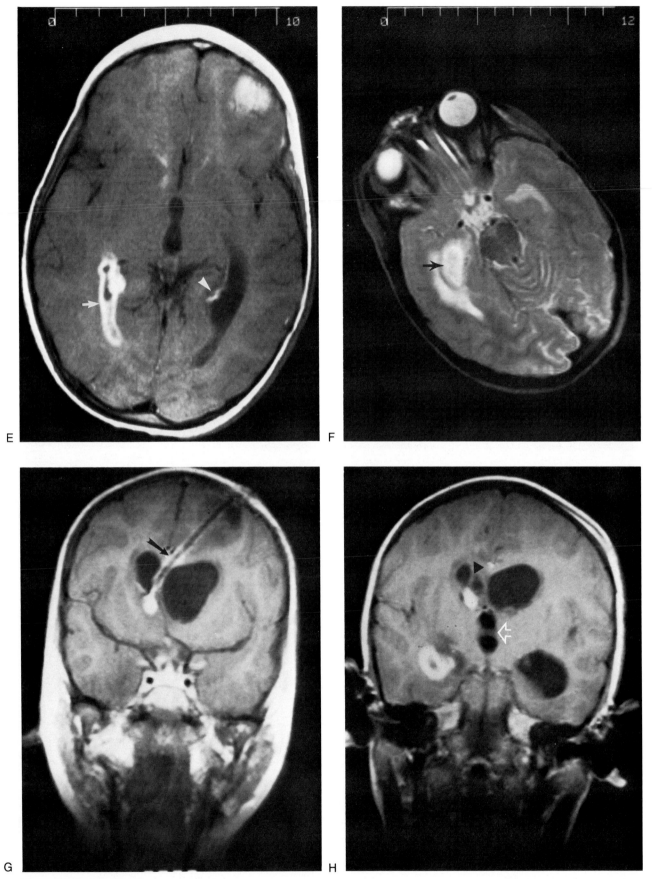

Figure 10–8. *Continued.*
G, H, Coronal postgadolinium T1 weighted images (600/26) after antimicrobial therapy and ventricular decompression demonstrate persistent enhancement of the right lateral ventricle. The abnormal enhancement also extends along the ventricular catheter (*arrow*). Septations within the ventricle are now also evident (*arrowhead*). The ventricular catheter is only draining the right lateral ventricle, while persistent dilatation of the left lateral ventricle and third ventricle (*open arrow*) remains.

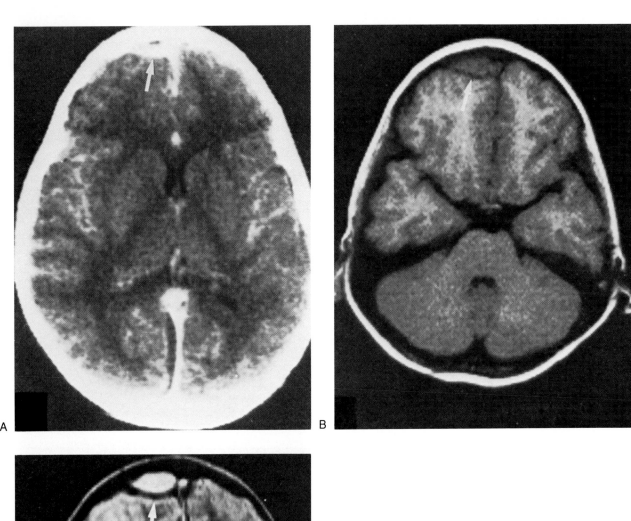

A

B

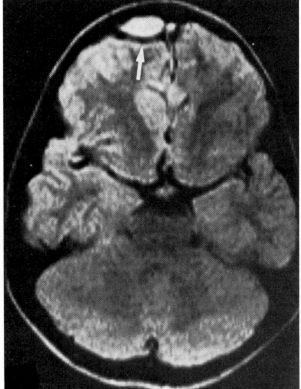

C

Figure 10–9. *Epidural abscess.* **A,** Postcontrast CT scan demonstrates an epidural lens-shaped collection in the right frontal region (*arrow*). Enhancement of the inner margin of the empyema is noted. **B,** Axial T1 weighted image without gadolinium-DTPA demonstrates the extra-axial collection in the right frontal region (*arrow*). **C,** Axial T2 weighted image superbly demonstrates the lens-shaped extra-axial collection. Marked hypointensity of the displaced dura (*arrow*) is appreciated. No abnormal signal is identified in the underlying brain parenchyma. (From Sze G, Zimmerman RD. The magnetic resonance imaging of infections and inflammatory diseases. Radiol Clin North Am 1988; 26:839–859.)

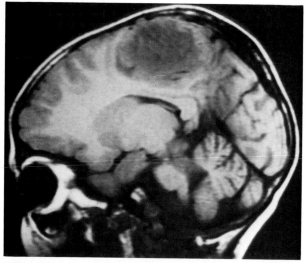
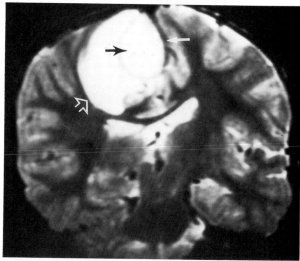

A   B

Figure 10–10. *Subdural empyema.* **A,** Sagittal T1 weighted image (600/20) demonstrates a focal area of decreased attenuation. From the sagittal projection alone, differentiation of a intra- or extra-axial location is not possible. **B,** Coronal T2 weighted image (2500/80) shows the subdural empyema (*black arrow*) adjacent to the falx (*white arrow*). The margin of the empyema is slightly hypointense (*arrowhead*). Underlying abnormal cortical signal indicative of adjacent edema and/or cerebritis is also identified (*open arrow*).

has been absent. Although effusions are far more common than empyemas, the severe neurologic sequelae of empyemas require that most enhancing extra-axial collections should be followed closely or aspirated to exclude infection. Treatment of the infected extra-axial collections generally involves surgical intervention and antimicrobial therapy. The noninfected subdural collections may be watched if the patient is stable or clinically improving.[31] Aspiration of the collection may be performed if the patient's condition worsens or if a prominent collection remains static. No difference with respect to neurologic damage has been identified between patients having noninfected subdural effusions and those without extra-axial collections.[32]

CEREBRITIS AND ABSCESS

Cerebritis and abscess in children may have a variety of causes. Most commonly the infection is related to trauma or otitis media. Congenital heart disease also is often associated with brain abscess.[33] In neonates the process may be related to skin or umbilical sepsis. Meningitis may also be a cause of cerebritis. In one study, no predisposing cause was found in up to 25 percent of patients.[34]

Cerebritis is the earliest stage of infection of the brain, and may or may not progress to abscess. Pathologically, cerebritis consists of an inflammatory infiltrate with vascular congestion and edema.[8] Minimal brain necrosis may also be present in this early stage. The focus of infection is generally poorly demarcated. In children, most foci of infection are solitary. In adults, approximately one-third of cases have multiple

foci of infection;[8] this relates to the increased incidence of hematogenous dissemination in adults. As the focus of cerebritis continues to evolve, a necrotic center begins to form. Surrounding this necrotic center are new blood vessels and fibroblasts. The brain attempts to encapsulate, with collagen, the focus of infection.[8] The formation of collagen and the granulation tissue, which attempts to wall off the infection, is dependent on many factors including host resistance, the organism present, and antibiotic therapy and corticosteroid administration. In children the infection is often in the temporal lobe (relating to otitic infections). Those cases that are hematogenous in origin, in addition to being multiple, tend to occur at the gray-white matter junction in the supratentorial space.[35] Associated septic thrombosis of the vessels and endothelial hyperplasia is also seen. Although the abscess phase of the infection delimits the infected focus, surrounding edema is almost always seen and is generally rather marked with respect to the size of the infected focus. The abscess may spread deeper into the white matter to produce daughter abscesses, or rarely may rupture into the ventricles, which is almost uniformly fatal.[36] The etiologic agents in infants are anaerobes and gram-negative organisms.[37] *E. coli* and *Proteus vulgaris* are most common. In older children and adults, streptococci and staphylococci are common as are anaerobes such as bacteroides.[37]

The symptoms of cerebritis and abscess are similar. In young children, most cases present with seizures, fever, meningitis, and symptoms of increased intracranial pressure.[37] In older children, as in adults, headache is the most frequent initial symptom. Other symptoms include altered mental status; seizures; and focal

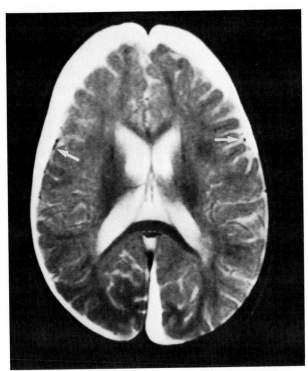

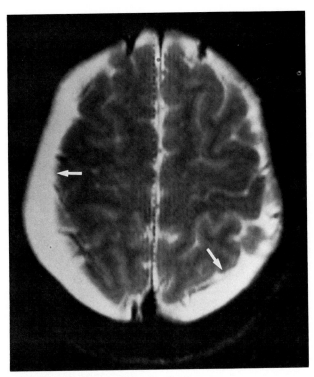

Figure 10–11. *Subdural effusions.* **A,** Bilateral convexity and posterior interhemispheric subdural collections are identified on this T2 weighted image (2500/80). The inward displacement of cortical veins (*arrows*) confirms the extra-axial nature of the fluid collections. This effusion was secondary to pneumococcal meningitis. No abnormal signal in the underlying cortex is identified. The lack of cortical abnormal signal helps to differentiate subdural effusion from subdural empyema. **B,** This case of *H. influenzae* meningitis demonstrates bilateral extra-axial collections (*arrows*) on this T2 weighted image (2500/80). No underlying cortical signal abnormalities are noted.

motor, sensory, or speech disorders. Fever is characteristic of the early phase of the disease, although the temperature may return to normal with abscess encapsulation. The WBC count is often normal, but in some cases is elevated with a neutrophil predominance. The erythrocyte sedimentation rate (ESR) is commonly elevated. CSF studies by lumbar puncture are usually contraindicated because the mass effect of the abscess increases the possibility of inducing brain herniation.

The pathologic basis for the CT appearance of cerebritis and abscess was described by Enzmann and colleagues,[38, 39] who divided the formation of abscess into four stages: early cerebritis, late cerebritis, early capsule formation, and late capsule formation. The CT appearance of the focal infection depends on which phase is imaged. In the cerebritis phase, CT shows a focus of low density with mass effect (Fig. 10–12). There may or may not be patchy enhancement. As the cerebritis phase continues, ring enhancement may be noted. The ring-enhancing lesion of cerebritis may be differentiated from frank abscess by delayed scanning. In the late cerebritis phase, contrast material appears to diffuse into the central portion of the lesion, which does not occur in encapsulated abscess. In the abscess stage, there is an area of decreased attenuation centrally surrounded by edema. Mass effect is present.

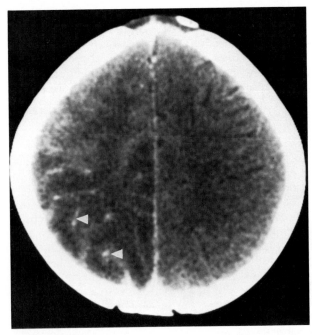

Figure 10–12. *Cerebritis.* This axial-enhanced CT scan demonstrates decreased attenuation in the right temporoparietal lobe. Patchy enhancement (*arrowheads*) is noted. The cerebritis was secondary to pneumococci.

With intravenous contrast administration the area of necrosis is typically surrounded by an enhancing ring (Fig. 10–13). The ring is generally thin and relatively smooth, but some abscesses may have thicker and irregular ring enhancement. The abscess capsule also is generally thicker adjacent to the gray matter. Abscesses with thicker or irregular capsules may be difficult to distinguish from necrotic tumors.

MRI has proved very useful in the evaluation of intracranial infection. The early cerebritis stage manifests itself as a focal area of decreased signal on T1 weighted images and increased signal on T2 weighted images (Figs. 10–14 to 10–16). Mass effect is also identified. No well-documented study relating patterns of gadolinium-DTPA enhancement to those seen and previously described in the CT literature has been published. In early cerebritis there is a patchy and somewhat irregular enhancement after gadolinium-DTPA injection (Fig. 10–15). The frank abscess stage on MRI is characterized by a focal area of markedly decreased signal on T1 and increased signal on T2

weighted images, consistent with the focus of necrosis (Fig. 10–17). The signal on T1 weighted images is greater than that of CSF but less than that of brain. Surrounding edema is noted as well as mass effect. MRI has demonstrated some irregularities in the signal of the capsule surrounding the necrotic focus. On T1 weighted images this capsule, representing the granulation and collagen layers, may have areas of irregular increased signal (Figs. 10–17, 10–18). On T2 weighted images foci of decreased signal may be present. Some authors have ascribed this to the presence of blood products secondary to oozing from the granulation layer; others have suggested that these findings are secondary to paramagnetic T1 effects or T2 shortening secondary to free radical formation.[5, 40] These capsular findings on MRI may be relatively specific for abscess and may help differentiate these from necrotic tumors. Enhancement of a mature abscess with gadolinium-DTPA demonstrates marked increased signal of the capsule wall on T1 weighted images (Fig. 10–18). Again, as in CT, the margins are relatively thin and smooth, although exceptions do occur.

The treatment of cerebritis and abscess relies on early diagnosis. If appropriately treated in the cerebritis phase by antibiotics, the focus of infection may not progress to the abscess stage. Well-formed abscesses generally require surgical drainage and antibiotic therapy. The data on adult mortality secondary to brain abscess show a rate of 15 to 20 percent.[41] The outcome in children, particularly infants, is worse than in adults. In survivors, at least 35 percent have neurologic sequelae.[42, 43]

TUBERCULOSIS

Although the incidence of tuberculosis in the United States has markedly decreased, occasional tubercular infection in children with intracranial involvement does occur. The cerebral involvement can be divided into two components: tuberculous meningitis and tuberculoma. The meningitis results from hematogenous dissemination from a primary source, most commonly the lung. Most cases are identified in children under 3 years old. Tuberculous meningitis is manifest as a marked thickening of the meninges, with significant thick exudate filling the basal cisterns in particular.[8] The convexities by comparison are less involved. Small tubercles are scattered over the base and convexities of the cerebral hemisphere and are similar to tubercles found elsewhere in the body, consisting of central caseation with surrounding granuloma cells, including giant cells. The exudate is composed of fibrin, plasma cells, and other mononuclear cells.[8] Extension of the inflammatory process into the ependyma and choroid plexus is also noted pathologically. The inflammatory exudate commonly spreads along the pial vessels to invade the underlying brain. The exudate inflames and may invade the arteries at the base of the brain, leading

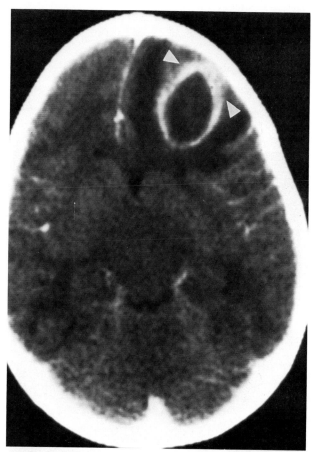

Figure 10–13. *Abscess.* Enhanced axial CT scan demonstrates a ring-enhancing lesion in the left frontal lobe. The wall is relatively uniform in thickness and is smooth along its inner margin. Some thickening of the abscess capsule adjacent to the gray matter (*arrowhead*) is identified. Surrounding edema and mass effect are also evident.

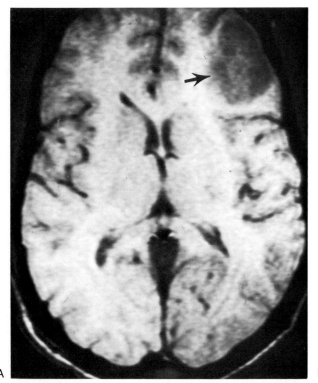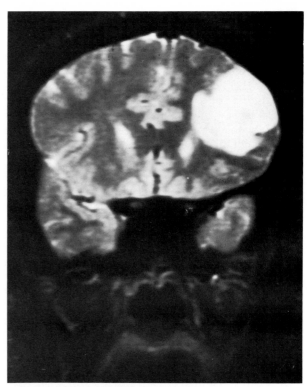

A | B

Figure 10-14. *Cerebritis.* **A,** Axial T1 weighted image (600/26) demonstrates a focal area of decreased signal in the left frontal lobe (*arrow*). Obliteration of gray-white matter distinction is seen in this area as well as effacement of the cortical sulci. Mild mass effect on the left frontal horn is also noted. **B,** Abnormal signal intensity on the T2 weighted image (2500/80) is identified. The margins are relatively well demarcated. The deep extent of the inflammation is better appreciated from the coronal view.

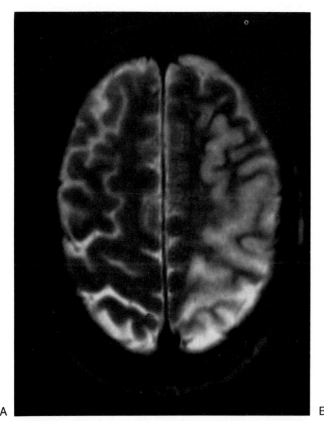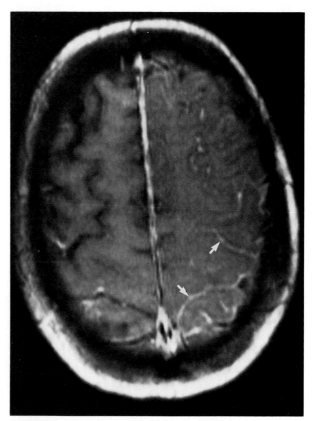

A | B

Figure 10-15. *Pnemococcal cerebritis.* **A,** Axial T2 weighted image (2500/80) demonstrates abnormal signal intensity in the gyri of the left cerebral hemisphere. Effacement of the sulci is also appreciated. **B,** Axial T1 weighted image (600/26) after intravenous gadolinium administration shows enhancement of the sulci and/or superficial cortex in the left cerebral hemisphere (*arrows*). Generalized effacement of the sulci over the left convexity is also noted.

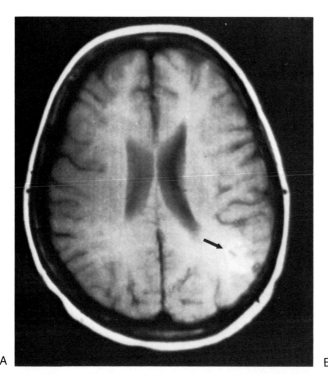
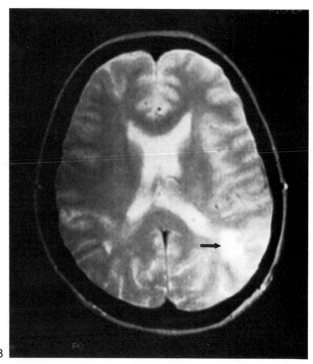

Figure 10–16. *Septic embolus with cerebritis.* ***A,*** Nonenhanced T1 weighted image (600/26) demonstrates a focal area of increased signal near the gray-white matter junction of the left parietal lobe (*arrow*). The increased signal is consistent with intracellular methemoglobin. ***B,*** T2 weighted image (2000/80) shows abnormal increased signal intensity in the left parietal lobe (*arrow*). The patient has staphylococcal bacterial endocarditis.

to thrombosis and resultant infarction. Hydrocephalus, either communicating or noncommunicating, is common. Clinically the patients present with headache, lethargy, and fever. Meningeal signs may also be present. In very young children apathy, irritability, vomiting, and seizures may also be noted. The clinical course of the disease is slower than that of bacterial meningitis.[12] Cranial nerve involvement, particularly ocular palsies, may be noted. CSF studies demonstrate increased pressure, leukocytosis with a lymphocytic predominance, and a moderately elevated CSF protein.[12] Glucose levels are decreased but rarely to the low values observed in bacterial meningitis. The presence of tubercle bacilli in the CSF is diagnostic.

The prognosis, even in adequately treated cases, remains somewhat poor because the incidence of retardation, seizures, and focal neurologic deficits is high.[12] Inadequate treatment is invariably fatal. Treatment with isoniazid (INH) for a prolonged period is generally effective.

Tuberculomas are tumor-like masses that form in the parenchyma of the brain. Multiplicity is frequent. They are round, with a necrotic center, and surrounding edema is common. Giant cells and collagen are seen in the capsule. Tuberculomas may appear before or subsequent to tuberculous meningitis. Clinically the symptoms relate to a space-occupying lesion and include focal neurologic signs, increased intracranial pressure, or seizures.[44] Treatment is similar to that of tuberculous meningitis, and the tuberculoma resolves

in many instances. Some cases, however, leave a residual small focus of calcification; if this area remains an irritant to the brain and is causing seizures, excision may be necessary.

CT examination of tuberculous meningitis often demonstrates ventricular enlargement consistent with hydrocephalus.[45] The thick exudate in the basal cisterns is evident by an increased density present in the basal cisterns without deforming the cisterns. Extension into the sylvian fissures is occasionally seen. Intravenous contrast administration generally demonstrates a marked enhancement of this basal meningitis (Fig. 10–19A).[45] Areas of infarction, particularly in the basal ganglia, are identified as low density on noncontrasted studies, with contrast enhancement in the subacute stage. Tuberculomas can vary in appearance from areas of decreased to increased attenuation on a nonenhanced study.[44] Calcification is relatively unusual, being present in approximately 5 percent of cases.[46] The lesion may be solitary or multiple. With intravenous contrast administration, most lesions enhance (Fig. 10–19B). Often a focal area of lucency in the center of the tuberculoma is identified consistent with the central caseation and necrosis.[44, 47] Surrounding edema is usually identified. Mass effect and associated hydrocephalus are also common.

MR evaluation of tuberculous meningitis has recently been reported by Schoeman and colleagues,[48] who demonstrate that the basal exudate is rarely identifiable on unenhanced MR studies. Several patients,

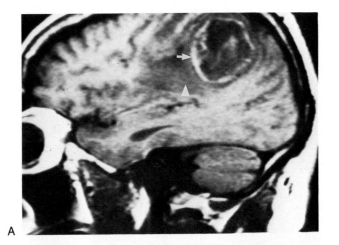

A

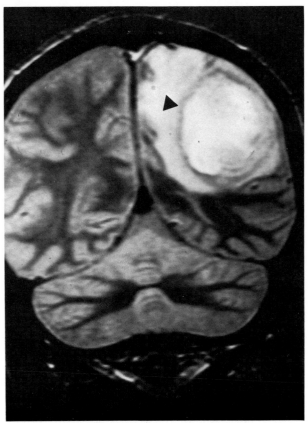

B

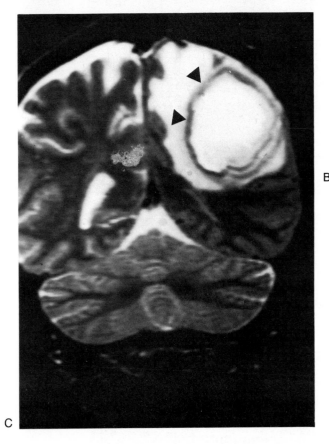

C

Figure 10–17. *Abscess.* **A,** Sagittal nonenhanced T1 weighted image (600/20) demonstrates an area of abnormal signal in the left parietal lobe (*arrow*). There is high signal along the margin of the lesion consistent with methemoglobin. The central portion of the lesion is very low in signal, suggesting necrosis. Signal surrounding the lesion is decreased on this T1 weighted image (*arrowhead*) consistent with edema. **B, C,** First and second echoes of the T2 (2500/20,80) coronal study show the lesion in the left parietal lobe. The central portion of the abnormality is high signal consistent with necrosis. The capsular margin shows progressive decreased signal with increased T2 weighting suggestive of deoxyhemoglobin or intracellular methemoglobin (*arrowheads*). Surrounding high-signal edema is also evident, as is associated mass effect.

however, did demonstrate decreased signal in the basal cisterns on T2 weighted images, presumably reflecting the presence of thick fibrous exudate. Further work may be useful in identifying the contribution of gadolinium-enhanced T1 weighted images in the evaluation of basal meningitis. Presumably this thick exudate will show marked enhancement that may even be more prominent than that seen on CT examination. The complications of tuberculous meningitis, however, are much better appreciated on MRI than on CT;[48] these include infarction in the basal ganglia and diencephalon. Abnormal signal on T2 weighted images is

seen in these regions consistent with the area of infarction. Abnormal signal is also identified on T2 weighted images in the areas of the pons, hypothalamus, and parahippocampal gyri. These probably represent other foci of early ischemic change. Hydrocephalus, either obstructive or communicating, will also be noted.

Tuberculomas appear to have a unique appearance on MRI (Figs. 10–19 to 10–21).[49, 50] The central core of caseation on T1 weighted images appears somewhat decreased in signal intensity, but markedly increased on T2 weighted images. The dense capsule is relatively

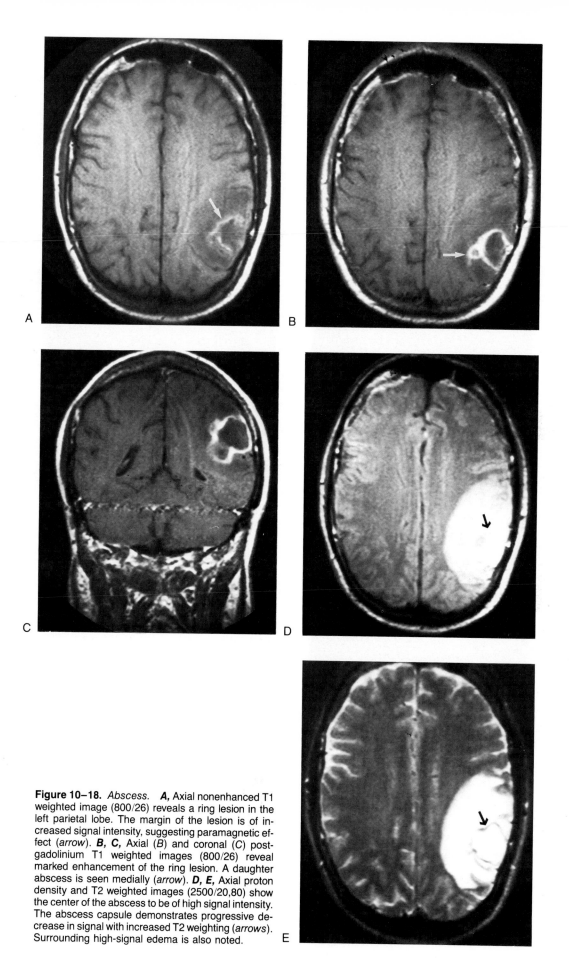

Figure 10–18. *Abscess.* **A,** Axial nonenhanced T1 weighted image (800/26) reveals a ring lesion in the left parietal lobe. The margin of the lesion is of increased signal intensity, suggesting paramagnetic effect (*arrow*). **B, C,** Axial (*B*) and coronal (*C*) post-gadolinium T1 weighted images (800/26) reveal marked enhancement of the ring lesion. A daughter abscess is seen medially (*arrow*). **D, E,** Axial proton density and T2 weighted images (2500/20,80) show the center of the abscess to be of high signal intensity. The abscess capsule demonstrates progressive decrease in signal with increased T2 weighting (*arrows*). Surrounding high-signal edema is also noted.

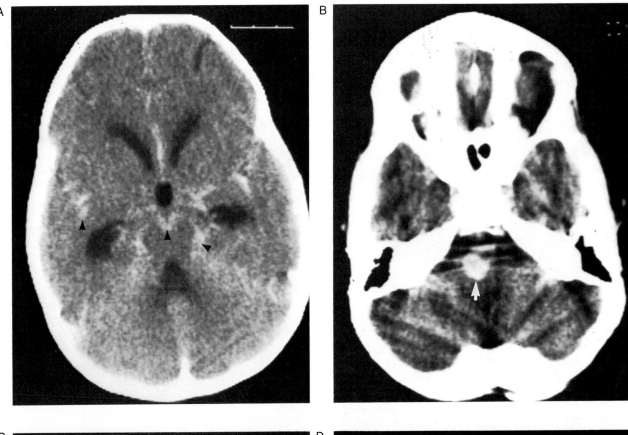

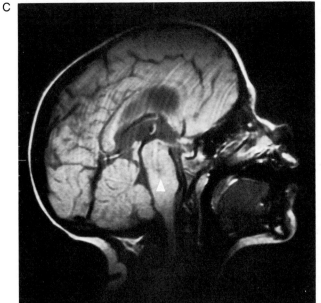

Figure 10–19. *Tuberculosis.* ***A,*** A section from the enhanced CT study demonstrates abnormal enhancement in the basal cisterns and fissures (*arrowheads*), consistent with tuberculous meningitis. Early ventricular prominence from communicating hydrocephalus is also noted. ***B,*** A lower section from the postcontrast CT scan shows a nodular area of enhancement in the pons (*arrow*). This tuberculoma shows no intrinsic inhomogeneity. Streak artifact partially obscures the margins of the tuberculoma and prevents assessment of associated edema and mass effect. ***C,*** Sagittal T1 weighted MR image (600/26) demonstrates intrinsic enlargement in the pons. Slight decreased signal intensity in the midportion of the pons (*arrowhead*) is noted and relates to edema. Prominence of the third ventricle is also seen. No abnormality with respect to the meninges is seen on this nonenhanced scan. ***D,*** Axial T2 weighted MR (2000/80) shows abnormal signal intensity in the pons (*arrow*). The fourth ventricle (*arrowhead*) is slightly prominent. The central area of decreased signal in the fourth ventricle relates to turbulence from increased flow through the cerebral aqueduct in this patient with communicating hydrocephalus. The tuberculous meningitis was not evident in this MR study. (From Smith RR. Brain stem tumors. Seminars in Roentgenol 1990; 25.)

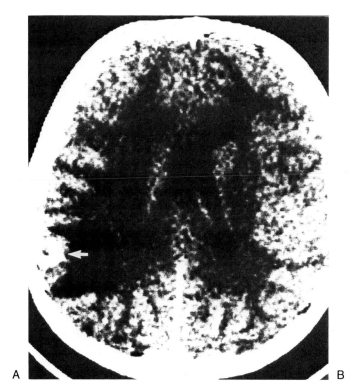

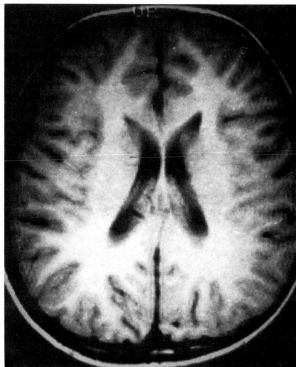

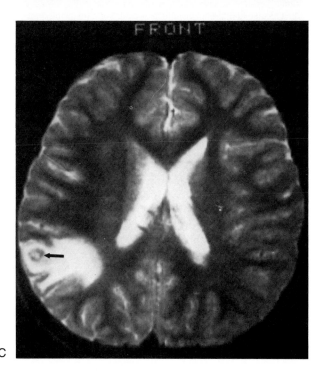

Figure 10–20. *Tuberculoma.* ***A,*** Enhanced CT scan vaguely demonstrates a ring-enhancing lesion near the convexity of the right parietal lobe (*arrow*). The central portion of the enhancing nodule is of decreased attenuation. ***B,*** Axial nonenhanced T1 weighted image (600/20) shows no definite abnormality in the region of the right parietal lobe. ***C,*** Axial T2 weighted image (2000/80) demonstrates the tuberculoma in the right parietal region (*arrow*). The central portion of the ring is of high signal, similar to that of CSF or edema. The capsule of the granuloma is decreased in signal intensity. Surrounding high-signal edema is also seen. (From Gupta RK, Jena A, Sharma A, et al. MR imaging of intracranial tuberculomas. J Comput Assist Tomogr 1988; 12:280–285.)

isointense on T1 weighted images and markedly hypo-intense on T2 weighted images. This leads to a target-like appearance on T2 weighted imaging. Presumably the capsular hypointensity is related to the significant fibrosis and compaction. Surrounding this capsule on T2 weighted images is high-signal edema. Signs of mass effect are also present. Calcification is not generally appreciated.

VIRAL INFECTIONS

Herpes Simplex Virus Encephalitis

In the United States herpes simplex encephalitis is the most common sporadic, acute, viral infection of the brain.[51] The diagnosis of herpes encephalitis is one area in which MRI is extremely useful. Since the prog-

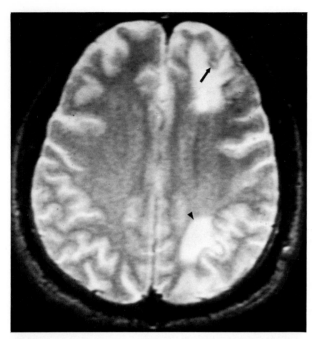

Figure 10–21. *Tuberculoma.* Axial T2 weighted image (2500/80) demonstrates a tuberculoma in the right frontal region (*arrow*). The lesion has a hyperintense center with a hypointense capsule. Surrounding edema is also noted. A second lesion in the left parietal lobe was also identified. Only the associated edema (*arrowhead*) is seen on this image.

nosis is intimately associated with the early institution of appropriate antiviral medication, the unique ability of MRI to demonstrate early water changes, particularly in the inferior temporal lobes, makes it the procedure of choice in evaluating these patients.[52] The herpes simplex virus itself can be divided into two types: type 1 causes an encephalitis in children and adults; type 2 is more common in congenital infection and newborn encephalitis.[53]

The congenital form of herpes encephalitis, part of the TORCH syndrome (toxoplasmosis, rubella, cytomegalovirus, and herpes simplex), leads to microcephaly, mental retardation, and other severe focal neurologic deficits.[54] Microphthalmia and chorioretinitis may also be noted. On pathology studies the brain demonstrates disordered architecture or areas of infarction and atrophy.[55] Foci of calcification are also commonly seen in the temporal lobes. CT examination demonstrates the brain atrophy and intracerebral calcifications. MR examination of these infants shows the sulcal prominence and ventricular enlargement consistent with brain atrophy. The intracerebral calcifications may be seen as foci of decreased signal, particularly on T2 weighted images. Unless the foci are relatively large, however, the calcification may be missed on MRI. New research relating to gradient-echo imaging in the evaluation of the presence of cal-

cification may have use in evaluating patients with the TORCH syndrome, since gradient-echo images have a greater sensitivity to the presence of calcification.[7]

Neonatal infection is often a systemic disease. In addition to the neurologic features of lethargy, seizures, and cranial nerve palsies, patients may have other systemic findings such as apnea, jaundice, hepatomegaly, lethargy, and poor feeding.[56] They generally become clinically symptomatic within the first week. Electroencephalographic (EEG) abnormalities also are commonly present. Mucocutaneous lesions, in the form of vesicles, are present in up to 50 percent of cases.

The prognosis is poor for these children; mortality rates, even with appropriate therapy, are high. If the patient survives, residual focal defects, seizures, mental retardation, and ophthalmic abnormalities are present.[57]

CT scans of neonatal herpes simplex encephalitis reveal a more aggressive and destructive infection than that usually seen in older children.[21, 58–60] Although the temporal lobes remain the most common foci of infection, the process can arise in other areas of the brain. Low attenuation consistent with edema and ischemia rapidly progresses to a destructive cystic encephalomalacia. Often, both hemispheres may be completely destroyed. Atrophy and periventricular calcification may also be seen. MRI demonstrates abnormal decreased signal on T1 weighted images and increased signal on T2 weighted images in the region of infection. The involvement of gray matter and associated mass effect is appreciated on MRI. Some cases may be very subtle, however. The watery nature of the neonatal brain, which is due to the lack of complete myelination at this age, may mask focal or diffuse edema on T2 weighted imaging. The progression to cystic encephalomalacia is seen on MRI as developing cavities filled with fluid identical to CSF intensity (Fig. 10–22).

The peak frequency for herpes simplex encephalitis is the second year. Clinically the patient presents with fever, vomiting, and headache. Seizures, behavioral changes, and speech difficulties generally occur several days after the onset of the infection.[56] In many cases the seizures are limited to one upper limb or the face. Alteration of consciousness becomes rapidly progressive. EEG studies show slowing of the basal activity. The CSF is sometimes hemorrhagic and demonstrates a mildly increased white blood cell count and protein elevation. The CSF usually does not contain infectious virus.[56] A normal CSF study during the first few days of the disease does not rule out the diagnosis. Brain biopsy is generally required for pathologic diagnosis.

The virus affects predominantly the temporal lobes. The insular cortex and inferior frontal lobes may also be involved. It has been speculated that the involvement of the temporal lobes is related to the virus remaining latent in the trigeminal ganglia.[19] With reac-

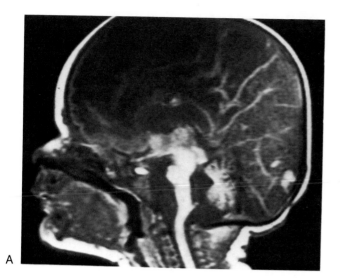

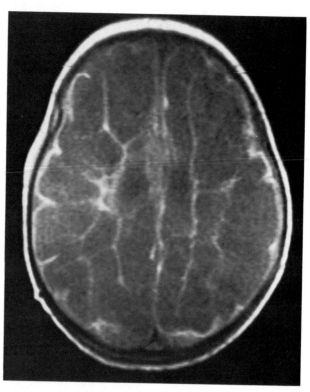

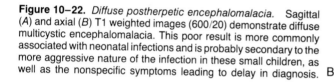

Figure 10–22. *Diffuse postherpetic encephalomalacia.* Sagittal (*A*) and axial (*B*) T1 weighted images (600/20) demonstrate diffuse multicystic encephalomalacia. This poor result is more commonly associated with neonatal infections and is probably secondary to the more aggressive nature of the infection in these small children, as well as the nonspecific symptoms leading to delay in diagnosis.

tivation the virus is presumed to migrate along the trigeminal nerve fibers that innervate the meninges of the anterior and middle cranial fossa. In addition to the necrotizing characteristics of the inflammation, hemorrhage generally is also present.

Current treatment includes acyclovir administration, but prompt institution of therapy is mandatory to reduce neurologic complications. CT examination results are commonly normal during the first few days of the disease (Fig. 10–23*A*).[61, 62] This is important in that treatment that may reduce significant neurologic sequelae will also be delayed if diagnosis is based on the CT results. The CT examination generally becomes positive several days after the clinical onset. The earliest abnormalities of herpes cerebritis on CT are focal areas of decreased attenuation, consistent with the edema from the infection in the temporal lobes. There may be extension into the insular cortex and the inferior frontal region. The putamen is usually spared by the infection.[19] Isolated frontal or parietal involvement is rare but does occur. After approximately 5 days the foci of hemorrhage may become evident on CT scanning.[63] Intravenous contrast administration is not usually useful early during the first week.[62] Most patients by 7 days demonstrate enhancement, which may be linear or gyral or involve the subarachnoid space (Fig. 10–23*E*). With treatment the infection wanes and residual foci of low attenuation are identi-

fied. This may be manifest in focal atrophy, porencephaly, or (less commonly) in multicystic encephalomalacia. The multicystic changes are more common in the neonatal infection, as described above. Calcification also may occasionally be noted.

The marked number of recent publications on MRI of herpes encephalitis is testimony to the advance that this modality brings in the evaluation of this disease.[2, 64–66] In several reports the MR results have been abnormal while CT results have been either normal or indeterminate.[2, 66] On MR examination the temporal lobe demonstrates decreased signal intensity on T1 weighted images and increased signal intensity on T2 weighted images (Figs. 10–23 to 10–25). Extension into the insular cortex and the inferior frontal region is also identified. The lentiform nucleus is usually spared. Acute hemorrhage is evident on MRI as well as areas of relative isointensity on T1 weighted images and marked hypointensity on T2 weighted images consistent with the presence of deoxyhemoglobin.[25] Gadolinium-DTPA enhancement is patchy and irregular (Fig. 10–26). MRI has been useful in monitoring the response to acyclovir therapy (Fig. 10–27).[67] MR examination in the long-term follow-up demonstrates the areas of brain necrosis or porencephaly as cystic collections of CSF within the brain parenchyma (Fig. 10–28). The fluid contents are similar to CSF in all pulse sequences. Severe multicystic encephalomalacia

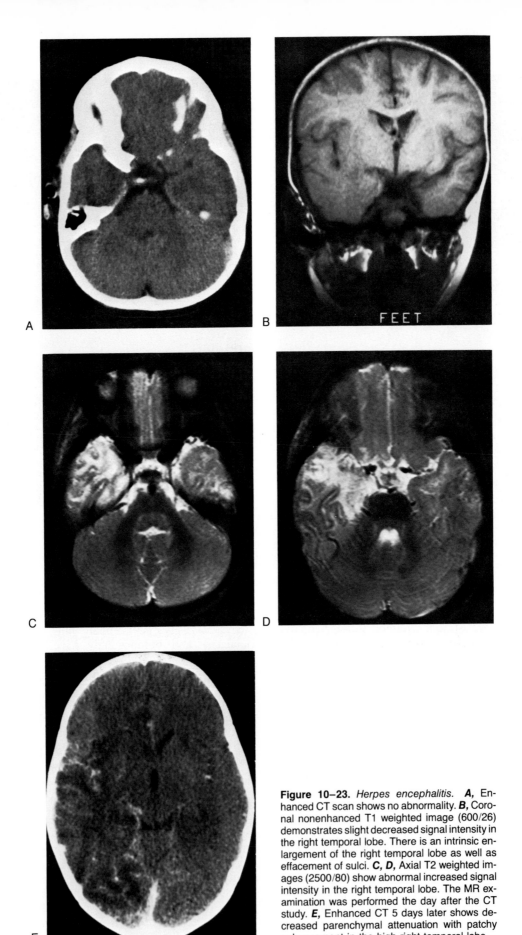

Figure 10–23. *Herpes encephalitis.* **A,** Enhanced CT scan shows no abnormality. **B,** Coronal nonenhanced T1 weighted image (600/26) demonstrates slight decreased signal intensity in the right temporal lobe. There is an intrinsic enlargement of the right temporal lobe as well as effacement of sulci. **C, D,** Axial T2 weighted images (2500/80) show abnormal increased signal intensity in the right temporal lobe. The MR examination was performed the day after the CT study. **E,** Enhanced CT 5 days later shows decreased parenchymal attenuation with patchy enhancement in the high right temporal lobe.

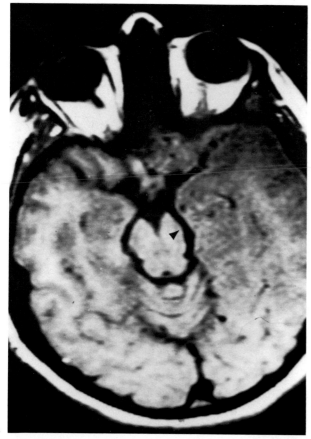

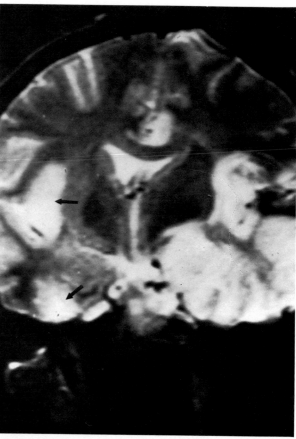

A   B

Figure 10–24. *Herpes encephalitis.* **A,** Axial T1 weighted image (600/20) demonstrates abnormal decreased signal in the left temporal lobe. There is swelling of the left temporal lobe and effacement of sulci. Slight flattening of the cerebral peduncle on the left (*arrowhead*) is also seen secondary to the swelling of the medial aspect of the temporal lobe. **B,** Coronal T2 weighted image (2500/80) shows abnormal increased signal intensity in the left temporal lobe as well as the left insular cortex. Foci of abnormal signal intensity are also identified on the right side in the inferior temporal and insular regions (*arrows*).

as described above is more common in the neonatal form of the disease and can also be readily identified by MRI.

Cytomegalovirus Infection

Congenital cytomegalovirus (CMV) infection is reported to occur in up to 0.5 percent of all live births.[68] The infection is generally transplacental. At birth patients have petechiae, jaundice, and hepatosplenomegaly.[69] Not all cases are associated with central nervous system (CNS) injury. Approximately 10 percent of patients have neural damage that generally consists of microcephaly, mental retardation, hearing loss, and optic abnormalities.[70] Seizures are also common. The presence of cytomegalovirus infection may also predispose to the development of bacterial meningitis. The isolation of the virus from the urine is diagnostic, but should be tested for in the neonatal period. Pathologically there are abnormalities with respect to normal brain development, including polymicrogyria and

pachygyria.[71] Hydranencephaly, multicystic encephalomalacia, and porencephaly have also been reported.[72] Intracerebral calcifications are relatively common and are seen in the subependymal or immediate periventricular region.[71]

CT examination demonstrates with great sensitivity the presence of periventricular calcification (Figs. 10–29, 10–30). The associated brain abnormalities such as hydranencephaly and porencephaly are also evident. Abnormalities of sulcation may be less well defined on CT than on MRI.

MRI may show diffuse white matter changes of increased signal (Fig. 10–30). Routine spin-echo MR studies may not demonstrate the presence of periventricular calcification that is readily evident on CT examination. Preliminary work with gradient-echo images, which are more sensitive to the magnetic susceptibility present in foci of calcification may help in the detection of such lesions, but this has not yet been proved in a large study.[7] Occasionally the calcification may be present on the MR examination and manifest as an area of decreased signal intensity, generally on

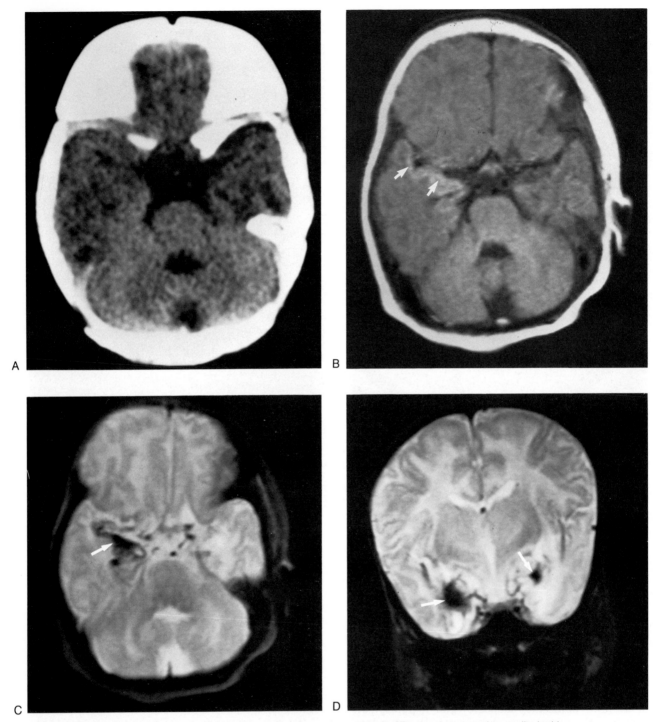

Figure 10–25. *Hemorrhagic herpes encephalitis.*   ***A,*** Axial nonenhanced brain CT scan shows no abnormality in this neonate with a diffuse vesicular rash. ***B,*** Axial unenhanced T1 weighted image (600/26) demonstrates abnormal signal intensity along the cortical margin of the right temporal lobe consistent with methemoglobin (*arrows*). ***C, D,*** Axial and coronal T2 weighted images (3000/100) demonstrate foci of decreased signal in the medial aspect of both temporal lobes (*arrows*), consistent with acute deoxyhemoglobin or intracellular methemoglobin. Foci of abnormal signal intensity in both temporal lobes are also noted. The CT and MR studies were performed on the same day.

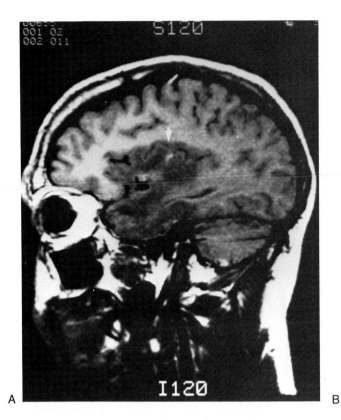

A

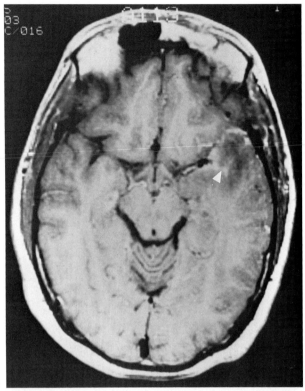

B

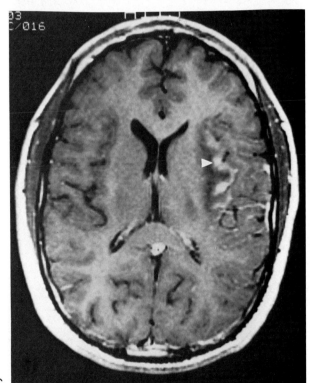

C

Figure 10–26. *Herpes encephalitis.* ***A,*** Sagittal nonenhanced T1 weighted image (600/20) demonstrates decreased attenuation in the temporal lobe and insular cortex (*arrow*). No abnormal increased signal intensity is identified. ***B, C,*** Axial T1 weighted images (600/20) after gadolinium-DTPA administration show patchy enhancement in the left temporal lobe and insular cortex (*arrowheads*). Enlargement of the temporal lobe is identified on the lower image. (Courtesy of Jeffery Reider, M.D., Indianapolis, IN.)

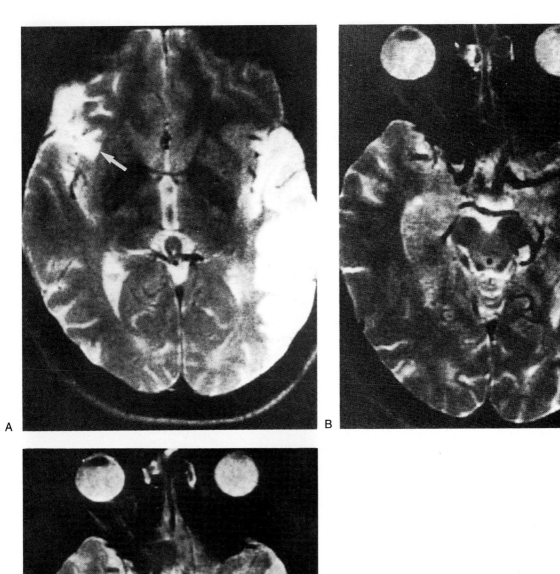

A

B

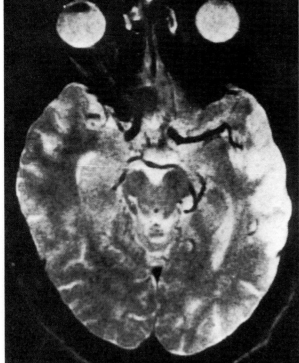

C

Figure 10–27. *Herpes encephalitis with acyclovir therapy.* **A,** T2 weighted image (2000/80) demonstrates increased signal in the left temporal lobe with a smaller focus of abnormal increased signal intensity in the posterior right frontal lobe (*arrow*). **B,** Axial T2 weighted image (2000/80) immediately after acyclovir therapy shows resolution of the left temporal lobe abnormality. **C,** Three months after treatment, a T2 weighted image (2000/80) demonstrates high signal in the left temporal lobe region consistent with postinfectious encephalomalacia. (From Lester JW, Carter MP, Reynolds TL. Herpes encephalitis: MR monitoring of response to acyclovir therapy. J Comput Assist Tomogr 1988; 12:941–943.)

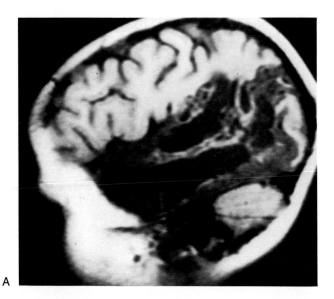

A

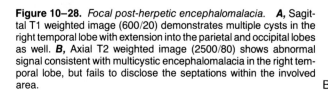

Figure 10–28. *Focal post-herpetic encephalomalacia.* **A,** Sagittal T1 weighted image (600/20) demonstrates multiple cysts in the right temporal lobe with extension into the parietal and occipital lobes as well. **B,** Axial T2 weighted image (2500/80) shows abnormal signal consistent with multicystic encephalomalacia in the right temporal lobe, but fails to disclose the septations within the involved area.

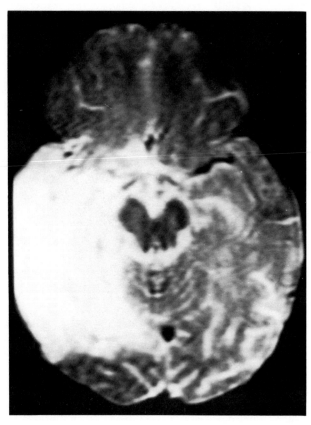

B

T2 weighted images. Rarely, other paramagnetic elements, perhaps manganese or copper, may be laid down with the calcium and lead to hyperintensity of the calcified focus on T1 weighted images. The hydranencephalic and porencephalic complications are well identified by MRI. The presence of pachygyria is also better appreciated on MR than on CT. Even though polymicrogyria is not commonly diagnosed on MRI, this sulcal abnormality is more likely to be seen on MRI than on CT.

Reports of foci of noncongenital CMV infection have also been published.[73] These areas of focal infection demonstrate increased signal intensity on T2 weighted images but remain relatively nonspecific. Gadolinium-DTPA injection may demonstrate enhancement consistent with the acute nature of the disease.

Rubella

Rubella is the last viral etiology associated with the TORCH syndrome. This infection is acquired during intrauterine life. Not all cases have neurologic sequelae. If neurologic manifestations are present, they may include hearing loss, alterations in globe size, and retinal abnormalities as well as retardation and microcephaly.[74] The neurologic manifestations may not be apparent for several years after birth.[75] Seizures, mental retardation, or focal neurologic deficits may also bring the patient to clinical attention. Chronic meningitis with periventricular foci of necrosis are identified at autopsy.[8] Delayed myelination is not uncommon. CT demonstrates a brain that is mildly atrophic but otherwise normal.[76] Cerebral calcifications are unusual.[76] MRI may also demonstrate mild diffuse atrophy. No reports of abnormal parenchymal signal have been published. The delay in myelination may be very well evaluated by MRI. Recent studies investigating the time, course, and pattern of normal white matter myelination have been undertaken and reported.[77] Deviations from this pattern can be detected.

Subacute Sclerosing Panencephalitis

Subacute sclerosing panencephalitis (SSPE) is thought to be related to the measles virus. It is a slow viral infection that commonly follows a measles infection, which may have been years earlier.[19] The infection begins clinically with language and behavioral changes.[78] Continued intellectual deterioration follows, with chorea, ataxia, seizures, and ocular problems.[79] SSPE can lead to death, although remissions are common. The CSF may demonstrate increased gammaglobulin content and the presence of neutraliz-

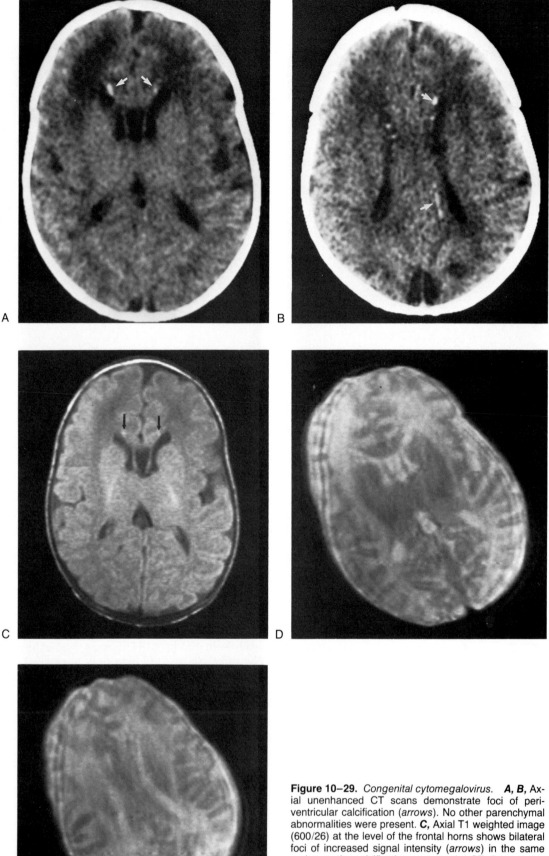

Figure 10–29. *Congenital cytomegalovirus.* **A, B,** Axial unenhanced CT scans demonstrate foci of periventricular calcification (*arrows*). No other parenchymal abnormalities were present. **C,** Axial T1 weighted image (600/26) at the level of the frontal horns shows bilateral foci of increased signal intensity (*arrows*) in the same region as the calcification seen on the CT. Presumably this relates to the deposition of paramagnetic elements with the calcium. **D, E,** Multiple axial T2 weighted images (3000/100) are partly degraded by patient motion, but fail to show any abnormal signal in the region of the periventricular calcifications.

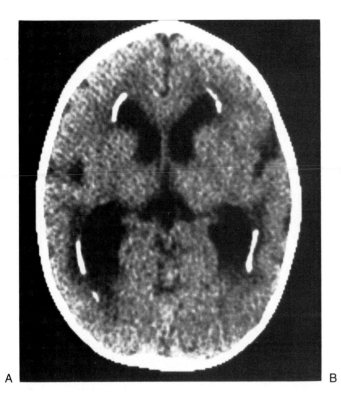

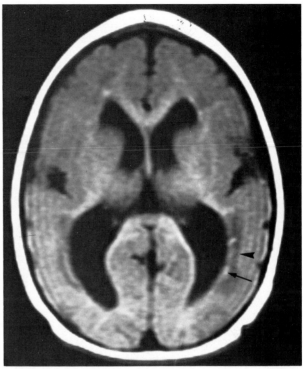

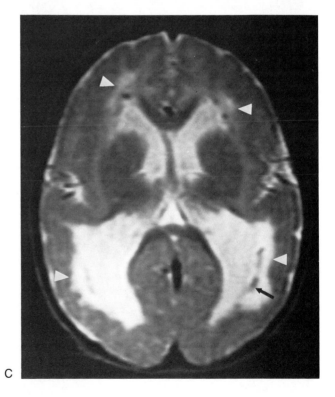

Figure 10–30. *Congenital cytomegalovirus.* **A,** Nonenhanced axial CT scan demonstrates foci of periventricular calcification. There is associated ventriculomegaly. No other abnormality was noted. **B,** Axial T1 weighted image (600/20) shows a focus of abnormal increased signal intensity in the periventricular region (*arrow*) consistent with the calcification seen on CT. Abnormal decreased signal intensity in the periatrial white matter (*arrowhead*) is noted but is not well defined on the T1 weighted image. **C,** T2 weighted axial MR (2500/80) demonstrates the foci of calcification to have low signal intensity (*arrows*). Marked white matter signal abnormalities are also identified (*arrowheads*) consistent with parenchymal infection that was not seen by CT. (Courtesy of Robert A. Zimmerman, M.D., Philadelphia, PA.)

ing antibody to measles virus.[80] Demyelination is a common pathologic finding. CT results are generally normal or may occasionally demonstrate mild-to-moderate cerebral edema (Fig. 10–31*A,B*).[81, 82] With continued progression of the disease, central and cortical parenchymal loss becomes evident.[83] MRI appears to be useful in the early evaluation of this disease. The

foci of demyelination and gliosis are identified as areas of decreased signal intensity on T1 and increased signal intensity on T2 weighted images (Fig. 10–31*C* to *F*).[78] These foci are periventricular or subcortical and may be confluent; they also may be seen in the basal ganglia. Lesions in the cerebellum have also been reported.

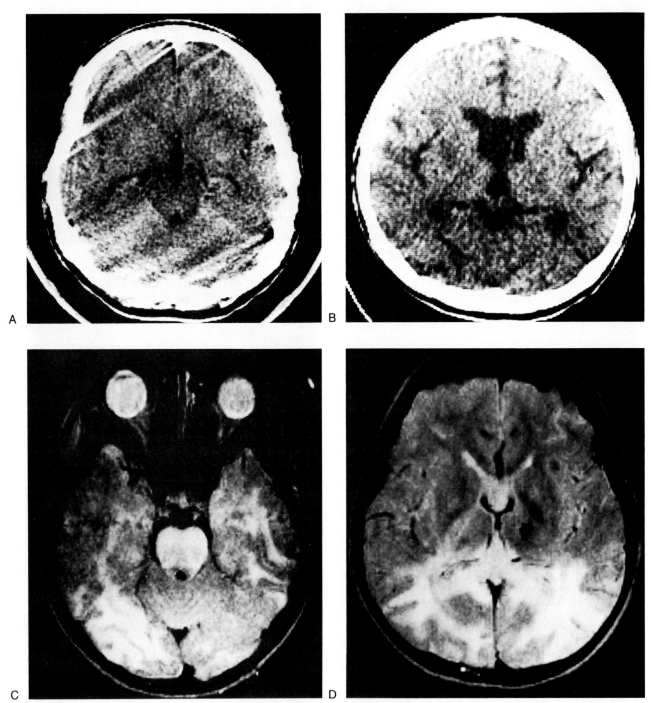

Figure 10-31. *Subacute sclerosing panencephalitis (SSPE).* **A, B,** Unenhanced CT scans show no abnormality although significant bone artifact is present. **C** to **F,** Axial T2 weighted images (2000/80) demonstrate multiple areas of abnormal signal intensity. These are seen predominantly in the white matter, particularly in the posterior half of the cerebral

Miscellaneous Viral Infections

MRI results have been reported to be abnormal in isolated cases of mumps encephalitis and Epstein-Barr virus (Figs. 10–32, 10–33).[2, 84] These lesions have all demonstrated abnormal signal intensity consistent with edema, but are nonspecific in their location and etiology.

Acute Disseminated Encephalomyelitis

Acute disseminated encephalomyelitis (ADEM) represents a postinfectious demyelinating disease in children, probably autoimmune in origin.[85, 86] Most typically the illness is seen 1 to 2 weeks after either a viral infection or vaccination. Clinically, patients may present with seizures, coma, papilledema, and ataxia.[87] The CSF is usually normal but an elevated opening pressure is relatively common.[88] Untreated, the disease may occasionally be fatal, although spontaneous resolution often occurs. Most children respond to corticosteroid therapy and have no residual neurologic deficits.[88] The CT scan is generally negative (Fig. 10–34A, B).[89, 90] Occasionally, CT may demonstrate focal hypodense areas in the white matter caused by focal demyelination or edema. MR examination has proved very helpful in the evaluation of ADEM. Multiple foci of abnormal increased signal intensity are identified on the T2 weighted images (Fig. 10–34C, D).[87, 88, 90] These may be in the white matter or involve the basal ganglia and thalamus. Cerebellar and brain stem lesions have also been documented. Presumably, gadolinium-enhanced studies will demonstrate increased signal around the margins of the foci of demyelination.[91] Follow-up studies have shown resolution of the lesions.

FUNGAL INFECTIONS

Most fungal infections are related to immunodeficient states in children. Frequently this is secondary to leukemia and its treatment.[12] Neurologic involvement may be manifest by progressive meningeal signs, seizures, focal deficits, and increased intracranial pressure. Pathologic involvement may be meningeal or parenchymal.

Candida is the most common cause of cerebral mycotic infection.[19] Most cases reach the CNS by hematogenous routes from primary lung or GI infections. Pathologically the fungus inflames vessels, leading to thrombosis and infarction.[8] Intraparenchymal abscess formation is also common. The pathology consists of noncaseating granulomas. Intraparenchymal abscess formation, vascular occlusion, leptomeningeal infection, and calcification may occur. The leptomeningitis is similar on CT and MRI to the meningeal processes previously described. Hydrocephalus may be noted.

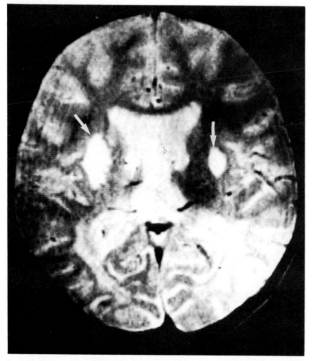

E

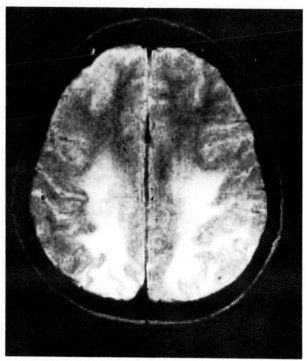

F

hemispheres. Foci of abnormal signal are also present in the lentiform nucleus bilaterally (*arrows*). Changes in the white matter of the cerebellum were also noted (*not shown*). (From Tsuchiya K, Yamauchi T, Furui S, et al. MR imaging vs CT in subacute sclerosing panencephalitis. AJNR 1988; 9:943–946. © by American Roentgen Ray Society.)

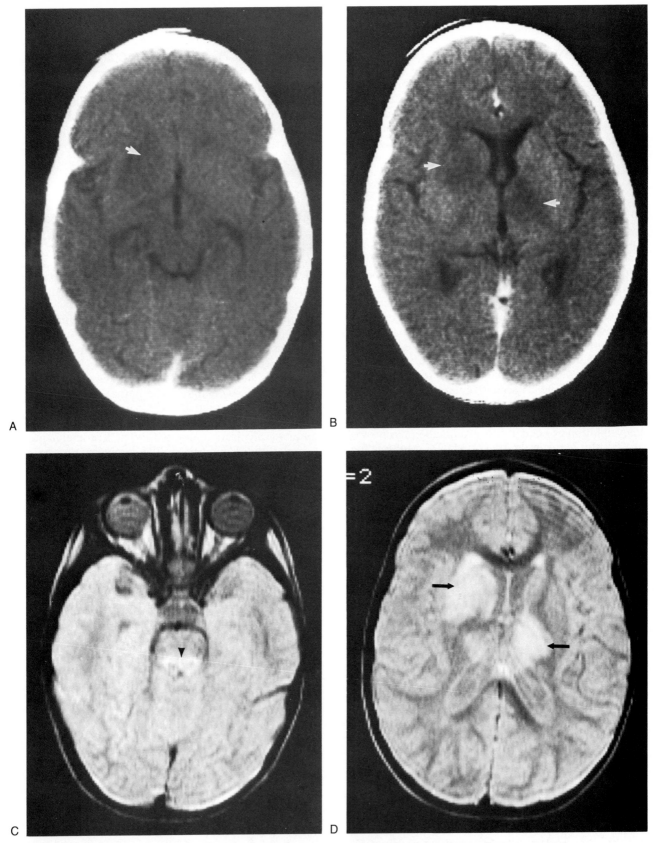

Figure 10–32. *Mumps encephalitis.* ***A, B,*** Axial enhanced CT scans demonstrate decreased attenuation without abnormal enhancement in the right anterior ganglionic area and in the left posterior ganglionic region (*arrows*). No abnormality is noted in the dorsal upper brain stem. ***C, D,*** Axial proton density weighted images (2000/20) demonstrate abnormal increased signal intensity in the right anterior ganglionic area and the left posterior ganglionic region (*arrows*). In addition, foci of abnormal increased signal intensity are seen in the right thalamus and dorsal upper midbrain (*arrowhead*). (From Tarr RW, Edwards KM, Kessler RM, Kulkarni MV. MRI of mumps encephalitis: comparison with CT evaluation. Pediatr Radiol 1987; 17:59–62.)

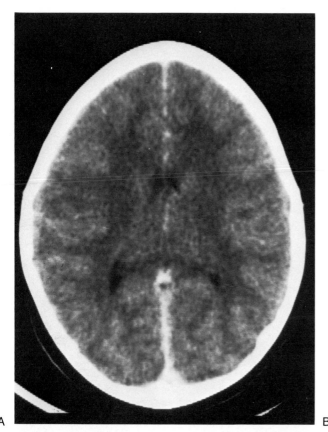
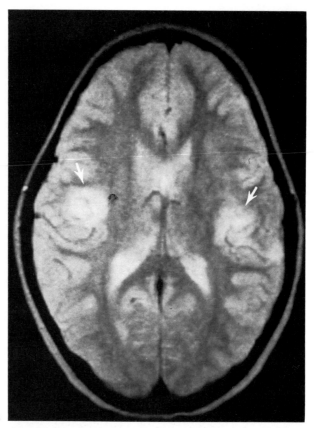

A   B

Figure 10–33. *Epstein-Barr virus encephalitis.* **A,** Enhanced axial CT scan is normal. **B,** Axial T2 weighted image (2000/80) demonstrates bilateral foci of increased signal intensity (*arrows*) in the area of the posterior sylvian fissure bilaterally. (From Bale JF, Andersen RD, Grose C. Magnetic resonance imaging of the brain in childhood herpesvirus infections. Pediatr Infect Dis J 1987; 6:644–647. © by Williams & Wilkins.)

Nodular or ring-enhancing parenchymal abscesses may be seen. *Candida* abscess formation may be associated with a relative absence of surrounding edema.

Aspergillosis also generally occurs secondary to hematogenous spread. Most commonly this is secondary to pulmonary involvement.[92] This fungus also invades arteries, resulting in ischemic infarction.[93] Foci of hemorrhage are commonly seen pathologically. Large abscesses may be present in the cerebral hemispheres. MRI has been reported to be more useful than CT, because it is able to demonstrate the early encephalitic stage, whereas CT cannot.[94] This early encephalitic stage appears before the multifocal enhancing lesions or large abscesses seen in later stages of the disease. Edema is relatively extensive with *Aspergillus* infection. On CT examination, decreased attenuation, with or without patchy irregular enhancement, is seen (Fig. 10–35A). A ring-enhancing focus may be seen (Fig. 10–36A, B). On MR examination, abnormal increased signal intensity on the T2 weighted images is identified with associated mass effect (Fig. 10–35B). Hemorrhage may be seen on both CT and MRI; smaller foci are better appreciated on MRI (Fig. 10–36C, D).

Histoplasmosis involving the CNS is rare without disseminated disease.[95] The appearance of histoplasmosis is similar to that of *Aspergillus* and *Candida* on both CT and MR examination (Fig. 10–37).[95] Like *Candida,* however, significant edema or mass effect is less common than with aspergillosis. Other fungal infections such as cryptococcosis, coccidioidomycosis, blastomycosis, nocardiosis, and mucormycosis may be seen but are even more rare.

CYSTICERCOSIS

Cysticercosis is a parasitic disease that has been recognized with increased frequency in the United States. The infection is caused by the larva of *Taenia solium.* The infection arises from eating poorly cooked infected pork. CNS involvement is seen in 60 to 90 percent of patients with cysticercosis.[96, 97] Intracranial involvement can include either the parenchyma, the ventricles, or the meningobasal system. Pathologically the nature of the infestation determines the CT and MR appearance. The embryo, which lodges in the CNS,

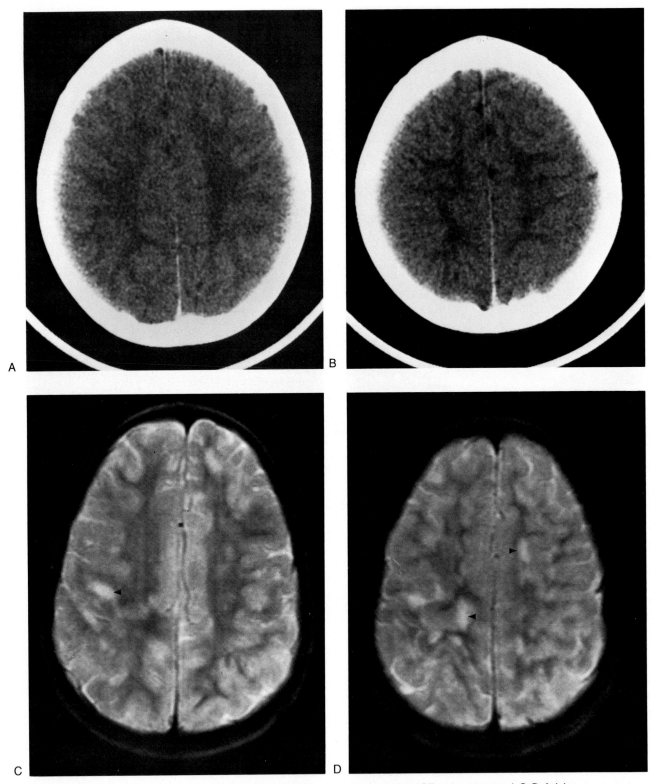

Figure 10–34. *Acute disseminated encephalomyelitis (ADEM).* **A, B,** Axial enhanced CT scans are normal. **C, D,** Axial T2 weighted images (2500/80) demonstrate multiple foci of abnormal increased signal intensity in the subcortical white matter (arrowheads).

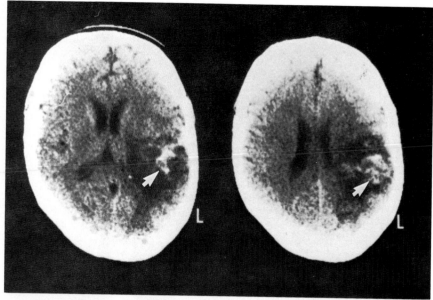

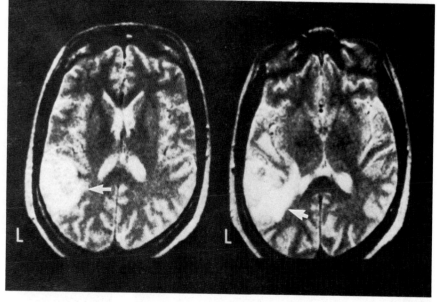

Figure 10–35. *Aspergillosis.* ***A,*** Axial CT examination, before (left) and after (right) contrast administration, demonstrates a hemorrhagic lesion in the left posterior temporal lobe (*arrows*) with associated enhancement of the adjacent parenchyma. ***B,*** Axial T2 weighted images (2000/60) show abnormal increased signal intensity in the left temporal lobe (*arrows*). Note that the left is reversed for the MR images. No hemorrhage was identifiable on MRI. (From Mikhael MA, Rushovich AM, Ciric I. Magnetic resonance imaging of cerebral aspergillosis. Comput Radiol 1985, Pergamon Press; 9:85–89.)

develops a cystic covering and scolex. The presence of the parasite produces an inflammation with fibroconnective tissue and granulation tissue as well as chronic inflammatory cells. Ultimately the organism dies, which leads to a more marked inflammatory response. The dead organism then calcifies. Symptoms may not arise for several years after the primary infection.[98] Symptoms include seizures, headache, dementia, and hydrocephalus. The hydrocephalus is generally related to obstruction of the ventricular system by an intraventricular cyst. Serologic tests have been reported to be 80 percent sensitive for detecting the antibody in serum in CSF.[99] Therapy includes praziquantel.[100]

With appropriate treatment, patients undergo symptomatic resolution.

Since the symptoms are rather nonspecific, and since the history of ingestion may not be obtained because of its remote occurrence and because of the relatively poor diagnostic markers for the disease, CT has represented the most reliable study for the diagnosis of cysticercosis in the brain. In the acute infestation, multiple foci of decreased attenuation are identified throughout the brain (Fig. 10–38A),[101] generally associated with edema. With intravenous contrast administration the lesions enhance as either dense nodules or small, ring-enhancing lesions (Fig. 10–39A). Over

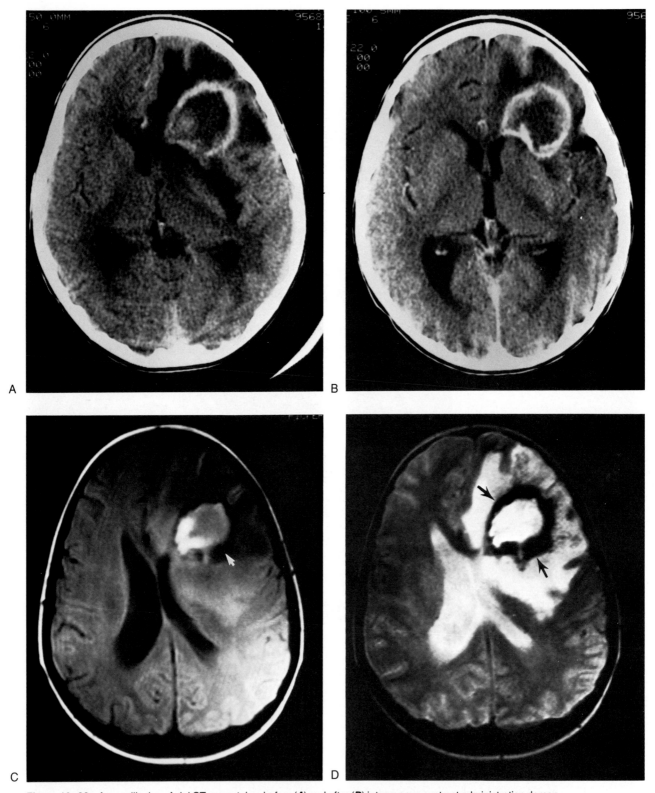

A

B

C

D

Figure 10–36. *Aspergillosis.* Axial CT scans taken before (*A*) and after (*B*) intravenous contrast administration demonstrate a ring lesion in the left frontal lobe. The margin of the lesion is hemorrhagic on the unenhanced study but does show some marginal enhancement. Surrounding edema with associated mass effect is also present. *C,* T1 weighted axial MR image (1000/20) demonstrates an area of increased signal intensity in the central portion of the lesion. This was thought to represent a proteinaceous fluid accumulation. A capsule of slightly decreased signal intensity is identified, suggesting a prominent effect of deoxyhemoglobin (*arrow*). Peripheral decreased signal consistent with surrounding edema is also seen, as is associated mass effect. *D,* Axial T2 weighted image (2500/80) shows marked increased signal intensity in the central portion of the aspergillous abscess. The capsule of the abscess shows marked decreased signal consistent with acute deoxyhemoglobin (*arrows*). Surrounding edema demonstrates high signal.

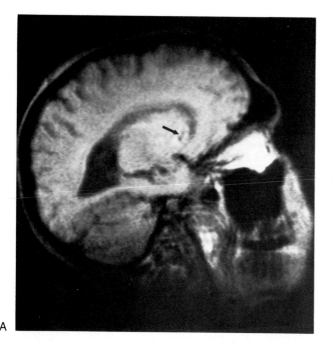

A

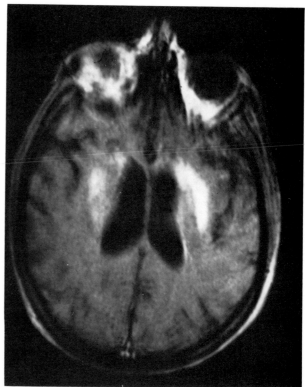

B

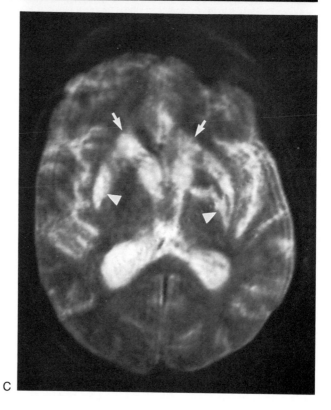

C

Figure 10–37. *Histoplasmosis.* **A,** Sagittal T1 weighted image (600/20) demonstrates no abnormal increased signal in the region of the anterior caudate head. A focus of decreased signal (*arrow*) may be present. **B,** Axial T1 weighted image (600/26) after gadolinium-DTPA administration shows enhancement in the periventricular region bilaterally. **C,** Axial T2 weighted image (2500/80) demonstrates abnormal increased signal intensity in the anterior periventricular region (*arrows*) with involvement also identified in the lentiform nuclei bilaterally (*arrowheads*). At biopsy the area of abnormal enhancement on the right periventricular region showed histoplasmosis infection. This was also documented at autopsy.

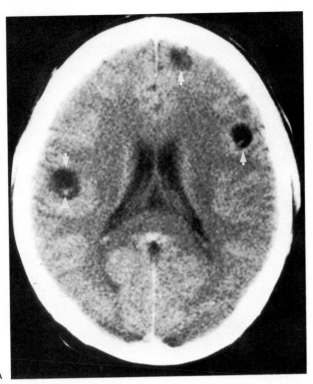
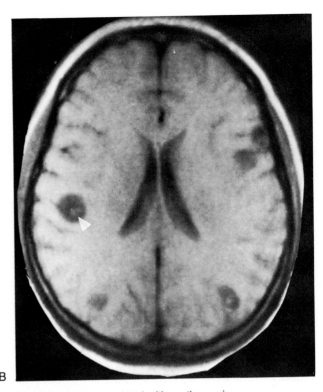

A

B

Figure 10–38. *Cysticercosis.* **A,** Axial enhanced CT scan demonstrates three cysts associated with cysticercosis (*arrows*). The lesion in the right parietal lobe is representative of the vesicle stage of the disease before significant capsule formation has occurred. The cyst itself is of CSF density with the scolex (*arrowhead*) present along the margin of the cyst. No marginal enhancement to suggest capsule formation is seen. **B,** Axial T1 weighted image (600/20) demonstrates multiple neurocysticercosis cysts. The intensity of the cyst fluid is slightly greater than that of CSF. The scolex (*arrowhead*) can again be identified. (From Zee C-S, Segall HD, Boswell W, et al. MR imaging of neurocysticercosis. J Comput Assist Tomogr 1988; 12:927–934.)

months the enhancement gradually disappears, with the edema persisting. Small calcifications are then identified consistent with parasitic death (Fig. 10–40A).[102] Cysts that occur in the ventricles are of the same absorption coefficient as CSF, which makes their detection difficult (Fig. 10–41A). The finding of obstructive hydrocephalus should be viewed with suspicion, however. Before the advent of MRI the diagnosis of intraventricular cysts required intraventricular contrast administration followed by CT scanning.

On MRI the parenchymal cysts have a low signal intensity on T1 weighted images and high intensity on T2 weighted images (Fig. 10–38B).[103, 104] The signal intensity within the cyst parallels that of CSF. Occasionally a small mural hyperintense nodule may be appreciated along the margin representing the scolex. On MRI, calcification may appear as a focus of decreased signal on both T1 and T2 weighted images if sufficiently large (Figs. 10–40B, C). The high-signal edema and reactive changes on the T2 weighted images are well outlined. The intraventricular cysts are particularly well visualized on MRI.[105] The intraventricular cysts are hyperintense to CSF on T1 weighted images (Fig. 10–41B). They are often of the same signal intensity as CSF on T2 weighted images (Fig. 10–41C). Although no reports of gadolinium-DTPA enhancement of the parenchymal cysticerci are currently available, presumably enhancement will be seen in the acute stage similar to that on CT scanning.

LYME DISEASE

Lyme disease is an illness caused by a tick-transmitted spirochete, *Borrelia burgdorferi,* which is endemic in the northeast and upper midwest United States. The illness generally begins within 1 month of the tick bite. A skin rash called erythema chronicum migrans quickly develops.[106] Other symptoms include fever, chills, headache, and stiff neck. The disease generally lasts 1 month, resolving even without treatment. Months later, however, neurologic dysfunction may begin. Some cases lead to death. The nervous system is involved in fewer than 15 percent of patients. Clinically they present with meningeal symptoms and cranial and peripheral neuropathies. Occasionally, seizures, dementia, and psychiatric symptoms also occur.[108] Diagnosis generally rests with serologic tests for specific

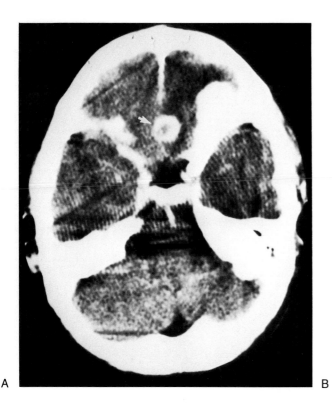

A

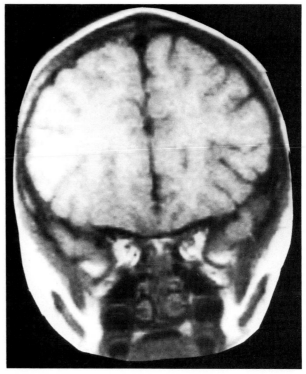

B

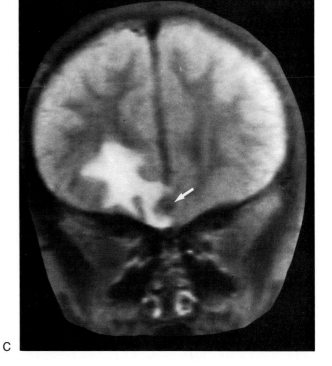

C

Figure 10–39. *Cysticercosis.* ***A,*** Axial enhanced CT scan demonstrates a ring-enhancing lesion in the inferior frontal gyrus (*arrow*), consistent with the capsular phase of the parenchymal reaction to the paracytic infection. ***B,*** Coronal nonenhanced T1 weighted image (600/20) shows no abnormality in the region of the inferior right frontal lobe. ***C,*** Coronal T2 weighted image (2250/80) demonstrates the lesion to have low signal intensity (*arrow*). A significant amount of associated abnormal increased signal intensity in the adjacent white matter is seen and is consistent with edema. (From Zee C-S, Segall HD, Boswell W, et al. MR imaging of neurocysticercosis. J Comput Assist Tomogr 1988; 12:927–934.)

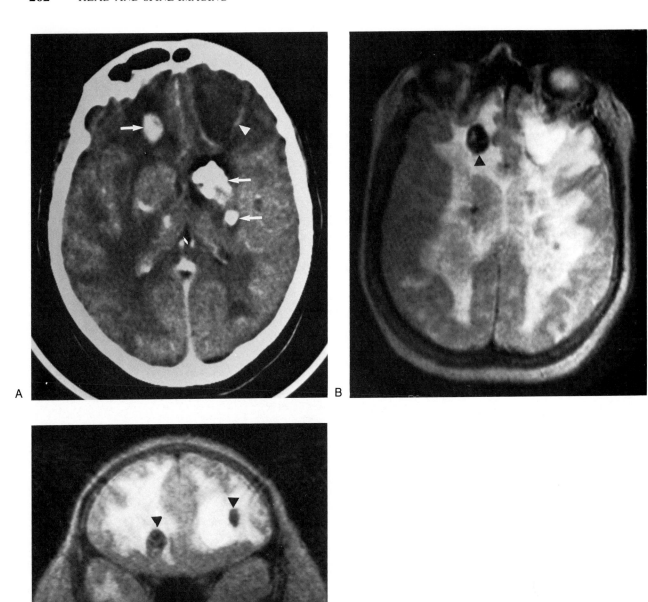

A

B

C

Figure 10–40. *Calcified cysticercosis.* ***A,*** Axial enhanced CT scan demonstrates three large foci of parenchymal calcification (*arrows*). Two smaller zones of calcification in the posterior right putamen and anterior right thalamus are also seen. Low attenuation in the white matter suggests reactive edema. A cyst is identified in the left frontal lobe (*arrowhead*). Axial (***B***) and coronal (***C***) T2 weighted images (2000/80) show the foci of calcification to be of markedly low signal intensity (*arrowheads*). Abnormal increased signal in the white matter is seen diffusely, consistent with reactive edema.

antibody to the spirochete. The best treatment for the CNS infection remains in doubt at this time. Penicillin appears to be the current prime therapeutic treatment, but some patients with neurologic abnormalities have failed to respond.[109] In such cases, chloramphenicol may be useful.

CT scanning has demonstrated small foci of decreased attenuation in the periventricular and subcor-

tical white matter.[106] Minimal contrast enhancement may be noted. The MR appearance of Lyme disease is relatively nonspecific.[110, 111] Small, generally punctate foci of increased signal intensity on T2 weighted images are identified in the periventricular and subcortical regions (Fig. 10–42). The appearance is similar to that of adult multiple sclerosis. Resolution of the MR abnormalities is seen with appropriate treatment.

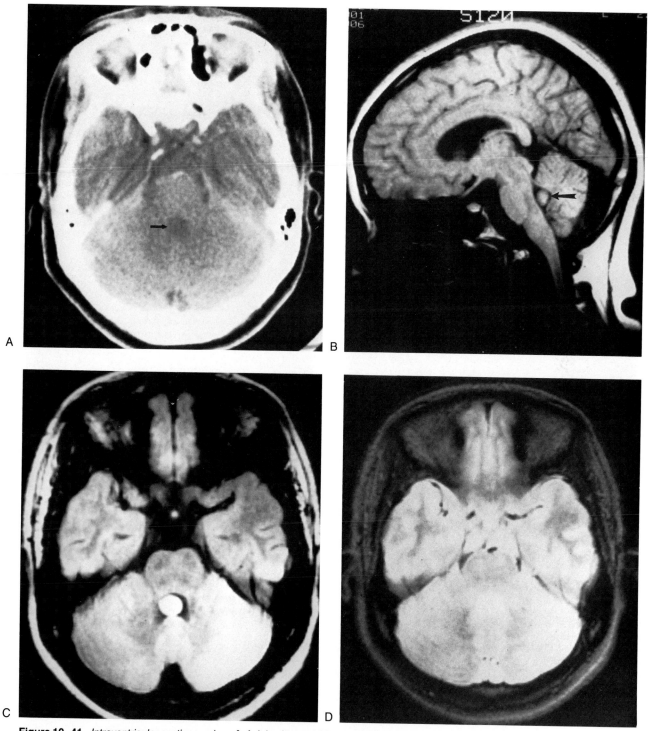

Figure 10–41. *Intraventricular cysticercosis.*   ***A,*** Axial enhanced CT scan fails to demonstrate an abnormality, although the CSF density within the fourth ventricle is somewhat greater than usually seen (*arrow*). ***B,*** Sagittal T1 weighted image (400/25) demonstrates a rounded cyst within the fourth ventricle (*arrow*). ***C, D,*** Axial proton density in T2 weighted images (2000/20,80) show the high signal cyst present in the fourth ventricle on the proton density weighted image only. On the more T2 weighted image, the high signal intensity of the cyst is averaged, with the high signal of the surrounding CSF obscuring the abnormality. (From Rhee RS, Kumasaki DY, Sarwar M, et al. MR imaging of intraventricular cysticercosis. J Comput Assist Tomogr 1987; 11:598–601.)

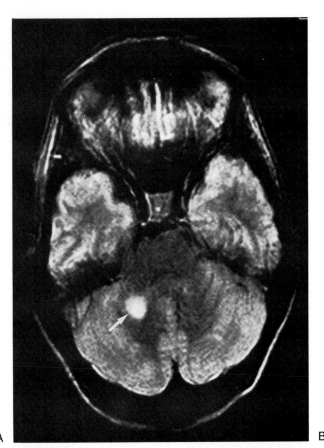
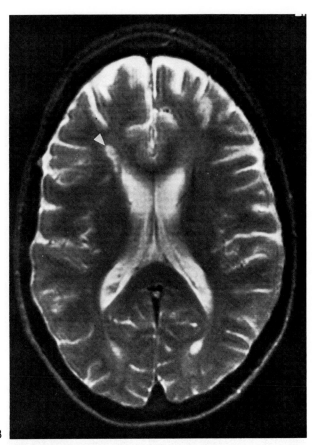

A

B

Figure 10–42. *Lyme disease in an adult.* **A, B,** Axial T2 weighted images (2208/100) show foci of increased signal in the right cerebellum (*arrow*) and right frontal periventricular zone (*arrowhead*). This patient had positive CSF and serum Lyme titers. (Courtesy of Susan B. Peterman, M.D., Atlanta, GA.)

TOXOPLASMOSIS

Toxoplasmosis, a protozoan infection, may be seen either as a congenital infection or as an acquired infection related to immune deficiency states, including AIDS. Congenital toxoplasmosis is the most frequent congenital brain infection.[76] In most cases the cysts are acquired by the mother from the specific host, the cat. Transplacental infection of the fetus then occurs. The frequency and severity of the cerebral lesions are most prominent when the disease is acquired early in pregnancy, as opposed to late.[76] The parasite produces a meningeal inflammation with areas of necrosis in the meninges and brain. The basal ganglia, white matter, and cerebral aqueduct are predominantly affected. Calcification in the areas of necrosis is common.

Clinically severe forms may present with symptoms related to meningoencephalitis or hydrocephalus. Microcephaly may also be present, as may orbital abnormalities. Seizures and mental retardation are also seen in these severe forms; in less severe forms, hydrocephalus may be the only clinical manifestation.

On CT, severe disease may include encephalomalacia or hydranencephaly.[112] Calcifications are multiple; these may, in most cases, be distinguished from CMV by the fact that CMV is periventricular in nature, whereas the *Toxoplasma* calcification is more parenchymal and particularly involves the basal ganglia. In less severe cases ventriculomegaly is seen, termed colpocephaly, involving the occipital horns.[76] In these less severe cases, calcification is frequently present but generally is not as exuberant as in severe cases. MR examination demonstrates similar findings in terms of gross cortical disruption. Abnormal increased signal is seen in the periventricular region on T2 weighted images. Calcification is less well identified on MRI.

The acquired form of toxoplasmosis usually occurs in children with AIDS.[113] This acquired form is discussed below.

ACQUIRED IMMUNODEFICIENCY SYNDROME

Between 30 and 50 percent of children with acquired immunodeficiency syndrome (AIDS) demonstrate a progressive encephalopathy.[113] The causative factor is a retrovirus termed human immunodeficiency virus (HIV). The encephalopathy appears to be caused by direct brain infection by the virus. The infection is thought to occur in utero or in the perinatal period.[114] The virus may be found within macrophages and multinucleated cells on electron microscopy.[115] Evidence of viral replication may also be seen. Inflammatory cell infiltrates are also identified on microscopic examination. White matter changes consisting of astrocytosis and pallor are noted. Calcification is relatively frequent in children. Overall, there is associated central and cortical parenchymal atrophy.[116]

Clinically, these patients demonstrate developmental delay. There may be a failure to achieve milestones or a regression from acquired milestones.[113] Cognitive impairment is also present in most cases. Dementia is common. Motor signs consist of bilateral pyramidal tract signs, including spastic paresis. Seizures are uncommon but can occur. Evidence of microcephaly may also be noted. The encephalopathy is generally progressive, although plateaus may be present for significant periods.[113] The onset of the encephalopathy is generally from months to several years after the initial infection, but is a very poor prognostic sign that invariably predicts a fatal outcome.[117]

CT scans most commonly demonstrate central and cortical parenchymal loss consistent with atrophy.[118, 119] The CT scan may demonstrate calcifications of the basal ganglia and frontal periventricular white matter (Fig. 10–43). MR examination also shows the central and cortical parenchymal loss consistent with atrophy (Fig. 10–44).[119] In addition, large irregular areas of abnormal increased signal on T2 weighted images are identified in the white matter, especially the periventricular and centrum semiovale areas (Fig. 10–45). This is presumed, in most cases, to be secondary to the HIV virus, but cases with a similar MR appearance have been found with CMV, herpes, and papovavirus infections (Fig. 10–46).[118] Calcification in the basal ganglia may be difficult to appreciate on MRI.

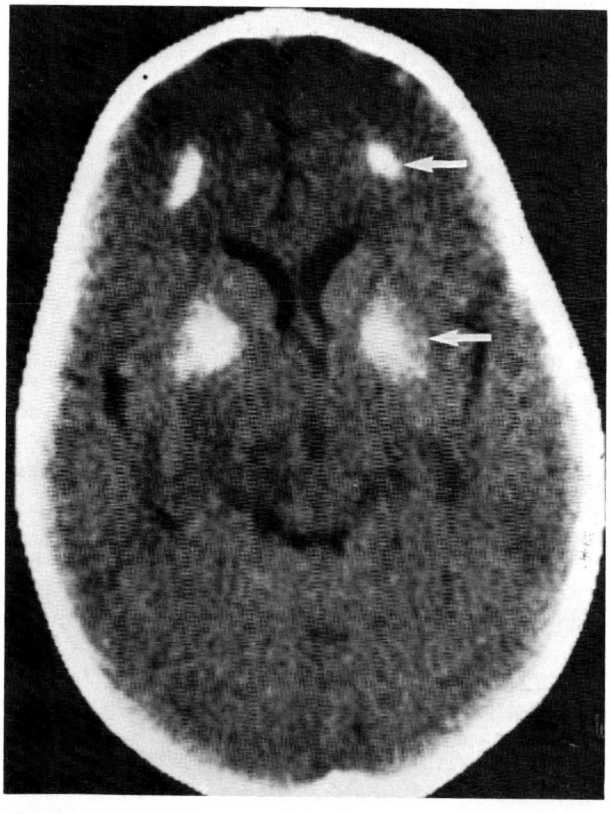

Figure 10–43. *AIDS-related atrophy and calcification.* This nonenhanced axial CT scan demonstrates calcifications in the basal ganglia bilaterally as well as in the periventricular white matter (*arrows*). Mild cerebral atrophy is also observed. (From Epstein LG, Sharer LR, Oleske JM, et al. Neurologic manifestations of human immunodeficiency virus infection in children. Pediatrics 1986; 78:678–687.)

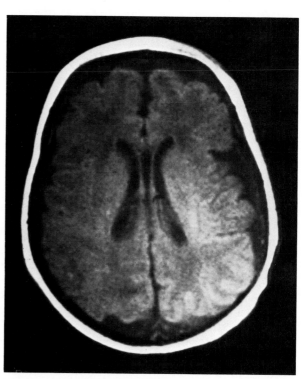

Figure 10–44. *AIDS-related atrophy.* Axial T1 weighted image (600/26) demonstrates prominence of the subarachnoid space and ventricles, consistent with AIDS-related atrophy.

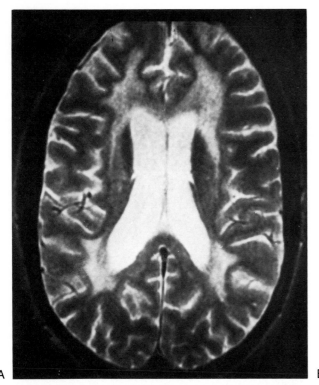
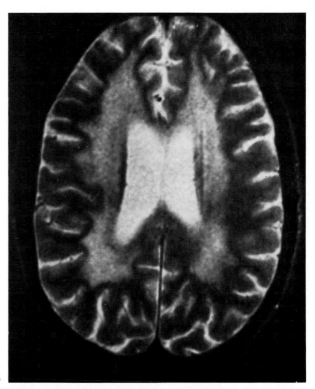

A   B

Figure 10–45. *HIV cerebritis in an adult.* ***A, B,*** Axial T2 weighted images (2500/80) demonstrate diffuse abnormal increased signal intensity in the periventricular and deep white matter. There is relative sparing of the white matter extending out into the gyri. A well-defined margin between the abnormal signal intensity and the ventricles is not present. These findings may help differentiate HIV cerebritis from progressive multifocal leukoencephalopathy (PML). (From Olsen WL, Longo FM, Mills CM, Norman D. White matter disease in AIDS: findings at MR imaging. Radiology 1988; 169:445–448.)

Mass Lesions Associated with AIDS

As in the adult population, mass lesions associated with pediatric AIDS do occur, but their incidence is much lower than in adults.[117] A mass lesion in the brain in a child with AIDS is more likely to be lymphoma than toxoplasmosis.[120] Lymphoma is also more commonly multicentric in children than in adults.

Children with AIDS-related lymphoma show a slightly different CT appearance than adults with AIDS. The children are more likely to show the more "classic" appearance of primary lymphoma,[120, 121] i.e., a mass that is slightly hyperdense on noncontrasted studies (Fig. 10–47A). Cyst formation or necrosis may also be present, and moderate enhancement is noted (Fig. 10–48A). Edema may or may not be significant. The lesions may be periventricular or peripheral and may be multiple.

On MRI the area of lymphoma is hypointense on T1 weighted images and hypo- or hyperintense on T2 weighted images (Figs. 10–47, 10–48).[119, 120] This hypointensity on the long TR studies may be related to the increased cellularity of these tumors or to their high nuclear-to-cytoplasmic ratio. The lesions may be central or peripheral, with associated mass effect and edema. Central cyst formation or necrosis is evident in many cases. Gadolinium-DTPA administration gives an enhancement pattern similar to that of CT. The use of gadolinium-DTPA may be very helpful in differentiating the margins of lymphoma from surrounding edema.

Acquired toxoplasmosis is seen less frequently in the pediatric population than is AIDS-related lymphoma. The CT appearance of toxoplasmosis in adults is that of single or multiple mass lesions with surrounding edema.[73, 122] The lesions are generally hypodense on CT and show nodular or ring enhancement. On MR examination the focus of toxoplasmosis is usually hypointense on T1 and hyperintense on T2 weighted images (Figs. 10–49, 10–50). Nodular or ring enhancement after gadolinium-DTPA administration is also seen. Significant surrounding edema is identified. Occasionally a focus of toxoplasmosis may be hemorrhagic. As in adults, it may be impossible to distinguish between lymphoma and toxoplasmosis on CT and MRI (Fig. 10–51).[124]

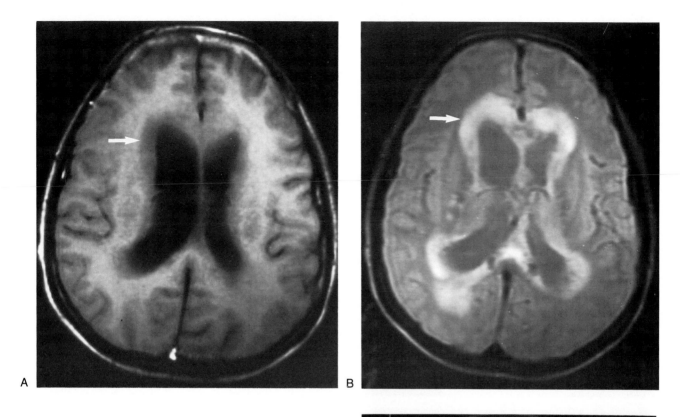

A

B

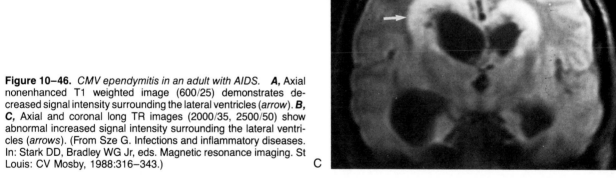

Figure 10–46. *CMV ependymitis in an adult with AIDS.* **A,** Axial nonenhanced T1 weighted image (600/25) demonstrates decreased signal intensity surrounding the lateral ventricles (*arrow*). **B, C,** Axial and coronal long TR images (2000/35, 2500/50) show abnormal increased signal intensity surrounding the lateral ventricles (*arrows*). (From Sze G. Infections and inflammatory diseases. In: Stark DD, Bradley WG Jr, eds. Magnetic resonance imaging. St Louis: CV Mosby, 1988:316–343.)

C

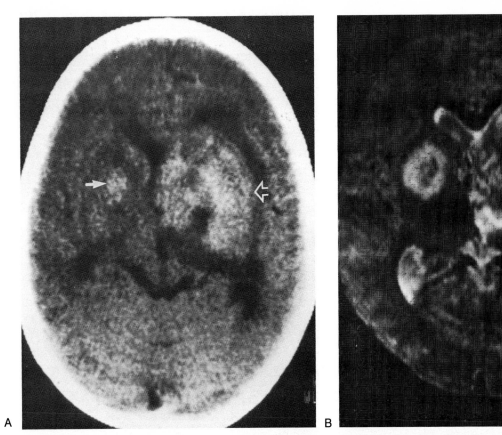

Figure 10–47. *AIDS-related lymphoma.* *A,* Unenhanced axial CT scan demonstrates a hyperdense mass involving the left ganglionic region, including the caudate head, lentiform nucleus, thalamus, and internal capsule (*open arrow*). A mild amount of surrounding edema is identified with associated mass effect. A focal area of increased attenuation in the right lentiform nucleus, without mass effect or surrounding edema, is also noted (*arrow*). *B,* Axial MR T2 weighted image (2000/80) shows most of the left-sided mass to be relatively hypointense (*arrow*). This may be secondary to the increased cellularity or high nuclear cytoplasmic ratio within the tumor. Surrounding edema and mass effect are again identified. The lesion in the right lentiform nucleus also demonstrates a somewhat hypointense central portion with surrounding high-signal edema. The left-sided lesion was biopsy-proven small cell lymphoma. No pathology on the right-sided lesion was available. (From Epstein LG, DiCarlo FJ, Joshi VV, et al. Primary lymphoma of the central nervous system in children with acquired immunodeficiency syndrome. Pediatrics 1988; 82:355–363.)

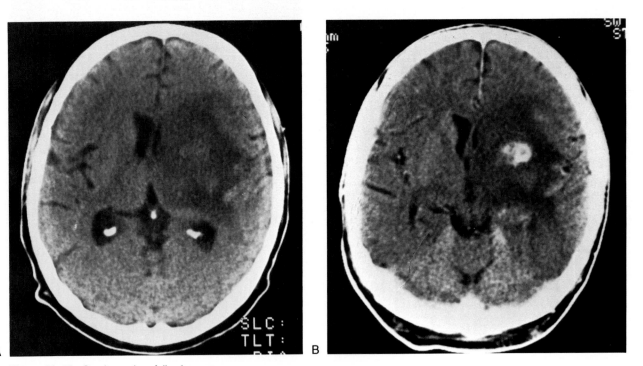

Figure 10–48. *See legend on following page.*

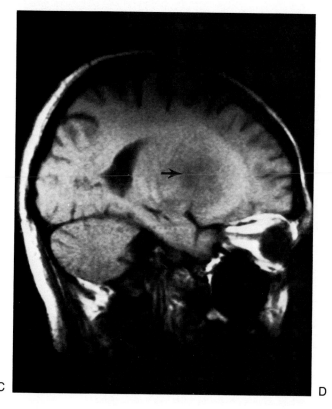

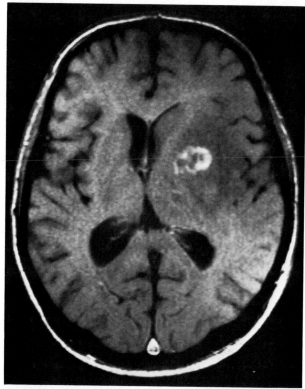

C

D

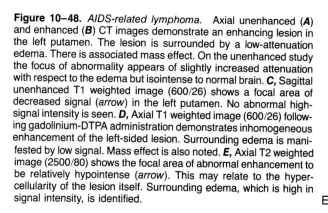

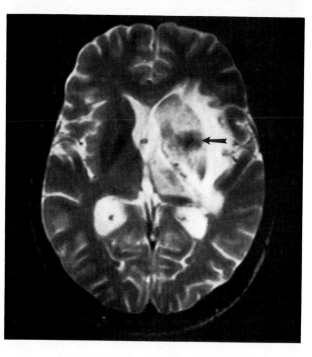

Figure 10–48. *AIDS-related lymphoma.*   Axial unenhanced (**A**) and enhanced (**B**) CT images demonstrate an enhancing lesion in the left putamen. The lesion is surrounded by a low-attenuation edema. There is associated mass effect. On the unenhanced study the focus of abnormality appears of slightly increased attenuation with respect to the edema but isointense to normal brain. **C,** Sagittal unenhanced T1 weighted image (600/26) shows a focal area of decreased signal (*arrow*) in the left putamen. No abnormal high-signal intensity is seen. **D,** Axial T1 weighted image (600/26) following gadolinium-DTPA administration demonstrates inhomogeneous enhancement of the left-sided lesion. Surrounding edema is mani-fested by low signal. Mass effect is also noted. **E,** Axial T2 weighted image (2500/80) shows the focal area of abnormal enhancement to be relatively hypointense (*arrow*). This may relate to the hyper-cellularity of the lesion itself. Surrounding edema, which is high in signal intensity, is identified.

E

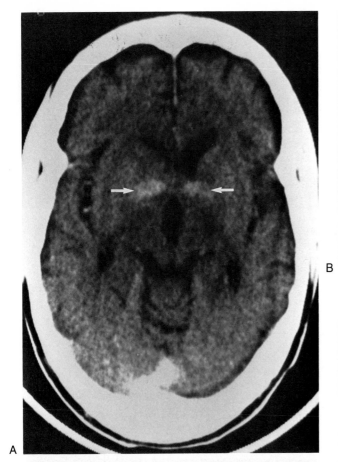

A

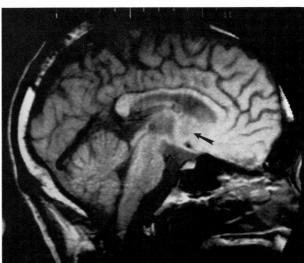

B

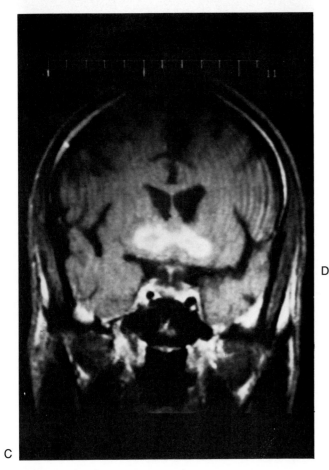

C

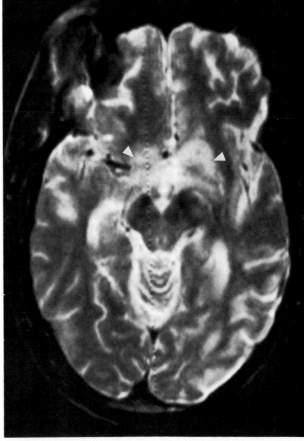

D

Figure 10–49. *Toxoplasmosis.* **A,** Axial enhanced CT scan demonstrates abnormal enhancement in the region of the anterior commissure with extension into both ganglionic regions (*arrows*). AIDS-related atrophic changes are also noted. **B,** Sagittal nonenhanced T1 weighted image (600/26) shows abnormal mass effect in the region of the anterior commissure (*arrow*) without abnormal increased signal intensity. **C,** Coronal T1 weighted image (600/26) after gadolinium-DTPA administration demonstrates a focal area of enhancement that bridges the anterior commissure, extending into both inferior ganglionic regions. **D,** Axial T2 weighted image (2500/80) shows abnormal signal intensity in the anterior commissure and inferior ganglionic region (*arrowheads*).

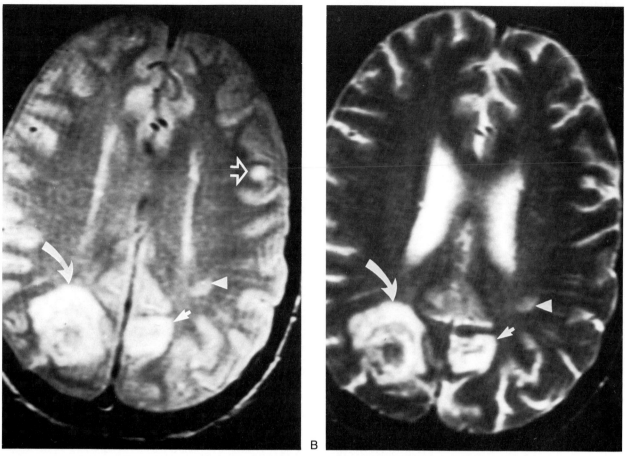

A   B

Figure 10–50. *Toxoplasmosis.*   Proton density (**A**) and T2 weighted (**B**) images (2500/20,80) demonstrate an area of abnormality in the right occipital lobe (*curved arrows*), of mixed signal intensity. Some decreased intensity in the central portion was found to represent deoxyhemoglobin. Other lesions are identified along the medial left occipital lobe (*arrows*), the deep white matter on the left (*arrowhead*), and the left posterior frontal subcortical region (*open arrow*).

Progressive Multifocal Leukoencephalopathy

Progressive multifocal leukoencephalopathy (PML) is another viral infection seen relatively often in adults with AIDS. Reports of the MR appearance of PML in the pediatric population are not available. The disease is caused by a papovavirus, producing demyelination and necrosis of the white matter.[125] It is seen most commonly as an area of decreased attenuation in the subcortical regions bilaterally on CT examination. It does not demonstrate mass effect, and contrast enhancement is uncommon.[125, 126] MRI better shows the white matter changes associated with this entity (Fig. 10–52).[127, 128] The peripheral nature of the abnormal signal intensity on T2 weighted images is better appreciated on MRI than on CT.

MR imaging is developing into the modality of choice in the evaluation of pediatric intracranial infection. Clearly, it is useful in patients in whom early subtle infection needs to be diagnosed. This is most evident in cases of herpes infection. MRI is also useful in cases of meningitis and in the diagnosis and followup of extra-axial collections. CT for the moment remains the procedure of choice for evaluating intracranial calcification associated with congenital infections. Further research into gradient-echo acquisition as a means of diagnosing intracranial calcification may lead to MRI becoming the procedure of choice in these cases as well, particularly since MRI is superior in evaluating the structural abnormalities often associated with these infections.

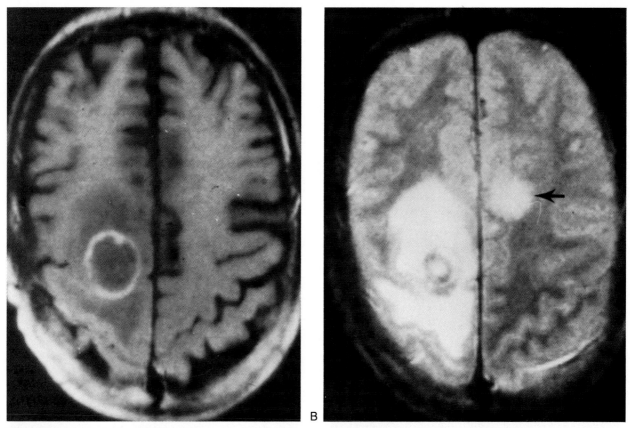

Figure 10–51. *Lymphoma and toxoplasmosis in an adult.* **A,** Axial T1 weighted (500/30) postgadolinium image demonstrates a ring-enhancing lesion in the high right parietal lobe. Surrounding low attenuation consistent with edema is noted. **B,** Axial T2 weighted image (2000/60) shows the lesion in the right parietal area surrounded by high-signal edema. A focus of abnormal signal intensity on the left (*arrow*) is now also identified. The lesion on the right was found to be lymphoma at biopsy; the lesion on the left was proved to be toxoplasmosis. (From Zimmerman RA, Bilaniuk LT, Sze G. Intracranial infection. In: Brant-Zawadzki M, Norman D, eds. Magnetic resonance imaging of the central nervous system. New York: Raven Press, 1987:235–257.)

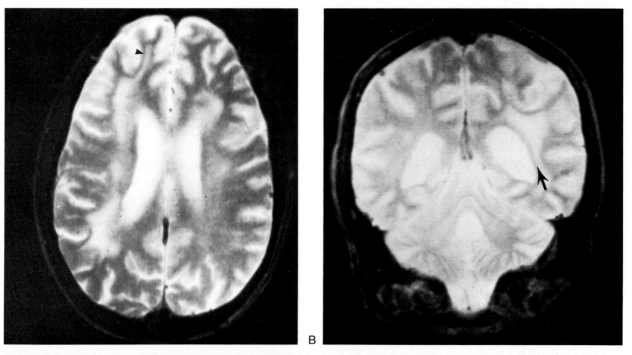

Figure 10-52. *Progressive multifocal leukoencephalopathy (PML).* Axial (**A**) and coronal (**B**) T2 weighted images (2500/80) demonstrate abnormal increased signal intensity in the subcortical and deep white matter. Extension of the abnormal signal into the white matter of the gyri (*arrowhead*) is noted. There is relative preservation of the immediate periventricular white matter (*arrow*). These findings help differentiate PML from simple HIV cerebritis.

REFERENCES

1. Brant-Zawadzki M, Davis PL, Crooks LE, et al. NMR demonstration of cerebral abnormalities: comparison with CT. AJNR 1983; 4:117–124.
2. Bale JF, Andersen RD, Grose C. Magnetic resonance imaging of the brain in childhood herpesvirus infections. Pediatr Infect Dis J 1987; 6:644–647.
3. Matthews VP, Smith RR, Kuharik MA, et al. Gd-DTPA enhanced MRI of meningitis: initial clinical experience. Scientific Presentation, American Society of Neuroradiology, Orlando, FL, March 19–24, 1989.
4. Holland BA, Perrett LV, Mills CM. Meningovascular syphilis: CT and MR findings. Radiology 1986; 158:439–442.
5. Goldberg HI, Titelbaum DS, Grossman RI, et al. High field MR of brain abscess (abstract). AJNR 1988; 9:1036.
6. Weingarten K, Zimmerman RD, Becker RD, et al. Subdural and epidural empyemas: MR imaging. AJNR 1989; 10:81–87.
7. Atlas SW, Grossman RI, Hackney DB, et al. Calcified intracranial lesions: detection with gradient echo acquisition rapid MR imaging. AJNR 1988; 9:253–259.
8. Schochet SS. Infectious diseases. In: Rosenberg RN, ed. The clinical neurosciences. New York: Churchill Livingstone, 1983:195–240.
9. Feldman WE. Relation of concentrations of bacteria and bacterial antigen in cerebrospinal fluid to prognosis in patients with bacterial meningitis,. N Engl J Med 1977; 296:433–435.
10. Moxon ER, Smith AL, Averill DR, et al. *Haemophilus influenzae* meningitis in infant rats after intranasal inoculation. J Infect Dis 1974; 129:154–162.
11. Gregorius FK, Johnson BL Jr, Stern WE, et al. Pathogenesis of hematogenous bacterial meningitis in rabbits. J Neurosurg 1976; 45:561–567.
12. McGee ZA, Kaiser AB. Acute meningitis. In: Mandell GL, Douglas RG Jr, Bennett JE, eds. Principles and practice of infectious diseases, 2nd ed. New York: John Wiley, 1985: 560–573.
13. Bell WE, McCormick WF. Neurologic infections in children, 2nd ed. Philadelphia: WB Saunders, 1981.
14. Payne WN, Chou SM. Arachnoid villitis and rapidly fatal outcome in pneumococcal meningitis. Neurology (Minn) 1981; 31:153.
15. Swartz MN, Dodge PR. Bacterial meningitis: a review of selected aspects. N Engl J Med 1965; 272:725–731.
16. Zimmerman RA, Patel S, Bilaniuk L. Demonstration of purulent bacterial intracranial infections by computed tomography. AJR 1976; 127:155–165.
17. Bilaniuk LT, Zimmerman RA, Brown L, et al. Computed tomography in meningitis. Neuroradiology 1978; 16:13–14.
18. Cockrill HH Jr, Dreisback J, Lowe B, et al. Computed tomography in leptomeningeal infections. AJR 1978; 130:511–515.
19. Grossman RI, Zimmerman RA. Infectious diseases of the brain. In: Latchaw RE, ed. Computed tomography of the head, neck and spine. Chicago: Year Book, 1985:119–136.
20. Sze G. Infections and inflammatory diseases. In: Stark DD, Bradley WG Jr, eds. Magnetic resonance imaging. St. Louis: CV Mosby, 1988:316–343.
21. Smith RR, Savolaine ER. Computed tomography evolution of multicystic encephalomalacia. J Comput Tomogr 1986; 10:249–254.
22. Grossman RI, Zimmerman RA. CNS abnormalities in the immunocompromised host. In: Latchaw RE, ed. Computed tomography of the head, neck, and spine. Chicago: Year Book, 1985:137–151.
23. Buonanno FS, Moody DM, Ball MR, Laster DW. Computed cranial tomographic findings in cerebral sinovenous occlusion. J Comput Assist Tomogr 1978; 2:281–290.
24. Crocker EF, Zimmerman RA, Phelps ME, et al. The effect of steroids on the extravascular distribution of radiographic contrast material and technetium pertechnetate in brain tumors as determined by computed tomography. Radiology 1976; 119:471–474.
25. Gomori JM, Grossman RI, Goldberg HI, et al. Intracranial hematomas: imaging by high-field MR. Radiology 1985; 157:87–93.
26. McMurdo SK, Brant-Zawadzki M, Bradley WG, et al. Dural sinus thrombosis: study using intermediate field strength MR imaging. Radiology 1986; 161:83–86.
27. Harris TM, Smith RR, Koch KJ. Gadolinium-DTPA enhanced MR imaging of septic dural sinus thrombosis. J Comput Assist Tomogr 1989; 13:682–684.
28. Rabe EF. Subdural effusions in infants. Pediatr Clin North Am 1967; 14:831–850.
29. Kaufman DM, Miller MH, Steigbigel NH. Subdural empyema: analysis of 17 recent cases and review of the literature. Medicine 1975; 54:485–498.
30. Handel SF, Klein WC, Kim YW. Intracranial epidural abscess. Radiology 1974; 111:117–120.
31. Syrogiannopoulos GA, Nelson JD, McCracken GH Jr. Subdural collections of fluid in acute bacterial meningitis: a review of 136 cases. Pediatr Infect Dis 1986; 5:343–352.
32. Benson P, Nyhan WL, Shimizu H. The prognosis of subdural effusions complicating pyogenic meningitis. J Pediatr 1960; 57:670–683.
33. Nielsen H, Gyldensted C, Harmsen A. Cerebral abscess. Aetiology and pathogenesis, symptoms, diagnosis and treatment. Acta Neurol Scand 1982; 65:609–622.
34. Garfield J. Brain abscesses and focal suppurative infections. In: Vinken P, Bruyn G, eds. Infections of the nervous system. Handbook of clinical neurology, Vol. 33, Part 1. Amsterdam, New York: North Holland, 1979:107–147.
35. Waggener JD. The pathophysiology of bacterial meningitis and cerebral abscesses: an anatomical interpretation. Adv Neurol 1974; 6:1–17.
36. Sze G, Zimmerman RD. The magnetic resonance imaging of infections and inflammatory diseases. Radiol Clin North Am 1988; 26:839–859.
37. Sutton DL, Ouvrier RA. Cerebral abscess in the under 6 month age group. Arch Dis Child 1983; 58:901–905.
38. Enzmann DR, Britt RH, Yeager AS. Experimental brain abscess evolution: computed tomographic and neuropathologic correlation. Radiology 1979; 133:113–122.
39. Britt RH, Enzmann DR, Yeager AS. Neuropathological and computerized tomographic findings in experimental brain abscess. J Neurosurg 1981; 55:590–603.
40. Haimes AB, Zimmerman RD, Morgello S, et al. MR imaging of brain abscesses. AJNR 1989; 10:279–291.
41. Gruszkiewicz J, Doron Y, Peyser E, et al. Brain abscess and its surgical management. Surg Neurol 1982; 18:7–17.
42. Garvey G. Current concepts of bacterial infections of the central nervous system. Bacterial meningitis and bacterial brain abscess. J Neurosurg 1983; 59:735–744.
43. Carey ME. Brain abscesses. Contemp Neurosurg 1982; 3:1–17.
44. Draouat S, Abdenabi B, Chanem M, Bourjat P. Computed tomography of cerebral tuberculoma. J Comput Assist Tomogr 1987; 11:594–597.
45. Kingsley DPE, Hendrickse WA, Kendall BE, et al. Tuberculous meningitis: role of CT in management of prognosis. J Neurol Neurosurg Psychiat 1987; 50:30–36.
46. Sibley WA, O'Brien JL. Intracranial tuberculomas: a review of clinical features and treatment. Neurology 1956; 6:157–165.
47. Whelan MA, Stern J. Intracranial tuberculoma. Radiology 1981; 138:75–81.
48. Schoeman J, Hewlett R, Donald P. MR of childhood tuberculous meningitis. Neuroradiology 1988; 30:473–477.
49. Venger BH, Dion FM, Rouah E, Handel SF. MR imaging of pontine tuberculoma. AJNR 1987; 8:1149–1150.
50. Gupta RK, Jena A, Sharma A, et al. MR imaging of intracranial tuberculomas. J Comput Assist Tomogr 1988; 12: 280–285.
51. Whitley RJ, Soong S-J, Linneman D Jr, et al. Herpes simplex encephalitis. Clinical assessment. JAMA 1982; 247:317–320.
52. Whitley RJ, Soong SJ, Dolin R, et al. Adenine arabinoside therapy of biopsy proven herpes simplex encephalitis. N Engl J Med 1977; 297:289–294.

53. South MA, Tompkins WA, Morris CR, et al. Congenital malformation of the central nervous system associated with genital type (type 2) herpes virus. J Pediatr 1969; 75:13–18.

54. Dublin AB, Merten DF. Computed tomography in the evaluation of herpes simplex encephalitis. Radiology 1977; 125:133–134.

55. Christie JD, Rakusan TA, Martinez MA, et al. Hydranencephaly caused by congenital infection with herpes simplex virus. Pediatr Infect Dis 1986; 5:473–478.

56. Hirsch MS. Herpes simplex virus. In: Mandell GL, Douglas RG Jr, Bennett JE, eds. Principles and practice of infectious diseases, 2nd ed. New York: John Wiley, 1985:945–952.

57. Smith JB, Groover RV, Klass DW, et al. Multicystic cerebral degeneration in neonatal herpes simplex virus encephalitis. Am J Dis Child 1977; 131:568–572.

58. Davis JM, Davis KR, Kleinman GM, et al. Computed tomography of herpes simplex encephalitis with clinical pathological correlation. Radiology 1978; 129;409–417.

59. Sage MR, Dubois PJ, Oakes J, et al. Rapid development of cerebral atrophy due to perinatal herpes simplex encephalitis. J Comput Assist Tomogr 1981; 5:763–766.

60. Sugimoto T, Woo M, Okazaki H, et al. Computed tomography in young children with herpes simplex virus encephalitis. Pediatr Radiol 1985; 15:372–376.

61. Enzmann DR, Ranson B, Norman D, et al. Computed tomography of herpes simplex encephalitis. Radiology 1978; 129:419–425.

62. Zimmerman RD, Russel EJ, Leeds NE, Kaufman D. CT in the early diagnosis of herpes simplex encephalitis. AJR 1980; 134:61–66.

63. Zimmerman RA, Bilaniuk LT, Sze G. Intracranial infection. In: Brant-Zawadzki M, Norman D, eds. Magnetic resonance imaging of the central nervous system. New York: Raven Press, 1987:235–257.

64. Davidson HD, Steiner RE. Magnetic resonance imaging in infections of the central nervous system. Am J Neuroradiol 1985; 6:499–504.

65. Schroth G, Gawehn J, Thron A, et al. Early diagnosis of herpes simplex encephalitis by MRI. Neurology 1987; 37:179–183.

66. Neils EW, Lukin R, Tomsick TA, Tew JM. Magnetic resonance imaging and computerized tomography scanning of herpes simplex encephalitis. J Neurosurg 1987; 67:592–594.

67. Lester JW, Carter MP, Reynolds TL. Herpes encephalitis: MR monitoring of response to acyclovir therapy. J Comput Assist Tomogr 1988; 12:941–943.

68. Stagno S, Reynolds D, Tsiantos A, et al. Comparative serial virologic and serologic studies of symptomatic and subclinical congenitally and natally acquired cytomegalovirus infections. J Infect Dis 1975; 132:568–577.

69. Panjvani ZF, Hanshaw JB. Cytomegalovirus in the perinatal period. Am J Dis Child 1981; 135:56–60.

70. Hanshaw JB. Developmental abnormalities associated with congenital cytomegalovirus infection. In: Woollam DHM, ed. Advances in teratology. New York: Academic Press, 1970:64–80.

71. Bignami A, Appiatole L. Micropolygyria and cerebral calcification in cytomegalic inclusion disease. Acta Neuropathol 1964; 4:127–137.

72. Bray PF, Bale JF, Anderson RE, et al. Progressive neurological disease associated with chronic cytomegalovirus infection. Ann Neurol 1981; 9:499–502.

73. Ramsey RG, Geremia GK. CNS complications of AIDS: CT and MR findings. AJR 1988; 151:449–454.

74. Bale JF, Reiley TT, Bray PF, et al. Cytomegalovirus and dural infection in infants. Arch Neurol 1980; 37:236–238.

75. Menser MA, Forrest JM. Rubella: high incidence of defects in children considered normal at birth. Med J Aust 1974; 1:123–126.

76. Diebler C, Dulac O, eds. Infectious diseases of the central nervous system. In: Pediatric neurology and neuroradiology. New York: Springer-Verlag, 1987:139–183.

77. McArdle CB, Richardson CJ, Nicholas DA, et al. Developmental features of the neonatal brain: MR imaging. Part I. Gray-white matter differentiation and myelination. Radiology 1987; 162:223–229.

78. Tsuchiya K, Yamauchi T, Furui S, et al. MR imaging vs CT in subacute sclerosing panencephalitis. AJNR 1988; 9:943–946.

79. Rish WS, Haddad FS. The variable natural history of subacute sclerosing panencephalitis. Arch Neurol 1979; 36:610–614.

80. Sever JL, Zeman W. Serological studies of measles and subacute sclerosing panencephalitis. Neurology 1968; 18:95–97.

81. Pedersen H, Wulff CH. Computed tomographic findings of early subacute sclerosing panencephalitis. Neuroradiology 1982; 23:31–32.

82. Jayakumar PN, Taly AB, Arya BYT, Nagara D. Computed tomography in subacute sclerosing panencephalitis: report of 15 cases. Acta Neurol Scand 1988; 77:328–330.

83. Duda EE, Huttenlocher PR, Patronas NJ. CT of subacute sclerosing panencephalitis. AJNR 1980; 1:35–38.

84. Tarr RW, Edwards KM, Kessler RM, Kulkarni MV. MRI of mumps encephalitis: comparison with CT evaluation. Pediatr Radiol 1987; 17:59–62.

85. Reik L. Disseminated vasculomyelinopathy: an immune complex disease. Ann Neurol 1980; 7:291–296.

86. Johnson KP, Wolinsky JS, Ginsberg AM. Immune mediated syndromes of the nervous system related to virus infection. In: Klawans HL, ed. Handbook of clinical neurology, Vol 34. New York: North Holland, 1978:391–434.

87. Atlas SW, Grossman RI, Goldberg HI, et al. MR diagnosis of acute disseminated encephalomyelitis. J Comput Assist Tomogr 1986; 10:798–801.

88. Dunn V, Bale JF, Zimmerman RA, et al. MRI in children with postinfectious disseminated encephalomyelitis. Magn Reson Imaging 1986; 4:25–32.

89. Lukes SA, Norman D. Computed tomography in acute disseminated encephalitis. Ann Neurol 1983; 13:567–572.

90. Kappelle LJ, Wokke JHJ, Huynen CHJN, van Gijn J. Acute disseminated encephalitis documented by magnetic resonance imaging and computed tomography. Clin Neurol Neurosurg 1986; 88:197–202.

91. Grossman RI, Gonzalez-Scarano F, Atlas SW, et al. Multiple sclerosis: gadolinium enhancement in MR imaging. Radiology 1986; 161:721–725.

92. Shapiro K, Tabaddor K. Cerebral aspergillosis. Surg Neurol 1975; 4:465–471.

93. Mikhael MA. Cerebral phycomycosis. J Comput Assist Tomogr 1979; 3:417–420.

94. Mikhael MA, Rushovich AM, Ciric I. Magnetic resonance imaging of cerebral aspergillosis. Comput Radiol 1985; 9:85–89.

95. Dion FM, Venger BH, Landon G, Handel SF. Thalamic histoplasmoma: CT and MR imaging. J Comput Assist Tomogr 1987; 11:193–195.

96. Acha PN, Aguilar FJ. Studies on cysticercosis in Central America and Panama. Am J Trop Med Hyg 1964; 13:48–53.

97. Pup PP. Cysticercosis of the nervous system: clinical manifestations. Rev Neuropsychiatr 1964; 27:70–82.

98. Dixon HBF, Lipscomb FM. Cysticercosis: an analysis and followup of 450 cases. In: Privy Council, Medical Research Council Special Report, No. 229. London: HM Stationery Office, 1961:1–59.

99. Nash TE, Neva FA. Recent advances in the diagnosis and treatment of cerebral cysticercosis. N Engl J Med 1984; 311:1492–1496.

100. Leblanc R, Knowles KF, Melanson D, et al. Neurocysticercosis: surgical and medical management with praziquantel. Neurosurgery 1986; 18:419–427.

101. Rodriguez-Carvajal J, Salgado P, Gutierrez-Alvarado R, et al. The acute encephalitic phase of neurocysticercosis: computed tomographic manifestations. AJNR 1983; 4:51–55.

102. Byrd SE, Locke GE, Biggers S, Percy AK. The computed tomographic appearance of cerebral cysticercosis in adults and children. Radiology 1982; 144:819–823.

103. Ramos OM, Stiebel-Chin G, Altman N, Duchowny M. Diagnosis of neurocysticercosis by magnetic resonance imaging. Pediatr Infect Dis 1986; 5:470–473.

104. Zee C-S, Segall HD, Boswell W, et al. MR imaging of neurocysticercosis. J Comput Assist Tomogr 1988; 12:927–934.
105. Rhee RS, Kumasaki DY, Sarwar M, et al. MR imaging of intraventricular cysticercosis. J Comput Assist Tomogr 1987; 11:598–601.
106. Feder HM, Zalneraitis EL, Reik L. Lyme disease: acute focal meningoencephalitis in a child. Pediatrics 1988; 82:931–934.
107. Steere AC, Broderick TF, Malawista SE. Erythema chronicum migrans and Lyme arthritis: epidemiologic evidence of a tick vector. Am J Epidemiol 1978; 108:312–321.
108. Reik L Jr, Steere AC, Bartenhagen NH, et al. Neurologic abnormalities of Lyme disease. Medicine 1979; 58:281–294.
109. Steere AC, Pachner AR, Malawista SE. Neurologic abnormalities of Lyme disease: successful treatment with high-dose intravenous penicillin. Ann Intern Med 1983; 99:767–772.
110. Halperin JJ, Luft BJ, Anand AK, et al. Lyme neuroborreliosis: central nervous system manifestations. Neurology 1989; 39:753–759.
111. Peterman SB, Hoffman JC. Lyme disease simulating multiple sclerosis (abstract). AJNR 1989; 10:884.
112. Friede RL. Developmental neuropathology. New York, Wien: Springer, 1975:159–162.
113. Belman AL, Diamond G, Dickson D, et al. Pediatric acquired immunodeficiency syndrome. AJDC 1988; 142:29–35.
114. Epstein LG, Sharer LR, Joshi VV, et al. Progressive encephalopathy in children with acquired immune deficiency syndrome. Ann Neurol 1985; 17:488–496.
115. Koenig S, Gendelman HE, Orentstein JM, et al. Detection of AIDS virus in macrophages in brain tissue from AIDS patients with encephalopathy. Science 1986; 233:1089–1093.
116. Sharer LR, Epstein LG, Cho E-S, et al. Pathological features of AIDS encephalopathy in children: evidence for LAV/HTLV-III infection of brain. Hum Pathol 1986; 17:271–284.
117. Epstein LG, Sharer LR, Goudsmit J. Neurological and neuropathological features of human immunodeficiency virus infection in children. Ann Neurol 1988; 23 (suppl):S23.
118. Epstein LG, Berman CZ, Sharer LR, et al. Unilateral calcification and contrast enhancement of the basal ganglia in a child with AIDS encephalopathy. AJNR 1987; 8:163–165.
119. Levy R, Rosenbloom S, Perrett LV. Neuroradiologic findings in AIDS: a review of 200 cases. AJNR 1986; 7:833–839.
120. Epstein LG, DiCarlo FJ, Joshi VV, et al. Primary lymphoma of the central nervous system in children with acquired immunodeficiency syndrome. Pediatrics 1988; 82:355–363.
121. Price DB, Inglese CM, Jacobs J, et al. Neuroradiologic and neurodevelopmental findings. Pediatr Radiol 1988; 18:445–448.
122. Kelly WM, Brant-Zawadzki M. Acquired immunodeficiency syndrome: neuroradiologic findings. Radiology 1983; 149:485–491.
123. Zee C-S, Segall HD, Rogers C, et al. MR imaging of cerebral toxoplasmosis: correlation of computed tomography and pathology. J Comput Assist Tomogr 1985; 9:797–799.
124. Smirniotopoulos JG, Murphy FM. Radiologic-pathologic correlation of CNS lymphoma (abstract). AJNR 1989; 10:878.
125. Carroll BA, Lane B, Norman D, Enzmann D. Diagnosis of progressive multifocal leukoencephalopathy by computed tomography. Radiology 1977; 122:137–141.
126. Conomy JP, Weinstein MA, Agamanolis D, Holt WS. Computed tomography in progressive multifocal leukoencephalopathy. AJR 1976; 127:663–665.
127. Federle MP. A radiologist looks at AIDS: imaging evaluation based on symptom complexes. Radiology 1988; 166:553–562.
128. Guilleux M-H, Steiner RE, Young IR. MR imaging in progressive multifocal leukoencephalopathy. AJNR 1986; 7:1033–1035.

Vascular Disorders
of the Brain

MARY K. EDWARDS, M.D.

The MR evaluation of pediatric vascular diseases deserves special consideration because of the profound difference between the responses of children and adults to ischemia. Significant physiologic and structural changes in the brain between birth and adulthood cause the brain to react differently to hypoxia at each age. Not only does the brain respond differently to ischemia at different ages, but the difference in water content of the brain, due to incomplete myelination, causes ischemia to appear quite different on MR images at different ages. The rich collateral circulation in the pediatric brain causes it to be resistant to regional ischemia, but the immature brain is quite susceptible to generalized hypoxia. Thrombotic venous infarcts are also more common in children, owing in part to their immature response to dehydration.

Because the parameters measured by MRI are different from those measured by CT, MRI has both advantages and disadvantages in the evaluation of pediatric vascular diseases. MRI is more sensitive than CT in the detection of lesions producing increased water content in the brain, such as ischemia and infarction.[1] MRI is also far more sensitive than CT in the detection of hemorrhage, both acute and chronic.[2,3] In the young infants, however, the undermyelinated brain has a physiologic increase in water content that may be confused with ischemia (Fig. 11–1). The problem of recognizing ischemia in infants mandates an understanding of the changing appearance of the neonatal brain through the myelination process up to 3 years of age.[4] Even given familiarity with the normal progression of myelination, MRI is less sensitive for detecting ischemic disease in children than in adults. The accuracy of detection of ischemic injury depends on the differences in signal characteristics between the injured tissue and surrounding normal brain. These dif-

ferences depend on the age of the injury and the normal signal intensity of white matter, which varies depending on the degree of myelination. The developmental changes in the brain are discussed more completely in the chapter on normal brain development.

For many reasons, MR scanning of pediatric ischemic disease is a more complicated process than in adults. Research elucidating the pathophysiologic causes of the MR appearance of pediatric vascular disease has understandably been slow. The logistics of scanning the sick neonate in a frequently hostile environment, the cost of the MR scan, and the confusing appearance of the undermyelinated brain on MR images have discouraged referring physicians from seeking MR studies. After increased experience with MR scanning, this is changing. Increased use of MRI in pediatric ischemic disease necessitates greater efforts to understand this complex disorder.

ISCHEMIA AND INFARCTION

In neonates the brain receives approximately 50 percent of the cardiac output, compared with 20 percent in adults.[5] Cerebral ischemia can result either from decreased flow of blood to the brain or from decreased oxygen content of the blood. In older children or adults, hypoxemia with normal cardiac output is rare, but a premature neonate with hyaline membrane disease may be severely hypoxic in spite of a normal cerebral blood flow.

Unlike the situation in adults, cerebral ischemia in children does not usually result from regional hypoperfusion, occurring in one of the branches of a major cerebral vessel. Rich collaterals available in children, both via the circle of Willis and through cortical anasto-

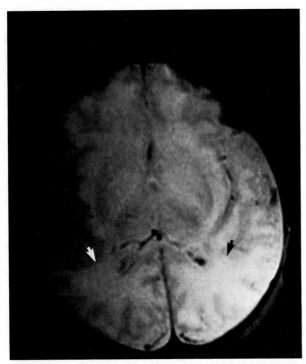

Figure 11-1. *T2 weighted axial image.* Extensive areas of ischemia (*arrows*) are difficult to detect in this hypoxic newborn owing to the increased water in the undermyelinated portions of the neonatal brain.

moses, protect against focal embolic and stenotic infarctions. Children are not prone to the small vessel, stenotic, or hypertensive conditions that contribute to most adult strokes.

Focal Ischemic Disease

Focal arterial infarctions occur so infrequently in children as to create disagreement about their cause. A congenital absence of anastomotic channels is one explanation for the large middle cerebral infarcts seen occasionally in children (Fig. 11-2). Regional cerebral susceptibility to ischemia has been suggested as a cause of focal bilateral infarcts in utero (Fig. 11-3).

When infarction occurs, a series of well-documented histologic changes may produce predictable patterns on MR examination. Within 30 minutes, hypoxia produces a series of biochemical cellular changes resulting in increased intracellular sodium and water, termed cytotoxic edema. There is an overall increase in water content in the affected area of 3 to 5 percent.[6] Irreversible damage to the brain and endothelial cells results from breakdown of the mitochondrial and cytoplasmic membranes, and by 6 hours there is breakdown in the blood-brain barrier. This produces leakage of water and protein from the intravascular compartment into the perivascular spaces. This phenomenon, termed va-

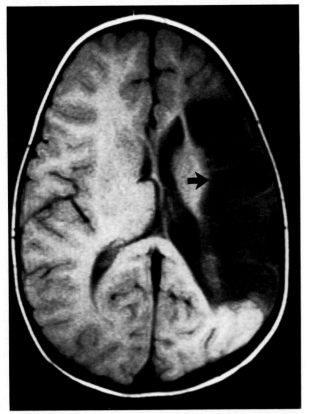

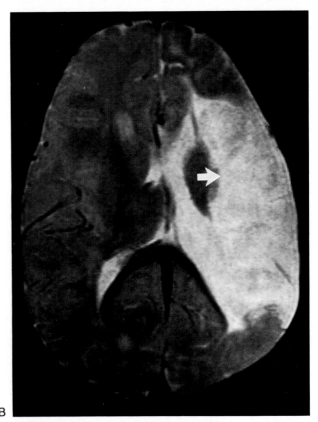

A   B

Figure 11-2. *2-year-old child with right hemiparesis.* **A,** T1 weighted axial image shows a right middle cerebral artery distribution infarct (*arrow*). **B,** T2 weighted axial sequence at the same level confirms spinal fluid density within the region of infarct (*arrow*).

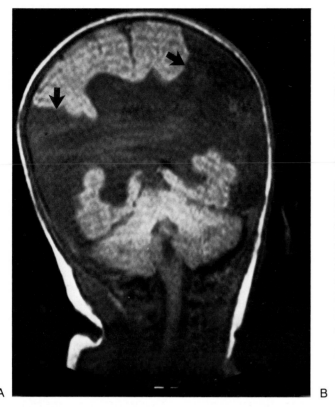

A

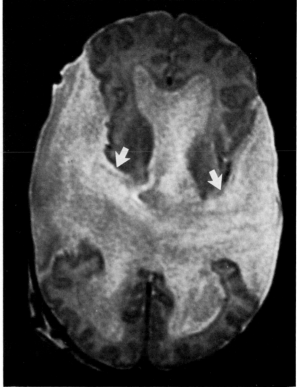

B

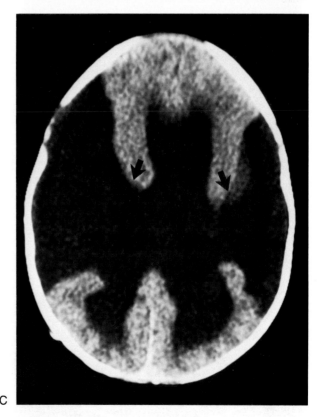

C

Figure 11–3. *12-month-old infant with developmental delay.* **A,** Coronal T1 weighted image demonstrates remote infarcts in the region of the middle cerebral artery bilaterally (*arrows*). This pattern may be termed schizencephaly. **B,** T2 weighted axial sequence confirms CSF within the large cavities (*arrows*). **C,** CT demonstrates the bilateral cavities creating a communication between the intraventricular and subarachnoid spaces (*arrows*).

sogenic edema, occurs only in the presence of reperfusion of the affected brain and is more common in generalized hypoxia than in embolic or stenotic infarcts. When reperfusion occurs in an area of damaged endothelium, the perfusion pressure of normal arterial flow can rupture the endothelium and result in hemorrhage.

A higher incidence of secondary hemorrhage in infarction is reported in the literature of pathology rather than in that of radiology.[7] This is probably due to the difficulty in detecting hemorrhage by CT unless scans are obtained soon after the time of hemorrhage, usually around 2 weeks following ischemia. Large embolic infarcts may develop frank hematomas earlier, within 1 week after the embolic episode. Smaller, irregular, and at times cortical petechial hemorrhages may occur 2 or more weeks after infarction and may be clinically insignificant (Fig. 11–4). MRI improves the ability to detect hemorrhage in infarction, both acutely and for a considerable time after the event (Fig. 11–5). The ability to demonstrate methemoglobin or hemosiderin in infarction long after the actual hemorrhage accounts for the significant improvement in the sensitivity of MRI compared with CT in the detection of intracranial hemorrhage. This is especially true in pediatric patients in whom generalized hypoxia is common, small

hemorrhages of the germinal matrix and cortex are typical, and other MR evidence of acute ischemia may be difficult to detect. Fast MR imaging techniques using advanced Fourier and partial flip scan parameters show promise in further improving the ability of MRI to detect small amounts of hemorrhage.[8] Typical fast scan parameters used at our institution are FE (field echo) = 18, TR = 500, 10-mm slice thickness, 20-degree flip angle, two repetitions, and 192 matrix. This sequence requires less than 3 minutes of scan time. If the acute signs of hemorrhage are not detected, ischemia and significant cerebral injury may be difficult to document until the child is much older. At 1 to 2 years of age the sequelae of white matter ischemia such as atrophy, decrease in overall white matter thickness, and cystic periventricular encephalomalacia can be shown (Fig. 11–6).

There is less controversy about the appearance than about the etiology of pediatric infarcts. In a pattern atypical for adult infarction, it is common to see areas of complete cavitation following infarction in pediatric patients. The younger the patient, the greater is the ability of the brain to remove the infarcted tissue, leaving only infrequent glial strands spanning the area of infarction (Fig. 11–7). On histologic examination, the reaction of the fetal nervous tissue to infarction is

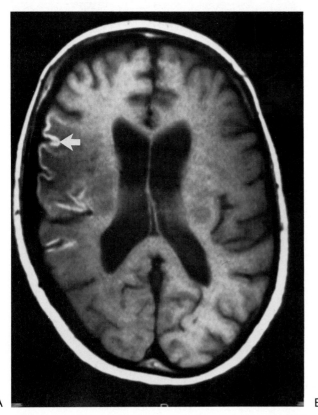

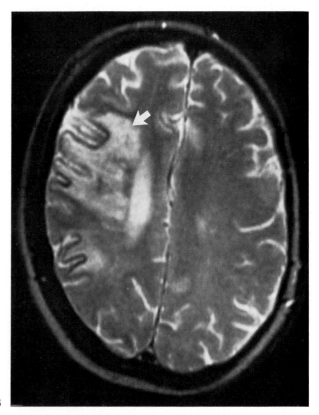

A   B

Figure 11–4. *Focal right middle cerebral artery infarct.* ***A,*** A thin rim of subacute hemorrhage is seen on the cortical surface on this axial T1 weighted image (*arrow*). ***B,*** T2 weighted axial sequence demonstrates extensive parenchymal injury associated with the hemorrhage (*arrow*).

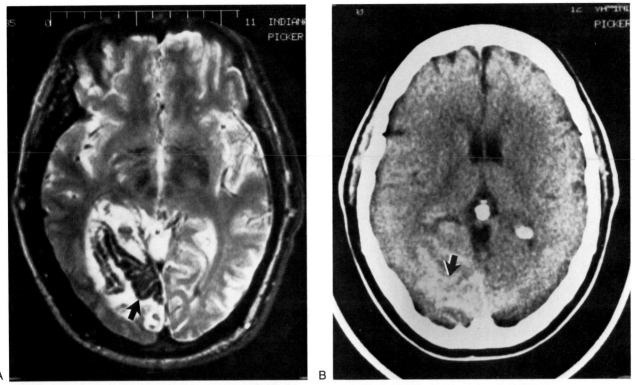

Figure 11–5. *Acute hemorrhagic infarct.* **A,** T2 weighted axial sequence illustrates with clarity the deoxyhemoglobin (*arrow*) related to blood-brain barrier breakdown within the center of an occipital cortical infarct. **B,** CT scan confirms the hemorrhage (*arrow*) but with less anatomic detail than in the MR scan.

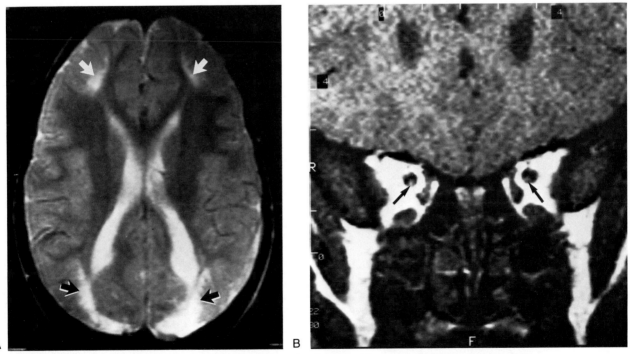

Figure 11–6. *5-year-old child who suffered a single hypoxic insult at age 14 months.* **A,** Global hypoxia results in symmetric multifocal bilateral ischemic lesions (*arrows*) and focal thinning of the white matter on this axial T2 weighted sequence. **B,** Coronal STIR (short tau inversion recovery) scan demonstrates bilateral optic nerve atrophy (*arrows*) related to the bilateral occipital lobe infarcts.

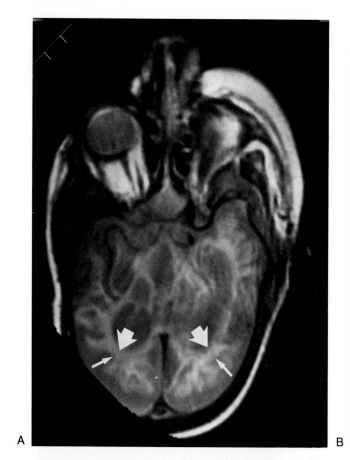

A

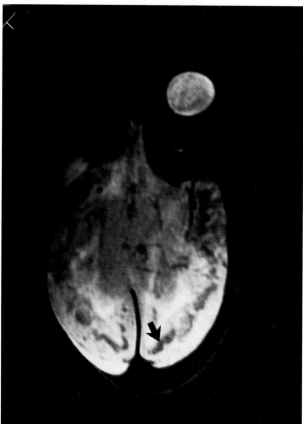

B

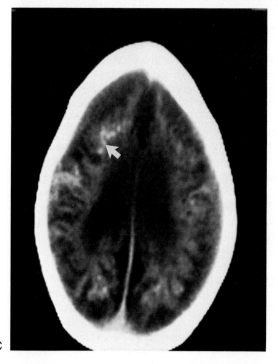

C

Figure 11–7. *Advanced bilateral encephalomalacia due to severe hypoxia.* ***A,*** T1 axial sequence shows shriveled, atrophic rim of remaining cortex (*arrows*). ***B,*** T2 weighted sequence shows very little anatomic detail owing to the high signal of the brain, which mimics the CSF within the ventricles and subarachnoid space. The only anatomic detail present is due to cortical hemosiderin staining (*arrow*) related to previous blood-brain barrier breakdown and hemorrhage. ***C,*** CT scan confirms severe bilateral encephalomalacia and provides the additional information of calcification within the brain parenchyma (*arrow*).

rapid, consisting of liquefaction and dissolution of the necrotic tissue. Unlike the adult brain, there is little or no proliferation of glial elements in response to infarction. The ability of the astrocytes to hypertrophy and proliferate, forming glial scars, begins to appear at the end of the fetal period. Because infarction is characterized by cavitation in the fetal period, prenatal infarcts present with the appearance of porencephaly or hydranencephaly.

Early porencephalic cysts occurring in the second trimester usually extend across the entire thickness of the cerebral cortex, creating a communication between the ventricles and subarachnoid space. They are commonly found in the middle cerebral artery territory (Fig. 11-8), associated with absence of the septum pellucidum and surrounded by abnormal gyral patterns, such as polymicrogyria.[9] Late porencephalic cysts, occurring in the third trimester, usually are smaller, spare the surface cortex, and occur in association with cerebral atrophy, frequently hemiatrophy or Dyke-Davidoff syndrome. A porencephalic cyst may become expansile, trapping cerebrospinal fluid (CSF) and presenting as a mass with cranial asymmetry.

The clinical appearance of porencephaly depends on the size, location, and severity of the associated lesions. Seizures, developmental delay, paresis, and microcephaly are common physical manifestations.

Focal infarcts do occur in the pediatric population in

the presence of predisposing conditions. For example, sickle cell anemia increases the risk of stroke in children under 15 years old.[10] In older children and adults there is an increased risk of intracranial hemorrhage (Fig. 11-9). MRI improves the ability to demonstrate the large-vessel occlusive changes of sickle cell disease.[10] Compared with CT, MRI increases sensitivity to ischemia and infarction in sickle cell disease.[11]

Meningitis is another common cause of focal infarction in children. Venous infarction due to thrombosis of cortical veins is the most common cause of infarction associated with meningitis. Basilar meningitis, however, predisposes to arterial infarcts in the basal ganglia, thalamus, and brain stem owing to arteritis of the perforating arteries (Fig. 11-10).

Nonfocal Ischemic Disease

Generalized, rather than focal, cerebral hypoperfusion occurs commonly in children. A reduction in blood flow, such as that due to placental insufficiency before birth or cardiac failure after birth, causes global cerebral hypoxia, even though compensatory collaterals are available in the pediatric brain. Many other factors may contribute to generalized hypoxia, including respiratory failure, apnea, congenital cardiac anomalies, arteriovenous shunting, hemorrhage, and anemia. Increased intracranial pressure of many causes, including Reye's syndrome, trauma, tumor, infection, and pseudotumor cerebri, also results in cerebral hypoperfusion and hypoxic brain injury.

The response of the brain to generalized hypoxic insult is dependent on the age of the patient and the duration and severity of the hypoxia. A premature infant not only is at increased risk of hypoxia owing to the immature lungs, but is at increased risk of cerebral injury because of the susceptibility of the immature brain to hypoxic insults. This increased susceptibility occurs both at the level of the germinal matrix and in the periventricular white matter. The arterial territories are different in the fetus and the newborn, with a progressive transition between meningocortical arterial anastomoses in the fetus to carotid and vertebrobasilar supply in the infant. In premature infants, meningocortical arterial anastomoses are numerous and the periventricular white matter represents a vascular border zone.[12] There is intense metabolic activity in the periventricular region, increasing susceptibility to hypoxia. The germinal matrix containing numerous fragile capillaries is especially prone to hemorrhage in response to hypoxia.[13] Germinal matrix hemorrhage, with the sequela of intraventricular extension, is the most frequent and severe complication of prematurity (Fig. 11-11).[14]

In premature infants with cardiorespiratory disturbance, the periventricular white matter is at risk of nonhemorrhagic infarction and resultant leukomalacia.[15] Periventricular leukomalacia was detected

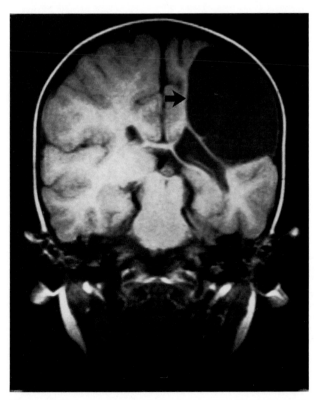

Figure 11-8. Large porencephalic cyst (*arrow*) with glial strand in the middle cerebral artery distribution on a coronal T1 weighted image.

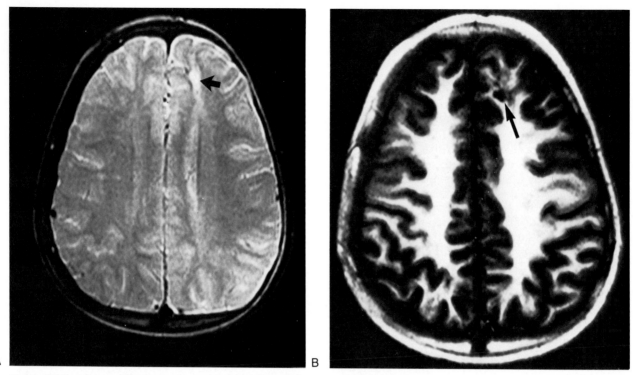

A   B

Figure 11–9. *14-year-old boy with sickle cell anemia.* **A,** T2 weighted axial sequence reveals subacute hemorrhage in the left frontal region (*arrow*). **B,** Axial inversion recovery sequence confirms hemorrhage (*arrow*).

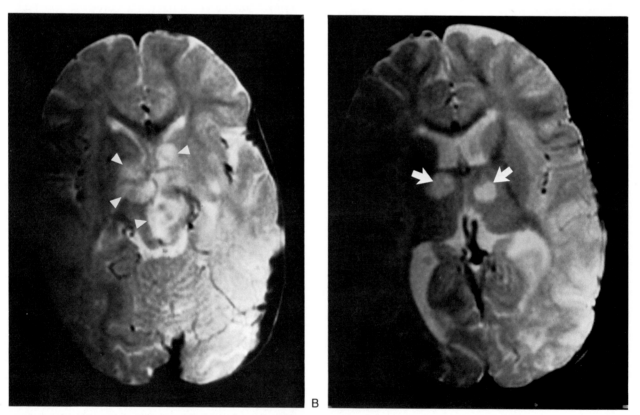

A   B

Figure 11–10. *6-year-old child with basilar meningitis.* **A,** T2 weighted axial sequence at the level of the midbrain shows extensive midbrain and basal ganglia ischemia (*arrowheads*). **B,** T2 weighted sequence at the level of the thalamus shows bilateral basal ganglia infarcts (*arrows*) due to arteritis of the lenticulostriate vessels.

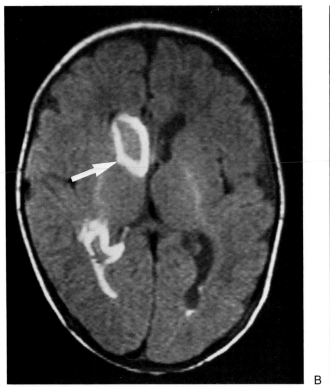 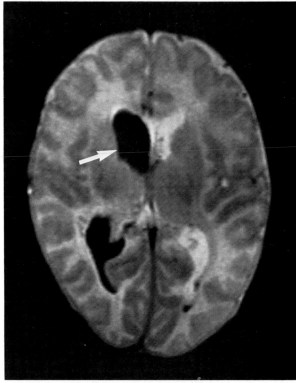

Figure 11–11. *Germinal matrix hemorrhage with intraventricular extension in a premature neonate.* **A,** T1 weighted axial sequence demonstrates evolution of a blood clot beginning at the periphery (*arrow*). **B,** T2 weighted axial sequences shows most of the clot to be deoxyhemoglobin (*arrow*).

in 88 percent of a group of high-risk premature infants and was found most frequently in infants weighing less than 2,200 g.[16] Prolonged or profound periods of hypoxia create more severe patterns of destruction, including multicystic encephalomalacia and severe atrophy.[17]

MR Appearance of Ischemia and Infarction

In children over 2 years of age, MRI is far more sensitive than CT in detecting ischemia and infarction (Fig. 11–12). The increased sensitivity to increases in the water content of tissues accounts for the improved ability of MRI to image areas of infarction that are smaller and earlier than can be seen on CT. Although gadolinium–DTPA is not generally necessary for the evaluation of ischemia or infarct, this contrast agent may improve the detection and characterization of ischemic areas in equivocal cases (Fig. 11–13). Enhancement with gadolinium–DTPA appears most pronounced in cases of embolic infarcts.[18] There is evidence that MR may be sensitive to areas of ischemia within 1 hour of the onset of hypoxia. Reversible and irreversible areas of ischemia cannot be distinguished by MR, since both appear isointense on T1 weighted sequences and hyperintense on T2 weighted sequences. CT, which is less sensitive to hypoxia, rarely

demonstrates reversible ischemia and may be of some value in determining the prognosis. In children under 2 years of age the undermyelinated appearance of the brain makes detection of areas of ischemia more difficult. Unless an area of ischemia is unilateral, accompanied by hemorrhage, or definitely abnormal in distribution compared with the normal pattern of myelination, the ischemic areas may blend imperceptibly with areas of immature myelinization that also have increased water content.

Chronic infarcts, commonly cavitary in children, appear as well-circumscribed cystic areas of low signal intensity on T1 weighted and high signal intensity on T2 weighted sequences, matching CSF in signal characteristics on all sequences. There typically is focal atrophy and compensatory enlargement of the adjacent ventricles. Old hemorrhage associated with the infarct appears as irregular areas of low signal on T2 weighted sequences, caused by the paramagnetic effects of hemosiderin. The appearance of hemosiderin may be somewhat difficult to distinguish from calcification. CT scans may help identify calcium within a lesion, and T1 weighted sequences would be expected to be somewhat darker in areas of calcification compared with areas of hemosiderin deposition. Chronic infarcts secondary to periventricular leukomalacia are especially well documented by MRI and appear as charac-

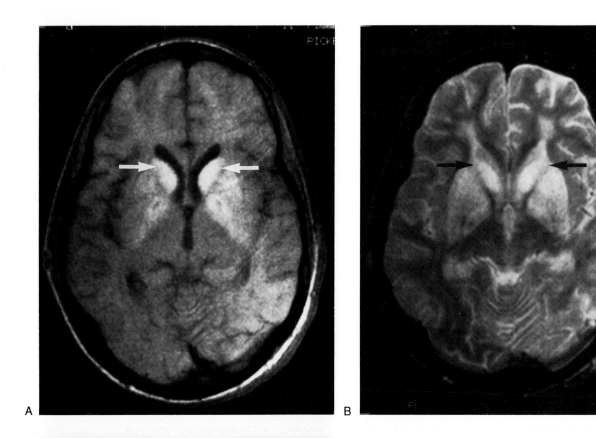

A

B

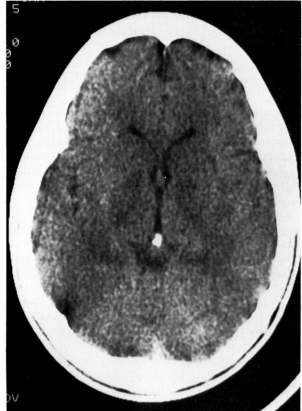

C

Figure 11–12. *Generalized hypoxia and near-drowning of a 17-year-old boy.* ***A,*** T1 weighted axial sequence shows subacute hemorrhage, which is symmetric and bilateral, involving the basal ganglia (*arrows*). ***B,*** T2 weighted axial sequence shows a more extensive area of hypoxia also involving the frontal white matter (*arrows*). ***C,*** CT scan done at the same time shows no evidence of injury.

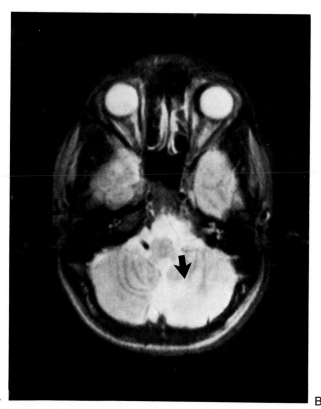
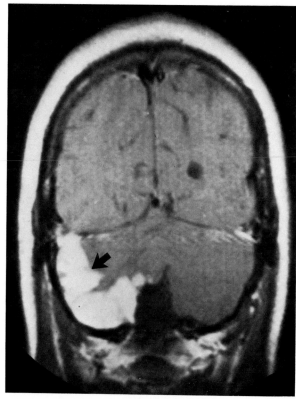

A   B

Figure 11–13. *Posterior fossa infarct.* **A,** T2 weighted axial sequence shows only subtle signs of infarction in the left cerebral hemisphere (*arrow*). **B,** Gadolinium-enhanced T1 weighted coronal sequence much better defines the extent of injury (*arrow*).

teristic lesions in the centrum semiovale and periatrial regions.

Sinus Thrombosis

Although arterial occlusion is uncommon in children, thrombosis of cortical veins and dural sinuses is more common in children than in adults. Thrombosis occurs in infants typically during a febrile illness when dehydration and malnutrition are present (Fig. 11–14). Other predisposing conditions include meningitis, mastoiditis, leukemia, head injury, and (rarely) ulcerative colitis.[19] A variable pattern of infarction results from venous thrombosis. The pattern of infarction depends on the extent and location of the thrombosis.[20, 21] Venous infarction does not follow any recognizable arterial distribution, is usually bilateral, and is commonly accompanied by parenchymal hemorrhage. Hemorrhage results from continued arterial pressure into an ischemic area with blood-brain barrier breakdown in which endothelial cell injury predisposes the vessels to rupture. In the months after sinus thrombosis, progressive atrophy and focal cavitation may be found, depending on the severity of the initial event. The use of MR imaging has improved the ability to detect sinus thrombosis and reveals that sinus throm-

bosis may be relatively common, especially in newborns, with a wide spectrum of severity, including a favorable outcome.[22]

MRI is sensitive to the presence of sinus thrombosis and to the secondary effects of the thrombosis, including infarction, hemorrhage, and atrophy.[23] Clot in the involved sinus has the characteristics of blood collections elsewhere, as described in the chapter on trauma and mechanical disorders of the brain. In the initial phase of sinus thrombosis, the clot is composed of deoxyhemoglobin and is isointense with brain on T1 weighted images and hypointense on T2 weighted images. In the subacute phase, at approximately 1 week, thrombi are characterized by an increased intraluminal signal on all planes of section and pulse sequences (Fig. 11–15). The change in signal intensity from the first to the second echo for thrombi is less than that found with slow flow.[23] In spite of careful observation of flow phenomena, very slow-flowing blood may mimic subacute clot in a sinus. Additional sequences using flow-related enhancement techniques may be necessary to exclude slow-flowing blood. The use of motion suppression techniques that routinely make venous blood appear bright should be discontinued in cases of suspected sinus thrombosis. Congestion of deep subcortical veins may also serve as a sign of dural sinus thrombosis on MRI.[21]

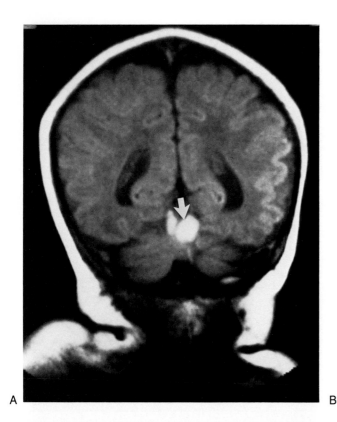

A

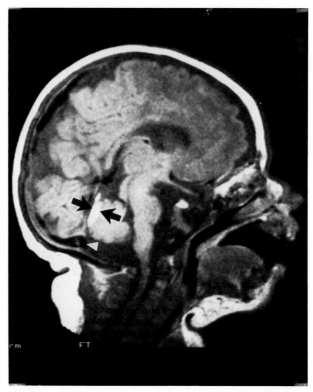

B

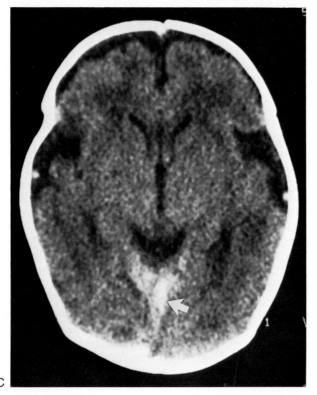

C

Figure 11–14. *Sinus thrombosis in an infant following a viral illness.* **A,** Coronal T1 weighted image shows bright thrombus within the straight sinus (*arrow*). **B,** Sagittal T1 weighted image confirms thrombus within the straight sinus (*arrows*) but shows sparing of the superior sagittal sinus and torcula (*arrowhead*). Cerebral atrophy is evident by widening of the subarachnoid spaces. **C,** CT scan shows density within the straight sinus (*arrow*) and again confirms the diffuse cerebral atrophy.

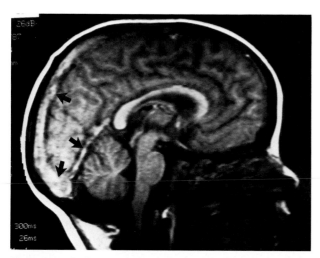

Figure 11-15. Extensive sinus thrombosis is present within the superior sagittal sinus, torcula, and straight sinus (*arrows*) on this sagittal T1 weighted image.

Arteritis

Arteritis in childhood may result from infection, autoimmune diseases, moyamoya, chemotherapy, or radiation therapy. The clinical presentation may be confusing owing to the multifocal nature of the disease process. Patients may experience seizures, headaches, confusion, and focal neurologic deficits. An elevated sedimentation rate and abnormal results on CSF studies may help suggest the diagnosis of arteritis.

Areas of arteritis appear similar to other ischemic lesions, except that foci of arteritis tend to be more patchy, bilateral, and more widespread than other ischemic processes (Fig. 11-16). As with other causes of hypoxic injury in children, hemorrhage is a common sequela to arteritis.

Arteritis due to autoimmune or allergic factors commonly produces reversible lesions that respond quickly to steroid administration. Arteritis secondary to moyamoya disease is commonly associated with hemorrhage, and flow void in dilated collaterals from lenticulostriate arteries is seen occasionally. On T2 weighted sequences, arteritis appears as patchy areas of bright signal in a nonsymmetric, bilateral distribution primarily within the white matter. Gray matter involvement may be seen but is much less common (Fig. 11-17). Hemorrhage, when present, appears as areas of bright or dark signal, reflecting the same properties and age of onset as hemorrhage elsewhere, as discussed in the chapter on hemorrhage and trauma. Focal ischemic lesions, which are usually reversible, may be caused by allergic or toxic reactions to many agents. The MR pattern of toxic and allergic arteritis on T2 weighted sequences may mimic multiple sclerosis (MS). The lesions in MS and arteritis are both patchy, bright, and variable with time. Because MS is uncommon in children, a thorough search for a history

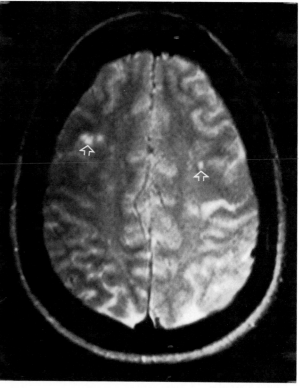

Figure 11-16. Migraine-induced arteritis in a 16-year-old girl is manifest as bilateral bright lesions in the white matter (*arrows*) on the T2 weighted axial sequence.

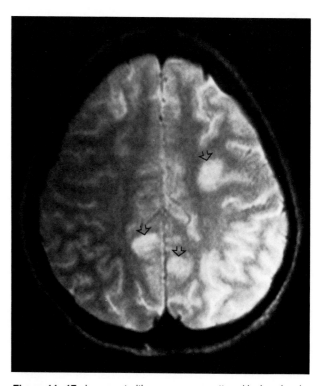

Figure 11-17. Lupus arteritis appears as scattered lesions involving both the gray and white matter (*open arrows*) on this T2 weighted axial sequence.

or clinical signs of arteritis should be made when patchy bilateral white matter lesions are found in such patients.

VASCULAR MALFORMATIONS

MRI has been of great value in detecting and characterizing the wide variety of vascular brain malformations. Vascular malformations vary in severity from those that are benign and occult to the highly aggressive and frequently fatal parenchymal arteriovenous malformations. Although each form of vascular malformation may demonstrate certain unique characteristics, there are features common to many different forms, including acute and chronic hematoma, flowing blood, ischemia, and edema.

Vascular malformations are found with increasing frequency with age, but at least 20 percent of arteriovenous malformations are found before the age of 20 years.[24] The incidence of the less severe and less symptomatic vascular malformations in children is not known, but is reported with increasing frequency in the CT and MR literature.[25]

Occult Vascular Malformations

The most benign form of vascular malformation, the occult vascular malformation (OCVM), also known as the cryptic malformation, is seen in both children and adults. By definition, these are malformations that cannot be demonstrated by routine cerebral angiography. On histologic examination, an OCVM may be found to be composed of any of the subtypes of vascular malformation, cavernous hemangioma, venous angioma, telangiectasia, and arteriovenous malformation.[26] All subtypes of vascular malformation may present an OCVM and are indistinguishable by CT or MR. An OCVM may cause seizures but is rarely of clinical significance otherwise (Fig. 11–18). Although the OCVM has long been recognized by CT, the increased sensitivity of MRI to chronic hemorrhage or clot has revealed far greater numbers of these lesions than was previously appreciated. An OCVM is commonly small, less than 2 cm in diameter, with little or no mass effect, although an occasional lesion can be quite large, as big as 4 to 5 cm. There is often some degree of calcification demonstrated on CT.

The MR appearance of OCVMs is so characteristic as to be almost pathognomonic. They appear as areas of mixed signal intensity on both T1 and T2 weighted sequences owing to the mixture of calcium, hemosiderin, and methemoglobin (Fig. 11–19). Enhancement to a variable degree is seen in most lesions. On CT these lesions may mimic slow-growing tumors, and MRI is now the preferred examination for the detection and characterization of OCVMs (Fig. 11–20).

Venous Malformations

Venous malformations, also known as venous angiomas or venous-venous malformations, are abnormal collections of veins draining in an atypical distribution. They are present in both children and adults. They are most commonly detected in older patients, however, because venous malformations are usually found as an incidental finding in a patient examined for unrelated symptoms. Symptoms due to venous malformations are uncommon, but patients rarely may present with seizures or headaches. Venous malformations are best understood as congenital, developmental anomalies in which the usual venous drainage did not develop normally, and anomalous collateral pathways formed to provide venous outflow.[27] When they occur in the supratentorial compartment, venous malformations rarely bleed or cause symptoms. In the posterior fossa, however, venous malformations may occasionally be associated with spontaneous hemorrhage. When present in the posterior fossa, a venous malformation may provide the only pathway for venous outflow in the region where they are located, and should not be excised (Fig. 11–21).

The anatomic demonstration of venous malformations is similar on angiography, CT, and MRI. All three studies show a dilated linear vein attached to a tangle of branching smaller venous tributaries, analogous to a tree trunk with its branches (Fig. 11–22).[27] These lesions were first described on angiography as an abnormal "arborization" of veins with the lesion seen only on the venous phase. Venous malformation was excluded in the face of any abnormality seen in an earlier phase of the angiogram, whether increased flow, abnormal arterial supply, or capillary blush. On MRI the venous pattern appears on either T1 or T2 weighted sequences as areas of signal void due to flowing blood.[27] Occasionally, paradoxical enhancement may be seen as areas of very bright signal in a linear pattern in association with the areas of flow void. Contrast enhancement is common and may help define the nidus of the venous malformation (Fig. 11–23). Although venous malformations are frequently seen with CT, MRI is better at detecting these lesions. The multiplanar capabilities of MRI also allow better anatomic display of the branching distribution of venous malformations. Gliomas with focal prominence of draining veins may mimic venous angiomas, and care should be taken to exclude the presence of focal parenchymal lesions in cases of suspected venous malformation.[27]

Arteriovenous Malformations

High-flow arteriovenous malformations (AVMs) are a common cause of hemorrhage and associated morbidity and mortality. They occur either as parenchymal lesions or pia-dural malformations. Although they may

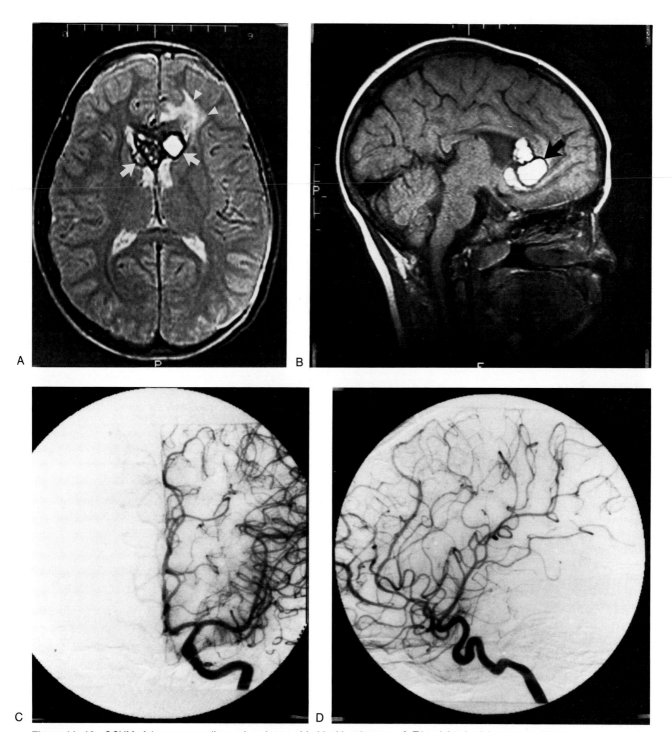

Figure 11–18. *OCVM of the corpus callosum in a 4-year-old girl with seizures.   **A,** T2 weighted axial sequence shows multiseptated OCVM filling both lateral ventricles (arrows) as well as left frontal edema (arrowheads). **B,** T2 weighted sagittal sequence shows methemoglobin within the center of the OCVM (arrow). **C, D,** Posteroanterior and lateral digital angiogram shows no filling of the vascular malformation.*

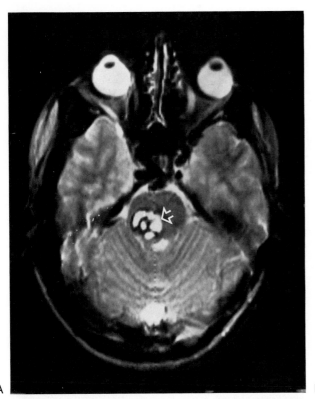
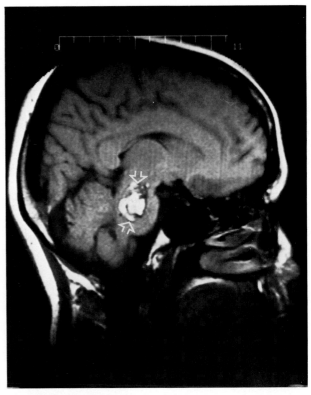

A   B

Figure 11–19. *Pontine OCVM. This is a typical location and appearance for OCVM.* ***A,*** *Axial images show a multiseptated lesion with a mixture of hemosiderin and methemoglobin (open arrow) on T2 weighted sequence.* ***B,*** *Coronal T1 weighted sequence better defines the cephalocaudal extent of the lesion (arrows).*

be present anywhere in the central nervous system, approximately two-thirds are found in the supratentorial space (Fig. 11–24).[28, 29] AVMs present with hemorrhage in approximately 50 percent of patients (Fig. 11–25).[25, 30, 31] The remainder present with symptoms of seizure or ischemia due to steal of blood by the AVM from the surrounding parenchyma.[30] Signs of ischemia typically are motor or visual disturbance. In neonates the AVM may shunt so much blood from the arterial to the venous system as to cause congestive heart failure.[32] This is especially true in children with vein of Galen aneurysms, in which the primary lesion is an AVM in the posterior circulation causing massive arteriovenous shunting, and subsequent dilatation of the vein of Galen.[33] The dilatation may extend to several centimeters, even as much as half the intracranial volume, by the large volume of high-pressure arterialized blood (Fig. 11–26). More accurately termed a varix, rather than an aneurysm, the vein of Galen dilatation is characteristically found in association with dilatation of the straight sinus, torcula, and other draining venous pathways. The vein of Galen will be the largest, because it is not confined by dural walls as are the venous sinuses. Steal from the cerebral hemispheres and posterior fossa is common.[34] Extreme cerebral ischemia, atrophy, and poor neurologic outcome are the usual result of AVMs presenting

in infancy as vein of Galen aneurysms. Hydrocephalus occurs because of venous hypertension or compression of the cerebral aqueduct. Generally, the earlier they present, and the greater the degree of cardiac compromise, the more devastating is the outcome of vein of Galen aneurysms, regardless of the heroic interventional and surgical measures used to try to control the AVM.

The hallmark of cerebral AVMs on MRI is a pattern of tangled areas of flow void in dilated blood vessels with variable associated hemorrhage, ischemia, and edema. In hemispheric and pia-dural malformations, more massively dilated cortical veins frequently are present on the surface, with smaller tangled arteries and the AVM nidus deep to the veins (Fig. 11–27). A pattern of increased flow within a dilated cavernous sinus has been reported with dural AVMs.[35] Calcium is a common feature of AVMs on CT scanning, but is frequently poorly demonstrated or missed entirely by MRI (Fig. 11–28). The less common central AVMs may cause dilatation of the internal cerebral vein and other deep veins, including the vein of Galen. When hemorrhage is present, the evolution of oxyhemoglobin through hemosiderin produces the characteristic T1 and T2 effects of hemorrhage discussed elsewhere. If rupture into the subarachnoid space has occurred remotely in the past, producing a large vol-

Text continues on page 300.

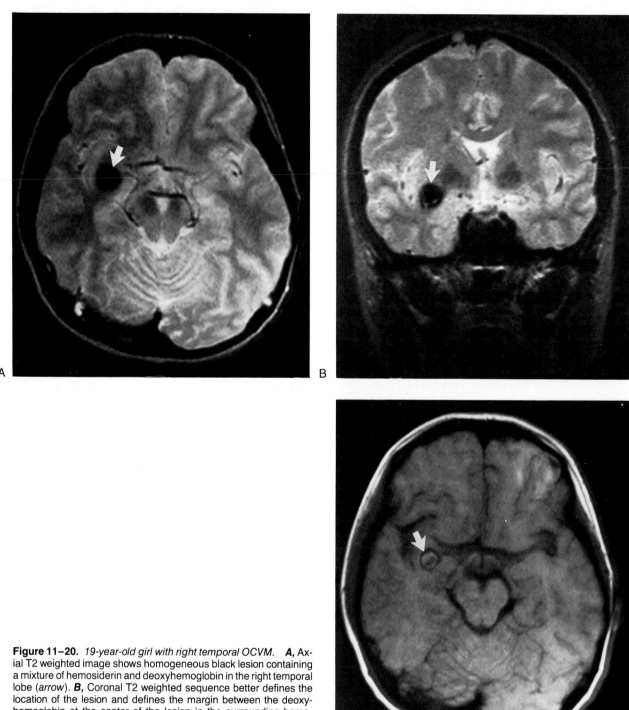

Figure 11–20. *19-year-old girl with right temporal OCVM.* ***A,*** Axial T2 weighted image shows homogeneous black lesion containing a mixture of hemosiderin and deoxyhemoglobin in the right temporal lobe (*arrow*). ***B,*** Coronal T2 weighted sequence better defines the location of the lesion and defines the margin between the deoxyhemoglobin at the center of the lesion in the surrounding hemosiderin (*arrow*). ***C,*** Axial T1 weighted sequence illustrates how this lesion can mimic an aneurysm with a hemosiderin rind surrounding deoxyhemoglobin (*arrow*).

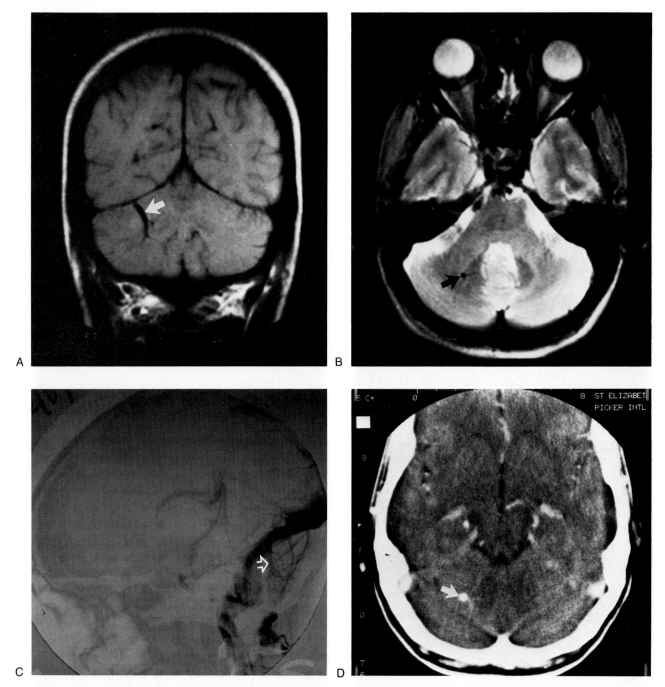

Figure 11–21. *Posterior fossa venous angioma.* ***A,*** Coronal T1 weighted sequence shows the classic appearance of flow void in an abnormal vascular location within the right cerebellar hemisphere (*arrow*). ***B,*** T2 weighted axial image confirms the flow void in the region of the dentate nucleus without evidence of surrounding ischemia (*arrow*). ***C,*** Angiography confirms venous angioma in the posterior fossa (*arrow*). ***D,*** Enhanced CT image with a punctate lesion in the right cerebellar hemisphere (*arrow*), consistent with venous angioma. MRI better demonstrates the entire extent of the lesion on the coronal sequence.

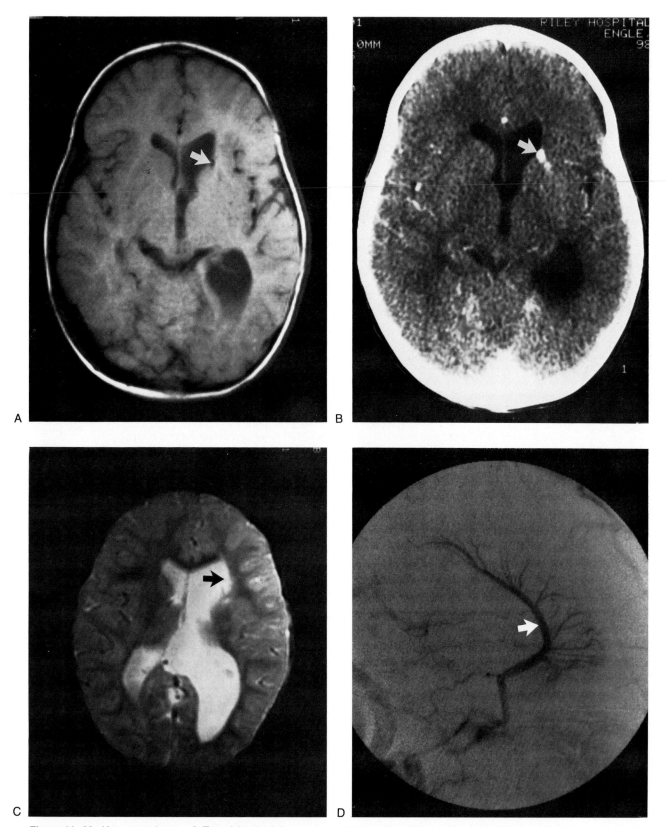

Figure 11–22. *Venous angioma.* ***A,*** T1 weighted axial sequence, axial projection. Flow void is present adjacent to the frontal horn of the left lateral ventricle (*arrow*). ***B,*** CT scan with enhancement shows vascular lesion in the same location (*arrow*). ***C,*** T2 weighted axial image demonstrates ischemia related to the venous angioma (*arrow*). ***D,*** Digital angiogram confirms venous angioma (*arrow*).

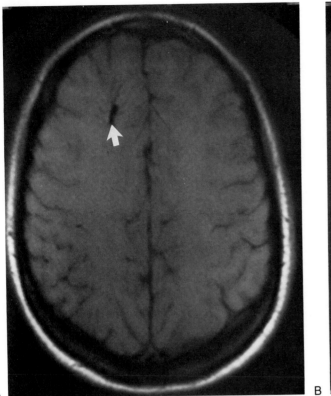

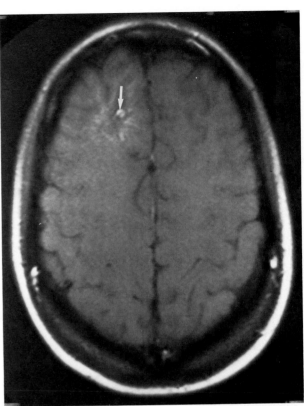

A   B

Figure 11–23. *Venous angioma.* ***A,*** Axial T1 weighted image shows flow void in a branching pattern with a central distended vein *(arrow).* ***B,*** Axial T1 weighted sequence with gadolinium–DTPA shows enhancement of the venous angioma *(arrow).*

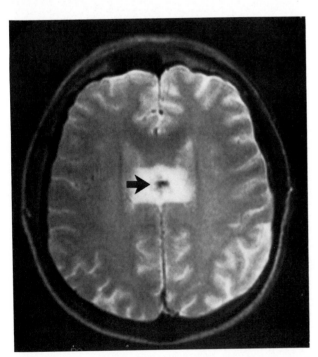

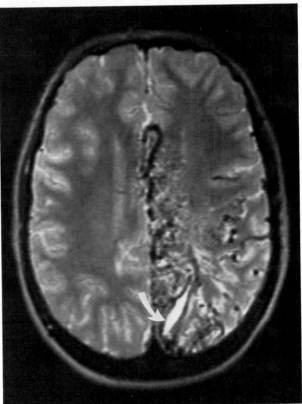

Figure 11–24. T2 weighted axial image of an arterial venous malformation of the corpus callosum shows extensive edema surrounding flow void within the central nidus of the vascular malformation *(arrow).*

Figure 11–25. Axial T2 weighted sequence shows hemorrhage *(arrow)* associated with a large callosal vascular malformation.

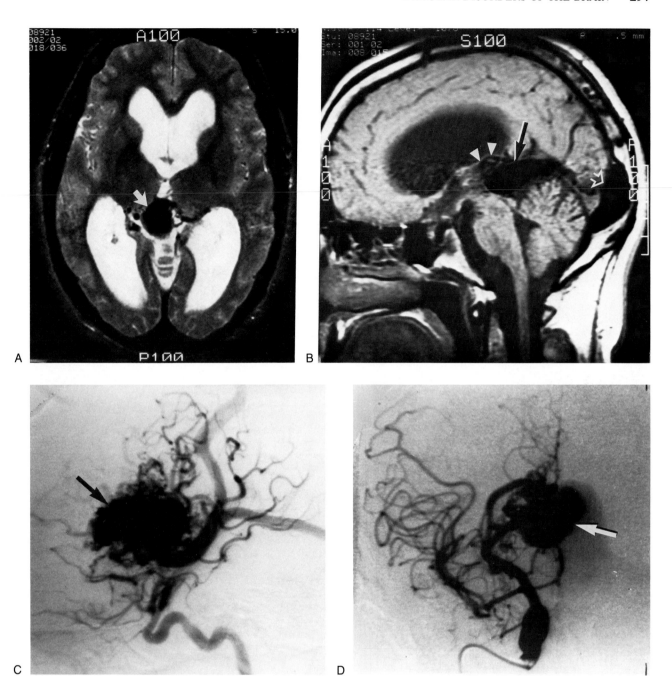

Figure 11–26. *Vein of Galen aneurysm.*   ***A,*** Axial T2 weighted sequence shows large flow void within a distended vein of Galen (*arrow*). ***B,*** Sagittal T1 weighted sequence confirms the distended vein of Galen (*arrow*) as well as dilated feeding arteries (*arrowhead*) and enlarged torcula (*open arrow*). ***C, D,*** Lateral and posteroanterior films from the angiogram show early arterial filling of the vein of Galen (*arrows*). (Courtesy of B. Mehta, M.D., Henry Ford Hospital.)

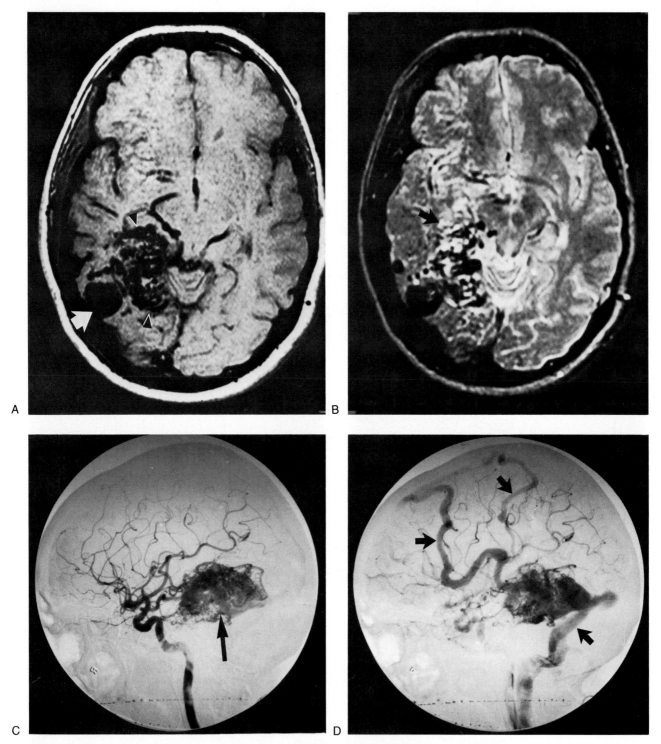

Figure 11–27. *Large arterial venous malformation.* **A,** T1 weighted axial sequence shows distended cortical veins (*arrow*) overlying the nidus of the vascular malformation (*arrowhead*). **B,** T2 weighted axial image shows "steal," manifest as a bright signal within the hypoxic temporal lobe on the right (*arrow*). **C,** Arterial phase of the angiogram confirms the malformation with multiple feeding vessels and prominent nidus (*arrow*). **D,** Venous phase of the angiogram demonstrates multiple dilated draining cortical veins (*arrows*).

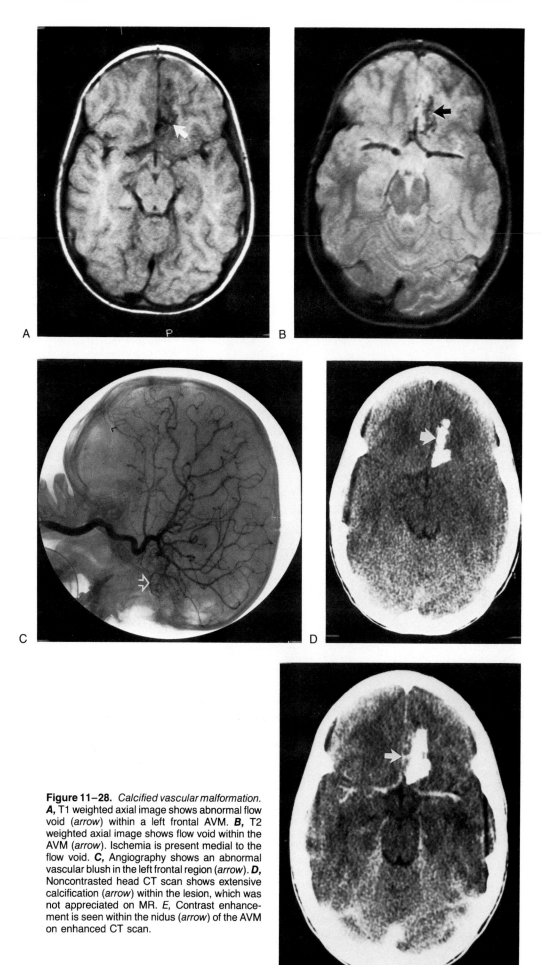

Figure 11–28. *Calcified vascular malformation.*
A, T1 weighted axial image shows abnormal flow
void (*arrow*) within a left frontal AVM. **B,** T2
weighted axial image shows flow void within the
AVM (*arrow*). Ischemia is present medial to the
flow void. **C,** Angiography shows an abnormal
vascular blush in the left frontal region (*arrow*). **D,**
Noncontrasted head CT scan shows extensive
calcification (*arrow*) within the lesion, which was
not appreciated on MR. *E,* Contrast enhancement is seen within the nidus (*arrow*) of the AVM
on enhanced CT scan.

ume of subarachnoid hemorrhage, superficial siderosis results. This is seen on MRI as linear black deposits of hemosiderin on the surface of the brain on T2 weighted sequences. MRI is far more sensitive than CT for the detection of subarachnoid hemorrhage, either acute or chronic (Fig. 11–29).[36]

The appearance of ischemia within the brain parenchyma surrounding an AVM depends on the severity and duration of symptoms. The clinical presentation of AVMs is one of unrelenting progression, originating long before they present clinically. Their exact origin is frequently impossible to establish. There is usually evidence of chronic ischemic changes. On MRI, these changes are seen as areas of bright signal within the parenchyma surrounding the AVM with variable degrees of associated atrophy and cavitary infarction. Contrast enhancement is seen both within the nidus of the AVM and within the area of ischemia in the surrounding brain parenchyma. MRI shows promise in following the response of AVMs to embolic therapy (Fig. 11–30).

ANEURYSMS

The usual form of berry aneurysm is uncommon in the pediatric population, probably because it develops in the postnatal period.[37] Aneurysms presenting in children are frequently induced by predisposing factors, including Ehler-Danlos syndrome, coarctation of the aorta, polycystic kidney disease, septic emboli, AVM, and trauma due to surgery or radiation.[38, 39] When found in children, aneurysms appear (as in adults) as areas of flow void on MR, with thrombosis seen when present in the arterial lumen. In adults 20 percent of aneurysms are multiple, but in children they are generally isolated lesions. They usually occur distally on the parent artery and tend to have irregular walls (Fig. 11–31).[40] Aneurysms in children are even more likely than those in adults to present with hemorrhage, and incidental demonstration of aneurysms is exceedingly rare. Thrombosis appears as concentric laminar areas of mixed signal, which are fairly characteristic for aneurysms.[41, 42] Subarachnoid and parenchymal hemorrhage secondary to aneurysms is well detected by CT, but MRI may help detect small amounts of hemorrhage when the CT scan is negative.

MR ANGIOGRAPHY

New techniques in subtraction MR imaging have been developed to create an angiographic depiction of the carotid and vertebral arteries.[43] The work is promising but still investigational. These techniques have been studied in arteriosclerotic stenosis of neck vessels and intracranial aneurysms. To date, no reports of angiographic techniques in the study of pediatric disease have appeared.

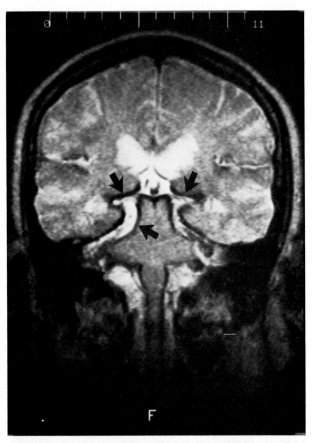

Figure 11–29. Coronal T2 weighted sequence shows superficial siderosis appearing as black staining of the meningeal surfaces (*arrows*) related to previous extensive subarachnoid hemorrhage.

Figure 11–30. *Pre- and postembolization MR study of a large, left frontal, parietal vascular malformation.* **A,** Preembolization sagittal T1 weighted image shows extensive flow void within dilated vessels in the nidus of the vascular malformation (*arrow*). **B,** Postembolization sagittal T1 weighted image shows marked decrease in the flow within the nidus of the vascular malformation (*arrow*). **C,** Preembolization sagittal T1 weighted image at the level of the dilated cortical veins shows extensive flow void in the draining veins (*arrow*). **D,** Postembolization T1 weighted sagittal image shows marked decrease in flow within the same cortical veins (*arrow*). **E,** Axial proton density image preembolization shows an extensive pulsation artifact from the large vascular malformation (*arrowheads*) and flow void within a prominent draining vein (*curved arrow*). **F,** Axial proton density image postembolization shows a clot within the draining cortical vein (*arrow*) and increasing edema surrounding the partially thrombosed vascular malformation (*arrowheads*). The pre- and postembolization MR images depict well the extent of residual malformation in preparation for definitive surgery after the embolization and postembolization MRI. (Courtesy of B. Mehta, M.D., Henry Ford Hospital.)

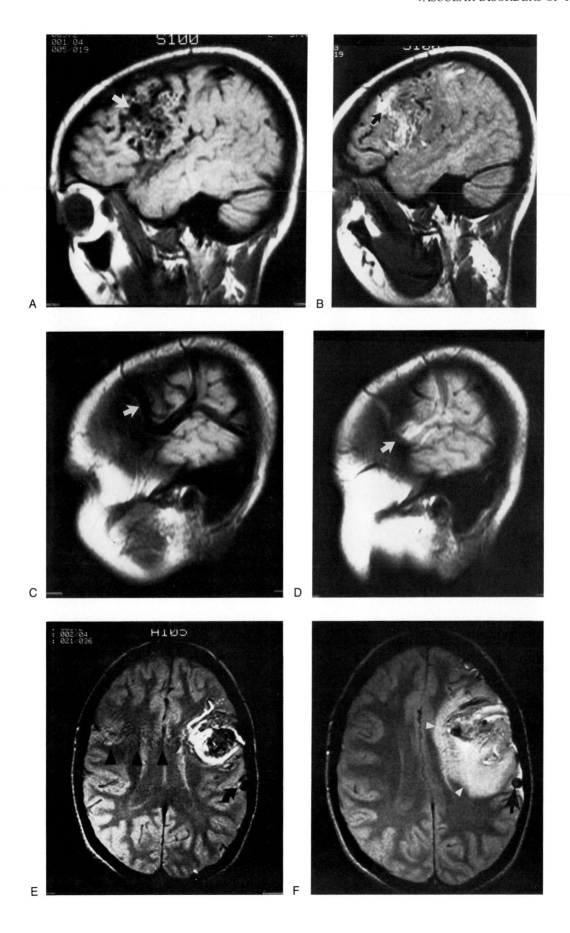

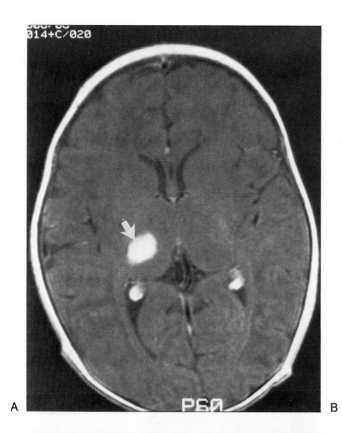

A

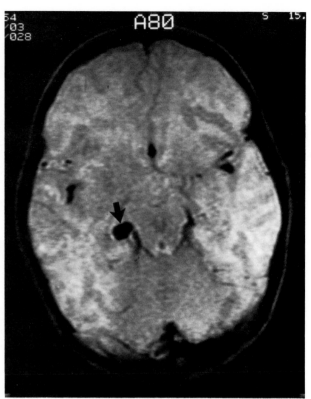

B

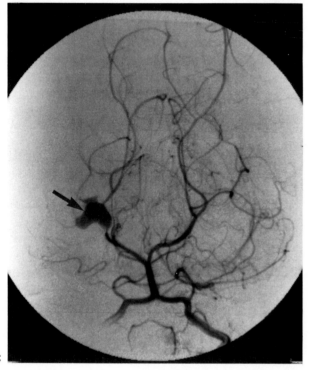

C

Figure 11–31. *Pediatric aneurysm in a 4-month-old infant presenting with mild paresis on the right.* ***A,*** Gadolinium-enhanced, T1 weighted axial image shows a small thalamic infarct with extension to the internal capsule on the right (*arrow*). ***B,*** Axial proton density image at the level of the midbrain shows flow void within an irregular posterior cerebral artery aneurysm (*arrow*). ***C,*** Left vertebral arteriogram confirms the large irregular aneurysm arising from the P2 segment of the right posterior cerebral artery (*arrow*).

MR imaging of vascular disease in children is challenging but promising. Many disease processes such as sinus thrombosis have been better demonstrated and even better understood since MRI has become available. Many other problems are far from solved, however. The difficulty of differentiating ischemia from normal undermyelination can be formidable in the infant. Imaging small children with MRI may require more sedation than CT, increasing the possible risk. The challenge exists to find the best pulse sequences to improve the diagnostic yield while decreasing scan time for the benefit of vulnerable hypoxic infants.

REFERENCES

1. Kertesz A, Black SE, Nicholson L, Carr T. The sensitivity and specificity of MRI in stroke. Neurology 1987; 37:1580–1585.
2. Zimmerman RD, Heier LA, Snow RB, et al. Acute intracranial hemorrhage: intensity changes on sequential MR scans at 0.5T. AJNR 1988; 9:47–57.
3. Gomori JM, Grossman RI, Hackney DB, et al. Variable appearances of subacute intracranial hematomas on high-field spin-echo MR. AJR 1988; 150:171–178.
4. Moore JB, Parker CP, Smith RJ, Goethe BD. Concealment of neonatal cerebral infarction on MRI by normal brain water. Pediatr Radiol 1987; 17:314–315.
5. Sankaran K, Peters K, Finer N. Estimated cerebral blood flow in term infants with hypoxic ischemic encephalopathy. Pediatr Res 1981; 15:1415–1418.
6. Gotoh O, Asano T, Koide T, Takakura K. Ischemic brain edema following occlusion of the middle cerebral artery in the rat. I: The time courses of the brain water, sodium and postassium contents and blood-brain barrier permeability to I-125-albumin. Stroke 1985; 16:101–109.
7. Leblanc R, O'Gorman AM. Neonatal intracranial hemorrhage: a clinical and serial computerized tomographic study. J Neurosurg 1980; 53:642–651.
8. Winkler ML, Olsen WL, Mills TC, Kaufman L. Hemorrhagic and nonhemorrhagic brain lesions: evaluation with 0.35-T fast MR imaging. Radiology 1987; 165:203–207.
9. Dekaban A. Large defects in cerebral hemispheres associated with cortical dysgenesis. J Neuropathol Exp Neurol 1965; 24:512–530.
10. El Gammal T, Adams RJ, Nichols FT, et al. MR and CT investigation of cerebrovascular disease in sickle cell patients. AJNR 1986; 7:1043–1049.
11. Adams RJ, Nichols FT, McKie V, et al. Cerebral infarction in sickle cell anemia: mechanism based on CT and MRI. Neurology 1988; 38:1012–1017.
12. Diebler C, Dulac O. Prenatal and perinatal vascular lesions of circulatory origin. In: Pediatric neurology and neuroradiology. New York: Springer-Verlag, 1987:185–211.
13. Babcock DS, Bove KE, Menke JA, et al. Intracranial hemorrhage in premature infants: sonographic-pathologic correlation. Am J Neuroradiol 1982; 3:308–317.
14. Hambleton K, Wigglesworth JS. Origin of intraventricular haemorrhage in the preterm infant. Arch Dis Child 1976; 51:651–659.
15. De Reuck J, Chatha AS, Richardson EP. Pathogenesis and evolution of periventricular leukomalacia in infancy. Arch Neurol 1971; 27:220–236.
16. Shuman RM, Selednik TK. Periventricular leukomalacia. A one year autopsy study. Arch Neurol 1980; 37:231–235.
17. Chutorian AM, Michener RC, Defendini R, et al. Neonatal polycystic encephalomalacia: 4 new cases and review of the literature. J Neurol Neurosurg Psychiatry 1979; 42:154–160.
18. Imakita S, Nishimura T, Naito H, et al. Magnetic resonance imaging of cerebral infarction: time course of Gd-DTPA enhancement and CT comparison. Neuroradiology 1988; 30:372–378.
19. David RB, Hadield MG, Vines FS, et al. Dural sinus occlusion in leukemia. Pediatrics 1975; 56:793–796.
20. Savino PJ, Grossman RI, Schatz NJ, et al. High-field magnetic resonance imaging in the diagnosis of cavernous sinus thrombosis. Arch Neurol 1986; 43:1081–1082.
21. Anderson SC, Shah CP, Murtagh FR. Congested deep subcortical veins as a sign of dural venous thrombosis: MR and CT correlations. J Comput Assist Tomogr 1987; 11:1059–1061.
22. Baram TZ, Butler IJ, Nelson MD, McArdle CB. Transverse sinus thrombosis in newborns: clinical and magnetic resonance imaging findings. Ann Neurol 1988; 24:792–794.
23. McArdle CB, Mirfakhraee M, Amparo EG, Kulkarni MV. MR imaging of transverse/sigmoid dural sinus and jugular vein thrombosis. J Comput Assist Tomogr 1987; 11:831–838.
24. Locksley HB. Natural history of subarachnoid hemorrhage, intracranial aneurysms and arterio-venous malformations. J Neurosurg 1966; 25:219–239.
25. Brunelle FO, Harwood-Nash DC, Fitz CR, et al. Intracranial vascular malformations in children: computed tomographic and angiographic evaluation. Radiology 1983; 149:455–461.
26. Rigamonti D, Drayer BP, Johnson PC, et al. The MRI appearance of cavernous malformations (angiomas). J Neurosurg 1987; 67:518–524.
27. Rigamonti D, Spetzler RF, Drayer BP, et al. Appearance of venous malformations on magnetic resonance imaging. J Neurosurg 1988; 69:535–539.
28. Celli P, Ferrante L, Palma L, et al. Cerebral arteriovenous malformations in children. Surg Neurol 1984; 22:43–49.
29. Harwood-Nash DC, Fitz CR. Abnormalities of the cerebral arteries. Vol III. In: Neuroradiology in infants and children. St. Louis: CV Mosby, 1976:902–964.
30. Humphreys RP, Hendrick EB, Hoffman HJ. Cerebrovascular disease in children. Can Med Assoc J 1974; 107:774–781.
31. Lagos JC, Riley HD. Congenital intracranial vascular malformations in children. Arch Dis Child 1971; 46:285–290.
32. Cronquist S, Grunholm L, Lundstrom NR. Hydrocephalus and congestive heart failure caused by intracranial arteriovenous malformation in infants. J Neurosurg 1972; 36:239–254.
33. Diebler C, Dulac O, Renier D, et al. Aneurysms of the vein of Galen in infants aged 2 to 15 months. Diagnosis and natural evolution. Neuroradiology 1981; 21:185–197.
34. Grossman RJ, Bruce DA, Zimmerman RA, et al. Vascular steal associated with the vein of Galen aneurysm. Neuroradiology 1984; 26:381–386.
35. Hirabuki N, Miura T, Mitomo M, et al. MR imaging of dural arteriovenous malformations with ocular signs. Neuroradiology 1988; 30:390–394.
36. Jenkins A, Hadley DM, Teasdale GM, et al. Magnetic resonance imaging of acute subarachnoid hemorrhage. J Neurosurg 1988; 68:731–736.
37. Sakai NK, Sakate K, Yomada H, et al. Familial occurrence of intracranial aneurysms. J Neurosurg 1966; 25:593–600.
38. Nagae K, Goka I, Udea K, et al. Familial occurrence of multiple intracranial aneurysms. J Neurosurg 1972; 37:364–367.
39. Sedzimir CB, Jones EW, Edwards R. Management of coarctation of aorta and bleeding intracranial aneurysm in paediatric cases. Neuropadiatrie 1973; 4:124–133.
40. Olsen WL, Brant-Zawadzki M, Hodes J, et al. Giant intracranial aneurysms: MR imaging. Radiology 1987; 163:431–435.
41. Eller TW. MRI demonstration of clot in a small unruptured aneurysm causing stroke. J Neurosurg 1986; 65:411–412.
42. Atlas SW, Grossman RI, Goldberg HI, et al. Partially thrombosed giant intracranial aneurysms: correlation of MR and pathologic findings. Radiology 1987; 162:111–114.
43. Alfidi RJ, Masaryk TJ, Haacke EM, et al. MR angiography of peripheral, carotid, and coronary arteries. AJR 1987; 149:1097–1109.

Metabolic, Endocrine, and Iatrogenic Lesions of the Brain

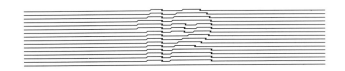

MARY K. EDWARDS, M.D.

The metabolic, endocrine, and iatrogenic diseases of the brain include a widely disparate, miscellaneous group of abnormalities. Although neurologic problems are common in these disorders, many do not show abnormalities on magnetic resonance (MR) or computed tomographic (CT) examinations. In this review, only those diseases that manifest MR abnormalities in the pediatric age group are discussed.

DEMYELINATING DISEASES

The ability of MR imaging (MRI) to detect white matter abnormalities and to demonstrate the extent of white matter diseases represents a dramatic improvement compared with CT (Fig. 12–1).[1–3] Only the largest areas of demyelination are apparent on CT scans. Demyelinating lesions of the spinal cord and optic nerves have long eluded CT. MRI, by contrast, has proved to be exquisitely sensitive to a myriad of white matter abnormalities, both reversible and irreversible. A major limitation of MR scanning may actually be the exceptional sensitivity to white matter pathology, coupled with a lack of specificity of white matter lesions. To increase the specificity of MR scanning of white matter diseases, one needs an adequate clinical history, a recognition of the different disease patterns on

MR scans, and an understanding of the different pulse sequences available.[4]

Multiple Sclerosis

Multiple sclerosis is the most common and most typical of the demyelinating diseases, also known as myelinoclastic diseases. These are diseases in which normally formed myelin is later destroyed. The causes of myelinoclastic diseases include infectious, postinfectious autoimmune, vascular, toxic, and idiopathic mechanisms. Although multiple sclerosis is poorly understood, there is a significant body of information that suggests a viral etiology in genetically susceptible individuals.[5]

The hallmark of the clinical presentation of multiple sclerosis is that of exacerbations and remissions of multifocal neurologic deficits. Patients commonly complain of impaired or double vision, weakness, numbness, tingling, and gait disturbances. As the disease progresses, loss of sphincter control, blindness, paralysis, and dementia may develop. Pain is an uncommon clinical feature. Although most patients present in the third and fourth decades, 15 percent present before the age of 20.[5]

The diagnosis of multiple sclerosis is frequently un-

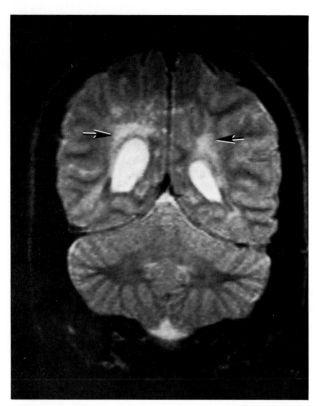

Figure 12–1. *Demyelination.* Coronal T2 weighted sequence (2000/80) demonstrates symmetric periventricular regions of demyelination (*arrows*). A CT scan performed at the same time was unremarkable.

certain, and elaborate criteria have been developed to establish the degree of certainty of the diagnosis.[6] Criteria based purely on the clinical picture have been employed, but have largely been replaced by criteria that include information from imaging studies and cerebrospinal fluid (CSF) analysis. The Bartel criteria, used at our institution, establish the diagnosis as possible, probable, or definite.[6] Using the Bartel method, three criteria must be met before the diagnosis of multiple sclerosis can be considered definite: (1) a history of neurologic symptoms with relapse and remission; (2) evidence of two or more anatomically separate lesions in the central nervous system (CNS) obtained by clinical examination, electrophysiologic tests, or imaging techniques; and (3) evidence of immunologic disturbance involving the CNS revealed by a demyelinative spinal fluid profile. The diagnosis of multiple sclerosis may be considered probable when there is evidence of two separate lesions in the CNS and when a patient satisfies only one of the two remaining essential criteria. Finally, patients showing evidence of a single lesion or clinical deficit, but satisfying one or both of the remaining essential criteria, are candidates for the diagnosis of possible multiple sclerosis.

Because many patients present with only one neurologic defect, MRI provides an excellent method of evaluating the neuraxis for clinically silent multifocal disease (see Fig. 12–3). Visual, auditory, and somatosensory evoked responses may also be used to help establish the multifocality of disease.[7] These are limited by the indirect nature of the examination, which requires intact hearing and vision in order to test the neurologic pathways.[8] The greatest limitation, though, is the narrow scope of the evoked responses, which measure only a fraction of the potentially affected pathways. Spinal fluid analysis, with attention to oligoclonal bands, myelin basic protein, and immunoglobulin G, is highly important in establishing the diagnosis of multiple sclerosis.[8]

On histologic examination, multiple sclerosis plaques demonstrate evolution from the acute to the chronic phase. Approximately 50 percent of plaques are present in the periventricular location, especially near the angles of the lateral ventricles.[9] Initially, lesions consist of inflammatory cells of microglial origin surrounding structural changes in the myelin sheaths. In the subacute phase occurring weeks after the acute inflammation, myelin is phagocytosed and the oligodendrocytes disappear. In the chronic phase, months after the initial event, fibrillary gliosis appears and atrophy and cavitation may develop. At this stage, the myelin sheaths are interrupted at the edge of the plaque of demyelination, where glial cells persist, indicating an active cellular margin even in old plaques.[10]

Multiple sclerosis may appear quite similar to many other white matter diseases, with scattered bright signal in the white matter on T2 weighted spin-echo sequences. Long TR inversion recovery sequences (TR = 3000, TI = 600, TE = 30) offer some promise of differentiating multiple sclerosis from other diseases affecting white matter (Fig. 12–2). Because of the extremely long T1 characteristics of plaques, they appear black on inversion recovery sequences, whereas ischemic disease and other white matter lesions appear a lighter gray (Fig. 12–3).[11]

The MR appearance of multiple sclerosis reflects the histologic findings. Acute inflammation appears as a rounded area of bright signal on T2 weighted sequences, appearing as a "snowball." Gadolinium–DTPA enhancement may be seen during the acute phase (Fig. 12–4).[10] With time the area of inflammation decreases in size but leaves a small residual plaque of bright signal, usually more linear or punctate in appearance than the initial lesion. Occasionally the plaque contains a cavity large enough to present as a CSF-containing cyst. With progression of disease, atrophy is apparent and increased iron deposition is present in the basal ganglia.[12] Plaques are common in the periventricular location, internal capsule, pons, and brachium pontis, but may appear throughout the myelinated white matter.

Spinal cord plaques can be demonstrated on MR scans, but MRI is not as sensitive in the detection of cord as it is of brain lesions. If a patient is suspected of having spinal cord multiple sclerosis, it is probably most reasonable to perform a head MR scan to screen for asymptomatic multifocal disease.[13]

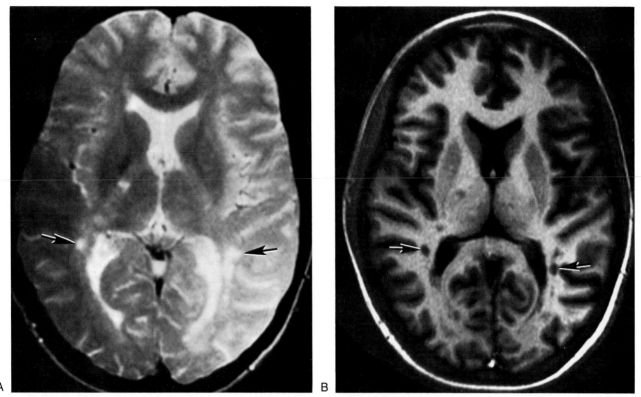

Figure 12–2. *Multiple sclerosis.* ***A,*** Axial T2 weighted images (2000/80) show multiple bright abnormalities consistent with white matter demyelination (*arrows*). ***B,*** These same areas appear black on inversion recovery axial images (3000/600/30) (*arrows*), confirming the long T1 characteristics of the multiple sclerosis plaques.

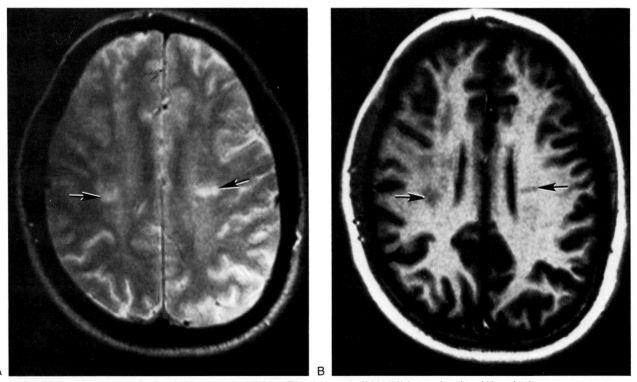

Figure 12–3. *Ischemia.* ***A,*** Ischemic areas appear bright on T2 axial images (2000/80) (*arrows*) and could be mistaken for multiple sclerosis plaques. ***B,*** These same areas appear gray on inversion recovery sequences (3000/600/30) (*arrows*), indicating that these lesions do not have long T1 characteristics typical of multiple sclerosis.

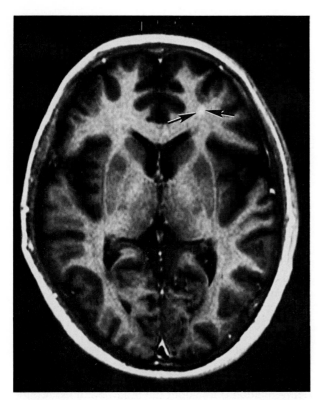

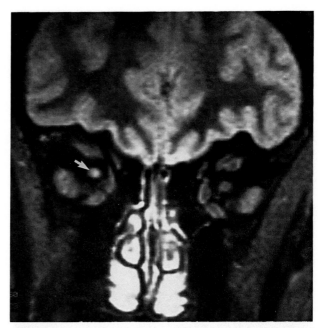

Figure 12–5. *Multiple sclerosis.* Coronal image through the optic nerves on a STIR sequence (2000/150/30) shows the right optic nerve to be bright compared with the left (*arrow*).

Figure 12–4. *Gadolinium–DTPA enhancement of multiple sclerosis plaque.* A small area of faint contrast enhancement is seen within an active multiple sclerosis plaque on an inversion recovery image (3000/600/30) (*arrow*). (Edwards MK. Multiple sclerosis and white matter diseases. Topics in MRI 1989; 2:41–48).

Optic nerve lesions are quite common clinically and at autopsy, but routine spin-echo sequences have failed to detect optic nerve involvement. Newer pulse sequences, especially STIR (short tau inversion recovery) show promise in detecting optic neuritis.[14] The STIR sequence shows the normal optic nerves to be isodense with brain tissue surrounded by black CSF. Optic neuritis appears as abnormal bright signal within the affected nerves (Fig. 12–5). The parameters of this sequence are TR = 2000, TI = 150, TE = 30, and two repetitions.

Virus-Induced Demyelination

Although many viruses infect and destroy brain and spinal cord tissue, some confine their effects almost entirely to white matter. Progressive multifocal leukoencephalopathy (PML), caused by the papovavirus, has become one of the most common viral demyelinating disorders. PML affects immunocompromised patients, and before the advent of the acquired immunodeficiency syndrome (AIDS) PML was found primarily in leukemia or lymphoma victims receiving immunosuppressive therapy. In recent years most patients with PML have been found to have AIDS. PML appears on MR as asymmetric, bilateral, patchy areas of demyelination with a preference initially for the subcortical white matter (Fig. 12–6).[15] The disease progresses quickly to involve greater amounts of white matter, becoming confluent in the later stages. At the acute margin of disease, gadolinium–DTPA enhancement may be noted. In patients with AIDS, other disease processes may affect white matter and mimic PML. These include lymphoma and infection with cytomegalovirus or the AIDS virus, HTLV-III. However, the papovavirus of PML is more aggressive, with a rapidly progressive course on MRI and a rapid downhill course clinically. Death occurs within months of the onset of symptoms.

Subacute sclerosing panencephalitis (SSPE) is now a rare disease resulting from infection with the measles virus. Probably because of widespread measles immunization in the United States, there has been a marked decrease in incidence.[16] A latency of several years may be present, the age of onset of SSPE being between 3 and 20 years. MR and CT findings are of edematous periventricular white matter lesions initially compressing the ventricles but progressing to marked cerebral atrophy. SSPE usually progresses to death in 6 months to 6 years.

Postviral Immune-Mediated White Matter Diseases

Occasionally after a viral illness a patient develops an autoimmune response to white matter, with variable and usually reversible demyelination. Guillain-Barré syndrome, Devic's syndrome, and acute dissem-

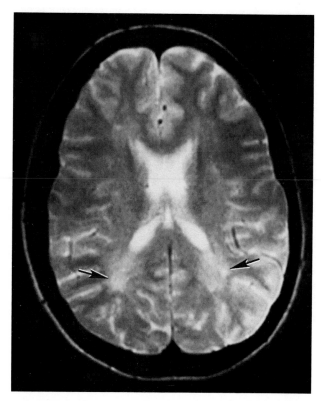

Figure 12–6. *Progressive multifocal leukoencephalopathy.* Scattered white matter lesions (*arrows*) are seen on this axial T2 image (2000/80) of a patient with AIDS.

inated encephalomyelitis (ADEM) are examples of virus-induced, immune-mediated white matter diseases. ADEM may present within weeks following varicella or influenza infection. White matter lesions on T2 weighted images show response to steroid therapy, and regress completely as the disease resolves (Fig. 12–7).[17] Devic's syndrome is similar to ADEM but includes optic nerve and spinal cord involvement.

Central Pontine Myelinolysis

Central pontine myelinolysis is a disorder of demyelination found commonly in alcoholics but also in children and other patients with electrolyte abnormalities.[18] The most commonly recognized etiologic factor is rapidly corrected hyponatremia. The symptoms of central pontine myelinolysis are quadriparesis, pseudobulbar palsy, and declining levels of consciousness, including coma and death.[19] A state of pseudocoma ("locked-in" syndrome) may precede death by a few days. Many patients progress to death, but with the improved detection of the disease by MR, many more have survived with varying degrees of residual neurologic deficits. The MR findings are of bright signal on T2 weighted sequences corresponding to the regions of demyelination throughout the brain, but most prominent in the pons (Fig. 12–8).[19, 20] The pontine lesion is central, with sparing of a rim of tissue peripherally in the pons. Extrapontine sites of myelinolysis may also

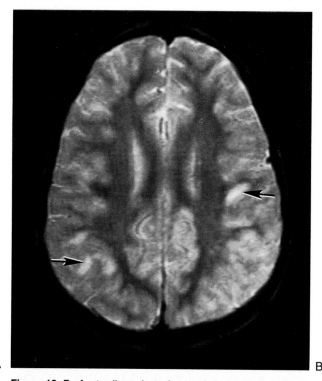

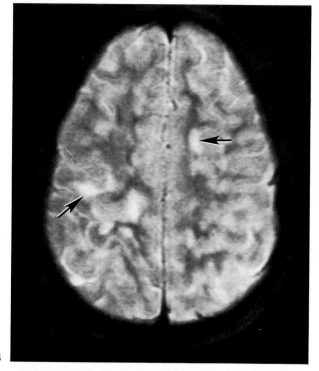

A   B

Figure 12–7. *Acute disseminated encephalomyelitis.* **A,** Scattered white matter lesions are seen in the subcortical region on a T2 weighted axial image (2000/80) (*arrows*). **B,** Additional lesions are seen in the high centrum semiovale on an axial T2 weighted sequence (2000/80) (*arrows*).

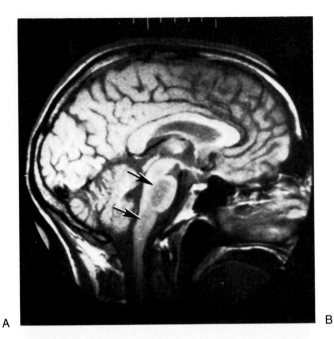

A

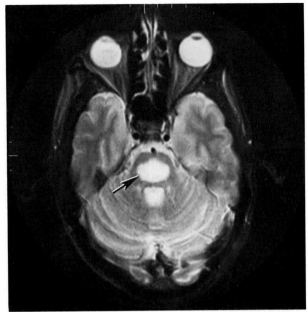

B

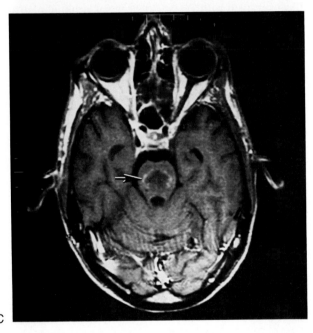

C

Figure 12–8. *Central pontine myelinolysis.* ***A,*** Sagittal T1 weighted image (800/26) demonstrates low signal lesions within the pons and medulla (*arrows*). ***B,*** T2 weighted axial image (2000/80) shows a characteristic bright lesion most prominently within the midpons (*arrow*) with a surrounding rim of normal-appearing pontine parenchyma. ***C,*** A thin rim of contrast enhancement appears at the periphery of the pontine lesion on a T1 weighted sequence (800/26), indicating an area of active demyelination (*arrow*) on this gadolinium-enhanced image. (Koch KJ, Smith RR. Gadolinium enhancement in central pontine myelinolysis on MRI. AJNR 1989; 10:558.)

be noted in association with electrolyte disturbance and its rapid correction.[21] The MR findings of myelinolysis are nonspecific, and when white matter lesions are seen beyond the pons, ischemia, tumor, multiple sclerosis, and radiation therapy effects may be confused with central pontine myelinolysis.

LEUKODYSTROPHIES

Leukodystrophies, also known as dysmyelinating diseases, are those in which an enzyme deficiency prevents normal formation or maintenance of white mat-

ter. This group of diseases is characterized by progressive destruction of the myelin of the white matter. The exact nature of the enzymatic defect is not equally clear in each of the disease processes. In general, the destruction of myelin is due to deficient catabolism of portions of the complex proteins in the myelin sheaths resulting in accumulation of different catabolites in the various diseases of this group. The clinical picture is that of progressive mental deterioration. Patients present with mental retardation, weakness, and long tract signs, as well as abnormal visual, auditory, and somatosensory evoked potentials.[22] The diseases progress to frank dementia, spasticity, and unresponsiveness. In most patients the disease is evident early in the first decade. The common leukodystrophies, metachromatic leukodystrophy, Krabbe's disease, and Canavan's disease, are transmitted by an autosomal recessive pattern of inheritance. Adrenoleukodystrophy, found only in boys, is inherited as a sex-linked recessive disease.

The MR picture is that of progressive white matter lesions eventually resulting in diffuse cerebral atrophy. Although the disease pattern on MRI is similar for all the leukodystrophies in the later stages, there are some distinguishing features early in the disease course.

Sudanophilic Leukodystrophies

The sudanophilic leukodystrophies include several poorly defined diseases that cause an accumulation of sudanophilic droplets containing cholesterol and triglycerides in the white matter. Pelizaeus-Merzbacher disease and Cockayne's syndrome are two of the sudanophilic leukodystrophies.[16] Widespread white matter lesions accompanied by a variable degree of calcification characterize the CT and MR appearance of these diseases (Fig. 12–9).

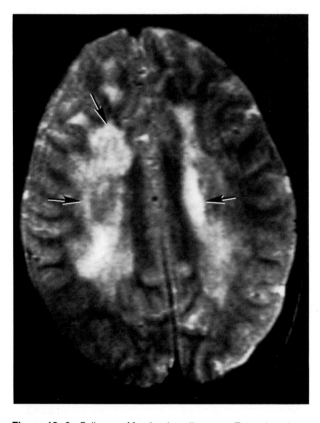

Figure 12–9. *Pelizaeus-Merzbacher disease.* Extensive abnormalities appear as bright lesions in the white matter (*arrows*) on this T2 weighted axial image (2000/80) through the level of the centrum semiovale.

Krabbe's Disease

In Krabbe's disease the histologic finding is that of large macrophages containing myelin breakdown products, called globoid cells.[16] The CT appearance is one of increased density within the thalami, caudate nuclei, and corona radiata. MR experience is limited in Krabbe's disease, but a distribution involving basal ganglia as well as white matter has been seen anecdotally (Fig. 12–10).

Metachromatic Leukodystrophy

Metachromatic leukodystrophy includes several disorders caused by deficiency of arylsulfatase A. Histologic examination reveals metachromasis of the white matter caused by accumulations of sulfatides.[16] Metachromatic staining implies that the tissue-dye complex has an absorption spectrum sufficiently different from the original dye to produce an obvious contrast in color. The principal forms are late infantile, presenting at age 2 to 3 years, and juvenile, presenting at 4 to 6 years. Unlike most of the other leukodystrophies, CT or MR studies reveal white matter lesions beginning in the frontal region and showing posterior progression (Fig. 12–11). Demyelination is diffuse but with emphasis on those tracts that myelinate during the latter part of infancy, resulting in the greater frontal involvement.

Adrenoleukodystrophy

In adrenoleukodystrophy, the enzyme defect, related to oxidation of long-chain fatty acids, results in characteristic cytoplasmic inclusions in the skin, adrenal gland, and conjunctiva, sites where biopsies seem to be specific.[23] The CT and MR appearance of adrenoleukodystrophy is somewhat specific, with symmetric areas of white matter abnormality surrounding the atria of the lateral ventricles, spanning the splenium of the corpus callosum. At the lateral margin of the zones of demyelination, contrast enhancement appears, corresponding to areas of active demyelination accompanied by inflammation (Schaumburg's zones 1 and 2) (Fig. 12–12). MR has been found to be more sensitive than CT in detecting the acute demyelinating lesions of adrenoleukodystrophy.[24] It has been suggested that MRI may be of some value in the screening of siblings of patients with the disease.[24]

Adrenoleukomyeloneuropathy

Variants of adrenoleukodystrophy also occur with less certain inheritance patterns and biochemical defects. One such variant, adrenoleukomyeloneuropathy, has been studied with MRI and CT.[25] In a patient

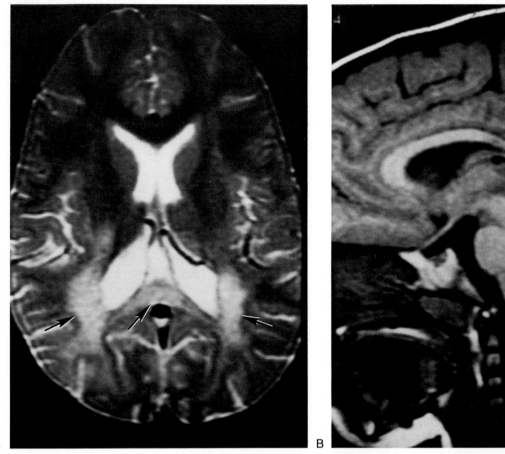

A   B

Figure 12–10. *Krabbe's disease.* **A,** Axial T2 weighted sequence (2000/80) demonstrates symmetric bilateral white matter lesions spanning the corpus callosum (*arrows*). **B,** T1 sagittal image (800/26) shows lesion of decreased signal within the splenium of the corpus callosum (*arrow*). (Edwards MK. Multiple sclerosis and white matter diseases. Topics in MRI 1989; 2:41–48).

with adrenoleukomyeloneuropathy the CT was normal, but MRI showed areas of abnormality on both T1 and T2 weighted sequences similar in appearance to that of adrenoleukodystrophy.[25] In addition, lesions characteristic of this disease were found in the pons and cervical spinal cord on MR examination.

Alexander's Disease

Alexander's disease usually is detected within the first year of life when the infant exhibits developmental delay, macrocephaly, spasticity, and seizures.[22] Eosinophilic material is deposited in the perivascular spaces and on the pial surface of the brain. The CT appearance of Alexander's disease is that of an evolving course beginning with normal scan results and progressing to generalized gray and white matter atrophy. In a single case of MRI in Alexander's disease, increased signal was present in the perivascular and pial

surfaces of the brain on a proton density sequence (Fig. 12–13).

ABNORMALITIES OF IRON METABOLISM

Iron deposition can be found within the brain in both children and adults when a high-field strength MR imaging system is used. Because of the exquisite sensitivity of MR to small amounts of iron deposition, this finding has become a significant indicator of many different disease processes.

Iron appears within the brain as a prominently decreased signal intensity on T2 weighted images. In a study comparing 150 normal individuals with autopsy specimens stained for iron, Drayer and colleagues reported patterns of normal iron deposition with age and stated that there is no detectable iron in the brain at birth.[12] Iron stains were first positive at 6 months in the

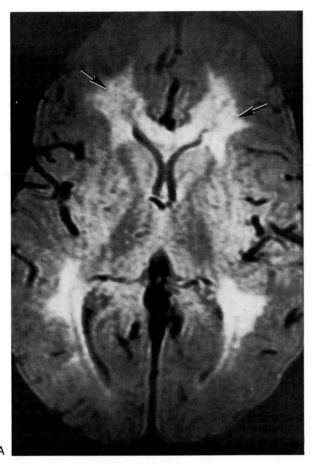
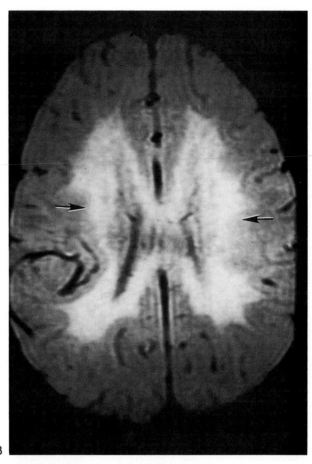

A   B

Figure 12–11. *Metachromatic leukodystrophy.* ***A,*** Extensive white matter lesions are seen symmetrically and more prominent anteriorly (*arrows*) on this axial proton density image (2000/20). ***B,*** White matter lesions appear bright and confluent on an axial image through the level of the roof of the lateral ventricles on this axial proton density image (2000/20) (*arrows*).

globus pallidum, followed by the substantia nigra at 9 to 12 months, the red nucleus at 18 to 24 months, and the dentate nucleus at 3 to 7 years. Moderate iron staining and decreased T2 signal were found in the putamen, the caudate, the Ammon's horn, and the thalamus. A thin rim of moderately intense staining and decreased T2 signal were found in the subcortical "U" fibers.

When increases in iron deposition occur in the brain, MRI reflects the disorder as areas of abnormally decreased signal on T2 weighted sequences. Many degenerative disorders of the brain have been found to cause increased iron deposition (Fig. 12–14).[26] In multiple sclerosis, increased iron deposition has been found adjacent to areas of demyelination.[27] In Huntington's disease, abnormal iron deposition has been found in the caudate and putamen.[28] Hemorrhage within the brain and subarachnoid space also results in abnormalities reflecting the regions of hemosiderin deposition. Hallervorden-Spatz disease is a rare disorder in which

iron deposition is severe. Several reports have described markedly abnormal signal in the globus pallidum and substantia nigra in this disease.[29–31]

Hemochromatosis

Hemochromatosis is caused by abnormal iron deposition in parenchymal cells, with eventual tissue damage and dysfunction of the involved organs. The disease may be primary (genetic) or secondary (acquired). Extreme iron overload of secondary hemochromatosis is associated with the disorders of erythropoiesis requiring frequent blood transfusions and iron therapy. Primary hemochromatosis results in the clinical manifestations of cirrhosis of the liver, diabetes, and increased skin pigmentation. Hypopituitarism is not uncommon, resulting from increased iron deposition in the anterior lobe of the pituitary gland.

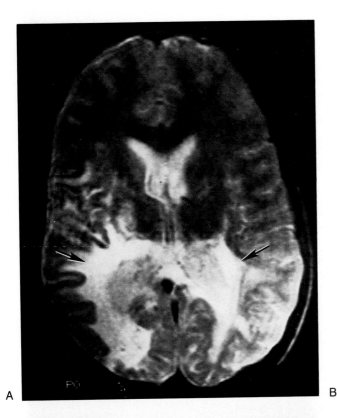

A

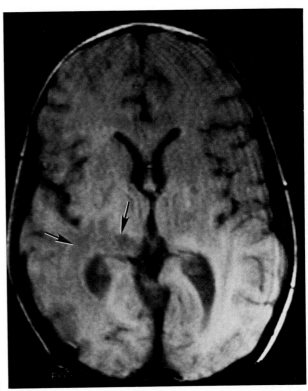

B

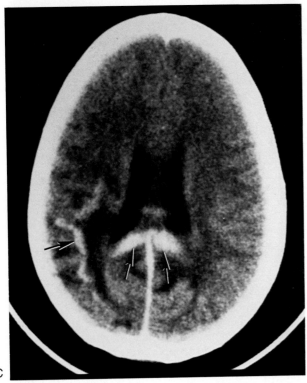

C

Figure 12–12. *Adrenoleukodystrophy.* **A,** Extensive bilateral white matter lesions appear bright on an axial T2 weighted sequence (2000/80) (*arrows*). **B,** The same areas appear slightly dark on an axial T1 weighted sequence (800/26) (*arrows*). **C,** Margin of demyelination shows contrast enhancement on an enhanced CT scan (*arrows*). (Edwards MK. Multiple sclerosis and white matter diseases. Topics in MRI 1989; 2:41–48).

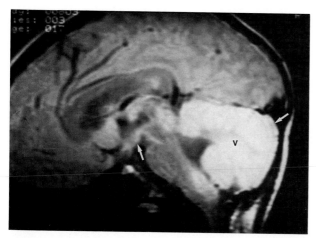

Figure 12–13. *Alexander's disease.* An abnormal signal is present on the pial surface on this sagittal proton density image (2000/20) (*arrows*). An increased signal is present throughout the cerebellar vermis (V).

MR findings in hemochromatosis include areas of decreased signal within the basal ganglia, thalamus, central white matter, and anterior lobe of the pituitary gland.[32]

Ischemic and Anoxic Insults in Children

Dietrich and Bradley described increased iron deposition in the basal ganglia in four children after severe ischemic or anoxic insults, with subsequent resuscitation.[33] The findings in all patients were similar: areas of hypointensity in the basal ganglia, thalami, and white matter on T2 weighted sequences (Fig. 12–15). Associated areas of hyperintensity were also seen in the periventricular and subcortical white matter, attributed to gliosis (Fig. 12–16).

METABOLIC DISEASES OF THE BASAL GANGLIA

Several of the inherited metabolic diseases have their predominant defects within the basal ganglia. These include Huntington's, Wilson's, Leigh's, and Fahr's diseases. The appearance late in the course of each of these diseases is that of generalized atrophy.[16] The early MR and CT pictures show the disease to be predominantly within the basal ganglia. In Huntington's disease, the lesion is within the caudate nucleus. The atrophy of the caudate nucleus is progressive with time, however, and is rarely abnormal on imaging studies in pediatric patients, even those who are symptomatic early. Other rare but related disorders classified as striatal degeneration have been re-

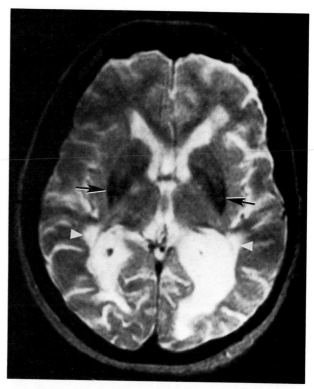

Figure 12–14. *Increased iron deposition after radiation therapy.* Symmetric areas of decreased signal are seen in the basal ganglia (*arrows*) on a T2 weighted sequence (2000/80). Scattered white matter lesions are also present (*arrowheads*).

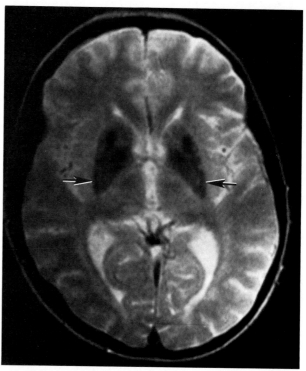

Figure 12–15. *Postanoxic iron deposition.* Marked iron deposition is present in a symmetric distribution on this axial T2 weighted sequence (2000/80) (*arrows*).

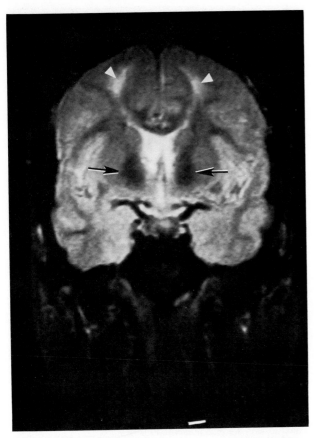

Figure 12–16. *Postanoxic iron deposition.* A coronal T2 weighted sequence (2000/80) shows iron deposition in the globus pallidum (*arrows*). Associated gliosis appears as areas of bright signal in the white matter (*arrowheads*).

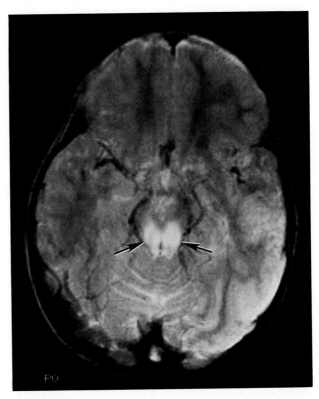

Figure 12–17. *Wilson's disease.* Symmetric areas of bright signal are seen within the midbrain on this axial T2 weighted sequence (2000/80) (*arrows*).

ported, and may show similar abnormality on MR images.[34]

Wilson's Disease

Wilson's disease is an uncommon metabolic disease in which large amounts of copper are deposited in the brain and liver, resulting in brain degeneration and cirrhosis of the liver. The disease is inherited by autosomal recessive transmission. The basal ganglia are affected early, and generalized cerebral atrophy develops as the disease progresses. Although the disease is rare, early diagnosis is particularly important because prompt therapy can prevent devastating neurologic sequelae.[35]

The MR appearance of Wilson's disease consists of bilaterally symmetric areas of bright signal within the globus pallidum, putamen, thalamus, and caudate and dentate nuclei. Symmetric lesions of the brain stem can also be found (Fig. 12–17). In a series by Aisen and colleagues, no progression of the disease was demonstrated in follow-up examination at 4 to 8 months in five patients in whom the disease had been detected and treated early.[35]

Leigh's Disease

Leigh's disease, or necrotizing encephalomyelopathy, is a rare disease resulting from poorly understood metabolic abnormalities, probably involving the pyruvate metabolism.[36] The disease is transmitted as an autosomal recessive. Symptoms usually appear before 2 years of age, and many cases are neonatal. Children with Leigh's disease commonly have developmental delay, and the more severely affected can present with respiratory and metabolic abnormalities.

MRI has shown great sensitivity in detecting the cerebral abnormalities of Leigh's disease. The lesions are symmetric, primarily within the gray matter of the basal ganglia and midbrain (Fig. 12–18).[36] The putamen and thalamus are the most severely affected regions. A thin rim of contrast enhancement is frequently demonstrated at the border of the active disease within the basal ganglia. White matter involve-

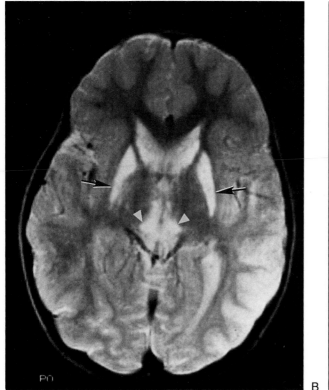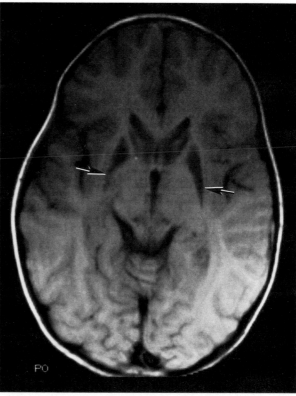

A   B

Figure 12–18. *Leigh's disease.* **A,** Symmetric basal ganglia lesions are seen most prominently within the putamen (*arrows*) and thalamus (*arrowheads*) appearing bright on this axial T2 weighted sequence (2000/80). **B,** T1 weighted axial image (800/26) shows the same areas as low signal lesions (*arrows*).

ment may develop, and generalized atrophy is common late in the disease.

Fahr's Disease

Fahr's disease is an inherited disorder with characteristic calcifications of the basal ganglia and dentate nuclei (Fig. 12–19).[37] No corresponding serum calcium or endocrinologic abnormalities have been detected. MR studies show a varied appearance, both bright and dark, on T2 sequences in the basal ganglia corresponding to the areas of calcification found on CT. Because calcification would be expected to cause signal void and a dark or isointense appearance, the varied signal on MR implies different stages of the disease with an abnormal increase in signal sufficient to overcome the dark signal of calcium in certain phases of the disease. Examination of the calcified regions shows mucopolysaccharide deposits and trace elements: zinc, phosphorus, chlorine, iron, aluminum, magnesium, and potassium.[37] It has not been worked out which elements are deposited and in what combinations to create the mixed patterns evident on the MR scans of Fahr's disease.

METABOLIC DISEASES WITH DIFFUSE GRAY MATTER DEGENERATION

Mitochondrial Encephalomyopathies

The mitochondrial encephalomyopathies are a heterogeneous group of disorders characterized by a defect in oxidative metabolism resulting in a multisystem degeneration with progressive cerebral involvement.[38] These disorders have been given several names including MELAS syndrome (for mitochondrial myopathy, encephalopathy, lactic acidosis, and strokelike episodes), familial poliodystrophy, Alpers' disease, and Toni-Debré-Fanconi syndrome.[39–42] The children develop normally for a variable period of 2 months to several years, then develop progressive mental retardation, seizures, dementia, and pyramidal and extrapyramidal disturbances. Vomiting and failure to thrive are common. The progression of the disease may be rapid and the patient may die in status epilepticus.

Laboratory studies may show electrocardiographic and electroencephalographic changes, elevation in lactate and pyruvate levels in the blood and CSF, and elevation in creatine kinase and lactate dehydrogenase blood levels.[38] Muscle biopsy demonstrates abnormal

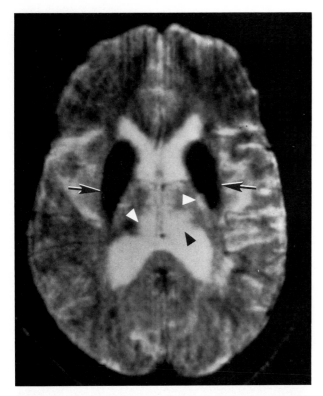

Figure 12–19. *Fahr's disease.* Dense calcification is seen within the basal ganglia and thalamus, appearing black (*arrows*) on T2 weighted sequence (2000/80). Scattered bright lesions appear in the thalamus and adjacent to the regions of calcification (*arrowheads*).

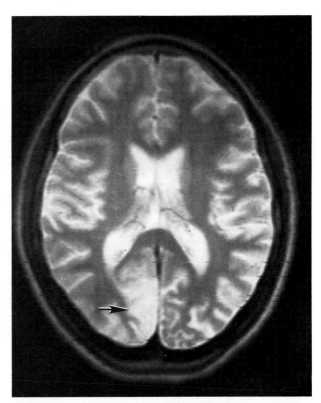

Figure 12–20. *Mitochondrial encephalomyopathy (MELAS).* Bright signal is seen within the occipital lobe confined to the gray matter on this axial T2 weighted sequence (2000/80) (*arrow*).

accumulations of mitochondria. At autopsy the brain shows focal atrophy of the gray matter, the ventricles are wide, and the corpus callosum is thin.[39] The white matter may be thinned but is generally of normal appearance. There are increased iron and calcium deposits in the basal ganglia.

The CT examination of patients with mitochondrial encephalomyopathy usually reveals ventricular dilatation and calcium deposits in the basal ganglia. Cortical lucencies with no enhancement may also be demonstrated on CT. MR studies have been shown to be much more sensitive to the extent of gray matter abnormalities, extensive areas of high signal being found within the cortex (Fig. 12–20).[38] Extension of edema to involve the underlying white matter may be present. The MR findings of bright signal in the cortex in patients with mitochondrial encephalopathy may be partially reversible, but the disease is progressive, eventually resulting in diffuse atrophy. The calcification of the basal ganglia is much better demonstrated on CT examination, however.[38]

Maple Syrup Urine Disease

Maple syrup urine disease is an unusual familial metabolic disease with an enzymatic defect resulting in the abnormal accumulation of ketoacids. These accumulate in the serum, CSF, and urine, causing the characteristic odor that gave rise to the name of the disease. MR findings in this disease have been reported to be those of abnormal bright signal within the white matter and globus pallidus on T2 weighted sequences.[43] Patients may be symptomatic by the first week of life, with poor feeding, vomiting, and lethargy. Unless a restricted diet is begun immediately, the children usually die within 1 year.

Lowe's Disease

Lowe's disease is a sex-linked recessive disorder with severe mental retardation, myopathy, and ocular abnormalities of glaucoma and/or cataract.[22] Generalized aminoaciduria, renal tubular acidosis, and rickets are also present. The biochemical defect is unknown. The disease is progressive and most patients die in childhood. The MR appearance early in the disease is that of abnormal bright signal lesions on T2 weighted sequences involving white and gray matter (Fig. 12–21). Later in the disease the MR appearance reflects the pathologic findings of severe bilateral encephalomalacia, advanced atrophy, and cavitation of the cerebral cortex.

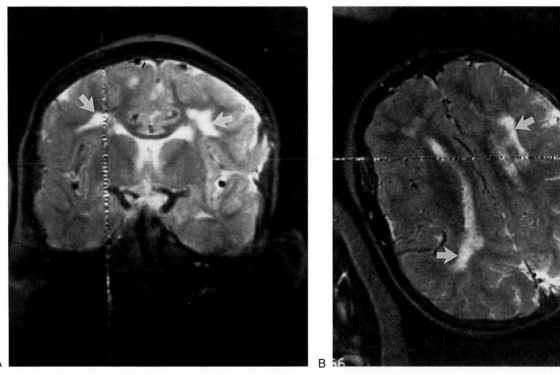

Figure 12–21. *Lowe's disease.* ***A,*** Bright lesions are seen within the periventricular white matter on a T2 weighted coronal image (2000/80) (*arrows*). ***B,*** Periventricular lesions are also present on this axial T2 weighted (2000/80) sequence through the centrum semiovale (*arrows*).

DISORDERS OF LIPID METABOLISM

This group of disorders includes a number of inherited diseases characterized by an abnormal sphingolipid metabolism, which in most instances leads to the intracellular deposition of lipid within the brain.[22] These disorders have a relentless, progressive course that cannot be altered and varies only in the rate of intellectual and visual deterioration. They include Tay-Sachs disease, Gaucher's disease, Neimann-Pick disease, Fabry's disease, and ceroid lipofuscinosis. Scattered reports have appeared of the common MR appearance of these disorders, revealing a periventricular bright signal on T2 weighted sequences.

Fabry's Disease

Fabry's disease is a rare, sex-linked systemic disorder, with symptoms appearing late in childhood but occasionally not recognized until the second or third decade of life. The first manifestation is usually a punctate angiectatic skin rash; later, fever, weight loss, and pain in the joints and abdomen develop.[22] The neurologic manifestations of periventricular vascular disease are a relatively late development. Vascular disease involving the small arteries and arterioles results in premature periventricular ischemia and infarcts. Cerebral

hemorrhage has also been reported. The MR appearance is that of periventricular high signal on T2 weighted sequences involving the entire periventricular region (Fig. 12–22).[44] Basal ganglia lacunar infarcts have also been found on MR examination in Fabry's disease.[44]

MUCOPOLYSACCHARIDOSIS

The mucopolysaccharidoses include a group of diseases in which there is an enzyme deficiency resulting in the inability of lysosomes to degrade mucopolysaccharides.[16] Hunter's disease is inherited by sex-linked transmission; all the other mucopolysaccharidoses are inherited by autosomal recessive transmission.

The clinical picture is one of variable skeletal, visceral, and CNS involvement. Morquio's disease, and the far less common Scheie's and Diferrante's diseases, are the only mucopolysaccharidoses in which patients are not mentally retarded or severely delayed in development.[16] Spinal cord compression is common, especially at the upper cervical level and foramen magnum. The cord compression results from skeletal narrowing and dural thickening from mucopolysaccharide deposits. MR findings include hydrocephalus, dural thickening, and periventricular white matter lesions (Fig. 12–23).[45] Spinal cord compression may be due to

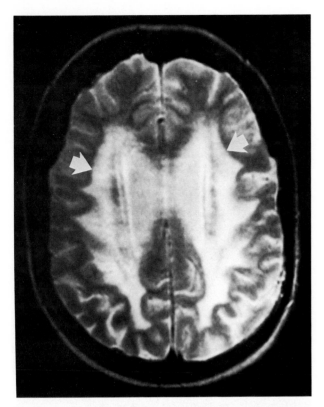

Figure 12–22. *Fabry's disease.* An extensive white matter abnormality throughout the periventricular region appears bright on a T2 weighted axial image (*arrows*) (2000/80).

atlantoaxial subluxation, thoracic gibbus, and dural thickening. Bone marrow transplant has been used as a means of therapy for the mucopolysaccharidoses. MRI has been used to follow the progress of two patients with Hurler's syndrome treated with bone marrow transplant.[45] In both cases, improvement in myelination and improved gray-white differentiation was found after bone marrow transplant.[45]

The following classification of the mucopolysaccharidoses is from Diebler and Dulac:[16]

| Type | Eponym | Lesions | | |
		Skeletal	Visceral	CNS
I H	Hurler's disease	+	+	+
I S	Scheie's disease	+	+	−
I H/S	Hurler-Scheide disease	+	+	+
II	Hunter's disease	+	+	+
III A–D	Sanfilippo's disease	−	−	+
IV A, B	Morquio's disease	+	−	−
VI	Maroteaux-Lamy disease	+	−	+
VII	Shy's disease	+	+	+
VIII	Diferrante's disease	+	−	−

IATROGENIC LESIONS OF THE BRAIN

Arteritis and secondary ischemic lesions of the brain may result from chemotherapy and radiation therapy. Determining whether the patient's symptoms are due to an exacerbation of the neoplasm or to the effects of therapy can be a confusing clinical problem. Symptoms of radiation- or chemotherapy-induced arteritis are similar to those of an intracranial mass: seizures, headaches, confusion, and focal neurologic deficits. MRI can be of great value in differentiating primary from secondary neurologic dysfunction. Most recurrent or residual tumors appear as focal areas of enhancement with surrounding edema. Areas of arteritis, on the other hand, appear similar to other ischemic lesions, except that foci of arteritis tend to be bilateral, more patchy, and more widespread than other ischemic processes. As with other causes of hypoxic injury, hemorrhage is a common sequela to arteritis.

The white matter lesions caused by radiation-induced arteritis may be transient or permanent.[46] The initial changes of transient white matter edema are of little clinical consequence. The chronic changes can be marked, with devastating clinical sequelae, including radiation necrosis, widespread leukomalacia, calcifying microangiopathy, and atrophy.[46] Focal atrophy can occur of any portion of the CNS including the optic nerves (resulting in optic atrophy) and the pituitary gland (resulting in panhypopituitarism) (Fig. 12–24). In children, the younger the patient at the time of radiation therapy, the more devastating is the result. In combination with chemotherapy, the effects of radiation may be even more severe. A subacute leukoencephalopathy is seen as a consequence of the combination of intrathecal methotrexate and irradiation of the CNS.[47]

Areas of radiation necrosis can be focal or disseminated within the white matter.[48] Radiation necrosis appears acutely as an area of abnormal signal brightness on T2 weighted sequences, with variable gadolinium–DTPA enhancement on T1 weighted sequences. Mass effect and edema are common findings in radiation necrosis. Later in the course, ventricular enlargement and atrophic changes predominate. The diffuse changes of radiation therapy on MR images appear as extensive, confluent white matter lesions, scalloped laterally, adjacent to the cortical gray matter, due to arcuate, U-fiber damage.[46] The corpus callosum is usually spared. The pattern is similar to that of multiple sclerosis on T2 weighted sequences, but can usually be differentiated using inversion recovery pulse sequences. As with other causes of white matter ischemia, radiation changes appear light gray on inversion recovery, compared with the plaques of multiple sclerosis, which appear black (Fig. 12–25). L-Asparaginase, an enzyme used in treating acute leukemia, has been associated with intracranial sinus thrombosis in 1 to 2 percent of children.[49] Hemorrhagic infarcts, the result of sinus thrombosis, present as seizures, obtundation, headache, or hemiparesis. MRI has been of great value in early detection of thrombosis in children treated with L-asparaginase.

Bone marrow transplantation has become one of the mainstays in the treatment of recurrent leukemia and other disseminated cancers, and of aplastic anemia and

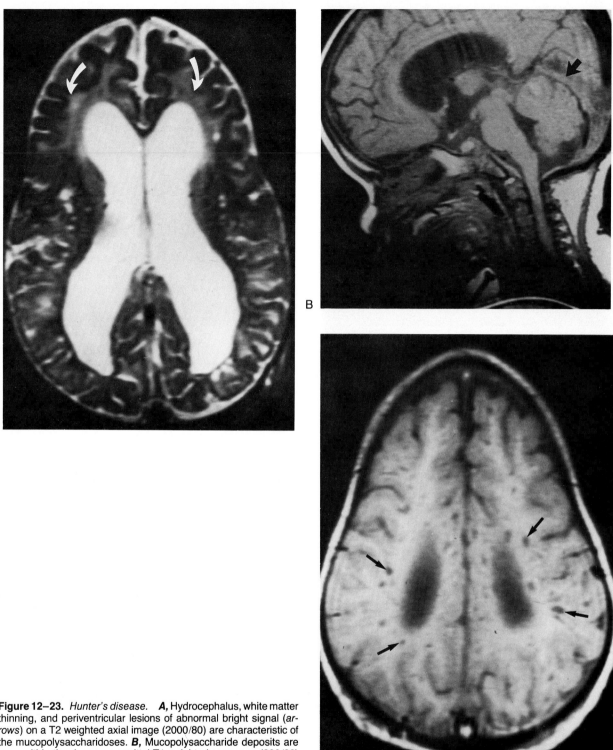

Figure 12–23. *Hunter's disease.* ***A,*** Hydrocephalus, white matter thinning, and periventricular lesions of abnormal bright signal (*arrows*) on a T2 weighted axial image (2000/80) are characteristic of the mucopolysaccharidoses. ***B,*** Mucopolysaccharide deposits are seen within the dura on a sagittal T1 weighted sequence (800/26) (*arrow*). ***C,*** Unusual punctate cavitary lesions are seen within the white matter on an axial T1 weighted sequence (800/26) (*arrows*).

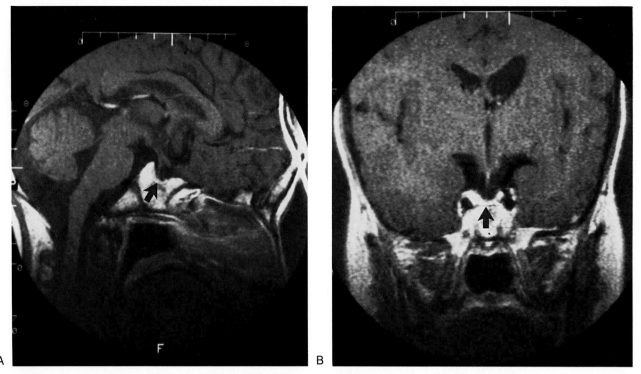

A

B

Figure 12–24. *Postradiation atrophy.* **A,** Focal pituitary atrophy (*arrow*) is demonstrated on this sagittal T1 weighted gadolinium-enhanced image (800/26). **B,** Coronal images confirm the pituitary atrophy (*arrow*) in this patient with panhypopituitarism on a T1 weighted sequence.

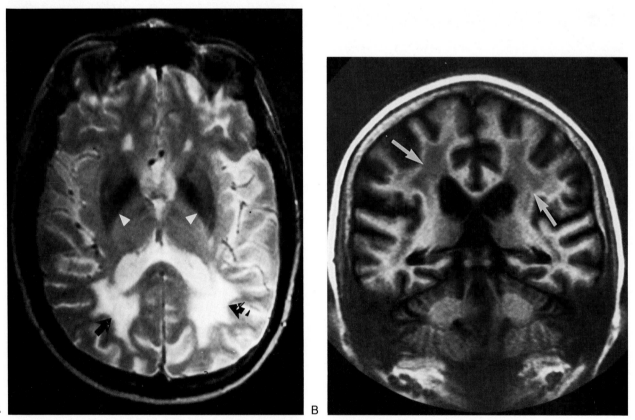

A

B

Figure 12–25. *Radiation effect.* **A,** Bright signal reflects radiation therapy effect in the periventricular regions (*arrows*) on a T2 weighted sequence (2000/80). Increased iron deposition is present in the globus pallidum (*arrowheads*). **B,** The gray appearance of the periventricular lesions on the inversion recovery sequence (3000/600/30) (*arrows*) indicates that multiple sclerosis is not a likely cause of the demyelination, but is consistent with radiation change.

a variety of inborn errors of metabolism. In one series, 59 percent of pediatric bone marrow recipients developed neurologic complications, including cerebral infarction, meningitis, and meningoencephalitis.[50] MRI is currently the best method of imaging these complications of bone marrow transplantation (Fig. 12–26).

ENDOCRINE ABNORMALITIES

Most cerebral complications of endocrine abnormalities are discussed elsewhere in this book. Pituitary dysfunction, for example, is well discussed in the chapter on brain tumors under the classification of pituitary adenomas. Adrenoleukodystrophy is discussed earlier in this chapter with the other leukodystrophies. The miscellaneous endocrine conditions resulting in brain abnormalities on MR examination are discussed below.

Hypothyroidism

The clinical presentation of hypothyroidism depends on the degree and duration of the thyroid insufficiency. When present at or before birth, hypothyroid-

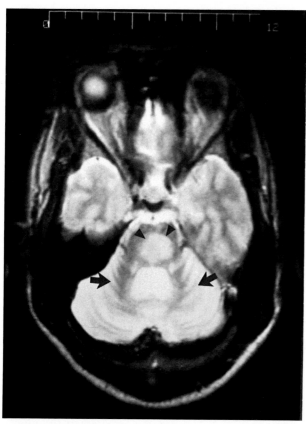

Figure 12–26. *Radiation therapy effect.* A pontine lesion (*arrowheads*) and cerebellar atrophy (*arrows*) reflect radiation therapy effects related to bone marrow transplantation on a T2 weighted sequence (2000/80).

ism may result in severe mental retardation and developmental delay, in spite of adequate hormone replacement therapy.[51] The diagnosis is considered in infants with the clinical presentation of developmental delay, protuberant abdomen, and dry hair and skin. The diagnosis is confirmed with low serum T4 and T3 determinations and elevated TSH. MRI and CT may be performed in children with developmental delay before the diagnosis of hypothyroidism is determined. The appearance on imaging studies is that of diffuse cerebral and cerebellar atrophy.

Diabetes

Although children with diabetes show many neurologic complications, it is unusual for abnormalities to be noted on imaging studies. Obviously, the common problems of peripheral neuropathy and polyradiculopathy cannot be studied by MRI, at least not with the current resolution of our scanners. Cranial nerve deficits and cerebrovascular disease are not encountered in diabetic children. Cerebral edema complicating diabetic ketoacidosis may be imaged as areas of increased water content in an edematous brain,[52] but these children are so acutely ill that MR studies are neither necessary nor appropriate. It is more likely that a child with diabetes may be studied on MRI for generalized or focal ischemia or infarction resulting from previous bouts of diabetic coma. During diabetic ketoacidosis, cerebral oxygen uptake is reduced by 40 percent and cerebral blood flow is decreased.[53] The result is that atrophy and focal ischemia lesions are common sequelae of repeated bouts of diabetic ketoacidosis.

The MR appearance of the myriad abnormalities making up the metabolic, endocrine, and iatrogenic lesions of the brain can be quite similar. In most of these diseases the early MR appearance is of scattered bright signal on T2 weighted sequences, and the late appearance is of diffuse cerebral atrophy. Attention to the distribution of lesions early in the course, and familiarity with the newer pulse sequences, may help improve the specificity of diagnosis. The clinical history and neurologic examination are invaluable, however. In these disorders in which MRI is sensitive to the detection of disease, but rarely specific, radiology and the clinical services must work closely together in order that the patient is best served.

REFERENCES

1. Jackson JA, Leake DR, Schneiders NJ, et al. Magnetic resonance imaging in multiple sclerosis: results in 32 cases. AJNR 1985; 6:171–176.
2. Jacobs L, Kinkel WR, Polachini I, et al. Correlations of nuclear magnetic resonance imaging, computerized tomography, and clinical profiles in multiple sclerosis. Neurology 1986; 36:27–34.
3. Scotti G, Scialfa G, Biondi A, et al. Magnetic resonance in multiple sclerosis. Neuroradiology 1986; 28:319–323.

4. Runge VM, Price A, Kirshner HS, et al. Magnetic resonance imaging of multiple sclerosis: a study of pulse-technique efficacy. AJR 1984; 143:1015–1026.

5. Batchelor JR: Histocompatibility antigens and their relevance to multiple sclerosis. Br Med Bull 1977; 33:72.

6. Bartel DR, Markand ON, Kolar OJ. The diagnosis and classification of multiple sclerosis: evoked responses and spinal fluid electrophoresis. Neurology 1983; 33:592–601.

7. Cutler JR, Aminoff MJ, Brant-Zawadzki M. Evaluation of patients with multiple sclerosis by evoked potentials and magnetic resonance imaging: a comparative study. Ann Neurol 1986; 20:645–648.

8. Farlow MR, Markand ON, Edwards MK, et al. Multiple sclerosis: magnetic resonance imaging, evoked responses, and spinal fluid electrophoresis. Neurology 1986; 36:828–831.

9. Holland BA. Diseases of white matter. In: Brant-Zawadski M, Norman D, eds. Magnetic resonance imaging of the central nervous system. New York: Raven Press, 1987:259–277.

10. Grossman RI, Gonzalez-Scarano F, Atlas SW, et al. Multiple sclerosis: gadolinium enhancement in MR imaging. Radiology 1986; 161:721–725.

11. Edwards MK, Smith RR, Farlow MR, et al. Clinical utility of inversion recovery in the diagnosis of multiple sclerosis. (Abstract.) AJNR 1989; 10:898.

12. Drayer B, Burger P, Darwin R, Riederer S, et al. MRI of brain iron. AJR 1986; 147:103–110.

13. Edwards MK, Farlow MR, Stevens JC. Cranial MR in spinal cord MS: diagnosing patients with isolated spinal cord symptoms. AJNR 1986; 7:1003–1005.

14. Smith RR, Edwards MK, Farlow MR, et al. Imaging of optic neuritis using STIR MR. (Abstract) AJNR 1989; 10:905.

15. Levy JD, Cottingham KL, Campbell RJ, et al. Progressive multifocal leukomalacia and magnetic resonance imaging. Ann Neurol 1986; 19:399–401.

16. Diebler C, Dulac O. Pediatric neurology and neuroradiology. Berlin: Springer-Verlag, 1987.

17. Saito H, Endo M, Takase S, et al. Acute disseminated encephalomyelitis after influenza vaccination. Arch Neurol 1980; 37:564–566.

18. Rippe DJ, Edwards MK, D'Amour PG, et al. MR imaging of central pontine myelinolysis. J Comput Assist Tomogr 1987; 11:724–726

19. Takeda K, Sakuta M, Saeki F. Central pontine myelinolysis diagnosed by magnetic resonance imaging. Ann Neurol 1985; 17:310–311.

20. Miller GM, Baker HL, Okazaki H, Whisnant JP. Central pontine myelinolysis and its imitators: MR findings. Radiology 1988; 168:795–802.

21. Dickoff DJ, Raps M, Yahr MD. Striatal syndrome following hyponatremia and its rapid correction. A manifestation of extrapontine myelinolysis confirmed by magnetic resonance imaging. Arch Neurol 1988; 45:112–114.

22. Menkes JH. Metabolic diseases of the central nervous system. In: Menkes JH, ed. Textbook of child neurology. 3rd ed. Philadelphia: Lea & Febiger, 1985:1–122.

23. Moser HW, Moser AE, Singh I, et al. Adrenoleukodystrophy: survey of 303 cases: biochemistry, diagnosis, and therapy. Ann Neurol 1984; 16:628–641.

24. Huckman MS, Wong PWK, Sullivan T, et al. Magnetic resonance imaging compared with computed tomography in adrenoleukodystrophy. Am J Dis Child 1986; 140:1001–1003.

25. Bewermeyer H, Bamborschke S, Ebhardt G, et al. MR imaging in adrenoleukomyeloneuropathy. J Comput Assist Tomogr 1985; 9:793–796.

26. Drayer BP, Olanow W, Burger P, et al. Parkinson plus syndrome: diagnosis using high field MR imaging of brain iron. Radiology 1986; 159:493–498.

27. Craelius W, Migdal MW, Luessenhop CP, et al. Iron deposits surrounding multiple sclerosis plaques. Arch Pathol Lab Med 1982; 106:397–399.

28. Klintworth GK. Huntington's chorea—morphologic contributions of a century. In: Advances in Neurology. New York: Raven Press, 1973:353–368.

29. Jankovic J, Kirkpatrick JB, Blomquist KA, et al. Late-onset Hallervorden-Spatz disease presenting as familial parkinsonism. Neurology 1985; 35:227–234.

30. Mutoh K, Okuno T, Ito M, et al. MR imaging of a group I case of Hallervorden-Spatz disease. J Comput Assist Tomogr 1988; 12:851–853.

31. Tanfani G, Mascalchi M, Dal Pozzo GC, et al. MR imaging in a case of Hallervorden-Spatz disease. J Comput Assist Tomogr 1987; 11:1057–1058.

32. Fujisawa I, Morikawa M, Nakano Y, et al. Hemochromatosis of the pituitary gland: MR imaging. Radiology 1988; 168:213–214.

33. Dietrich RB, Bradley WC. Iron accumulation in the basal ganglia following severe ischemic-anoxic insults in children. Radiology 1988; 168:203–206.

34. Seidenwurm D, Novotny E Jr, Marshall W, Enzmann D. MR and CT in cytoplasmically inherited striatal degeneration. AJNR 1986; 7:629–632.

35. Aisen AM, Martel W, Gabrielsen TO, et al. Wilson disease of the brain: MR imaging. Radiology 1985; 157:137–141.

36. Geyer CA, Sartor KJ, Prensky AJ, et al. Leigh disease (subacute necrotizing encephalomyelopathy): CT and MR in five cases. J Comput Assist Tomogr 1988; 12:40–44.

37. Scotti G, Scialfa G, Tampieri D, Landoni L. MR imaging in Fahr disease. J Comput Assist Tomogr 1985; 9:790–792.

38. Taverni N, Dal Pozzo G, Arnetoli G, et al. Diagnosis and follow-up of mitochondrial encephalomyopathy: CT and MR studies. J Comput Assist Tomogr 1988; 12:696–697.

39. Shapira Y, Cederbaum SD, Cancilla PA, et al. Familial poliodystrophy, mitochondrial myopathy, and lactate acidemia. Neurology 1975; 25:614–621.

40. Heiman-Patterson TD, Bonilla E, Di Mauro S, et al. Cytochrome-c-oxydase in a floppy child. Neurology 1982; 32:898–900.

41. Sandbank U, Lerman P. Progressive cerebral poliodystrophy—Alpers' disease. Disorganized giant neuronal mitochondria on electron microscopy. J Neurol Neurosurg Psychiatry 1972; 35:749–755.

42. De Volder A, Ghilain S, de Barsy T, Goffinet AM. Brain metabolism in mitochondrial encephalomyopathy: a PET study. J Comput Assist Tomogr 1988; 12:854–857.

43. Uziel G, Savoiardo M, Nardocci N. CT and MRI in maple syrup urine disease. Neurology 1988; 38:486–488.

44. Boothman BR, Bamford JM, Parsons MR. Magnetic resonance imaging in Fabry's disease. J Neurol Neurosurg 1988; 51:1240–1241.

45. Johnson MA, Desai S, Hugh-Jones K, Starer F. Magnetic resonance imaging of the brain in Hurler syndrome. AJNR 1984; 5:816–819.

46. Hecht-Leavitt C, Grossman RI, Curran SJ, et al. MR of brain radiation injury: experimental studies in cats. AJNR 1987; 8:427–431.

47. Peylan-Ramu N, Poplack DG, Pizzo PA, et al. Abnormal CT scans in asymptomatic children with acute lymphocytic leukemia after prophylactic treatment of the central nervous system with radiation and intrathecal chemotherapy. N Engl J Med 1978; 298:815–818.

48. Robain O, Dulac O, Dommergues JP, et al. Necrotising leukoencepahlopathy complicating treatment of childhood leukaemia. J Neurol Neurosurg Psychiatry 1984; 47:65–72.

49. Priest JR, Ramsay NKC, Steinherz PG, et al. A syndrome of thrombosis and hemorrhage complicating L-asparaginase therapy for childhood acute lymphoblastic leukemia. J Pediatr 1982; 100:984–989.

50. Wiznitzer M, Packer RJ, August CS, Burkey ED. Neurological complications of bone marrow transplantation in childhood. Ann Neurol 1984; 16:569–576.

51. Fisher DA. Thyroid function in the fetus. In: Fisher DA, Furrow GN, eds. Perinatal thyroid physiology and disease. New York: Raven Press, 1975:21.

52. Rosenbloom AL, Riley WJ, Weber FT, et al. Cerebral edema complicating diabetic ketoacidosis in childhood. J Pediatr 1980; 96:357–361.

53. Kety SS, Polis BD, Nadler CS, Schmidt CF. The blood flow and oxygen consumption of the human brain in diabetic acidosis and coma. J Clin Invest 1948; 27:500–510.

The Orbit

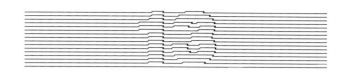

RICHARD R. SMITH, M.D.

Magnetic resonance (MR) imaging has supplanted computed tomography (CT) in nearly all areas of neuroradiology, but MRI of the orbit has not yet gained widespread acceptance. This is primarily due to the superb contrast differentiation present on CT scans of the orbit. The low attenuation of orbital fat prominently highlights most orbital pathology. Pathologic processes involving the bony orbit are also well identified on CT.

This continued clinical preference for orbital CT was augmented by the relatively poor quality of early orbital MR images during the introduction of MR into clinical imaging. Early imaging was particularly hampered by motion. This was secondary to prolonged imaging times, which were necessary to achieve sufficient signal-to-noise ratios. The lack of surface coils also contributed to this problem. Thick slices, a large field of view (FOV), and large matrix sizes also led to poor resolution. Long TR–long TE (so-called T2 weighted) images were degraded by chemical shift artifacts.[1,2]

The development of high magnetic fields, surface coils, and new pulse sequences has for the most part resolved many of the early problems associated with orbital MR imaging. The inherent increased signal to noise associated with high-field imaging coupled with the increased signal provided by surface coils has allowed a decrease in imaging time and an improvement in resolution. Software upgrades with anti-aliasing have allowed small field of view imaging with resultant improved resolution.[3-8] New pulse sequences, such as short T1 inversion recovery (STIR), which are based primarily on fat suppression, have minimized chemical shift and allowed imaging of the additive effects of prolonged T1 and T2 present in most pathologic processes.[9]

These developments have led to an improvement in orbital imaging, particularly in areas difficult to study with CT. These include improved detection and differentiation of intraocular disease; increased sensitivity to lesions affecting the optic nerve, particularly in the intracanalicular region; and improved visualization of chiasmatic masses.[10-16]

These advantages are augmented by the multiplanar capability of MRI. The ability to obtain direct sagittal images has been of significant help in evaluating orbital apex and chiasmatic lesions. Also, MRI does not entail an ionizing radiation delivery to the orbit, and in particular the lens. This is of great importance, because many patients require long-term follow-up studies.

As experience with orbital MRI grows, it likely will become the procedure of choice in orbital imaging.

ORBITAL IMAGING TECHNIQUE

Patient motion severely degrades orbital MRI. As a result, techniques must be used that can be performed quickly and therefore result in less patient motion. The goal in orbital imaging is to achieve sufficient signal and resolution in the shortest amount of time. An increased signal-to-noise ratio (SNR) is provided by a high field unit and by the routine use of an orbital surface coil. In addition, the use of a surface coil de-

325

creases any degradation that may be contributed by noise outside the effective margin of the coil.[7] The improved signal-to-noise ratio present with high-field and surface coil imaging allows thinner sections to be acquired while imaging acquisition time is decreased.[3–7]

Most orbital surface coils are large enough to allow imaging of both orbits simultaneously. Some monocular coils have been used for detailed evaluation of known unilateral processes.[12] In most cases the use of a binocular coil allows diagnosis of pathologic conditions in either orbit and also allows comparison of normal with abnormal when pathology is unilateral. A variety of surface coils are available, including some mask-type coils that are directly applied to the patient.[17] At our institution we currently use a rectangular coil, approximately 15×10 cm, which is held in place just anterior to both orbits. This coil gives satisfactory coverage relating to the craniocaudad and lateral margins of both orbits. The margins of coverage related to surface coils are generally not a problem, but the imaging depth provided by the coil may be critical.[5–7] With our rectangular coil we are able to achieve sufficient signal for successful imaging of the orbital apex and the optic chiasm. The surface coil is used to obtain short TR (T1 weighted) and STIR images. Because of the signal dropoff associated with the surface coil and the decreased SNR inherent in T2 weighted images, we generally use the head coil for the acquisition of T2 weighted images. We have found that in most cases the information provided by the STIR images exceeds that provided by the long TR images in the orbit; however, chiasmatic and optic tract abnormalities may remain best visualized by the long TR images in the head coil.

Currently, all MR examinations of the orbit include short TR (T1 weighted), STIR, and long TR (T2 weighted) sequences. By combining multiple pulse sequences, combinations of signal intensity can be used to provide differentiation of orbital lesions rather than just anatomic localization.

Spin-echo T1 weighted images are acquired with a TR between 600 and 800 msec and a TE between 20 and 30 msec. To provide optimal resolution a matrix size of 256×256 pixels and a 12- to 16-cm field of view is used as well as a slice thickness of 3 mm. An interslice gap of up to 1 mm may be used, but we currently do not employ an interslice gap. However, it may be useful if images are degraded secondary to interslice cross-talk, or if interleaving the images leads to an increase in imaging time. To prevent a prolonged imaging time, one repetition is utilized. Using these parameters, the imaging sequence requires approximately 2.5 minutes to perform. Just before the acquisition of this sequence, the patient, if old enough, is requested to fix his or her gaze upon an area within the magnet and keep eye motion and lid motion to a minimum. In all cases axial images parallel to the course of the intraorbital optic nerve are obtained as well as coronal images, which extend through the chiasm.

Recent reports relating to STIR imaging have led to our including this in our routine orbital study.[9, 18] The purpose of this imaging sequence is to eliminate chemical shift artifact as well as signal from intraorbital fat. This sequence allows the additive effects of prolonged T1 and T2 to be imaged. By choosing an appropriate TI (inversion time), fat will be at the null point (TI_{null}) and have no signal. The TI_{null} can be calculated by the equation $TI_{null} = T1 \times \ln 2$, if TR is greater than T1.[19–21] Using a T1 for fat of 225 msec at 1.5T, $TI_{null} = 150$ msec. For our STIR studies we use a TR of 2,000 msec/TI 150 msec/TE 40 msec. Again employing the surface coil, images are acquired at 4-mm slice thickness, 12- to 16-cm field of view, and one repetition. We do not currently use an interslice gap. We believe that the STIR sequence allows the easiest and most reliable acquisition of fat-suppressed images. However, other methods are available and have shown clinical promise.[22–23]

The last imaging sequences obtained in the orbit are long TR spin-echo images. These are acquired through the entire head, including the orbits. The longer imaging time associated with this technique precludes the fixed gaze technique used in short TR and STIR imaging. As a result, patients are generally instructed only to try to keep as still as possible with the eyes closed. We use T2 weighted images with a TR of 2,500 msec and a TE of 20 and 80 msec and gradient moment nulling. Using a single repetition the scan acquisition time is approximately 8 minutes. An imaging matrix of 192×256 pixels, 20-cm field of view, and 5-mm thick sections without an interslice gap are used. In most cases axial acquisition of the T2 weighted images is performed.

The wide variety and location of orbital pathology often necessitate alteration of the usual scanning projections. For instance, apical lesions may be best visualized by oblique sagittal images, and chiasm lesions require true sagittal projections. One of the advantages of MRI is the ease with which multiple planes can be acquired. Lesions that are both intraorbital and intracranial may require a combination surface coil and head coil T1 weighted imaging.

At this time, the effectiveness of gadolinium–DTPA (Gd–DTPA), a paramagnetic contrast agent, remains unproven in the evaluation of orbital lesions. This contrast agent shortens T1 and T2 times,[24] resulting in an increased signal intensity on short TR, short TE images. We have used intravenous contrast-enhanced MRI primarily to study orbital masses. On T1 weighted images, however, enhancement may be difficult to appreciate, as the enhancing mass blends in with the hyperintense orbital fat. T1 weighted fat suppression images with gadolinium enhancement are currently being investigated, however, and appear promising.[25] Gadolinium injection does not play a role in conventional T2 weighted spin-echo or STIR imaging.

Photography of the acquired images is very important. If narrow window widths are chosen, the high signal from the retro-orbital fat on short TR images may obscure small lesions.[26] If a wide window width is employed, however, signal dropoff in the orbital apex is accentuated. Some MR units now have available surface coil corrections that allow a more uniform intensity throughout the field of view, thereby eliminating some of these problems.[27]

GROSS ANATOMY OF THE ORBIT

Orbital anatomy has been well described in the literature.[28] The major structures present within the orbit include the globe, extraocular muscles, optic nerve sheath complex, intracanalicular and intracranial optic nerves and chiasm, intraorbital vessels, lacrimal gland, and orbital fat. All these structures are contained by a bony margin.

The bony orbit is shaped like a four-sided pyramid. The neurovascular structures enter from the apex. The globe is located at the base. The orbital roof is made up of the frontal bone anteriorly and the lesser wing of the sphenoid posteriorly. The lateral orbital wall is formed by the frontal and zygomatic bones as well as the greater wing of the sphenoid. The orbital floor is formed by the maxilla and portions of the zygomatic and palatine bones. The medial wall is composed of the maxilla, the lacrimal, and the ethmoid bones. The junction of the bones leads to the formation of fissures. The superior orbital fissure is demarcated laterally by the greater wing of the sphenoid and medially by the lesser wing. The cranial nerves III, IV, V-1, and VI, the superior ophthalmic vein, and sympathetic fibers traverse this fissure. The inferior orbital fissure is demarcated laterally by the greater wing of the sphenoid and medially by the maxillary bone. The inferior ophthalmic vein, cranial nerve V-2, and the infraorbital artery traverse this fissure. The optic canal perforates the lesser wing of the sphenoid and contains the optic nerve, the ophthalmic artery, and sympathetic fibers.

The globe fills the anterior third of the orbit. It is somewhat ovoid in shape. The external surface of the globe is fibrous and is made up of the sclera posteriorly and the cornea anteriorly. The middle layer of the globe is highly vascular and includes the choroid posteriorly and the iris and ciliary body anteriorly. The internal layer is the retina. The lens is present in the anterior aspect of the globe. It separates the anterior chamber, filled with aqueous humor, from the posterior chamber, filled with the gelatinous vitreous body. The radius of curvature of the anterior chamber is smaller than that of the posterior chamber. The posterior two-thirds of the globe sits in a socket made up of a fibrous sheath called Tenon's capsule. The capsule is pierced by the optic nerve and extraocular muscles.

The optic nerve is a continuation of the diencephalon. It enters the orbit through the optic canal and continues anteriorly to enter the posterior aspect of the globe. Its neurons are continuous with the retina. The optic nerve is somewhat redundant in its course, curving laterally and inferiorly as it passes from the canal to the globe. The pia is intimately applied to the circumference of the optic nerve. Surrounding this is a thin subarachnoid space filled with cerebrospinal fluid (CSF) that is in continuity with the intracranial CSF. The arachnoid and dura make up the outer aspect of this optic nerve sheath complex. The dura as it approaches the orbital apex merges with the periosteal lining of the optic canal.

The extraocular muscles include the superior rectus and adjacent levator palpebrae superioris (the combination sometimes referred to as the superior muscle group), medial rectus, lateral rectus, inferior rectus, and superior and inferior oblique muscles. In the orbital apex, attached to the periorbital tissues around the optic foramen, is a fibrous ring, the annulus of Zinn. Arising from this fibrous ring and extending anteriorly are all the extraocular muscles except the superior and inferior oblique and levator palpebrae superioris muscles. The superior oblique and levator palpebrae superioris muscles arise individually from the periorbital tissues near the apex, while the inferior oblique muscle arises from the anteromedial aspect of the orbit. All the rectus muscles directly insert into the sclera in the anterior half of the globe. The oblique muscles insert into the posterior half of the globe, the superior oblique having made an acute turn through the trochlea in the anterosuperior aspect of the orbit. Between the extraocular muscles is a thin fascial plane that defines a muscle cone. Processes within this muscle cone are termed intraconal, while processes outside it are defined as extraconal.

The lacrimal gland lies within the lacrimal gland fossa in the superolateral aspect of the orbit. The gland is posterior to the orbital septum and extraconal.

The remainder of the intraorbital contents are retrobulbar fat, arteries, veins, and nerves. Structures relatively often visualized include the superior ophthalmic vein, which enters the orbit through the superior orbital fissure and runs just inferior to the superior muscle group. The ophthalmic artery may occasionally be visualized. It enters through the optic canal and courses parallel to the optic nerve sheath complex.

The orbital septum is a thin connective tissue membrane. It is an extension of the periosteum around the anterior orbital margin, which extends centrally into the tarsal plates. This connective tissue membrane acts as a barrier to separate the preseptal soft tissues from the postseptal orbital contents.

MAGNETIC RESONANCE IMAGING ANATOMY OF THE ORBIT

An understanding of orbital anatomy as demonstrated on MRI is mandatory for evaluating orbital pathology (Figs. 13-1 to 13-5).

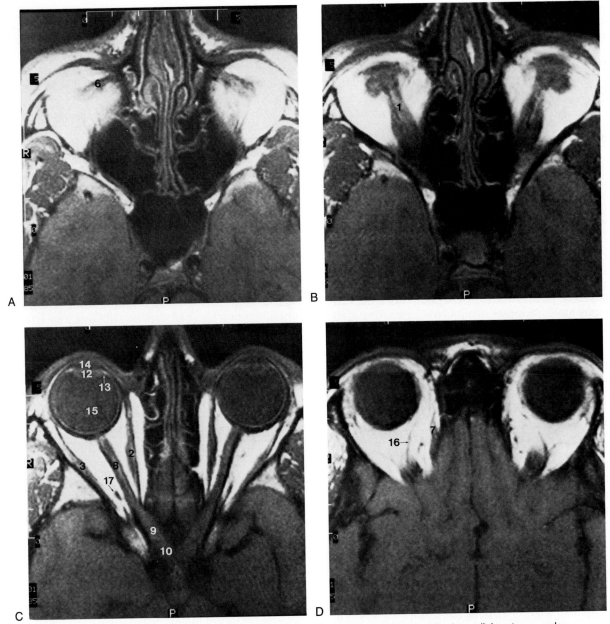

Figure 13–1. *A* to *F,* Normal anatomy, axial projection (600/26). 1, Inferior rectus muscle; 2, medial rectus muscle; 3, lateral rectus muscle; 4, superior rectus muscle; 5, levator palpebrae superioris muscle; 6, inferior oblique muscle; 7, superior oblique muscle; 8, optic nerve sheath complex; 9, intracanalicular optic nerve; 10, intracranial optic nerve; 11, optic chiasm; 12, lens; 13, ciliary body; 14, anterior chamber; 15, posterior chamber; 16, superior ophthalmic vein; 17, ophthalmic artery; 18, lacrimal gland.

The globe and retrobulbar fat are the dominant features within the orbit. Earlier studies used high resolution to study the ultrastructure of the globe.[29] The aqueous and vitreous humors are of low signal intensity on short TR images and high signal intensity on long TR and STIR images. The anterior and posterior chambers are separated by the crystalline lens. By means of high-resolution techniques, MRI is able to distinguish the external lens cortex from the lens nu-

cleus.[30] On short TR images the capsule appears of somewhat higher intensity than the lens nucleus. The ciliary body may occasionally be identified on routine orbital MR along the lateral margins of the lens. The choroidal and retinal layers of the globe can be differentiated from the sclera on short TR images by the increased intensity of the choroid and retina secondary to their vascular nature.

The optic nerve sheath complex appears as a homo-

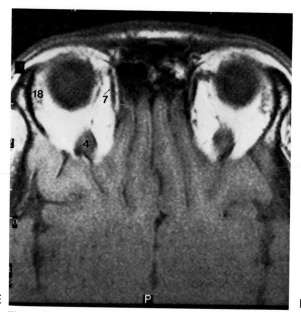 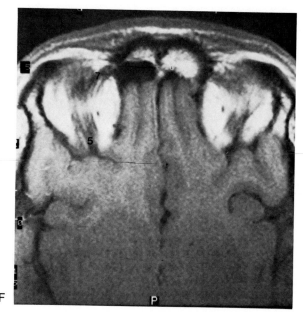

Figure 13–1. *Continued.*

geneous low signal structure within the high signal retro-orbital fat. Occasionally the optic nerve may be discerned from the surrounding hypointense subarachnoid space on short TR images. The intracanalicular portion of the optic nerve is generally visible because it is isointense to brain but surrounded by low-intensity cortical bone. With STIR imaging, particularly in the coronal projection, the high intensity of the CSF present within the subarachnoid space is seen to encircle the optic nerve entirely, which appears isointense to normal white matter. This is less obvious on T2 weighted images because of the chemical shift effect. The two optic nerves join to form the optic chiasm, which is well identified on coronal and sagittal images and somewhat less well seen on axial images.

The extraocular muscles are well visualized on MRI and appear hypointense to fat on short TR images. They appear slightly hyperintense on long TR and STIR images because of the relative decreased signal of retro-orbital fat. The margins of the extraocular muscles are smooth and regular and their insertions are tapered.

The superior ophthalmic vein is identified as a signal void just inferior to the superior muscle group. It runs from lateral to medial as it goes anteriorly. On some MR images, particularly coronal images, the superior ophthalmic vein may have high signal secondary to flow-related enhancement. The ophthalmic artery may occasionally be identified as a signal void adjacent to the optic nerve sheath complex.

The lacrimal gland is seen as an area slightly more hyperintense than the extraocular muscles but less intense than orbital fat. It is identified in the anterior superolateral aspect of the orbit. It is a crescentic shape and appears adjacent to the globe.

CLASSIFICATION AND DESCRIPTION OF ORBITAL LESIONS

The anatomic borders present within the orbit define certain compartmentalized spaces. Most pathologic processes within the orbit tend to arise within one of these compartments. Differential diagnosis may then be approached by knowing which lesions arise in which compartment. Probably the most useful delineation of orbital compartments was that provided by Bryan and Craig,[31] who divided the orbit into the following compartments:
1. Ocular
2. Intraconal with optic nerve involvement
3. Intraconal without optic nerve involvement
4. Muscular
5. Extraconal
6. Extraorbital

Table 13–1 lists the relatively common pathologic processes arising within each orbital component.

Ocular Lesions

This category includes congenital abnormalities of size and shape of the globe, a wide variety of tumors (of which retinoblastoma is the most common), and some other acquired ocular abnormalities that may mimic retinoblastoma clinically.

Congenital
Congenital lesions of the globe are generally associated with the globe either being too large or too small, or having some sort of defect.

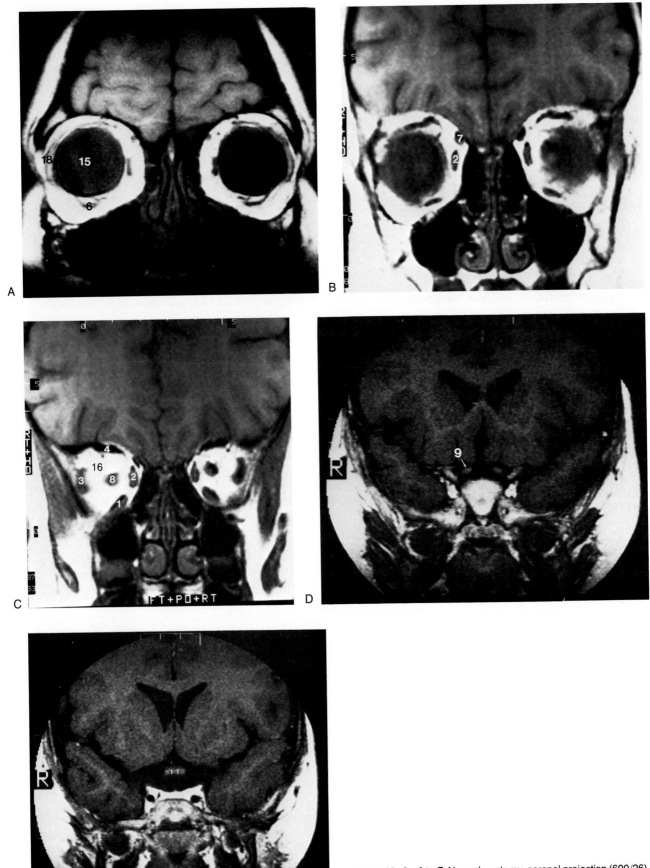

Figure 13–2. *A* to *E,* Normal anatomy, coronal projection (600/26). See legend to Figure 13–1.

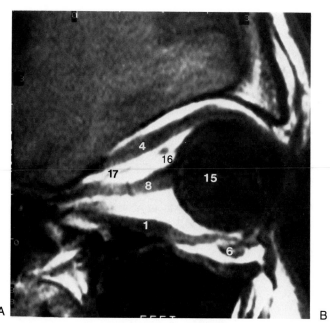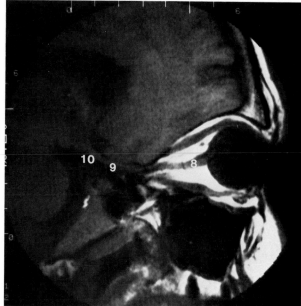

Figure 13–3. A, B, Normal anatomy, oblique-sagittal (600/26). See legend to Figure 13–1.

Table 13–1. CLASSIFICATION OF PEDIATRIC ORBITAL ABNORMALITIES BY ANATOMIC LOCATION

Ocular
  Microphthalmos
  Buphthalmos
  Coloboma
  Retinoblastoma
  Medulloepithelioma
  Choroidal hemangioma
  Melanoma
  Retinal detachment
Intraconal with optic nerve or sheath involvement
  Optic nerve glioma
  Meningioma
  Optic atrophy (septo-optic dysplasia)
  Optic neuritis
Intraconal without optic nerve or sheath involvement
  Capillary-cavernous hemangioma
  Leukemia
  Neurofibroma
  Schwannoma
  Pseudotumor
  Varices
Muscular
  Graves' disease
  Pseudotumor
  Rhabdomyosarcoma
Extraconal
  Rhabdomyosarcoma
  Lymphoma
  Lymphangioma
  Lacrimal gland lesions
  Neurofibroma
  Schwannoma
  Capillary hemangioma
  Infection
Extraorbital
  Neuroblastoma
  Ewing's tumor
  Fibrous dysplasia
  Craniofacial anomalies
  Facial–skull base tumors

ANOPHTHALMOS AND MICROPHTHALMOS. Anophthalmos, a congenital absence of the eye, is rare.[32] It occurs either as an isolated failure of the normal development of the optic pit or in association with a forebrain neural tube malformation. It may be familial. It has been associated with trisomy 13, Klinefelter's syndrome, and cerebral maldevelopments. Microphthalmos is more common than anophthalmos.[33] A retrobulbar cyst may or may not be associated with the small malformed globe.[34] Approximately 70 percent are unilateral. If an intraocular lens has developed, cataracts are common. Detachment and gliosis of the retina are also commonly associated with the abnormality. When the process is bilateral, it is often associated with CNS, cardiac, facial, or skeletal abnormalities.

The etiology of the lesion appears to be secondary to defective closure of the embryonic orbital fissure. Treatment generally consists of excision with the placement of prostheses through puberty to promote bony orbital development. CT shows rudimentary globe formation with irregular soft tissue density in the area of the globe (Fig. 13–6).[35] The MR appearance depends on the degree of development of the globe. In severely affected cases, only a small amount of irregular tissue is seen in the usual region of the globe. It is isointense to muscle on T1 weighted images and may be minimally hyperintense to retro-orbital fat on T2 weighted images (Fig. 13–7). When the globe is minimally affected, it appears normal on both short and long TR images except for a mild but generalized decrease in size. If proliferation of neural ectoderm at the margin of the embryonic fissure develops, a second cavity can develop that may form a cyst. In cases with associated cyst formation, only about 25 percent are bilateral. In a case reported by Wright and colleagues, the globes were

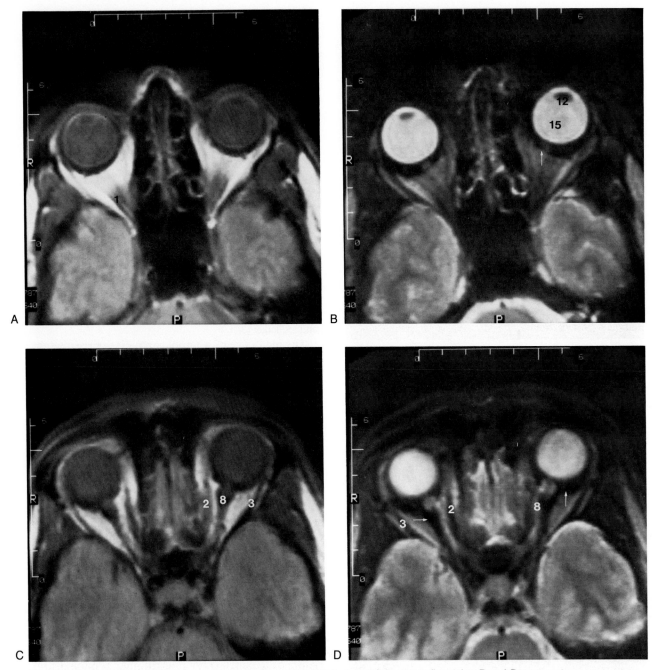

Figure 13–4. *A* to *D,* Normal anatomy, axial projection (2500/20,80). *A* and *C* represent first echo; *B* and *D* represent second echo. Note the chemical shift artifact (*arrows*).

bilaterally small in size but relatively normal in their architecture and signal intensity.[34] Bilateral retrobulbar cysts were present that had signal intensity consistent with water (Fig. 13–8).

CONGENITAL GLAUCOMA.   An enlarged globe is present in congenital glaucoma (buphthalmos).[36] This diffuse globe enlargement appears secondary to an abnormal trabecular meshwork in the angle of the anterior chamber leading to an obstruction of aqueous outflow. Increased intraocular pressure and optic nerve damage may result. Approximately 80 percent of cases are diagnosed within the first year. About 80 percent are bilateral. There is some evidence for inheritance through an autosomal recessive gene. Symptoms include photophobia, epiphora, corneal enlargement with a deep anterior chamber, and optic nerve cupping secondary to the severe increase in intraocular pressure. The optic nerve may ultimately be damaged.

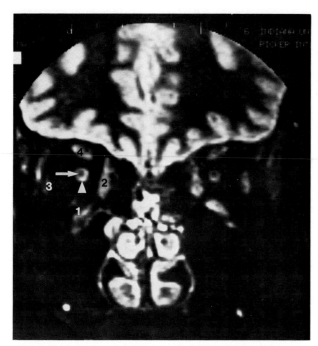

Figure 13–5. Normal anatomy, coronal STIR (2500/150/30). The normal optic nerve is seen as a central area of hypointensity (*arrow*) surrounded by hyperintense CSF (*arrowhead*). The normal optic nerve signal is similar to that of normal brain white matter.

Cases of globe rupture have also been reported. With MR, the intrinsic globe architecture and signal intensity generally appear normal, with only diffuse globe enlargement. Buphthalmos may also be associated with plexiform neurofibromas (Fig. 13–9).

COLOBOMA AND STAPHYLOMA. Coloboma is a congenital defect in a portion of the globe.[37] The coloboma may be anterior or posterior and may involve

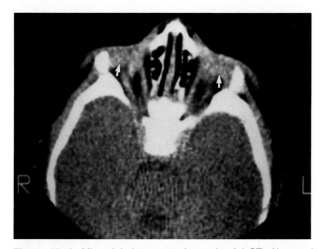

Figure 13–6. Microphthalmos, unenhanced axial CT. Abnormal irregular tissue (*arrows*) is seen in the region of the globe bed bilaterally.

the optic nerve head. The lesion is associated with incomplete closure of the choroidal fissure. Association with retinal detachment and congenital cataract is known. MRI easily demonstrates the outpouching of the globe margin (Fig. 13–10). The associated retinal detachment is also well identified, along with the congenital cataract. Coloboma may be differentiated from staphyloma, which is an acquired outpouching of the globe margin. This can occur anteriorly near the ciliary body, along the globe equator, or in a posterior location between the equator and optic nerve. This may be secondary to prolonged increased intraocular pressure or to a local decrease in resistance of the sclera by injury or infection.

Tumors

RETINOBLASTOMA. Retinoblastoma is the most common intraocular malignancy in children.[38] The tumor arises from precursor cells in the retinal photoreceptor line. These neural ectodermal cells may be similar to those seen in other primitive neural ectodermal cell lines.

The incidence of retinoblastoma is approximately 1 in 20,000.[38] Although the tumor is congenital in origin, it usually is not recognized at birth. The average age at diagnosis is approximately 18 months, and 90 percent of all diagnoses are made in children under 3 years old.[39] No sex preference or preference with respect to the right or left eye has been noted.

Approximately 70 percent of the tumors are unilateral; 30 percent of patients have tumors in both eyes.[39] About 30 percent of orbital tumors are multifocal within one eye. The presence of a bilateral lesion is a manifestation of the genetic transmission of this disease.[40] All patients with bilateral retinoblastoma, and approximately 15 percent of those with unilateral disease, carry a retinoblastoma gene.[39] These genetic forms are centered on the long arm of chromosome 13, generally autosomal dominant, and have a 95 percent penetrance.[41] These genetically transmitted tumors are diagnosed at an earlier age than are nonheritable tumors; thus, a child diagnosed with retinoblastoma before 1 year of age needs to be followed very carefully for the probable development of bilateral disease. Patients with genetically transmittable retinoblastoma also appear to have a propensity for the development of second malignancies, usually osteogenic sarcomas, remote from the orbit, which may appear years after the retinoblastomas.[42] These same patients are also susceptible to radiation-induced tumors.[42] An associated pineal tumor, the so-called trilateral retinoblastoma, has also been described. The tumor shares a neural ectodermal origin, and indeed retinoblastoma and pinealoma may be indistinguishable pathologically.

The most common clinical sign in retinoblastoma is a white pupillary reflex, leukokoria, which is present in approximately 60 percent of patients.[39] A whitish-pink fundus mass is noted at examination. Exophthalmos

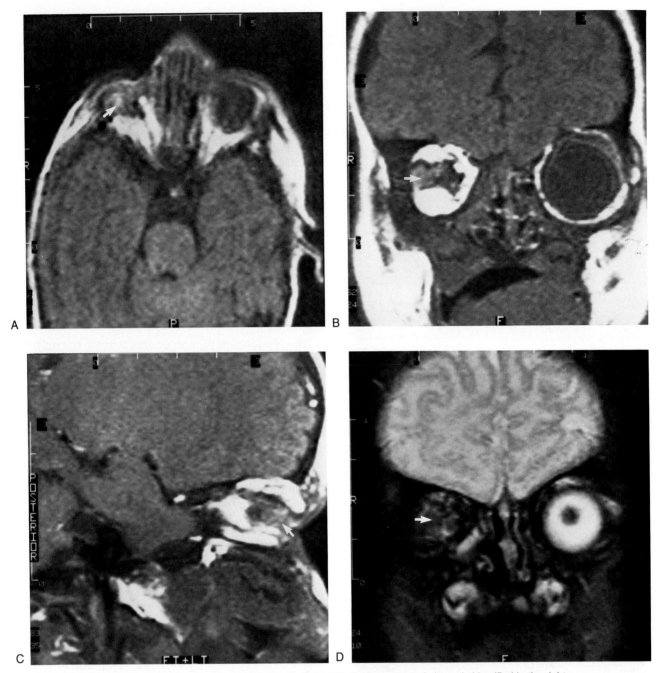

Figure 13–7. *Right microphthalmos.* ***A*** to ***C,*** (600/26); ***D,*** (2500/80). Rudimentary soft tissue is identified in the right globe bed (*arrows*). A normal left globe is evident.

may be present and occurs when the tumor has extended into the orbit. Most cases, however, demonstrate only intraocular extension into the vitreous, which is termed endophytic. Exophytic extension may be identified as the tumor extends into the region of the sclera, commonly causing an associated retinal detachment. Extension into the optic nerve, and particularly into the subarachnoid space surrounding the optic nerve, is a pathway for intracranial extension and is the most common cause of death in these patients. Ap-

proximately 13 percent of patients demonstrate this extraocular extension at presentation.[43] Hematogenous metastases may develop secondary to tumor seeding through choroidal blood vessels, and about 40 percent of deaths related to retinoblastoma are secondary to these distant metastatic lesions.[43] Interestingly, 50 cases of complete and spontaneous regression of tumor, similar to that seen in neuroblastoma, have been documented.[44]

The tumor consists of undifferentiated, small,

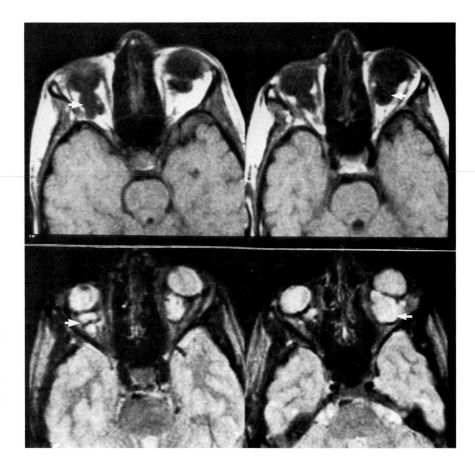

Figure 13–8. Bilateral microphthalmos with retro-orbital cyst. Upper row, 600/20; lower row, 2500/80. Bilateral microphthalmos is identified. Bilateral retro-orbital cysts are seen (*arrows*). The cysts have signal intensity similar to that of vitreous. (From Wright DC, Yah WTC, Thompson HS, Nerad JA: Bilateral microphthalmos with orbital cysts: MR findings. J Comput Assist Tomogr 1987, 11:727–729.)

round, densely packed cells with hyperchromatic nuclei and scant cytoplasm.[43] Necrosis may be present as well as tumor blood vessels. Flexner-Winterstiner pseudorosettes are specific for retinoblastoma and represent viable tumor cells surrounding the lumen of a blood vessel.[43]

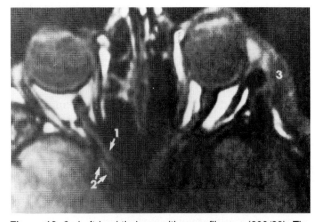

Figure 13–9. Left buphthalmos with neurofibroma (600/20). The left globe is enlarged. There is an associated plexiform neurofibroma present (3). The intracanalicular optic nerve (1) is well delineated from the anterior clinoid (2) on the opposite side. (From Atlas SW, Grossman RI, Axel L, et al. Orbital lesions: proton spectroscopic phase dependent contrast MR imaging. Radiology 1987; 64:510–514.)

CT markedly aids the diagnosis of retinoblastoma and remains the primary imaging modality, because of its superb ability to detect calcification. Over 90 percent of retinoblastomas demonstrate calcification on CT (Figs. 13–11, 13–12).[45] The calcification may be small, large, single, or multiple. The tumors enhance minimally with intravenous contrast material. Noncalcified tumors may be difficult to differentiate from retinal detachment or subretinal effusion on CT.[30] Extrascleral spread is demonstrated by tumor masses present within the orbit, with thickening along the optic nerve, commonly identified when there is optic nerve invasion.

On MRI the tumor may have variable signal intensities. Most cases demonstrate a mass extending from the retina into the vitreous that is hyperintense to the vitreous on short TR images (Figs. 13–11, 13–12).[30, 46] The tumor generally appears hypointense to vitreous on long TR images. Calcification is not generally appreciated on MRI, although some large calcifications may occasionally be noted as markedly hypointense foci on all pulse sequences. The tumor, however, may appear of markedly high signal on short TR images secondary to paramagnetic elements that may be deposited with the calcium.[30] The tumor, on occasion, also appears bright on long TR images secondary to tumor necrosis. MRI is superior to CT in the diagnosis of noncalcified retinoblastoma, which may be clinically

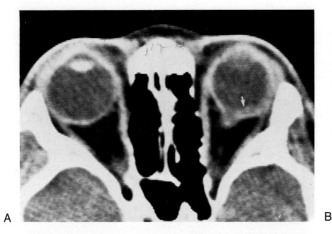

A

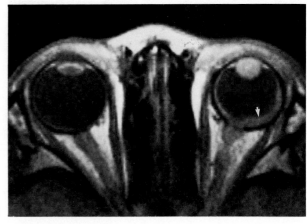

B

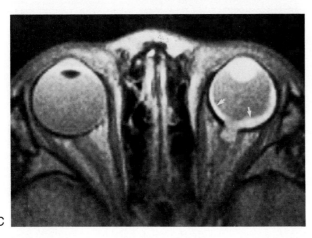

C

Figure 13–10. *Left coloboma.* ***A,*** Unenhanced axial CT scan. Note the posterior outpouching of the globe margin. A suggestion of minimal increased density along the posterior aspect of the vitreous is also noted (*arrow*). ***B, C,*** Axial MR scan (***B,*** 600/20; ***C,*** 2000/60). The coloboma is again identified. The associated retinal detachment is better appreciated on MRI (*arrows*). The vitreous fluid is hyperintense on both short and long TR images consistent with proteinaceous or hemorrhagic components. The left lens is also abnormal. (From Tonami H, Nakagawa T, Yamamoto T, et al. MR imaging of morning glory syndrome. J Comput Assist Tomogr 1987; 11:529–531.)

misdiagnosed or obscured on CT by retinal detachment.[30] Such detachment is most commonly hyperintense on both T1 and T2 weighted images owing to the presence of methemoglobin. The retinoblastoma is then seen as hypointense to blood on T1 and T2 weighted images. There so far is no experience with gadolinium enhancement of retinoblastoma. Orbital extension may be better appreciated on short TR images because it appears of lower signal than retrobulbar fat. Extension along the optic nerve should be demonstrated on STIR imaging as an intrinsic enlargement of the nerve. Foci of intracranial metastases have been reported to be of mixed signal intensity on short and long TR images and are not, by themselves, pathognomonic of retinoblastoma.[47] Intracranial subarachnoid spread should be identified as foci of linear or nodular enhancement on short TR gadolinium-enhanced images. The pineal region tumor, trilateral retinoblastoma, is seen as a mass relatively isointense to brain on T1 and hyperintense on T2 weighted images (Fig. 13–13).

For endophytic tumors, treatment consists of radiation therapy. Cure rates now approach 90 percent. When exophytic extension into the orbit is noted, resection of the globe and intraorbital mass is generally performed in association with radiation therapy, although cure rates are lowered. An intraorbital prosthesis is usually placed for cosmesis (Fig. 13–12A, E). In cases of widespread metastatic disease or subarachnoid spread, chemotherapy is generally added.

The differential diagnosis of retinoblastoma includes several disorders that clinically mimic retinoblastoma. CT is superior in the detection of calcified retinoblastoma, but MRI can still play a role in imaging these patients. MRI appears to differentiate other causes of leukokoria from retinoblastoma. This is significant in that one study from a large referral eye hospital found that in most patients referred to them for evaluation of retinoblastoma, leukokoria was caused by conditions other than retinoblastoma.[48] These included persistent hyperplastic primary vitreous, Coats' disease, retrolental fibroplasia, and *Toxocara* infection. These are discussed below. In addition, MRI may better evaluate optic nerve extension and intracranial subarachnoid extension. The MR evaluation of extension may require fat suppression techniques and the use of gadolinium.

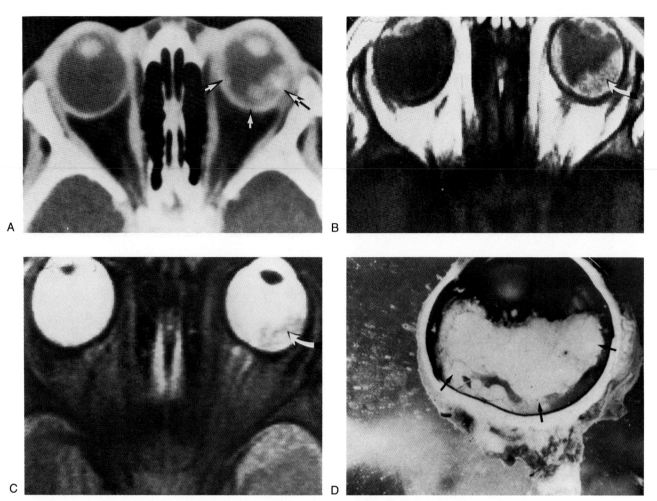

Figure 13–11. *Retinoblastoma.* ***A,*** Enhanced axial CT demonstrates a mass extending into the vitreous of the left globe. Foci of calcification are seen. The mass may be multicentric (*arrows*). ***B*** (500/30), A hyperintense mass (*arrow*) is seen extending into the vitreous. Calcification is not identified. ***C*** (2000/120), The tumor (*arrow*) is now seen to be hypointense with respect to normal vitreous. ***D,*** Sagittal section of the gross specimen demonstrates a large mass (*arrows*) extending into the vitreous. (From Sullivan JA, Harms SE. Characterization of orbital lesions by surface coil MR imaging. Radiographics 1987; 7:9–28.)

RARE TUMORS.   Melanoma of the globe is rare in children (personal communication, JJ Augsburger, 1989). The appearance of melanoma of the globe has been well described in the adult literature.[12] On CT the melanoma is seen as a soft tissue density projecting into the vitreous. Associated retinal detachment may obscure the mass (Fig. 13–14). The melanin pigment is paramagnetic and results in a shortened T1. This leads to the appearance of a markedly hyperintense mass on the short TR images (Fig. 13–15*A*). The lesion is generally hypointense to vitreous on long TR images. Separation of melanoma from associated retinal detachment is possible (Fig. 13–15*B,C*).[49]

Medulloepithelioma is a congenital nonpigmented ciliary epithelial tumor usually arising in the ciliary body.[43] Malignant degeneration can occur. Portions may be cystic. It is diagnosed at a mean age of 5 years and is almost always unilateral.[43] Reported CT findings are of a small mass of soft tissue density.[50] Occasional calcification may be present. MR findings have been reported to show a hyperintense mass on both T1 and T2 weighted images.[51]

Choroidal hemangioma is a benign vascular tumor. It is moderately hyperintense to vitreous on T1 weighted images and slightly hyperintense on T2 weighted studies (Fig. 13–16).[51]

The astrocytic hamartoma is a benign lesion of the retina or optic nerve head associated with tuberous sclerosis.[52] The MR findings of this tumor have not been described.

Ocular metastasis is not common in adults and is very rare in children.

Miscellaneous Ocular Lesions

PERSISTENT HYPERPLASTIC PRIMARY VITREOUS (PHPV).   PHPV represents a persistence of the primitive hyaloid artery and the primary vitreous. The hy-

Text continues on page 340.

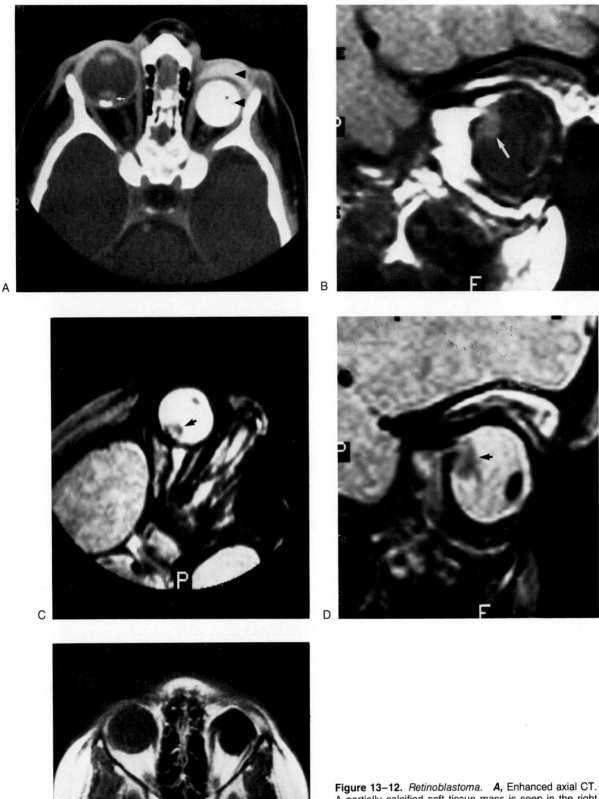

Figure 13–12. *Retinoblastoma.* ***A,*** Enhanced axial CT. A partially calcified soft tissue mass is seen in the right globe (*arrow*). The patient had previous left globe enucleation for retinoblastoma. An orbital prosthesis is in place (*arrowheads*). ***B*** (600/26), A sagittal image demonstrates a slightly hyperintense mass (*arrow*) extending into the vitreous. No calcification is seen. ***C, D*** (2500/80), Axial and sagittal images demonstrate the retinoblastoma (*arrow*) as hypointense with respect to vitreous. ***E,*** Orbital prosthesis (600/26). The left prosthesis can be imaged without difficulty by MRI. The remainder of the left orbit can also be evaluated in most cases.

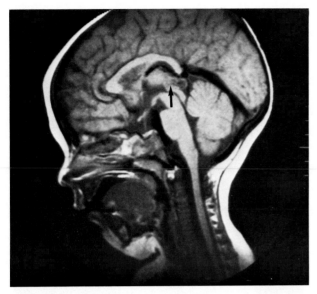

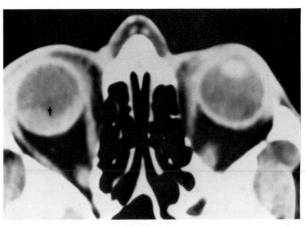

Figure 13–14. Melanoma. Enhanced axial CT. A soft tissue density mass is seen extending into the vitreous of the right globe (*arrow*). With CT alone, the mass may occasionally be obscured by retinal detachment.

Figure 13–13. Trilateral retinoblastoma (600/26). Sagittal image demonstrates a mass (*arrow*) in the region of the pineal gland. This pineal tumor was present in a patient who had had previous bilateral orbital retinoblastomas.

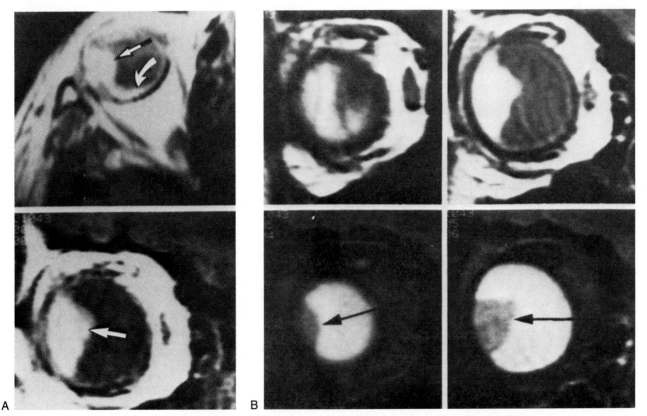

A   B

Figure 13–15. *Melanoma.* **A** (500/20), Axial (*top*) and coronal (*bottom*) T1 weighted images demonstrate an area of marked hyperintensity extending into the vitreous (*straight arrow*). Subretinal fluid (*curved arrow*) can be seen as a lens-shaped collection on the axial image but cannot be separated from the tumor on the coronal image. **B** (top, 2000/20; bottom, 2000/80), On the T2 weighted images the tumor (*arrow*) is hypointense with respect to the normal vitreous. The signal intensity of the subretinal fluid remains hyperintense on the T2 weighted images and cannot be distinguished from the vitreous. (Peyster RG, Augsburger JJ, Shields JA, et al. Intraocular tumors: evaluation with MR imaging. Radiology 1988; 168:773–779.)

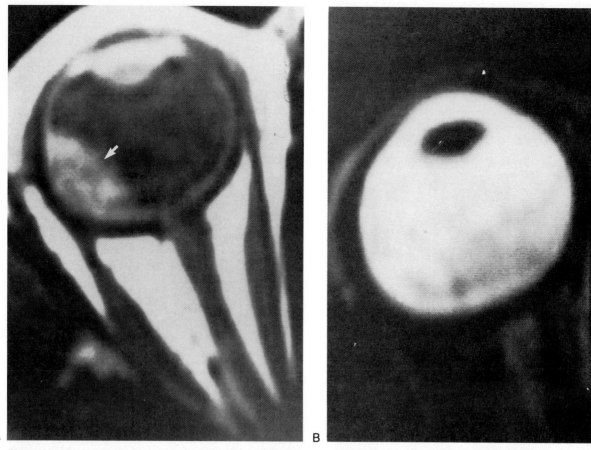

A   B

Figure 13–16. *Choroidal hemangioma.* ***A*** (500/20), Hyperintense mass (*arrow*) is identified extending into the vitreous of the right globe. ***B*** (2000/80), The hemangioma becomes isointense to the surrounding vitreous. (From Peyster RG, Augsburger JJ, Shields JA, et al. Intraocular tumors: evaluation with MR imaging. Radiology 1988; 168:773–779.)

aloid artery is an embryologic vessel that runs from the ophthalmic artery to the posterior aspect of the lens. By the 8th month of gestation the hyaloid vascular system has regressed. During this same time, the primary vitreous, which is vascular in nature, is replaced by the secondary vitreous or adult vitreous, which is more gelatinous. Cloquet's canal represents the collapsed residual primary vitreous and regressed vessels. This thin canal runs between the optic nerve head and the posterior surface of the lens.

Clinically, this lesion is generally diagnosed early in life.[53] It is the second most common cause of leukokoria in children.[54] Ninety percent are unilateral. Associated findings are macular hypoplasia, cataracts, glaucoma, and retinal detachment. Norrie's disease is also associated with retrolental vascular masses and is considered by some to be an X-linked recessive form of PHPV.

On CT, PHPV is generally diagnosed by the finding of increased attenuation within a small globe.[55] The increased attenuation is diffuse within the vitreal chamber. Occasionally a tubular intravitreal density

consistent with Cloquet's canal can be visualized (Fig. 13–17A). There may be minimal enhancement. A blood level may also be noted with dependent imaging. It is particularly noteworthy that no calcification is present. This, along with the decreased globe size, helps to differentiate most cases of PHPV from retinoblastoma.

MR imaging of PHPV has demonstrated abnormal increased signal on the short TR images in a microphthalmic eye (Figs. 13–17B, C, 13–18, 13–19). This increased signal intensity is related to the proteinaceous nature of the vascular primary vitreous. Occasionally Cloquet's canal can be visualized as a curvilinear, thin, low-signal structure. On T2 weighted imaging, the vitreous remains hyperintense (Fig. 13–17D); this helps differentiate PHPV from retinoblastoma, which is generally hypointense to vitreous on T2 weighted images. If free blood is also noted, a blood fluid level may be seen, with the signal intensity of the blood determined by the hemoglobin breakdown product that is present.

COATS' DISEASE. Coats' disease is a vascular ab-

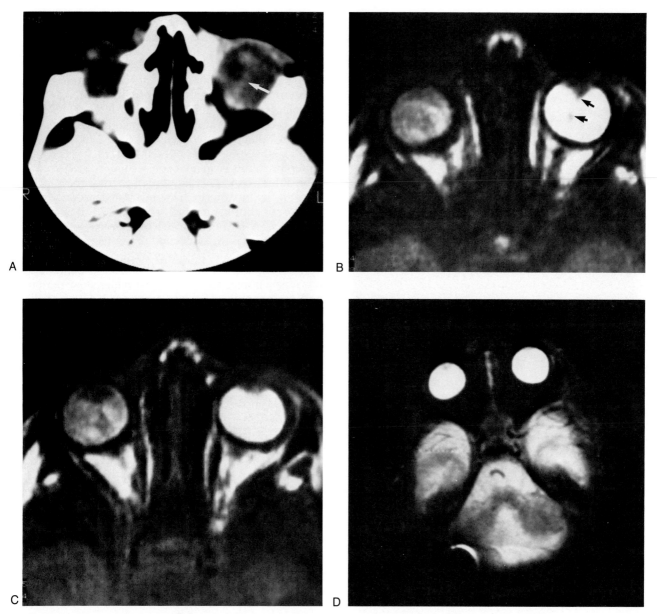

Figure 13–17. *Persistent hyperplastic primary vitreous (PHPV).*   ***A,*** Unenhanced axial CT. This image, part of a routine head examination, demonstrates increased density in the left globe. There is a suggestion of a linear density (*arrow*) extending from the lens to the posterior aspect of the globe (Cloquet's canal). ***B, C,*** Axial MRI (600/26). Marked hyperintensity is identified in the vitreous of the left globe. There is a suggestion of a linear strand extending from the region of the lens toward the posterior aspect of the globe (*arrows*). The signal intensity of the right vitreal chamber is also abnormally increased. This patient was found to have bilateral PHPV. ***D,*** Axial MRI (2500/80). The vitreous demonstrates normal hyperintense signal intensity on this pulse sequence.

normality of the retina.[56] Aneurysmal and telangiectatic retinal vessels, which resemble those seen in von Hippel-Lindau disease, leak serum and lipid into the intraretinal and subretinal space. This lipoprotein exudate causes retinal detachment in approximately two-thirds of patients. No systemic abnormality is identified. Ten to 15 percent of cases are bilateral.[39] There is a 3 to 1 male predominance. Symptoms generally do not develop until there is retinal detachment. In those cases diagnosed before the patient reaches 4 years of age, all vision is generally lost in the affected eye.[56] Of patients in whom the condition is diagnosed after 4 years of age, approximately 50 percent are legally blind, but some vision is retained. Therapy is aimed at photocoagulation to obliterate the abnormal vessels.

CT scanning demonstrates diffuse increased density

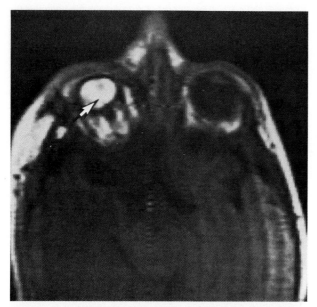

Figure 13–18. PHPV (500/30). Abnormal increased signal intensity is within the right globe. The globe itself is smaller in size than the left. (From Sullivan JA, Harms SE. Characterization of orbital lesions by surface coil MR imaging. RadioGraphics 1987; 7:9–28.)

in the vitreous chamber in a normal-sized eye (Fig. 13–20). Differentiation between Coats' disease and retinoblastoma without calcification may be very difficult.

MR imaging demonstrates increased intensity on the short TR images consistent with the presence of the proteinaceous and lipid exudate (Fig. 13–21).[46] The globe is of normal size. On T2 weighted imaging the vitreous remains hyperintense.

SCLEROSING ENDOPHTHALMITIS. Sclerosing endophthalmitis is an infection secondary to *Toxocara canis* infestation. This infestation is from the second stage of the larva form. The infection causes a severe chorioretinal inflammation. The mass itself is granulomatous. A fecal-oral route of transmission is presumed. There is an associated proteinaceous subretinal exudate.[57] Calcification is frequent; globe size is normal; and associated physical findings are fever and hepatosplenomegaly. Laboratory values show peripheral eosinophilia. The long-term progression of the disease in the orbit is toward the formation of intravitreal bands and cataracts. Final diagnosis is made with radioimmunoassay.[57]

The CT appearance of this infection is a calcified

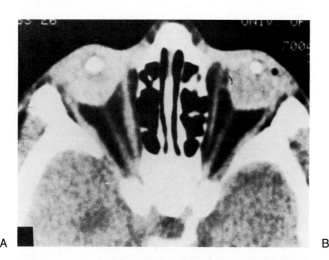

A

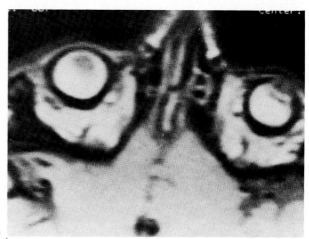

B

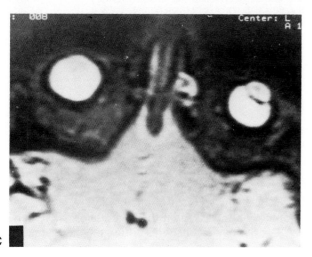

C

Figure 13–19. *Norrie's disease with bilateral PHPV.* **A,** Axial CT demonstrates abnormal increased intensity in the vitreous chambers bilaterally. The globes are also small bilaterally. **B** (2000/20), Abnormal increased intensity in the vitreous is seen. The small globes are again noted. **C** (2000/80), The vitreous signal remains hyperintense on this T2 weighted scan. (From Mafee MF, Goldberg MF, Greenwald MJ, et al. Retinoblastoma and simulating lesions: role of CT and MR imaging. Radiol Clin North Am 1987; 25:667–682.)

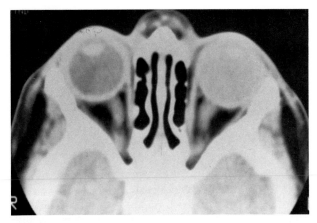

Figure 13-20. Coats' disease. Unenhanced axial CT demonstrates diffuse abnormal attenuation in the posterior chamber of the left globe, which is of normal size.

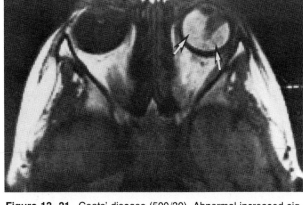

Figure 13-21. Coats' disease (500/30). Abnormal increased signal is seen in the posterior chamber of the left globe (*arrows*). The globe is normal in size. (From Sullivan JA, Harms SE. Characterization of orbital lesions by surface coil MR imaging. RadioGraphics 1987; 7:9-28.)

mass in the uveoscleral region of the globe.[57] There may be enhancement. This lesion most closely resembles retinoblastoma on CT examination. In one series from a major eye hospital, *Toxocara* infection was the most likely diagnosis in patients referred with possible retinoblastoma.[48]

With MRI the focal vitreal mass appears of high signal intensity on the short T1 image consistent with the presence of the proteinaceous subretinal exudate (Fig. 13-22A).[58] The granuloma appears markedly hyperintense on long TR images, even greater in intensity than the remainder of the vitreous (Fig. 13-22B). The high signal on the T2 weighted images helps differentiate this lesion from retinoblastoma.[58]

RETROLENTAL FIBROPLASIA. Retrolental fibroplasia is a retinopathy that occurs in premature infants

requiring prolonged oxygen therapy. Leukokoria may be seen unilaterally or bilaterally.[58] In most patients the history allows diagnosis of this condition. The increased oxygen stimulates new vascular proliferation, which may regress.[59] With continued therapy, however, intraretinal membranes and folds as well as vascular masses form that do not regress. Ultimately, lensectomy and vitrectomy may be necessary.

On CT the involved globe is generally small.[60] There is scattered increased attenuation in the posterior chamber, with some linear densities that probably represent scar formation.

On MR examination the involved globe demonstrates an abnormal increased signal on the short TR images consistent with the neovascular stromal proliferation (Fig. 13-23).[60] This is generally diffuse but can

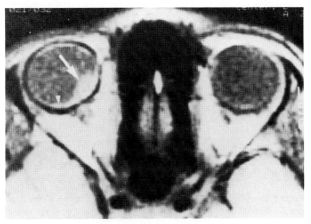

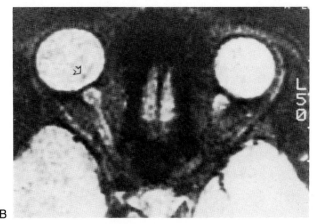

A   B

Figure 13-22. *Ocular toxocariasis.* **A** (2000/20), There is a hyperintense mass (*arrow*) along the posterior and medial aspect of the globe. An associated subretinal effusion (*arrowhead*) is also seen. **B** (2000/80), The mass and subretinal effusion are isointense on this sequence to normal vitreous. A small amount of scar tissue (*open arrow*) may be present. The increased signal of the mass on a T2 weighted image helps to differentiate it from retinoblastoma, which is hypointense to vitreous. (From Mafee MF, Goldberg MF, Greenwald MJ, et al. Retinoblastoma and simulating lesions: role of CT and MR imaging. Radiol Clin North Am 1987; 25:667-682.)

be more focal. The involved globe is small. On T2 weighted images the vitreous remains hyperintense.

HEMORRHAGE.   Hemorrhage within the globe can be exquisitely diagnosed by MRI. The pathogenesis of hemorrhage and its resultant MR appearance have been eloquently described by Gomori and colleagues previously and are detailed elsewhere in this book.[61] Retinal detachment (RD) is more common than choroidal hematoma (CH). Choroidal hemorrhage may be difficult to differentiate from RD except for the fact that CH extends into the region of the ciliary body (Fig. 13–24).[62] The blood does not extend into the region of the ciliary body in RD. MRI has proved valuable in making it possible to diagnose tumors within areas of RD or CH. Nonhemorrhagic effusions can also occur in the retina and choroid. Traumatic intraocular hemorrhage is discussed in the section on trauma.

Intraconal Lesions with Optic Nerve or Sheath Involvement

This category includes lesions of the optic nerve and the optic nerve sheath. Lesions of the optic nerve can be divided into tumoral and nontumoral. The tumor is the optic nerve glioma. Nontumoral conditions are optic nerve hypoplasia, as most commonly evidenced in septo-optic dysplasia, and optic neuritis. The primary optic nerve sheath lesion is the meningioma.

Tumors

OPTIC NERVE GLIOMAS.   Gliomas can affect the optic nerve, the chiasm, or both. These tumors repre-

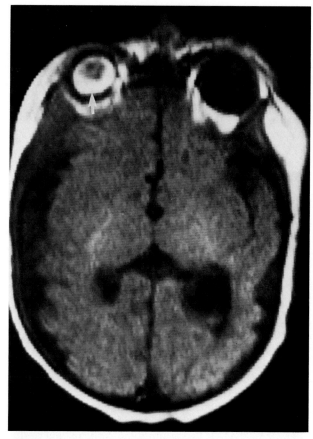

Figure 13–23. Retrolental fibroplasia (600/20). An abnormal increased signal is seen in the posterior chamber of the right globe (*arrow*). The globe is also small. No definite abnormality was identified in the left globe. (McArdle CB, Richardson CJ, Hayden CK, Nicholas DA, Amparo EG. Abnormalities of the neonatal brain: MR imaging. Part II. Hypoxic-ischemic brain injury. Radiology 1987; 163:395–403.)

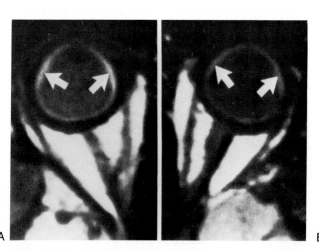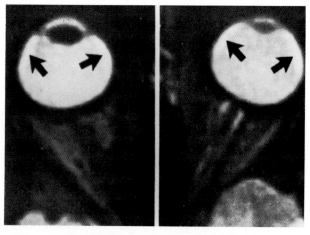

A   B

Figure 13–24. *Choroidal effusion.*   *A* (2000/20), Bilateral choroidal effusion is seen as a hyperintense layer around the periphery of the vitreous (*arrows*). *B* (2000/80), The choroidal effusion becomes similar in intensity to the vitreous. It may still be differentiated by its slight residual increased intensity (*arrows*). The hyperintense ring reaches the region of the ciliary body. Retinal detachment does not extend into this region. (Mafee MF, Linder B, Peyman GA, et al. Choroidal hematoma and effusion: evaluation with MR imaging. Radiology 1988; 168:781–786.)

sent approximately 6 percent of orbital tumors and 1 percent of intracranial tumors.[43] Some groups separate the intraorbital from the intracranial variety. Eighty-five percent present below the age of 15; the peak incidence is between ages 4 and 6 years.[43] There is a strong association with neurofibromatosis. The lesion can be unilateral or bilateral. Sixty to 70 percent of lesions have an intraorbital and an intracranial component.[43]

Extension of the chiasmatic lesions along the optic tracts is often noted. This is particularly true in cases associated with neurofibromatosis.

Pathologically these lesions are seen as a fusiform expansion of the nerve in any part of its course. The nerve is expanded by the tumor growth, but a significant portion of the identified swelling may be due to extension into the surrounding meningeal sheath.[43] Three different patterns of tumor growth have been described.[43] In the first there is glial hypercellularity with a slightly disordered arrangement; in the second the tumor may be cystic; the last resembles a juvenile astrocytoma. All three patterns found in children are different from the more malignant astrocytomas identified in adults. Malignant change in a child with optic nerve glioma is rare.[43] The association with neurofibromatosis is well described.[63] There appears to be no microscopic difference between the gliomas that are associated with neurofibromatosis and those that are not.[43] The tumors are exceedingly slow-growing. This has led to very conservative management, particularly for tumors purely intraorbital in location. Surgery appears to be reserved for the atypical progressively growing tumor. Serial radiographic imaging is performed to follow the tumor closely. Treatment of chiasmatic lesions generally consists of radiation therapy.

The tumors present clinically with visual loss and proptosis,[64] the former generally preceding the latter. Lesions in the optic chiasm may also present with symptoms secondary to hydrocephalus and diabetes insipidus.

CT was a tremendous advance in the diagnosis of optic nerve gliomas of both the intraorbital and the intracranial type. With pure intraorbital lesions the tumor may symmetrically enlarge the optic nerve in a fusiform fashion or may arise as a nodular exophytic extension (Fig. 13-25). The tumor itself is inseparable from the normal nerve tissue. Some lesions enhance after administration of intravenous contrast material, although the degree of enhancement is less than that associated with meningiomas and neurofibromas.[65] Calcification is unusual. The extension of the tumor into the optic canal can be demonstrated as well as chiasmatic extension, but this may be difficult in some cases because of severe bone artifact. Usually, with intracranial extension, enlargement of the involved optic foramen is noted on bone window images. The differentiation of glioma from meningioma can usually be made on CT examination. The optic nerve glioma is inseparable from the optic nerve itself, particularly on

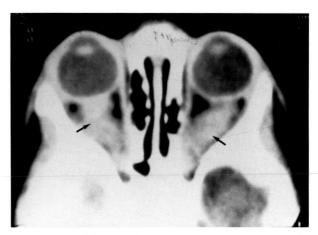

Figure 13–25. Bilateral optic nerve glioma. An enhanced axial CT scan demonstrates bilateral enlargement of the optic nerves (*arrows*). The optic nerves also become redundant within the intraorbital component.

coronal views. The meningioma, in contradistinction, tends to arise along the outside of the dural sheath. This leads to a "tramtrack" appearance of an enhancing tumor surrounding a relatively intact optic nerve. Differentiation of optic nerve glioma from optic nerve enlargement secondary to retrobulbar neuritis or pseudotumor may be difficult on CT.[66] Optic chiasm glioma presents as a mass in the suprasellar cistern. Without intravenous contrast enhancement the intensity is similar to that of the brain; with intravenous contrast there generally is marked enhancement (Fig. 13–26). Cystic portions may be present. Mass effect upon the third ventricle may also be noted, as may hydrocephalus. Extension of the tumor into the optic tracts may be difficult to appreciate on CT, particularly when there is associated neurofibromatosis.

MRI has been very helpful in the evaluation of optic nerve glioma, both in the intraorbital region and intracranially. Lesions in the orbit are relatively isointense to normal nerve tissue on short TR images, but can be markedly hyperintense on long TR studies (Figs. 13–27 to 13–31). In some cases the glioma remains isointense to brain on T2 weighted images.[66] Their gross morphologic appearance is the same as that seen on CT. The intrinsic nature of the optic nerve swelling may be better appreciated on MRI than on CT. STIR imaging of the orbit has been useful in evaluating these lesions. The prolonged T1 and T2 times associated with the tumors lead to a very hyperintense lesion within the optic nerve (Fig. 13–31*F, H*). Meningioma is often better differentiated by MRI than by CT because the direct imaging of the subarachnoid space on MRI serves to separate the normal nerve from the surrounding dural tumor. In most optic gliomas the intracanalicular spread is also well identified by MRI. We have had variable results with gadolinium enhancement in these patients. Most cases have been associated with neurofibromatosis and have shown no signifi-

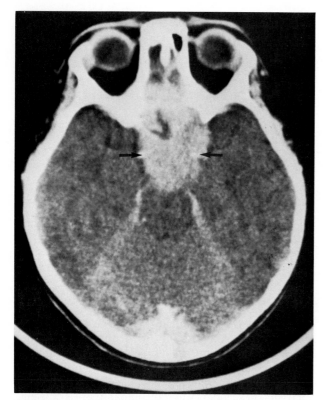

Figure 13–26. Chiasmatic glioma. Enhanced axial CT scan of the head demonstrates a rather homogeneously enhancing mass (*arrows*) arising in the region of the optic chiasm. The margins are relatively sharp. No definite extension along the optic tracts is seen.

cant enhancement with gadolinium (Fig. 13–32). One case, also associated with neurofibromatosis, did demonstrate enhancement (Fig. 13–31). Whether enhancing tumors are more aggressive remains to be seen. The chiasmatic lesions are generally of decreased intensity with respect to normal white matter on short

TR images (Fig. 13–33A). Cystic portions may show marked hypointensity. On T2 weighted images the tumor is very hyperintense (Fig. 13–33B). Marked enhancement of the tumor is generally seen on short TR images after gadolinium injection (Fig. 13–33C, D). The extension along the optic tracts is exquisitely identified by MRI. This is generally seen best on the long TR images, which demonstrate this extension as hyperintensity extending back toward the lateral geniculate bodies.[67]

MRI is the procedure of choice in the evaluation of optic nerve tumors, whether they be intraorbital, chiasmatic, or a combination of both.

MENINGIOMA. Intraorbital meningiomas are most frequently seen in middle-aged women, but can be identified in children. The tumors are generally associated with neurofibromatosis when they occur in the first or second decades.[43] Some meningiomas are primarily intraorbital and apparently arise from arachnoid cells in the optic nerve sheath.[43] Most orbital meningiomas, however, appear to arise in the region of the optic canal or sphenoid ridge and extend along the optic nerve sheath into the orbit. Pathologically the tumors are divided into three major categories: syncytial, transitional, and fibrous.[43] Some texts distinguish angioblastic meningiomas from the above three categories.

Clinically, patients present with visual loss and proptosis. Papilledema or optic atrophy may also be noted as well as motility disorders. Lesions that involve the superior orbital fissure may also demonstrate other cranial nerve abnormalities.

CT examination of intraorbital meningiomas demonstrates a mass that encircles the optic nerve sheath complex, giving rise to the "tramtrack" appearance (Fig. 13–34).[68] The mass may be mildly hyperdense and calcified on the noncontrasted study and demonstrate significant contrast enhancement after the injec-

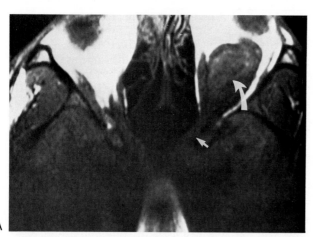

A

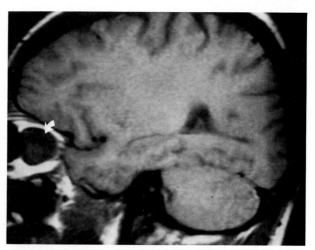

B

Figure 13–27. *Left optic nerve glioma (600/20).* **A,** Axial and **B,** sagittal T1 weighted images demonstrate an intrinsic enlargement of the optic nerve (*curved arrows*). The tumor appears slightly more exophytic than usual. No definite extension into the intracanalicular portion of the optic nerve is seen (*straight arrow*).

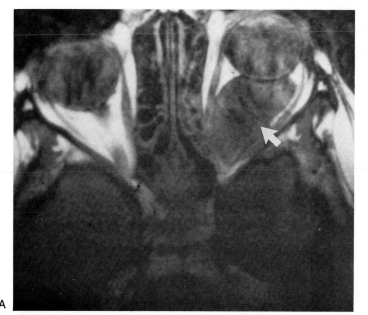
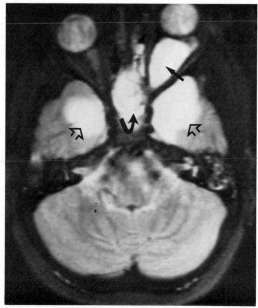

A   B

Figure 13–28. *Optic nerve glioma with intracranial extension.*   *A* (600/20), A large retrobulbar mass (*arrow*) is identified. On other images this could not be separated from the optic nerve. Globe motion causes some artifacts in the phase encoding direction. *B* (2500/80), The optic nerve glioma is hyperintense on the T2 weighted images (*straight arrow*). Extension into the region of the chiasm (*curved arrow*) and the middle cranial fossa (*open arrows*) bilaterally is noted.

tion. In some cases the CSF-containing space between the dural sheath and the optic nerve is evident. Intracanalicular extension may be difficult to appreciate on CT.

Similar morphologic findings are identified on MRI, with the exception that extension into intracanalicular region is better appreciated.[16, 69] The ability to separate the dural sheath meningioma from the optic nerve also appears better delineated by MRI than by CT. The mass is hypointense to fat on T1 weighted images and may have a variable appearance on T2 weighted studies (Fig. 13–35).[16, 69] The tumor may be iso- or hyperintense to fat on these images. Although no examples have yet been published, these tumors presumably also show significant gadolinium enhancement after the injection. Because of the enhancement, the tumors may actually be less well appreciated on routine T1 imaging because of similar signal intensity to that of retrobulbar fat. This may be a case in which fat-suppressed T1 weighted gadolinium-enhanced imaging is clinically useful.

The treatment of intraorbital meningiomas may involve surgical resection, but this remains controversial. Radiation therapy may also be employed. In many cases an expectant approach is undertaken, sequential imaging being performed and treatment reserved for significant enlargement or acute clinical deterioration.

Optic Nerve Hypoplasia

Optic nerve hypoplasia may occur alone or in association with other congenital abnormalities. With true optic nerve hypoplasia there is a decreased number of

axons within the optic nerve itself.[70] This may be secondary to failure of the ganglion cells in the retina and their axons to develop, or may be secondary to the degeneration of these ganglion cells. There may be an associated microphthalmos. Unilateral and bilateral abnormalities occur with equal frequency. Symptoms include blindness, strabismus or nystagmus, seizures, and hydrocephalus.[71] There may be visual findings ranging from decreased peripheral vision to complete blindness. Certain drugs can be associated with this entity, including phenytoin, quinine, meperidine, and steroids. Many metabolic neurodegenerative diseases can also be associated with this progressive atrophy.

Septo-optic dysplasia (de Morsier syndrome) consists of agenesis of the septum pellucidum with hypoplasia of the optic nerves and chiasm.[72] Pituitary infundibular hypoplasia is also present. In these cases there may also be associated short stature in addition to the visual symptomatology. Septo-optic dysplasia may also be associated with partial or complete absence of the corpus callosum, or schizencephaly.[71]

CT may show the hypoplastic nerves within the optic nerve sheath complexes, although this is not uniformly demonstrable. Septo-optic dysplasia on CT is manifested by absence of the septum pellucidum, a squaring of the frontal horns in the axial projection, and "pointing" of the inferior margins of the lateral ventricles on coronal images.[73]

MRI now appears to be the procedure of choice in the evaluation of congenital anomalies of the brain,[74, 75] and the evaluation of septo-optic dysplasia is no excep-

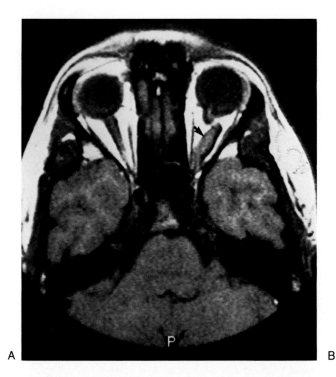

A

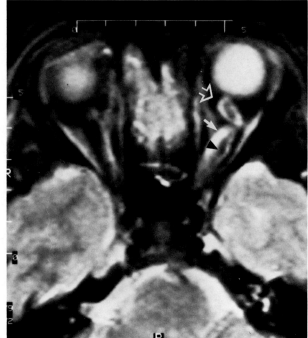

B

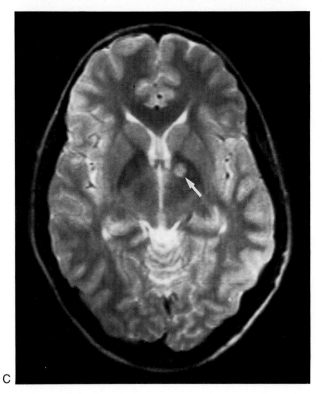

C

Figure 13–29. *Left optic nerve enlargement.* ***A*** (600/26), Abnormal enlargement is seen in the intraorbital portion of the left optic nerve (*arrow*). ***B,C*** (2500/80), At least a portion of the enlarged left optic nerve is not hyperintense on the T2 weighted image (*arrowhead*). Some of the hyperintensity may represent surrounding CSF (*straight arrow*). A chemical shift artifact also partially obscures detail (*open arrow*). The T2 weighted image of the head (***C***) demonstrates a focal area of increased signal intensity in the region of the genu of the left internal capsule (*arrow*). These lesions are commonly seen in association with neurofibromatosis.

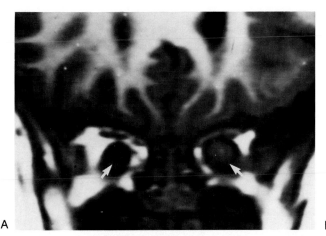
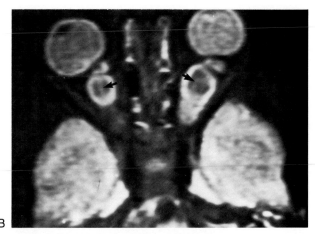

A   B

Figure 13–30. *Bilateral optic nerve enlargement.* **A** (600/20), A coronal T1 weighted image demonstrates bilateral enlargement of the intraorbital optic nerves (*arrows*) in this patient with neurofibromatosis. **B** (2500/80), The abnormal optic nerves remain relatively hypointense on the T2 weighted images (*arrows*).

tion. Similar findings are identified on MRI as on CT (Fig. 13–36).[71] The optic nerve and certainly the optic chiasm hypoplasia are better evaluated by MRI than by CT. STIR imaging of the orbit is particularly useful in differentiating the optic nerve itself from the surrounding CSF within the optic nerve sheath complex.

Optic Neuritis

Optic neuritis is much less common in children than in adults. Presumably this is secondary to the high incidence of optic neuritis in patients with multiple sclerosis, an adult disease.[76] No pathologic process other than demyelination has been noted in pathologically evaluated cases. The inflammation may be either in the retrobulbar portion or in the papillary portion of the nerve. In children it most commonly is associated with postviral encephalomyelitis.[77] It can also occur following bacterial meningitis, as a manifestation of disseminated sclerosis, or secondary to exogenous toxin or drug effects such as lead poisoning or chloramphenicol treatment.

The clinical symptom is an acute onset of visual loss that usually is rapidly progressive. Associated findings may be central scotoma and loss of color vision. Most cases of retrobulbar disease are funduscopically normal. Visual evoked response results may show decreased amplitude and prolonged conduction, but are commonly difficult to perform in children. The disease is generally self-limited, with improvement beginning after approximately 4 weeks; steroids may be useful in shortening this time. CT examination may rarely demonstrate an enlarged optic nerve in the acute setting, but most imaging results are normal.[31]

Recent studies using STIR imaging of the optic nerve have shown great sensitivity in the evaluation of optic neuritis.[18, 78] There is an abnormal increased sig-

nal within the optic nerve on STIR images (Fig. 13–37). The findings are similar to those of an optic nerve glioma except for the absence of mass effect. Preliminary evidence with gadolinium enhancement has shown a case of enhancement in the area of demyelination.[25]

Miscellaneous Lesions

Schwannomas or neurofibromas (discussed under Extraconal Lesions) may involve the optic nerve sheath. Extension of retinoblastoma and rarely metastatic disease may also affect the nerve or sheath. Inflammatory lesions (pseudotumor) and traumatic lesions that may affect the nerve sheath are discussed under separate categories.

Intraconal Lesions Without Optic Nerve or Sheath Involvement

Hemangioma

Hemangiomas can be divided into capillary and cavernous varieties. Capillary hemangiomas generally occur during the first year of life. The cavernous hemangioma is more common in adults but may occur occasionally in children. Although capillary hemangiomas usually extend onto the face and are extraconal in location, intraconal extension is not infrequent.[79] For this reason and because of the propensity for cavernous hemangiomas to occur intraconally, capillary hemangiomas are discussed under this heading.

Capillary hemangiomas often grow in size during the first year of life and then undergo spontaneous regression.[79] In most cases no treatment is necessary. These lesions are composed of a tangle of small, formed capillaries. The vascular supply is often from a combination

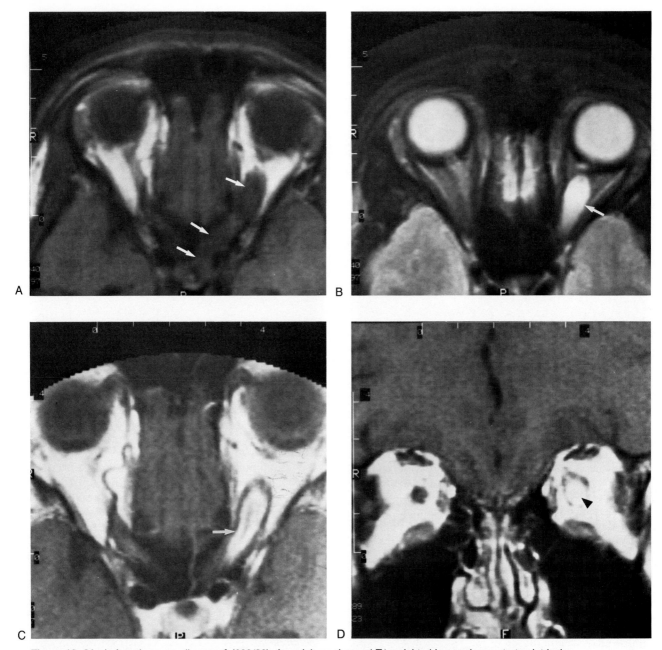

Figure 13–31. *Left optic nerve glioma.* **A** (600/26), An axial unenhanced T1 weighted image demonstrates intrinsic enlargement of the left optic nerve involving the intraorbital, intracanalicular, and intracranial portions of the optic nerve (*arrows*). **B** (2500/80), The axial T2 weighted image demonstrates markedly hyperintense signal within the optic nerve mass (*arrow*). This was seen to extend into the region of the chiasm on higher sections. **C** (600/26), This enhanced axial T1 weighted image demonstrates marked hyperintensity of the mass (*arrow*). **D,E,** Coronal enhanced T1 weighted images

of external and internal carotid artery branches.[79] As noted above, the lesion usually involves the skin surface. Extension may also be seen intracranially. These lesions are most commonly seen in the superior nasal quadrant. In many cases their margination is poor, with rather irregular borders.

CT demonstrates soft tissue density on unenhanced

studies with significant contrast enhancement after the injection.[79] Intracranial extension may be difficult to identify by CT.

MRI demonstrates a soft tissue mass that is isointense to muscle on T1 weighted images and very hyperintense on T2 weighted studies (Figs. 13–38, 13–39).[80] The signal characteristics are comparable

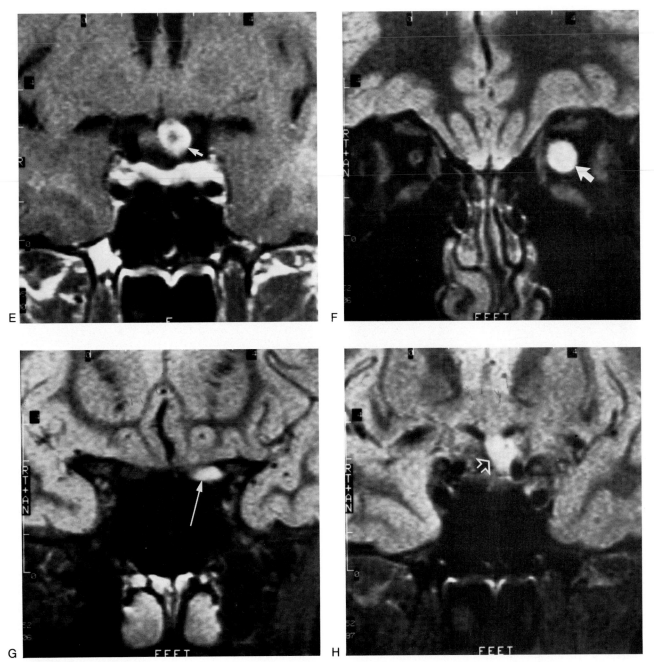

Figure 13–31. *Continued.*
again demonstrate the marked enhancement of the optic nerve tumor (*arrowhead*) with extension into the chiasm (*arrow*). *F* to *H* (2500/150/30), Coronal STIR images demonstrate marked hyperintensity of the optic nerve extending from the intraorbital portion (*thick arrow*) through the intracanalicular portion (*thin arrow*) and into the chiasmatic portion (*open arrow*) of the left optic nerve.

with those of cavernous hemangiomas in the orbit, although the capillary lesion does not share the smooth margination.

Cavernous hemangiomas are generally intraconal in location but can be extraconal or may bridge both spaces. The pathologic lesion consists of dilated vascular spaces without capillary formation and without sig-

nificant intervening parenchyma.[80] The lack of intervening parenchyma often leads to spontaneous intratumoral hemorrhage. Calcification is not infrequent.[66] Capillary hemangiomas generally come to attention because of the associated facial involvement, whereas cavernous hemangiomas generally present because of the mass effect.[81] Proptosis and blurred vision are the

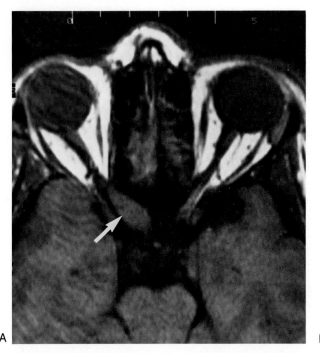
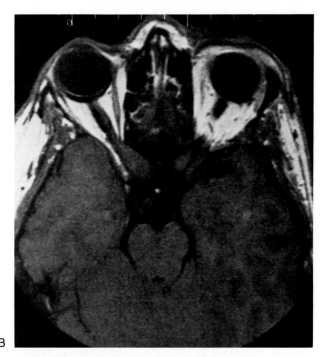

A   B

Figure 13–32. *Nonenhancing optic nerve enlargement (600/26).* **A,** The image before gadolinium administration shows an abnormal enlargement of the right intracanalicular and intracranial optic nerve (*arrow*). **B,** After intravenous gadolinium administration, no evidence of enhancement is seen.

most common clinical findings. Surgery is performed for those lesions with significant clinical symptomatology.

CT scanning demonstrates a well-defined and smoothly marginated mass, usually in the intraconal space (Fig. 13–40A).[66] This lesion may be isointense to muscle or slightly hyperdense. Foci of calcification may also be seen. Variable degrees of enhancement are present owing to the slow circulation present within the tumor.

MR imaging demonstrates a smoothly marginated mass that is relatively isointense to muscle on T1 weighted images (Fig. 13–40B, C).[49, 82] T2 weighted images demonstrate significant hyperintensity (Fig. 13–41). STIR imaging has also been used to evaluate this lesion and also demonstrates high signal intensity of the cavernous hemangioma (Fig. 13–42).[9] There is no experience at this time with gadolinium enhancement of these lesions.

Miscellaneous Lesions

HEMANGIOPERICYTOMA. Hemangiopericytomas are benign tumors arising from the pericytes of Zimmermann that surround the capillaries. This is a slowly progressive mass lesion that presents with proptosis and blurred vision. On both CT and MR imaging these lesions may appear identical to cavernous angiomas, although the margins may not be as sharp.[79, 82] It is atypical, however, for calcification to be present within the mass.

VASCULAR DISORDERS. Various abnormalities associated with the blood vessels may be seen in the intraconal location. Thrombosis of the superior ophthalmic vein can be identified by the lack of normal flow void within the structure.[78] The appearance of the signal within the veins depends on the hemorrhagic breakdown products that are present.

With cavernous carotid fistulas an increase in the size of the superior ophthalmic vein associated with increased flow may be identified.[30] There may also be associated enlargement of the extraocular muscles, and asymmetry in the size of the cavernous sinus, with accentuated flow void.

Orbital varices are a congenital proliferation of venous elements. These may present with proptosis and pain. The lesions enlarge upon maneuvers designed to increase venous pressure, such as the Valsalva maneuver or compression of the jugular vein. Both CT and MR results may be normal without a provocative maneuver to distend the varices. MRI demonstrates dilated veins with flow void during the provocative test.

UNCOMMON TUMORS. Schwannoma and neurofibroma can occur in the intraconal compartment but are more generally seen in the extraconal compartment. Other lesions, such as pseudotumor and metastases, have a similar predisposition for other compartments but can involve the intraconal region. Extension of ocular tumors can also lead to an intraconal mass.

Text continues on page 357.

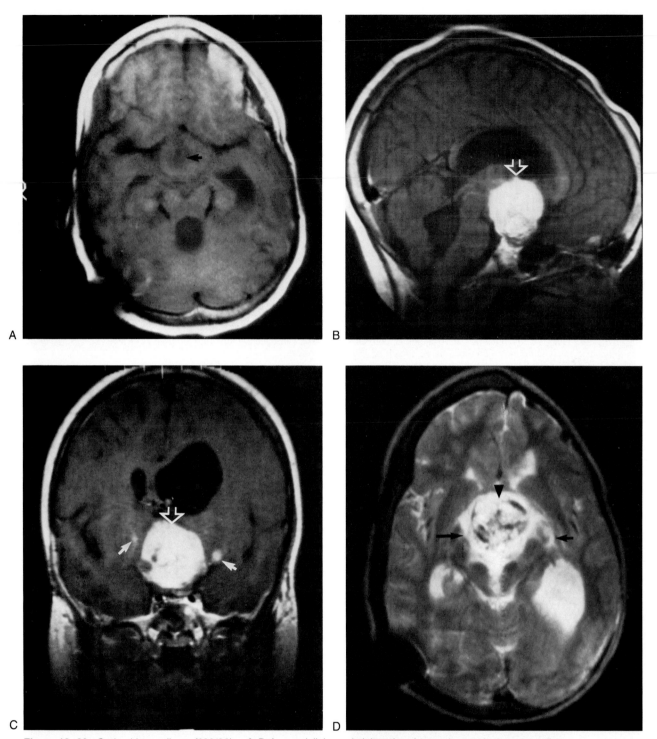

Figure 13–33. *Optic chiasm glioma (600/26).* **A,** Before gadolinium administration. A mass is seen in the suprasellar cistern with probable central necrosis (*arrow*). Obstructive hydrocephalus is identified involving the temporal horns and fourth ventricle. Artifact from a ventricular shunt is seen in the region of the right cerebellar hemisphere. **B** (sagittal) and **C** (coronal) views are taken after intravenous gadolinium administration. There is marked enhancement of the optic chiasm glioma (*open arrows*). There is mild extension of the enhancement into the optic tracts bilaterally as seen on the coronal view (*closed arrows*). **D** (2500/80), This unenhanced T2 weighted image demonstrates an inhomogeneous tumor (*arrowhead*). Extension of abnormal signal intensity along both optic tracts is identified (*arrows*).

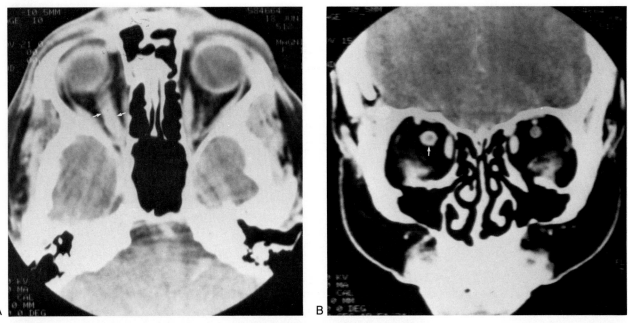

Figure 13–34. *Perioptic meningioma.* ***A,*** Axial and ***B,*** coronal enhanced CT images demonstrate a partially calcified and enhancing mass surrounding the optic nerve sheath on the right (*arrows*).

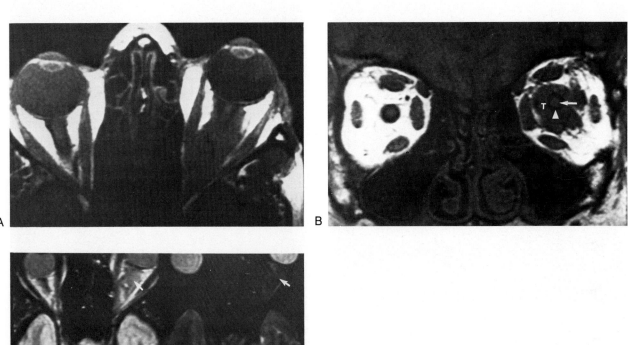

Figure 13–35. *Perioptic meningioma.* ***A,B*** (600/20), A mass is identified surrounding the optic nerve on these T1 weighted images. The perioptic nature of the process is best identified on the coronal view. The tumor (T) can be separated from the optic nerve (*arrow*) and the surrounding CSF (*arrowhead*). ***C*** (2500/20,80), Proton density and T2 weighted images demonstrate no increased signal intensity of the meningioma (*arrows*).

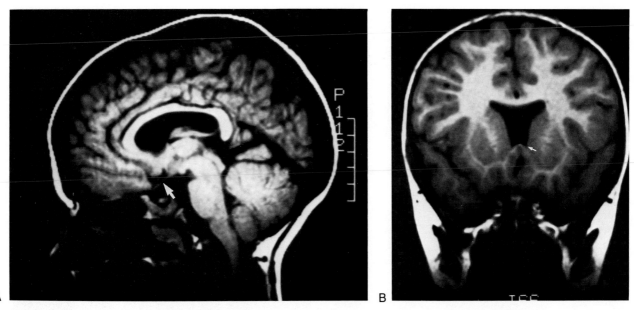

Figure 13–36. *Septo-optic dysplasia (600/20).* The sagittal view (*A*) of the head demonstrates a hypoplastic optic chiasm (*arrow*). The coronal image (*B*) shows the lack of septum pellucidum. Slight inferior pointing of the frontal horns is also seen (*arrow*). (Courtesy of Sharon Byrd, M.D., Chicago.)

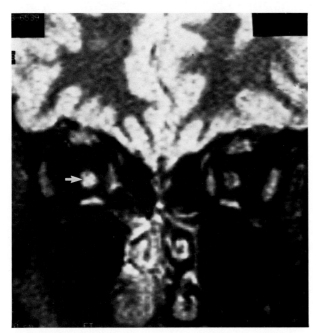

Figure 13–37. Right optic neuritis (2500/150/30). This STIR image demonstrates abnormal signal intensity within the right optic nerve (*arrow*). The left optic nerve is normal.

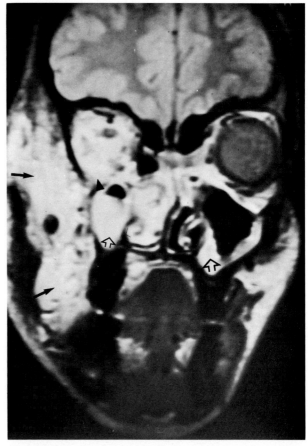

Figure 13–38. Capillary hemangioma (2500/20). A large hyperintense mass is seen over the right face (*closed arrows*). There is extension into the right retrobulbar region (*arrowhead*). Paranasal sinus disease is also seen bilaterally (*open arrows*).

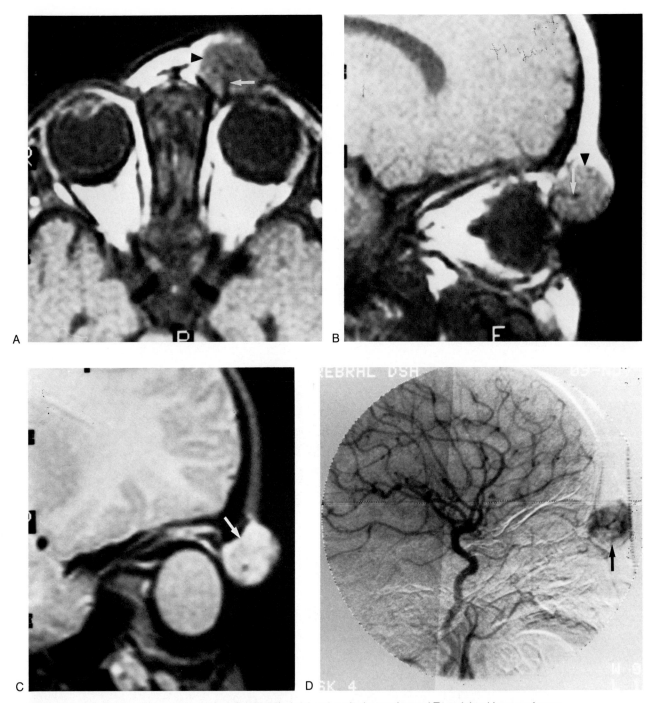

Figure 13–39. *Cavernous hemangioma.* ***A,B*** (600/26), Axial and sagittal nonenhanced T1 weighted images demonstrate a well-demarcated mass anterior and medial to the globe (*arrowheads*). There is a prominent feeding vessel in the posterior half of the mass (*arrow*). ***C*** (2500/80), Sagittal T2 weighted image demonstrates marked hyperintensity of the hemangioma (*arrow*). ***D,*** Lateral intra-arterial digital subtraction angiography (DSA) demonstrates a blush of the tumor (*arrow*). This is slightly atypical for cavernous hemangioma, but the pathologic examination was consistent with that diagnosis.

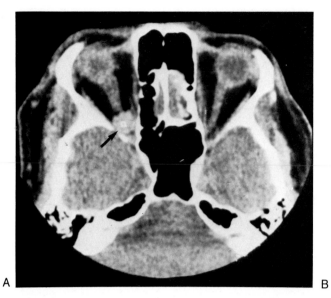

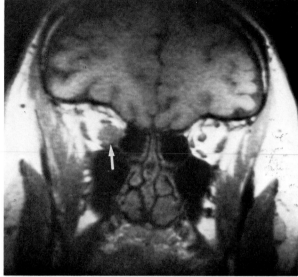

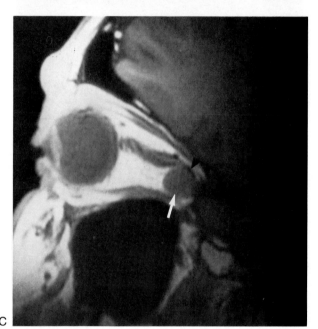

Figure 13–40. *Cavernous hemangioma.* ***A,*** Enhanced axial CT demonstrates a rounded, homogeneously enhancing mass (*arrow*) near the right orbital apex. A cursor overlies the mass. ***B,C*** (600/20), Coronal (***B***) and oblique (***C***) sagittal images identify the mass, which is isointense with muscle. The oblique sagittal view is particularly useful in demonstrating impingement of the mass on the optic nerve sheath complex.

Muscular Abnormalities

The two main abnormalities involving the intrinsic musculature of the orbit are Graves' disease and pseudotumor. Other lesions occasionally occur within the muscle, such as rhabdomyosarcoma, lymphoma, or metastatic disease, but because these more commonly originate in the extraconal space, they are described under that heading.

Graves' Disease

Approximately 2.5 percent of all cases of Graves' disease occur in children and adolescents.[83] The incidence of the ophthalmologic changes in pediatric pa-

tients with Graves' disease has been reported to range from 48 to 82 percent.[84, 85] Graves' ophthalmopathy was the most common cause of proptosis in children in a study from the Toronto Hospital for Sick Children.[86] The clinical course is more benign than in adults. In one study no cases of ophthalmoplegia, optic neuropathy, or corneal involvement were seen.[87] The ophthalmologic changes noted in Graves' disease can be seen as the first manifestation of this disorder.[66] The entity may also occur after successful treatment of hyperthyroidism. Most cases, however, occur at the time of or shortly after the discovery of the systemic thyroid abnormality.

It is presumed that the long-acting thyroid stimulat-

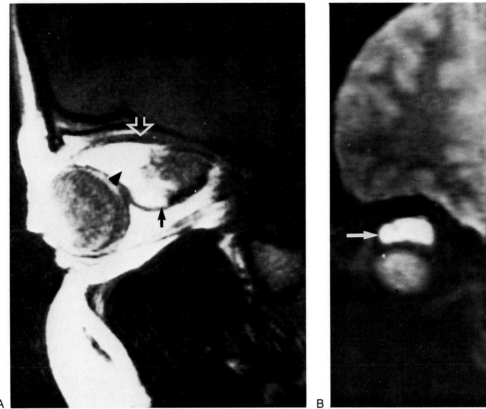

A   B

Figure 13–41. *Hemorrhagic cavernous hemangioma.* **A** (600/20), A well-circumscribed mass (*closed arrow*) is identified in the retrobulbar region just inferior to the superior muscle group (*open arrow*). There is increased signal intensity in
the anterior portion of the mass consistent with methemoglobin formation (*arrowhead*). **B** (2500/80), Coronal T2 weighted
imaging demonstrates the hemangioma as markedly hyperintense (*arrow*). This hyperintensity may be accentuated by the
presence of extracellular methemoglobin.

ing factors (LATS) cause an accumulation of collagen, glycoprotein, and mucopolysaccharides in the muscles as well as an increase in the amount of retro-orbital fat.[84] The treatment is primarily aimed at returning the patient to a euthyroid state. As stated above, studies suggest that most ophthalmologic complications that occur in adults are not seen in children; therefore, surgery to decompress the optic nerve in the orbital apex, as an example, is not generally necessary in children.

The CT findings of thyroid ophthalmopathy are well described.[66] There is an intrinsic swelling of the extraocular muscles. This enlargement is in a fusiform pattern with relative sparing of the insertions of the muscles on the globe. The medial and inferior rectus muscles are the most commonly affected. It has been reported that isolated lateral rectus muscle enlargement does not occur in this disease. It is common for the superior muscles also to be involved in the process. Although symmetry is not necessary for the diagnosis, most cases are bilateral. The muscles may demonstrate mild enhancement with intravenous contrast administration. The increased amount of retro-orbital fat is

evident by the degree of proptosis with associated stretching of the extraocular muscles and optic nerve sheath complex.

The MR findings in thyroid ophthalmopathy are similar to those of CT (Fig. 13–43).[16] No definite signal abnormalities on T1 or T2 weighted images are identified within the muscles themselves. The outline of the muscles, particularly in the orbital apex, may be better delineated on MRI than on CT.

Idiopathic Orbital Pseudotumor

Orbital pseudotumor is an idiopathic inflammation that is related to lymphoma. It occurs most commonly in middle-aged adults, but 6 to 16 percent of patients with this disease are under 20 years of age.[88] Pathologically, there is a polymorphic cellular pattern of inflammatory lymphocytes.[89] This inflammation always involves the orbital fat. Other intraorbital structures such as the extraocular muscles, optic nerve sheath, lacrimal gland, and episcleral region may also be affected. Approximately 53 percent of pediatric patients have significant constitutional symptoms, including headache, fever, vomiting, pharyngitis, and an-

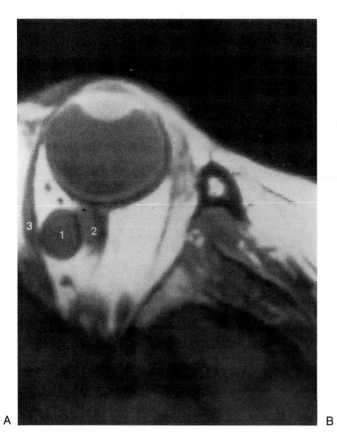

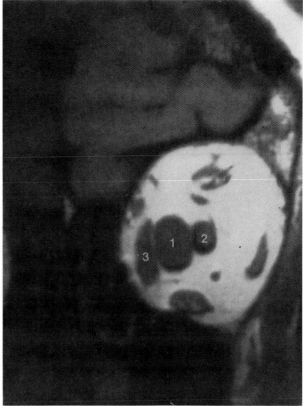

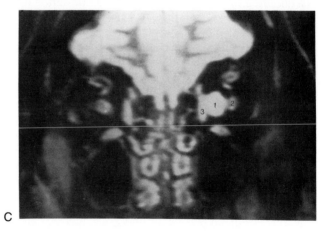

Figure 13–42. *Intraconal cavernous hemangioma.* ***A,B*** (600/20), A well-demarcated mass is seen between the medial rectus and the optic nerve sheath complex. 1, Mass; 2, optic nerve sheath complex; 3, medial rectus. ***C*** (2500/150/30), Coronal STIR imaging demonstrates the hemangioma as markedly hyperintense. (From Atlas SW, Grossman RI, Hackney DB, et al. STIR MR imaging of the orbit. AJNR 1988; 9:969–974.)

orexia.[90] These constitutional symptoms are generally absent in adults. Local pain, swelling, and ptosis are commonly found. Ophthalmoplegia, proptosis, and photophobia may also be present. Bilaterality of the process is more common in children than in adults.[91] The administration of prednisone leads to an abrupt cessation of symptoms and resolution of radiologic abnormalities. Imaging studies are aimed both at diagnosing pseudotumor and at excluding other more se-

rious causes that can mimic pseudotumor clinically, including lymphoma, rhabdomyosarcoma, neuroblastoma, and orbital cellulitis.

The CT appearance of pseudotumor depends on the main area of involvement.[45, 92, 93] In our experience, most cases have involved the extraocular muscles, so-called orbital myositis. The CT findings demonstrate enlargement of the extraocular muscles, especially the insertions (Fig. 13–44*A*). The involvement of the in-

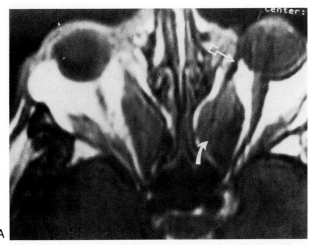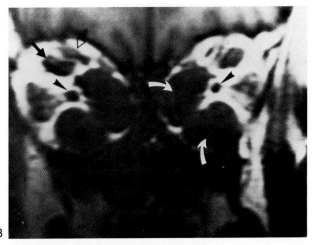

Figure 13–43. *Graves' ophthalmopathy (600/20).*   **A,** Axial and **B,** coronal T1 weighted images demonstrate marked enlargement of the rectus muscles. Predominantly involved are the medial and inferior rectus muscles (*curved arrows*). The optic nerve sheath complexes are well delineated (*arrowheads*). The superior muscle group, made up of the superior rectus (*solid arrow*) and levator palpebrae superioris (*open arrow*), is also seen. Sparing of the tendinous insertions is noted (*straight white arrow*). (Bilaniuk LT, Atlas SW, Zimmerman RA. Magnetic resonance imaging of the orbit. Radiol Clin North Am 1987; 25:509–528.)

sertion of the rectus muscles helps differentiate pseudotumor from Graves' disease. The muscle is uniform in intensity and may demonstrate mild enhancement; the margins may be smooth or somewhat shaggy. A second area of involvement is along the posterior aspect of the globe, episcleritis. This can occur alone or in association with muscular involvement. The abnormality may coat the posterior and lateral aspects of the globe, effacing all intervening fat. This finding is characteristic of pseudotumor as well as of lymphoma and leukemia. Pseudotumor may also extend along the optic nerve sheath. In the retrobulbar region it may form a rather well-defined mass that can at times mimic hemangioma. This idiopathic inflammation may also involve the lacrimal gland as its only manifestation; this generally appears as a homogeneous enlargement of the lacrimal gland. Bilateral involvement may be present in systemic diseases such as Wegener's granulomatosis, polyarteritis nodosa, or sarcoidosis. Lastly, the intraorbital fat may be the only area involved. This may be seen as a diffuse, mild, increased density of the fat with respect to the orbit on the opposite side.

MRI has been useful in the diagnosis of inflammatory pseudotumor.[26] In comparison with normal retrobulbar fat signal, pseudotumor is hypointense on T1 weighted images and relatively isointense on T2 weighted images (Figs. 13–44, 13–45). The findings on T2 weighted images help differentiate pseudotumor from other lesions such as metastatic disease. Lymphoma, however, may have a similar appearance on MRI; this may be secondary to the hypercellularity of these two entities. The morphologic characteristics are otherwise similar to those noted on CT. Recently, STIR imaging has been applied to pseudotumor and

demonstrates an increased signal intensity to the lesion with respect to the intraorbital fat.[9]

Extraconal Lesions

Lymphangioma

Lymphangiomas are tumors that usually occur in infants and children and are composed of endothelium-lined channels filled with a clear lymphlike fluid.[82] Septa with foci of lymphoid tissue are common. These tumors generally present with lid swelling, exophthalmos, and diplopia. These lesions slowly enlarge with time.[81] Because of the presence of lymphoid tissue, they may increase in size during various systemic infections.[81] They also have a propensity to hemorrhage, causing a sudden increase in tumor size and clinical symptomatology.[82] These lesions most commonly arise along the medial aspect of the orbit. Surgical excision is often necessary.

CT examination of lymphangiomas generally demonstrates a soft tissue density mass with relatively sharp margins (Fig. 13–46).[82] Small cysts and areas of acute hemorrhage may be seen. Contrast enhancement is inhomogeneous secondary to the cystic nature of these lesions. Calcification is unusual.

MRI demonstrates lymphangiomas as either iso- or slightly hypointense to fat on T1 weighted studies (Fig. 13–47).[82] On T2 weighted images the lesions are markedly hyperintense to fat. Hemorrhagic products are sometimes identified on MRI.[22]

Epidermoid and Dermoid

Both these developmental lesions result from the inclusion of extra elements during neural tube closure.

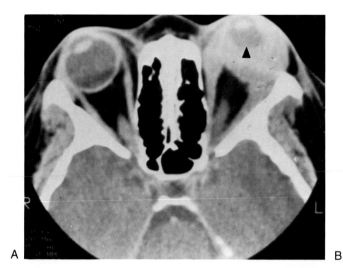

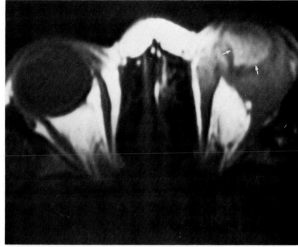

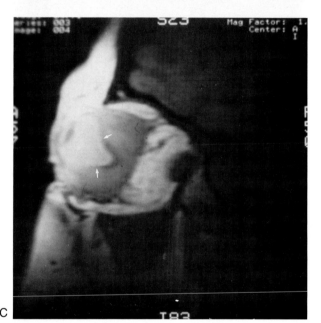

Figure 13–44. *Orbital pseudotumor.* **A,** Enhanced CT demonstrates marked thickening of the insertions of the medial and lateral rectus muscle on the left. There is coating of the globe margin by the mass. The globe (*arrowhead*) is anteriorly displaced and compressed. **B,C** (600/20), The intrinsic muscle abnormality is well identified on sagittal and axial T1 weighted images. The margins of the globe (*arrows*) are better delineated than on CT. The marked compression of the globe is evident. The signal intensity of the muscles is not significantly altered from normal, allowing for some surface coil artifact.

Dermoid tumors are relatively frequent, but epidermoid lesions are generally uncommon.[94] Approximately 25 percent are noticeable at birth; the remainder become apparent during childhood.[81] Epidermoid tumors contain keratin and epithelial debris. Dermoid tumors contain sebaceous material in addition to the keratin and epithelial debris. Hair may also be present in dermoids. Teratomas are rare lesions and include all three embryologic layers. These lesions occur along the anterior margin of the orbits, and are most commonly seen laterally and superiorly. There is usually a painless proptosis and a palpable mass on clinical examination. Hemorrhage may occur within the lesions, and associated bone defects may be present.

CT scanning demonstrates these masses to be of low signal intensity (Figs. 13–48A, 13–49A). The signal intensity is that of fat and is secondary to the lipid nature of the contents. No enhancement is present after intravenous contrast injection. The margins are well demarcated, with a sharp interface.

MRI is diagnostic of these lesions, as is CT. On short TR images the lesions demonstrate a high signal intensity similar to that of fat (Figs. 13–48B, 13–49B).[69, 95] The lesions decrease in signal intensity on long TR images (also similar to intraorbital fat). Fluid-fat levels may be present (Fig. 13–48C).

Lymphoma

Grades of lymphomatous infiltration of the orbit range from relatively benign to malignant. Seventy-

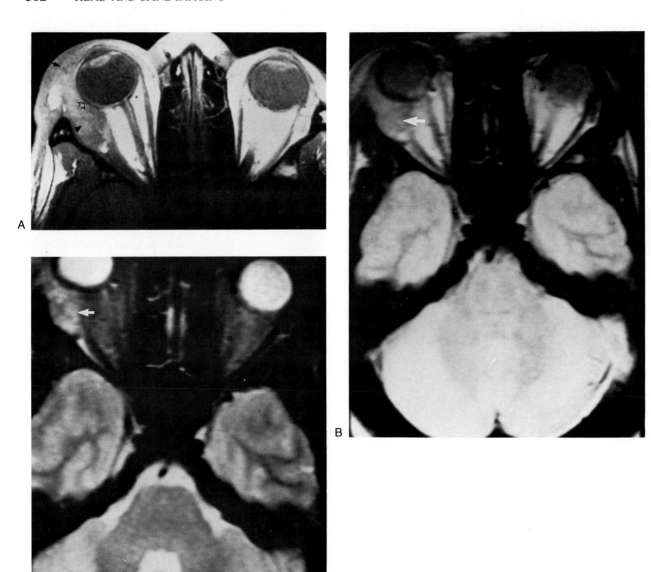

Figure 13–45. *Orbital pseudotumor.* **A** (600/20), Marked enlargement of the right lateral rectus muscle is seen. There is both a pre- (*arrow*) and a postseptal (*arrowhead*) component. Coating of the lateral globe margin is identified (*open arrow*). **B,C** (2500/20,80), Proton density and T2 weighted images demonstrate the mass (*arrows*) to be only minimally hyperintense to fat with increased T2 weighting. This relative lack of marked hyperintensity is characteristic of pseudotumor and lymphoma.

five percent of patients with orbital lymphoma ultimately develop systemic lymphoma.[96] Involvement in children is far less common than in adults. Most cases are non-Hodgkin's type.[31] Bilateral involvement is not infrequent and is more consistent with non-Hodgkin's lymphoma. The tumor may involve the extraconal space as a well-defined mass, may primarily or secondarily involve the extraocular muscles, or may involve solely the lacrimal gland.[97] As discussed under

inflammatory pseudotumor, lymphomas tend to have blurred margins and to coat the contour of the globe. Involvement of the eyelids and conjunctiva is common. Because of this anterior involvement, these lesions are usually palpable and appear early. Decreased ocular motility is also common. For most lesions, radiation therapy is curative.

CT examination shows a spectrum of findings (Fig. 13–50*A, B*).[97] The lesions may be well defined or

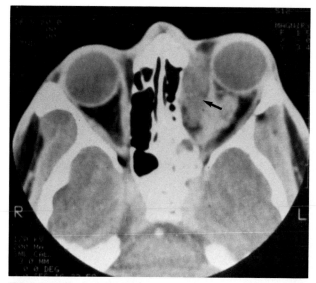

Figure 13–46. Lymphangioma. Enhanced CT scan demonstrates an extraconal mass on the left (*arrow*). The tumor is relatively homogeneous and sharply marginated.

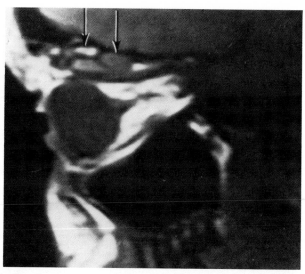

Figure 13–47. Lymphangioma (600/20). Sagittal T1 weighted image demonstrates an extraconal mass in the superior orbit. One area of increased intensity within the mass is identified (*anterior arrow*). This is consistent with methemoglobin. The remainder of the lesion (*posterior arrow*) was hyperintense on the T2 weighted images (not shown). (From Bilaniuk LT, Atlas SW, Zimmerman RA. Magnetic resonance imaging of the orbit. Radiol Clin North Am 1987; 25:509–528.)

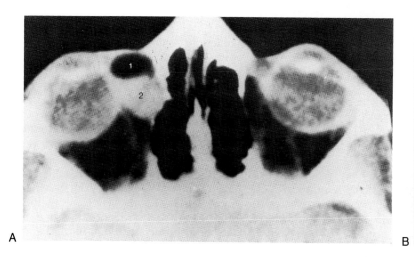

A

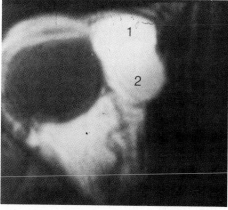

B

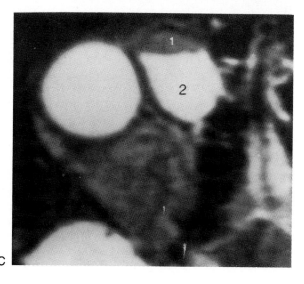

C

Figure 13–48. *Dermoid.* ***A,*** Axial CT scan demonstrates a fat-fluid level. The fat is of low attenuation, while the fluid is of increased attenuation (1, fat; 2, fluid). ***B,*** Axial MRI (600/20). The fat is hyperintense on the T1 weighted image. ***C,*** Axial MRI (2500/80). The fat decreases with increased T2 weighting. The intensity of the fluid increases. (From Atlas SW, Bilaniuk LT, Zimmerman RA, et al. Orbit: initial experience with surface coil spin-echo MR imaging at 1.5T. Radiology 1987; 164:501–509.)

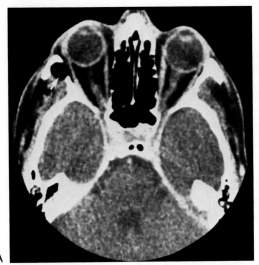
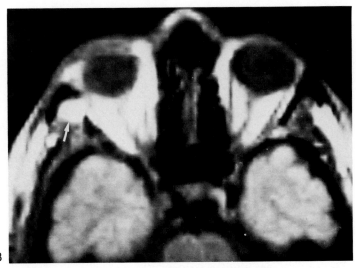

A   B

Figure 13–49. *Dermoid.* ***A,*** Enhanced CT scan demonstrates the characteristic low attenuation of the fatty tumor (*arrow*) arising in the right lateral orbital wall. ***B,*** Axial MRI (600/20). This T1 weighted image demonstrates the tumor to be of high signal intensity consistent with fat (*arrow*). (From Sobel DF, Kelly W, Kjos BO, et al. MR imaging of orbital and ocular disease. AJNR 1985; 6:259–264.)

diffuse in nature. They tend to involve the anterior orbit more than the posterior.[97] Involvement of the extraocular muscles is common. The lesions may or may not enhance with intravenous contrast administration.

On MR, lymphoma shows a variable appearance.[46] The lesion is generally of decreased signal intensity to fat on T1 weighted images and iso- or slightly hyperintense to fat on T2 weighted images (Figs. 13–50C, D, 13–51). It may be difficult to differentiate lymphoma from pseudotumor. Presumably the decreased signal intensity on the long TR images seen in both lymphoma and pseudotumor is secondary to the hypercellularity of these lesions and the relative lack of interstitial free water.

Neurofibroma

Neurofibromas can occur solely in the orbit or as part of a generalized neurofibromatosis. Of those neurofibromas presenting in the orbit in children, the most frequent is the plexiform neurofibroma, which commonly involves the orbit and the eyelid. Craniofacial anomalies are not uncommon, particularly dysgenesis of the greater wing of the sphenoid; this may be associated with pulsatile exophthalmos.[82] Neurofibromas are composed of Schwann cells and axons. They have a predilection for the superior aspect of the orbit. In cases of neurofibromatosis there is an association of buphthalmos with the presence of the neurofibroma.[22] Solitary neurofibromas are not usually treated unless significant complications from mass effect arise. However, an attempt at removal of large lesions may be made for cosmetic reasons.

CT scanning generally demonstrates these lesions as dense masses with relatively sharp margins.[98] With intravenous contrast administration there is marked enhancement. Associated findings of buphthalmos, bony expansion or dysplasia of the greater wing of the sphenoid, may be present (Fig. 13–52).

On MRI, neurofibromas appear hypointense to fat on T1 weighted images and markedly hyperintense on T2 weighted images (Fig. 13–53).[99] These lesions enhance with intravenous gadolinium. On STIR imaging these lesions have demonstrated a very high signal characteristic (Fig. 13–54). The associated findings of orbital expansion and dysplasia of the greater wing of the sphenoid have been appreciated on both MRI and CT.

Schwannomas of the orbit appear similar in signal intensity to that of neurofibromas (Fig. 13–55). They also enhance with gadolinium.

Rhabdomyosarcoma

Rhabdomyosarcoma is the most common primary malignant orbital tumor in children.[66] This embryonic mesenchymal tumor has been histologically divided into four types: embryonal, alveolar, botryoid, and differentiated.[100] The tumors are highly malignant and invasive; extension into adjacent bone or sinuses is common. The lesion affects children at the end of the first decade. The clinical history is generally that of a very rapidly progressive exophthalmos.[81] An associated palpable mass, periorbital edema, and ophthalmoplegia are common findings; decreased visual acuity may also be seen. Rhabdomyosarcoma is also a common cause of congenital proptosis.

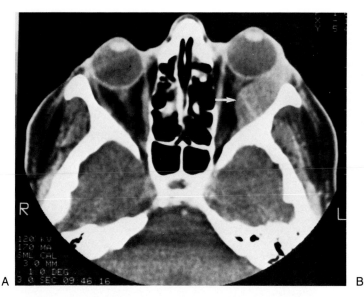

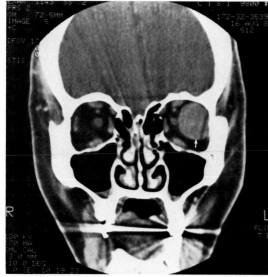

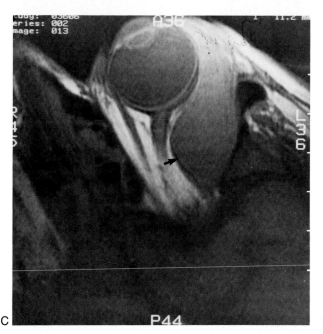

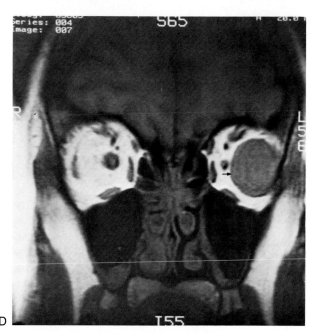

Figure 13–50. *Lymphoid lesion of the lateral rectus muscle.* **A,B,** Unenhanced CT demonstrates marked enlargement of the lateral rectus muscle (*arrow*) including the insertion. **C,D** (600/20), MR imaging also demonstrates the intrinsic enlargement of the lateral rectus muscle (*arrow*) extending into the insertion. No significant signal alteration is seen in the mass with respect to normal extraocular muscles. (From Curtin HD. Pseudotumor. Radiol Clin North Am 1987; 25:583–599.)

CT examination discloses a soft tissue density mass within the orbit (Fig. 13–56).[101] These lesions commonly are seen in the superior nasal quadrant. Preseptal and intracranial extension is common. The lesions are generally homogeneous. Destruction of bone or invasion of sinuses also is often seen on CT. With intravenous contrast administration most tumors demonstrate a diffuse enhancement. Intracranial extension may also be evident.

MR examination has demonstrated lesions of decreased signal intensity with respect to orbital fat on T1 weighted images (Fig. 13–57). The lesions have been slightly hyperintense to fat on the T2 weighted images. In our experience, these lesions do show inhomogeneous enhancement. Invasion of bone appears as loss of the usual cortical low signal and loss of the usual high marrow signal on T1 weighted images. Invasion of the paranasal sinuses may also be demonstrated.

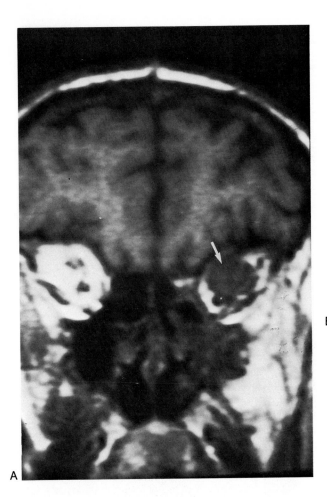

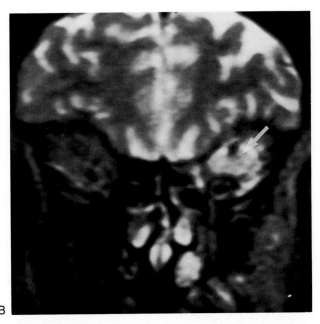

Figure 13–51. *Lymphoma.* **A** (600/20), A mass (*arrow*), isointense to muscle, is identified in the left orbit. It is well marginated. **B** (2500/80), On T2 weighted imaging the mass (*arrow*) is mildly hyperintense to fat.

Metastases

Three major groups of metastatic lesions are seen in the pediatric orbit: neuroblastoma, Ewing's sarcoma, and leukemia.[81] Over 20 percent of patients with neuroblastoma have orbital metastases.[102] Metastases are commonly bilateral.[66] Both neuroblastoma and Ewing's sarcoma have a propensity to metastasize to the orbital walls. Soft tissue components, therefore, are generally extraconal. Leukemic infiltration of the orbit can be extraconal but generally is diffuse in nature. Leukemia may also demonstrate retinal or optic nerve sheath involvement.

Neuroblastoma on CT generally demonstrates bony destruction with an associated soft tissue mass (Fig. 13–58A, B). This mass on unenhanced studies is often slightly hyperdense, which may help to differentiate it from rhabdomyosarcoma.[101] Patchy contrast enhancement may be noted as well as foci of calcification. On MRI these lesions have demonstrated a decreased signal with respect to fat on T1 weighted images and increased signal on T2 weighted images (Fig. 13–58C to E). Our results have shown rather marked gadolinium enhancement. Ewing's tumor has a similar appearance to that of neuroblastoma (Fig. 13–59).

Orbital leukemia generally demonstrates a diffuse increased attenuation on CT imaging and does not show significant contrast enhancement (Fig. 13–60A).[97] The margins are usually irregular and blend in with the soft tissue structures within the orbit. On T1 weighted MR imaging the fat demonstrates a diffuse decrease in its usual signal (Fig. 13–60B, C).[97] No well-defined mass is evident. On T2 weighted imaging the leukemic infiltrates are generally iso- to minimally hyperintense to fat. Again, as in pseudotumor and lymphoma, the leukemic infiltrate has a tendency to coat the posterior and lateral aspects of the globe.

Lacrimal Gland Abnormalities

Lacrimal gland abnormalities in the pediatric population are rare, and no well-defined studies relating to pediatric lacrimal gland pathology are available. In the adult literature 50 percent of lacrimal masses are

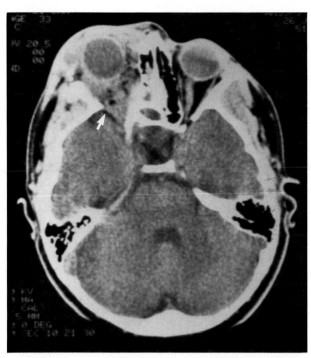

Figure 13–52. Orbital neurofibroma. Axial nonenhanced CT scan through the orbit demonstrates a plexiform neurofibroma of the right orbit. There is associated dysplasia of the greater wing of the sphenoid on the right (*arrow*).

epithelial tumors.[103] Most of these are benign mixed adenomas; the remainder are malignant tumors, generally adenoid cystic carcinoma. The remaining 50 percent of lacrimal gland masses are of the lymphoid or inflammatory type. Most benign lesions present as a painless mass in the lacrimal fossa.[81] A painful or progressively enlarging mass tends to be associated with a more malignant lesion. Secondary bony invasion may be present in these malignant tumors.

CT examination generally demonstrates a well-defined extraconal mass involving the lacrimal gland; little enhancement is generally seen in benign lesions (Fig. 13–61A).[31] Malignant tumors show variable enhancement patterns.[66] In many cases the mass may appear more invasive, involving the rectus muscles and even extending intraconally to displace the optic nerve.

MR examination has demonstrated the benign lesions to be relatively isointense to the usual lacrimal gland signal on T1 weighted images (Fig. 13–61). Benign lesions tend to be well marginated and noninvasive. T2 weighted images show variable signal in the mass. Some lesions may be hyper- and others isointense to the normal gland (Fig. 13–62).[69]

Inflammatory conditions may be unilateral or bilateral. Unilateral involvement is typically seen in orbital pseudotumor and has been described previously. Bilat-

eral lacrimal gland enlargement may be seen in sarcoidosis, Sjögren's syndrome, amyloidosis, and lymphoid hyperplasia. Lymphoma may be seen either bilaterally or unilaterally. T2 weighted images show variable lacrimal gland signal intensity.[69] Another inflammatory condition that can present with unilateral involvement is infection; no MR reports of lacrimal gland infection have been published. In the absence of abscess with focal necrosis and cyst formation, the increased signal present on T2 weighted images in a case of lacrimal gland infection may be indistinguishable from that of benign tumors.

Infection of the Orbit

Inflammation or infection of the orbit can be separated into two major components: preseptal and postseptal. As discussed in the anatomy section, a reflection of periosteum extends from the bony margins onto the tarsal plates. This tough membrane, the orbital septum, defines the preseptal and postseptal spaces. Lesions anterior to this membrane are preseptal, whereas lesions posterior to the membrane are postseptal. Inflammatory lesions that are anterior to the orbital septum have a more benign course than lesions involving the postseptal region.[81] Most cases of preseptal inflammation arise locally from cellulitis or abscess.[81] Occasionally, preseptal inflammation may arise from sinusitis, although this is a more common cause of postseptal inflammation.

The CT findings of preseptal inflammation are a soft tissue swelling involving the tissues anterior to the orbital septum.[104] Unless an abscess is present, there is usually little enhancement after intravenous contrast administration. MR examination demonstrates increased signal in the preseptal tissues on T2 weighted images with associated swelling of these tissues.[30]

Postseptal inflammation can be subdivided into three components: intraconal, extraconal, and subperiosteal. Most cases of postseptal inflammation are a result of paranasal sinus disease, particularly in the ethmoid sinuses. Most cellulitis is extraconal, while most abscesses are subperiosteal. Bony defects are present in the medial wall of the orbit that allow communication between the ethmoid sinuses and the orbit. The periosteum of the bone can act as a barrier to the spread of inflammation. The inflammatory process, however, may breach the periorbital region and extend into the retrobulbar region.[104] This direct spread is more consistent with higher-grade inflammatory lesions such as osteomyelitis. Frequent symptoms include lacrimation, edema, proptosis, decreased extraocular muscle motion, and episcleritis.[81] In some patients antibiotics may be sufficient to clear the inflammatory process, but some may require open drainage.

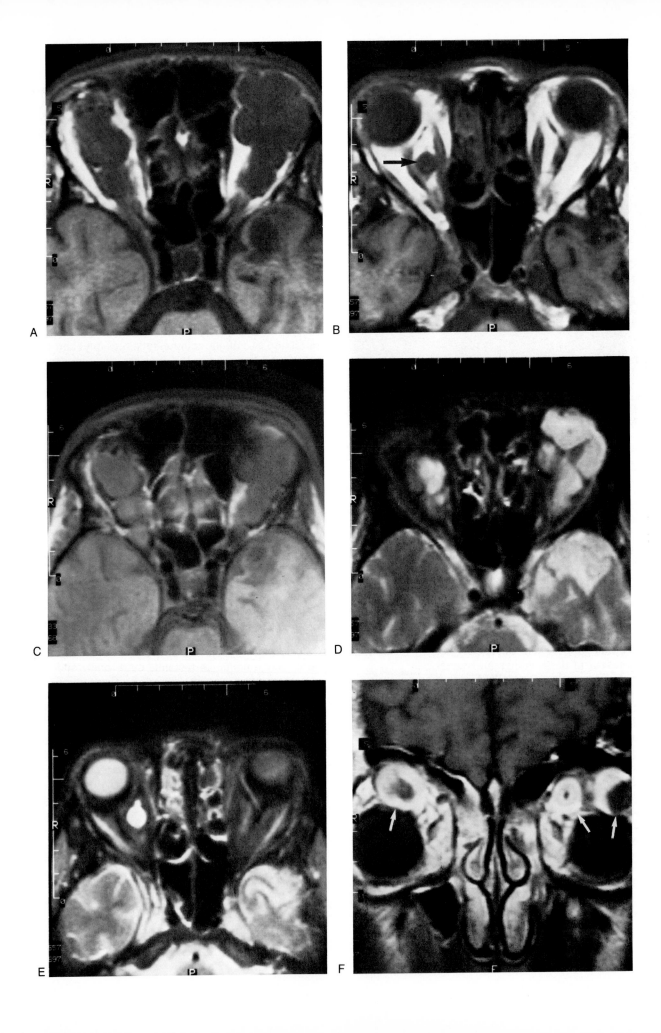

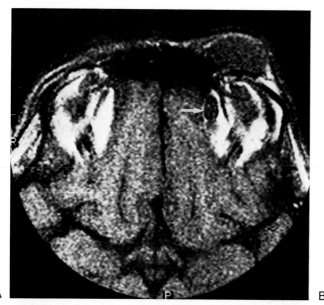 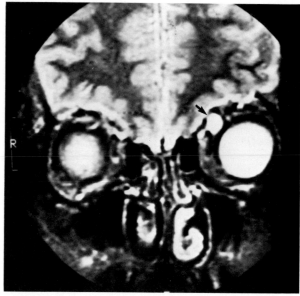

Figure 13–54. *Neurofibroma.* ***A*** (600/26), This axial T1 weighted image demonstrates prominent neurofibroma just anterior to the superior orbital rim. A second neurofibroma is seen along the superior and medial aspect of the left orbit (*arrow*). ***B*** (2500/150/30), This coronal STIR image through the orbit shows the neurofibroma to be markedly hyperintense (*arrow*).

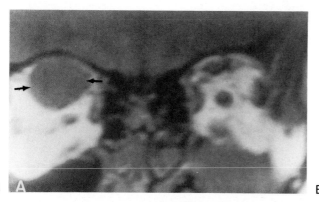 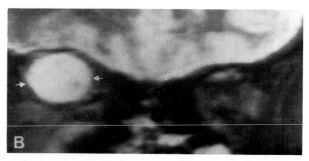

Figure 13–55. *Schwannoma.* ***A*** (600/20), The schwannoma (*arrows*) in the superior right orbit is isointense to the extraocular muscles. It is sharply marginated. ***B*** (2500/80), The schwannoma is markedly hyperintense on T2 weighted imaging. (From Atlas SW. Magnetic resonance imaging of the orbit: current status. Mag Res Q 1989; 5:39–96.)

On CT, subperiosteal lesions demonstrate a sharp border at the interface of the inflammatory process and the orbit (Fig. 13–63).[81] Soft tissue density with partial or complete opacification of the adjacent sinuses is seen. This same density material appears to extend into this subperiosteal region. There may be enhancement, particularly of the subperiosteal tissue.

MRI demonstrates abnormal signal intensity within the paranasal sinus and the subperiosteal region (Fig. 13–64). This is generally hypointense to fat on T1 weighted images and hyperintense on T2 weighted images. STIR imaging may be more valuable than T1 or T2 weighted images and nicely demonstrates the abnormal increased signal intensity associated with this process. The margin of the subperiosteal infection is sharp. Abnormal increased signal may also be identi-

◀ **Figure 13–53.** *Bilateral neurofibromas.* ***A,B*** (600/26), Axial images through the orbit demonstrate bilateral neurofibromas. The neurofibromas in the superior orbits are markedly lobular. A neurofibroma is also seen between the medial rectus and optic nerve sheath complex on the right (*arrow*). ***C*** (2500/20), This proton density weighted image also shows the bilateral orbital neurofibromas. ***D,E*** (2500/80), T2 weighted images through the orbit demonstrate marked hyperintensity of the neurofibromas. ***F*** (600/26), This coronal T1 weighted image following gadolinium administration shows inhomogeneous enhancement of the bilateral orbital neurofibromas (*arrows*).

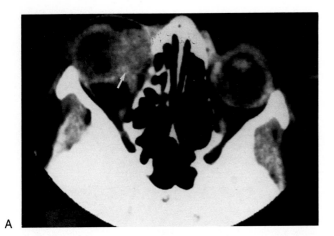

A

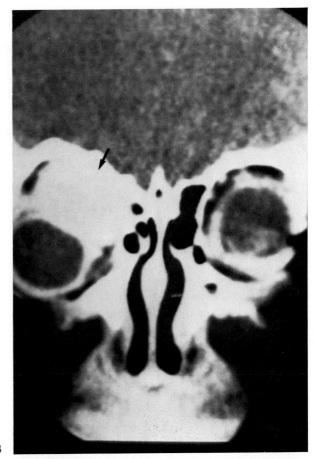

B

Figure 13–56. Rhabdomyosarcoma. Axial nonenhanced (**A**) and coronal enhanced (**B**) CT scans demonstrate a large mass (*arrows*) in the right orbit, in the superior and medial aspects. The margins are relatively sharp. No gross sinus invasion is identified.

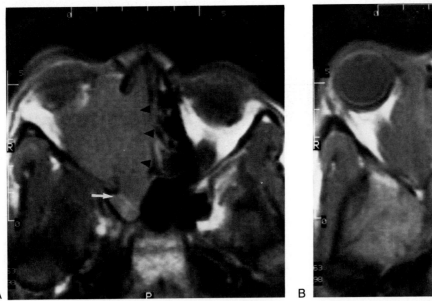

A

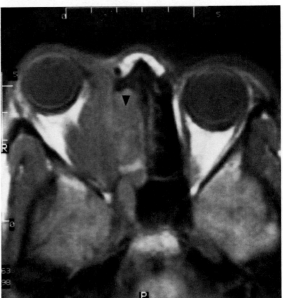

B

Figure 13–57. *Rhabdomyosarcoma.* **A,B** (600/26), Axial T1 weighted images demonstrate a large mass invading the right orbit. There is associated sinus invasion as well (*arrowheads*). The medial orbital wall is destroyed. A question is

fied within the adjacent extraocular muscles, presumably on an inflammatory basis. Extraconal lesions have a similar appearance to that of subperiosteal lesions, although the margin may be less well demarcated because of the absence of any limiting membrane. Intraconal abnormalities appear rather diffuse. The signal intensity of the fat is generally decreased on T1 weighted images and increased on T2 weighted images secondary to the presence of increased free water.[26] Orbital emphysema may be present and appears as

Text continues on page 374.

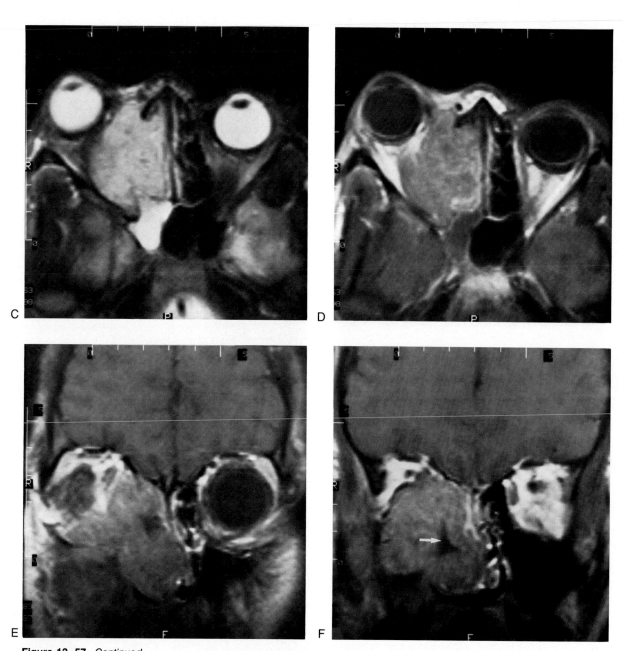

Figure 13–57. *Continued.*
raised of extension of tumor into the right side of the sphenoid sinus *(arrow)*. **C** (2500/80), The tumor is hyperintense to orbital fat on the T2 weighted image. The density seen in the sphenoid sinus on the T1 weighted images is now very hyperintense, and seen to represent an occluded sphenoid air cell. **D** to **F** (600/26), Postgadolinium T1 weighted images in the axial and coronal projections demonstrate mild enhancement of the tumor. The coronal images also show a focal area of central necrosis *(arrow)*. The extent of the lesion is well demonstrated by using the multiplanar capability of MRI.

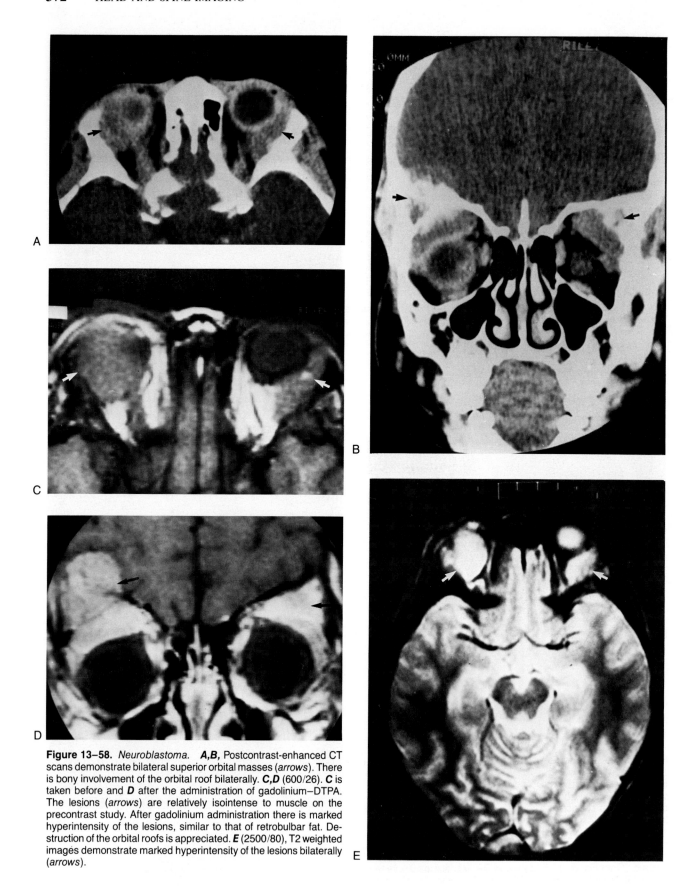

Figure 13–58. *Neuroblastoma.* ***A,B,*** Postcontrast-enhanced CT scans demonstrate bilateral superior orbital masses (*arrows*). There is bony involvement of the orbital roof bilaterally. ***C,D*** (600/26). ***C*** is taken before and ***D*** after the administration of gadolinium–DTPA. The lesions (*arrows*) are relatively isointense to muscle on the precontrast study. After gadolinium administration there is marked hyperintensity of the lesions, similar to that of retrobulbar fat. Destruction of the orbital roofs is appreciated. ***E*** (2500/80), T2 weighted images demonstrate marked hyperintensity of the lesions bilaterally (*arrows*).

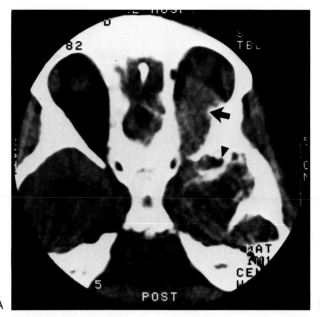

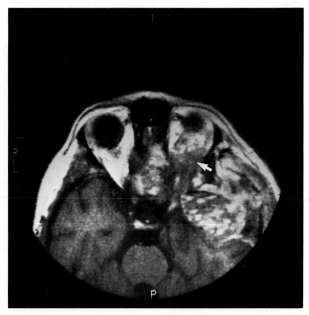

Figure 13–59. *Ewing's tumor.* **A,** Axial enhanced CT demonstrates a soft tissue mass surrounding the greater wing of the sphenoid on the left. The mass extends into the orbit (*arrow*) as well into the middle cranial fossa (*arrowhead*). **B** (600/26), Axial gadolinium-enhanced MRI shows the mass extending into the left orbit (*arrow*). The mass shows inhomogeneous enhancement.

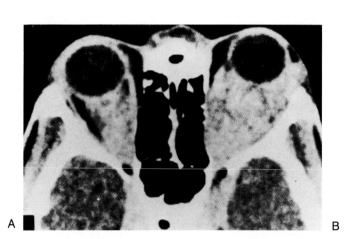

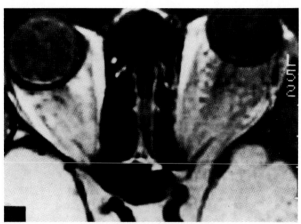

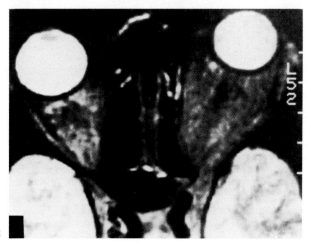

Figure 13–60. *Leukemic infiltration.* **A,** Axial CT scan demonstrates poorly marginated infiltrative masses. They are primarily intraconal with some extraconal involvement. **B** (2000/20), The usual hyperintensity from the retrobulbar fat is not present. Decreased signal consistent with the leukemic infiltrate is identified bilaterally. **C** (2000/80), The bilateral masses show relatively low signal intensity. This decreased signal intensity can be seen in pseudotumor and lymphoma as well as in leukemia. Other metastatic lesions are generally hyperintense on these T2 weighted images. (From Flanders AE, Espinosa GA, Markiewicz DA, Howell DD. Orbital lymphoma. Role of CT and MRI. Radiol Clin North Am 1987; 25:601–613.)

373

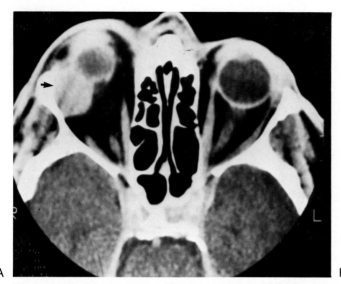
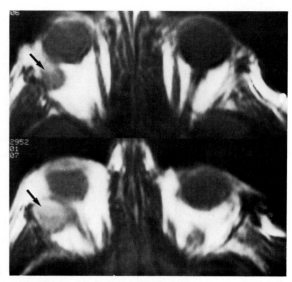

Figure 13–61. *Benign adenoma of the lacrimal gland.* **A,** Enhanced CT scan of the lacrimal gland (*arrow*) demonstrates intrinsic enlargement. No inhomogeneity is identified and no invasive margin is seen. **B** (600/20), Axial MR imaging shows a well-defined lesion (*arrows*) involving the lacrimal gland. It is decreased in signal intensity with respect to retro-orbital fat.

sharply demarcated foci of marked hypointensity. The complications of orbital infection can also be identified on MRI. This generally involves vascular thrombosis. Lack of flow void is noted in the involved vascular structure. The signal intensity depends on the hemoglobin breakdown product that is present at the time of imaging. Bony destruction may also be identified as an interruption of the hypointense intact cortical bone

margin. Extension into the intracranial structures in the form of an epidural abscess can also be appreciated on MRI.

Extraorbital Lesions

Extraorbital lesions with orbital involvement include primary bone lesions, secondary bone lesions, and soft

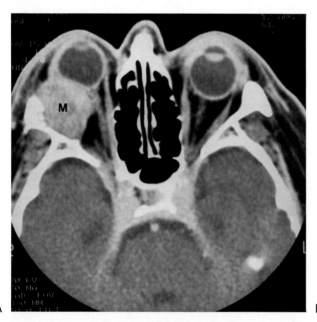
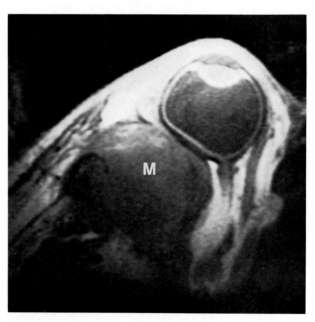

Figure 13–62. *Lacrimal gland adenoid cystic carcinoma.* **A,** A large mass (M) is seen arising from the lacrimal gland on enhanced CT. The intraorbital margins are relatively sharp. Three is destruction of the greater wing of the sphenoid, and the globe is deformed. **B,C** (600/20), The mass is relatively isointense to the extraocular muscles. The cortical bone (*black arrows*) is seen intact in the superior and inferior aspects of the lateral orbit. The lateral bony wall, however, shows

Figure continues on following page.

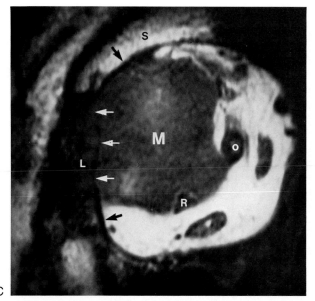

C

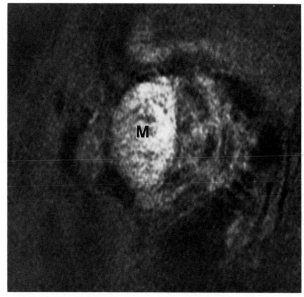

D

Figure 13–62. *Continued.*
permeation of the cortex by tumor (*white arrows*). The lateral rectus muscle (R) is markedly inferiorly and medially deviated. The optic nerve sheath complex (o) is also medially displaced. ***D,*** (2000/80), The T2 weighted image of the orbit demonstrates marked hyperintensity of the mass with respect to retro-orbital fat. (Hendrix LE, Massaro BM, Daniels DL, et al. Surface coil MR evaluation of a lacrimal gland carcinoma. J Comput Assist Tomogr 1988; 12:866–868.)

tissue tumors. Craniofacial anomalies also fall into this category in terms of alteration of the bony orbit itself or the relationship of the bony orbits with each other.

The most common primary bone lesion in children is fibrous dysplasia.[31] This entity is associated with a marked thickening of the cortical bone in the orbital region. This exuberant cortical bone may cause compression of the orbital fissures and optic canal. There may be impingement on the orbital contents. MR examination demonstrates a signal void consistent with the dense cortical bone present in the orbital area on CT (Figs. 13–65, 13–66). Osteoblastoma has also been reported (Fig. 13–67).[46] Secondary bone lesions include the metastatic lesions associated with neuroblastoma and Ewing's sarcoma, as described previously. Eosinophilic granuloma may also occur.[102]

Soft tissue tumors such as esthesioneuroblastoma can involve the orbit (Fig. 13–68).[105] Juvenile angiofibroma may also be associated with orbital invasion (Fig. 13–69).

Craniofacial abnormalities such as Crouzon's disease and Treacher Collins syndrome are associated with shallow orbits and globe proptosis. Craniosynostoses may produce bony orbit asymmetries. Nasal encephaloceles are associated with hypertelorism (Fig. 13–70). Mucoceles are seen to expand into the orbit (Fig. 13–71).

Trauma to the Orbit

At our institution, acute orbit trauma is generally evaluated by CT. This is in part due to the possibility of orbital penetration by metallic fragments.[106] In addition, CT exquisitely demonstrates the bony anatomy and superbly identifies periorbital fractures. The study is quickly and easily performed, although coronal imaging is much easier to perform with MRI. In some cases, MRI may be useful in the evaluation of post-traumatic complications such as vascular thrombosis, which was discussed earlier. Hematomas of the orbit involve ocular, retrobulbar, muscular, and optic sheath structures.

Text continues on page 381.

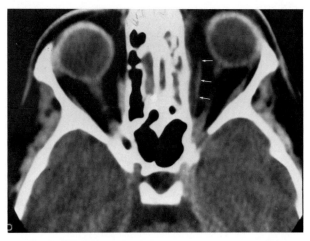

Figure 13–63. Subperiosteal abscess. Axial enhanced CT scan demonstrates opacification of the left ethmoid air cells. There is some low-density material extending between the medial orbital wall on the left and the medial rectus muscle (*arrows*).

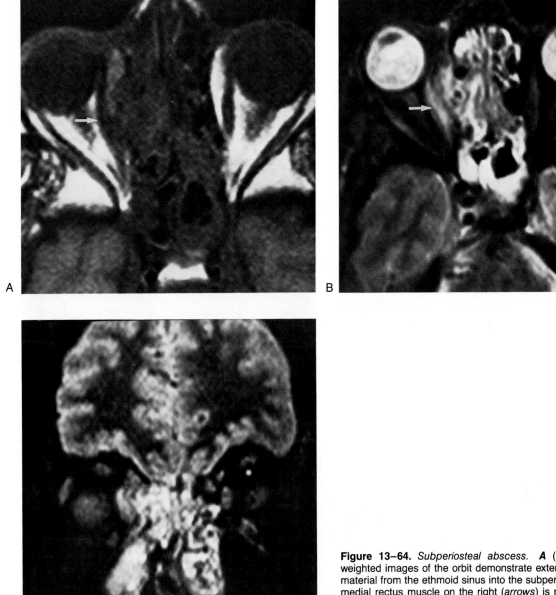

Figure 13–64. *Subperiosteal abscess.* **A** (600/26), Axial T1 weighted images of the orbit demonstrate extension of soft tissue material from the ethmoid sinus into the subperiosteal region. The medial rectus muscle on the right (*arrows*) is medially displaced. **B,C** (2500/150/30), Axial and coronal STIR imaging of the orbit shows the inflammatory debris to be hyperintense to fat. Some abnormal increased signal within the medial rectus (*arrows*) is also identified.

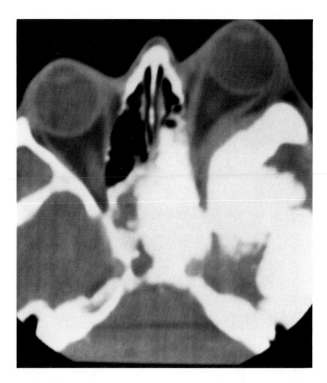

Figure 13–65. Fibrous dysplasia. Axial CT scan demonstrates marked cortical thickening consistent with fibrous dysplasia surrounding the left orbital apex.

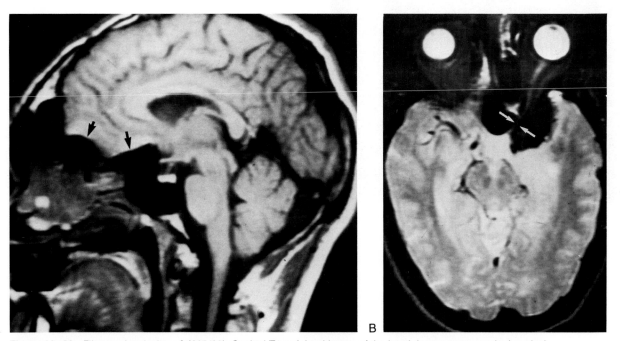

A   B

Figure 13–66. *Fibrous dysplasia.* **A** (600/20), Sagittal T1 weighted image of the head demonstrates marked cortical thickening, manifest by marked decreased signal intensity (*arrows*). **B** (2500/80), Axial T2 weighted image also shows marked cortical thickening. The optic nerve can be seen extending through the markedly narrowed optic canal (*arrows*).

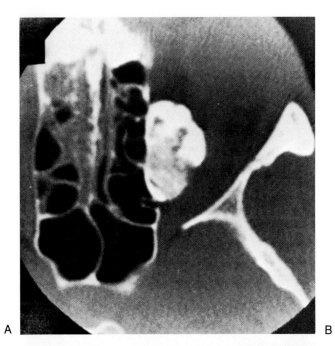

A

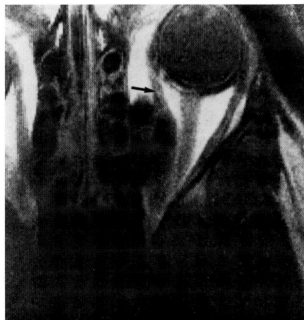

B

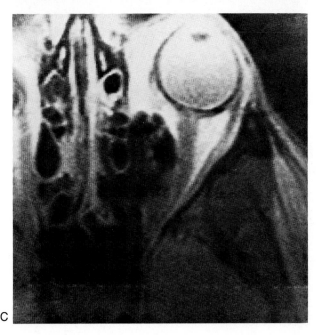

C

Figure 13–67. *Osteoblastoma.* ***A,*** Axial CT scan demonstrates an expansile bony lesion arising along the medial aspect of the left orbit. ***B*** (500/30), There is an area of signal loss consistent with cortical bone along the medial portion of the left orbit. The medial rectus (*arrow*) is seen draped around the mass. ***C*** (1000/30), On this more T2 weighted image, no significant signal alteration is identified within the osteoblastoma itself, consistent with its bony nature. (Sullivan JA. Surface coil MR imaging of orbital neoplasms. AJNR 1986; 7:29–34.)

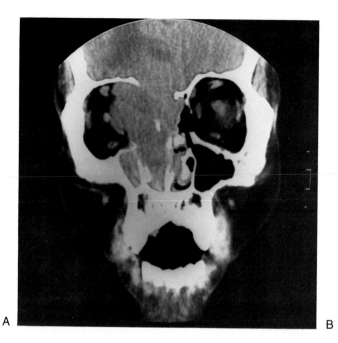

A

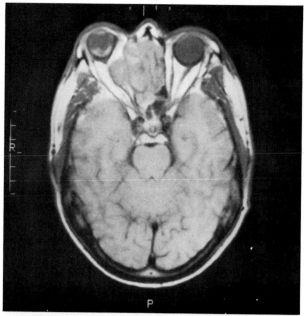

B

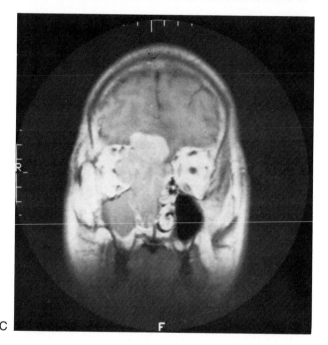

C

Figure 13–68. *Esthesioneuroblastoma.* **A,** Coronal enhanced CT shows a large mass involving the right ethmoid sinus, maxillary sinus, orbit, and nasal cavity. The tumor has extended intracranially, although the demarcation of tumor and normal brain is not evident. **B** (600/26), Axial nonenhanced MRI shows a homogeneous mass in the ethmoid sinus with extension into the surrounding structures. **C** (600/26), Coronal postgadolinium MRI shows the mass and its extension. The demarcation of intracranial tumor and normal brain is superb.

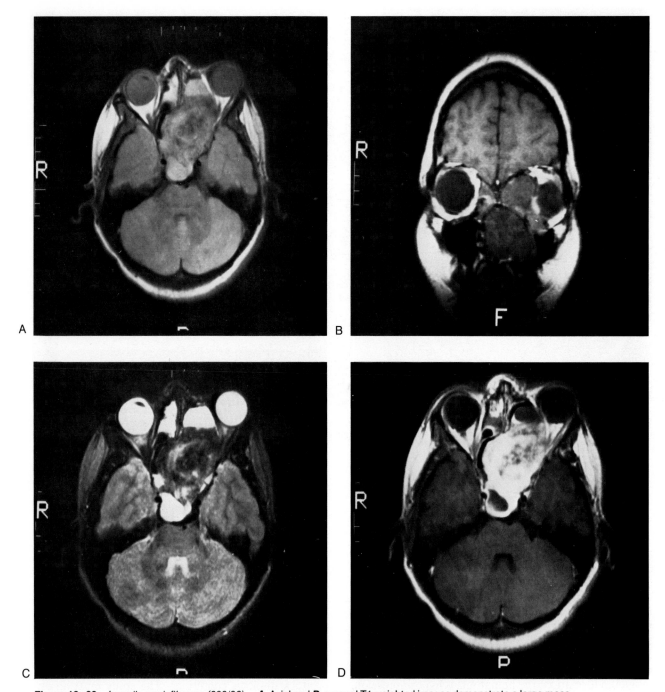

Figure 13–69. *Juvenile angiofibroma (600/26).* **A,** Axial and **B,** coronal T1 weighted images demonstrate a large mass extending into the nasopharynx and paranasal sinuses, and also into the left orbit. The lesion is inhomogeneous in character. **C** (2500/80), Most of the lesion is hypointense on T2 weighted imaging. Hyperintense foci both anteriorly and posteriorly probably represent obstructed sinus chambers. **D** (600/26), After gadolinium–DTPA administration most of this vascular tumor shows marked increased signal. The areas of sinus obstruction do not enhance.

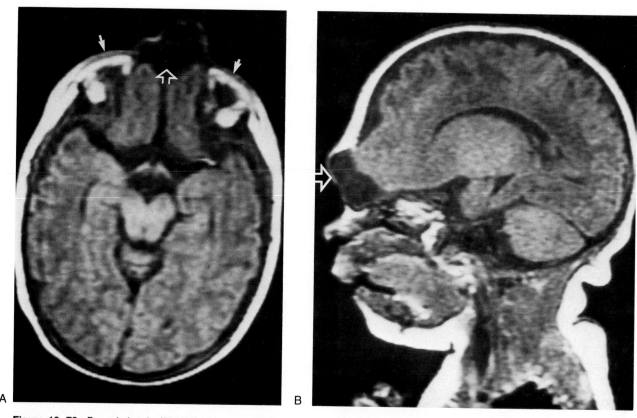

Figure 13–70. *Encephalocele (600/20).*   **A,** Axial and **B,** sagittal images demonstrate a nasofrontal encephalocele (*open arrow*). The CSF is seen to extend into the defect. This caused hypertelorism (*arrows*).

CT examination shows a soft tissue density in the postseptal space;[104] there is often preseptal edema. MR imaging allows a precise evaluation of hemorrhage (Fig. 13–72). The signal intensity in the area of hemorrhage depends on the hemoglobin breakdown products present at the time of imaging.[61] Acute hemorrhagic products are relatively isointense to muscle on short TR images and hypointense on long TR images, consistent with the presence of deoxyhemoglobin. In the subacute stage, the hallmark of which is methemoglobin formation, the hematoma is hyperintense on both T1 and T2 weighted images. The hyperintensity may be difficult to appreciate on T1 weighted images because of the high signal from adjacent fat. No study has been reported relating to long-term hemosiderin deposition in the orbit. Presumably the macrophages that convert the methemoglobin into hemosiderin are able to exit from the orbital structures. This may lead to only a transient appearance of hemosiderin, which is manifest on T2 weighted images as a very hypointense focus.

Early work with MRI to evaluate periorbital fractures has recently been undertaken.[107] In the evaluation of medial and inferior blowout fractures, MRI was found to have an exquisite ability to define the nature of the fracture (Fig. 13–73). In addition, MRI may be better able than CT to delineate muscular or fatty entrapment, the presence of which generally requires surgical intervention.

By appropriately tailoring orbital MR examinations, the radiologist can image a wide variety of pediatric orbital pathologic conditions. The study must be obtained as quickly as possible, yet without sacrificing resolution. In many patients, multiple pulse sequences are necessary for optimal differentiation of orbital lesions. This may require a longer examination time than CT, but many of these differential considerations cannot be made from the CT scan alone. In addition, multiple imaging planes that may be impossible with CT are easily obtained with MRI. Further development of improved surface coils and rapid pulse sequences will lead to even further increased use of MRI

Text continues on page 384.

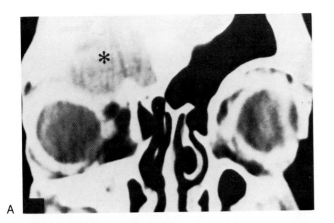

A

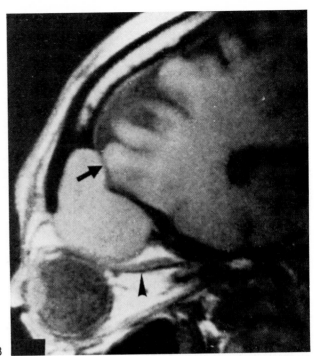

B

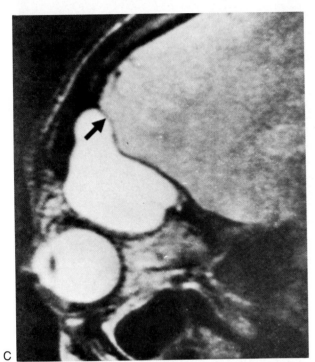

C

Figure 13–71. *Mucocele.* **A,** Coronal enhanced CT demonstrates soft tissue density within the right frontal sinus (*asterisk*). Bony destruction is also appreciated. The globe is displaced inferiorly and laterally. **B** (500/19), A parasagittal section nicely outlines the extent of the mucocele. Extraconal extension is also seen. The superior muscle group (*arrowhead*) is inferiorly displaced. Bony destruction of the posterior wall of the frontal sinus (*arrow*) is also noted. **C** (1000/75), On this more T2 weighted image, there is increased signal intensity in the mucocele. Again noted is the lack of signal void in the posterosuperior sinus wall. (Bilaniuk LT, Atlas SW, Zimmerman RA. Magnetic resonance imaging of the orbit. Radiol Clin North Am 1987; 25:509–528.)

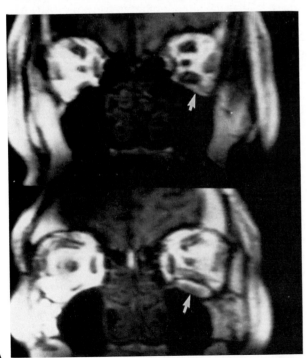

A

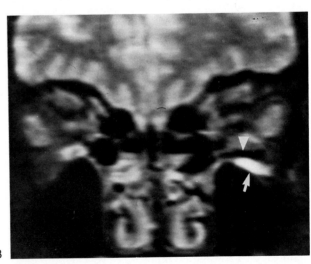

B

Figure 13–72. *Orbital hemorrhage.* **A** (600/20), Coronal T1 weighted images of the orbit demonstrate an area of increased signal intensity in the subperiosteal region of the floor of the left orbit (*arrows*). The high signal is consistent with methemoglobin. **B** (2500/20), Hyperintensity of the hematoma is again shown (*arrow*). This is consistent with extracellular methemoglobin. A presumed chemical shift artifact is seen superior to the subperiosteal hematoma (*arrowhead*).

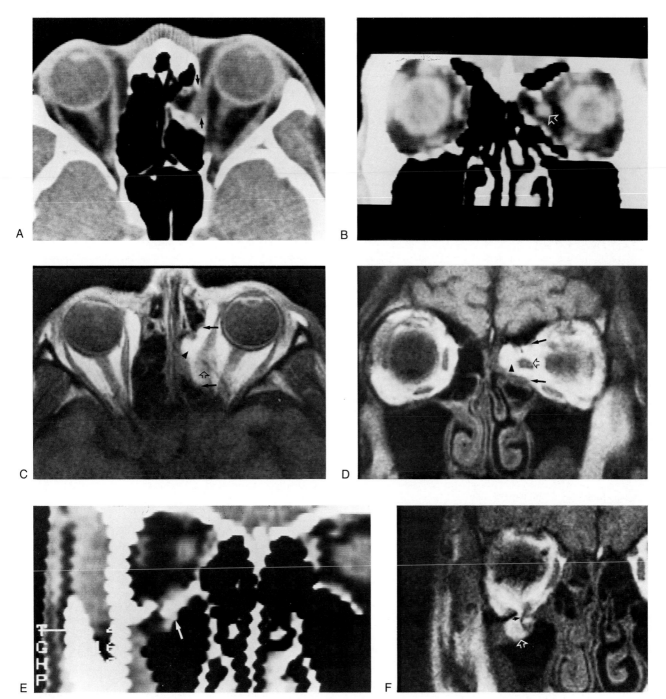

Figure 13–73. *Orbital wall fractures.* ***A,B,*** Axial and coronal reformatted CT images demonstrate a medial orbital wall fracture (*arrows*) with entrapment of the medial rectus muscle (*open arrow*). ***C,D*** (600/20), Axial and coronal MR images of the same patient demonstrate the extension of extraconal fat (*arrowhead*) into the medial orbital fracture defect (*arrows*). The medial rectus muscle (*open arrow*) is seen to be displaced into the fracture defect. ***E,*** Coronally reformatted CT demonstrates a right inferior orbital wall fracture, a trapdoor fracture (*arrow*). ***F*** (600/20), A direct coronal T1 weighted MR image shows the extension of intraorbital fat through the floor fracture (*open arrow*). The inferior rectus muscle (*arrow*) is seen to extend into the fracture defect. (From Kelly WM, Paglen PG, Pearson JA, et al. Ferromagnetism of intraocular foreign body causes unilateral blindness after MR study. AJNR 1986; 7:243–245.)

in the orbit. It is our conviction that ultimately most orbital imaging will be performed with MRI rather than with CT.

REFERENCES

1. Brateman L. Chemical shift imaging: a review. AJR 1986; 146:971–980.
2. Pusey E, Lufkin RB, Brown RKJ, et al. Magnetic resonance imaging artifacts: mechanism and clinical significance. RadioGraphics 1986; 6:891–911.
3. Wehrli FW, Breger RK, MacFall JR, et al. Quantification of contrast in clinical MR brain imaging at high magnetic field. Invest Radiol 1985; 20:360–369.
4. Wehrli FW, Kanal E. Orbital imaging: factors determining magnetic resonance imaging appearance. Radiol Clin North Am 1987; 25:419–427.
5. Axel L. Surface coil magnetic resonance imaging. J Comput Assist Tomogr 1984; 8:381–384.
6. Schenck JF, Hart HR, Foster TH, et al. Improved MR imaging of the orbit at 1.5T with surface coils. AJNR 1985; 6:193–196.
7. Schenck JF, Hart HR, Foster TH, et al. High resolution magnetic resonance imaging using surface coils. In: Kressel HY, ed. Magnetic resonance annual 1986. New York: Raven Press, 1986:123–160.
8. Kneeland JB, Hyde JS. High-resolution MR imaging with local coils. Radiology 1989; 171:1–7.
9. Atlas SW, Grossman RI, Hackney DB, et al. STIR MR imaging of the orbit. AJNR 1988; 9:969–974.
10. Penning BJ, Cheng HM, Barnett P, et al. MR imaging of enucleated human eyes at 1.4 Tesla. J Comput Assist Tomogr 1986; 10:551–559.
11. Mafee MF, Peyman G. Retinal and choroidal detachments: role of magnetic resonance imaging and computed tomography. Radiol Clin North Am 1987; 25:487–507.
12. Gomori JM, Grossman RI, Shields JA, et al. Choroidal melanomas: correlation of NMR spectroscopy and MR imaging. Radiology 1986; 160:773–780.
13. Albert A, Lee BC, Saint-Louis L, et al. MRI of optic chiasm and optic pathways. AJNR 1986; 7:255–258.
14. Daniels DL, Herfkins R, Gager WE, et al. Magnetic resonance imaging of the optic nerves and chiasm. Radiology 1984; 152:79–83.
15. Azar-Kia B, Mafee MF, Horowitz SW, et al. CT and MRI of the optic nerve and sheath. Semin Ultrasound CT MR 1988; 9:443–454.
16. Bilaniuk LT, Atlas SW, Zimmerman RA. Magnetic resonance imaging of the orbit. Radiol Clin North Am 1987; 25:509–528.
17. Lenkinski RE, Kressel HY, Atlas SW, et al. A flexible surface coil for high-resolution MR imaging of the orbits. Presented at the Radiological Society of North America annual meeting, Chicago, Nov 29–Dec 4, 1987.
18. Miller DH, Newton MR, van der Poel JC, et al. Magnetic resonance imaging of the optic nerve in optic neuritis. Neurology 1988; 38:175–179.
19. Wehrli FW, MacFall JR, Glover GH, et al. Dependence of nuclear magnetic resonance (NMR) image contrast on intrinsic and pulse sequence timing parameters. Magn Reson Imaging 1985; 2:3–16.
20. Bottomley PA, Foster TH, Arsinger RE, Pfeifer LM. A review of normal tissue hydrogen NMR relaxation times and relaxation mechanisms from 1–100 MHz: dependence on tissue type, NMR frequency, temperature, species, excision, and age. Med Phys 1984; 11:425–448.
21. Newman R. Operator's pulse sequence data notes. Milwaukee: General Electric, 1987.
22. Atlas SW, Grossman RI, Axel L, et al. Orbital lesions: proton spectroscopic phase dependent contrast MR imaging. Radiology 1987; 64:510–514.
23. Simon J, Szumowski J, Totterman S, et al. Fat-suppression MR imaging of the orbit. AJNR 1988; 9:961–968.
24. Kilgore DP, Breger RK, Daniels DL, et al. Cranial tissues: normal MR appearance after intravenous injection of Gd-DTPA. Radiology 1986; 160:757–761.
25. Simon JH, Szumowski J, Totterman S, et al. Paramagnetic enhancement accentuation by chemical shift imaging. Presented at the American Society of Neuroradiology annual meeting, Orlando, FL, March 19–24, 1989.
26. Atlas SW, Grossman RI, Savino PJ, et al. Surface coil MR of orbital pseudotumor. AJNR 1987; 8:141–146.
27. Axel L, Constini J, Listerud J. Intensity correction in surface-coil MR imaging. AJR 1987; 148:418–422.
28. Gardner E, Gray DJ, O'Rahilly R. Anatomy, 4th ed. Philadelphia: WB Saunders, 1975.
29. Gomori JM, Grossman RI, Shields JA, et al. Ocular MR imaging and spectroscopy: an ex vivo study. Radiology 1986; 160:201–205.
30. Atlas SW. Magnetic resonance imaging of the orbit: current status. Magn Res Q 1989; 5:39–96.
31. Bryan RN, Craig JA. The eye. CT of the orbit. In: Bergeron RT, Osborn AG, Som PM, eds. Head and neck imaging excluding the brain. St. Louis: CV Mosby, 1984:575–618.
32. Pearce WG, Nigam S, Rootman J. Primary anophthalmos: histological and genetic features. Can J Ophthalmol 1974; 9:141–145.
33. Makley TA, Battles M. Microphthalmos with cyst. Surg Ophthalmol 1969; 13:200–206.
34. Wright DC, Yuh WTC, Thompson HS, Nerad JA. Bilateral microphthalmos with orbital cysts: MR findings. J Comput Assist Tomogr 1987; 11:727–729.
35. Weiss A, Martinez C, Greenwald M. Microphthalmos with cyst: clinical presentations and computed tomographic findings. J Pediatr Ophthalmol Strab 1985; 22:6–12.
36. Walton DS. Primary congenital open angle glaucoma: a study of the anterior segment abnormalities. Trans Am Ophthalmol Soc 1979; 77:746–768.
37. Brown G, Tasman W, eds. Congenital anomalies of the optic disc. New York: Grune & Stratton, 1983:97–191.
38. Danziger A, Price HI: CT findings in retinoblastoma. AJR 1979; 133:695–697.
39. Abramson DH. Retinoblastoma: diagnosis and management. CA 1982; 32:130–140.
40. Zimmerman LE, Bilaniuk LT. CT in the evaluation of patients with bilateral retinoblastomas. J Comput Tomogr 1979; 3:251–257.
41. Tso MOM, Zimmerman LE, Fine BS, et al. A cause of radio-resistance in retinoblastoma: photoreceptor differentiation. Trans Am Acad Ophthalmol Otolaryngol 1970; 74:959–969.
42. Abramson DH, Ronner HJ, Ellsworth RM. Second tumors in nonirradiated bilateral retinoblastoma. Am J Ophthalmol 1979; 87:624–627.
43. Russell RS, Rubinstein LJ. Tumours of specialized tissues of central neuroepithelial origin. In: Russell RS, Rubinstein LJ, eds. Pathology of tumours of the nervous system, 5th ed. Baltimore: Williams & Wilkins, 1989.
44. Khoudadoust AA, Roozitalab HM, Smith RE, Green WR. Spontaneous regression of retinoblastoma. Surv Ophthalmol 1977; 21:467–478.
45. Hilal SK, Trokel SL. Computerized tomography of the orbit using thin sections. Semin Roentgenol 1977; 12:137–147.
46. Sullivan JA, Harms SE. Characterization of orbital lesions by surface coil MR imaging. RadioGraphics 1987; 7:9–28.
47. Atlas SW, Kemp SS, Rorke L, et al. Hemorrhagic intracranial retinoblastoma metastases: MR-pathology correlation. JCAT 1988; 12:286–289.
48. Shields JA. Diagnosis and management of intraocular tumors. St. Louis: CV Mosby, 1983:437–496.
49. Bilaniuk LT, Schenck JF, Zimmerman RA, et al. Ocular and orbital lesions: surface coil MR imaging. Radiology 1985; 156:669–674.

50. Peyman GA, Mafee MF. Uveal melanoma and similar lesions: the role of magnetic resonance imaging and computed tomography. Radiol Clin North Am 1987; 25:471–486.

51. Peyster RG, Augsburger JJ, Shields JA, et al. Intraocular tumors: evaluation with MR imaging. Radiology 1988; 168:773–779.

52. Brown GC, Shields JS. Tumors of the optic nerve head. Surv Ophthalmol 1985; 29:239–264.

53. Reese AB. Persistent hyperplastic primary vitreous. Am J Ophthalmol 1955; 40:317–331.

54. Howard GM, Ellsworth RM. Differential diagnosis of retinoblastoma. A statistical survey of 500 children. I. Relative frequency of the lesions which simulate retinoblastoma. Am J Ophthalmol 1965; 60:610–618.

55. Mafee MF, Goldberg MF, Valvassori GE, Capek V. Computed tomography in the evaluation of patients with persistent hyperplastic primary vitreous (PHPV). Radiology 1982; 145:713–717.

56. Ridley ME, Shields JA, Brown GC, Tasman WS. Coats' disease, evaluation of management. Ophthalmology 1982; 82:1381–1387.

57. Margo CE, Katz NNK, Wertz FD, Dorwart RH. Sclerosing endophthalmitis in children: computed tomography with histopathologic correlation. J Pediatr Ophthalmol Strab 1983; 20:180–184.

58. Mafee MF, Goldberg MF, Greenwald MJ, et al. Retinoblastoma and simulating lesions: role of CT and MR imaging. Radiol Clin North Am 1987; 25:667–682.

59. Kushner BJ, Essner D, Cohen IJ, et al. Retrolental fibroplasia. II. Pathologic correlation. Arch Ophthalmol 1977; 95:29–38.

60. Nolan JP, Mafee MF, Johnson G, et al. MR imaging characterization of intraocular lesions. Scientific exhibit at the Radiological Society of North America annual meeting, Chicago, Nov 27–Dec 2, 1988.

61. Gomori JM, Grossman RI, Goldberg HI, et al. Intracranial hematomas: imaging by high-field MR. Radiology 1985; 157:87–93.

62. Mafee MF, Linder B, Peyman GA, et al. Choroidal hematoma and effusion: evaluation with MR imaging. Radiology 1988; 168:781–786.

63. Lewis RA, Gerson LP, Axelson KA, et al. von Recklinghausen neurofibromatosis. II. Incidence of optic gliomata. Ophthalmology 1984; 91:929–935.

64. Spencer WH. Diagnostic modalities and natural behavior of optic nerve gliomas. Ophthalmology 1979; 86:881–885.

65. Azar-Kia B, Naheedy MH, Elias DA, et al. Optic nerve tumors: role of magnetic resonance imaging and computed tomography. Radiol Clin North Am 1987; 25:561–581.

66. Peyster RG, Hoover ED. The orbit and neuro-ophthalmology. In: Rosenberg RN, ed. The clinical neurosciences. New York: Churchill Livingstone, 1984:687–755.

67. Bognanno JR, Edwards MK, Lee TA, et al. Cranial MR imaging in neurofibromatosis. AJNR 1988; 9:461–468.

68. Johns TT, Citrin CM, Black J, et al. CT evaluation of perineural orbital lesions: evaluation of the "tram-track" sign. AJNR 1984; 5:587–590.

69. Atlas SW, Bilaniuk LT, Zimmerman RA, et al. Orbit: initial experience with surface coil spin-echo MR imaging at 1.5T. Radiology 1987; 164:501–509.

70. Frisen L, Holmegaard L. Spectrum of optic nerve hypoplasia. Br J Ophthalmol 1978; 62:7–15.

71. Barkovich AJ, Fram EK, Norman D. Septo-optic dysplasia: MR imaging. Radiology 1989; 171:189–192.

72. deMorsier G. Etudes sur les dysraphies cranioencephaliques. III. Agenesie du septum lucidum avec malformation du tractus optique: la dysplasie septo-optique. Schweiz Arch Neurol Psychiatr 1956; 77:267–292.

73. Manelfe C, Rochiccioli P. CT of septo-optic dysplasia. AJR 1979; 133:1157–1160.

74. Barkovich AJ, Chuang SH, Norman D. MR of neuronal migration anomalies. AJNR 1987; 8:1009–1017.

75. Atlas SW, Zimmerman RA, Bilaniuk LT, et al. Corpus callosum and limbic system: neuroanatomic MR evaluation of developmental anomalies. Radiology 1986; 160:355–362.

76. Cohen MM, Lessell S, Wolf PA. A prospective study of the risk of developing multiple sclerosis in uncomplicated optic neuritis. Neurology 1979; 29:208–213.

77. Dunn V, Bale JF, Zimmerman RA, et al. MRI in children with postinfectious disseminated encephalomyelitis. Magn Reson Imaging 1986; 4:25–32.

78. Smith RR, Farlow MR, Edwards MK, et al. Imaging of optic neuritis utilizing STIR MR. Presented at the American Society of Neuroradiology annual meeting, Orlando, FL, March 19–24, 1989.

79. Mafee MF, Putterman A, Valvassori GE, et al. Orbital space-occupying lesions: role of computed tomography and magnetic resonance imaging. An analysis of 145 cases. Radiol Clin North Am 1987; 25:529–559.

80. Rafto SE, Gefter WB. MRI of the upper aerodigestive tract and neck. Radiol Clin North Am 1988; 26:547–571.

81. Ruchman MC, Stefanyszyn MA, Flanagan JC, et al. Orbital tumors. In: Gonzalez CF, Becker MH, Flanagan JC, eds. Diagnostic imaging in ophthalmology. New York: Springer-Verlag, 1986:201–238.

82. Armington WG, Bilaniuk LT. The radiologic evaluation of the orbit: conal and intraconal lesions. Semin Ultrasound CT MR 1988;9:455–473.

83. Bram I. Exophthalmic goiter in children: comments based upon 128 cases in patients of 12 and under. Arch Pediatr 1937; 54:419–424.

84. Young LA. Dysthyroid ophthalmopathy in children. J Pediatr Ophthalmol Strab 1979; 16:105–107.

85. McKendrick T, Newns GH. Thyrotoxicosis in children: a follow-up study. Arch Dis Child 1965; 40:71–76.

86. Department of Ophthalmology, Toronto Hospital for Sick Children. The eye in childhood. Chicago: Year Book Medical Publishers, 1967:333.

87. Uretsky SH, Kennerdell JS, Gutai JP. Graves' ophthalmopathy in childhood and adolescence. Arch Ophthalmol 1980; 98:1963–1964.

88. Blodi FC, Gass J. Inflammatory pseudotumour of the orbit. Br J Ophthalmol 1968; 52:79–93.

89. Henderson JW, ed. Orbital tumors. Philadelphia: WB Saunders, 1973.

90. Mottow-Lippa L, Jakobiec F, Smith M. Idiopathic inflammatory orbital pseudotumor in childhood. II. Results of diagnostic tests and biopsies. Ophthalmology 1981; 88:565–574.

91. Mottow L, Jakobiec F. Pseudotumor in children. Arch Ophthalmol 1978; 96:1410–1417.

92. Enzmann D, Donaldson SS, Marshall WH, Kriss JP. Computed tomography in orbital pseudotumor (idiopathic orbital inflammation). Radiology 1976; 120:597–601.

93. Curtin HD. Pseudotumor. Radiol Clin North Am 1987; 25:583–599.

94. Youssefi B. Orbital tumors in children: a clinical study of 62 cases. J Pediatr Ophthalmol 1969; 6:177–181.

95. Sobel DF, Kelly W, Kjos BO, et al. MR imaging of orbital and ocular disease. AJNR 1985; 6:259–264.

96. Jakobiec FA, Bibralter RA, Knowles DM, et al. Lymphoid tumors of the lid. Ophthalmology 1974; 87:1058–1064.

97. Flanders AE, Espinosa GA, Markiewicz DA, Howell DD. Orbital lymphoma. Role of CT and MRI. Radiol Clin North Am 1987; 25:601–613.

98. Forbes GS, Earnest F, Waller RR. Computed tomography of orbital tumors, including late-generation scanning techniques. Radiology 1982; 142:387–394.

99. Atlas SW, Bilaniuk LT, Zimmerman RA. Orbit. In: Stark DD, Bradley WG, eds. Magnetic resonance imaging. St. Louis: CV Mosby, 1988:570–613.

100. Jakobiec FA, Jones IS. Mesenchymal and fibro-osseous tumors. In: Jones IS, Jakobiec FA, eds. Diseases of the orbit. Hagerstown, MD: Harper & Row, 1979:461–502.

101. Vade A, Armstrong D. Orbital rhabdomyosarcoma in childhood. Radiol Clin North Am 1987; 25:701–714.

102. Hopper KD, Haas DK, Sherman JL. The radiologic evaluation of congenital and pediatric lesions of the orbit. Semin Ultrasound CT MR 1988; 9:413–427.

103. Hesselink JR, Davis KR, Dallow RL, et al. Computed tomography of masses in the lacrimal gland region. Radiology 1979; 131:143–147.

104. Rothfus WE. Orbital trauma and infection. In: Latchaw RE, ed. Computed tomography of the head, neck and spine. Chicago: Year Book Medical Publishers, 1985:369–377.

105. Regenbogen VS, Zinreich SJ, Kim KS, et al. Hyperostotic esthesioneuroblastoma: CT and MR findings. J Comput Assist Tomogr 1988; 12:52–56.

106. Kelly WM, Paglen PG, Pearson JA, et al. Ferromagnetism of intraocular foreign body causes unilateral blindness after MR study. AJNR 1986; 7:243–245.

107. Tonami H, Kakagawa T, Ohguchi M, et al. Surface coil MR imaging of orbital blowout fractures: comparison with reformatted CT. AJNR 1987; 8:445–449.

Central Nervous System: Ear, Nose, Throat, and Skull

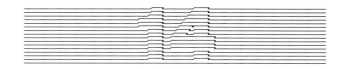

THEODORE R. HALL, M.D.

IMAGING TECHNIQUES

In the evaluation of pathologic conditions involving the skull or the ear, nose, and throat region, imaging techniques must be tailored to the particular clinical problem. In the pediatric population, routine protocols are less applicable. Generally, magnetic resonance imaging (MRI) spin-echo pulse sequences provide the necessary diagnostic and preoperative planning information for most problems. Partial saturation, or T1 weighted scans are best for anatomic resolution. Short TR-TE pulse sequences emphasize the T1 characteristics of tissues that lead to improved definition of tissue planes; this is particularly true for muscle and fat. However, lymphoid tissue and mucosal membranes are better defined on long TR-TE pulse sequences.[1-3] For this reason, T2 weighted scans may provide subtle information concerning infiltration of tumor through fascial planes and in the lymph nodes. The signal characteristics of the normal structures of the head and neck are summarized in Table 14–1.

Selection of imaging planes is solely dependent on the region to be analyzed and on the clinical problem. The nasopharynx can be best evaluated in the sagittal and axial imaging planes. The sagittal plane is best for evaluation of the clivus, sphenoid sinus, and posterior pharyngeal wall. The axial plane provides visualization of the skull base and the pharyngobasilar fascia. For evaluation of pathology in the infratemporal fossa, the coronal imaging plane should be added to rule out invasion of the skull base. The axial plane is also useful to determine tumor extension into adjacent anatomic compartments and evaluate the mastication muscles. The pterygopalatine fossa is also best analyzed in this plane. Lesions involving the oral and nasal cavities can be assessed in any of the three planes. The choice of which combination of imaging planes to use is based on the extent of the pathology. For the reasons cited above, tumors of the tongue require a T2 weighted pulse sequence to determine the extent of the pathology accurately.

The complex anatomic relationships in the neck usually make the axial the initial plane of choice to assess pathologic conditions in the region. Both the coronal and sagittal planes can be useful supplemental imaging planes. For lesions involving the midline, the sagittal plane may provide global information concerning the superoinferior extension of a lesion. The same is true of the coronal plane for lesions that are off the midline.

Improvement of the signal-to-noise ratio (SNR) (i.e., resolution) requires the use of surface coils for all head and neck imaging. In newborns and very small infants, a head coil may be employed to achieve resolution comparable with that achieved with solenoid band coils. The use of surface coils allows images to be produced with a pixel size of 0.5 × 0.5 mm. This also translates into fewer averages or decreased scanning time necessary to achieve high-resolution images than if imaging were performed without a surface coil.

Although there is improved contrast resolution on MRI compared with that obtainable on computed tomography (CT), the ability to separate many tumors

Table 14–1. SIGNAL CHARACTERISTICS OF STRUCTURES IN THE HEAD AND NECK

	T1	T2	Gadolinium-DTPA Enhancement
1. Mucosa	Low-moderate	Increases	Yes
2. Turbinates	Variably high	High	Yes
3. Tonsils	Low-moderate	Increases	Yes
4. Muscle	Low	Low	No
5. Salivary glands	High	Decreases	Yes
6. Fat	High	Decreases	No
7. Cartilage	Low	Low	No
8. Hyoid bone	Marrow-high	Marrow-high	
9. True cords	Moderate	Moderate	No
10. False cords	High	High	No
11. Epiglottis	Moderate	Moderate	No
12. Thyroid	Moderate	Increases	Yes

Adapted from Crawford SC, Harnsberger HR, Lufkin RB et al. Role of Gadolinium-DTPA in the evaluation of extracranial head and neck mass lesions. Radiol Clin North Am 1989; 27:219–242.

from surrounding normal structures is less than optimal when muscles are invaded or there is intracranial tumor extension. For this reason, a paramagnetic contrast agent such as gadolinium-DTPA can accentuate the differences among tissues in which it accumulates. Gadolinium-DTPA accomplishes improvement in contrast resolution by shortening the T1, and to a lesser extent T2, relaxation times of the tissues in which it is deposited. This effect is more noticeable for fluids or tissues with long T1 and T2 values.[4-6]

The routine use of gadolinium-DTPA requires an intravenous injection at a dose of 0.1 mmol per kilogram of body weight, administered over a 6- to 8-second interval with a 5-ml saline flush. Postgadolinium T1 weighted scans are obtained in the best planes to show the pathology. All patients have T2 weighted scans before the gadolinium-DTPA injection. The normal distribution of gadolinium-DTPA in the tissues is shown in Table 14–1.

For MRI of head and neck pathology the most useful applications for gadolinium-DTPA include tumor evaluation in the tongue area, perineural tumor infiltration, and evaluation of leptomeningeal spread of tumor. In the sinonasal region the differentiation of tumor from pockets of inspissated secretions is less than adequate on CT because of the lack of density difference between them. MR signal characteristics of tumor and inspissated secretions are also similar on both short and long pulsing sequences. T1 weighted gadolinium-DTPA scans provide superior definition of tumor interfaces and mucosa.

Similarly, early perineural extension of tumor cannot be detected by CT with or without iodinated contrast material. CT cannot reliably identify cranial nerves that are routinely demonstrated on unenhanced T1 weighted MR images. Gadolinium-DTPA enhancement can show early perineural tumor extension.

Recent observations have shown that even though the meninges normally enhance with the gadolinium-DTPA administration, pathologic and transient postoperative enhancement may be reliably detected on contrast-enhanced T1 weighted scans.[7] Contrast-enhanced MRI is more sensitive than contrast-enhanced CT for the evaluation of normal and abnormal meninges.

NORMAL ANATOMY

The ear, nose, and throat region is one of the most challenging areas of human anatomy for radiologic imaging. This is largely because of the complex and intimate relationships of structures within this region. Reconstructive x-ray CT imaging has improved the mapping and staging of lesions. The limits of lesion operability are more clearly defined with image reconstruction. Direct tomographic imaging and improved tissue contrast resolution have made MRI the imaging procedure of choice for the evaluation of most head and neck diseases. Sound interpretation of MR images of the ear, nose, and throat region requires a thorough knowledge of normal anatomy (Figs. 14–1 to 14–6).

Nasopharynx

The anatomy of the nasopharyngeal region can be best understood by defining the boundaries of the nasopharynx. The roof of the nasopharynx is formed by

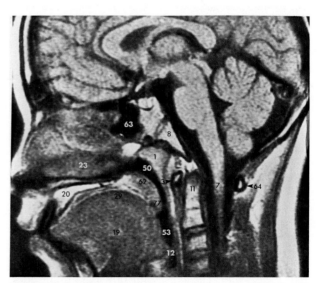

Figure 14–1. *Normal anatomy.* A midline sagittal MR image (480/30). Key: adenoid (1), arch of C1 (3), cervical cord (7), clivus (8), dens (11), epiglottis (12), genioglossus m. (19), hard palate (20), inferior turbinate (23), longitudinal muscle (29), nasopharynx (50), oropharynx (53), soft palate (62), sphenoid sinus (63), spinous process (64), uvula (77).

the adenoid, an aggregate of lymphoid tissue, which has low to intermediate signal intensity on partial saturation or T1 weighted pulse sequences (Fig. 14–1). Differences in the signal intensity of mucosal and lymphoid tissue lining the nasopharynx surface from underlying muscle layers are minimal on short TR-TE pulse sequences. The pharyngobasilar fascia lies between the mucosal and muscular layers of the nasopharynx. This tough fascial layer maintains the patency of the nasopharynx. On axial T1 weighted images the fascial layer appears as a thin line of relative hypointensity (Fig. 14–2).[1] It may be outlined over several slices from its origin at the pterygoid plate between the levator and tensor palatini muscles. The fascia is attached to the torus tubarius, a small mound of cartilaginous tissue that forms the opening of the eustachian tube. From the lateral recess (the fossa of Rosenmüller) the fascia is reflected medially over the longus colli and rectus capitis muscles (Fig. 14–3). The anterior boundary of the nasopharynx is formed by the nasal turbinates, while the posterior margin is defined by a fascial plane covering the longus colli muscles and the anterior longitudinal ligament. The inferior boundary is a free margin opening into the oropharynx.

Infratemporal Fossa

The infratemporal fossa is an irregularly shaped cavity lying medial or deep to the zygomatic arch. The lateral boundary is formed by the infratemporal surface of the maxilla and the ridge from the zygomatic process. The osseous boundaries include the great wing of the sphenoid, the inferior surface of the temporal squama, the alveolar border of the maxilla, the spine of the sphenoid, and the lateral pterygoid plate. This compartment contains the maxillary vessels, the mandibular and maxillary nerves, the pterygoid venous plexus, and the temporalis and both medial and lateral pterygoid muscles. The high-signal-intensity buccal fat pad surrounds the anterior, posterior, and medial margins of the pterygoid muscles (Fig. 14–2). The deep lobe of the parotid gland lies in the posterolateral portion of the fossa. It is easily differentiated from the surrounding muscle by its slightly higher signal on short TR-TE pulse sequences (Figs. 14–4, 14–5).[2]

Retropharyngeal Space

The retropharyngeal space is in reality only a potential space. The anterior boundary is a thin superficial layer of glandular and lymphoid tissue covering the longus colli muscle and the pharyngeal constrictors. The anterior longitudinal ligament descends along the anterior margin of the vertebral column between the parallel longus colli muscles. The glandular and lymphoid tissue layer can best be identified on long TR-TE pulse sequences where the relatively short T2 of muscle contrasts with the higher signal intensity of the thin superficial layer.

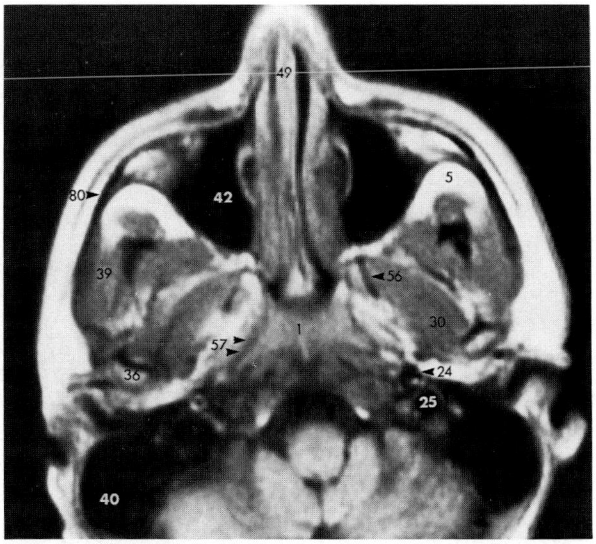

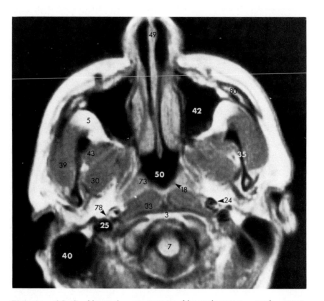

Figure 14–2. *Normal anatomy.*   Adenoid and infratemporal fossa. Axial image (649/22). Key: adenoid (1), buccal fat pad (5), internal carotid artery (24), internal jugular vein (25), lateral pterygoid m. (30), mandibular condyle (36), masseter m. (39), mastoid antrum (40), maxillary sinus (42), nasal septum (49), pterygoid plate (56), pharyngobasilar fascia (57), zygomatic arch (80).

Figure   14–3. *Normal anatomy.* Nasopharynx and parapharyngeal space. Axial image (649/22). Key: arch of C1 (3), buccal fat pad (5), cervical cord (7), fossa of Rosenmüller (18), internal carotid artery (24), internal jugular vein (25), lateral pterygoid m. (30), longus colli m. (33), mandible (35), masseter m. (39) mastoid antrum (40), maxillary antrum (42), medial pterygoid m. (43), nasal septum (49), nasopharynx (50), torus tubarius (73), vagus nerve (78), zygomatic arch (80).

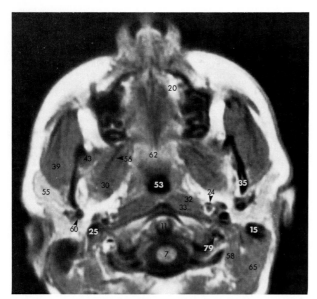

Figure 14–4. *Normal anatomy.* Hard palate and maxilla. Axial image (649/22). Key: cervical cord (7), dens (11), external jugular vein (15), hard palate (20), internal carotid artery (24), internal jugular vein (25), lateral pterygoid m. (30), longus capitis m. (32), longus colli m. (33), mandible (35), masseter m. (39), medial pterygoid m. (43), oropharynx (53), parotid gland (55), pterygoid plate (56), posterior belly of digastric m. (58), retromandibular vein (60), soft palate (62), sternocleidomastoid m. (66), vertebral artery (79).

Tongue and Oral Cavity

The nine paired muscles that make up the tongue are divided into extrinsic and intrinsic muscle groups. The extrinsic muscles that originate outside the tongue include the genioglossus, the hyoglossus, the chondroglossus, the styloglossus, and the palatoglossus muscles. These muscles control movement of the tongue. The intrinsic muscle group, which are four in number, include the superior and inferior longitudinal muscles and the transverse and vertical muscles. These muscles change the shape of the tongue. Individual bundles of muscle fibers have characteristic orientations that appear on MR images as low-signal striations surrounded by high-signal fat (Fig. 14–1).[8]

The oral cavity is divided into two distinct compartments: an outer part, the vestibule, and a inner portion, the mouth cavity proper. The vestibule is bounded externally by the lips and the cheeks, and internally by the gums and teeth. The reflection of the mucous membrane over the lips, cheeks, and gums to the upper and lower alveolar arch forms the superior and inferior boundaries of the vestibule. Secretions from the parotid gland are received in this compartment. Communication between the oral cavity proper and the vestibule is established via its free posterior end and between the teeth.

The mouth cavity proper is bounded laterally and anteriorly by the alveolar arches and teeth. The hard and soft palates form the roof, with communication to the pharynx at the posterior margin. The tongue forms the majority of the floor. The mouth cavity receives secretions from the sublingual and submandibular

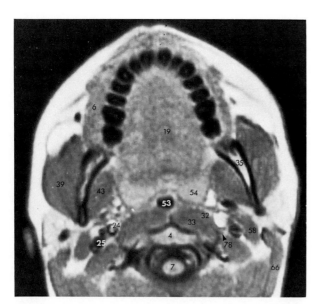

Figure 14–5. *Normal anatomy.* Oral cavity. Axial image (649/22). Key: axis (4), buccinator m. (6), cervical cord (7), genioglossus m. (19), internal carotid artery (24), internal jugular vein (25), longus capitis m. (32), longus colli m. (33), mandible (35), masseter m. (39), medial pterygoid m. (43), oropharynx (53), palatine tonsil (54), posterior belly of digastric m. (58), sternocleidomastoid m. (66), vagus nerve (78).

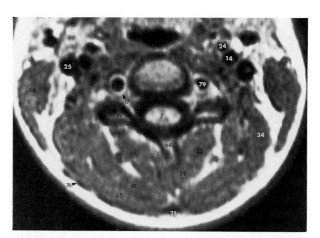

Figure 14–6. *Normal anatomy.* Nuchal region. Axial image (800/30). Key: cervical cord (7), external carotid artery (14), foramen transversarium (17), inferior oblique m. (22), internal carotid artery (24), internal jugular vein (25), ligamentum nuchae (31), longissimus capitis m. (34), rectus capitis posterior major m. (59), semispinalis capitis m. (61), spinous process (64), splenius capitis m. (65), sternocleidomastoid m. (66), transverse process (75), trapezius m. (76), vertebral artery (79).

glands. The hard palate contains marrow that produces a high signal because of the short T1 relaxation of fat surrounded by the lower signal cortical bone. The soft palate is normally of equal or slightly lower signal intensity than the marrow of the hard palate on T1 weighted scans (Fig. 14–1).

Neck

The regional anatomy of the neck can be described in relation to its different anatomic compartments. The anterior and posterior cervical triangles in the neck contain important nerves and blood vessels.

The anterior cervical triangle's posterior margin is defined by the sternocleidomastoid muscle. The superior boundary is defined by a line drawn along the lower margin of the mandible extending to the mastoid process, and the anterior boundary is the midline. The sternum resides at the apex of the triangle.

The anterior cervical triangle can be further subdivided into four smaller triangles: the inferior and superior carotid triangles and the suprahyoid and the submandibular triangles. The inferior or muscular triangle is bounded by the superior belly of the omohyoid muscle, the sternocleidomastoid muscle, and the midline of the neck. The isthmus of the thyroid gland, larynx, and trachea lie within this region. Other vital structures contained within the muscular triangle include the lower portion of the common carotid artery in the carotid sheath with the internal jugular vein and the vagus nerve.

The superior or carotid triangle is bounded at its inferior margin by the superior belly of the omohyoid muscle, the upper margin of the sternocleidomastoid muscle, and the posterior belly of the digastric muscle. Its floor is formed by pharyngeal constrictor muscles, and the thyrohyoid and hyoglossus muscles. Important structures contained within this region are the bifurcation of the carotid artery, the branches of the external carotid artery, and the hypoglossal and superior laryngeal nerves.

The submandibular triangle is bounded superiorly by the lower margin of the body of the mandible, and posteriorly by the stylohyoid and posterior belly of the digastric muscles and the anterior belly of the digastric muscle. The floor is formed by the mylohyoid and hyoglossus muscles. Both the submandibular and parotid glands lie in this space as well as the external carotid and the facial nerve.

The suprahyoid triangle is formed by the anterior belly of the digastric muscle, the hyoid bone, and the midline. Lymph nodes and branches of the anterior jugular vein are located in this region.

The posterior cervical triangle is defined by the posterior margin of the sternocleidomastoid muscle and the trapezius muscle, with the middle third of the clavicle forming the base of the triangle. This triangle can be divided into smaller ones: the occipital and the subclavian triangles. The occipital triangle is bounded below by the omohyoid, anteriorly by the sternocleidomastoid, and posteriorly by the trapezius muscle. The subclavian triangle is formed by the omohyoid, the lower border of the sternocleidomastoid, and the clavicle. In general, pathology in the posterior triangle is limited by a chain of lymph nodes behind the sternocleidomastoid and the brachial plexus.

CONGENITAL DISORDERS

In general the evaluation of congenital lesions of the head and neck region requires superior anatomic resolution for definition of vital structures that may be involved in a future reconstructive procedure. Because detailed bone anatomy is better demonstrated by CT, and soft tissue structure is better portrayed by MRI, the two modalities complement each other. Three-dimensional reconstruction algorithms can be adapted to both CT and MR scanning techniques. Soft tissue contrast differentiation is best appreciated on short TR-TE pulse sequences. The use of multiple imaging planes can provide invaluable information concerning the relationships of vital structures.

Most developmental and genetic anomalies are readily recognized by their clinical features and phenotypic characteristics. Therefore, the role of the radiologist is to suggest appropriate imaging procedures that may both narrow the differential possibilities and refine the diagnosis.

Facial Clefts

Midline facial clefts may range from a mild form such as cleft uvula to an extreme form such as bilateral facial cleft, in which the cleft runs from the corner of the mouth to the tragus of the ear. Cleft lip, with or without cleft palate, is not a rare anomaly. Isolated cleft lip is bilateral 20 percent of the time.[9] Cleft lip without cleft palate occurs with greater frequency in boys. Approximately 80 percent of bilateral cleft lips are associated with cleft palate, and 70 percent of unilateral cleft lips are associated with cleft palate.[9] The cleft may be complete (with extension into the nostril) or incomplete. A number of syndromes have associated cleft lip and/or cleft palate (Table 14–2). Various manifestations of the lobster claw deformity (ectrodactyly) associated with nasolacrimal duct obstruction, cleft lip/palate, and alterations of the skin and hair constitute a well-recognized syndrome referred to as ectrodactyly–ectodermal dysplasia–clefting syndrome.[10] The patients are also characterized by a paucity of scalp, eyebrow, and eyelash hair. The other ectodermal manifestations include syndactyly, clinodactyly, and nail dystrophy of the hands and feet.

Table 14–2. SYNDROMES ASSOCIATED WITH FACIAL CLEFTING

Ectrodactyly–ectodermal dysplasia–clefting syndrome
Frontonasal dysplasia
Kneist's syndrome*
Meckel's syndrome*
Paramedian lower lip pit syndrome
Popliteal pterygium syndrome†
Robert's syndrome†
Pierre Robin anomalad*
Stickler's syndrome*
4q-syndrome*
Trisomy 13

*Cleft palate; †cleft lip.

Frontonasal dysplasia (median clefting syndrome)[11,12] is phenotypically characterized by facial malformation, which may be mild or severe (Fig. 14–7). Severe hypertelorism, a flat nose with widely spaced nares, and clefting of the lip and palate are generally found in this developmental aberration. Other associated findings include preauricular tags, low-set ears, congenital cataracts, conductive hearing deficit, umbilical hernia, and cryptorchidism. The radiologic features, which may lead to a specific diagnosis, are cranium bifidum and hypoplastic frontal sinus. Patients may also have coronal craniosynostosis, anterior encephalocele, absence of the corpus callosum, and hydrocephalus. The cause of this condition is unknown; most cases occur sporadically.

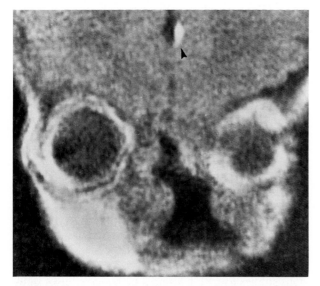

Figure 14–7. *Frontonasal dysplasia.* The association of congenital cataracts, low-set ears, and cleft lip and palate shown in this coronal MR image (480/28) led the neonatologists to suspect cranial abnormalities. A lipoma of the corpus callosum is demonstrated in this child with absence of the corpus callosum.

Pierre Robin Anomalad

The Pierre Robin anomalad is a triad of findings that include micrognathia, glossoptosis, and cleft palate.[13] It is not a specific disorder but contains features that may be found in association with other conditions. The mandible is small and recessed but by age 6 years it has usually achieved a normal size. Acyanotic congenital heart disease may be seen in up to 20 percent of infant deaths from this anomaly.[13] The infants often manifest respiratory difficulty very early. The basic defect is arrested development of the mandible, which then prevents the normal descent of the tongue between the palatine shelves. Micrognathia such as cleft lip and cleft palate may be seen in a number of other developmental anomalies (Table 14–3) (Fig. 14–8).

Beckwith-Wiedemann Syndrome

A discussion of craniofacial anomalies cannot be complete without inclusion of the Beckwith-Wiedemann syndrome, which is one of the more common entities (Figs. 14–9, 14–10).[14,15] Its classic features include macroglossia, omphalocele, postnatal somatic gigantism, and neonatal hypoglycemia. These infants are often large at birth, weighing on average approximately 3.9 kg. The estimated frequency is one per 15,000 births, with no sex predilection. Approximately 15 percent of infants born with omphalocele have this syndrome.[14] Generalized visceromegaly is a frequent occurrence. Hemihypertrophy may be seen in up to 15 percent of patients.[15] Other frequent associated findings are mental retardation, facial birthmarks (90 percent),[14] malrotation, inguinal hernia, and eventration of the diaphragm.

The cause of Beckwith-Wiedemann syndrome is presently unknown. Most cases are sporadic occurrences. Amniocentesis shows an elevated alpha-fetoprotein level in patients with an omphalocele. There is an increased incidence of both Wilms' tumor and adrenocortical carcinoma in patients with this syndrome.

Table 14–3. SYNDROMES ASSOCIATED WITH MICROGNATHIA

Cerebrocostomandibular syndrome
Cerebrohepatorenal syndrome
Dubovitz's syndrome
Hypoglossia-hypodactylia spectrum
Mandibular dysostosis
Melnick-Needles syndrome
Menkes' syndrome
Oculomandibulofacial syndrome
4q-syndrome
Pierre Robin anomalad
Russell's syndrome

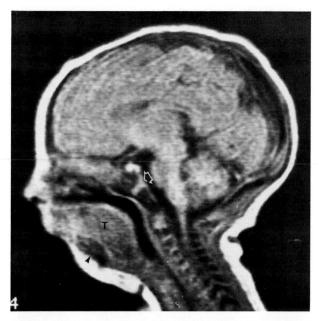

Figure 14–8. *Micrognathia.* This newborn child was transferred from another hospital for further evaluation of multiple congenital anomalies. The clinical findings were consistent with arthrogryposis multiplex congenita, a crippling disorder characterized by limitation of range of joint motion and contractures present at birth. The sagittal MR image (500/28) demonstrates mandibular hypoplasia (*arrowhead*) with an overhanging tongue (T). Note the lower-signal hematopoietic marrow in the clivus and the higher-signal cartilage of the spheno-occipital synchondrosis (*open arrow*).

Encephaloceles

Congenital defects of the calvarium include herniation of the brain (encephalocele) or only the meninges (meningocele) (Fig. 14–11). The classification of encephaloceles is based on the site of origin: occipital, parietal, or anterior. Occipital encephaloceles occur most frequently and make up 75 percent of all encephaloceles.[16] The anterior defects may be visible (sincipital) or hidden, occurring at the skull base (basal). The frontoethmoidal variety of anterior encephalocele includes an increased incidence of associated mental retardation.

Thornwaldt's Cyst

Thornwaldt's cysts result from an adhesion between the notochord and pharyngeal ectoderm. A persistent pouch is formed as the notochord regresses dorsally. The location of the pouch, or nasopharyngeal bursa, is always midline at the roof of the nasopharynx. A Thornwaldt cyst is formed when the opening of the bursa is occluded and fluid accumulates within the sac. The cyst is usually 2 to 3 cm in diameter. Although

Thornwaldt's cyst can occur at any age, it most often appears between the ages of 15 and 30 years. MR signal characteristics are similar to those of uninfected fluid collections, with low or intermediate signal intensity on partial saturation sequences and high signal intensity on long TR-TE pulsing sequences.

Thyroglossal Duct Cyst

Thyroglossal duct cysts are described by their location in relationship to the hyoid bone; the most common is infrahyoid.[17] Nearly two-thirds occur in this location; suprahyoid is the next most frequent site, followed by hyoid. The cyst may be eccentric in location. Previous infection of the cyst is most often the cause of an associated fistula, which may drain into the pharynx or out to the skin.

Histologic sections of a thyroglossal duct cyst typically show a squamous cell lining. These cysts typically have intermediate signal intensity on T1 weighted images and high signal intensity on long TR-TE pulsing sequences (Fig. 14–12). They characteristically demonstrate a gradual increase in size requiring surgical excision. Removal of the entire cyst and tract together with the middle one-third of the hyoid bone is most important to prevent recurrence.

INFECTION

Sinusitis

Radiologic evaluation of disease in the paranasal sinuses is based on plain film demonstration of findings such as air-fluid interfaces, mucosal thickening, or complete opacification. The presence of an air-fluid interface is indicative of acute sinus disease. MRI has very little to contribute in this clinical setting. However, various degrees of partial opacification and mucosal thickening may present a problem in interpretation when a partially opacified sinus is noted on routine plain films.

In the past the incorrect diagnosis of sinus opacification has been generally accepted to be due to the technical difficulties of obtaining diagnostic quality films in young children. The technical factors often referred to include positioning, motion artifact, the small size of paranasal sinuses, and overlying soft tissue disease. Opacification in children under 10 months old has often been linked to redundant mucous membranes and passive congestion in crying children. Previous studies using CT found a high incidence of sinus abnormalities in children with and without evidence of recent upper respiratory infection.[18, 19] A recent study by McAlister and colleagues found a 35 percent false-positive rate of disease and a 45 percent false-negative

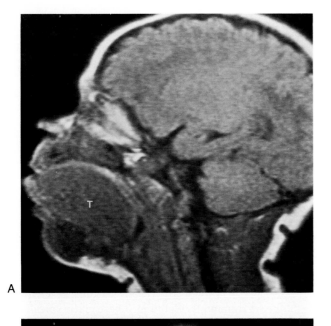

A

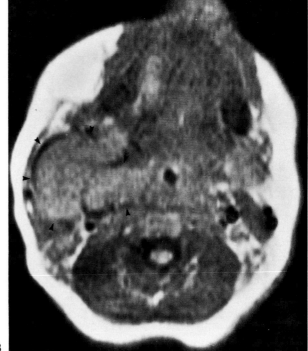

B

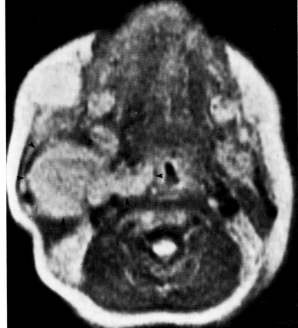

C

Figure 14–9. *Beckwith-Wiedemann syndrome.* Hemihypertrophy, macroglossia, and airway obstruction with an enlarging mass in the right submandibular region were the presenting signs in this 15-month-old boy. *A,* Midline sagittal MR image (500/28) shows preservation of the intrinsic muscle fiber pattern in the hypertrophied tongue (T). *B,* T1 weighted axial image (480/28) shows the location of the mass (*arrowheads*) to be in the anterior cervical triangle. *C,* Moderate increase in signal intensity is noted on the T2 weighted axial image (2000/84). A fine-needle aspiration biopsy showed lymphoid follicle formation and metastatic Wilms' tumor.

rate with plain film radiography when these films were compared with a CT examination of the paranasal sinuses in the same patient.[20]

MRI offers an improved method of evaluation of the paranasal sinuses. The ability to distinguish between mucosal disease and partial pneumatization of a sinus is made possible with long TR-TE pulse sequences. Both mucosal disease and bone marrow in the nonpneumatized portion of a sinus have short T2 signal characteristics. Marrow within nonpneumatized por-

tions of a sinus has high signal on T1 weighted images (Fig. 14–13). This is in contrast to mucosal disease, which typically has intermediate signal intensity with short TR-TE pulse sequences.

There is significant overlap in the opacification owing to sinus disease and various degrees of anatomic development.[21] Data derived from a retrospective study of 80 pediatric patients without upper respiratory tract symptoms, in the age range of 2 months to 17 years, showed that various degrees of pneumatiza-

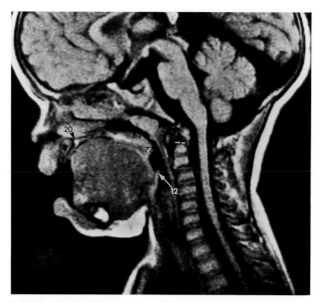

Figure 14-10. *Macroglossia.* After a partial glossectomy this 2-year-old girl continued to have difficulty swallowing. A sagittal MR image (500/28) clearly shows the line of resection, with a hypertrophied tongue filling the entire oral cavity. The soft palate is displaced superiorly and the vallecula is completely obliterated. Key: epiglottis (12), hard palate (20), soft palate (62), uvula (77).

tion may exist in the ethmoid sinuses up to age 2 years and in the maxillary sinuses up to age 4 years.[21] Routine sinus radiographs alone are inadequate to determine the presence or absence of sinus disease at these younger ages.

Chronic inflammatory disease involving the paranasal sinuses is best assessed by either CT or MRI. Both of these modalities offer more detailed evaluation of the extent of disease; better soft tissue contrast resolution is achieved with MRI (Figs. 14-14, 14-15, 14-16). T1 weighted pulse sequences are preferred for the anatomic definition necessary to define the extent of disease. Long TR-TE pulse sequences can reliably separate fluid in an obstructed sinus from soft tissue disease affecting the sinus. MRI can also be used in the follow-up period after treatment to document resolution of disease, or to image the possible sequelae of inflammatory or allergy-related disease of the paranasal sinuses, such as retention cysts or polyps (Fig. 14-17). Retention cysts typically are intermediate in signal intensity on T1 weighted images, with very short T2 characteristics manifested by a marked increase in signal intensity on T2 weighted images. The signal intensity increase with long TR-TE pulse sequences is not as dramatic in polyps.

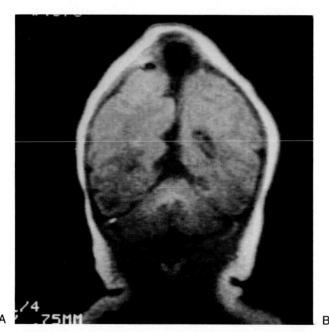

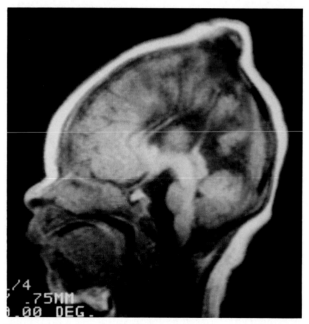

A   B

Figure 14-11. *Meningocele.* A prenatal ultrasound examination in this newborn infant diagnosed a cranial defect. **A, B,** Both coronal (600/28) (**A**) and sagittal (500/28) (**B**) images show an extracranial mass with signal intensity similar to that of cerebrospinal fluid. No evidence of gray matter was found at surgery.

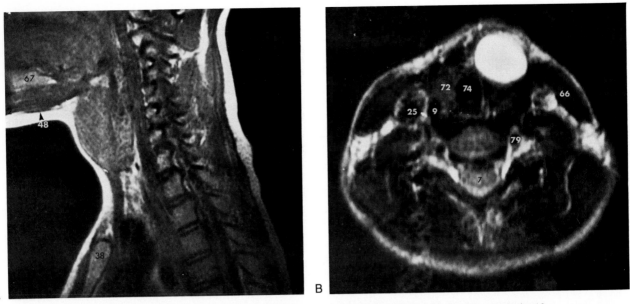

Figure 14–12. *Thyroglossal duct cyst.* This 17-year-old boy complained of a rapidly enlarging lump in the neck in the 10 days before this MR study.   **A,** Sagittal image (480/30) depicts an ovoid mass of intermediate signal intensity, palpable to the left of midline. **B,** Marked increase in signal intensity on the axial image (2000/85) is consistent with highly proteinaceous fluid. The borders are smooth and well defined. Key: anterior belly of digastric m. (2), cervical cord (7), common carotid artery (9), foramen transversarium (17), internal jugular vein (25), manubrium (38), mylohyoid m. (48), spinous process (64), sternocleidomastoid m. (66), sublingual gland (67), thyroid gland (72), vertebral artery (79).

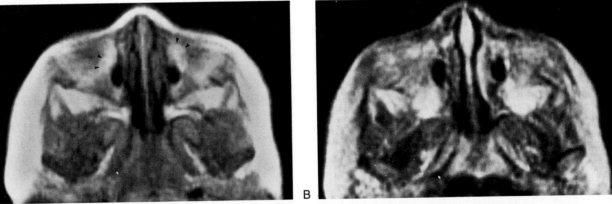

Figure 14–13. *Normal sinus development.*   Sinus films in the eight-month-old infant were reported as mucosal thickening from chronic inflammation. A magnetic resonance scan of the brain was obtained for an unrelated problem. **A,** An axial (649/22) MR image shows a partially pneumatized maxillary antrum with high signal marrow (*arrowheads*) in the anterior portion of the sinus. **B,** The same area is also high in signal intensity on the axial (3000/85) image.

Soft Tissue Infection

The first signs of inflammation or infection in the hypopharynx are usually fever, stiff neck, and dysphagia. Retropharyngeal abscess is uncommon in newborn infants and is most often associated with perforation of the hypopharynx following instrumentation. In the first year of life the most common cause of retropharyngeal abscess is *Haemophilus influenzae.*

The radiographic findings of prevertebral soft tissue swelling and on occasion retropharyngeal emphysema are enough to suggest the diagnosis in the proper clini-cal setting. However, when the abnormalities are more subtle, an MR scan may define a focal area of inflammation more clearly. MRI cannot differentiate cellulitis from a drainable fluid collection. For detection of tiny amounts of gas, CT is more reliable than MRI.[3, 22, 23] Widening of the prevertebral space with intermediate-signal-intensity soft tissue is characteristic on T1 weighted images. The long TR-TE pulsing sequences best demonstrate obliteration of the fascial planes and infiltration of the underlying glandular tissue in the prevertebral region. Signal intensity of the infiltrated region is increased on T2 weighted scans (Fig. 14–18).

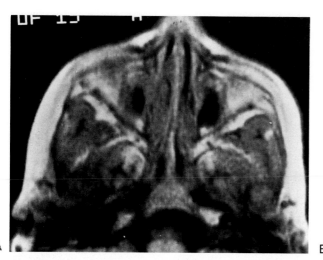
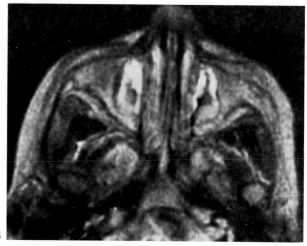

Figure 14–14. *Sinusitis.* **A,** The maxillary sinuses are filled with intermediate signal intensity in this axial (649/22) image. **B,** A uniform increase in signal intensity is noted in the axial (3000/85) image.

TUMOR AND TUMOR-LIKE DISORDERS

Benign

Angiofibroma

Angiofibromas are the most common benign nasopharyngeal tumors. Predominantly occurring in teenagers, they have been referred to as juvenile angiofibroma. There is a pronounced male predominance. The lesions typically are slow-growing masses that cause pressure erosion of the regional osseous structures such as the pterygoid plate and the posterior wall of the antrum. Intracranial spread into the middle cranial fossa via the inferior and superior orbital fissures is not uncommon. On occasion the lesions may invade the sphenoid sinus. Because of the slow growth pattern, bone destruction is uncommon with these lesions.

Juvenile angiofibromas tend to be highly vascular

lesions. Patients may present with epistaxis in addition to a nasal mass, which may be mistaken clinically for a polyp. The lesions show marked contrast enhancement on CT scans after a bolus injection of intravenous contrast material. Both intermediate signal intensity and a salt-and-pepper appearance on T1 weighted images are typical for this tumor (Fig. 14–19).[24] Gradient-echo imaging may enhance visualization of the vascular channels in the lesion. Because of the highly vascular nature of these tumors, transnasal biopsy is contraindicated. The clinical presentation and imaging appearance of the tumors are enough to suggest the diagnosis prior to therapy. Embolization before surgical resection may lead to a more satisfactory operative result with less intraoperative hemorrhage.

Nasal Polyps

In the pediatric population nasal polyps are rare before the age of 5 years. Most of these lesions occur in

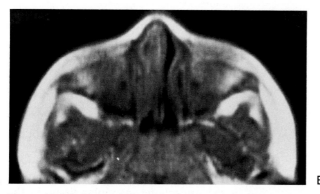
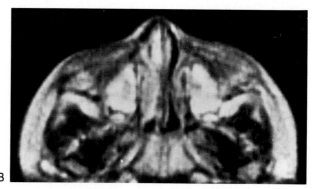

Figure 14–15. *Mucosal disease.* **A,** Intermediate signal intensity mucosal thickening is demonstrated in this axial (649/22) image at the level of the maxillary antra. This is contrasted to a partially aerated sinus with marrow. **B,** There is uniform increased signal intensity of the mucosal disease in the axial (3000/85) image.

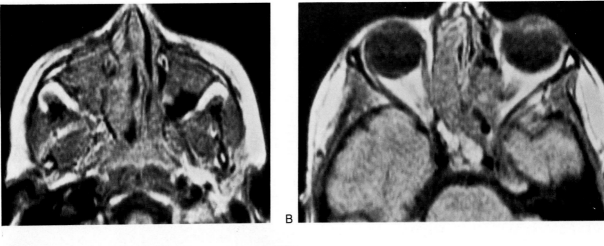

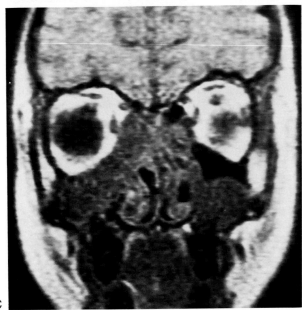

Figure 14–16. *Fungal sinusitis.* Extensive infiltration of the paranasal sinuses in this patient resulted from an indolent fungal infection. ***A, B*** Axial (800/28) and ***C,*** coronal (600/28) images show the aggressive nature of this difficult-to-eradicate infection. There is extensive abnormality in the maxillary and ethmoid sinuses, with penetration through the sinus walls.

teenagers and young adults. Both asthmatics and patients with cystic fibrosis have historically been considered to be at risk for the development of nasal polyps. In point of fact the incidence of nasal polyps in asthmatic patients has been reported to be only 0.1 percent.[25] Patients with negative results from allergy skin tests and inhalants have a greater association with nasal polyps than those patients whose results are positive. In patients with cystic fibrosis the incidence of polyps ranges from 6 to 25 percent.[26] Most of these are detected in patients from 4 to 13 years of age in association with mucoid impaction of the paranasal sinuses, particularly the ethmoid and frontal sinuses. Polypoid masses may be associated with both allergic rhinitis and chronic infections. MRI probably has little role to play in the evaluation of nasal polyps. They may be seen incidentally as well-defined, nonspecific masses on images obtained for other reasons.

Lipoma

Lipomatous masses are uncommon in the head and neck region. When they do occur, the buccal mucosa is the most common site; over 50 percent of lipomas involve this region.[27] The tongue, floor of the mouth, lips, perioral tissues, and hypopharynx may also be involved in descending order of frequency. The tumor is well encapsulated, subcutaneous, and submucous in location. Sudden enlargement may be the result of hemorrhage into the tumor. Signal intensity on both short and long TR-TE pulsing sequences is equal to that of normal subcutaneous fat. Thin fibrous septations may be demonstrated throughout the tumor (Fig. 14–20).

Hamartoma

Hamartomas are simple, spontaneous growths composed of local soft tissue components. The tumor mass

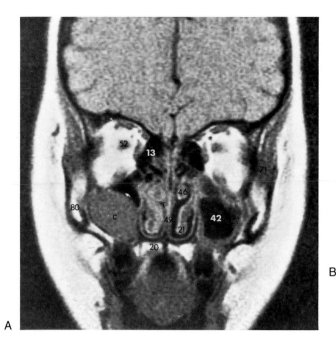

A

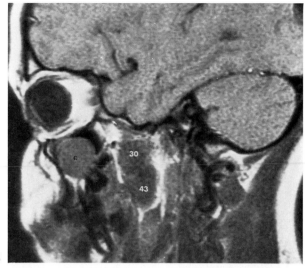

B

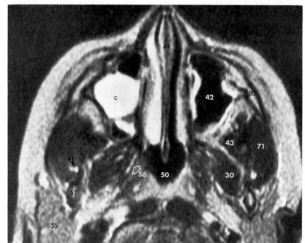

C

Figure 14–17. *Retention cyst.* An abnormal dental radiograph prompted further study in this asymptomatic 11-year-old boy. **A, B,** Coronal (587/30) and sagittal (480/30) MR images clearly define the margins of the intermediate-signal-intensity right maxillary sinus retention cyst (c). The mass is resting on the floor of the maxillary sinus just superior to a tooth. **C,** Axial (2000/85) image demonstrates uniform signal enhancement. Endoscopic exploration and resection confirmed the diagnosis of a retention cyst. Key: ethmoid sinus (12), hard palate (20), inferior concha (21), lateral pterygoid m. (30), longus colli m. (33), maxillary artery (41), maxillary antrum (42), medial pterygoid m. (43), middle concha (46), nasal septum (49), nasopharynx (50), optic nerve (52), parotid gland (55), pterygoid plate (56), temporalis m. (71), zygomatic arch (80).

is self-limiting. MRI characteristics vary according to the histologic components of the tumor. Areas of high signal intensity on T1 and T2 weighted images most likely represent fat; other components, such as muscle, fibrous tissue, or cartilage may have low or intermediate signal intensity (Fig. 14–21).

Neurogenic Tumors

The benign tumors of neurogenic origin differ in their clinical and pathologic presentation. Schwannomas tend to be solitary and encapsulated tumors without association with von Recklinghausen's disease. Necrosis and hemorrhage are often present. Neurofibromas tend to be multiple and nonencapsulated and are considered the hallmark tumor of neurofibromatosis (Fig. 14–22). Although solitary neurofibromas and multiple neurofibromas without neurofibromatosis do occur, they are much less com-

mon (Fig. 14–23). Less than 10 percent of neurofibromas undergo malignant change.[28]

Neurofibromas are typically asymptomatic unless the mass presses on a nearby nerve. Although café au lait spots are reported in association with neurofibromatosis, more than half of the cases do not have pigmented skin lesions. Neurogenic tumors typically demonstrate intermediate signal intensity on T1 weighted and proton density images with either high signal or a salt-and-pepper appearance on T2 weighted pulse sequences (Fig. 14–24).[24]

Hemangioma

Hemangiomas are the most common tumor of the head and neck region in children; with lymphangiomas they constitute 30 percent of all childhood oral tumors.[29] Cutaneous, mucosal, and invasive varieties of hemangioma all have different locations and different

Text continues on page 402.

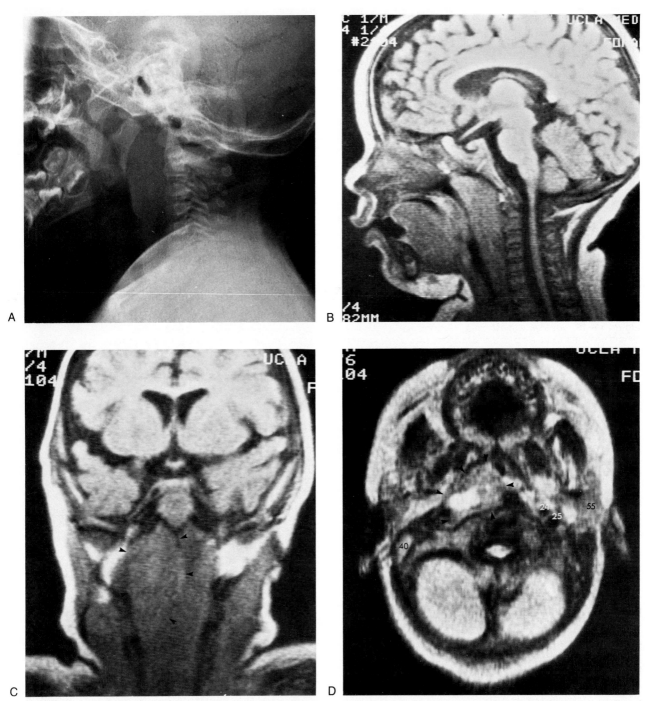

Figure 14–18. *Retropharyngeal abscess.*   Fever and excessive drooling were the presenting manifestations of infection in this 14-month-old boy. *A,* After the preliminary lateral neck radiograph, which demonstrates pharyngeal soft tissue swelling, he developed right-sided facial weakness. Follow-up sagittal (*B*) and coronal (*C*) MR images (500/28) confirmed the radiograph findings. The pharyngeal soft tissue is asymmetrically thickened (*arrowheads*) with intermediate signal intensity. *D,* Axial MR image (2000/84) shows focal high signal intensity involving the right side of the pharynx. Additional soft tissue (*arrowheads*) is noted filling the right side of the pharynx, with high signal intensity in the right mastoid antrum secondary to eustachian tube obstruction. Key: internal carotid artery (24), internal jugular vein (25), mastoid antrum (40), parotid gland (55).

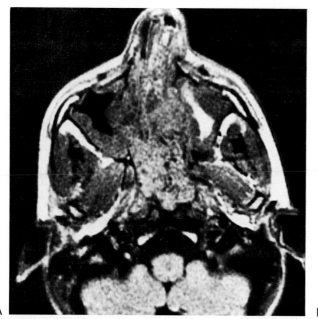
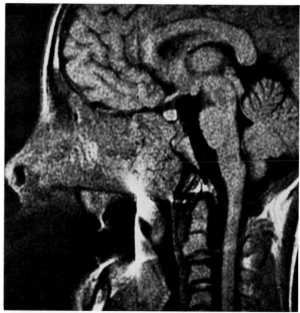

A   B

Figure 14–19. *Juvenile angiofibroma.* Chronic nasal congestion in this 15-year-old boy prompted further study after films of abnormal sinus were obtained to rule out polyps. *A,* Axial MR image (800/30) demonstrates a lesion with a salt-and-pepper appearance filling the nasal cavity and nasopharynx. The ostium of the left maxillary sinus is obstructed, as evidenced by the high-signal fluid within the sinus. Prominent mucosal thickening is noted in the right maxillary sinus. *B,* The mass completely fills the nasopharynx and extends into the sphenoid sinus in this midline sagittal MR image (500/30). Angiography confirmed the highly vascular nature of the lesion.

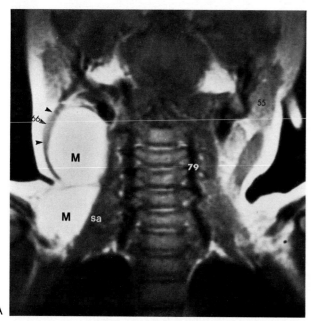
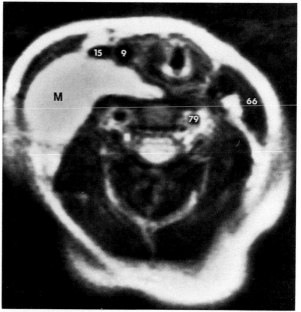

A   B

Figure 14–20. *Lipoma.* The mother of this 2-year-old girl noticed a lump in her daughter's neck that had increased in size over a 4-week interval and was soft to palpation. *A,* Coronal image (587/30) shows a lobulated high-signal-intensity mass (M) arising from the posterior cervical triangle and extending down to the supraclavicular area. *B,* T2 weighted (2300/85) axial scan shows that the signal intensity of the mass (M) is equal to that of the subcutaneous fat. Key: common carotid artery (9), external jugular vein (15), foramen transversarium (17), parotid gland (55), sternocleidomastoid m. (66), vertebral artery (79), scalenus anterior m. (sa).

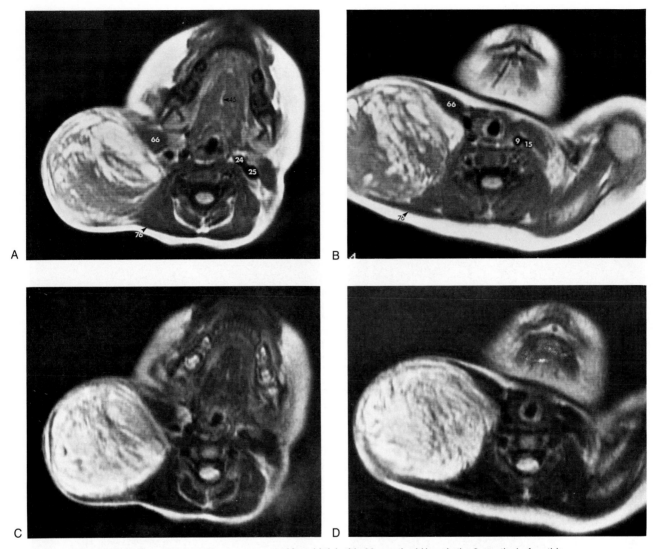

Figure 14–21. *Hamartoma.* A right neck mass was noted from birth in this 20-month-old boy. In the 2 months before this evaluation, the mass had doubled in size. *A, B,* Axial MR images (778/28) define a large, mixed-signal-intensity mass arising behind the sternocleidomastoid muscle in the posterior cervical triangle. Fascial planes are preserved. *C, D,* Axial T2 weighted scans (2000/84) show increased signal intensity in the entire mass. Excisional biopsy showed a proliferation of mature lobules of adipose tissue with fibrous septa. Key: common carotid artery (9), external jugular vein (15), internal carotid artery (24), internal jugular vein (25), median raphe (45), sternocleidomastoid m. (66), trapezius m. (76).

clinical behavior patterns. Cutaneous hemangiomas occur primarily in infants and young children. Two forms of this lesion are capillary and cavernous types. The capillary type may involute spontaneously without therapy. Histologic specimens of capillary hemangiomas are characterized by numerous variably sized, but predominantly small, closely packed capillaries that are usually separated by thin reticulin fibers. The endothelial cells lining the capillaries are large and prominent, with only a small potential space as a lumen.

Spontaneous regression of the cavernous variety is typical only of lesions that are present at birth, and less likely than in lesions occurring later in life. Cavernous hemangiomas are histologically characterized by large,

blood-filled spaces due to dilatation and thickening of the capillary walls.

The other two types of cutaneous hemangiomas are mucosal and invasive. The mucosal variety typically arise in the mucosa of the oropharynx and upper respiratory tract. The invasive variety are usually more deeply situated than either cutaneous or mucosal types. They occur in the deep fascial layers and muscles. Although the invasive form may be seen in adults, they are much less common than in the pediatric population.

Typical MR scan features of hemangiomas include an intermediate-signal-intensity mass on T1 weighted and proton density images. Long TR-TE pulsing se-

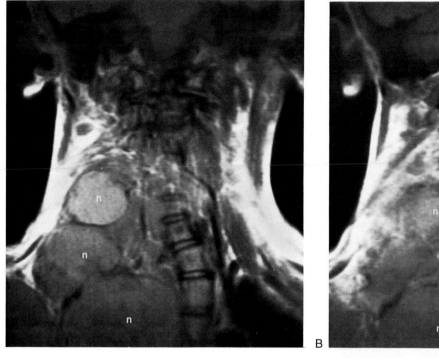

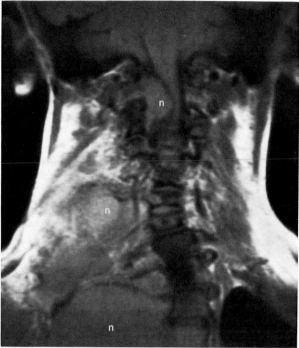

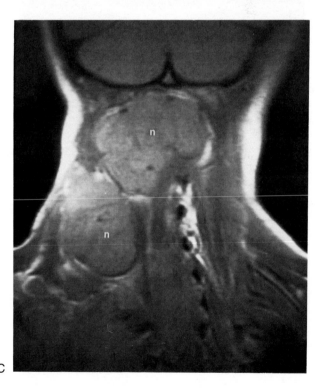

Figure 14–22. *Neurofibromatosis.* An increase in pain involving the right arm and forearm prompted this 15-year-old girl to seek medical attention. *A–C,* Coronal MR images (800/30) clearly show the multilobulated tumor in the region of the brachial plexus, which was compressed by mass effect from these large neurofibromas (n). Tumor extension into the neural foramen is also clearly demonstrated at the C1–C2 level. This finding required a neurosurgical consultation to plan the resection.

quences often demonstrate a marked increase in signal intensity, which may be greater than the signal arising from fat in the same scan (Fig. 14–25). The degree of signal intensity increase is inversely proportional to the amount of fibrous tissue in the lesion.[30] Signal void secondary to tumor vessels or phleboliths may also be seen on T1 weighted images.[24, 30] Partial saturation sequences may demonstrate large sinusoids with occasional fluid-to-fluid levels.

For lesions that are present at birth, therapy is usu-

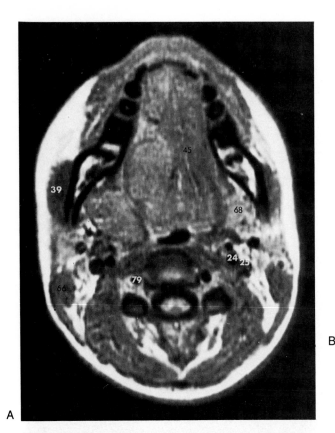

A

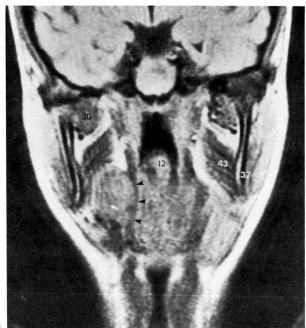

B

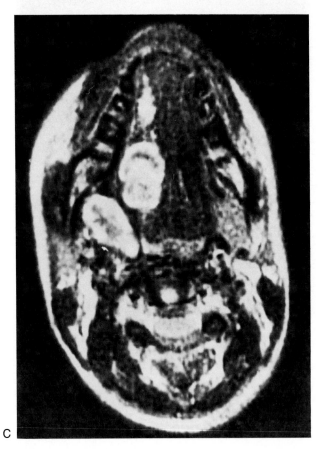

C

Figure 14–23. *Plexiform neurofibroma.* This 15-year-old girl had noted "lumps" on her tongue since childhood. A recent increase in the size of the masses prompted this MR study. *A,* Axial image (800/30) defines three well-circumscribed intermediate-signal-intensity masses in the distribution of the lingual nerve along the right side of the tongue. The medial margin of the most anterior lesion is indistinguishable from the muscle fibers of the tongue. *B,* Coronal image (587/30) clearly shows that the more posterior mass is separate from the tongue (*arrowheads*). *C,* T2 differences between muscle and the abnormal neural tissue are accentuated in this axial MR image (2000/85). Key: epiglottis (12), internal carotid artery (24), internal jugular vein (25), lateral pterygoid m. (30), mandibular ramus (37), masseter m. (39), medial pterygoid m. (43), sternocleidomastoid m. (66), vertebral artery (79).

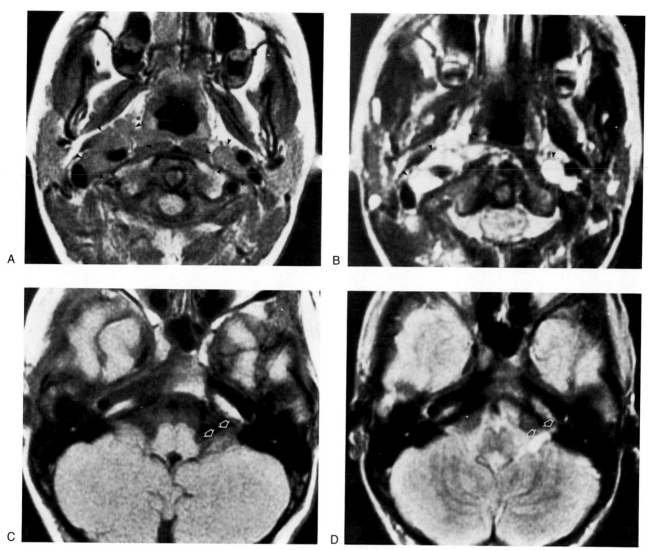

Figure 14–24. *Neurofibromatosis.* A routine chest radiograph for a positive tuberculin test in this 8-year-old boy showed a mass in the apical region of the left thorax. A needle biopsy was consistent with a benign neurofibroma. Both axial (800/30) (**A**) and the corresponding axial (2000/84) (**B**) MR images demonstrate bilateral intermediate signal masses (*arrowheads*) of the 9th, 10th, and 11th cranial nerves. Extension of neuroma through the left jugular foramen (*open arrows*) is clearly shown on T1 (**C**) and T2 (**D**) weighted pulse sequences. T2 weighted axial images demonstrate signal enhancement typical of neuromas.

ally unnecessary since they undergo spontaneous regression. Radiation therapy, injection of sclerosing agents, and surgical excision have been used in the management of these lesions. Radiologic embolization before surgery may dramatically improve the operative outcome. Therapy is often individualized. A multitude of factors, including patient size and age, site of lesion, extent of lesion, and associated clinical manifestations, determine the appropriate therapeutic course for each case.

Lymphangioma

Lymphangiomas are generally present at birth or appear shortly thereafter (Fig. 14–26). Most congenital lymphangiomas arise in the neck in the posterior cervical triangle. Occasionally, tumor may extend beyond the sternocleidomastoid muscle that forms the anterior margin of the posterior triangle. Masses that arise anteriorly usually involve the floor of the mouth and the tongue base (Fig. 14–27). Lymphangiomas involving the tongue are particularly important be-

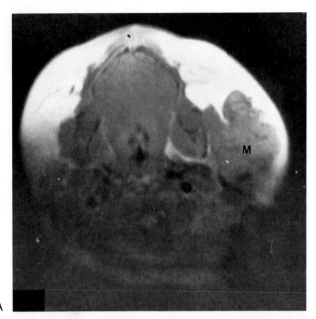
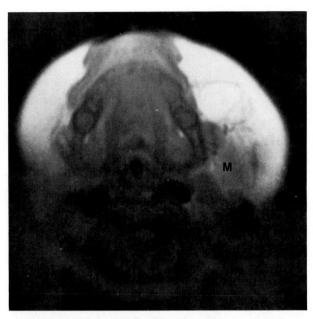

A   B

Figure 14–25. *Juvenile hemangioendothelioma.* History on admission showed that this child had experienced 3 weeks of the left cheek swelling. *A, B,* A multilobulated soft tissue mass (M) was identified on axial images (500/28). Surgical resection and histologic examination showed a highly vascular tumor containing multiple sinusoids.

cause of possible hemorrhage, which may be fatal. Masses beginning in the neck may extend medially to involve the parotid gland or caudad into the lung apex and the mediastinum. Compression of the brachial plexus because of tumor size may result in pain or hyperesthesia. The histologic appearance of these tumors is typical, with large, dilated, endothelium-lined lymphatic channels. Hemangiomatous elements are commonly associated with tumors of the upper neck, pharynx, and parotid gland.

The term cystic hygroma refers to a congenital form of lymphangioma with thin-walled cysts. The neck is a typical location. Signs and symptoms may include distortion of facial architecture, stridor, and a sudden increase in size, usually from acute hemorrhage.

The MR appearance of lymphangiomas is similar to that of hemangiomas.[31, 32] Short TR-TE pulsing sequences may resolve the dilated lymphatic channels, which appear as lobules (Fig. 14–28). Focal areas of high signal intensity on T1 weighted images may represent hemangiomatous elements or sites of hemorrhage within the lesion.

Histiocytosis

Of the benign tumor-like disorders, the histiocytosis Langerhans cell syndrome has the most malignant clinical presentation. Histiocytosis is classified into three forms of disease that vary in clinical severity and prognosis. A proliferation of histiocytes occurs in all three forms.

The mildest presentation in the spectrum of this disease is eosinophilic granuloma of bone. The lesions are limited to bone and may be single or multiple lytic defects. The rib is the most common flat bone involved, with lesions occurring in the skull, extremities, spine, and pelvis. The temporal bone is a favored site of involvement in the skull. Lytic lesions involving the mandible or maxilla may lead to painful swellings and can dislodge teeth in young children (Fig. 14–29). This radiographic sign is commonly referred to as the "floating" tooth.

The MR appearance of these lesions is relatively nonspecific, with low to intermediate signal intensity on T1 weighted images that increases on long TR-TE pulsing sequences. An excisional biopsy can initiate therapy and establish the diagnosis. For multifocal lesions or other forms of the disease with visceral involvement, chemotherapy with cyclophosphamide (Cytoxan) is the treatment of choice.

Fibrous Dysplasia

Of the benign lesions that may involve the head and neck region, fibrous dysplasia may be the most disfiguring. Craniofacial manifestations of fibrous dysplasia are common. Skull lesions frequently involve the convexities of the calvarium and the floor of the anterior cranial fossa (Fig. 14–30). The term fibro-osseous aberration is an acceptable but nonspecific description of the underlying pathology of this lesion. Normal bony architecture is replaced by connective tissue, fibroblasts, and varying amounts of osteoid and calcified matrix bone. The lesions may be grossly lytic, bone forming, or more likely a combination of the two processes. The leontiasis ossea variation of this dysplasia

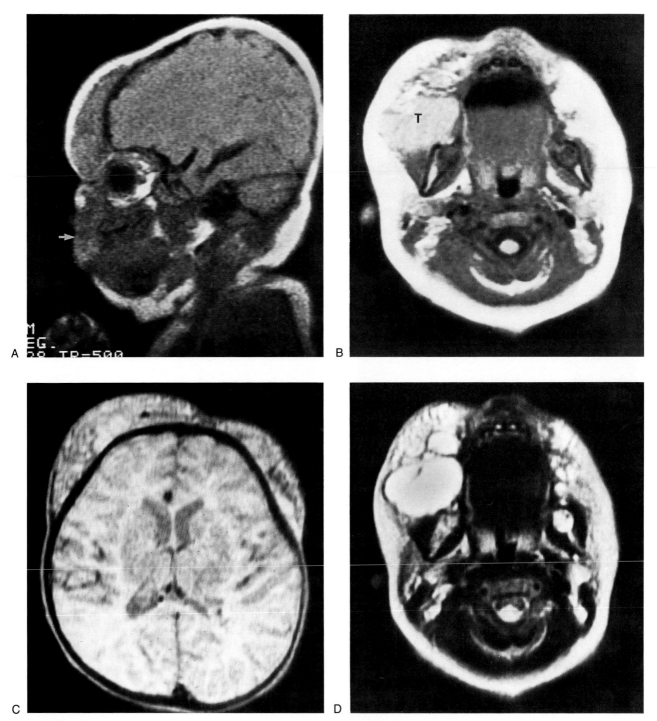

Figure 14–26. *Congenital lymphangioma.* The workup on this 2-day-old girl included an MR scan to determine the extent of tumor involvement. *A,* Sagittal MR image (500/28) through the right hemisphere and orbit shows the intermediate-signal-intensity mass extrinsic to the calvarium with tumor infiltration of the paranasal soft tissue structures (*arrow*). *B,* Corresponding axial MR image (2000/84) again demonstrates the intact cortical margin with high-signal-intensity loculations within the tumor (T). *C, D,* Corresponding axial images (800/30, 2000/84) show signal changes characteristic of hemangiomatous and lymphangiomatous lesions. Multiple loculations within the lesions are also typical, particularly of the lymphangiomatous lesions.

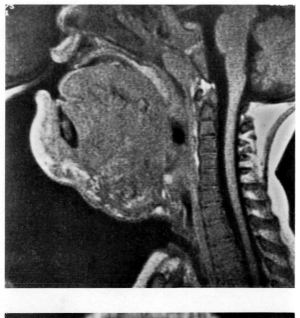

A

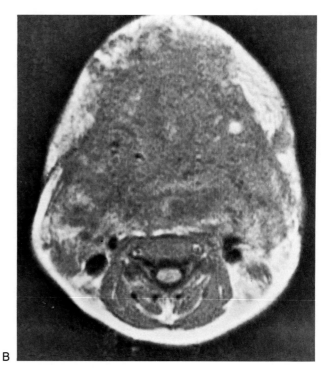

B

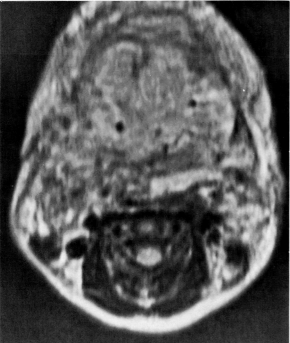

C

Figure 14–27. *Cystic hygroma.* This 5-year-old boy has received radiotherapy for an unresectable congenital lymphangioma. *A,* Midline sagittal image (472/20) shows the infiltrative features of the lesion. The tongue is displaced superiorly. Obliteration of both the nasal and oral segments of the pharynx necessitated a tracheostomy. *B, C,* Transaxial images (550/20, 2000/85) demonstrate marked distortion and obliteration of the fascial planes. The lack of signal change in the T2 weighted scan may be due to replacement of the lymphangiomatous components with fibrous tissue.

presents with overgrowth of the facial bones and the base of the skull, causing asymmetry and lion-like facies.

The association of precocious puberty, pigmented skin lesions, and polyostotic disease is commonly referred to as Albright's syndrome. The polyostotic manifestations are frequently unilateral. Although the syndrome predominantly affects females, males may be affected in rare instances. Radiologically, small flecks of calcium may be seen in the lesions. The MR appearance is characterized by expansion of the marrow or diploic spaces, which exhibit a heterogeneous signal on T1 weighted scans. Involvement of the skull base at the foramen magnum may lead to cord compression. Orthogonal imaging planes are useful for preoperative planning of decompression.

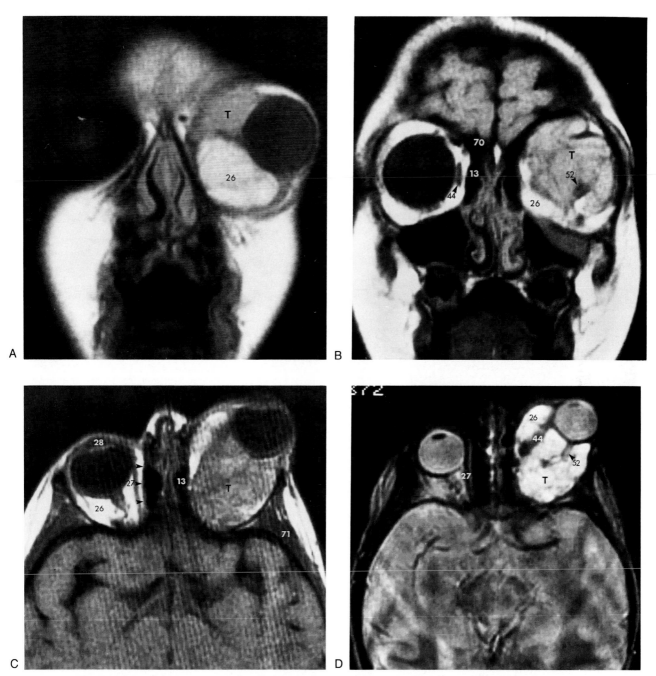

Figure 14–28. *Orbital lymphangioma.*   A large infiltrating orbital mass resulted in progressive proptosis in this 5-year-old girl. *A, B,* Coronal MR images (800/30) clearly demonstrate encasement of the optic nerve and expansion of the orbit because of slow growth of the infiltrating tumor (T). T1 weighted images demonstrate the tumor with intermediate signal intensity and multiple lobulations. The intraconal fat of the left orbit is displaced into both the anterior and inferior parts of the orbit. *C,* Axial image (600/30) shows the tumor filling the orbital cavity without extension into the intracranial compartment. *D,* T2 weighted axial image (2000/85) suggests the presence of loculations within the tumor. Key: ethmoid sinus (13), intraconal fat (26), lamina papyracea (27), lens (28), medial rectus m. (44), optic nerve (52), superior oblique m. (70), temporalis m. (71).

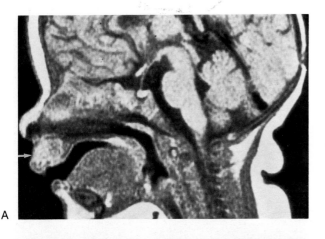

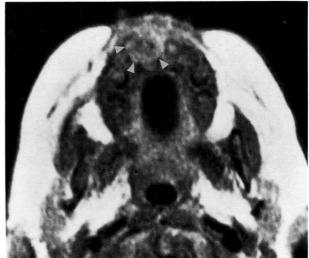

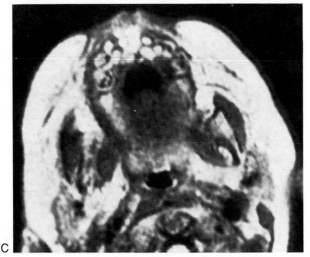

Figure 14–29. *Langerhans cell histiocytosis (eosinophilic granuloma).* Focal swelling and erythema of the hard palate behind the front incisors were noted by the mother of this 3-month-old girl. Despite resolution of the erythema after a full course of antibiotic therapy, the soft tissue lump remained. *A,* Sagittal MR image (587/30) shows disruption of the cortical margin of the anterior portion of the hard palate with focal expansion of the bone. The lesion has signal intensity higher than that of skeletal muscle, but only slightly less than that of fat. *B, C,* Infiltration of the gum (*arrowheads*) and the hard palate is also shown on axial T1 weighted scan (800/30). The lesion (*arrow*) has enhanced signal intensity on T2 weighted axial scan (1500/60). An excisional biopsy with histologic sections showed Langerhans cells and histiocytes typical of eosinophilic granuloma.

Malignant

The seven most common malignant tumors of childhood, measured by incidence or mortality rates, include leukemia, tumors of the central nervous system, lymphoma, neuroblastoma, Wilms' tumor, bone cancer, and rhabdomyosarcoma.[33] Retinoblastoma is the eighth most common malignancy, but because of its high cure rate (80 percent of cases)[34] mortality rates are no guide to its relative frequency. With the exclusion of the CNS tumors, lymphoma and rhabdomyosarcoma more often involve the head and neck region than any of the other malignant lesions of childhood.

Lymphoma

Lymphoma of the head and neck most frequently involves the cervical lymph node chain. The next most common sites of involvement are the structures around Waldeyer's ring, the nasopharynx, and the lymphoid tissue at the tongue base. When disease presents in the head and neck region, occult disease below the diaphragm may often occur simultaneously. Extranodal lymphomas of the head and neck region are usually the histiocytic and lymphocytic types. Hodgkin's and nodular lymphomas rarely involve extranodal sites.

MR signal characteristics of lymphomas are generally the same regardless of the histologic composition of the tissues. They generally exhibit intermediate signal intensity on T1 weighted pulse sequences and moderately high signal intensity on long TR-TE pulse sequences.[24, 35–38] For the evaluation of lymphadenopathy in the neck, size is a relatively unimportant criterion since a good examiner can detect anything greater than 1 cm.[3, 22, 23, 29, 39, 40] MRI in neck lymphadenopathy is useful (1) to determine the extent of pathology; (2) to differentiate abnormal lymph nodes from normal fat, muscle, vessels, and thyroid; and (3) to distinguish end-stage fibrosis from recurrent disease in the posttherapy patient.

Neuroblastoma

Neuroblastomas in the head and neck region may be either primary or secondary and represent the fourth

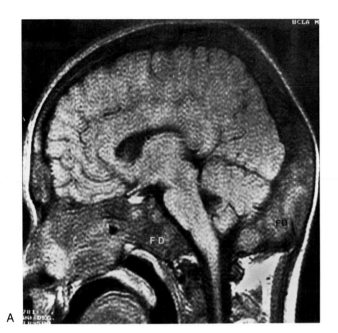

A

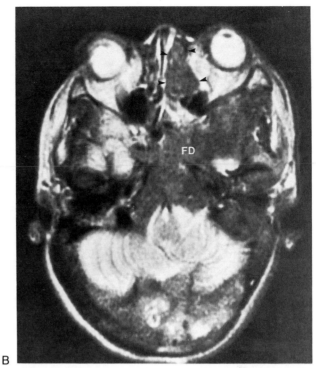

B

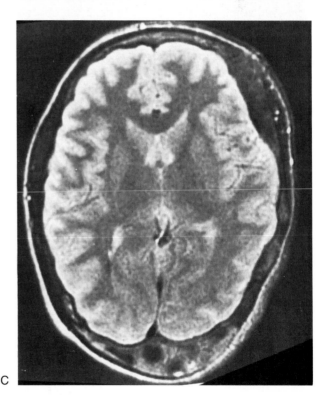

C

Figure 14–30. *Fibrous dysplasia.* A recent complaint of headaches brought this 22-year-old woman to her physician's office. An MR scan was requested for evaluation. *A,* Sagittal T1 weighted image (500/30) shows the typical appearance of bone overgrowth in the clivus (FD) and the occipital bone. The signal intensity is mixed and heterogeneous. *B, C,* Axial images (2000/85). The base of the skull and floor of the anterior cranial fossa are filled with the abnormal proliferation of fibrous and nonmineralized osteoid tissue (FD). There is extension into the left ethmoid sinus (*arrowheads*) with subsequent expansion of the sinus, and proptosis. Focal expansion of the diploic space is also noted on the T2 weighted image of the brain.

most common malignancy in childhood. Approximately two-thirds of all neuroblastomas arise within the abdomen. The more common presentation of neuroblastoma in the head and neck region is that of a metastasis to the dura (Fig. 14–31). Dural metastases invade the suture region and cause suture widening. A palpable mass appears in many patients when the invasion is focal. Skull radiographs are usually diagnostic. Metastatic lesions to the calvarium may present radiographically as osteolytic, osteoblastic, or a combination of these patterns.

Primary lesions may arise in the cervical region from

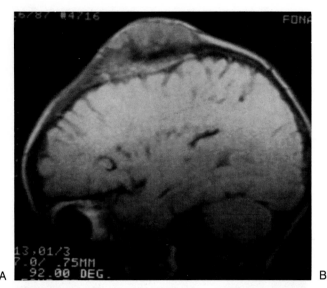
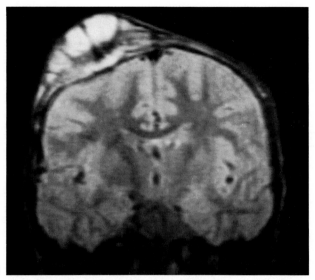

Figure 14–31. *Metastatic neuroblastoma.* A primary neuroblastoma of the left adrenal gland was found in this 5-year-old boy with a lump on the head. The tumor mass involves both the inner and outer tables of the skull. Infiltration of the diploic space is demonstrated on both sagittal (800/28) (*A*) and coronal (2000/84) (*B*) MR images.

the sympathetic nervous system[41] or in the olfactory region as a neurogenic tumor (Fig. 14–32). This latter variety has been referred to as esthesioneuroblastoma, a rare form of neuroblastoma. Documentation of the rarity of this lesion is provided by the published experience at the M.D. Anderson Hospital in Houston, Texas, where only one example was found in 40,000 surgical specimens over a 13-year period.[42]

Masses in the cervical sympathetic area present with symptoms related to the esophagus, larynx, or pharynx. Dysphagia, hoarseness, dyspnea, apnea, and stridor are the usual presenting symptoms. Tumors often grow rapidly and may become invasive. Vascular encasement, which is common within the abdominal primaries, may also be seen in the neck, involving the carotid sheath and its contents. In general, neuroblastoma tends to be an aggressive primary lesion with hematogenous and lymphogenous metastases already present at the time of diagnosis (Fig. 14–33).[43–45]

MRI is now considered the primary imaging modality for evaluation of neuroblastoma at initial presentation and for post-therapy evaluation of possible recurrent tumors.[46] The tumors are typically isointense to skeletal muscle on T1 weighted and proton density images, with moderately high signal intensity on long TR-TE pulse sequences (Fig. 14–34).[46] Lesions with hemorrhage or necrosis may have areas of high signal on short TR-TE pulse sequences and low signal areas on both short and long TR sequences when calcification is grossly macroscopic.

Rhabdomyosarcoma

Rhabdomyosarcoma makes up 5 to 15 percent of all malignant solid tumors in the pediatric population.[33]

Most patients present in the first decade of life. The head and neck region, including the orbit (38 percent of all locations), is the most common site of origin for this tumor.[47] Approximately one-third of rhabdomyosarcomas of the head and neck involve the pharynx.[48] Up to 35 percent of patients with head and neck disease have skull base invasion, usually through the sphenoid sinus.[1] The overall survival rate has risen from less than 20 percent to approximately 70 percent,[47] largely on the basis of early identification of large groups of patients at risk for relapse. Signs and symptoms relate to the location of the primary tumor or metastatic disease. Proptosis is common with orbital tumors. Tumors of the nasopharynx may go undetected for unusual lengths of time.

Epistaxis, obstruction of the airways, sinusitis, and dysphagia have all been described in association with nasopharyngeal involvement.

Two major groups of rhabdomyosarcoma exist when they are grouped according to anatomic location: parameningeal and nonparameningeal. Parameningeal sites include the nasopharynx, nasal cavity, paranasal sinuses, pterygopalatine and infratemporal fossae, and middle ear and mastoid. There is an increased incidence of extension into the meninges and CNS (35 percent of patients) when lesions arise in a parameningeal location.[47] The mortality rate for these patients is 90 percent.[49]

The nonparameningeal sites include the eyes, orbits, scalp, parotids, oral cavity, larynx, oropharynx, and cheek. This group of patients has an excellent prognosis:[49] approximately 90 percent are relapse free 2 years after postoperative radiation and chemotherapy.[47]

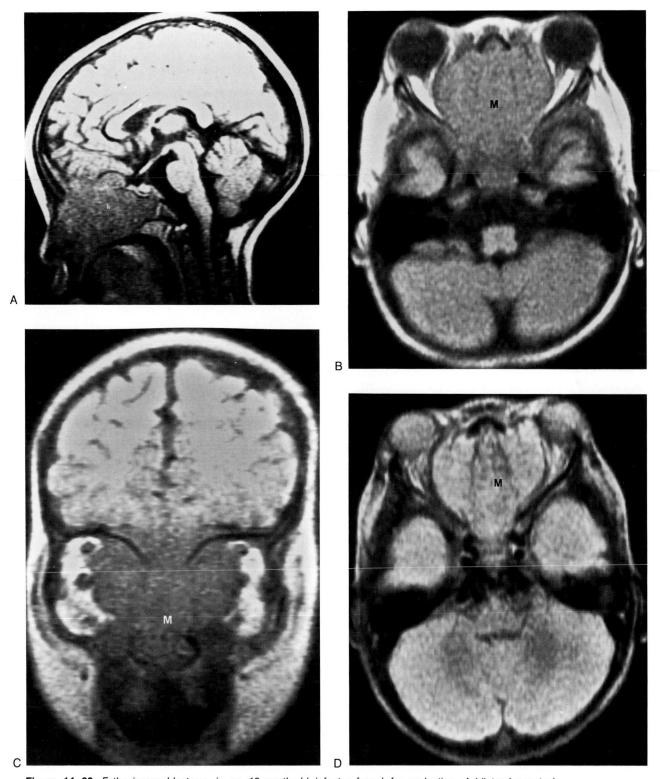

Figure 14–32. *Esthesioneuroblastoma in an 18-month-old infant referred for evaluation of bilateral proptosis.* ***A,*** Sagittal MR image (500/28) shows a large, intermediate-signal-intensity tumor mass (M) invading the sphenoid sinus. Both axial (***B***) and coronal (***C***) images (778/28) show the epicenter of the tumor in the area of cribriform plate and ethmoid sinuses. Destruction of the cribriform plate is clearly demonstrated on the coronal image. ***D,*** Focal areas of high signal are present on the axial (2000/85) image, with a moderate increase in the signal intensity of the lesion.

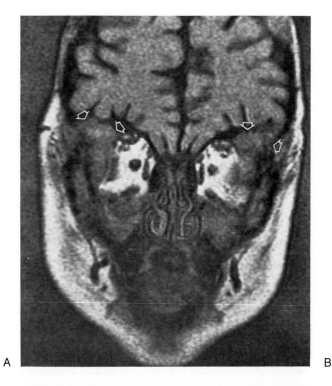

A

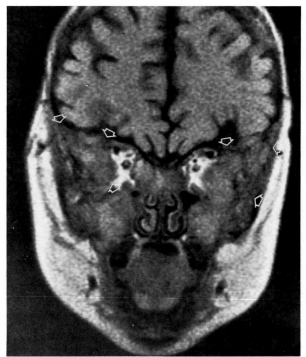

B

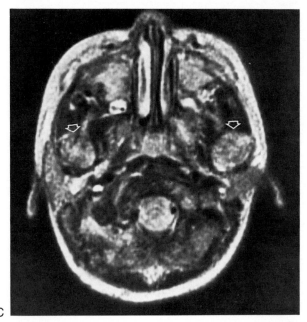

C

Figure 14–33. *Metastatic neuroblastoma.* This 4-year-old girl was diagnosed as having stage IV disease. The passive nasal congestion was originally thought to be related to chronic sinusitis. MR images in the coronal plane (800/30) (***A, B***) demonstrate infiltration of the paranasal sinuses (maxillary and ethmoid) by an intermediate-signal tumor mass. Extension of lobulated tumor into the temporal and infratemporal fossae (*arrows*) is clearly shown on the coronal and axial (***C***) MR images (2000/85).

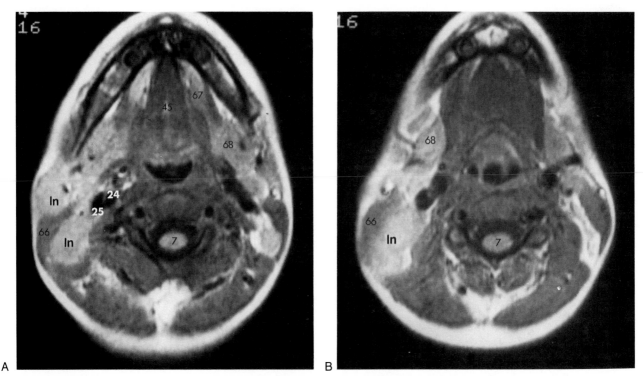

A   B

Figure 14–34. *Metastatic neuroblastoma.*   Prominent soft tissues along the right side of the neck were noted on the physical examination of this 5-year-old boy. *A, B,* Axial MR scans (500/28) show infiltration and enlargement of the lymph nodes (In) in the anterior and posterior cervical triangle. The MR scans helped to define the local soft tissue anatomy before the aspiration biopsy. Key: cervical cord (7), internal carotid artery (24), internal jugular vein (25), median raphe (45), sternocleidomastoid m. (66), sublingual gland (67), submandibular gland (68).

MRI with CT is the primary modality for assessing intracranial extension; MRI is the best tool to evaluate the soft tissues of the neck. The tumor has a similar appearance to lymphoma, with intermediate signal intensity on short TR-TE pulse sequences and moderately high signal intensity on T2 weighted images.[24] MRI is better than CT in differentiating the tumor from the surrounding musculature and the deep soft tissue structures of the neck.[2, 13, 22, 31]

Fibrosarcoma

Of the primary mesenchymal malignancies, fibrosarcoma is a distant second in frequency behind rhabdomyosarcoma.[33] The principal sites of origin in the head and neck, in descending order of frequency, include the soft tissues of the face and neck, the maxillary antrum, other paranasal sinuses, and the nasopharynx. Fibrosarcoma of the jaw arising from endosteum or periodontal membranes is a debated entity among some pathologists, although most agree on the category of periosteal fibrosarcoma arising from periosteum or periosteal tissues.[50] This latter group of lesions is more malignant and has a greater tendency to

invade bone than fibrosarcoma of the jaw arising from periodontal membranes.[51] The less common fibrosarcomas of the perioral soft tissues occur in the subcutaneous tissues, especially in the chin and the angle of the mandible. These fibrosarcomas occur particularly in children or young adults and tend to be more malignant than the periosteal fibrosarcomas (Fig. 14–35).

Nasopharyngeal Carcinoma

Other primary malignant tumors of the head and neck region are rare in the pediatric population. Nasopharyngeal carcinoma has a reported incidence of 0.25 to 0.5 percent of all malignant tumors.[1, 52, 53] The peak age of occurrence is in the fifth decade, with tumors occurring rarely in the pediatric population from the middle to late teens. Lesions may be asymptomatic, resulting in delayed diagnosis. A palpable neck mass from nodal metastases occurs in over 50 percent of patients.[54] The tumor mass is characteristically homogeneous and isointense to skeletal muscle on short TR-TE pulse sequences. Increased signal occurs on T2 weighted images (Fig. 14–36).[1, 40, 55]

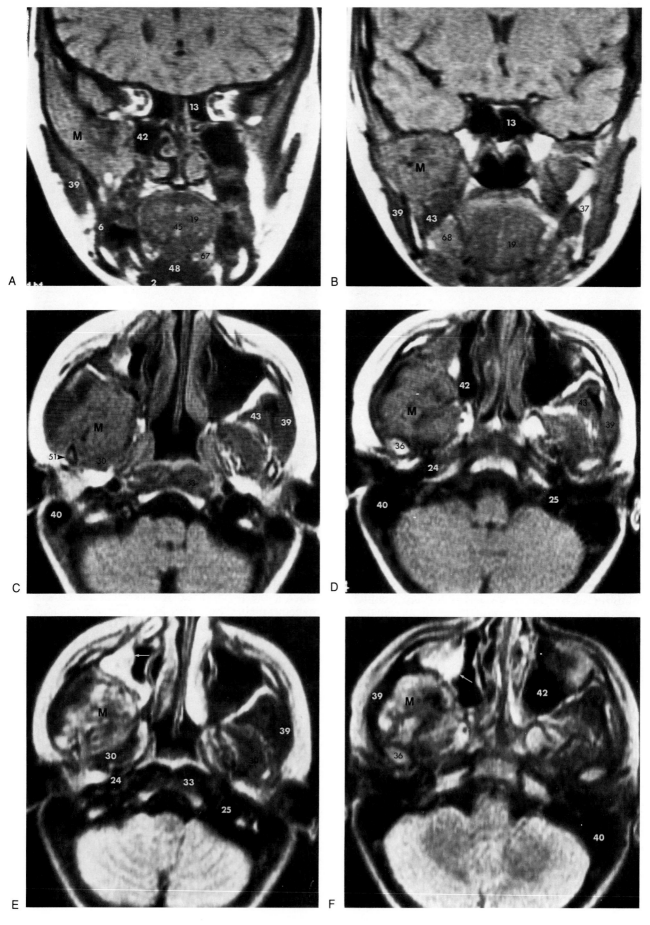

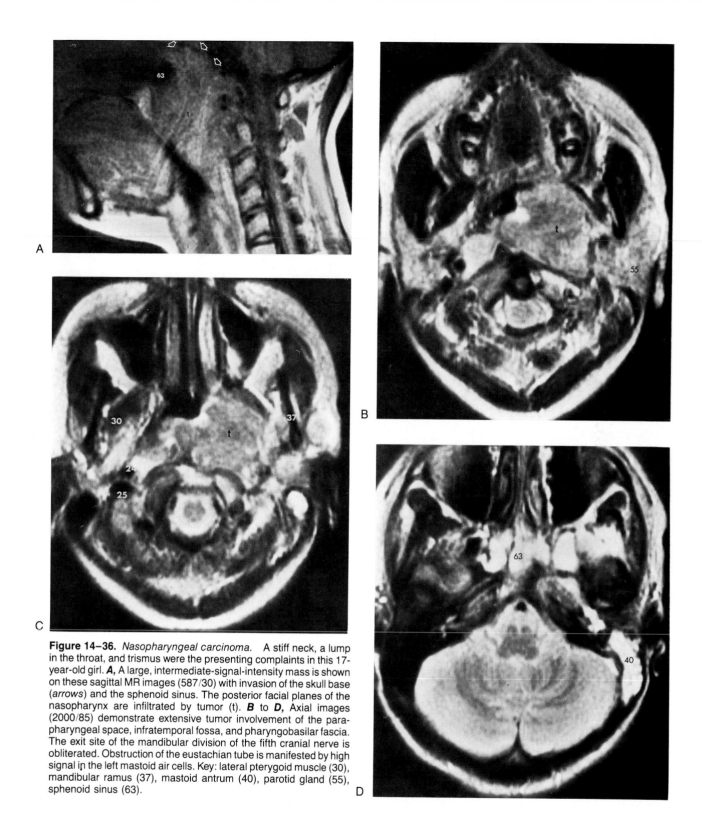

Figure 14–36. *Nasopharyngeal carcinoma.* A stiff neck, a lump in the throat, and trismus were the presenting complaints in this 17-year-old girl. *A,* A large, intermediate-signal-intensity mass is shown on these sagittal MR images (587/30) with invasion of the skull base (*arrows*) and the sphenoid sinus. The posterior facial planes of the nasopharynx are infiltrated by tumor (t). *B* to *D,* Axial images (2000/85) demonstrate extensive tumor involvement of the parapharyngeal space, infratemporal fossa, and pharyngobasilar fascia. The exit site of the mandibular division of the fifth cranial nerve is obliterated. Obstruction of the eustachian tube is manifested by high signal in the left mastoid air cells. Key: lateral pterygoid muscle (30), mandibular ramus (37), mastoid antrum (40), parotid gland (55), sphenoid sinus (63).

◄ **Figure 14–35.** *Fibrosarcoma in a 10-year-old girl who presented with a firm, swollen right cheek.* An intermediate signal intensity mass (M) in the temporal and infratemporal fossae is shown on the coronal (*A, B*) and axial (*C, D*) images (556/28). The mass is centered in the mandible, with compression of the adjacent masseter and lateral pterygoid muscles, which have lower signal intensity on both T1 and T2 weighted images. Note the signal intensity of the neck of the mandible (*arrowhead*), lower on the right than that of the left side. *E, F,* Axial (2000/84) MR images help to differentiate mucosal disease in the right maxillary sinus from tumor infiltration. The inflamed mucosa is of very high signal (*arrow*), greater than that of tumor mass (m). The increased signal intensity within the mastoid air cells is due to obstruction of the left eustachian tube. Key: anterior belly of the digastric m. (2), buccinator m. (6), coronoid process (10), ethmoid sinus (13), genioglossus m. (19), lateral pterygoid m. (30), longus colli m. (33), mandibular condyle (36), mandibular ramus (37), masseter m. (39), mastoid antrum (40), maxillary sinus (42), medial pterygoid m. (43), median raphe (45), mylohyoid m. (48), neck of mandible (51), sublingual gland (68), submandibular gland (68), zygomatic arch (80).

417

REFERENCES

1. Braun IF. MR of the nasopharynx. Radiol Clin North Am 1989; 27:315–330.
2. Dillon WP, Mills CM, Kjos B, et al. Magnetic resonance imaging of the nasopharynx. Radiology 1984; 152:731–738.
3. Glazer HS, Neimeyer JH, Balfe DM, et al. Neck neoplasms: MR. Parts I and II. Initial evaluation and post-treatment evaluation. Radiology 1986; 160:343–354.
4. Bydder GM. Clinical applications of gadolinium-DTPA. In: Stark DD, Bradley WG Jr., eds. Magnetic resonance imaging. St Louis: CV Mosby, 1987:182–200.
5. Gadian DG, Payne JA, Bryant DJ, et al. Gadolinium-DTPA as a contrast agent in MR imaging—theoretical projections and practical observations. J Comput Assist Tomogr 1985; 9:242–251.
6. Goldstein EJ, Burnett KR, Hansell JR, et al. Gadolinium-DTPA (an NMR proton imaging contrast agent): chemical structure, paramagnetic properties and pharmacokinetics. Physiol Chem Med NMR 1984; 16:97–105.
7. Sze G, Soletsky S, Bronen R, Wol G. MR imaging of the cranial meninges with emphasis on contrast enhancement and meningeal carcinomatosis. AJNR 1989; 10:965–975.
8. Lulkin RB, Worhtam DG, Dietrich RB, et al. Tongue and oropharynx: findings on MR imaging. Radiology 1986; 161:69–75.
9. Lynch HT, Kimberling WJ. Genetic counseling in cleft lip and cleft palate. Plast Reconstr Surg 1981; 68:800–815.
10. Rosenmann A, Shapira T, Cohen MM. Ectrodactyly, ectodermal dysplasia and cleft palate (ECC syndrome): report of a family and review of the literature. Clin Genet 1976; 9:347–353.
11. De Myer W. The median cleft face syndrome: differential diagnosis of cranium bifidum occultum, hypertelorism and median cleft nose, lip and palate. Neurology 1967; 17:961–971.
12. Sedano HO, Cohen MM, Jirasek JE, et al. Frontonasal dysplasia. J Pediatr 1970; 76:906–913.
13. Cohen MM Jr. The Robin anomaly—its nonspecificity in associated syndromes. J Oral Surg 1976; 34:587–593.
14. Cohen MM Jr. Macroglossia, omphalocele, visceromegaly, cytomegaly of the adrenal cortex and neonatal hypoglycemia. Birth Defects 1971; 7:226–232.
15. Roe TF, Kershnar AK, Weitzman JJ, et al. Beckwith syndrome with extreme organ hyperplasia. Pediatrics 1973; 52:372–381.
16. McLaurin RL. Parietal cephaloceles. Neurology 1964; 14:764–772.
17. Ward GE, Hendrick JW, Chambers RG. Thyroglossal tract abnormalities—cysts and fistulas. Surg Gynecol Obstet 1949; 89:727–737.
18. Diament MJ, Senac MO, Gilsanz V, et al. Prevalence of incidental paranasal sinuses opacification in pediatric patients: a CT study. J Comput Assist Tomogr 1987; 11:426–431.
19. Glasier CM, Ascher DP, Williams KD. Incidental paranasal sinus abnormalities on CT of children: clinical correlation. AJNR 1986; 7:861–864.
20. McAlister WH, Lusk R, Muntz HR. Comparison of plain radiographs and coronal CT scans in infants and children with recurrent sinusitis. AJR 1989; 153:1259–1264.
21. Duerinckx AJ, Hall TR, Boechat MI, et al. Differentiation of mucosal disease from partial development of paranasal sinuses by MRI in pediatric patients. Presented at 75th Scientific Assembly and Annual Meeting of the RSNA, Nov–Dec 1, 1989, Chicago. Radiology 1989 (P): 77 (abstract).
22. Dooms GC, Hricak H, Crooks LE, et al. Magnetic resonance imaging of the lymph nodes: comparison with CT. Radiology 1984; 153:719–728.
23. Stark DD, Moss AA, Gamsu G, et al. Magnetic resonance imaging of the neck. Parts I and II. Normal anatomy and pathologic findings. Radiology 1984; 150:455–461.
24. Som PM, Braun IF, Shapiro MD, et al. Tumors of the parapharyngeal space and upper neck: magnetic resonance imaging characteristics. Radiology 1987; 164:823–829.
25. Settipane A, Chafee FH. Nasal polyps in asthma and rhinitis. A review of 6,037 patients. J Allergy Clin Immunol 1977; 59:17–21.
26. Berman JM, Colman BH. Nasal aspects of cystic fibrosis in children. J Laryngol Otol 1977; 91:133–139.
27. Hatziotis JC. Lipoma of the oral cavity. Oral Surg Oral Med Oral Pathol 1971; 31:511–524.
28. D'Agostino AN, Soule EH, Miller RH. Sarcomas of the peripheral nerves and somatic soft tissues associated with multiple neurofibromatosis (von Recklinghausen's disease). Cancer 1963; 16:1015–1027.
29. Bhaskar SN. Oral tumors of infancy and childhood: a survey of 293 cases. J Pediatr 1963; 63:195–202.
30. Itoh K, Nishimura K, Togoshi K, et al. Magnetic resonance imaging of cavernous hemangioma of the face and neck. J Comput Assist Tomogr 1986; 10:831–835.
31. Mancuso AA, Dillon WP. The neck. Radiol Clin North Am 1989; 27:407–431.
32. Siegel MJ, Glazer HS, St Amour TE, et al. Lymphangiomas in children: MR imaging. Radiology 1989; 170:467–470.
33. Young JL, Miller RW. Incidence of malignant tumors in US children. J Pediatr 1975; 86:254–258.
34. Jensen RD, Miller RW. Retinoblastoma: epidemiologic characteristics. N Engl J Med 1971; 285:307–311.
35. Han JS, Huss RG, Benson JE, et al. Magnetic resonance imaging of the skull base. J Comput Assist Tomogr 1984; 8:944–952.
36. Olsen WL, Jeffrey RB, Sooy CD, et al. Lesions of the head and neck in patients with AIDS: CT and MR findings. AJNR 1988; 9:693–698.
37. Shapiro MD, Sze G, Charles J, et al. Magnetic resonance imaging of central nervous system lymphoma. AJNR 1988; 9:1013.
38. Silver AJ, Mawad ME, Hilal SK, et al. Computed tomography of the carotid and related cervical spaces. Part I. Anatomy. Radiology 1984; 150:723–728.
39. Gefter WB, Spritzer CE, Eisenberg B, et al. Thyroid imaging with high-field-strength surface-coil MR. Radiology 1987; 164:483–490.
40. Mancuso AA, Hanafee WN. Computed tomography and MR of the head and neck. Baltimore: Williams & Wilkins, 1985.
41. deLorimier AA, Bragg KU, Linden G. Neuroblastoma in childhood. Am J Dis Child 1969; 118:441–450.
42. Aldave A, Gallager HS. Olfactory esthesioneuroblastoma: report of a case and review of the literature. Arch Pathol 1959; 67:43–47.
43. Young LW, Rubin P, Hanson RE. The extra-adrenal neuroblastoma: high radiocurability and diagnostic accuracy. Am J Roentgenol 1970; 108:75–91.
44. Koop CE. The role of surgery in resectable, non-resectable and metastatic neuroblastoma. JAMA 1968; 205:157–158.
45. King RL, Stornasli JP, Bolande RP. Neuroblastoma: review of 28 cases and presentation of two cases with metastases and long survival. Am J Roentgenol 1961; 85:733–748.
46. Dietrich RB, Kangarloo H, Lenarsky C, et al. Neuroblastoma: the role of MR imaging. AJR 1987; 148:937–942.
47. Malogolowkin MH, Ortega JA. Rhabdomyosarcoma of childhood. Pediatr Ann 1988; 17:251–268.
48. Dito WR, Batsakis JG. Intraoral, pharyngeal and nasopharyngeal rhabdomyosarcoma. Arch Otolaryngol 1963; 77:123–127.
49. Teft M, Fernandez C, Donaldson M, et al. Evidence of meningeal involvement by rhabdomyosarcoma of the head and neck in children. Cancer 1978; 42:253–258.
50. Batsakis JG. Tumors of the head and neck. Clinical and pathological considerations. 2nd ed. Baltimore: Williams & Wilkins, 1979:252–279.
51. Reade PC, Radden BG. Oral fibrosarcoma. Oral Surg 1966; 22:217–224.
52. Godfredsen E. Ophthalmologic and neurologic symptoms of malignant nasopharynx tumors: a clinical study comprising 454 cases, with special references to histopathology and the possi-

bility of early recognition. Acta Psychiatr Neurol 1944; 34:1–7.

53. Schnohr P. Survival rates of nasopharyngeal cancer in California. A review of 516 cases from 1942 to 1965. Cancer 1970; 25:1099–1106.

54. Wang CC, Meyer JE. Radiotherapeutic management of carcinoma of the nasopharynx: an analysis of 170 patients. Cancer 1971; 28:566–570.

55. Teresi LM, Lufkin RB, Vineula F, et al. Magnetic resonance imaging of the lymph nodes: comparison with CT. Radiology 1987; 164:811–821.

Spinal Dysraphism

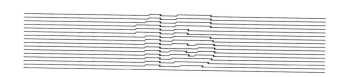

GORDON CHEUNG, M.D.
GORDON SZE, M.D.
JAMES ABRAHAMS, M.D.

DEFINITIONS*

SPINAL DYSRAPHISM. An all-encompassing term meaning failure of fusion of the vertebral osseous and neural structures in the median dorsal plane. The dysraphism may be of the open or closed type, i.e., spina bifida aperta or occult spinal dysraphism, respectively.

NEURAL TUBE DEFECT. A nonspecific term that refers to the nonfusion and subsequent malformation of the neural tube secondary to a neurulation disorder.

Myelocele and myelomeningocele are forms of neural tube defects. The term is often used interchangeably with neural placode or spina bifida aperta.

SPINA BIFIDA APERTA. Used interchangeably with spina bifida cystica and includes myelocele and myelomeningocele. These are open lesions with midline vertebral defects, deficient skin covering, and exposed neural tissue, with or without protrusion.

MENINGOCELE. A herniation of a cystic, CSF-filled, meninges-lined, midline mass that does not contain any neural elements. These herniations occur through a defect in the posterior elements, with a propensity for the occipital and lumbosacral regions.

---

* In order of usage in this chapter.

MYELOMENINGOCELE. The most common form of spina bifida aperta. The midline neural tissue is exposed with underlying expansion of the subarachnoid space. This causes a visible bulge because of the raised open neural placode above the skin.

MYELOCELE. Structurally identical to a myelomeningocele with exposed midline neural tissue, except that the neural plate is flush with the surface of the skin.

MYELOCYSTOCELE (SYRINGOMYELOCELE). A rare form of spina bifida aperta caused by localized dilatation of the central canal or hydromyelia. A cystic mass, which actually represents a markedly dilated spinal cord, results. Most of these lesions are skin covered. Sensory and motor deficits are common.

RACHISCHISIS. Used with a variable meaning, ranging from a mild form of dysraphism in which only bony vertebral defects exist to a severe form in which there is a large, exposed neural placode.

MYELOSCHISIS. Often used synonymously with rachischisis. Strictly, however, myeloschisis refers to the exposed neural placode, which is a dorsally split spinal cord. If there is complete myeloschisis or splitting of the cord, it is called diastematomyelia.

NEURAL PLACODE. The exposed midline dorsal neural tissue. In fact, it consists of a spinal cord that has been filleted open (dorsally split) with a central groove that embryologically would have formed the central canal. This midline groove is contiguous with the intact central canal superiorly; CSF is often seen emanating from the ostium.

SPINA BIFIDA OCCULTA. In recent years this term has been used to describe simple nonfusion of the posterior vertebral arches, as diagnosed on plain radiographs, without underlying soft tissue abnormalities.

OCCULT SPINAL DYSRAPHISM. Used to describe a form of spinal dysraphism covered by skin, without exposure of the underlying neural tissue or meninges. Occult spinal dysraphism includes entities such as diastematomyelia, tight filum terminale, split notochord syndrome, dermal sinus, epidermoid and dermoid tumors, and lipomyelomeningocele.

LIPOMYELOMENINGOCELE. The most common form of occult spinal dysraphism. Lipomatous tissue inserts onto the dorsal spinal cord with an associated meningocele causing a visible protrusion. Since the lipomatous tissue is extradural and extra-arachnoid, the nerve roots do not traverse any fatty tissues.

DIASTEMATOMYELIA. An anomaly of the spine characterized by complete splitting of the cord to form two hemicords. A bony or fibrocartilaginous cleft may or may not be present.

DIPLOMYELIA. Used by some authors synonymously with diastematomyelia. Strictly, however, diplomyelia refers to a complete duplication of the cord in which each hemicord has paired ventral and dorsal nerve roots.

TIGHT FILUM TERMINALE SYNDROME. Caused by tethering of the spinal cord as a result of a short, thick filum terminale.

CONGENITAL DERMAL SINUS. A congenital defect characterized by an epithelium-lined tract extending from the skin inward, often connecting with the central nervous system.

EPIDERMOID AND DERMOID. Heterotopic formations composed of elements of the skin. They may be congenital developmental tumors, secondary to misplacement of normally developing somatic cells, but there are also acquired etiologies.

TERATOMA. A true maldevelopmental lesion that displays neoplastic growth and arises from misplacement of multipotential germinal cells early in embryonic development. It is very rare.

HAMARTOMA. Composed of well-differentiated mesodermal elements, a true hamartoma is a rare lesion that usually presents in the newborn period. However, other hamartomatous masses may also be seen in association with spinal lipomas.

SYNDROME OF CAUDAL REGRESSION. A complex congenital malformation characterized by a spectrum of anomalies involving the distal spine and the corresponding segments of the spinal cord. Mild forms are asymptomatic; severe forms are associated with disabling neurologic, muscular, and other deficits.

SPLIT NOTOCHORD SYNDROME. A term that encompasses a wide spectrum of anomalies, all of which result from abnormal development of the notochord to form persistent connections between the dorsal skin and the gut.

NORMAL EMBRYOLOGY

In order to grasp the various theories of pathogenesis of spinal dysraphism and the complex anatomy involved, some understanding of the embryologic formation of the spinal cord is needed.[1-7] Development of the spinal cord and axial skeleton begins in the second week of embryonic life, with the embryo as a circular, bilaminar embryonic disc composed of a layer of dorsal epiblast overlying the hypoblast. By the end of the third week the bilaminar embryo is transformed into a trilaminar embryo consisting of the three primary germ layers: ectoderm, mesoderm, and endoderm.[1-4] This transformation process, known as gastrulation, is dependent on the primitive streak.[1]

The dorsal linear primitive streak is a proliferating band of epiblast in the caudal midline that appears on about day 15 (Fig. 15-1).[14] Some of the proliferating cells migrate to form the third germ layer, the embryonic mesoderm. At this stage, the epiblast is referred to as embryonic ectoderm and the hypoblast as embryonic endoderm. In addition, active growth causes the primitive streak to elongate and develop a thickening at the cephalic end known as the primitive knot, or Hensen's node (Fig. 15-1).[1,4]

Hensen's node is the origin of the notochordal process, a midline cylindric rod of cells that lies between the ectoderm and endoderm. The notochordal process

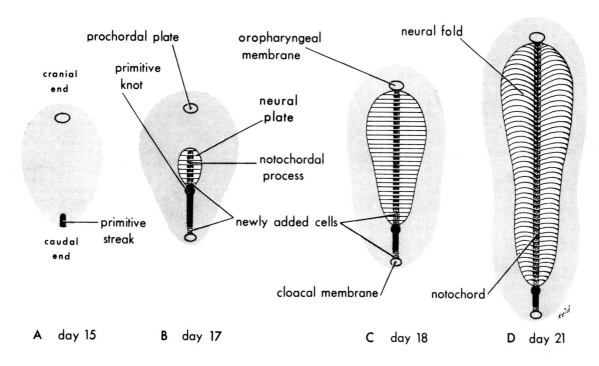

cranial end

prochordal plate

primitive knot

oropharyngeal membrane

neural fold

neural plate

notochordal process

primitive streak

caudal end

newly added cells

cloacal membrane

notochord

A   day 15   B   day 17   C   day 18   D   day 21

Figure 15–1. *Changes in the embryonic disc during the third week.* ***A*** *to* ***D,*** *Dorsal views of the embryonic disc during the third week. Lengthening of the primitive streak is by proliferation of cells at its caudal end. Formation of the notochordal process is a result of cell migration from the primitive knot. Inducement of neural plate formation is related to the underlying notochordal process and adjacent mesoderm. (From Moore KL. The developing human—clinically oriented embryology. Philadelphia: WB Saunders, 1988:52.)*

migrates cephalad from Hensen's node to the prochordal plate (endodermal cells).

The prochordal plate is fused with the overlying ectoderm to form the future buccopharyngeal membrane. This region of the embryonic disc remains bilaminar. Similarly, the caudally located cloacal membrane is bilaminar. This means that the fused endoderm and ectoderm is not separated by the mesoderm. The third location where mesoderm is not found is in the midsagittal plane because of the insinuation of the notochordal process between the ectoderm and endoderm.

By the latter half of the third week, canalization of the solid notochordal process occurs by formation and extension of the primitive pit, thus forming the notochordal canal (Fig. 15–2).[1,4] Shortly thereafter, the ventral wall of the notochordal canal degenerates by extensive fenestration to form the notochordal plate. At this time, a temporary canal is established between the amniotic cavity and the yolk sac cavity, called the neurenteric canal. Eventually the true solid notochord is formed by infolding and fusion of the notochordal plate during the fourth week (Fig. 15–2).

Mesoderm surrounds the notochord to form the future axial skeleton. The trapped notochord degenerates to become the future nucleus pulposus of the intervertebral disc.

Paralleling the development of the notochord is the appearance of the neural plate, a midline thickening of the ectodermal germ layer, during the beginning of the third embryonic week (Fig. 15–2).[1] Since the neural plate is formed from ectoderm, it consists of "neuroectoderm." The neural plate develops just cephalad to the primitive knot, and enlarges by widening and extending in a cranial direction to the future buccopharyngeal membrane level, corresponding in dimension to the underlying notochord. This process is believed to be induced by the adjacent paraxial mesoderm and underlying notochordal tissue.[1-4] The cranial two-thirds of the neural plate and neural tube represents the primordial brain, whereas the remaining caudal portion (distal to the fourth pair of somites) represents the primordial spinal cord.[1]

Initially, the neural plate is a flat, thickened portion of the ectoderm, but within days, generally on the 18th day, the edges of the neural plate elevate to form neural folds and the central portion deepens to form the neural groove.[4] The subsequent closing and fusion of the neural folds into a neural tube is called neurulation (Fig. 15–2). Fusion of the neural folds begins in the

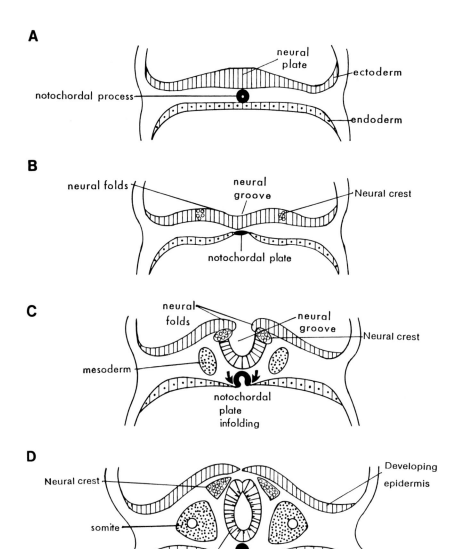

A

neural plate

notochordal process

ectoderm

endoderm

B

neural folds

neural groove

Neural crest

notochordal plate

C

neural folds

neural groove

Neural crest

mesoderm

notochordal plate infolding

D

Neural crest

Developing epidermis

somite

neural tube

notochord

Figure 15–2. *Formation of the neural tube.* **A** to **D,** Schematic cross-sectional diagram through successively older embryos illustrates the process of neurulation and disjunction. The development and differentiation of the neural tube, notochord, and neural crest begins with the neural plate and are complete by the end of the fourth week.

cervical region, proceeding in the cephalic direction and shortly thereafter in the caudal direction.[4] The anterior neuropore closes first at the level of the lamina terminalis, and the posterior neuropore closes 2 to 3 days later in the lumbar region.[2] The process of neurulation thus begins during the start of the third embryonic week with the neural plate, and terminates at the end of the fourth week (26 to 28 days) with the closure of the caudal or posterior neuropore.[1,3,4]

During neurulation, certain neuroectodermal cells along the crest of the neural folds (edge of the neural plate) become independent, separate, and then migrate dorsolateral to the neural tube (Fig. 15–2). Lying between the superficial ectoderm and the neural tube (Fig. 15–1), these cells form bilateral masses

constituting the neural crests. Much of the peripheral nervous system is derived from the neural crest cells. This includes the dorsal root ganglia and autonomic ganglia.

Immediately after complete fusion of the neural folds and formation of the neural tube, the dorsally situated ectoderm separates from the neural tube in a process called disjunction. The free edges of the interrupted superficial ectoderm fuse across the midline to form a continuous layer. Ectodermal fusion occurs only if a complete neural tube has formed. It is this combined process of neurulation and disjunction that forms the functioning spinal cord.

After completion of neurulation the embryo must go into marked flexion by forming a head fold cranially and a tail fold caudally.[7] This is related to differential rates of growth of different embryonic structures, with the longitudinal axis growing more rapidly.

The distalmost portion of the neural tube is formed by a different process called canalization and retrogressive differentiation. Just beyond the posterior neuropore lies a conglomerate mass of undifferentiated cells in the coccygeal region, which eventually develops and transforms into an ependymally lined lumen in a process called canalization.[5] Subsequent involution by cell necrosis of this caudal cell mass is termed retrogressive differentiation. This process forms the nonfunctioning portion of the spinal cord, namely, the ventriculus terminalis, a focal dilatation of the distal central canal and a glioependymal strand or filum terminale.[6,7] Accessory lumina normally can be seen adjacent to the true lumen in one-third of embryos.[5] The process of canalization is complete by the end of 7 weeks, but retrogressive differentiation continues until some time after birth.[5]

SPINA BIFIDA APERTA: MYELOCELE AND MYELOMENINGOCELE

Incidence

The incidence of spina bifida aperta is approximately one per 1,000 live births.[8–10] The incidence varies greatly depending on the geographic location, ranging from two per 10,000 births in Japan to four per 1,000 births in regions of the United Kingdom, especially Ireland and Wales.[11,12] In North America, there is a slightly higher incidence in the eastern states than in the western states. Approximately 10 percent of spina bifida aperta lesions represent meningoceles; the remainder consist of myelomeningoceles.[6]

A steady, slow decline in the prevalence of spinal dysraphism over the past three to four decades has been witnessed in North America and Great Britain.[11] The reason for the decline is yet to be determined but is only partially related to prenatal screening.

Etiology

Although the exact etiology of spinal dysraphism and the subgroup of spina bifida aperta is unknown, it is safe to say that multiple factors are involved, with heredity and genetics playing a major role.[11] Neural tube malformations are increased in patients who have consanguineous parents.[12] If one sibling is affected, the subsequent sibling has a 5 percent chance of spinal dysraphism. If two siblings are affected, the risk to a subsequent child is two to three times that of a singly affected child.[3,12,13] Some studies suggested that there is an increased incidence of spina bifida occulta in the parents of children with spina bifida aperta;[14] however, a more recent study does not show any such correla-

tion.[15] The general consensus is that the hereditary factor is polygenic; rarely, however, some families have shown autosomal recessive, autosomal dominant, and even X-linked transmission of neural tube defects.[16] In most series there is a slight female predominance, with a female-to-male ratio of 1.3:1.0.[2] Females also tend to be more severely affected.[17]

Migrating populations tend to take their inherent risk of neural tube defects with them. However, the risk factor is modified after migration, suggesting that environmental factors are significant.[2]

Various teratogens, most of which are dietary, have been suggested as an etiology for neural tube defects.[3,12,18]

Although many of the above factors are correlative, a direct causal relationship between these factors and neural tube malformations is difficult to establish. Thus, although most cases of neural tube malformations appear to be sporadic in nature, there is a complex interaction of multifactorial genetic and environmental influences.

Prenatal Diagnosis

Routine screening of pregnant women for maternal serum alpha-fetoprotein can detect neural tube defects. False-negative results may occur because this test is unable to detect the closed type of spinal dysraphism. When high levels of maternal serum alpha-fetoprotein are discovered, fetal ultrasonography is performed to confirm the diagnosis.[19] The sagittal plane is ideal for demonstrating the soft tissue protrusion of a myelomeningocele. Splaying of the posterior elements is best seen in the axial plane and constitutes a finding essential to the diagnosis.[20] The intracranial structures of the fetus can also be easily evaluated for evidence of associated hydrocephalus.[21]

Embryogenesis

There is as much controversy as there are theories regarding the pathogenesis of the various types of spinal dysraphism. It is presumed that any derangement during the formation of the spinal cord, which includes the processes of neurulation, disjunction, canalization, and retrogressive differentiation, may lead to the clinically known forms of spinal dysraphism.

The most prominent theory (the nonclosure theory) is that myelomeningocele and myelocele are due to failures of neurulation.[22–26] When the neural folds fail to fuse dorsally and the ectoderm consequently fails to separate from the neuroectoderm, the neural plate remains flat. The result is a midline defect with exposure of the reddish neural plate. According to the nonclosure theory, spinal dysraphism must occur during the first 4 weeks of gestation before neural tube closure. Experiments in rats have produced spina bifida aperta lesions (myeloceles) in support of the nonclosure theory.[25]

Another major theory of embryogenesis of these malformations involves the reopening or rupture of a neural tube that has already closed.[27] By definition, this process must occur after the closure of the posterior neuropore or after the 26th day of gestation.[28–30] Once the neural tube closes, pressure within the neural tube increases owing to cerebrospinal fluid (CSF) secretion. Because of disturbed permeability of the roof of the fourth ventricle, embryonal hydrocephalomyelia ensues. This ballooning is most prominent at the ends of the neural tube where the tissue is less mature as a result of recent closures. Rupture of the caudal neural tube will form a myelomeningocele.[29]

A third hypothesis, the overgrowth theory, was developed by Patten (1952), who demonstrated excess neural tissue at the defect site. He suggested that this overgrowth prevents neural tube closure.[31, 32]

None of the above theories adequately explains all the nuances and intrinsic abnormalities of spinal dysraphism. Perhaps a combination of theories is needed to produce the end product of spinal dysraphism.[33]

Any proposed etiology or theory must also take into account the close relationship of intracranial anomalies with spina bifida aperta. Both anencephalus and spina bifida aperta are often considered to be derived from the same embryologic etiology at the neurulation stage.[3] Indeed, they have similar incidences in the same population. A Chiari II malformation is invariably associated with a myelomeningocele; however, it forms separately at a later time in fetal life via an unknown mechanism. The traction theory postulated that a myelomeningocele could pull the brain stem into the upper cervical canal, with subsequent obstruction and hydrocephalus, and was an initially attractive hypothesis. We now know, however, that the stress on the cord extends only to the upper thoracic region. Thus, the Chiari II malformation is not considered to be secondary to the myelomeningocele, but is part of the spectrum of anomalies secondary to a common insult.[34]

Clinical Findings

Most myelomeningoceles occur in the lower spine, and less than 10 percent involve the cervical or thoracic region without involvement of the lumbar spine.[17] Simple meningoceles show a similar concentration of cases in the lumbar and lumbosacral regions. However, in contrast to myelomeningoceles, simple meningoceles are more than twice as likely to occur in the cervical or thoracic region.[17]

The clinical symptoms of myelomeningocele and related forms of abnormality are highly variable, depending on the type, location, and severity of the lesion. Symptoms may range from flaccid paralysis in patients with spina bifida aperta to no symptoms at all in patients with meningocele.

The highest level of spinal cord involvement is broadly suggested by the highest level of the spinal dysraphism. Foot deformities and dislocated hips are often present. Urinary dribbling and rectal prolapse are suggestive of future incontinence. Over 90 percent of patients with myelomeningocele have some degree of neurogenic bladder.

Infants with meningomyeloceles commonly have associated anomalies of the central nervous system (CNS). Associated lesions such as diastematomyelia and lipomas may be difficult to detect clinically, but may present as a marked side-to-side asymmetry in the level of neurologic function. Since myelomeningoceles and Chiari II malformations are associated, brain stem dysfunction including central apnea, stridor, and swallowing difficulties from bulbar palsies, ataxia, and spastic paralysis are not uncommon.

The predominant intracranial finding is that of a Chiari II malformation (Figs. 15–3, 15–4). Zimmerman and colleagues demonstrated an abnormally low

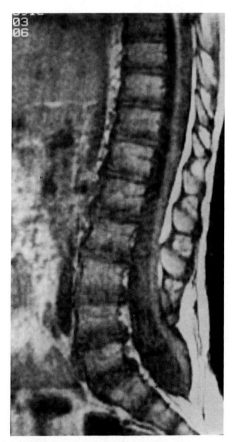

Figure 15–3. Normal postoperative myelomeningocele repair. T1 weighted (600/20) midsagittal image demonstrates a repaired lumbosacral myelomeningocele with dilatation of the thecal sac. There is no evidence of retethering since the distal spinal cord is completely surrounded by CSF and there is no posterior angulation of the spinal cord under the last lamina.

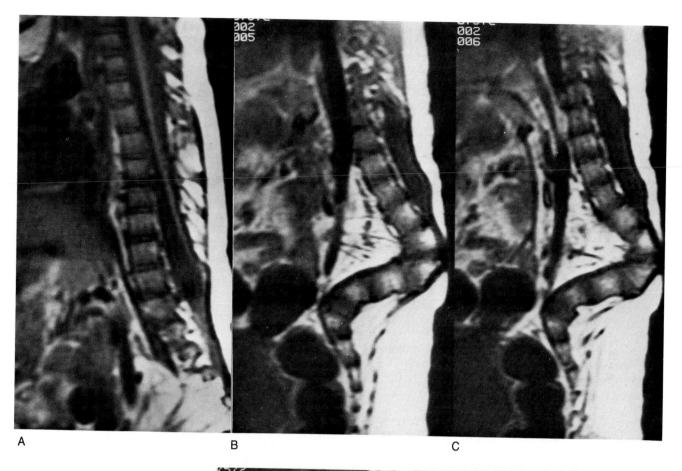

A   B   C

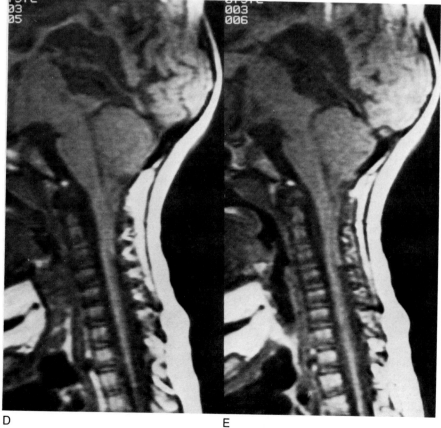

Figure 15–4. *Postmyelomeningocele repair.* **A,** T1 weighted (600/20) mid-sagittal scan demonstrates a low-lying stretched cord that is posteriorly angulated under the last lamina, consistent with retethering. **B, C,** T1 weighted (600/200) parasagittal scan of the same patient illustrates the typical "jackknife" lumbar kyphosis seen with widely everted laminae. **D, E,** T1 weighted (600/20) sagittal scan of the craniovertebral junction shows the associated Chiari II malformation. Low posterior fossa contents are illustrated, including pointed cerebellar tonsils that extend to the C2–C3 level.

D   E

fourth ventricle in 92 percent and hydrocephalus in 85 percent of patients with myelomeningocele.[35]

The vertebral bodies may exhibit congenital hemivertebra, butterfly vertebra, and fusion anomalies separate from the myelomeningocele. Diastematomyelia is seen in up to 46 percent of patients.[36,37]

The incidence of scoliosis associated with myelomeningocele has been reported as 9 to 90 percent.[38-40] One reason for the discrepancy may be that scoliosis is highly dependent on the patient's age and the severity of the myeloschisis.[40-42] Scoliosis may be due to congenital vertebral abnormalities or a developmental problem.[43]

Hydromyelia is one cause of developmental scoliosis and should be suspected when accelerated progression of scoliosis and neurologic dysfunction are noticed.[44] Thus, rapid scoliosis necessitates a prompt radiologic workup, including magnetic resonance imaging (MRI), because a syrinx potentially is a surgically treatable lesion. Associated hydromyelia and syringomyelia are seen in up to 85 percent of patients with spina bifida aperta.[36,37]

An acute congenital lumbar kyphosis is seen in up to 30 percent of patients with myelomeningocele.[45,46] The apex of the kyphos is normally at the level of the most widely everted laminae.

Pathologic Anatomy

With frequent usage, the term myelomeningocele has almost become synonymous with spina bifida aperta; however, the latter term also includes myelocele. The two types of spina bifida aperta are anatomically identical except that the neural plate protrudes in myelomeningocele but is flush with the skin in myelocele. The predominant osseous vertebral abnormality consists of failure of fusion combined with absence of the neural arches, resulting in a large defect. The remaining laminae, hypoplastic and malformed, become widely everted. This results in a markedly narrowed spinal canal in the anteroposterior dimension. In severe cases there may be orientation of the laminae into the coronal plane, with the posterior surface now facing anteriorly. This causes the paraspinal muscles to rotate anteriorly, augmenting the pull of the psoas muscles, to produce a "jackknife" kyphosis (Fig. 15–4).[6] Posterior fusion defects remote from the myelomeningocele are often seen, especially at the C1 vertebral body. Superimposing severe kyphosis with wide laminal eversion maximizes a situation for possible neural tissue compromise and skin ulceration.

The dorsal neural placode, visible at birth as raw, reddish, often bleeding tissue, actually represents the innards of the spinal cord. On the exposed surface of this flattened neural tissue, a median furrow, continuous with the intact central canal above, may be identified. Escaping CSF may be seen. In an attempt to heal itself, rapid encrustation of scar and epithelial tissue on the dorsal plate surface may begin in utero and may form a secondary covering of "skin" within a few weeks to months if left untreated surgically.[9] The initial surface scar tissue at birth is a potential barrier to infections.

Immediately surrounding the neural placode is a thin zone of pia, fibrous connective tissue, and partial epithelialization, which acts as a bridge between the neural tissue and the adjacent normal skin. At this junction the dural attachment is found. Thus, the dorsal region is durally deficient.

Enlargement of the ventral subarachnoid space forms a meningeal sac, which transforms a myelocele into a myelomeningocele. The neural placode then forms the dorsal wall of the meningocele, and the nerve roots become elongated and stretched. Normal nerve roots descend as the cauda equina in the lumbar region, but in myelomeningocele a radiating "sunburst" appearance of nerve roots emanating from a low-lying neural plate can be seen. The nerve roots may course cephalad, transversely, or caudally to exit from their respective neural foramina.[2,6]

Caudal to the myelomeningocele, a normal spinal cord may re-form with attachment to the sacrum. At the craniocervical junction, findings of a Chiari II malformation may be noted.

Imaging

With the exception of plain films, any radiologic study of the spine before surgery is probably contraindicated, since little useful information is gained and the exposed neural tissue is subjected unnecessarily to the risk of trauma and infection. On the other hand, the cranium may be effectively assessed with sonography to identify hydrocephalus and evidence of a Chiari II malformation.

Although not useful at the time of presentation at birth, MRI is an ideal imaging tool for screening and delineating the various causes of late neurologic deterioration after surgery. After myelomeningocele repair, the untethered conus medullaris remains low-lying, even if there is no clinical evidence of the tethered cord syndrome (Fig. 15–3). While this may be partially related to an overextended cord and to an insufficient follow-up period to allow for cord ascent,[47] another explanation is provided by Tamaki and colleagues.[48] Using MRI, they noted that all patients after surgery had potential conus fixation at the site of previous repair, presumably related to postoperative scarring. Thus, the normal MR appearance of a repaired myelomeningocele is that of a low-lying conus medullaris (Fig. 15–3) that has no clear separation from the posterior thecal sac at the operative site. The remainder of the neural tissue should be free from the rest of the posterior thecal sac. No posterior angulation of the neural tissue should be seen.

Patients with the tethered cord syndrome may show

the additional finding of adhesions just below the last laminae, the level of the cephalad fibrovascular band.[48] Retethering on MRI may be documented by demonstrating a low-lying conus medullaris with adhesion at the surgical site, associated with posterior kinking and angulation of neural tissue under the last laminae (Fig. 15–4). No CSF cleavage plane is seen between the cord and the two levels of the posterior dura tethering (Fig. 15–5).[48, 49] If cord atrophy is seen on MRI, cord infarction related to the previous surgery is the prime consideration.

Ultrasonography may be useful in infants, because a sonographic window is often present at the repair site. After surgery, the absence of normal cord pulsation is suggestive of retethering.

Treatment

The aim of initial surgery in all patients is to reconstruct the normal anatomic barriers. The encrusted neural tissue is first debrided and sterilized. The neural placode is then dissected away from the surrounding tissues and folded to reconstruct the neural tube. The dura must be freed and closed in a watertight fashion to prevent CSF leakage and to provide a capacious subdural space in which the spinal cord can reside. For large defects, Silastic, fascia lata, or cadaveric substitutes for dura may be used. Finally, proper closure of the overlying skin will guard against infections. The bony canal is not reconstructed; on the contrary, a laminectomy or even a kyphectomy (removal of a ver-

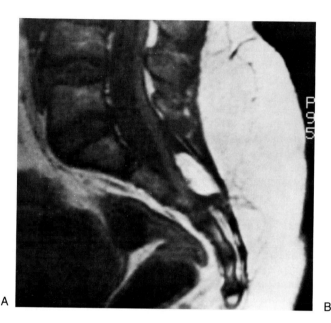

A

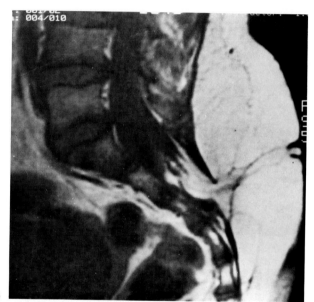

B

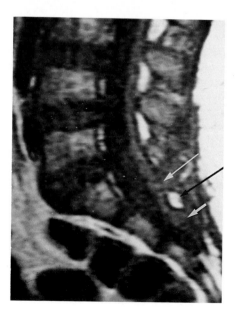

C

Figure 15–5. *Pre- and postoperative lipomyelomeningocele.* ***A,*** T1 weighted (600/20) midsagittal image demonstrates the tethered spinal cord secondary to the dorsally attached hyperintense lipoma. ***B,*** T1 weighted (600/20) paramedian sagittal image illustrates extension of the lipoma into the subcutaneous tissues, resulting in a lumbosacral mass. Note the cutaneous stigmata of a sacral skin tag and skin dimple. ***C,*** T1 weighted (400/20) sagittal image postoperatively demonstrates subtotal resection of the lipoma (*low black arrow*). There is no cleavage plane identified between the low-lying spinal cord and the posterior thecal sac at the distal surgical site, which can be a normal postoperative appearance (*short white arrow*). However, a second level of adhesion just caudal to the last lamina (*long white arrow*) is suggestive of retethering.

tebral body) may be necessary to reduce pressure on the overlying skin.

There has been some debate over the immediate treatment of myelomeningocele.[50] The general consensus at this time is that early aggressive treatment and surgery yield the best results.[51-55]

In the past, some centers selected severe cases for nontreatment, on the grounds that the poor prognosis would lead to a markedly reduced quality of life. On the contrary, it has been found that neither favorable nor unfavorable results can be predicted at birth. This has been borne out in a series of "unselected" patients who were all given the opportunity of early surgery (McLane and associates).[53] The results in these individuals are similar to the best results in selected patients in terms of mortality, although their IQs were slightly lower.

The extent of disability after surgery varies with respect to the severity of the lesion. Ambulation is essentially an impossibility in all thoracic and high lumbar lesions.[42] Of all patients, only 20 percent at school age are confined to a wheelchair.[53]

Symptoms may be secondary to the primary neural tube lesion, but the culprit may often be a concomitant abnormality such as syringohydromyelia or Chiari II malformation. Posterior fossa decompression has been used with some success in patients with signs of brain stem compression.[56, 57]

Relatively normal intelligence (IQ > 80) is seen in three-quarters of all survivors, although learning disabilities are common: one-half of survivors need special schooling.[53, 58]

Postoperative and long-term care includes attention to the urinary system, orthopedic deformities, hydrocephalus, and associated anomalies.[53, 59]

Late Complications

Once a patient has stabilized neurologically after a myelomeningocele repair, there should be no further change in the neurologic status with aging. Any late progressive neurologic deterioration is an indication of a complication that may be amenable to surgery; clinical and radiologic evaluation, including MRI, should assess the possibility of shunt malfunction, syringohydromyelia formation, arachnoid cyst, inclusion cyst, spinal cord retethering, and traction bands or adhesions. Likewise, associated anomalies, such as diastematomyelia or Chiari II malformation with hindbrain compression, may be present.[53] Several complications may occur simultaneously.[59, 60]

Cord retethering is the most common cause of late neurologic deterioration, with a 3 to 15 percent incidence after a myelomeningocele repair.[48, 59, 60] The actual incidence of retethering increases with the patient's age. The clinical presentation is identical to that of patients with primary cord tethering related to occult spinal dysraphism. Eight to 10 years is the average

age when symptoms begin, since this is a period of rapid growth.[48] Progressive scoliosis is a common symptom that may be seen with either retethering of the cord or syringohydromyelia.[47, 59, 60]

OCCULT SPINAL DYSRAPHISM: SPINAL LIPOMA AND LIPOMYELOMENINGOCELE

Occult spinal dysraphisms are skin-covered lesions that include spina bifida occulta, diastematomyelia, tight filum terminale syndrome, dorsal dermal sinus, intraspinal lipoma, and lipomyelomeningocele; most are lipomyelomeningoceles.

Incidence

Spina bifida occulta (posterior fusion defect) occurs most commonly in the lumbosacral region, especially the first sacral segment or the first and second sacral segments combined. This anomaly is best regarded as a normal variant. Spina bifida occulta is extremely common in the normal population, with an incidence ranging from approximately 1 to over 30 percent.[61-64]

Lipomatous spinal lesions account for 35 percent of all skin-covered lumbosacral masses; most are lipomyelomeningoceles (20 percent).[6, 65, 66]

Embryogenesis

A defect in disjunction, a subcategory of neurulation, is thought to produce lipomyelomeningocele, other CNS lipomas, and the dorsal dermal sinus.[6, 67] If the dorsal ectoderm separates from the underlying neural tube before completion of neural tube closure, the adjacent mesenchyme is allowed to come into contact with the open dorsal surface of the neural plate. When mesenchyme is exposed to the interior of the neural tube, it appears to be induced to form lipomatous tissues, which prevent neural tube closure. The lipoma can easily track superiorly into the central canal formed by the closed portion of the neural tube.

The other theories on the pathogenesis of spinal cord lipomas include overgrowth of normal fat cells within the leptomeninges, fatty differentiation of multipotential mesenchymal cells, and inclusions or ectopic rests of fatty cells during neural tube closure.[68, 69]

Clinical Findings

The signs and symptoms of occult spinal dysraphism are highly variable.[70] Patients are often asymptomatic for many years and may present late in life.[71, 72] In patients with lipomyelomeningoceles, approximately half present before 6 months of age. The most common manifestations are cutaneous stigmata.[73] With increasing age, neurologic dysfunction becomes the predominant symptom. Almost 90 percent of patients over 2 years of age have a neurologic deficit.[74] The most common symptoms, all of which are long-standing,[75] are urinary incontinence, foot deformities, unilateral limb atrophy, and sensory deficits in the lower extremities. If left untreated, these problems can eventually produce severe peripheral neuropathies with trophic ulcers, paraplegia, and surgically irreparable orthopedic deformities.[76–78] Less commonly, back or leg pain may be experienced. The neurologic symptoms are presumably related to cord tethering, angulation around a fibrovascular band, and mass effect from the lipoma. It has been noted that an acceleration of neurologic deficits may occur with puberty, weight gain, or relatively insignificant injury to the spine.

On examination the most evident finding is a skin-covered lumbosacral mass above the intergluteal cleft (Fig. 15–6). Masses at or caudal to the intergluteal cleft are usually sacrococcygeal teratomas. Thirty-five percent of all skin-covered lumbosacral lesions eventually prove to be spinal lipomas.[6, 65] On palpation, these lesions have a fatty consistency. They are not as large and do not extend as far cephalad as myelomeningoceles. If the skin-covered bulge is asymmetric,

one can predict that the lipoma is likely to be associated with a meningocele.[79] If there is no dorsal protrusion, the lesion is termed a lipomyelocele. A palpable laminal defect may be present. Up to two-thirds of patients have some cutaneous stigmata, including skin tags, subcutaneous fat, a long patch of abnormal hair, angioma, hyperpigmentation, pilonidal cysts, dermal sinus tracts, and dermal dimples (Figs. 15–5, 15–7).[66, 76, 80–83]

Associated anomalies include Klippel-Feil syndrome, pseudohermaphroditism, cataracts, harelip, absent kidney, and cloacal exstrophy.[68, 81, 84, 85] With the use of MRI as a screening modality, it is expected that subtle cases of Chiari I malformation will be revealed.[67, 86]

Pathologic Anatomy

In 1969 Emery and Lendon attempted to classify the various types of fatty tumors related to spinal dysraphism.[87] Six different categories of fat-containing lesions were identified. Three of these are not generally recognized as being true lipomatous lesions: they consist of hamartomas associated with diastematomyelia, heterotopic tissues of which fat is a small component,

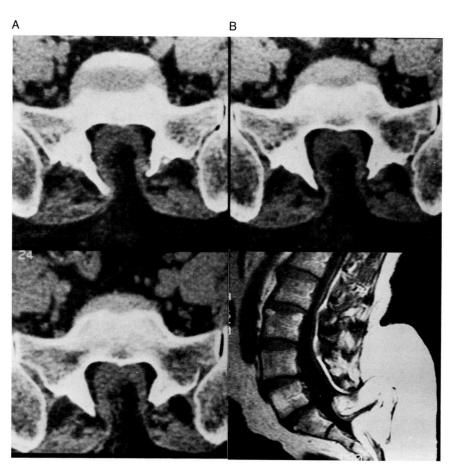

Figure 15–6. *Lipomyelomeningocele in an asymptomatic patient who was evaluated for a lumbosacral mass.* **A** to **C,** Noncontrast axial CT scan through S1 demonstrates a lumbosacral lipoma, extending into the subcutaneous tissues through a large posterior element defect. **D,** T1 weighted (600/20) sagittal scan confirms the lumbosacral lipoma. The lipomatous tissue mushrooms into a large subcutaneous component by passing beneath the cephalad fibrovascular band. Note the tethered and thinned spinal cord.

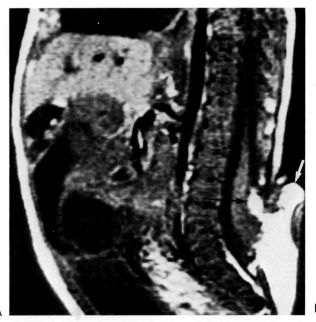
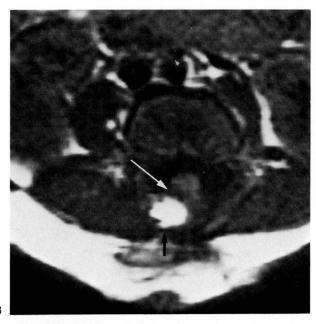

A

B

Figure 15–7. *Lumbosacral lipomyelomeningocele.* ***A,*** T1 weighted (500/20) sagittal scan demonstrates the high-signal lipoma and its dorsal relationship to the tethered neural placode. There is cephalad tracking of the lipoma dorsal to the placode and central canal (*long arrow*). A lipomatous skin appendage is depicted (*short arrow*). ***B,*** T1 weighted (400/20) axial scan shows rotation of the low-lying spinal cord caused by the dorsal lipoma. There is a band of slight hypointensity relative to the neural tissue at the liponeural junction (*long arrow*); this may represent dense fibrous connective tissue. Chemical shift artifact is seen posterior to the lipoma (*short arrow*). Note the characteristic flattened shape of the neural placode.

and implantation fat associated with trauma or previous surgery. The other three categories consist of (1) lipoma of the filum terminale, (2) intradural lipoma, and (3) lipomyelomeningocele. These latter three categories are accepted by most authors. Pathologically the fat is identical in all three types and is composed of normal adult adipose tissue, which is partially encapsulated and attached both to the meninges and to the spinal cord. The fat is divided into lobules by dense collagen.[54, 88]

Hamartomatous elements may be seen in the various types of lipomas associated with spina bifida, but this association is distinctly unusual (Fig. 15–8).[87–91] Malignant degeneration of the lipomatous tissue into carcinoma or malignant teratoma is an extremely rare event.[92–94]

Lipoma or Fibrolipoma of the Filum Terminale

Lipoma or fibrolipoma of the filum terminale is a relatively common lesion (Fig. 15–9).[87] When the lipoma is confined to the thecal sac, it tends to be encapsulated with a sausage shape; extrathecal fibrolipoma is typically larger with less distinct margins. The lesion may have both an intrathecal and an extrathecal component. These lesions do not expand above the ventriculus terminalis and are associated with central canal duplication within the filum.[87] Occasionally, un-

usual ectodermal and mesodermal tissues such as neuroglial tissue, striated muscle, cartilage, and bone may be seen within the fibrous tract that joins the lipoma to the conus medullaris.[88]

Intradural Lipoma

Intradural lipomas make up less than 1 percent of all spinal cord tumors (Fig. 15–8).[91] Two-thirds of these lesions occur in the cervical or thoracic region. Patients often are asymptomatic or have mildly progressive symptoms that typically relate to cord compression or tethering. The spinal canal is most often normal or exhibits minimal posterior fusion defects. Occasionally, it may be widened with evidence of pedicular or vertebral body erosion.

Although these encapsulated lesions have a seemingly clear cleavage plane, surgical removal of intradural lipomas can be hazardous because of the capsular attachment at the fibrous liponeural interface,[90, 95] and the close association of the lipoma with the dorsal half of the neural placode. If the lipoma is asymmetric to one side, it may cause rotation of the spinal cord, which stretches the contralateral nerve roots and places them in a position for increased surgical risk.

Although the lipoma may have a subpial extension with thickened overlying pia, it is never truly intramedullary, i.e., completely surrounded by neural tis-

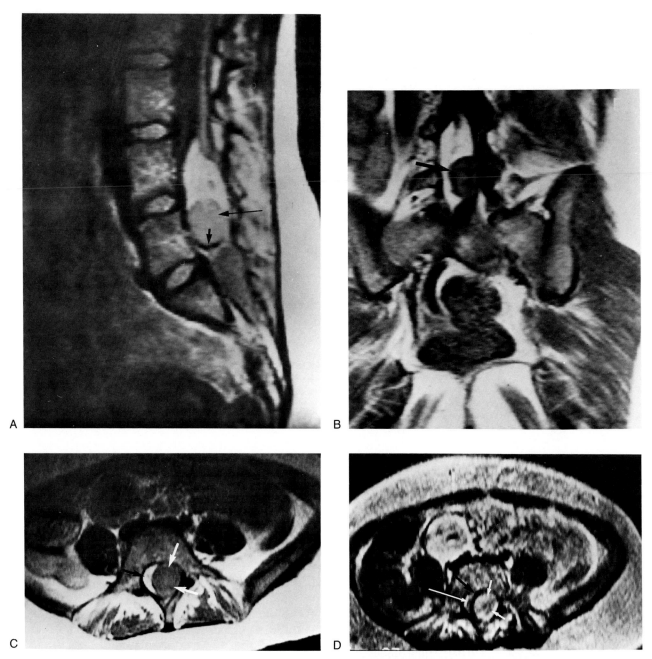

Figure 15–8. *Intradural lipoma with hamartomatous component.* **A,** Spin-density (2300/40) midsagittal image shows a lumbar intradural lipoma and an associated tethered spinal cord. Characteristically, the laminae are nearly normal with no or minimal extracanalicular fat. The rounded isointense lesion within the lipoma represents the hamartomatous component (*long arrow*). A prominent chemical shift artifact is seen in the frequency encoding direction (*short arrow*). **B,** T1 weighted (500/21) coronal image demonstrates the hamartomatous component (*arrow*), easily seen within the lipoma. **C,** T1 weighted (652/22) axial section shows the isointense hamartomatous tissue (*white arrows*) predominantly to the left of the lipoma (*black arrow*). **D,** T2 weighted (2000/70) axial section shows that the hamartomatous tissue signal remains isointense with the adjacent soft tissues (*short white arrows*). The lipoma has become hypointense (*long white arrow*). Note the chemical shift artifact (*black arrow*).

sue.[91] However, radiographically it may appear to be intramedullary. The dura is attached to the lateral aspect of the neural placode (between the dorsal nerve roots and lipoma) without extension across the dorsum, creating a dural defect posteriorly.[95] Thus the lipoma, besides being extramedullary, is actually extradural as well, making the term intradural lipoma a misnomer. The ventral CSF sac is enclosed by the dura and a pia-arachnoid layer. The dorsal wall of the sac is formed by the ventral neural placode. Because the

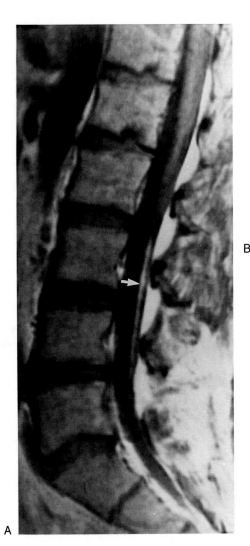

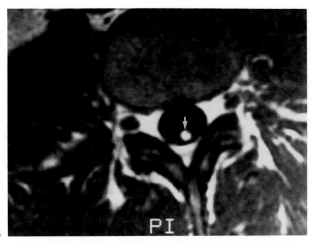

Figure 15–9. *Lipoma of the filum terminale.* **A** to **B,** T1 weighted (1000/20) midsagittal and axial images show a thickened fatty filum terminale (*arrow*). (From Raghavan N, Barkovich AJ. MR imaging in the tethered spinal cord syndrome. AJNR 1989; 10:27–36. © by American Society of Neuroradiology.)

nerve roots reside within the subarachnoid space, they have no contact with the extradural lipoma.

Lipomyelomeningocele

Among the various forms of fatty tumors related to spinal dysraphism, lipomyelomeningocele is the most common type. According to Naidich and colleagues, the anatomy of a lipomyelomeningocele is identical to that of an intradural lipoma, except that the lipoma and neural plate herniate through a wide laminal defect.[95] The lipomatous tissue is free to extend from the subcutaneous region through the bony and dural defect and insert into the dorsal neural cleft. Since the cleft extends deep into the central canal, it is possible for lipomatous tissue to track superiorly within this canal (Fig. 15–7). Just lateral to the entrance into the cleft is the dural attachment onto the placode. Because of the position of this dural attachment, the fatty tissue is completely extradural, whereas the anterior nerve roots travel within the subarachnoid space, having no

contact with the fat.[95] Previous authors, however, have suggested that there is intermixing of the fat with the nerve roots.[54, 69, 74, 75, 77] The large ventral subarachnoid CSF space and associated CSF pulsations result in thinning of the neural tissue and herniation of it posteriorly through the laminal defect.

Again, as with intradural lipomas, the fat is completely separated from the neural tissue at the so-called liponeural junction by dense irregular connective tissue, making the lipoma tightly adherent to the placode. The lipoma itself is encapsulated.

The fundamental characteristics of the localized osseous defect have been elegantly defined by Naidich and colleagues.[6] Superiorly, the posterior arches progress from an intact bony arch to a mild spina bifida defect to widely everted laminae. This sequence is then reconstituted in reverse order as one progresses caudally. In addition, Naidich and colleagues state that a constant fibrovascular band, stretched between the most superior, widely bifid laminae, kinks and notches the superior surface of the spinal cord and meningocele in all cases of lipomyelomeningocele.[95] The cephalad fibrovascular band in conjunction with the adherent lipoma causes cord tethering, and results in a low-lying conus with horizontally oriented nerve roots. A similar fibrovascular band may be seen in the caudal portion of the spinal bifida defect.

Imaging

Various diagnostic modalities are available for evaluation of occult spinal dysraphism. Plain radiographs are useful for revealing associated vertebral anomalies and predicting the level of meningocele sac herniation by noting the location of the most cephalad widely bifid spinous process, which marks the fibrovascular band. In the past, conventional myelography, gas myelography, and digital myelography have all been used to document the low-lying conus medullaris, traction bands, associated intra- and extradural masses, and Chiari malformations.[96-98] Ultrasonography has also been studied as a potential screening modality because of its low cost, easy accessibility, and good visualization of anatomic details,[99, 100] but inherent problems such as poor soft tissue lesion specificity and acoustic shadowing from calcified and bony lesions have restricted ultrasound from being the ideal screening tool. Conventional computed tomography (CT) and CT myelography were the imaging modality of choice before the advent of MRI.[101-104] CT myelography is more accurate than either CT or myelography alone in assessing the complex bony and soft tissue abnormalities.[104, 105]

In recent years, MRI has become the diagnostic tool of choice for screening patients with suspected occult spinal dysraphism.[106-114] The sensitivity and accuracy of MRI compare favorably with myelography and CT myelography.[107, 109] At the authors' institution, all patients with lumbosacral masses and cutaneous stigmata suggestive of occult spinal dysraphism undergo an MR study at the earliest age possible, before the development of neurologic symptoms.

If MRI is compared with CT myelography, the former can be performed faster and less expensively. In addition, MRI is noninvasive, does not use ionizing radiation, has superior soft tissue differentiation (no bone signal to give interference), and has multiplanar capability. The position of the conus and the presence of associated soft tissue tumors and syrinxes are easily assessed. MRI is also ideal for rapidly assessing the entire spine for concomitant lesions. Use of MRI in conjunction with plain radiographs eliminates the need for myelography, although CT scan may still play a supplemental role in elucidating complex bony vertebral anomalies.

The disadvantages of MRI include poor bony and cartilaginous detail, poor visualization of the nerve roots, and inability to assess the possibility of adhesive bands. The problem with bony detail may be overcome by additional plain radiographs in the screening process. Imaging patients with severe kyphoscoliosis may be difficult, but by increasing the sagittal slice thickness and including coronal views in addition to the axial images, a diagnostic study can be obtained. Three-dimensional reconstructions may also prove beneficial.

Routine short TR, short TE thin-section images (3 mm) of the lumbosacral region using sagittal and axial views are initially obtained. Coronal images are a useful adjunct for diastematomyelia, vertebral anomalies, and kyphoscoliosis. If the initial screening scans are normal, no other sequences are needed. If an occult lesion such as a lipomyelomeningocele is discovered, it is necessary to image the remainder of the spine and posterior fossa region to exclude a concomitant syrinx or other vertebral or neural anomalies. Use of a coil holder that allows the spine surface coil to slide underneath sedated infants or children without disturbing them facilitates the screening process.

Lipomyelomeningoceles are readily diagnosed by MRI (Figs. 15-6, 15-7).[111, 112] Although bony detail is not as well seen as on CT, the posterior fusion defects and laminal inversion are easily assessed on sagittal and axial views. With careful observation, even the superiormost minimally bifid lamina can be identified. The dorsally cleft neural placode can be identified by its flattened configuration instead of the normally rounded or oval shape of the conus medullaris and distal thoracic spinal cord.

The extradural lipoma and its subcutaneous extension are seen as a hyperintense lesion on T1 weighted images. Since they are composed of mature adipose tissue, their signal intensity is identical to that of the surrounding epidural and subcutaneous fat.[113] The appearance is diagnostic, especially when seen in conjunction with the chemical shift artifact in the frequency encoding gradient direction. If necessary, to distinguish fat from blood, a T2 weighted image may also be taken (Fig. 15-8).

A low-signal band is often seen at the liponeural junction (anterior to the lipoma) (Figs. 15-5, 15-7, 15-8) and may represent a chemical shift artifact or the dense fibrous tissue that gives tight adhesion to the neural and fatty components. The lipoma is always dorsal to the neural tissue. However, when it is large, the lipomatous tissue may appear to be intradural and intermixed with the nerve roots because of partial voluming artifact. This appearance should not be confused with normal nerve roots, which travel within the caudalmost epidural fat after they leave the subarachnoid space. The lipoma itself may also cause vertebral scalloping, unilateral thinning, and decrease in size of the pedicles and laminae. When the lipoma is asymmetric, the meningocele bulges to the contralateral side, and rotation of the placode occurs.[95] Stretching of the contralateral nerve roots may sometimes be documented.

Enlargement of the ventral subarachnoid space

causes neural tissue thinning and herniation of the meningocele under the fibrovascular band. The resultant notch in the superior aspect of the sac and in the low-lying tethered conus is easily assessed on sagittal images.

Treatment

Occult spinal dysraphism with cord tethering is best treated by preventive microsurgery before symptoms develop. Surgery is simplified with the use of evoked potentials by electronic stimulation. The primary goal is to release the conus medullaris and free the neural tissue from all surrounding adhesions and masses.[82, 115] A more complex surgical approach is needed when dealing with a lipomyelomeningocele. First, the fibrovascular band where the neural placode is tethered must be resected. The dorsal lipoma and its liponeural junction must then be identified. Careful dissection of the lipoma and neural tissue from the epithelial tissue is important to prevent the development of inclusion dermoids and to prevent future retethering. Because of the tight adherence of the lipoma to the neural tissue, total removal of the fatty tissue may not be possible without injury to the neural placode. As long as the decompression is adequate, even if only subtotal resection of the lipoma is possible, results will be favorable since lipomatous recurrence is rare.[68] With larger lipomyelomeningoceles, a filum terminale may not be found, but if one is visible it must be transected. Once the spinal cord has been untethered, there may be relaxation with slight ascent. Lastly, the dura must be freed from its attachment to the lipoma and cord in order to reconstruct a watertight thecal sac.

Postsurgically, improvement of gait and of bladder function is seen in 20 and 25 percent of patients, respectively.[76] Surgical repairs on asymptomatic patients carry the best prognosis.

DIASTEMATOMYELIA

Diastematomyelia is an anomaly of the spine characterized by a sagittal cleft that separates the cord into two hemicords (Fig. 15–10). It is usually associated with vertebral column abnormalities and varying degrees of cord tethering. A bony or fibrocartilaginous septum may or may not be present within the cleft. The definition of diplomyelia is somewhat more confusing. Some authors use the terms diastematomyelia and diplomyelia synonymously;[116] others reserve the term diplomyelia to describe a more complete duplication of the cord in which each hemicord has paired ventral and paired dorsal nerve roots.[117–119] In most cases of diastematomyelia, however, each hemicord has only a single ventral and dorsal nerve root, and indeed it is extremely rare for each hemicord to have two paired roots. Naidich and colleagues question whether true

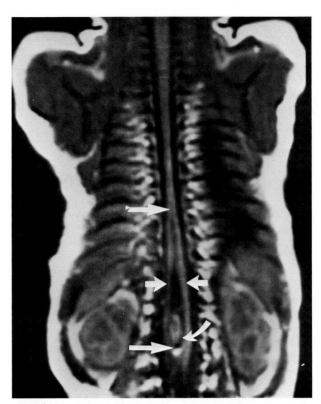

Figure 15–10. *Diastematomyelia.* T1 weighted (500/20) coronal image illustrates the bony spur (*curved arrow*) and unequal hemicords (*short arrows*). Note that the cleft (*long arrows*) is longer than the actual spur and that the spur is situated in the caudal aspect of the cleft. Each hemicord is smaller than the normal cord.

diplomyelia really exists.[6] To add to the confusion, Hori and associates use the term dimyelia to describe diplomyelia, and use the term diplomyelia to describe an accessory lumbar spinal cord that has no nerve roots and is situated ventral to the true cord.[120] In general, the term diastematomyelia should be used in a general sense, and the term diplomyelia should be reserved for a form of diastematomyelia in which there is a more perfect duplication of the cord, each hemicord containing two ventral and two dorsal nerve roots.

Ollivier is given credit for first using the term diastematomyelia in 1837.[121] During the 1800s there were several other sporadic reports of diastematomyelia.[22, 122] The first comprehensive review, however, was provided by Herren and Edwards (1940) with a report of the pathology in 42 cases.[116] Pickles (1949) described the first case to be diagnosed preoperatively and treated surgically.[123] Matson and colleagues (1950) discussed the surgical strategies from their experience with 11 patients.[124] They stressed the fact that the progressive symptoms noted in these patients were related to traction of the fixed cord during spinal growth. They further stated that the goal of surgery should be a "prophylactic rather than a curative one" and warned that "parents should understand that surgical treatment is undertaken in order to permit normal growth and maturation of the nervous system and thus prevent, if possible, subsequent increase in loss of function." Several other series have since appeared in the literature.[125-135]

Imaging advances have improved our understanding of diastematomyelia. CT has allowed a more detailed evaluation of the bony spur and associated vertebral anomalies, and CT myelography has permitted better evaluation of the two hemicords and surrounding thecal sac. Undoubtedly, however, MRI has provided the greatest breakthrough in imaging of diastematomyelia and has allowed evaluation of the cord in a completely noninvasive fashion.

Embryogenesis

The true etiology of diastematomyelia is not known. Genetic factors are not very important.[6] Many theories have developed over the years[29, 79, 116, 136, 137] and can be broken down into two main groups: (1) an intrinsic abnormality of the neuroectoderm and (2) an extrinsic abnormality causing secondary splitting of the cord. In the former there is a primary splitting of the cord, which subsequently causes the abnormalities of the vertebral column; in the latter the vertebral column abnormalities are thought to cause the splitting of the cord.

Clinical Findings

Diastematomyelia is more prevalent in females than in males: 70 to 94 percent of patients are female.[127, 132, 138] Typically, the diagnosis is made during childhood, but occasionally it is made in adult life.[138-142] In one series of 25 children, seven were diagnosed during the first year of life, ten between the first and fifth years, and eight between the fifth and 15th years.[118]

The clinical presentation has been well described in the literature.[6, 118, 124, 125, 132, 142, 143] Typically, patients present with a dorsal cutaneous abnormality, scoliosis, or a neurologic deficit. The neurologic deficit, not the cutaneous abnormality, is the most frequent presenting complaint.[124, 125, 143] Since the defect may present as a lower extremity deformity, these children are often initially referred to an orthopedic surgeon. Foot deformities reported include pes planus, pes cavus, talipes equinovarus, calcaneovalgus, and congenital vertical talus.[127] The neurologic deficit may also express itself with muscular atrophy, extremity shortening, bowel and urinary incontinence, paresthesia, paresis, reflex abnormalities, and gait disturbances. During the first year of life, gait disturbances and bowel and urinary incontinence may not be recognized, but when the child begins to walk and toilet train these findings become more apparent.

The cause of the neurologic deficit demonstrated in these patients has been an issue of question for some time. Matson and colleagues believed it related to traction of the cord by the bony or fibrocartilaginous spur.[124] Since the spine grows at a more rapid rate than the cord, the normal cord appears to migrate cephalad during growth and development. The conus is naturally the region of greatest migration, since the cephalad portion of the cord is fixed to the brain. Fixing the cord in the caudal aspect results in traction during spinal growth. Supporting evidence for this theory is provided by the fact that the neurologic symptoms in these children no longer progress after the tethered area is released. The actual physical splitting of the cord seems not to be the major cause of symptoms, as suggested by reports of completely asymptomatic patients diagnosed incidentally during scoliosis screening or autopsy.[144, 145]

Humphreys and associates suggested that the explanation is not quite so simple, and consider it likely to be multifactorial.[142] Since the conus reaches the adult level between birth and 2 months of age, these authors question why symptoms progress throughout life rather than presenting at a maximum by 2 months. Other possible contributing factors may be the scoliosis itself; a tight filum; bands; compression ischemia by the spur; associated abnormalities such as meningocele, dermal sinus, or lipoma; and possible inherent myelodysplasia at the ultrastructural level.

Of the cutaneous stigmata, hypertrichosis (hairy patch) is the most common, seen in 26 to 81 percent of patients.[118, 127, 138, 142, 144] The hypertrichosis typically lies in the midline and over the area of diastematomyelia, and may or may not be associated with a pigmented nevus. The hairy patch has often been referred to as a horse's tail because of its triangular shape and apex, which points inferiorly. The hair typically is quite long and coarse and different in appearance from that of normal body hair. Occasionally the hair may be of a finer texture. Although hypertrichosis is often a sign of diastematomyelia, there are many other anomalies in which this finding may be noted. In a series of 39 cases of occult spinal dysraphism with hypertrichosis, 51 percent had diastematomyelia.[144]

Other cutaneous findings that may be seen with diastematomyelia are lipomas, sacral dimples, hemangiomas, dermal sinuses, and atretic meningoceles. In the series of Hood and colleagues, physical examination revealed a dorsal cutaneous abnormality in 39 of 60 patients.[143]

Scoliosis is the third most common finding, demonstrated in 39 of the 60 patients reported by Hood and colleagues[143] and in 19 of the 34 reported by Hilal and associates.[132] Hilal and associates noted that the more severe cases of scoliosis were observed in older children, and concluded that the longer the patients were left undiagnosed, the greater chance they had of developing scoliosis. These authors further state that the length and location of the spur influence the development of scoliosis.

Pathologic Anatomy

Cleft, Septum, and Meninges

In diastematomyelia, each of the two hemicords is surrounded by its own pial membrane.[126, 146] The

arachnoid and dura, however, form either a single or a double tube.[126]

TYPE 1: CASES WITH A SINGLE DURAL TUBE. In this type the two hemicords lie within a common subarachnoid space and are surrounded by a single arachnoid and dural membrane. No osseous or fibrocartilaginous spur is present and the space between the two hemicords contains CSF.

TYPE 2: CASES WITH SEPARATE DURAL TUBES.

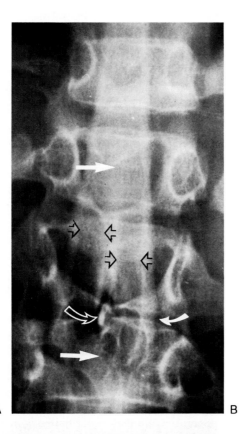

A

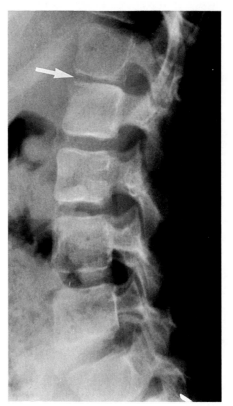

B

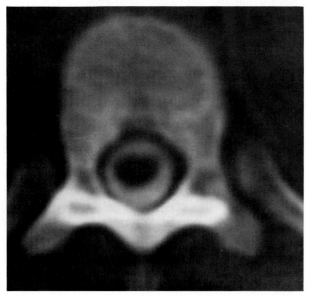

C

Figure 15–11. *Diastematomyelia extending from T12 to L2.* ***A,*** Myelogram demonstrates a bony spur (*curved open arrow*) in the caudal aspect of the cleft (*bold white arrows*). The two hemicords, outlined by short open arrows, reunite at the conus below the spur. Note the narrowed intervertebral space (*curved solid arrow*) and widened interpediculate space. ***B,*** Lateral plain radiograph illustrating the narrow intervertebral space (*arrow*). ***C*** to ***G,*** CT myelogram in a cephalad to caudal direction demonstrating the normal cord above the cleft (***C***), the cleft and septum (***D, E***), the reunited conus (***F***), and the cauda equina (***G***). The pedicles (*short bold arrows*) are widened (***D***) and the lamina (*long bold arrow*) is thickened where the spur (*open arrow*) attaches posteriorly (***E***). Note that at the same level the lamina forms a complete neural arch, and the spinous process (*curved arrow*) is poorly developed. Anteriorly, where the spur attaches to the vertebral body (***D, E***), there is a radiolucent line (*long thin arrow*), which some believe represents a synchondrosis. Note also the narrowed anteroposterior diameter of the vertebral body (***D*** to ***F***). On ***D*** and ***E***, two leaves of dura sandwich the bony spur and form separate dural tubes.

The dura and arachnoid split and form two tubes that surround each hemicord separately. The space between the two hemicords is therefore lined by two layers of dura. Between these layers and within the cleft is a septal spur of osseous or fibrocartilaginous material (Figs. 15–10, 15–11). No CSF is present in this space. The two dura-arachnoid tubes unite to form a single tube above and below the cleft at a level where the two hemicords unite to form a single cord again. Type 2 diastematomyelia has been reported in 29 to 100 percent of cases, but the average is approximately 50 percent.[6, 118, 126, 133]

Although the sagittally oriented cleft usually extends through the full thickness of the cord, it occasionally may not. When it does not, it is referred to as partial ventral or dorsal diastematomyelia.[126, 146] The cleft varies in length and location and in type 2 is usually somewhat longer than the septum itself; it ranges from 1 to 9.5 cm long (Figs. 15–10, 15–11).[116, 126]

The septum or spur that lies within the cleft may occur at any level, but is most often between T12 and L5.[138] It may be as small as 1 mm or may span four vertebral bodies.[132] In the thoracic spine the septum

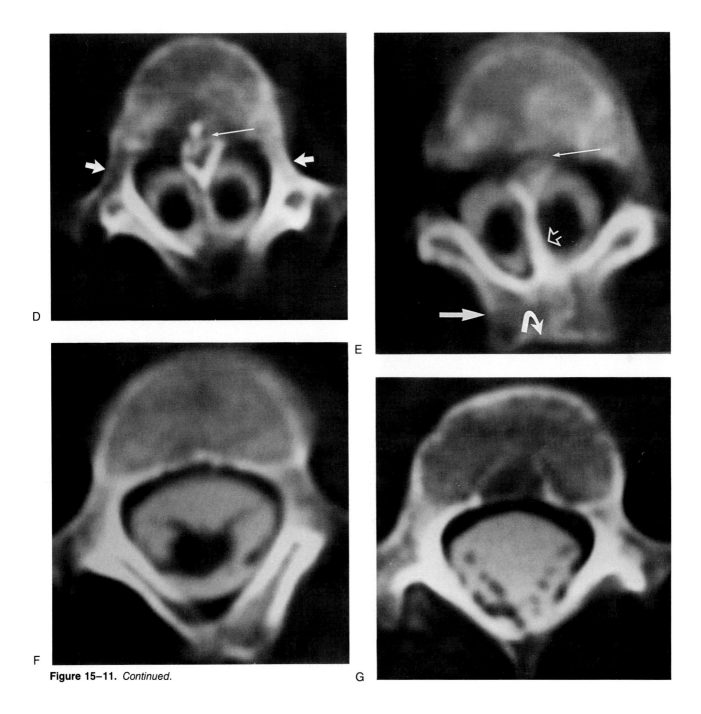

Figure 15–11. Continued.

tends to be longer than in the lumbar region.[118, 132] Occasionally, patients may have two or more septa.[132] Most septa are osseous rather than fibrocartilaginous.[118, 144] The spur may lie in the midline or cross the canal obliquely, depending in part on the degree of scoliosis.[6] A radiolucency seen on CT between the spur and its attachment may represent a synchondrosis (Fig. 15–11).[132, 146] Typically the spur attaches to the lamina posteriorly and to the vertebral body anteriorly. At the site where the septum attaches posteriorly, the neural arch is usually complete, but the spinous process may not be well formed (Fig. 15–2).[144] The septum is usually at the lower end of the cleft,[132] and there may be evidence of pressure necrosis of the cord in this region (Figs. 15–10, 15–11).[144] If the spur is not at the lower end of the cleft, one should look for a second spur more inferiorly.

Cord, Nerve Roots, and Bands

The hemicords lie lateral to each other and are rotated approximately 90 degrees. This rotation causes the ventral gray columns and ventral median sulcus of each hemicord to face each other and assume a medial instead of a ventral position. The anterior spinal artery, which splits along with the cord, also assumes a medial position.[132] There often is asymmetry of the two hemicords, one being larger than the other and both being narrower than the normal cord above or below the cleft (Figs. 15–10, 15–12).[118] The gray matter within the hemicord, although disorganized, tends to

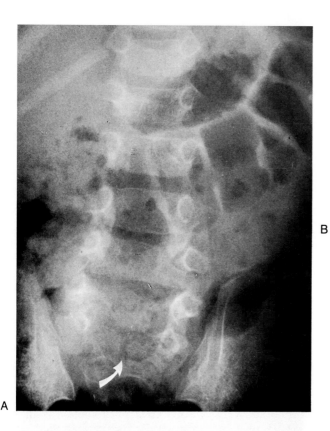

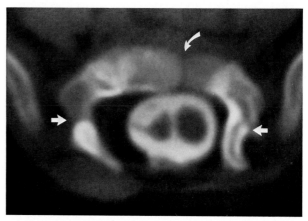

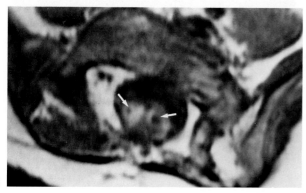

Figure 15–12. *Diastematomyelia with cord tethered at S1.* **A,** Anteroposterior plain radiograph demonstrating widened pedicles in the lumbosacral region and a sagittal cleft (*curved arrow*) of the S1 vertebral body. **B,** CT myelogram shows the sagittal cleft (*curved arrow*), widened interpediculate distance (*bold arrows*), and decreased vertebral body anteroposterior diameter. Note the unequal diameter of the two hemicords. **C,** A syrinx (*arrows*) is seen on T1 weighted (500/20) axial MR image in each hemicord.

form a dorsal and ventral column. The ipsilateral segmental dorsal and ventral nerve roots will arise from each of these columns.[6] Herren and Edwards stated that the fundamental structure of well-formed hemicords is similar to that of a normal cord, with each hemicord containing a central canal and four gray columns (two ventral and two dorsal) arranged in the typical H configuration.[116]

Commissural bands may cross from one hemicord, through the cleft, and into the other hemicord. These bands, which are up to 5 mm in diameter, are composed of either aberrant dorsal nerve roots or strands of dense fibrous tissue. The latter are thought to represent atrophied nerve roots. Occasionally, they may actually penetrate through a bony spur. In addition, fibers may cross from one hemicord to the other in thickened bundles of nerves that run on the cranial or caudal end of the cleft.[126, 144, 146] The bands are often accompanied by blood vessels and run from the intradural space, extradurally.[144] They are believed to play some role in the tethering process and should therefore be severed at surgery.[142]

The conus medullaris is often low.[132] If the cord does not reunite below the cleft, it will end in two prominent fila terminale. A prominent filum terminale (2 mm or more in diameter) was identified in 14 of 34 children.[132] The cord above the cleft is usually normal, except in hydromyelia, which may rarely be seen.

Vertebral Column

Abnormalities of the vertebral column are seen in almost all patients with diastematomyelia and can be divided into three groups: those of curvature, those of the vertebral bodies, and those of the posterior elements. Scoliosis is a fairly common feature reported in 56 to 90 percent of patients with diastematomyelia.[127, 132, 143] In 392 patients with congenital scoliosis, 23 (4.9 percent) had diastematomyelia.[127] The severity or degree of scoliosis appears to increase with age.[132]

Vertebral body anomalies are also seen relatively frequently and have been reported in 85 percent of 34 patients.[132] The abnormalities of the vertebral bodies are quite varied and include simple narrowing of the intervertebral space (Fig. 15–11)[119, 132] and failure of segmentation with block vertebrae involving one or multiple segments.[127, 132] The latter has been reported in 56 percent of 27 patients.[127] Narrowing of the anteroposterior diameter of the vertebral body at the level of the spur also appears to be seen quite commonly (Fig. 15–12).[132] Sagittal clefts or hemivertebra have been reported in 30 to 45 percent of patients (Fig. 15–12).[127, 143]

Associated anomalies of the posterior elements are typically seen (91 percent) and may involve multiple levels (81 percent).[132] The interpediculate distance is widened quite frequently (Figs. 15–11, 15–12).[119, 127, 132, 138] The region where the pedicles are the widest is often the region where the spina bifida is the widest. The actual septum, however, may be one or several segments above or, less often, below this region.[118, 132] The region of involvement may be small or quite extensive, affecting several vertebral segments.[127] Spina bifida has been reported in 50 to 93 percent of patients.[116, 127, 143] The laminae are often thickened and fused in two or more vertebral segments (Fig. 15–11). The combination of an abnormal lamina and spina bifida at the same level appears to be common, reported in 59 percent of 34 patients.[132] At the level of the spur the lamina typically forms a complete neural arch (Fig. 15–11).

Since scoliosis is a relatively common finding on plain film radiography, the diagnosis of diastematomyelia should be suspected when scoliosis is accompanied by widening of the pedicles, spina bifida, or abnormal laminae.

Unusual Features and Associated Anomalies

Some unusual or less common features of diastematomyelia have also been noted.[147, 148] Nine cases of double diastematomyelia and two of triple diastematomyelia have been reported.[132, 145, 147, 149] The exact definition of double or triple diastematomyelia is somewhat vague; it should not be used to describe doubling or tripling of the spur. Double diastematomyelia refers to two sagittal clefts separated by a normal segment of cord regardless of the number of spurs present. Multiple spurs, which can also be seen, are usually less than three vertebral bodies apart. However, one case was reported in which the spurs were at T2 and L3.[147]

Diastematomyelia in the cervical spine is extremely rare.[116, 144, 146, 150–153] It appears to have some association with adult presentation,[150] which by itself is quite rare.[139, 141, 150, 151] Cervical diastematomyelia may produce less tethering than the lumbar form, and thus may cause symptoms later in life.

Other anomalies associated with diastematomyelia include Klippel-Feil syndrome and Chiari malformation.[153] Diastematomyelia has also been associated with teratomas[154] and Wilms' tumor.[155] Hydromyelia has been reported in six of 13 patients (Fig. 15–12).[156] This can affect the segment above the diastematomyelia or may extend into each hemicord. An unusual and rare postoperative phenomenon is the regrowth of a previously excised spur, described in three patients in whom the spur was excised but the two dural sleeves were left intact.[157] It therefore is now recommended that the two-layered dural cleft be excised to permit formation of a single dural tube. Another case of regrowth of a fibrous spur was thought to be caused by scar formation.[148]

Imaging

In the past, myelography, CT myelography, or both were the final imaging modalities used to evaluate patients suspected of having diastematomyelia. MRI has replaced myelography in many situations and therefore has become the final imaging tool for evaluating these patients. The importance of a complete and thorough MR examination cannot be overstated.

Plain films can be extremely useful in suggesting the level of the lesion and thus the level of study for MRI. They may reveal widened pedicles, deformed laminae, a spur, spina bifida, or scoliosis. If this information is not available, a screening MR scan can be performed. Since most cases of diastematomyelia occur in the lumbar or thoracic spine, a complete study should image both of these regions. We recommend first performing a T1 weighted sagittal sequence of the lumbar spine to determine the level of the conus and to exclude other associated anomalies such as dermoids or lipomas. Since the cleft in diastematomyelia has a sagittal orientation, it may be difficult to see on sagittal images. Therefore, a coronal T1 weighted sequence is most important (Fig. 15–10); it allows a large segment of the cord to be scanned and permits easy visualization of the cleft and hemicords. If an abnormality is identified, axial T1 weighted images should be taken above and below the lesion to exclude an associated syrinx (Fig. 15–12). Since diastematomyelia in the cervical spine is extremely rare and usually occurs in adults, imaging of the cervical spine need not be done in children.

The findings on MRI correlate well with the anatomic abnormalities described previously. The two hemicords should be readily apparent and separated by a spur or CSF. The spur itself may be low in signal if it is composed of cortical bone, or may have a central high signal if it contains fatty marrow. Since bone is not optimally visualized on MRI, a CT scan is recommended to delineate the bony abnormalities in this lesion (Figs. 15–11, 15–12).

In summary, if a high degree of suspicion for this lesion exists from the clinical examination (hypertrichosis, scoliosis, foot deformities, neurologic deficits) and the plain films (scoliosis, widened pedicles, deformed laminae, spina bifida, spur), the MR study can be designed specifically for optimal evaluation. In general, a screening T1 weighted examination that images the thoracic and lumbar spine in the sagittal and coronal planes, with axial images through the cord itself, should be sufficient.

Treatment

Treatment of diastematomyelia consists of surgery.[118, 124, 125, 142, 144, 157, 158] Occasionally a more conservative approach may be considered, especially if the patient is asymptomatic and has a spur situated in the middle of the cleft rather than in the caudal portion.[142]

The goal of surgery is to form a single dural tube by excising the spur and adjacent dura of the two dural tubes. A laminectomy that extends one to two levels above and below the lesion is carried out and the spur is gradually removed. Dura or bands that adhere to the spur are released. Some authors also advocate sectioning the filum terminale, although others believe that this procedure, which requires more extensive surgery, offers little benefit.[158, 159]

The results of surgery in most series are similar. Of 19 patients in one series, three were slightly improved, two were slightly worse, and 14 were unchanged.[127] In another series, similar results with 25 patients were encountered: six improved, none were made worse, and the rest remained unchanged, without progression of disease.[118] Since the natural history of diastematomyelia is one of gradual deterioration, surgery should be prophylactic and aimed at preventing further progression of the deficits.[124]

TIGHT FILUM TERMINALE SYNDROME

The tight filum terminale syndrome, also known as the tethered conus, tethered filum, and cord traction syndrome, is defined as a condition in which a spinal cord is tethered with the conus in low position by a short, thick filum terminale.[6, 49, 160–162] The syndrome is specific and excludes cases in which the cord is tethered as a result of other conditions, such as diastematomyelia, lipomyelomeningocele, spinal cord tumor, or fibrous bands, or after meningomyelocele repair.[6, 49, 163] These other conditions are discussed elsewhere. Of patients with symptoms of tethered cord, 12[164] to 70 percent[165] have a tight filum terminale.[164–168]

Embryogenesis and Pathology

The neural tube becomes atrophic caudal to the 32nd somite to form the filum.[169] As the embryo grows, there is rapid ascent of the conus, owing to the lumbar vertebrae growing faster than the cord. The filum lengthens as the result of degeneration of the primitive conus and the intrinsic increase in the length of its nerve fibers.[169] If the terminal cord fails to involute or if the nerve fibers fail to lengthen, the tight filum terminale syndrome may result.[170, 171]

The syndrome is usually sporadic but there may be hereditary forms.[166, 172] It occurs equally in males and females.[6, 164, 165]

Clinical Findings

Patients present with symptoms due to stretching of the cord. These symptoms increase during periods of rapid growth and are also aggravated by exercise. Most patients become symptomatic as children. Symptoms are often progressive and accentuated in adolescence; this may be explained by the growth of the spine.[161, 169] In infants, only one mild curve is normally present in the spine, which is concave ventrally. When the child ambulates, a lumbar curve develops and lengthens the canal. At puberty, growth of the spine is faster than that of the cord. In all these developments, increased tension on the cord occurs if tethering is present.[169]

In most cases, patients present with progressive motor difficulties and/or sensory loss in the lower extremities. Motor symptoms range from a sensation of stiffness to actual weakness and wasting.[161, 163, 169] Initially, only mild limping may be seen, particularly on exertion.[172] Later, more profound weakness and atrophy may occur. Often, the development of the foot on the affected side is decreased. Pes cavus deformities are common. Abnormal stretch reflexes are noted.

Bladder dysfunction is common but generally is not the sole symptom.[161, 163, 169] In infants and young children, absence of dry periods between diaper changes and continuous dribbling is often noted.[165] There may be a delay in toilet training. Older children are frequently enuretic, despite daytime continence. Some experience frequency and urgency and a few may even experience constant incontinence. Bowel dysfunction is uncommon.

Low back pain or leg pain is a frequent complaint.[161, 162, 169, 172] Radiation down the legs is comparatively unusual. The back pain intensifies with exercise and coughing.[172] Tightness of the hamstring tendons may be so severe that the child cannot sit upright in a chair.[172]

Bony abnormalities are common.[6, 160–165, 169, 172] All patients have spina bifida.[160, 161, 169] In addition, scoliosis is often seen, generally progressive and associated with motor weakness and/or bladder dysfunction.[162] Cutaneous abnormalities are seen in approximately one-half of the patients and include hypertrichosis, angiomas, subcutaneous lipomas, dimples, and sinus tracts.[163]

Imaging

Plain films show spina bifida in all patients.

In the tight filum terminale syndrome, the filum is thicker than its normal 2-mm diameter.[98] The conus also lies below the normal level, which is at mid L2 or above by 2 months postnatally. Fitz and Harwood-Nash suggested that a conus tip below L2–L3 in a child over 5 years old is abnormal.[163]

Traditionally, myelography demonstrates the low-lying conus.[160, 161, 163] The thecal sac is displaced backward, necessitating supine myelography.[163] Tubular widening of the filum is often seen, especially near its termination. The filum passes posteriorly and tents the arachnoid. CT confirms these findings and CT can provide additional information in some cases. Occasionally, the filum is so tightly applied to the posterior surface of the arachnoid that it cannot be identified as a discrete structure. CT can delineate this situation. In addition, CT can better show the extradural component of a filum after it pierces the thecal sac and passes inferiorly to insert on the dorsal surface of the coccyx.

MRI provides further delineation of the findings in the tight filum terminale syndrome. T1 weighted sagittal and axial sequences are optimal to determine the morphology. T2 weighted sagittal images, particularly with cardiac gating and gradient moment nulling techniques, can provide information regarding the status of the cord itself. Raghavan and associates suggested measuring the filum at the L5–S1 interspace, excluding any lipomatous tissue that may be present.[164] In the tight filum terminale syndrome the filum can usually be measured, although in other pathologic abnormalities that may lead to a tethered cord the filum often is not measurable owing to its lack of visualization and adjacent abnormalities.

The level of the conus is also well delineated on MRI.[164] Generally, both sagittal and axial views are necessary. In the series of 19 patients of Raghavan and associates, measurements of the level of the conus were concordant in 17 patients.[164] However, if sections are slightly off midline, it may be hard to identify the tip of the conus in the sagittal section. In general, axial sections are best for identifying the conus level.

In patients with the filum terminale syndrome, 25 percent have lipomas of the filum terminale. Fatty content of the filum is easily delineated on both sagittal and axial scans, owing to the high intensity of the fat on T1 weighted images.[164] The extent of the lipoma in the thickened filum is well demarcated. However, a fatty filum terminale is not necessarily an indication of a tethered cord, because it may be seen in normal individuals.

MRI is also useful because it can visualize associated changes in the lower cord,[164] changes probably due to myelomalacia or syringohydromyelia. Best assessed on T2 weighted scans, myelomalacia may appear as an area of high signal in the cord. Syrinxes are seen as low-intensity linear defects in the substance of the cord. Confirmation in the axial plane is necessary, since sagittal images often suffer from artifacts, particularly the Gibbs artifacts, which may resemble a syrinx. The finding of these abnormalities within the cord substance itself may be useful in two ways. First, these changes may be permanent and thus important for the prognosis. Second, these changes may be useful in the unusual case of tight filum terminale syndrome in which the cord is not low-lying. Raghavan and associates noted that the tethered cord syndrome may occur with a normal conus position.[164] They also noted the tethered cord syndrome with a normal filum thickness at L5–S1.

Treatment

Surgery is generally indicated for these patients, especially when symptoms progress.[161–163, 165, 166, 169] Early diagnosis is important since some of the changes may be permanent. In the tight filum terminale syndrome, laminectomy is performed, followed by division of the filum terminale. Often, upward movement of the cord is seen after division of the filum. The cord may retract 0.5 to 2.5 cm.[162, 163, 168] In some patients the cord appears to extend to the lower end of the dural sac without a filum; in these the cord terminates in a small lipoma attached to the sac. Section of the cord at the dural attachment may also provide improvement.

In general, results of surgery are good. In nearly all patients, pain disappears with division of the filum. Motor capabilities usually improve. However, many patients have residual motor and sensory loss. Bladder function may or may not recover.[161]

CONGENITAL DERMAL SINUS

Congenital dermal sinuses are congenital defects consisting of an epithelium-lined tract extending from the skin inward.[173–183] They frequently connect the central nervous system or its coverings with the surface of the body.

Embryogenesis

Embryologically, these anomalies arise between the third and fifth weeks of intrauterine life.[174] Incomplete cleavage between the epithelial ectoderm and neuroectoderm is thought to be the mechanism by which a dermal sinus tract is produced.

The most frequent location for congenital dermal sinuses is sacrococcygeal. Wright found 72 in the lumbosacral region, 30 in the occipital region, 12 in the thoracic region, and only 2 in the cervical region.[174] Embryology explains this distribution. Fusion of the primitive neural tube begins in the cervical region and progresses toward each end.[1, 182] Areas of later closure have a higher incidence of dermal sinus.

Congenital dermal sinus tracts extend to the neuroectodermal segmental level corresponding to the epithelial ectodermal level (dermatome) of origin.[179] Therefore, a dermal sinus tract arising in the lumbosacral region extends inward to its embryologic level in the cord, i.e., the conus medullaris. The sinus tract ascends past many vertebral segments. In the cervical and upper thoracic region, the sinus usually travels obliquely downward to enter the spinal canal a segment or two below the external opening of the sinus.[174] Cranial sinus tracts pass inward in a caudal direction. In all cases the sinus enters the spinal canal through a neural arch defect or through an opening in the intraspinous ligament, with approximately equal frequency.[174]

Clinical Findings

Congenital dermal sinuses present in two ways.[174, 175, 177] First, the sinus itself can be detected. A small dimple or sinus opening can be seen although it may be passed over as nonsignificant. Tufts of hair may be present at the sinus opening. The sinus opening may also be associated with an area of pigmentation or a capillary hemangioma. If infection occurs, drainage or an inflammatory reaction may surround the sinus. Second, associated CNS symptoms may occur.[173–176, 179, 180, 182] These include infection of nervous structures secondary to the spread of microorganisms from the skin through the sinus, and symptoms of an associated mass, since up to 50 percent of dermal sinuses are associated with congenital cell rest tumors or cysts.[181, 182] Depending on the extent of the sinus tract into the CNS, a variety of infections may occur, including subdural abscess, meningitis, intramedullary abscess, and epidural abscess.[173–176, 178–180, 182, 183] Congenital tumors associated with dermal sinuses consist of epidermoids, dermoids, and teratoid tumors. The inner end of the sinus is often expanded to form a dermoid or an epidermoid cyst.

The sex distribution of congenital dermal sinuses is either equal or slightly in favor of a male preponderance. They may be familial. Haworth and Zachary noted that several of the relatives of their patients also had congenital dermal sinuses.[177]

Patients generally present in childhood.[173–180, 182, 183]

The most frequently seen congenital dermal sinus is the pilonidal sinus, which occurs in the sacrococcygeal region. It generally extends cephalad for a short distance and ends blindly.[174] Although it may become inflamed, since it is filled with squamous debris and hair, communication with the spinal canal is very rare. However, extension of infection may occur to create an epidural abscess.

One-half to two-thirds of sinuses above the sacrococcygeal region extend intraspinally.[174] Since many superficial congenital dermal sinuses are not reported, accurate assessment of the percentage that actually involve the CNS is difficult. However, Wright suggested that half or more of the congenital dermal sinuses enter the cranial cavity or the spinal canal.[174]

Often, lesions occurring in the lower half of the spine present with infectious complications. Meningitis may be bacterial in origin or may be aseptic from spontaneous leakage of keratinous material into the subarachnoid space. Lesions occurring over the upper half of the spine present with signs and symptoms typical of a cord tumor.[175] Of the 12 cases occurring in the thoracic region reported by Wright, 11 had sinuses that terminated in intradural tumors.[174] Of the 72 congenital dermal sinuses in the lumbosacral region, 31 terminated in intraspinal congenital tumors.[174]

Of the associated local congenital anomalies, spina bifida occulta is the most common, although it is not invariable, since the tract can pass either through the spina bifida or pierce the spinous ligaments.[174-176, 180] Hypoplastic or bifid spinous processes may be seen. In addition, congenital dermal sinuses have been associated with diastematomyelia.[174]

Imaging

Radiographically, plain film findings include evidence of spina bifida, widening of the interpedicular distance, thinning of one or more pairs of pedicles, or any other congenital abnormality of the vertebra.[179] Traditionally, myelography and postmyelography CT pinpoint the presence of an intraspinal mass. Instillation of contrast material into the sinus tract is contraindicated, since it may introduce infection.

On MRI, congenital dermal sinuses are generally best seen on T1 weighted images (Figs. 15-13, 15-14). They appear as a low-intensity band cleaving the high-intensity subcutaneous fat. If the entire sinus is visible, its connection to the epidermis can generally be determined. Detection of congenital dermal sinuses may be difficult, however, owing to their small size. If the sinus lies between two slices within an intersection gap, it may not be seen. In addition, the sinus may be visible only on multiple contiguous slices: e.g., on axial images taken at a different angle from the sinus. Finally, congenital dermal sinuses in the thoracic or cervical spine are particularly difficult to detect because of the paucity of subcutaneous fat in these regions. Attention must be paid to the underlying spinal structures to rule out associated complications such as tumors or abscesses; these are easily demonstrated by MRI.

Treatment

Treatment consists of excision of the congenital dermal sinus tract as soon as it is detected. Prophylactic surgery can prevent further complications of the disease such as infection. The entire tract must be removed, including any extension to the CNS.[179] If previous infection has occurred, the sinus tract may be found closely adherent to the nerve roots of the cauda. If dermoid or epidermoid cysts are present, the contents are thoroughly evacuated.[179]

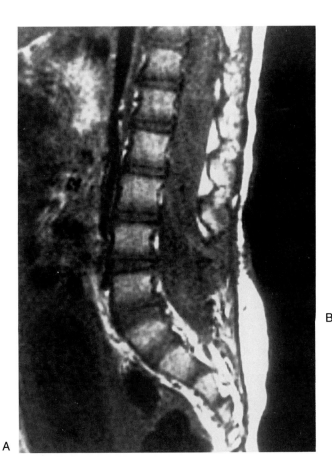

A

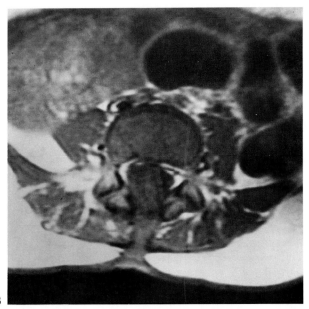

B

Figure 15–13. *Dermal sinus and epidermoid.* ***A, B,*** T1 weighted (600/20) sagittal and axial scans demonstrate a large dermal sinus extending from the skin into the spinal canal. In addition, a poorly defined area of minimally increased signal intensity, compared with normal CSF, is noted to extend superiorly from the dermal sinus. At surgery this proved to be a large epidermoid. Spinal dysraphism is also noted. (From Barkovich AJ. Congenital anomalies of the spine. In: Barkovich AJ, Naidich TP, eds. Contemporary neuroimaging. Pediatric neuroimaging. New York: Raven Press, Vol. 1. 1990.)

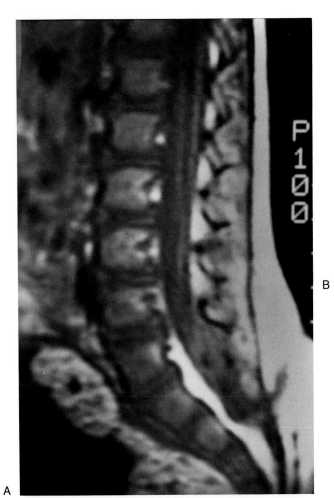

A

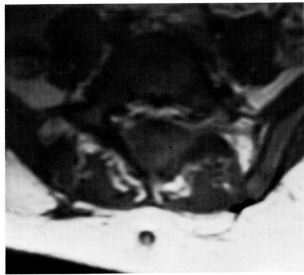

B

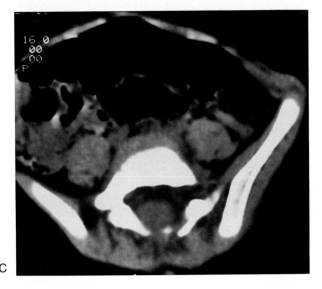

C

Figure 15–14. *Dermoid.* *A,* T1 weighted (500/20) sagittal MR image demonstrates a prominent dermal sinus extending into a heterogeneous intraspinal mass that is primarily somewhat hyperintense to CSF. *B,* T1 weighted (500/20) axial MR image depicts the mass and the associated spina bifida. Also noted is the dermal sinus tract in the subcutaneous fat. *C,* Axial CT scan confirms the presence of the mass, the spina bifida, and the dermal sinus. (Courtesy of Eugene Brown, M.D., and Sharon Byrd, M.D., Chicago)

EPIDERMOID AND DERMOID CYSTS

Epidermoids and dermoids are heterotopic formations composed of elements of the skin.[184-194] They are hamartomas rather than true neoplasms.[184] They form 10 percent of spinal cord tumors in patients under 15 years of age.[190] About 20 percent have an associated dermal sinus.[184]

These cysts are usually single and lie posteriorly in the canal.[184] Approximately 20 to 40 percent invaginate into the cord and are intramedullary, about to 60 to 67 percent are intradural extramedullary, and the rest are extradural.[184,187]

Embryogenesis and Pathology

Dermoids and epidermoids may arise from congenital rests,[184] from focal expansion of a dermal sinus,[194] or from implantation of viable epidermal elements during a spinal puncture or during surgery.[190-192] For example, inadvertent incorporation of epidermal tissue into the surgical closure of myelomeningoceles or other dysraphic states may result in epidermoids.

Epidermoids are cystic tumors lined by a membrane composed of superficial (epidermal) layers of the skin.[184,187-189] The viable cells form a thin capsule, while the interior consists of dead, cornified epithelial cells and debris.

Dermoids are uni- or multilocular cystic tumors.[184-189,193] They are lined by epithelium that contains all layers of the skin, epithelial and mesenchymal, and also the accessory cutaneous organs such as sebaceous and sweat glands and hair follicles.[184] As in epidermoids, the viable cells form a thin capsule. In dermoids, however, the contents include not only sloughed epithelial debris but also sebaceous matter and hair. Pathologic differentiation of epidermoids and dermoids may be difficult since only small areas of the cyst wall may possess those structures, such as hair follicles, that characterize the tumor as a dermoid rather than an epidermoid. On gross inspection, dermoids appear smooth and white, although slightly less bright and glistening than epidermoids.

Clinical Findings

Both types of tumors present with symptoms typical of mass lesions.[184,189] The degree of motor and sensory impairment may be very minor in comparison with the amount of anatomic damage.

Although epidermoids are congenital tumors and can produce symptoms in young children, they more often manifest later in life.[184,187,189] They grow extremely slowly, and the time from the onset of symptoms to diagnosis may be 10 years or more. There is a slight male preponderance.[187]

Dermoids usually cause symptoms before the age of 20. List suggested that their earlier age of presentation may be due to the contribution of additional elements, such as secretion from sebaceous glands, in addition to the accumulation of dead epithelial cells seen with epidermoids.[184] They occur equally in males and females.

When dermoids or epidermoids occur in the cauda equina, they often cause a severe radicular and local meningeal irritation.[184,185] Marked spasm of the back muscles may be seen. These symptoms are probably due to chemical arachnoiditis from leakage of the tumor contents.[184] Both epidermoids and dermoids have remissions of their clinical symptoms, often making the diagnosis of tumor more difficult.[184] Lumbar puncture may inadvertently puncture the tumor and verify the lesion.[186]

Spina bifida is seen in half of the patients who have typical histories, and suggests the diagnosis of a developmental type of tumor.[185-187] In addition, cutaneous abnormalities associated with spina bifida are seen.

Imaging

Epidermoids are mass lesions that may expand the spinal canal, although perhaps less so than dermoids and other tumors. Therefore, pedicle erosion and scalloping of the vertebral bodies may be seen. Epidermoids may be either extramedullary or intramedullary, but List noted that epidermoids in the thoracic region are especially prone to lie within the spinal cord.[184] Seventeen percent of spinal epidermoids lie in the upper thoracic spine, 26 percent in the lower thoracic spine, 22 percent in the lumbosacral region, and 35 percent in the cauda equina.[184]

Like epidermoids, dermoids act as a spinal canal mass. However, expansion of the canal, with erosion of the pedicles and scalloping of the vertebrae, is more common. This may be because epidermoids tend to be softer and more pliable than dermoids.

Dermoids are most common in the lumbosacral spine (60 percent). Twenty percent occur in the cauda equina, with only 5 percent cervical, 10 percent upper thoracic, and 5 percent lower thoracic in location.[184]

For both dermoids and epidermoids a total spinal block is seen in 80 to 90 percent of cases by the time of presentation.[185,187] Myelography shows the lesion to be smooth and ovoid or to have a frondlike appearance.[184]

On MRI, epidermoids of the spinal canal have a similar appearance to those in the CNS elsewhere (Fig. 15-13). Because they may be subtle, both short and long TR sequences are indicated. Spin-density images (long TR, short TE) provide the most information in some cases. Generally, they have a signal intensity equal to or slightly higher than that of CSF. The increase in signal may be due to their proteinaceous contents or to the absence of CSF pulsations within them. If the MR results are suboptimal, they may be difficult to detect, since they resemble CSF. In these cases, myelography may still be appropriate, although cine MR or diffusion imaging may be of use in the future.

On MRI, dermoids may vary from slightly to markedly hyperintense, the signal intensity being dependent on the relative proportions of epithelial debris and sebaceous material. In some patients the tumors may demonstrate signal intensities that approach those of subcutaneous adipose tissue (Fig. 15–14). The differential diagnosis in these cases includes intraspinal lipomas. Intrinsic calcifications may be detected as hypointense regions.

Treatment

Treatment consists of surgical removal.[184–189] Because epidermoids and dermoids are benign, encapsulated tumors, total removal results in cure. Caution is necessary during the surgical procedures so as not to spill the contents of the tumors, which could lead to a chemical arachnoiditis. If fragments are adherent to vital structures and must be left behind, recurrence is a possibility. Nevertheless, evacuation of the cystic contents alone may help in relieving symptoms.[185] Improvement may not be marked but surgery will prevent further deterioration.[185]

TERATOMA

Primary teratomas of the spinal canal, as opposed to sacrococcygeal teratomas, are very rare tumors: fewer than 50 have been reported.[188,195–220] Discussion of spinal teratomas is complicated by the variety of terms under which they have been reported and by confusion between the diagnosis of this entity and other entities, such as enterogenous cysts. Willis defined teratoma as "a true tumor or neoplasm composed of multiple tissues of kinds foreign to the part in which it arises."[214] A true tumor displays a degree of progressive uncoordinated growth, unlike enterogenous cysts, dermoids, and epidermoids, which contain heterotopic tissues but do not exhibit neoplastic growth. Common components of teratomas include skin, teeth, CNS tissue, respiratory and gastrointestinal mucosa, and glands.

Structural differences distinguish dermoids, epidermoids, and enterogenous cysts from teratomas. Teratomas contain components of tissues that originate from each of the three embryonic layers.[188,200,201,207,208] They differ from epidermoids and dermoids, which involve only tissues of ectodermal or ectodermal and mesodermal origin, respectively.[201] In addition, teratomas are usually differentiated from enterogenous cysts, which arise exclusively from the foregut or endoderm. Therefore, epidermoids, dermoids, and enterogenous cysts are simple developmental tumors, secondary to misplacement of normally developing somatic cells. In contrast, teratomas are true mal-

developmental lesions arising from the misplacement of some multipotential germinal cells early in embryonic development (Fig. 15–15).[197,202,203,207,208,215,216] They contain elements that do not have an embryologic relationship to the nervous system.

The origin of these lesions is still obscure, although a number of theories do exist.[210,214,217]

Spinal teratomas are rare tumors. Ingraham and Bailey found seven teratomas and teratoid tumors of the spine among 231 neoplasms of the CNS in patients under 16 years old.[203]

Spinal teratomas can occur at any age but are probably more common in childhood than in adulthood,[200,204] although some authors suggest a peak in early adulthood.[210]

Teratomas may occur anywhere along the spinal axis, although they are most common in the cervical spine or lower thoracic and upper lumbar spine.[204,212] They usually occur on the dorsal surface of the cord.[211,212,215,216] They may be associated with abnormalities of the vertebral bodies, such as spina bifida and block vertebrae,[200,202–204,207,210,212] spina bifida occulta, syrinxes,[200,209] scoliosis,[199] diastematomyelia,[154,205,210] or lipomyelomeningoceles.[91]

Teratomas are generally intradural extramedullary but may occur at other sites.[200,205,208,219] Fifty percent

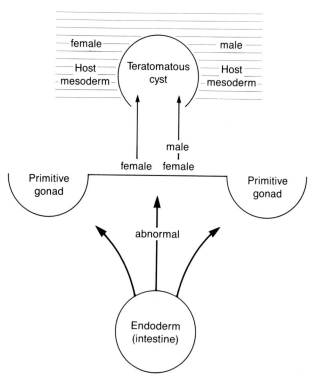

Figure 15–15. The failure of germ cells to complete their normal migrations from the endoderm to the primitive gonads is represented in this diagram. The germ cells come to lie in a midline dorsal position and can subsequently produce a teratoma. (From Rewcastle MB, Francoeur J. Teratomatous cysts of the spinal cord. Arch Neurol 1964; 11:91–99. © 1964, American Medical Association.)

are connected by pedicles to the cord or are adherent to the cord.[207]

Pathologically, teratomas usually contain cystic areas. The cysts may be grossly white, yellow, or chocolate.[203]

Mesodermal derivatives are often associated with a cyst and include muscle, bone, cartilage, and fat.[200, 215, 216] Also, ectodermal derivatives such as neurologic tissue may be seen.

Clinical Findings

Symptoms and signs include localized back pain and posterior cord or nerve root compression.[195, 207, 215] The symptoms may be intermittent and reversible or progressive.[200, 215] Exacerbations may be caused by increasing secretory activity of the tumor's glandular elements.[195] Recurrent chemical meningitis has also been described.[204]

Imaging

Radiologically, the most common findings on plain films are thinning of the laminae and pedicles.[207, 210, 215] Associated spina bifida or other vertebral anomalies may also be seen. Myelography generally shows a significant degree of cord compression, often associated with a high degree of block.

To date, there has been only one case report of the MR appearance of intraspinal teratomas. Smoker and colleagues described a case in which a cystic lesion appeared of intensity slightly higher than that of CSF (Fig. 15–16). Presumably, however, teratomas may have a variety of signals, depending on whether any hemorrhagic, lipid, calcified, or ossified components are present.

Treatment

The treatment for teratomas is surgical. These tumors may be very adherent to the cord and surrounding structures[200, 210] or may be easy to remove.[212] Even if they are intramedullary, total removal can be accomplished in some cases.[154] The tumors are usually benign,[203] and removal often offers long-term relief.[201, 203, 208] However, they are occasionally malignant.[85, 200, 205]

HAMARTOMA

A dorsal midline skin-covered mass is most commonly a sacrococcygeal teratoma or an occult spinal dysraphic lesion. Rarely, it is a hamartomatous mass. The hamartoma appears to be a distinct clinico-pathologic entity unrelated to the lipomas of occult spinal dysraphism that may have associated hamartomatous tissues.[88, 221]

Clinical Findings

Hamartomas usually present in the newborn period as a thoracic or a lumbar skin-covered mass. The location easily differentiates them from sacrococcygeal teratomas, which are usually at the level of the intergluteal cleft or below. There is no sex predilection.[221] At this young age patients exhibit no neurologic symptoms. Visibly the lesion most closely resembles a meningocele or lipomyelomeningocele; however, upon examination, most of the lesions, instead of being soft and fluctuant, have a hard component corresponding to the intrinsic bone and cartilage.

Pathologic Anatomy

Pathologically, hamartomas are composed of well-differentiated mesodermal elements, namely, fat, muscle, cartilage, and bone. Neural elements and blood vessels may also be seen. Unlike teratomas, hamartomas have absolutely no neoplastic potential. Reported associated abnormalities include laminar defects, fibrous tracts penetrating the dura, and articulations between ectopic bone and the laminae.[221]

Imaging

Because hamartomas consist of normal mesodermal elements in an abnormal mixture and location, the MR signal characteristics are equivalent to those of normal tissues. For example, if a significant bony component is present, it is hypointense relative to soft tissues on both T1 and T2 weighted images. The fatty and soft tissue components behave similarly to the normal surrounding tissues. Laminal defects or widening of the spinal canal may also be seen with hamartomas.

Treatment

Surgical removal of a hamartoma is a relatively simple procedure, since the lesion has no spinal cord attachment.[221] Treatment should be performed before the development of neurologic symptoms.

SYNDROME OF CAUDAL REGRESSION

The syndrome of caudal regression, also known as caudal dysplasia, consists of a congenital malformation characterized by a spectrum of anomalies involving the lumbar, sacral, and coccygeal vertebrae and the corresponding segments of the spinal cord.[222–241] Varying

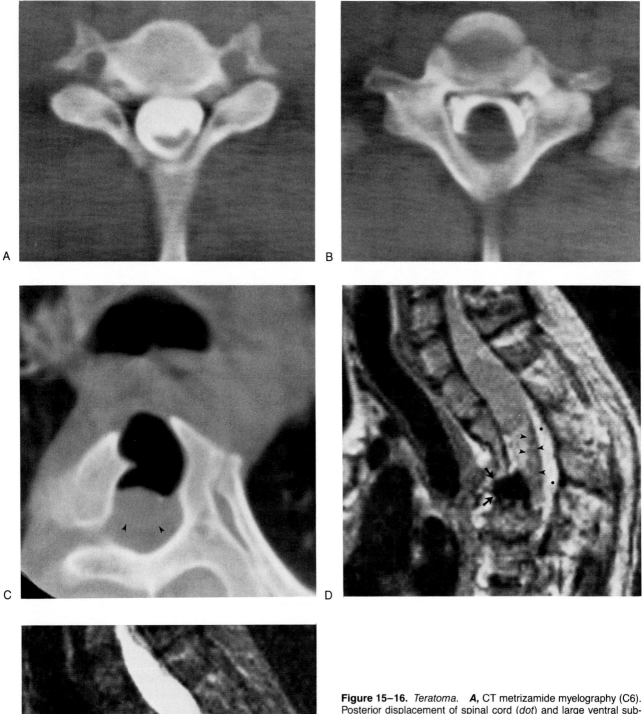

Figure 15–16. *Teratoma.* ***A,*** CT metrizamide myelography (C6). Posterior displacement of spinal cord (*dot*) and large ventral subarachnoid space. ***B,*** CT metrizamide myelography (C7–T1 disc space). The posterior aspect of the subarachnoid space is obliterated by an intradural lesion. ***C,*** CT metrizamide myelography (midbody of T5). Air instilled at myelography is identified in the anterior subarachnoid space filling a cleft in the T5 vertebral body. There is a suggestion of the cord outline (*arrowheads*). ***D, E,*** T1 and T2 weighted sagittal MR images more clearly show the craniocaudad extent of the tumor extending from C7–T1 to T5–T6. Most of the lesion is cystic, but a smaller solid component is located at T4 (*arrowheads*). The spinal cord is displaced posteriorly (*dots*). Air fills a cleft of the T5 vertebral body (*arrows*). (From Smoker W. Intradural spinal teratoma. AJNR 1986; 7:905–909. © American Society of Neuroradiology.)

combinations of anomalies and differing degrees of developmental failure may occur. Defects of the spine range from asymptomatic absence of the coccyx to aplasia of the sacrum and coccyx to agenesis of sacral, lumbar, and occasionally thoracic vertebrae. The more severe bony malformations are almost invariably associated with disabling neurologic and muscular deficits.[223–245] In addition, severe visceral anomalies of the genitourinary tract, gastrointestinal system, and respiratory system may form part of this syndrome.[225,227,232–234,237–239,246–248]

The first case of sacral aplasia was reported by Hohl in 1852.[231] Sporadic reports appeared until comprehensive reviews were presented in the 1950s.[227–230,233,241,244]

Etiology

The syndrome appears sporadically. Genetic factors are probably relatively unimportant.[227,236,249–252]

The role of extrinsic factors is clearer. Maternal diabetes mellitus is associated with the syndrome. Sacral agenesis is estimated to occur in 1 percent of infants of diabetic mothers.[238] Of infants with caudal regression, 14 to 19 percent have diabetic mothers.[224,253,254] Pang and Hoffman suggested a role for paternal diabetes.[235] Possible teratogenic effects of insulin on the embryo have been suggested.[227,255,256] Other teratogens have also been suspected.[224,240,254] Most likely, the cause of caudal agenesis is multifactorial, with extrinsic factors supplying an outside teratogenic influence on a genetically susceptible system.[235,250]

Embryogenesis

The inciting event or events must be present early in fetal life,[225,232,235,237,246,249,252] possibly before the fourth week of embryonic life.[249,252,256,257]

Pathology

Price and associates studied the neuropathology of a 10-day-old infant with caudal regression syndrome.[258] They found extreme hypoplasia and dysplasia of the cord in the region normally occupied by the lumbosacral enlargement. The cord ended abruptly at L2 without a suggestion of a tapered conus. Extreme atrophy of the related spinal nerves and roots was seen. Defective innervation of the distal lower extremity musculature was present. Other authors also reported atrophy of the lumbosacral roots.[242,254] The level of dysplasia is generally, but not necessarily, related to the level of the vertebral anomaly.[242,244]

Clinical Findings

The syndrome of caudal regression has been estimated to occur in one in 7,500 births, if all forms are included.[259] The fully developed syndrome, however, is not often seen and occurs only in one in 20,000 to 110,000 births.[237,242,259]

Clinically, the anatomic abnormalities cover a wide spectrum of malformations. In the syndrome's most mild form, solitary coccygeal absence is seen;[260] these cases are asymptomatic.[245] Progressing craniad, multiple varieties of sacral involvement including hemisacrum may occur. Several classification systems have been proposed, differing primarily in how they deal with the sacrum.[236,260,261] There may be partial or total agenesis of one side or both sides of the sacrum.

Varying degrees of lumbar and lower thoracic agenesis may occur. Mongeau and Leclaire and Barkovich and Raghaven report agenesis below T9, but survival of patients with regression at this level is extremely rare.[234,262] However, agenesis from T11 or T12 down is not rare.

The clinical appearance of the patient is primarily dependent on the degree of involvement of the spine and of associated neurologic changes. Patients with absence of the coccyx or of the very distalmost portions of the sacrum may appear normal.[240] Patients with hemisacral abnormalities often have secondary elevation of the ilium and congenital defect of the hip.[240] When subtotal agenesis occurs, S1 is often preserved. In these patients, the iliac bones articulate normally with the sacrum, and stance and gait are preserved.[229] In total sacral agenesis, the pelvis articulates with one of the lumbar vertebrae so that weightbearing is fairly normal. However, the iliac bones often form the bony pelvic ring by articulating with each other. These patients are often unable to stand or walk since the iliac bones assume a more vertical configuration, resulting in dislocation of the hips.[229] In severe cases the hips are flexed, abducted, externally rotated, and fixed, resulting in a Buddha-like or froglike appearance.[236,237] Flexion contractures of the knees and hips are common, resulting in arthrogrypotic deformities.[223]

Atrophy of the muscles supplied by nerves of the affected segments occurs.[229] The involved muscles generally correspond to the levels of the bony abnormalities.[232,236] Thus, the muscles most often affected are those of the perineum (S2–S5) and legs and buttocks (L5–S1).

Since the thigh muscles are normal, there is a characteristic cone shape to the lower limbs. Atrophy of the muscles of the buttocks contributes to a characteristic flattening of the buttocks and a short intergluteal cleft. Prominent popliteal webbing is seen in severe cases.[224] In the most extreme cases, fusion of the lower extremities occurs, termed "sirenomelia," or "mermaid."[226,263] The limbs are rotated and fused along their *outer* borders, resulting in a leg that flexes anteriorly rather than posteriorly. The single limb often articulates with a single acetabulum. Bones range from the normal number to none at all.[230]

Neurologic abnormalities seen in the caudal regression syndrome almost always include bladder incontinence.[237] Bowel incontinence is less often seen. Sensory changes occur less frequently than motor and are invariably less severe.[223,238]

Associated bony anomalies are common and include scoliosis, clubfoot, kyphosis, hemivertebrae, congenital bars, hypoplastic vertebrae, and spina bifida.[225,229,235,236]

Other neural anomalies are often associated with the syndrome of caudal regression. Myelomeningocele and spina bifida are common[244] and tethered cords have been seen.[245] In most of these cases a thick and tight filum terminale is present. However, tethering may also occur when a lipoma attached to the surrounding dura penetrates the conus.[246,264] Dermoids rarely coexist with sacral agenesis.[235] Diastematomyelia has been reported.[241]

Imaging

Radiographically, the diagnosis is easily made by plain films.[265] The level of vertebral column termination is generally readily identified. Plain films and CT can also identify the associated bony abnormalities, such as spina bifida or spinal canal stenosis.

MRI provides additional information.[262] The level of vertebral column termination is easily determined on MRI (Figs. 15–17, 15–18). Associated hypoplasia of the terminal first or second vertebrae is easily seen. MRI is particularly accurate in demonstrating the cord terminus, which generally occurs above the last intact vertebral body,[242,262] and in determining its level and shape (Fig. 15–18). In patients with the syndrome of caudal regression, the distal end of the spinal cord often appears blunted and angulated.[262,265] The dorsal aspect of the cord extends further distally than the ventral portion. In addition, the distal end often appears bulbous.

Patients with the syndrome of caudal regression often have central spinal stenosis. Associated spinal canal stenosis can be accurately determined on MRI. These patients also often have abnormalities of the thecal sac. In some patients, high termination of the subarachnoid space is seen; in others, there is a widened subarachnoid space.[242,243,245]

MRI accurately identifies associated lesions. For example, associated tumors, such as lipomas, can be precisely delineated. Because these lesions often tether the cord, the association of the tumor with the cord is important. Abnormalities of the filum can also be identified, such as thickened filum.

The imaging evaluation of these patients may be important. Pang and Hoffman separated the neurologic deficits associated with the syndrome of caudal regression into two categories: those that are static and those that are progressive.[235] Of course, the difficulty

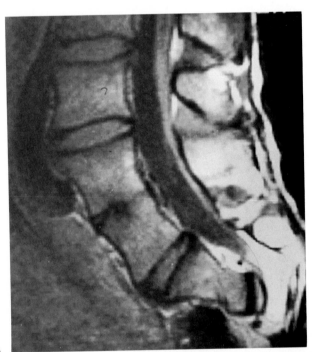

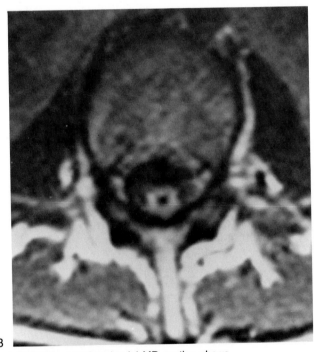

A   B

Figure 15–17. *Syndrome of caudal regression.* **A, B,** T1 weighted (500/20) sagittal and axial MR section shows agenesis of the distal sacrum. Tethering of the cord also appears to be present. Note the associated syrinx, seen in the region of the conus and verified on the axial scan. (From Barkovich AJ. MR of the syndrome of caudal regression. AJNR, 1989; 10:1223–1231. © American Society of Neuroradiology.)

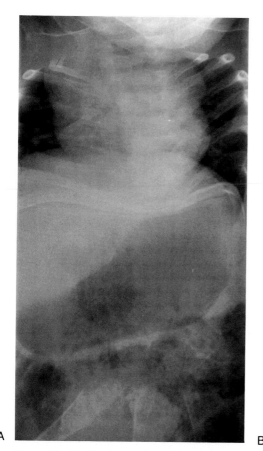

A

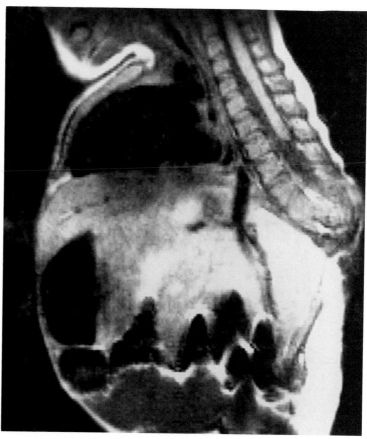

B

Figure 15–18. *Syndrome of caudal regression.* ***A,*** Plain film demonstrates agenesis of the spine distal to T9. ***B,*** T1 weighted (600/20) sagittal MR scan confirms the termination of the spine at T9. In addition, termination of the spinal canal and of the cord at the abnormally high level are seen. Note the blunted appearance of the distal cord, typical of this syndrome. (From Barkovich AJ. MR of the syndrome of caudal regression. AJNR, 1989; 10:1223–1231. © American Society of Neuroradiology.)

associated with this condition is largely due to the existing neurologic deficits. However, in some patients, specific neuropathologic lesions can be identified that are amenable to operative therapy. For example, Brooks reported a patient with a thickened and tight filum associated with adhesive arachnoidal bands who benefited from surgical release of filum and lysis of the adhesions.[265] Therefore, careful baseline neurologic evaluation is suggested, along with consistent follow-up using available imaging modalities. Treatment of dural sac stenosis, tethered cord, and intrathecal or extrathecal masses can offer significant improvement in the neurologic condition of these patients.

SPLIT NOTOCHORD SYNDROME

In 1960 Bentley and Smith suggested a common basis for a wide spectrum of anomalies believed to result from an abnormal splitting or deviation of the notochord with persistent connection between the gut and the dorsal skin.[137] They grouped together under the term "split notochord syndrome" many individual malformations that previously had separate names. This syndrome includes lesions that have previously been called anterior and combined spina bifida, accessory or persistent neurenteric canal, dorsal intestinal fistula, enteric duplication, neurenteric cysts, ependymal cysts of the spinal canal, gastrocytoma, and various other anomalies.[137, 218, 266–287] Some authors also suggested a common basis for diastematomyelia-diplomyelia and teratomas.

Embryogenesis

If the notochord develops with a partial separation, a gap may occur through which the ventral yolk sac or gut anlage may herniate and adhere to the dorsal ectoderm or skin anlage. Alternatively, a previous adhesion between the ectoderm and endoderm may prevent the notochord from growing normally in the midline (Fig. 15–19).[285] It then splits to surround the adhesion or deviates around the adhesion to one side.[267, 278]

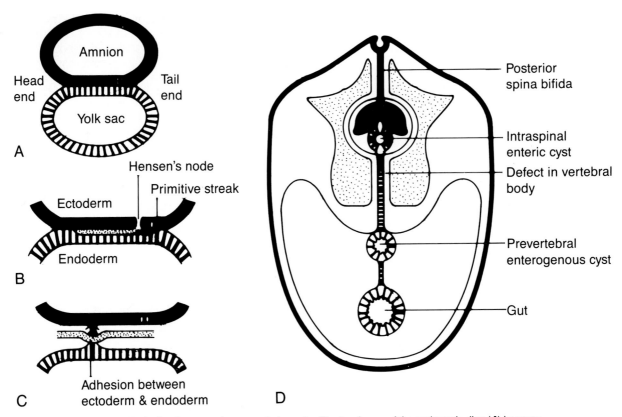

Figure 15–19. *The embryologic development of a neurenteric cyst.*   The two layers of the embryonic disc (*A*) become separated by mesoderm except in the midline, because of the notochordal process (*B*). If a midline adhesion develops between ectoderm and endoderm, the notochordal process may be deflected (*C*), resulting in vertebral defects associated with enteric cysts (*D*). (Modified from Bale PM. A congenital intraspinal gastroenterogenous cyst in diastematomyelia. J Neurol Neurosurg Psychiat 1973; 36:1011–1017.)

Pathologic Anatomy

In the most severe form of split notochord syndrome (dorsal enteric fistula), the entire tract between the gut and the skin surface remains open. The other less severe anomalies are thought to arise when portions of the dorsal enteric fistula become obliterated (Figs. 15–20, 15–21).[137] Depending on which remnant persists, isolated diverticula, duplications, cysts, or sinuses may be found. Because of differential growth rates, the defects may become long and connect distant sites (e.g., diverticula originating within the abdomen may pass through in the diaphragm to a high thoracic vertebral attachment).[137, 269] Persisting remnants of the yolk sac or gut anlage may differentiate into tissues characteristic of any part of the gut (including gastric or pancreatic mucosa) or of its embryologic derivatives, such as the lung.

In posterior enteric diverticulum, only the anterior portion of the tract persists, forming a blind outpouching in communication with the intestines.[137] A fibrous adhesion to the spine documents the previous existence of the tract.[269]

If only the central portion of the embryonic fistula persists, dorsal enteric cysts are formed.[137] These are the most common manifestation of the split notochord syndrome and form 2 to 9 percent of all primary mediastinal tumors or cysts.[286] The remnants of the fistula form fibrous bands anteriorly and posteriorly. These enteric lined cysts may be prevertebral, postvertebral, or intraspinal.

The extent of spinal and CNS malformations depends on the persistence of the embryonic fistula. If the fistula persists, the spine typically demonstrates wide anterior and posterior spina bifida that can cause meningoceles.[283] The spine usually rejoins below the level of the communication to form a ring defect. The left and right hemiarches often fuse longitudinally to form laminar ridges. Deformed continued growth of the hemivertebrae results in distortion of the spine. The vertebrae are still separated by disc spaces, indicating previous clefting of the notochord.[6] Most of the vertebral anomalies involve the cervical and upper thoracic vertebrae.[269, 286] Scoliosis may develop.[281]

Cysts may also occur within the spinal canal.[267, 271, 275–281] These intraspinal enteric cysts pres-

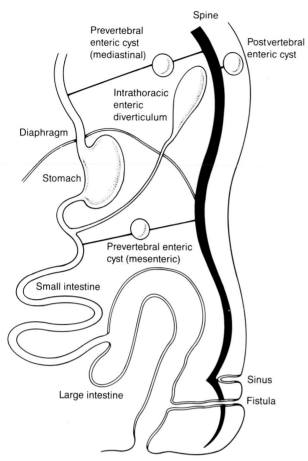

Figure 15–20. Split notochord syndrome. Diagrammatic representation of developmental posterior enteric remnants. Varying segments of the prototypical dorsal enteric fistulas leave diverse posterior enteric remnants. Each of these types may happen at any segmental level. (From Bentley JFR, Smith JR. Developmental posterior enteric remnants and spinal malformations. Arch Dis Child 1960; 35:76–86.)

ent either in young adults or in the pediatric population.[267] Males are affected more often than females. Intraspinal enteric cysts typically are located in the lower cervical–upper thoracic region and initially cause sharp local and radicular pain.[267] As they grow, signs of cord compression become more prominent. The cysts are generally smooth and unilocular. The cyst contents and walls may vary; in some cases their contents strongly resemble CSF. In others the cysts are filled with gelatinous or xanthochromic debris. Similarly, the cyst walls may be thin and transparent or thick, similar to normal gut.[267] They are usually ventral or ventral-lateral to the cord.[267,276]

Clinical Findings

A dorsal enteric fistula passes posteriorly from the gut through the mesentery or mediastinum, traversing the vertebral bodies, spinal canal, and posterior vertebral elements to open on the dorsal skin surface. In extreme cases the bowel herniates through the communication into a skin- or membrane-covered dorsal sac to create a dorsal bowel hernia.[270] These patients are usually newborns on presentation. The dorsal skin opening passes meconium or feces.[268,285]

Posterior enteric diverticuli and enteric cysts usually present in infancy or early childhood with abdominal pain, abdominal or intrathoracic masses, or gastrointestinal hemorrhage.[269,274] Large masses in the chest cavity may produce dyspnea, cyanosis, and other respiratory symptoms.[273] In cases that communicate with the subarachnoid space, meningitis may result.[277]

Intraspinal cysts cause mass effect on the spinal cord. Other symptoms include infections due to the connections with the gut. Meningitis may occur. In

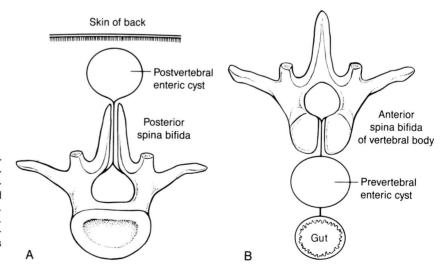

Figure 15–21. *Diagrammatic representation of the dorsal enteric cyst.* **A,** Enteric cyst dorsal and **B,** ventral to the vertebral column. Both may be associated with splitting of the vertebral elements. (Adapted from Bentley JFR, Smith JR. Developmental posterior enteric remnants and spinal malformations. Arch Dis Child 1960; 35:76–86.)

addition, intramedullary abscesses have been recorded.[279]

Imaging

Plain films may show widening of the spinal canal with thinning of the pedicles. Vertebral anomalies are often seen.[267, 271, 275–281] If intrathoracic duplications are present, plain films of the chest may reveal soft tissue masses, often with contained air or fluid.[269]

MR findings vary, depending on the entity involved. The cysts have an extremely varied appearance with well-defined margins, strong signal on T2 weighted images, and variable signal on T1 weighted images, depending on the presence of mucus or blood in the cyst fluid. Spinal and CNS anomalies are well documented on MRI (Fig. 15–22).[288] T1 weighted sagittal

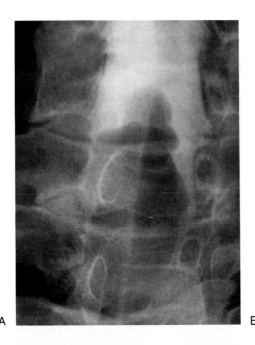

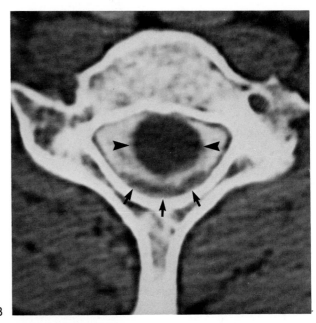

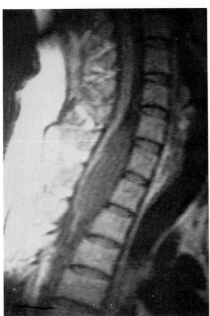

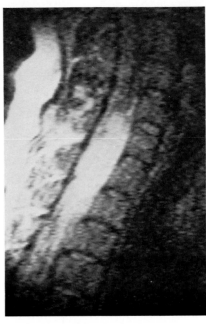

Figure 15–22. *Split notochord syndrome.* **A,** Cervical metrizamide myelogram, anteroposterior view. Partial obstruction to caudal flow of contrast is demonstrated at C6. **B,** Axial CT myelographic image of the cervicothoracic spine. Metrizamide outlines a relatively low-attenuation lesion (*arrowheads*) ventral to the spinal cord. The cord is flattened posteriorly (*arrows*). **C, D,** MR images of the cervicothoracic spine employing a flat surface coil for sagittal imaging. T1 weighted (350/30) sagittal image (**C**) shows that the ventral mass is relatively hypointense relative to the compressed spinal cord, but hyperintense relative to CSF. Note the erosive nature of the mass evidenced by widening of the spinal canal and posterior scalloping of the vertebral bodies. The T2 weighted (2120/120) sagittal image (**D**) shows that the mass is relatively hyperintense relative to the spinal cord and CSF, a reversal of the mass-cord relationship seen with the T1 weighted sequence. (From Geremia GK. MR imaging characteristics of a neurenteric cyst. AJNR 1988; 9:978–980. © American Society of Neuroradiology.)

and axial images are generally sufficient. As with other cystic lesions, however, intraspinal enteric cysts may sometimes be subtle and better delineated on spin-density sequences. Ultimately, cine MR or diffusion imaging may prove more effective for lesions of near-CSF intensity, such as epidermoids and some teratomas, in addition to intraspinal enteric cysts. MRI may not be as effective as CT in documenting open connections with bowel, although the use of oral contrast agents may improve this capability in the future.

Although it may not show bony detail to the same extent as CT, MRI can also demonstrate associated bony anomalies. Anterior or posterior spinal bifida is generally easily identified. Fibrous remnants of fistulas may occasionally be seen as low-intensity bands traversing higher-intensity fat.

Treatment

Surgical extirpation of enterogenous cysts generally results in permanent cure.[280, 284] If the cyst lies outside the spine but has an intraspinal extension, care must be taken to remove the intraspinal portion. Successful removal of cysts that are purely intraspinal has been reported.[289, 290] Similarly, for diverticula, the entire diverticulum is removed. Remaining portions are prone to acid secretion or infection.

REFERENCES

1. Moore KL. The developing human—clinically oriented embryology. Philadelphia: WB Saunders, 1988:50–59.
2. Brocklehurst G. Spina bifida for the clinician. Spastics International Medical Publications. London: Heinemann; Philadelphia: JB Lippincott, 1976:562–572.
3. Warkany J. Congenital malformations. Notes and comments. Chicago: Year Book, 1971:189–352.
4. Pattern BM. Human embryology. New York: McGraw-Hill, 1968:51–77.
5. Lemire RJ, Loeser JD, Leech RW, Alvord EC Jr. Normal and abnormal development of the human nervous system. Hagerstown, MD: Harper & Row, 1975:71–83.
6. Naidich TP, McLone DG, Harwood-Nash DC. Spinal dysraphism. In: Newton TH, Potts DG, eds. Modern neuroradiology. Vol 1. Computed tomography of the spine and spinal cord. San Anselmo, CA: Clavadel Press, 1983:299–353.
7. McLone D. Embryonic deformation and caudal suppression. Concepts Pediatr Neurosurg 1987; 7:169–171.
8. Carter CO, Evans K. Spina bifida and anencephalus in greater London. J Med Genet 1973; 10:209–234.
9. Bamforth S, Baird P. Spina bifida and hydrocephalus: a population study over a 35-year period. Am J Hum Genet 1989; 44:225–232.
10. Jansen J. Spina bifida: epidemiological data from a pilot study. Acta Neurol Scand 1978; 57:193–197.
11. Elwood JM, Elwood JH. Epidemiology of anencephalus and spina bifida. Oxford: Oxford University Press, 1980.
12. Carter CO. Clues to the aetiology of neural tube malformations. Dev Med Child Neurol 1974; 16(Suppl 32):3–15.
13. Fraser F. Genetic counseling in some common paediatric diseases. Am J Hum Genet 1974; 26:636–659.
14. Lorber J, Levick K. Spina bifida cystica. Incidence of spina bifida occulta in parents and in controls. Arch Dis Child 1967; 42:171–173.
15. Carsin A, Journel H, Roussey M, Le Marec B. Fréquence du spina-bifida occulta lombo-sacré chez les parents d'enfants porteurs d'un spina-bifida. J Genet Hum 1986; 34:285–292.
16. Jensson O, Arnason A, Gunnarsdottir H, et al. A family showing apparent X-linked inheritance of both anencephaly and spina bifida. J Med Genet 1988; 25:227–229.
17. Doran PA, Guthkelch AN. Studies in spina bifida cystica. I. General survey and reassessment of the problem. J Neurol Neurosurg Psychiatry 1961; 24:331–345.
18. Lammer E, Sever L, Oakley G Jr. Teratogen update: valproic acid. Teratology 1987; 35:465–473.
19. Allanson J. Spina bifida: prenatal diagnosis and genetic counseling. BNI Q 1988; 4:5–8.
20. Gray D, Crane J, Rudloff M. Prenatal diagnosis of neural tube defects: origin of midtrimester vertebral ossification centers as determined by sonographic water-bath studies. J Ultrasound Med 1988; 7:421–427.
21. Nicolaides KH, Gabbe SG, Campbell S, Guidetti R. Ultrasound screening for spina bifida: cranial and cerebellar signs. Lancet 1986; 2:72–74.
22. Von Recklinghausen F. Untersuchungen über die Spina bifida. Virchows Arch 1886; 105:243–373.
23. Osaka K, Matsumoto S, Tanimura T. Myeloschisis in early human embryos. Childs Brain 1978; 4:347–359.
24. Osaka K, Tanimura T, Hirauama A, Matsumoto S. Myelomeningocele before birth. J Neurosurg 1978; 49:711–724.
25. Lendon RG. The embryogenesis of trypan-blue induced spina bifida aperta and short tail in the rat. Dev Med Child Neurol 1975; 17(Suppl. 35):3–10.
26. Lemire RJ, Shepard TH, Alvord EC Jr. Caudal myeloschisis (lumbo-sacral spina bifida cystica) in a five millimeter (horizon XIV) human embryo. Anat Rec 1965; 152:9–16.
27. Morgani JB. The seats and causes of diseases investigated by anatomy, translated by Benjamin Alexander. Vol 3. London: A Millar and T Cadell, 1769.
28. Padget DH. Neuroschisis and human embryonic maldevelopment: new evidence on anencephaly, spina bifida and diverse mammalian defects. J Neuropathol Exp Neurol 1970; 29:192–216.
29. Gardner WJ. Myelomeningocele, the result of rupture of the embryonic neural tube. Cleve Clin Q 1960; 27:88–100.
30. Epstein F, Marlin A, Hochwald G, Ransohoff J. Myelomeningocele: a progressive intra-uterine disease. Dev Med Child Neurol 1976; 18(Suppl 37):12–15.
31. Patten BM. Overgrowth of the neural tube in young human embryos. Anat Rec 1952; 113:381–393.
32. Patten BM. Embryological stages in establishing of myeloschisis with spina bifida. Am J Anat 1953; 93:365–395.
33. Oi S, Saya H, Matsumoto S. A hypothesis for myeloschisis: overgrowth and reopening: an experimental study. J Neurosurg 1988; 68:947–954.
34. Gilbert JN, Jones KL, Rorke LB, et al. Central nervous system anomalies associated with meningomyelocele, hydrocephalus, and the Arnold-Chiari malformation: reappraisal of theories regarding the pathogenesis of posterior neural tube closure defects. Neurosurgery 1986; 18:559–564.
35. Zimmerman R, Breckbill D, Dennis M, Davis D. Cranial CT findings in patients with meningomyelocele. AJR 1979; 132:623–629.
36. Cameron AH. The Arnold-Chiari and other neuro-anatomical malformations associated with spina bifida. J Pathol Bacteriol 1957; 73:195–211.
37. Sherk H, Charney E, Pasquariello P, et al. Hydrocephalus, cervical cord lesions, and spinal deformity. Spine 1986; 11:340–342.
38. Raycroft JF, Curtis BH. Spinal curvature in myelomeningocele. Natural history and etiology. In: The American Academy of Orthopedic Surgeons Symposium on Myelomeningocele. St Louis: CV Mosby, 1972:186–201.
39. Shurtleff DB, Goiney R, Gordon LH, Livermore N. Myelodysplasia: the natural history of kyphosis and scoliosis. A preliminary report. Dev Med Child Neurol 1976; 18(Suppl 37):126–133.

40. Piggott H. The natural history of scoliosis in myelodysplasia. J Bone Joint Surg 1980; 62B:54–58.

41. Hall P, Lindseth R, Campbell R, et al. Scoliosis and hydrocephalus in myelocele patients: the effects of ventricular shunting. J Neurosurg 1979; 50:174–178.

42. Samuelsson L, Eklof O. Scoliosis in myelomeningocele. Acta Orthop Scand 1988; 59:122–127.

43. Samuelsson L, Eklof O. Conventional spinal radiography as a supplement to the neurologic assessment in myelomeningocele. Acta Radiol 1987; 28:615–619.

44. Hall PV, Campbell RL, Kalsbeck JE. Meningomyelocele and progressive hydromyelia: progressive paresis in myelodysplasia. J Neurosurg 1975; 43:457–463.

45. Barson AJ. Radiological studies of spina bifida cystica: the phenomenon of congenital lumbar kyphosis. Br J Radiol 1965; 38:294–300.

46. Hoppenfeld S. Congenital kyphosis in myelomeningocele. J Bone Joint Surg 1967; 49B:276–280.

47. Hall WA, Albright AL, Brunberg JA. Diagnosis of tethered cords by magnetic resonance imaging. Surg Neurol 1988; 30:60–64.

48. Tamaki N, Shirataki K, Kojima N, et al. Tethered cord syndrome of delayed onset following repair of myelomeningocele. J Neurosurg 1988; 69:393–398.

49. Heinz ER, Rosenbaum AE, Scarff TB, et al. Tethered spinal cord following meningomyelocele repair. Radiology 1979; 131:153–160.

50. Charney EB, Weller SC, Sutton LN, et al. Management of the newborn with myelomeningocele. Time for a decision-making process. Pediatrics 1985; 75:58–64.

51. McLaurin R, Warkany J. Management of spina bifida and associated anomalies. Comprehensive Therapy 1986; 2:60–65.

52. Knox EG. Spina bifida in Birmingham. Dev Med Child Neurol 1967; (Suppl 13):14–22.

53. McLone D, Dias L, Kaplan W, Sommers M. Concepts in the management of spina bifida. Concepts Pediatr Neurosurg 1985; 5:97–106.

54. Dubowitz V, Lorber J, Zachary RB. Lipoma of the cauda equina. Arch Dis Child 1965; 40:207–213.

55. Rickham PP, Mawdsley T. The effect of early operation on the survival of spina bifida cystica. Dev Med Child Neurol 1966; 10(Suppl 11):20–26.

56. Venes JL, Black KL, Latack JT. Preoperative evaluation and surgical management of the Arnold-Chiari II malformation. J Neurosurg 1986; 64:363–370.

57. Hoffman HJ, Henrik EB, Humphreys RP. Manifestations and management of Arnold-Chiari malformation in patients with myelomeningocele. Childs Brain 1975; 1:255–259.

58. Mawdsley T, Rickham PP. Further follow-up study of early operation for open myelomeningocele. Dev Med Child Neurol 1969; 11(Suppl 20):8–12.

59. McLone DG, Naidich TP. Myelomeningocele: outcome and late complications. In: McLaurin RL, Schut L, Venes JL, Epstein F, eds. Pediatric neurosurgery: surgery of the developing nervous system. 2nd ed. Philadelphia: WB Saunders, 1989:53–70.

60. Nelson M, Bracchi M, Naidich T, McLone D. The natural history of repaired myelomeningocele. Radiographics 1988;8:695–706.

61. Fidas A, MacDonald HL, Elton RA, et al. Prevalence and patterns of spina bifida occulta in 2707 normal adults. Clin Radiol 1987; 38:537–542.

62. Boone D, Parsons D, Lachmann SM, Sherwood T. Spina bifida occulta: lesion or anomaly? Clin Radiol 1985; 36:159–161.

63. Southworth JD, Bersack SR. Anomalies of the lumbosacral vertebrae in 550 individuals without symptoms referable to the low back. Am J Roentgenol 1950; 64:624–634.

64. Friedman MM, Fischer FJ, VanDemark RE. Lumbosacral roentgenograms of 100 soldiers: a control study. Am J Roentgenol 1946; 55:292–298.

65. Lemire RJ, Graham CB, Beckwith JB. Skin-covered sacrococcygeal masses in infants and children. J Pediatr 1971; 79:948–954.

66. Villarejo FJ, Blazquez MG, Gutierrez-Diaz JA. Intraspinal lipomas in children. Childs Brain 1976; 2:361–370.

67. McLone DG, Mutluer S, Naidich TP. Lipomeningoceles of the conus medullaris. In: Concepts in pediatric neurosurgery. Vol 3. American Society for Pediatric Neurosurgeons. Basel: S Karger, 1982.

68. Rogers HM, Long DM, Chou SN, French LA. Lipomas of the spinal cord and cauda equina. J Neurosurg 1971; 34:349–354.

69. Swanson HS, Barnett JC Jr. Intradural lipomas in children. Pediatrics 1962; 29:911–926.

70. Schut L, Bruce DA, Sutton LN. The management of the child with a lipomyelomeningocele. In: Weiss MH, ed. Clinical neurosurgery. Vol 30. Baltimore: Williams & Wilkins, 1983:464–476.

71. Sostrin R, Thompson J, Rouche S, Hasso A. Occult spinal dysraphism in the geriatric patient. Radiology 1977; 125:165–169.

72. Balagura S. Late neurological dysfunction in adult lumbosacral lipoma with tethered cord. Neurosurgery 1984; 15:724–725.

73. Hoffman HJ, Taecholarn C, Hendrick BE, Humphreys RP. Management of lipomyelomeningoceles. J Neurosurg 1985; 62:1–8.

74. Pierre-Kahn A, Lacombe J, Pichon J, et al. Intraspinal lipomas with spina bifida. J Neurosurg 1986; 65:756–761.

75. Giuffe R. Intradural spinal lipomas: review of the literature (99 cases) and report of an additional case. Acta Neurochir 1966; 14:69–95.

76. Anderson FM. Occult spinal dysraphism: a series of 73 cases. Pediatrics 1975; 55:826–835.

77. Bassett RC. The neurologic deficit associated with lipomas of the cauda equina. Ann Surg 1950; 131:109–116.

78. Burrows FGO, Sutcliffe J. The split notochord syndrome. Br J Radiol 1968; 41:844–847.

79. Lassman LP, James CCM. Lumbosacral lipomas: critical survey of 26 cases submitted to laminectomy. J Neurol Neurosurg Psychiatry 1967; 30:174–181.

80. Lichtenstein BW. Spinal dysraphism: spina bifida and myelodysplasia. Arch Neurol Psychiatry 1940; 44:792–810.

81. Caram P, Scarcella G, Carton C. Intradural lipomas of the spinal cord with particular emphasis on the "intramedullary" lipomas. J Neurosurg 1952; 14:28–42.

82. James CCM, Lassman LP. Spinal dysraphism: an orthopaedic syndrome in children accompanying occult forms. Arch Dis Child 1960; 35:315–327.

83. Bruce DA, Schut L. Spinal lipomas in infancy and childhood. Childs Brain 1979; 5:192–203.

84. Anderson FM. Occult spinal dysraphism. Diagnosis and management. J Pediatr 1968; 73:163–177.

85. Gorey MT, Naidich TP, McLone DG. Case report. Double discontinuous lipomyelomeningocele: CT findings. J Comput Assist Tomogr 1989; 9:584–591.

86. Hoffman HJ, Taecholarn C, Hendrick EB, Humpheys RP. Lipomyelomeningoceles and their management. Concepts Pediatr Neurosurg 1985; 5:107–117.

87. Emery JL, Lendon RG. Lipomas of the cauda equina and other fatty tumours related to neurospinal dysraphism. Dev Med Child Neurol 1969; 11(Suppl 20):62–70.

88. Walsh JW, Markesbery WR. Histological features of congenital lipomas of the lower spinal canal. J Neurosurg 1980; 52:564–569.

89. Bouton JM, Martin CH, Rickham PP. Hamartoma and spina bifida. J Pediatr Surg 1966; 1:559–565.

90. Ammerman BJ, Henry JM, De Girolami U, Earle KM. Intradural lipomas of the spinal cord: clinicopathological correlation. J Neurosurg 1976; 44:331–336.

91. Ehni G, Love JG. Intraspinal lipomas: report of cases, review of the literature, and clinical and pathologic study. Arch Neurol Psychiatry 1945; 53:1–28.

92. Mickle JP, McLennan JE. Malignant teratoma arising within a lipomeningocele. J Neurosurg 1975; 43:761–763.

93. Love JG. Delayed malignant growth of a congenital teratoma with spina bifida. J Neurosurg 1968; 29:532–534.

94. Thorp RH. Carcinoma associated with myelodysplasia. J Neurosurg 1967; 27:446–448.

95. Naidich TP, McLone DG, Mutluer S. A new understanding of dorsal dysraphism with lipoma (lipomyeloschisis): radiologic evaluation and surgical correction. AJNR 1983; 4:103–116.

96. Swedberg M. Meningo- and myelomeningocele studied by gas myelography. Acta Radiol 1963; 1:796–803.

97. Barnes PD, Reynolds AF, Galloway DC, et al. Digital myelography of spinal dysraphism in infancy: preliminary results. AJNR 1984; 5:208–211.

98. Gryspeerdt GL. Myelographic assessment of occult forms of spinal dysraphism. Acta Radiol [Diagn] 1963; 1:702–717.

99. Naidich TP, McLone DG, Shkolnik A, Fernbach SK. Sonographic evaluation of caudal spine anomalies in children. AJNR 1983; 4:661–664.

100. James HE, Scheible W, Kerber C, et al. Comparison of high resolution real time ultrasonography and high resolution computed tomography in an infant with spinal dysraphism. Neurosurgery 1983; 3:301–305.

101. Wolpert SM, Scott RM, Carter BL. Computed tomography in spinal dysraphism. Surg Neurol 1977; 8:199–206.

102. Scatliff JH, Bidgood WD Jr, Killebrew K, Staab EV. Computed tomography and spinal dysraphism: clinical and phantom studies. Neuroradiology 1979; 17:71–75.

103. Scatliff JH, Kendall BE, Kingsley DPE, et al. Closed spinal dysraphism: analysis of clinical, radiological and surgical findings in 104 consecutive patients. AJNR 1989; 10:269–277.

104. Rappaport ZH, Tadmor R, Shaked I, Robinson S. Computer assisted myelography in spinal dysraphism. Neurochirugia 1982; 25:190–194.

105. Resjo IM, Harwood-Nash DC, Fitz CR, Chuang S. Computed tomographic metrizamide myelography in spinal dysraphism in infants and children. J Comput Assist Tomogr 1978; 2:549–558.

106. Sutterlin CE, Grogan DP, Ogden JA. Diagnosis of developmental pathology of the neuraxis by magnetic resonance imaging. J Pediatr Orthop 1987; 7:291–297.

107. Altman NR, Altman DH. MR imaging of spinal dysraphism. AJNR 1987; 8:533–538.

108. Roos RAC, Vielroye GJ, Voormoten JHC, Peters ACB. Magnetic resonance imaging in occult spinal dysraphism. Pediatr Radiol 1986; 16:412–416.

109. Barnes PD, Lester PD, Yamanashi WS, Prince JR. Magnetic resonance imaging in infants and children with spinal dysraphism. AJNR 1986; 7:465–472.

110. Doyon D, Sigal R, Poylecut G, et al. MRI of spinal cord congenital malformations. J Neuroradiol 1987; 14:185–201.

111. Cecchini A, Locatelli D, Bonfanti N, et al. Lipomyelomeningoceles: a neuroradiological approach. J Neuroradiol 1988; 15:49–61.

112. Wippold FJ, Citrin C, Barkovich AJ, Sherman JS. Evaluation of MR in spinal dysraphism with lipoma: comparison with metrizamide computer tomography. Pediatr Radiol 1987; 17:184–188.

113. Komiyama M, Hakuba A, Inoue Y, et al. Magnetic resonance imaging: lumbosacral lipoma. Surg Neurol 1987; 28:259–264.

114. Walker HS, Dietoich RB, Flannigan BD, et al. Magnetic resonance imaging of the pediatric spine. Radiographics 1987; 7:1129–1152.

115. Chapman P. Congenital intraspinal lipomas. Childs Brain 1982; 9:37–47.

116. Herren RJ, Edwards JE. Diplomyelia (duplication of the spinal cord). Arch Pathol 1940; 30:1203–1214.

117. Cohen J, Sledge CB. Diastematomyelia: an embryological interpretation with report of a case. Am J Dis Child 1960; 100:257–263.

118. Sheptak PE. Diastematomyelia-diplomyelia. In: Vinken PJ, Bryun GW, eds. Handbook of clinical neurology. Vol. 32. New York: North Holland, 1978:239–254.

119. Arrendondo F, Haughton VM, Hemmy DC, et al. The computed tomographic appearance of the spinal cord in diastematomyelia. Radiology 1980; 136:685–688.

120. Hori A, Fischer G, Dietrich-Schott B, Ikeda K. Dimyelia, diplomyelia, and diastematomyelia. Clin Neuropathol 1982; 1:23–30.

121. Ollivier CP. Traite de maladies de la moelle epiniere. 3rd ed. Vol I. Paris: Mequignon-Marvis, 1837.

122. Humphrey GM. The anatomy of spina bifida. J Anat Physiol 1885; 19:500.

123. Pickles W. Duplication of spinal cord (diplomyelia): account of clinical example with consideration of other reports. J Neurosurg 1949; 6:324–331.

124. Matson DD, Woods RP, Campbell JB, Ingraham FD. Diastematomyelia (congenital clefts of the spinal cord). Pediatrics 1950; 6:98–112.

125. Sheptak PE, Susen AF. Diastematomyelia. Am J Dis Child 1967; 113:210–213.

126. James JCC, Lassman LP. Diastematomyelia: a critical survey of 24 cases submitted to laminectomy. Arch Dis Child 1964; 39:125–130.

127. Winter RB, Haven JJ, Moe JH, Lagaard SM. Diastematomyelia and congenital spine deformities. J Bone Joint Surg 1974; 56A:27–39.

128. Neuhauser EBD, Wittenborg MH, Dehlinger K. Diastematomyelia: transfixation of the cord or cauda equina with congenital anomalies of the spine. Radiology 1950; 54:659–664.

129. Holman CB, Svien HJ, Bickel WH, et al. Diastematomyelia. Pediatrics 1955; 15:191–194.

130. Liliequist B. Diastematomyelia: report of a case examined by gas myelography. Acta Radiol [Diagn] 1965; 3:497–502.

131. Ritchie GW, Flanagan MN. Diastematomyelia. Can Med Assoc J 1969; 100:428–433.

132. Hilal SK, Marton D, Pollack E. Diastematomyelia in children. Radiographic study of cases. Radiology 1974; 112:609–621.

133. Scott G, Musgrave MA, Harwood-Nash DC, et al. Diastematomyelia in children: metrizamide and CT metrizamide myelography. AJR 1980; 135:1225–1232.

134. Tadmor R, Davis KR, Roberson GH, Chapman PH. The diagnosis of diastematomyelia by computed tomography. Surg Neurol 1977; 8:434–436.

135. Weinstein MA, Rothner AD, Duchesneau P, Dohn DF. Computed tomography in diastematomyelia. Radiology 1975; 118:609–611.

136. Bremer JL. Dorsal intestinal fistula; accessory neurenteric canal; diastematomyelia. Arch Pathol 1952; 54:132–138.

137. Bentley JFR, Smith JR. Developmental posterior enteric remnants and spinal malformations. Arch Dis Child 1960; 35:76–86.

138. Kennedy PR. New data on diastematomyelia. J Neurosurg 1979; 51:355–361.

139. English WJ, Maltby GL. Diastematomyelia in adults. J Neurosurg 1967; 27:260–264.

140. Baldi PG, Paini GP, Bertolino GC, Cusmano F. Diastematomyelia in adults. Surg Neurol 1986; 25:501–504.

141. Chehrazi B, Haldeman S. Adult onset of tethered spinal cord syndrome due to fibrous diastematomyelia: case report. Neurosurgery 1985; 16:681–685.

142. Humphreys RP, Hendrick EB, Hoffman HJ. Diastematomyelia. In: Sano K, ed. Clinical neurosurgery. Baltimore: Williams & Wilkins, 1982:436–456.

143. Hood RW, Riseborough EJ, Nehme A-M, et al. Diastematomyelia and structural spinal deformities. J Bone Joint Surg 1980; 62A:520–528.

144. James CCM, Lassman LP. Spinal dysraphism, spina bifida occulta. New York: Appleton-Century-Crofts, 1972: 61–76.

145. Keim HA, Greene AF. Diastematomyelia and scoliosis. J Bone Joint Surg 1973; 55A:1425–1435.

146. Naidich TP, Harwood-Nash DC. Diastematomyelia: hemicord and meningeal sheaths; single and double arachnoid and dural tubes. AJNR 1983; 4:633–636.

147. McClelland RR, Marsh DG. Double diastematomyelia. Radiology 1977; 123:378.

148. Guthkelch AN. Diastematomyelia with median septum. Brain 1974; 97:729–742.

149. Gilmor RL, Batnitzky S. Diastematomyelia—rare and unusual features. Neuroradiology 1978; 16:87–88.

150. Wolf AL, Tubman DE, Seljeskog EL. Diastematomyelia of the cervical spinal cord with tethering in an adult. Neurosurgery 1987; 21:94–98.

151. Beyerl BD, Ojemann RG, Davis KR, et al. Cervical diastematomyelia presenting in adulthood. J Neurosurg 1985; 62:449–453.

152. Levine RS, Geremia GK, McNeill TW. CT demonstration of cervical diastematomyelia. J. Comput Assist Tomogr 1985; 9:592–594.

153. Simpson RK. Cervical diastematomyelia: report of a case and review of a rare congenital anomaly. Arch Neurol 1987; 44:331–335.

154. Ugarte N, Gonzalez-Crussi F, Sotelo-Avila C. Diastematomyelia associated with teratomas. J Neurosurg 1980; 53:720–725.

155. Fernbach SK, Naidich TP, McLone DG, Leestma JE. Computed tomography of primary intrathecal Wilms' tumor with diastematomyelia. J Comput Assist Tomogr 1984; 8:523–528.

156. Schlesinger AE, Naidich TP, Quencer RM. Concurrent hydromyelia and diastematomyelia. AJNR 1986; 7:473–477.

157. Pang D, Parrish RG. Regrowth of diastematomyelic bone spur after extradural resection. J Neurosurg 1983; 5:887–890.

158. French BN. Midline fusion defects and defects of formation. In: Youmans JR, ed. Neurological surgery. 2nd ed. Philadelphia: WB Saunders, 1982:1236–1380.

159. Moes CAF, Hendrick EB. Diastematomyelia. J Pediat 1963; 63:23–248.

160. Kaplan JO, Quencer RM. The occult tethered conus syndrome in the adult. Radiology 1980; 137:387–391.

161. Hendrick EB, Hoffman HJ, Humphreys RP. Tethered cord syndrome. In: McLavrin RL, ed. Myelomeningocele. New York: Grune & Stratton, 1977:369–376.

162. Garceau GJ. The filum terminale syndrome. J Bone Joint Surg 1953; 35A:711–716.

163. Fitz CR, Harwood-Nash DC. The tethered conus. AJR 1975; 125:515–523.

164. Raghavan N, Barkovich AJ, Edwards M, Norman D. MR imaging in the tethered spinal cord syndrome. AJNR 1989; 10:27–36.

165. Pang D, Wilberger JE. Tethered cord syndrome in adults. J Neurosurg 1982; 57:32–47.

166. Simon RH, Donaldson JO, Ramsby GR. Tethered spinal cord in adult siblings. Neurosurgery 1981; 8:241–244.

167. James CCM, Lassman LP. Diastematomyelia and tight filum terminale. J Neurol Sci. 1970; 10:193–196.

168. Hoffman HJ, Hendrick EB, Humphreys RP. The tethered spinal cord: its protean manifestations, diagnosis, and surgical correction. Childs Brain 1976; 2:145–155.

169. Jones PH, Love JG. Tight filum terminale. Arch Surg 1956; 73:556–566.

170. Sarwar M, Crelin ES, Kier L, Virapongse C. Experimental cord stretchability and the tethered cord syndrome. AJNR 1983; 4:641–643.

171. Yamada S, Zinke DE, Sanders D. Pathophysiology of "tethered cord syndrome." J Neurosurg 1981; 54:494–503.

172. Love JG, Daly DD, Harris LE. Tight filum terminale. Report of condition in three siblings. JAMA 1961; 176:31–33.

173. Mount LA. Congenital dermal sinuses. JAMA 1949; 18:1263–1268.

174. Wright RL. Congenital dermal sinuses. Progr Neurol Surg 1971; 4:175–191.

175. Kooistra HP. Pilonidal sinuses occurring over the higher spinal segments with report of a case involving the spinal cord. Surgery 1942; 11:63–74.

176. Walker AE, Bucy PC. Congenital dermal sinuses: a source of spinal meningeal infection and subdural abscesses. Brain 1934; 57:401–421.

177. Haworth JC, Zachary RB. Congenital dermal sinuses in children. Their relation to pilonidal sinuses. Lancet 1955; 2:10–14.

178. Noise TS. Staphylococcus meningitis secondary to congenital sacral sinus. Surg Gynecol Obstet 1926; 42:394–397.

179. Matson DD, Jerva MJ. Recurrent meningitis associated with congenital lumbo-sacral dermal sinus tract. J Neurosurg 1966; 25:288–297.

180. Cardell BS, Laurance B. Congenital dermal sinus associated with meningitis. Br Med J 1951; 2:1588–1561.

181. Sachs E, Horrax G. A cervical and a lumbar pilonidal sinus communicating with intraspinal dermoids. J Neurosurg 1949; 6:97–112.

182. Perloff MM. Congenital dermal sinus complicated by meningitis. J Pediatr 1954; 44:73–76.

183. Bean JR, Walsh JW, Blacker HM. Cervical dermal sinus and intramedullary spinal cord abscess: case report. Neurosurgery 1979; 5:60–62.

184. List CL. Intraspinal epidermoids, dermoids, and dermal sinuses. Surg Gynecol Obstet 1941; 73:525–538.

185. Bailey IC. Dermoid tumors of the spinal cord. J Neurosurg 1970; 33:676–681.

186. Boldrey EB, Elvidge AR. Dermoid cysts of the vertebral canal. Ann Surg 1939; 110:273–284.

187. Guidetti B, Gagliardi FM. Epidermoid and dermoid cysts. J Neurosurg 1977; 47:12–18.

188. Black SP, German WJ. Four congenital tumors found at operation within the vertebral canal: with observations of their incidence. J Neurosurg 1950; 7:49–61.

189. Schwartz HG. Congenital tumors of the spinal cord in infants. Ann Surg 1952; 136:183–192.

190. Choremis C, Economos D, Papadatos C, Gargoulas A. Intraspinal epidermoid tumours (cholesteatomas) in patients treated for tuberculous meningitis. Lancet 1956; 2:437–439.

191. Gibson T, Norris W. Skin fragments removed by injection needles. Lancet 1958; 2:983–985.

192. Van Gilder JC, Schwartz HG. Growth of dermoids from skin implants to the nervous system and surrounding spaces of the newborn rats. J Neurosurg 1967; 26:14–20.

193. Hamby WB. Tumors in the spinal canal in childhood. J Nerv Ment Dis 1935; 81:24–42.

194. Sachs E Jr, Horrax G. A cervical and a lumbar pilonidal sinus communicating with intraspinal dermoids: report of 2 cases and review of the literature. J Neurosurg 1949; 6:97–112.

195. Azariah R. Teratoma of the spinal cord. Br J Surg 1967; 54:658–660.

196. Biggs CR, Quinlivan WF, Raymond JE. Cystic teratoma of the spinal cord. J AOA 1969; 69:64–67.

197. Bucy P, Buchanan DN. Teratoma of the spinal cord. Surg Gynecol Obstet 1935; 60:1137–1144.

198. Desousa AL, Kalsbeck JE, Mealey J, et al. Intraspinal tumors in children: a review of 81 cases. J Neurosurg 1979; 51:437–445.

199. Enestrom S, von Essen C. Spinal teratoma. Report of one case. Acta Neurochir 1977; 39:121–126.

200. Furtado D, Marques V. Spinal teratoma. J Neuropathol Exp Neurol 1951; 10:384–393.

201. Harrington ES, Kell JF. Intraspinal teratoma with report of a case. J Neuropathol Exp Neurol 1955; 14:214–221.

202. Hosoi K. Intradural teratoid tumors of the spinal cord. Report of a case. Arch Pathol 1931; 11:875–883.

203. Ingraham FD, Bailey OT. Cystic teratomas and teratoid tumors of the central nervous system in infancy and childhood. J Neurosurg 1946; 3:511–532.

204. Larbrisseau A, Renevey F, Brochu P, et al. Recurrent chemical meningitis due to an intraspinal cystic teratoma. J Neurosurg 1980; 52:715–717.

205. Lemmen LJ, Wilson CM. Intramedullary malignant teratoma of the spinal cord. Arch Neurol Psychiatry 1951; 61–68.

206. Masten MG. Teratoma of the spinal cord. Arch Pathol 1940; 30:755–761.

207. Padovani R, Tognetti F, Sanpaolo P, et al. Intramedullary cystic teratomas. Acta Neurochir (Wien) 1982; 62:101–108.

208. Padovani R, Tognetti F, Laudadio S, Manetto V. Teratoid cyst of the spinal cord. Neurosurgery 1983; 13:74–77.

209. Pickens JM, Wilson J, Myers GG, Grunnet ML. Teratoma of the spinal cord. Report of a case and review of the literature. Arch Pathol 1975; 99:446–448.

210. Rosenbaum TJ, Sokule EH, Onofrio BM. Teratomatous cyst of the spinal canal. J Neurosurg 1978; 49:292–297.

211. Teng P, Gordon J. Teratoma of the conus medullaris. Report of a case. J Neurosurg 1958; 15:569–571.

212. Smoker WRK, Biller J, Moore SA, et al. Intradural spinal teratoma: case report and review of the literature. AJNR 1986; 7:905–909.

213. Willis RA. The borderland of embryology and pathology. London: Butterworths, 1962:442–462.

214. Willis RA. Teratomas. In: Atlas of tumor pathology. Sect 3, part 9. Washington, DC: AFIP, 1951:9–58.

215. Hoefnagel D, Benirschke K, Durate J. Teratomatous cysts within the vertebral canal. Observations on the occurrence of sex chromatin. J Neurol Neurosurg Psychiatry 1962; 25:159–164.

216. Rewcastle MB, Francoeur J. Teratomatous cysts of the spinal cord. Arch Neurol 1964; 11:91–99.

217. Kubie LS, Fulton JF. A clinical and pathological study of two teratomatous cysts of the spinal cord, containing mucus and ciliated cells. Surg Gynecol Obstet 1928; 47:297–311.

218. Rhaney K, Barclay GPT. Enterogenous cysts and congenital diverticula of alimentary canal with abnormalities of vertebral column and spinal cord. J Pathol Bacteriol 1959; 77:457–471.

219. Garrison JE, Kasdon DI. Intramedullary spinal teratoma: case report and review of the literature. Neurosurgery 1980; 7:509–512.

220. Fabinyi GCA, Adams JE. High cervical spinal cord compression by an enterogenous cyst. J Neurosurg 1979; 51:556–559.

221. Tibbs PA, James HE, Rorke LB, et al. Midline hamartomas masquerading as meningomyeloceles or teratomas in the newborn infant. J Pediatr 1976; 89:928–933.

222. Silverman FN. The pelvis. In: Silverman FN, Kuhn J, Girdany B, et al, eds. Essentials of Caffey's pediatric x-ray diagnosis. Chicago: Year Book, 1990.

223. Andrish J, Kalamchi A, MacEwen GD. Sacral agenesis: a clinical evaluation of its management, heredity, and associated anomalies. Clin Orthopaed 1979; 139:52–57.

224. Banta JV, Nichols O. Sacral agenesis. J Bone Joint Surg 1969; 51A:693–703.

225. Berdon WE, Hochberg B, Baker DH, et al. The association of lumbosacral spine and genitourinary anomalies with imperforate anus. Am J Roentgenol 1966; 98:181–191.

226. Bloch B. Sirenomelia (sympodia or mermaid deformity): a case report. S Afr Med J 1977; 52:196–200.

227. Blumel J, Evans EB, Eggers GWN. Partial and complete agenesis or malformation of the sacrum with associated anomalies. Etiologic and clinical study with special reference to heredity: a preliminary report. J Bone Joint Surg 1959; 41A:497–518.

228. Duhamel B. From the mermaid to anal imperforation: the syndrome of caudal regression. Arch Dis Child 1961; 36:152–155.

229. Grand MJH, Eichenfeld S, Jacobson HG. Sacral aplasia (agenesis). Radiology 1960; 74:611–618.

230. Hendry DW, Kohler HG. Sirenomelia ("mermaid"). J Obstet Gynaecol Br Emp 1956; 63:865–870.

231. Hohl AF. Zur Pathologie des Beckens (I. Das schrage-ovale Becker). Leipzig: Wilhelm Engelman, 1852:61–74.

232. Ignelzi RJ, Lehman RAW. Lumbosacral agenesis: management and embryological implications. J Neurol Neurosurg Psychiatry 1974; 37:1273–1276.

233. Kampmeier OF. On sireniform monsters, with a consideration of the causation and the predominance of the male sex among them. Anat Rec 1927; 34:365–389.

234. Mongeau M, Leclaire R. Complete agenesis of the lumbosacral spine. J Bone Joint Surg 1972; 54A:161–164.

235. Pang D, Hoffman HJ. Sacral agenesis with progressive neurological deficit. Neurosurgery 1980; 7:118–126.

236. Renshaw TS. Sacral agenesis: a classification and review of 23 cases. J Bone Joint Surg 1978; 60A:373–383.

237. Rubenstein MA, Bucy JG. Caudal regression syndrome: the urologic implications. J Urol 1975; 114:934–937.

238. Sarnat HB, Case ME, Graviss R. Sacral agenesis: neurologic and neuropathologic features. Neurology (Minneap.) 1976; 26:1124–1129.

239. Say B, Coldwell JG. Hereditary defect of a sacrum. Hum Genet 1975; 27:231–234.

240. Stanley JK, Owen R, Koff S. Congenital sacral anomalies. J Bone Joint Surg 1979; 61B:401–409.

241. Williams DI, Nixon HH. Agenesis of the sacrum. Surg Gynecol Obstet 1957; 105:84–88.

242. Abraham E. Lumbosacral coccygeal agenesis. J Bone Joint Surg 1976; 58A:1169–1171.

243. Lourie H. Sacral agenesis. Case report. J Neurosurg 1973; 38:90–95.

244. Smith GD. Congenital sacral anomalies in children. Aust NZ J Surg 1959; 29:165–176.

245. Zeligs II. Congenital absence of the sacrum. Arch Surg 1940; 41:1220–1228.

246. Campbell JB. Neurosurgical treatment of bladder and bowel dysfunction resulting from anomalous development of the sacral neural axis. Clin Neurosurg 1962; 8:133–156.

247. Barnes JC, Smith WL. The VATER association. Radiology 1978; 126:445–449.

248. Scott MR, Wolpert SM, Bartoshesky LE, et al. Segmental spinal dysgenesis. Neurosurgery 1988; 22:739–744.

249. Frye FL, McFarland LZ, Enright JB. Sacrococcygeal agenesis in Swiss mice. Cornell Vet 1964; 54:487–495.

250. Stewart JM, Stoll S. Familial caudal regression anomaly and maternal diabetes. J Med Genet 1979; 16:17–20.

251. Finer NN, Bowen P, Dunbar LG. Caudal regression anomalad (sacral agenesis) in siblings. Clin Genet 1978; 13:353–358.

252. Davies J, Chazen E, Nance WE. Symmelia in one of monozygotic twins. Teratology 1970; 4:367–378.

253. Passarge E, Lenz W. Syndrome of caudal regression in infants of diabetic mothers: observations of further cases. Pediatrics 1966; 37:672–675.

254. Rusnak SL, Driscoll SG. Congenital spinal anomalies in infants of diabetic mothers. Pediatrics 1965; 35:989–995.

255. Danforth CH. Artificial and hereditary suppression of sacral vertebrae in the flow. Proc Soc Exp Biol Med 1932; 30:143–145.

256. Landauer W. Rumplessness of chick embryos produced by the injection of insulin and other chemicals. J Exp Zool 1945; 98:65–77.

257. Ho NK, Lo DSC. Sympodia. Am J Dis Child 1974; 128:391–393.

258. Price DL, Dooling EC, Richardson EP Jr. Caudal dysplasia (caudal regression syndrome). Arch Neurol 1970; 23:212–220.

259. Kallen B, Winberg J. Caudal mesoderm pattern of anomalies: from renal agenesis to sirenomelia. Teratology 1974; 9:99–112.

260. Shands AR, Bundens WD. Congenital deformities of the spine. An analysis of the roentgenograms of 700 children. Bull Hosp Joint Dis 1956; 17:110–133.

261. Foix C, Hillemand P. Dystrophie cruro-vesico-fessiere par agenesie sacro-coccygienne. Rev Neurol (Paris) 1924; 42:450–468.

262. Barkovich AJ, Raghavan N. MR imaging of the caudal regression syndrome. AJNR 1989; 10:1223–1231.

263. Kohler HG. An unusual case of sirenomelia. Teratology 1972; 6:295–302.

264. Diaz Lira E. Agenesia sacro-coccigea. Rev Ortop Traumatol 1938; 7:231–237.

265. Brooks BS, El Gammal T, Hartlage P, Beveridge W. Myelography of sacral agenesis. AJNR 1981; 2:319–323.

266. Adams RD, Wegner W. Congenital cyst of the spinal meninges as cause of intermittent compression of the spinal cord. Arch Neurol Psychiatry 1947; 58:57–69.

267. Bale PM. A congenital intraspinal gastroenterogenous cyst in

diastematomyelia. J Neurol Neurosurg Psychiatry 1973; 36:1011–1017.

268. Burrows FGO, Sutcliffe J. The split notochord syndrome. Br F Radiol 1968; 41:844–847.

269. Davis JE, Barnes WA. Intrathoracic duplications of the alimentary tract communicating with the small intestine. Ann Surg 1952; 136:287–295.

270. Denes J, Nonti J, Leb J. Dorsal herniation of the gut: a rare manifestation of the split notochord syndrome. J Pediatr Surg 1967; 2:359–363.

271. Fabinyi GCA, Adams JE. High cervical spinal cord compression by an enterogenous cyst. J Neurosurg 1979; 51:556–559.

272. Gleeson JA, Stovin PGI. Mediastinal enterogenous cysts associated with vertebral anomalies. Clin Radiol 1961; 12:41–48.

273. Fallon M, Gordon ARG, Lendrum AC. Mediastinal cysts of fore-gut origin associated with vertebral abnormalities. Br J Surg 1954; 41:520–533.

274. Gross RE, Neuhauser EBD, Longino LA. Thoracic diverticula which originate from the intestine. Ann Surg 1950; 131:363–375.

275. Harriman DGF. An intraspinal enterogenous cyst. J Pathol Bacteriol 1958; 75:413–419.

276. Hyman I, Hamby WB, Sanes S. Ependymal cyst of the cervicodorsal region of the spinal cord. Arch Neurol Psychiatry 1938; 40:1005–1012.

277. Jackson FE. Neurenteric cysts: report of a case of neurenteric cyst with associated chromic meningitis and hydrocephalus. J Neurosurg 1961; 18:678–682.

278. Klump TE. Neurenteric cyst in the cervical spinal canal of a 10-week-old boy. J Neurosurg 1971; 35:472–475.

279. Millis RR, Holmes AE. Enterogenous cyst of the spinal cord with associated intestinal reduplication, vertebral anomalies, and a dorsal dermal sinus. J Neurosurg 1973; 38:73–77.

280. Mohanty S, Rao CJ, Shukla PK, et al. Intradural enterogenous cyst. J Neurol Neurosurg Psychiatry 1979; 42:419–421.

281. Moore MT, Book MH. Congenital cervical ependymal cyst. J Neurosurg 1966; 24:558–561.

282. Neuhauser EDB, Harris GBC, Berrett A. Roentgenographic features of neurenteric cysts. AJR 1958; 79:235–240.

283. Odake G, Yamaki T, Naruse S. Neurenteric cyst with meningomyelocele. J Neurosurg 1976; 45:352–356.

284. Piramoon AM, Abbassioun K. Mediastinal enterogenic cyst with spinal cord compression. J Pediatr Surg 1974; 9:543–545.

285. Saunders RL de CH. Combined anterior and posterior spina bifida in a living neonatal human female. Anat Rec 1943; 87:255–278.

286. Sabiston DC, Scott HW. Primary neoplasms and cysts of the mediastinum. Ann Surg 1952; 136:777–797.

287. Veeneklaas GMH. Pathogenesis of intrathoracic gastrogeneic cysts. Am J Dis Child 1952; 83:500–507.

288. Geremia GK, Russell EJ, Clasen RA. MR imaging characteristics of a neurenteric cyst. AJNR 1988; 9:978–980.

289. Knight G, Griffiths T, Williams I. Gastrocytoma of the spinal cord. Br J Surg 1955; 42:635–638.

290. Scoville WB, Manlapaz JS, Otis RD, Cabieses F. Intraspinal entrogenous cyst. J Neurosurg 1963; 20:704–706.

Spinal Tumors

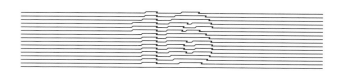

MICHAEL TWOHIG, M.D.
GORDON SZE, M.D.

EXTRADURAL TUMORS
  Neuroblastoma
  Ganglioneuroma and Ganglioneuroblastoma
  Osteochondroma
  Osteoid Osteoma
  Osteoblastoma
  Chordoma
  Aneurysmal Bone Cyst
  Vertebral Hemangioma
  Giant Cell Tumor
  Sacrococcygeal Teratoma
  Ewing's Sarcoma
  Eosinophilic Granuloma
  Osteosarcoma

Chondrosarcoma
  Leukemia
  Non-Hodgkin's Lymphoma
  Hodgkin's Disease
INTRADURAL EXTRAMEDULLARY TUMORS
  Neurofibroma
  Meningioma
  Spinal Subarachnoid Tumor
INTRAMEDULLARY TUMORS
  Astrocytoma
  Ependymoma
  Hemangioblastoma

Tumors of the spine are extremely uncommon in children. They represent less than 1 percent of all childhood malignancies and less than 10 percent of all central nervous system (CNS) malignancies in children.[1] Brain tumors are four to 20 times as common as intraspinal tumors in children.[2,3]

Spinal tumors may be extradural, intradural extramedullary, or intramedullary in location. Sixty percent are extradural in adults, but in children there is an equal distribution among the three categories. In the extradural space, various lesions can be seen and any one individually represents a small percentage of the total number of spinal lesions. This group includes leukemias; lymphomas; bony metastases (especially from neuroblastoma and rhabdomyosarcoma); malignant primary bone tumors such as osteosarcoma, Ewing's, and chondrosarcoma; and numerous benign bony lesions such as aneurysmal bone cyst, osteoid osteoma, osteoblastoma, and hemangioma.[4] Intraspinal extension of paraspinal lesions such as neuroblastoma and ganglioneuroma can also occur.[4] In the intradural extramedullary space, leptomeningeal (drop) metastases are the most common (roughly 10 percent of all pediatric spinal tumors), and medulloblastoma (6.3 percent) and retinoblastoma (3.1 percent) are some of the more common lesions.[4] Other intradural extramedullary lesions seen in children include nerve sheath tumors (7.8 percent) and tumors associated with spinal dysraphism. In the intramedullary space, Rand and Rand found that astrocytoma occurred in 14 percent of all pediatric spinal tumors, while ependymoma represented 12.5 percent of all cases.[5]

Age plays an important role in the differential diagnosis of a spinal tumor. If the patient is under 5 years of age, developmental neoplasms, such as sacrococcygeal teratoma and neuroblastoma, should be considered.[6] Astrocytomas, ependymomas, and dermoids usually present after 8 years of age, commonly in the second decade.[6] Bony metastases and spinal subarachnoid metastases can occur in the first or second decade. Most of the primary osseous lesions occur in the second decade or later.

Similarly, location within the spinal canal is pertinent and some generalities apply, as shown by Harwood-Nash and Fitz.[6] An intramedullary tumor in the cervical region is usually an astrocytoma or a hydromyelia. In the thoracic region, a teratoma, a dermoid, or an astrocytoma should be considered. In the lumbar region, two subcategories exist based on whether there is spinal dysraphism or not: if there is spinal dysraphism, the lesion is most likely to be a dermoid, teratoma, or lipoma; if there is no dysraphism, an ependymoma, astrocytoma, or dermoid should be considered.

Similarly, an intradural extramedullary lesion in the cervical region is most likely to be a neurofibroma; in the thoracic region, a leptomeningeal tumor; and in the lumbar region, a dermoid or lipoma if there is dysraphism and an ependymoma or leptomeningeal tumor if there is no dysraphism.[6]

Finally, extradural lesions in the cervical spine are likely to be neurofibromas; in the thoracic and lumbar region, neuroblastomas, metastases, or extradural sarcomas are most common.[6]

When a child has a spinal tumor, the symptoms can

be present for a long time before the diagnosis is eventually considered.[7] In one series the average duration of symptoms was 1.5 years.[7] Frequently the reason for the delay can be attributed to the nonspecific nature of the symptoms as well as the child's inability to convey complaints accurately.

Pain is the initial complaint in roughly 40 to 50 percent of patients.[2,7–9] Often the pain is poorly defined in nature and can increase in intensity with activity or postural changes. Initially a definite cause of the child's pain cannot be determined. Changes in gait posture or motor weakness can be seen in 50 to 62 percent of cases.[7,9] Decreased activity may result.[7,8] Other symptoms include fatigue, scoliosis, weight loss, and a change in bowel or bladder habits, especially if a trained child regresses and develops incontinence, enuresis, or urgency.[7,9] Later symptoms include increased gait disorder, urinary incontinence, pain, stiffness, and orthopedic abnormalities such as torticollis, scoliosis, or kyphosis.[7–9] Principal signs include abnormal reflexes with hyper- or hypoactive deep tendon reflexes, a positive Babinski sign or ankle clonus, and diminished sensory or motor capabilities.[7,8]

EXTRADURAL TUMORS

Neuroblastoma

Neuroblastoma is a disease of infancy and childhood that occurs in one in every 10,000 births.[10] Rarely, this tumor can be familial.[10] Excluding CNS tumors, neuroblastoma is the most common solid tumor of children.[11–13] The lesions are more common in white children than black children, with roughly seven cases per million population.[14,15] There is a slight male predilection, 56 percent of cases being reported in males in some studies.[11,14–17] Children under 5 years of age are most often affected;[11,15,18] 50 percent of patients are under 2 years of age.[11,15,17] Congenital and fetal forms of neuroblastoma have been described.[15]

Neuroblastoma originates from primitive cells called neuroblasts, which are of neural crest origin.[11,15] In the fetus, some neural crest cells separate and embryologically form the adrenal medulla and the paravertebral sympathetic chain.[14] These tumors can therefore be found within the adrenal medulla (36 to 40 percent) or in the paravertebral sympathetic chain.[18] The adrenal medulla and upper abdominal parasympathetic chain are the primary site of 65 percent of neuroblastomas.[11,14,15,18] Neuroblastoma can occur anywhere along the sympathetic chain, including paraspinal locations, the carotid ganglia, the aortic bodies, and the organ of Zuckerkandl.[15] Overall, the abdomen is the most common location of these tumors (54 to 68 percent).

Clinical Findings

Symptomatology can vary tremendously according to the location and extent of disease.[19] Frequently, patients present with constitutional symptoms such as anemia, vomiting, fever, or general malaise.[17,18] Interestingly, patients can present with chronic diarrhea secondary to catecholamine production.[14,17] Lesions in the abdomen and pelvis tend to present later; lesions in the neck are visible earlier and tend to be smaller at the time of diagnosis.[18]

Up to 35 percent of patients present with complaints referable to metastatic disease.[11] Metastatic disease at the time of initial presentation is common, the reported incidence being up to 74 percent.[20] The sites of metastatic foci differ with the age of the patient. Children under 1 year of age tend to have metastases to liver, skin, and bones; older children have metastases to bones and local lymph nodes.[18,20] Actual brain and spinal cord parenchymal metastases from neuroblastoma are rare, although leptomeningeal tumor spread is not unusual.

Since neuroblastoma occurs in a paraspinal location, it can extend through the neural foramina to form a dumbbell-shaped lesion with an epidural component.[18] Epidural extension occurred in 17 of 129 cases in a study from the Hospital for Sick Children.[12] It can be symptomatic or asymptomatic, although spinal cord compression as an initial symptom is rare, seen in less than 4 percent of patients.[12,20] Punt and colleagues reported 21 children with neuroblastoma who had spinal cord compression as the initial complaint.[20] They ranged in age from 1 day to 11 years, with a median age of 1 year; in four children, spinal cord compression was present at birth.[20]

With intraspinal involvement, the most common presenting symptoms include local pain and spinal cord dysfunction.[17,19] The patient may notice a paraspinal mass or may have signs of spinal cord compression.[21] In one series, impaired motor and sphincter function was seen in eight of 11 patients, weakness of the lower extremities in six of 11, and weakness of the arms in two of 11.[17]

Harwood-Nash and other investigators found that of all intraspinal neoplasms, 7 to 8 percent are the result of intraspinal extension of a paraspinal neuroblastoma.[6,7,9,22] Involvement of the spine occurs most frequently in the thoracic and lumbar regions, and is rare in the cervical area.[6] In the series of 21 cases with spinal cord compression (Punt and colleagues) the distribution was as follows: nine in the thoracic, five in the thoracolumbar, six in the lumbosacral, and only one in the cervical region.[20]

Pathology

Histologically, neuroblastomas are composed of small round cells with hyperchromatic dense nuclei.[11,14,15] These can be confused with Ewing's sarcoma, rhabdomyosarcoma, lymphoma, and Wilms' tumor.[11,18] Neuroblastoma is composed primarily of primitive cells and lacks more mature elements.[14] Histologic changes that indicate further maturation of the cellular elements include increased size of nuclei, increased amount of cytoplasm, and production of fibrillar elements.[11] Neuroblastomas are frequently hemorrhagic, with groups or nests of cells separated by fibrovascular septa.[11] Calcifications are not common (10 percent).

Imaging

As tumor extends through the neural foramina, there may be erosion of the pedicle, widening of the foramina, scalloping of the vertebral body, thinning of the ribs, or widening of the spinal canal.[17,20,23] The intraspinal component of the tumor may spread through the epidural space over several levels, resulting in cord block remote from the site of the paravertebral mass.[6] Rarely, these lesions may directly invade the intradural space.[6]

Magnetic resonance imaging (MRI) allows ready demonstration of the intraspinal extension of tumor, since multiplanar imaging can easily show extension into the spinal canal through the intervertebral foramina.[12] Frequently, this can be best shown with coronal imaging.[13] On unenhanced MRI, the mass is evident displacing the thecal sac and spinal cord.[12] Areas of necrosis have low signal intensity on T1 weighted images and increased signal intensity on T2 weighted images. Focal areas of hemorrhage may have a varied appearance. Acute hemorrhage is evident by decreased signal intensities on both T1 and T2 weighted images. Subacute hemorrhage tends to have increased signal on T1 weighted images and decreased signal on T2 weighted images, and slowly progresses to increased signal on both T1 and T2 weighted images. Large areas of calcification can be seen as areas of signal void. MRI clearly demonstrates the relationship of the paraspinal portion of the mass to adjacent vascular structures, i.e., the aorta and vena cava. Encasement of these structures is evident when the signal void of the vascular structures is encircled by the tumor. Finally, with contrast administration these tumors tend to enhance. Contrast often helps separate the epidural component from the normal thecal sac and spinal cord on T1 weighted images.

Treatment

It is extremely important for the purposes of initial preoperative diagnosis that any intraspinal extension of paravertebral masses such as neuroblastoma be ascertained, since symptoms referable to spinal cord compression may become permanent if not treated.[12,20] In addition, when debulking a paraspinal mass, it is helpful to remove epidural tumor, since significant blood loss can occur at the time of resection if an unsuspected epidural component remains within the spinal canal.[12,20]

Prognostic factors in neuroblastoma depend on the patient's age at diagnosis, the extent of the disease, the site of the primary tumor, and the degree of maturation of the cells. Factors consistent with a favorable outcome include a younger age at diagnosis, extra-adrenal location, more differentiated histology, and more localized disease.[11,17] Overall, there is a better prognosis for children presenting with spinal cord compres-

sion.[17,20] Of 21 children in this category, 11 of 13 survivors were long-term survivors at the time of the report.[20]

Ganglioneuroma and Ganglioneuroblastoma

Ganglioneuromas and ganglioneuroblastomas arise from the same cells as neuroblastomas. Ganglioneuromas are more common in girls, whereas ganglioneuroblastomas occur with equal frequency in the two sexes. They tend to present later than neuroblastomas and are most often seen in the 5- to 8-year-old age group.[6] The most common location for ganglioneuromas is the posterior mediastinum (38 percent), with the adrenal gland second in incidence (30 percent). Commonly they are located at the thoracolumbar junction, followed by the lumbar spine and finally the cervical spine. They are most frequently extradural in location, although intradural extramedullary extension can occur. These lesions tend to be elongated, with tapered superior and inferior margins. Intramedullary spread is very rare. Neuroblastomas may differentiate into ganglioneuroma. In fact, neuroblastoma metastases may have ganglioneuroma elements within the lesions. Two percent of all intraspinal lesions result from intraspinal extension of paravertebral ganglioneuroma.[6]

Pathology

Ganglioneuroblastoma is a mixture of immature neuroblastoma and more mature elements. The nuclei are large and there is more cytoplasm present within the cells than in neuroblastoma. As the axonal processes develop, more mature fibrillary structures will be present.[14,18] Ganglioneuroma is the most differentiated lesion and is composed almost entirely of mature ganglia cells. Here a sheath cell surrounds the axon. The cells have larger nuclei and more abundant cytoplasm. Calcifications are seen in 20 percent.[11,14]

Imaging

Radiography shows a paraspinal mass. There may be widening of the neural foramina and the interpedicular distance, as well as erosion of the ribs. An associated scoliosis may be present, frequently convex toward the side of the mass.

MRI can show the paravertebral mass and the intraspinal extent (Fig. 16–1) and is extremely important in relation to the treatment of patients, since it can show epidural disease readily. As mentioned previously, early decompressive laminectomy preserves spinal cord function and decreases the amount of blood loss at surgery when a paravertebral mass is removed.

Osteochondroma

The most common benign bone tumor is the osteochondroma, making up 40 percent of all benign bone tumors.[25-27] Three-fourths of osteochondromas appear in patients under 20 years of age. There is a slight male predilection.[27,28] Any bone preformed in car-

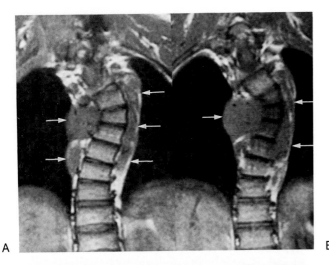

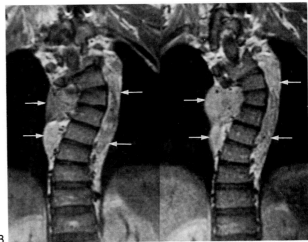

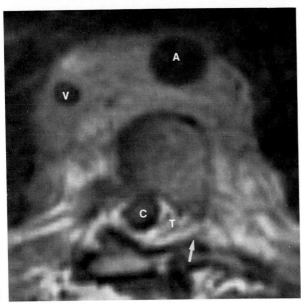

Figure 16–1. *Ganglioneuroma in a 10-year-old girl.* **A,** Coronal T1 weighted image (600/20) reveals a large inhomogeneous paraspinal mass (*arrows*) associated with thoracic scoliosis. **B,** Coronal T1 weighted image (600/20) after gadolinium-DTPA administration shows enhancement of the mass (*arrows*). **C,** Axial T1 weighted image (700/20) after gadolinium-DTPA shows that there is encasement of the aorta (A) and the vena cava (V). There is also extension of the mass through the neural foramen on the left (*arrow*). Epidural tumor (T) displaces the spinal cord (C) to the right.

tilage may be involved with this lesion; the knee is the most common site.[26, 29] These lesions may be solitary or multiple; the latter is seen in multiple hereditary exostosis.

Although the precise incidence of vertebral osteochondroma is unknown, roughly 3 percent of solitary and 7 percent of multiple osteochondromas occur within the spine.[27, 30, 31] Osteochondromas of the vertebral column almost always exclusively involve the posterior elements, with a predilection for the spinous processes.[27, 32] Frequently, these lesions bridge multiple vertebral segments,[27] which can result in fusion and restricted motion, most evident in the cervical region.[33]

Clinical Findings

Signs and symptoms are nonspecific. Pain is often present. There may or may not be associated swelling or a palpable soft tissue mass.[27] The lesions are usually large by the time they are symptomatic and come to medical attention.[26] Neurologic symptoms are rare,

being seen in less than 1 percent of all patients.[23] However, there is a greater incidence of spinal cord symptoms in the teenage years, which suggests that growth spurts could compromise a marginally narrowed canal.[31] Thoracolumbar lesions may present with bowel or bladder dysfunction; cervical lesions have a varied presentation, including paresthesias and even dysphagia.[30, 34]

Pathology

These lesions are composed of cancellous bone surrounded by cortical bone.[30, 34] They have a gracile pedicle that attaches to the adjacent bone, usually at the site of ligamentous insertions.[26, 27] Marrow is present within them.[27] A thin layer of cartilage covers the tumor.

Imaging

Plain films show a pedunculated or sessile lesion with its cortex in direct contiguity with the cortex of the adjacent bone, connected by a thin pedicle.[29] These lesions generally originate from the posterior elements. Computed tomography (CT) often can show better the exact site of attachment of the lesion to the adjacent bone, the presence of the cartilaginous cap, and any compromise of the spinal canal.[26, 27] In addition, CT can be helpful in distinguishing between benign osteochondromas and malignant degeneration into an osteosarcoma. Factors favoring benignity include cortical margins contiguous with the adjacent bone, well-defined lobular surfaces, lack of adjacent bone destruction, and a thin cartilaginous cap (usually less than 1 cm).[29]

These tumors have a heterogeneous appearance on MRI. The cartilaginous portions of these lesions show increased signal intensity on T2 weighted images, while the osteoid or calcified portions show low signal intensity.

Treatment

Since these lesions are benign, no treatment is required unless they are large and compress adjacent structures.[28] In this instance surgery can be performed and is usually curative, with only a 5 percent recurrence rate.[29] Obviously, tumors with malignant degeneration require additional therapy.

Osteoid Osteoma

Osteoid osteoma is a common benign bone tumor.[8, 35, 36] The etiology of these lesions is controversial and includes post-traumatic conditions and infection.[37] This tumor has been reported in virtually every bone. The most common location is the lower extremity, especially around the knee.[38] Ten to 15 percent occur in the spine.[35, 38-40] The most common sites in the spine are the lumbar region (59 percent), followed by the cervical (27 percent), thoracic (12 percent), and sacral (2 percent) regions.[39] This lesion involves the posterior elements in 75 percent of patients.[41] Thirty percent of cases involve the laminae; 20 percent affect the articular facets and pedicles.[39, 40] The vertebral body is affected in 7 percent.[39, 41, 42]

Osteoid osteomas are more common in males than in females (2:1 to 5:1).[37, 38, 43] The peak incidence (50 percent of cases) occurs between 10 and 20 years of age.[43] This tumor is rare after age 30; 87 percent of cases occur before this age.[38] Jackson and colleagues reported a series of nine patients with an average age of 19.9 years.[38] When data concerning osteoid osteoma of the spine were compiled from the literature, 36 cases occurred at an average age of 16.7 years; 72 percent occurred in patients between 10 and 20 years of age.[43]

Clinical Findings

The lesions are almost always symptomatic, although rarely they are symptom free (1.6 percent).[38] Initial symptoms are often vague and nonspecific. Classically, the chief complaint is pain, worse at night

and relieved by aspirin.[40] Radicular pain can occur if the lesion encroaches on the neural foramina.[40, 41, 43]

There may be a significant delay in evaluation and diagnosis until the symptoms increase in severity.[40, 42] The average delay from initial symptoms to diagnosis in Jackson's series was 11.3 months.[38] Back pain without a history of trauma is very unusual in a child and should prompt evaluation.[44]

Osteoid osteoma may cause certain signs, focal tenderness being the most common.[45] Also frequently seen are scoliosis due to muscle spasm, and a resultant pelvic tilt.[40-45] Scoliosis was seen in 29 of 36 patients in one study.[43] If a child presents with painful scoliosis, the possibility of a structural lesion should be entertained. Other bone lesions to be considered in the differential diagnosis with osteoid osteoma include osteoblastoma, eosinophilic granuloma, osteomyelitis, and aneurysmal bone cyst.[23]

Pathology

Grossly, this tumor has a central, vascular nidus that is reddish-gray in color. Histologically, the tumor contains multinucleated giant cells.[45] The nidus consists of very vascular fibrous connective tissue with surrounding osteoid matrix.[23, 36, 44, 45] It may be calcified in an irregular fashion. The size of the nidus is less than 1.5 cm (if greater than 1.5 cm, the lesion would be classified as an osteoblastoma) with an average size of 0.9 cm.[37] The nidus is surrounded by sclerotic bony reaction.[23, 44] The extent of sclerosis is extremely variable.[44]

Imaging

In young patients with painful scoliosis, it is paramount to search for subtle areas of sclerosis involving the bony spine, especially the posterior elements.[41] Delays (an average of 27 months) in the diagnosis of osteoid osteoma can frequently be attributed to overlooked areas of subtle sclerosis on plain films.[43] Plain films, which demonstrate the classic findings in 66 percent of cases, show a lucent nidus.[44, 46] A small amount of calcium is often present in the nidus.[23, 40] Surrounding bony sclerosis can be seen but is variable in extent.[23, 40] If there is extensive bony sclerosis, the exact location of the nidus may be difficult to discern on plain films and may not even be apparent at surgery.[23] Other imaging is frequently required preoperatively to localize the nidus precisely and ensure complete removal.[40, 47]

If results on initial plain films are negative and there is still a high clinical suspicion of an osteoid osteoma, further imaging is required. A nuclear medicine bone scan is generally recommended. Osteoid osteomas are focally "hot" on bone scan.[40, 46, 47] Once this level is localized with the bone scan, further cross-sectional imaging may be performed either with CT or MRI to confirm the precise location of the nidus preoperatively.[40, 46]

Frequently, the nidus can be seen only on cross-sectional imaging.[40, 47, 48] CT shows a small rounded area of low attenuation, with or without calcification.[40,48] Surrounding sclerosis is evident and may be extensive.[40,47] CT may show intense enhancement, which may help not only to localize the nidus but also to differentiate it from a nonenhancing lytic lesion such as Brodie's abscess.[40]

On MRI the lesion has a heterogeneous appearance, with the calcification within the nidus as well as the surrounding bony sclerosis of low signal intensity on T1 and T2 weighted images.[36] The noncalcified portions of the nidus itself are of increased signal intensity on T2 weighted images (Fig. 16–2).[36] Finally, the administration of gadolinium-DTPA, like that of iodinated contrast material, shows intense enhancement within the very vascular nidus. Because of the sensitivity of CT to bone detail, it is unlikely that MRI will supplant CT in the evaluation of suspected osteoid osteomas.

Osteoblastoma

Osteoblastoma is an uncommon benign bone tumor accounting for 1 percent of all primary bone tumors.[49–52] It has been described in almost every bone.[51] Three-quarters of cases occur in the spine, femur, mandible, or tibia.[52] There is a particular predilection for the spine, which accounts for 35 to 50 percent of cases.[35,50,53–57] In the Mayo Clinic series, 39 of the 123 tumors were in the spine.[52] The most common location is the lumbar region, followed by the thoracic and cervical regions.[50,52,56]

Osteoblastoma occurs most often in the posterior elements. Myles and MacRae reported ten cases of spinal osteoblastoma in children and found that nine were located in the posterior elements.[50] Infrequently,

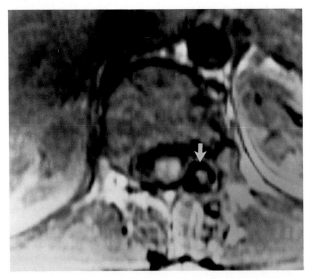

Figure 16–2. *Osteoid osteoma.* An 18-year-old male with back pain. Axial T1 weighted image shows a left thoracic pedicular mass (*arrow*) with a hypointense cortical rim and central signal nidus. (Pomerantz S. Craniospinal magnetic resonance imaging. Philadelphia: WB Saunders, 1989.)

this lesion can involve the vertebral body (14 percent).[50–52] The vertebral body and dorsal elements are involved 24 percent of the time.[52] Epidural extension of tumor may be seen.[50]

Osteoblastoma is more common in males.[38,50,56,57] In the Mayo Clinic series, 87 of 123 cases were found in males.[52] Ninety percent of cases occur before the age of 30.[38,52] This lesion usually presents in patients within the first two decades of life.[50,53,58] Myles and MacRae's study of ten children reported an age range of 2 to 16 years, with an average of 11 years.[50]

Clinical Findings

Osteoblastomas are symptomatic, with pain and local tenderness as common complaints.[38,50,51] Sometimes the symptoms occur before the lesion becomes evident on plain films. There is often a delay in diagnosis (an average of 9.3 to 12.3 months).[38,50,57,59]

Pathology

Grossly these masses are soft, hemorrhagic, and very friable.[38] They have a granular appearance because of the osteoid trabeculae present.[52] They are very vascular and contain osteoid and bone-forming elements.[60] Histologically the tumor appears very similar to osteoid osteoma;[38,56] the two lesions are differentiated by their size. Osteoblastomas have a nidus larger than 1.5 cm; the average size of the nidus in one study was 2.5 cm.[38] Osteoblastomas contain fibrovascular stroma, osteoid tissue, mature bone, and giant cells.[38,49,50,56,57] There may be patchy calcification within the osteoid, and areas of hemorrhage may be noted.[38,53,57]

Imaging

On plain films these lesions are mixed, with both lytic and sclerotic areas, and involve the posterior elements.[50,51,57] In 75 percent of cases there is an eccentric lytic lesion with cortical expansion.[52,57] Twenty percent of patients show cortical destruction mimicking a malignant lesion.[52] A dense periosteal reaction may be associated with these lesions.[52,57]

CT may show associated soft tissue masses as well as epidural extension.[50,51,61] The central nidus may be lucent or dense, as it is often ossified.[52,61] There is a tendency for the bone to be expanded.[49] MRI readily shows the lesion and any associated soft tissue mass. These lesions are inhomogeneous if areas of hemorrhage or calcification are present. T2 weighted images show lesions of high signal intensity (Fig. 16–3). On T1 weighted images after the administration of contrast material, osteoblastomas demonstrate enhancement.

Treatment

Treatment is aimed at total excision of the lesion.[49,50,52] If the lesion is completely removed, there usually is complete disappearance of symptoms and relatively little risk of recurrence.[49,50,57,62] Overall, a 10 percent recurrence rate is seen, this event being

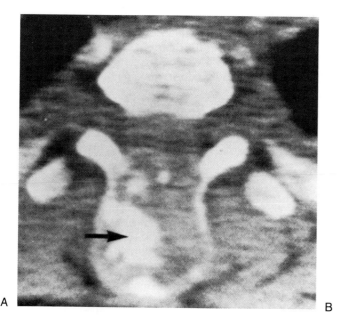

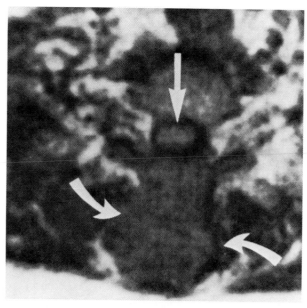

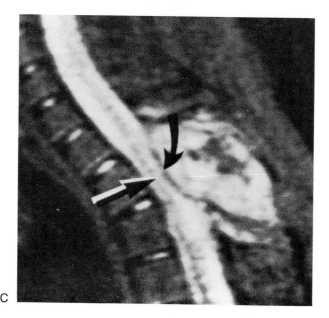

Figure 16–3. *Osteoblastoma of the spinous process of T2.* ***A,*** Axial CT scan shows an expanded spinous process of the second thoracic vertebra with internal amorphous calcifications (*arrow*). The anterior extent of the tumor and its relationship with the cord cannot be established. ***B, C,*** Axial SE (600/25) and midline sagittal (2500/80) MR images show the cord (*straight arrows*) and its relationship with the tumor (*curved arrows* in ***C***). Note the partial obliteration of the posterior subarachnoid space (*curved arrow* in ***B***) on the sagittal MR image. (Beltran J, Noto AM, Chakeres DW, Christoforidis AJ. Tumors of the osseous spine: staging with MR imaging versus CT. Radiology 1987; 162:565–569.)

more common in lesions involving the spine and pelvis.[62] Recurrences as long as nine years after surgery have been reported, so long-term follow-up is essential.[62] Radiation therapy may be given for incompletely removed recurrent lesions.[50] Rarely, these benign tumors may undergo malignant degeneration.[38, 63]

Chordoma

Chordomas are malignant tumors of the skeleton that represent 3 to 4 percent of all primary bony tumors.[64, 65] They arise from primitive remnants of the notochord,[66] which forms the early fetal skeleton and extends from the clivus to the sacrum. Consequently, chordomas may occur anywhere along the skull base and spine. With ossification of the skeleton, the notochord eventually forms the nucleus pulposus of the intervertebral disc.[67]

The distribution of lesions is 50 percent in the sacrum, 35 percent in the clivus, and 15 percent in the vertebrae.[64, 68] There is definite male predominance: in a large series of 155 patients from the Mayo Clinic, 103 were male and 52 female.[65] These figures agree with other reports, which show roughly a 2:1 male-to-female ratio. In the Mayo Clinic study the age range was 8 to 83 years, with an average age at diagnosis of 48 years.[65] One patient in a study of 46 was 2½ years old.[68]

In the spine, 14 percent of all reported chordomas were seen to involve the vertebrae.[64] The areas most commonly involved are the cervical, lumbar, and thoracic spine in descending order of frequency.[69]

The most common symptom is pain, usually localized to the site of origin. Vertebral tumors may show signs and symptoms of cord compression. When chordomas involve the vertebral column, symptoms are frequently progressive and include motor abnormalities, radicular symptoms, vertebral collapse, and finally paralysis. In one series of 46 patients, the average duration of symptoms to the time of diagnosis was almost 1 year; there was an average survival of 3 years after the time of diagnosis.[68] This slow-growing lesion invades adjacent structures but rarely metastasizes, although one series reported metastases in 10 to 15 percent of patients.[68] Distant metastases occur to lymph nodes, liver, lungs, thyroid, and skin. In 80 percent of cases involving the vertebral body, there are eventual distant metastases.[38] As a result, it appears that chordomas involving the vertebral bodies are more malignant than their counterparts in the sacrum or the clival region.

Pathology

These lesions are composed of large, vacuolated, physaliphorous cells. The cells are usually arranged in cords and contain abundant glycogen.

Imaging

Plain films show bony destruction with areas of amorphous calcification in 50 to 70 percent of patients.[69] In one study of 16 patients, involvement of two or more adjacent vertebral bodies and the intervening intervertebral disc was seen in seven.[69] This plain film finding is generally associated with infectious etiologies and is unusual in the case of neoplasms. In addition, paravertebral masses may be seen.

CT can better show the calcification and paravertebral soft tissue masses. CT scans performed after intravenous contrast administration or after myelography may show an associated epidural component.

MRI is inferior to CT in showing bony destruction or calcification.[67] However, MRI is better able to show epidural disease and the true extent of disease involving the bone. In a series of 20 intracranial and upper cervical chordomas, the MR characteristics were reviewed.[67] Seventy-five percent of chordomas are isointense on T1 weighted images and 25 percent are hypointense. The lesions are of high signal intensity on T2 weighted images.[67] Seventy percent of cases show internal septations and a surrounding capsule of low signal intensity. Areas of hemorrhage and cystic change are readily demonstrated if present.

Treatment

Treatment consists of surgical resection with radiation therapy.[65] Overall, the prognosis is fairly dismal, only 10 percent of patients surviving 5 years free of disease.[38] Although metastases are not common, local recurrence is the major problem, usually within 2 to 4 years after initial surgery and radiation therapy.

Aneurysmal Bone Cyst

Aneurysmal bone cyst is a benign disorder of bone of unknown etiology.[70] This uncommon tumor was found to represent 1.4 percent of bone tumors in a study of 2,000 primary bone tumors. The lesions may arise de novo in bone or may be associated with other lesions such as giant cell tumor, hemangioma, chondroblastoma, chondromyxoid fibroma, fibrous dysplasia, and nonossifying fibroma.[71-73] There is either a slight female predilection or no sexual predominance.[71-75] Patients are usually in their first two decades; 66 to 78 percent of cases occur in patients under 20 years of age. In a study evaluating 81 cases in the literature, the peak incidence of aneurysmal bone cyst was seen at 16 years of age, and most occurred in patients between 10 and 25 years of age.[73, 74, 76, 77] In contradistinction, giant cell tumor is usually seen in patients over 30 years of age.[72, 73, 75, 78]

This lesion has been found in almost every bone.[74] One-half involve the long bones, the lower extremity being more commonly affected than the upper.[71-73] The spine is frequently involved. In the Mayo Clinic series of 134 cases, 27 were in the spine. Various other studies report between 3 and 20 percent involving the spine.[35, 72-74, 76] Sixty percent of these lesions involve the posterior elements;[35, 70, 74] 40 percent arise in the vertebral bodies.[74] There is a greater incidence of these tumors in the lumbar spine. They may cross the intervertebral disc space and involve an adjacent vertebral body.[35, 72, 74, 76] About 22 percent have extension into the paraspinal soft tissues. There may or may not be an associated soft tissue mass.

Clinical Findings

The symptoms vary tremendously depending on the size and degree of differentiation of the lesion. A small lesion may be entirely asymptomatic. When symptoms are present, they usually consist of localized pain or swelling.[7, 72-74]

Symptoms are often long-standing. The average duration of symptoms in one series was 8 months.[74] If the lesion is large enough, there may be impingement on the spinal cord, with resultant focal neurologic defect or long tract signs.[74] In one study of 15 patients, compression fracture contributed to symptoms in four patients.[77] Neural foraminal narrowing may result in radiculopathy. Extremely large lesions may result in displacement or compression of paravertebral structures with variable symptoms, including paraplegia.[74]

Pathology

These tumors are composed of large cavernous spaces filled with unclotted blood.[75, 78-80] The linings of these spaces are not typical for blood vessels; i.e., they do not contain endothelium, muscle fibers, or elastic laminae.[4, 73, 75, 77, 79, 81, 82] These benign lesions also have solid portions that frequently are composed of osteoid material, sometimes intermixed with fibrous tissue.[72, 77] Histologically, these lesions may be confused with other entities, such as a telangiectatic osteosarcoma. Giant cells are present within the trabeculae of these lesions, which may lead to a confusing histologic picture and an erroneous diagnosis of giant cell tumor.[72]

Imaging

Plain films show an expansile lytic lesion usually involving the posterior elements.[4, 74, 83] An eggshell-thin cortical margin is often seen.[74] When the vertebral body is destroyed, there may be resultant collapse and vertebra plana.[74, 77] CT confirms these findings and better defines any soft tissue extension of the tumor.[78, 84] In addition, multiple small fluid levels can be seen on CT.[80] Often, to best visualize these fluid levels, the patient must remain motionless for 10 minutes before scanning to allow the different components of blood to settle out within the cavernous spaces of the tumor.[4, 80]

MRI imaging exhibits similar findings to those seen on CT. Again seen on MRI are multiple small fluid-fluid levels and internal septations.[4, 70, 80] This finding is not pathognomonic; it is also seen in telangiectatic osteosarcoma. The fluid may have varying signal intensities based on the phase of blood present within the cavities, varying from high to low signal on T1 and T2 weighted images.[80] These levels have been shown to be more evident on T1 weighted images.[70, 86] The superior fluid represents plasma and is of low signal intensity on T1 weighted images; the lower portion is of high signal intensity secondary to red cell content and T1 shortening by methemoglobin.[4, 70, 80, 86] This is not as apparent on T2 weighted images.[80] If only T2 weighted images are obtained, the fluid-fluid levels may not be readily apparent.[4] A rim of low signal intensity may surround the lesion and has been reported as a helpful sign of the benignity of this bony lesion. Often any paravertebral extension of the mass is better demonstrated on MRI. Any epidural extension or spinal cord compression is also better shown on MRI than on CT (Fig. 16-4).

The finding of a lesion involving the posterior elements of the spine, with a rim of low signal intensity and fluid levels within it of various signal intensities, is highly suggestive of an aneurysmal bone cyst.

Treatment

Curettage is the initial treatment employed. If the lesion recurs several times, radiation therapy may be used. Very large lesions may be treated by embolization.

Vertebral Hemangioma

Vertebral hemangioma is the most common benign lesion in the spinal column. These vascular tumors are present in 10 to 12 percent of all patients.[79, 87, 88] Vertebral hemangiomas tend to increase in incidence with age.[88] These lesions are solitary in 66 percent and multiple in 34 percent of patients.[89] There is a slight female predilection.

Vertebral hemangiomas may involve either the thoracic or lumbosacral region. Cervical involvement is rarely seen.

Clinical Findings

Vertebral hemangiomas tend to be asymptomatic and found incidentally.[87] They occasionally cause symptoms. Symptomatic lesions tend to occur in the thoracic region. In one study, 93 percent of cases (13 of 14) of symptomatic vertebral hemangiomas were in the thoracic region, specifically between T3 and T9.[90] Symptoms include pain, tenderness, radiculopathy, and spinal cord compression. Motor and/or sensory abnormalities may be seen with cord compression. These lesions usually cause slowly progressive compression of the cord, which may occur secondary to (1) mechanical compression of the spinal cord by the enlarged vertebral body and/or posterior elements as a result of the angiomatous tumor, (2) actual invasion of the epidural space by the tumor itself, or (3) rarely, compression fracture of the involved vertebral body.[88, 89, 91] The last-named is unusual, since hemangiomas have thickened vertical trabeculae that tend to prevent axial collapse.

Pathology

Grossly, these lesions are dark red.[91] Histologically, they consist of vascular structures within bony sinuses lined by endothelium and filled with blood. These angiomatoid tumors may grow, with resultant destruction of some bony trabeculae; there is compensatory thickening of the remaining vertical trabeculae.

Imaging

The thickened vertical trabeculae cause parallel linear densities in the vertebral body, yielding the classic findings on plain film of the "corduroy cloth" or "jail bar" appearance.[87] These sclerotic lines not only involve the vertebral body but may extend into the posterior elements, i.e., the laminae, the transverse or spinous processes, and the pedicles.[88] On CT images, the thickened trabeculae give a dotted appearance to the vertebral bodies.

Since these lesions are so common, they are usually seen incidentally and are of no clinical significance. On both T1 and T2 weighted noncontrast images, these lesions have increased signal intensity. This high signal reflects the fatty component of this lesion, not a hemorrhagic component. Portions of the tumor within the bony confines may have a somewhat mottled appear-

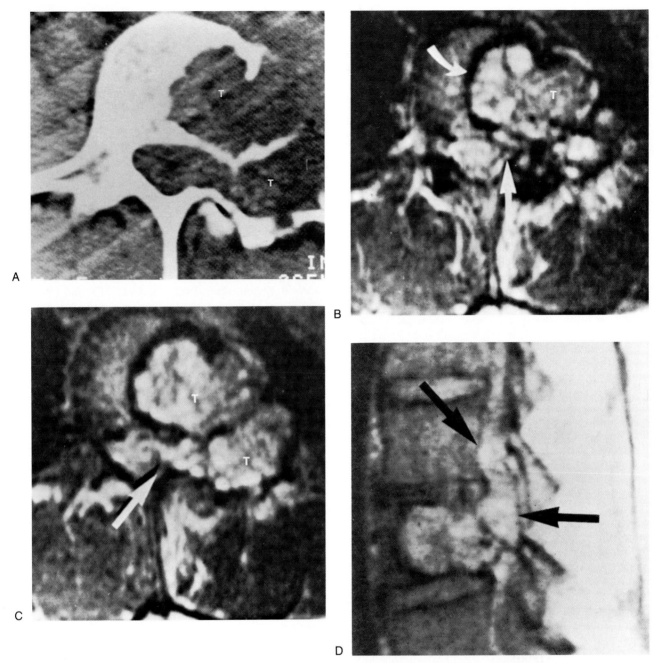

Figure 16–4. *Aneurysmal bone cyst of L3 with paraspinal extension.* ***A,*** Axial CT scan obtained without intrathecal contrast material. This shows osseous extension of the tumor (T), but spinal canal invasion cannot be confirmed. ***B, C,*** Axial MR images (SE 1500/60) at two different levels of L3 demonstrate the relationship between the tumor (T) and the thecal sac (*straight arrows*). Note the bubbly appearance of the tumor, with small cysts of different signal intensity. The interface between the psoas muscle and the tumor is better demonstrated on MRI imaging than on CT. Observe the band of decreased signal intensity (*curved arrow* in ***B***) between the tumor and vertebral body, representing the rim of sclerosis. ***D,*** Left parasagittal MR image (SE 1500/20) shows the superior extension of the tumor into the spinal canal (*arrows*). (Beltran J, Noto AM, Chakeres DW, Christoforidis AJ. Tumors of the osseous spine: staging with MR imaging versus CT. Radiology 1987; 162:565–569.)

ance.[87] MRI shows paravertebral extension of the mass as well as any epidural tumor. Spinal cord or thecal sac compression or displacement is readily identified.

Treatment

Asymptomatic lesions are left untreated. Therapy for symptomatic lesions with cord compression is controversial. They may be treated with surgical decompressive laminectomy, but since this procedure frequently leads to much blood loss, radiation therapy is another consideration.

Giant Cell Tumor

Giant cell tumors represent 3 to 7 percent of all primary bone tumors.[92–94] These lesions are uncommon in young children and usually occur in patients after epiphyseal closure.[94, 95] In a study of 218 patients, 74 percent were between 13 and 39 years of age.[96] Specifically, 38 of 218 patients were 13 to 19 years old, 74 were 20 to 29, and 51 were 30 to 39.[96] There is a slight female predominance: 125 of 218 patients.[94–96]

These tumors are most common around the knee (98 of 209 cases).[96, 97] Besides the long bones, other sites include the skull, talus, pelvis, spine, and sacrum.[93, 95, 96] This lesion is the most common benign tumor to involve the sacrum (11 of 209 patients).[96, 97] Giant cell tumors less often involve spine (two of 25 patients and three of 209).[95, 96]

Clinical Findings

Overall, pain and an enlarging mass are the most common symptoms.[94, 96–98] Initially the pain is intermittent and relieved by rest, but it eventually becomes persistent.[96] Pain can be present weeks to months before diagnosis.[94, 96–98]

Pathology

Giant cell tumor is characterized by multinucleated giant cells.[93, 96] Giant cells are not specific to this lesion but are found in numerous lesions including chondroblastoma, chondromyxoid fibroma, aneurysmal bone cyst, and osteosarcoma.[94] The malignant portion of the tumor, however, is composed of spindle-shaped mononuclear fibroblastic mesenchymal cells.[96] In their review of giant cell tumors McInerney and colleagues state that the aggressiveness of this lesion is determined by the stromal cells.[94]

Imaging

Plain films show a lytic lesion with a "soap-bubble" appearance; rarely, the border of this lesion is sclerotic.[94] There is thinning of the cortex.[94] Plain films show a soft tissue mass in 48 percent of patients. Since these lesions are usually very vascular, arteriography can be used to demonstrate an associated soft tissue component, but this study is invasive and can be falsely

negative in nonvascular tumors.[94] CT may show an associated soft tissue mass regardless of its vascularity.[99]

MRI is noninvasive and is better able to demonstrate the bony and soft tissue components of the lesion. Unenhanced T1 weighted images may show the extent of the tumor within the bone, since the lesion displaces the normal higher signal of fat-containing marrow.[100] Enhanced T1 weighted images show the high signal enhancing soft tissue mass separate from adjacent low-signal bony structures (Fig. 16–5). MRI also helps to demonstrate tumor recurrence after curettage.[98]

Treatment

The usual treatment for this tumor is curretage.[94, 97] If surgery is not optimal owing to the location or to numerous recurrences, radiation therapy may be employed.[97]

Sacrococcygeal Teratomas

Sacrococcygeal teratomas are rare tumors of childhood that occur in one in 40,000 births.[101] They arise from multipotential cells of Hensen's node, which comes to lie within the coccyx.[101, 102] As a result, the soft tissue mass is frequently accompanied by bony abnormalities of the coccyx. The surgical section of the American Academy of Pediatrics has devised the following grading system: type 1 tumors are almost always completely external; type 2 have a pelvic portion, but again almost all of the tumor is external; type 3 are predominantly intrapelvic; type 4 have no external portion, and almost all of the tumor is intrapelvic.[103]

Overall, there is a 4:1 female predominance.[101, 103, 104] Most sacrococcygeal teratomas are benign and identified at birth.[23] Malignant lesions tend to be more common in males.[103] Malignancy is also more common in lesions with a greater internal component (types 3 and 4), with a long delay in diagnosis and treatment, and finally with more solid and fewer cystic components.[23, 102, 103]

Pathology

Grossly, these tumors can be cystic, cystic and solid, or solid. They are derived from all three germ layers and most frequently contain neural, squamous, or intestinal epithelium. They may contain skin, appendages, teeth, or calcification.

Imaging

Plain films show an abnormal or absent coccyx with an adjacent soft tissue mass. The mass may lie in a presacral location and displace the urinary bladder or bowel loops.[103] The solid portions of this tumor are calcified in 60 percent of patients. Calcification is more common in benign lesions.[104, 105]

CT and MRI again show the lesion in close proximity

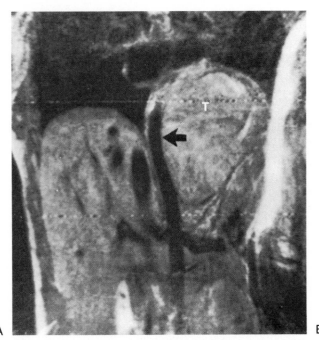
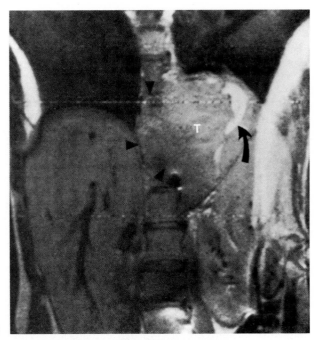

A
B

Figure 16–5. *Recurrent giant cell tumor involving T12 and L1 with large left paraspinal extension.* ***A, B,*** Coronal MR images (SE 2000/25) at the level of the abdominal aorta and vertebral bodies, respectively. Note the displacement of the aorta *(straight arrow)* by the tumor (T). Vertebral invasion is seen in ***B*** *(arrowheads)*. High-intensity signal *(curved arrow)* is due to areas of necrosis and hemorrhage within the tumor (T). (Beltran J, Noto AM, Chakeres DW, Christoforidis AJ. Tumors of the osseous spine: staging with MR imaging versus CT. Radiology 1987; 162:565–569.)

to the coccyx and disclose the intrapelvic or external components of the lesion. Calcifications may be present. The lesion may be entirely solid or may have cystic components. While cysts generally appear of decreased intensity on T1 weighted images and increased intensity on T2 weighted images, some variability may exist, depending on the cyst contents (Fig. 16–6). Solid portions of the tumor may enhance.

Treatment

Treatment of benign lesions consists of immediate surgical excision. Expeditious therapy is required since these tumors have increased malignant potential with age. Ninety percent contain malignant tissue at 2 months of age compared with 10 percent at birth.[23] The prognosis for benign lesions is excellent, although there may be morbidity secondary to surgical damage of the sacral plexus[106] or to severe blood loss at the time of surgery, owing to the vascular nature of these tumors.[105]

Malignant sacrococcygeal teratomas are initially excised, but can metastasize to the lungs, to vertebral bodies, and to regional lymph nodes.[106] They then carry an extremely poor prognosis, since there is very limited response to chemotherapy or radiation therapy.[103]

Ewing's Sarcoma

Ewing's sarcoma is a primary malignancy of bone affecting children and young adults. It is the second most common primary malignant bone tumor after osteosarcoma in younger individuals, and represents 7 to 15 percent of all primary bone malignancies.[35] There is a definite racial predilection: this lesion is rarely seen in black children.[107] Overall, Ewing's sarcoma has an incidence of 3.04 cases per million people per year in the Caucasian population. These tumors most commonly occur in individuals 15 to 25 years of age;[35, 58, 108–110] 66 percent are seen in the first two decades. The youngest patient from the Mayo Clinic series of 229 patients was 14 months old.[111] Ewing's sarcoma is rarely seen in children under 5 years of age.[58, 108, 109] There is a male predominance of 54 to 72 percent.[58, 108–110]

Any bone in the body may be involved. Long bones are most frequently affected, especially the femur;[110–112] other common locations include the iliac bone, the scapula, and the ribs.[108–110] These lesions do not often occur in the spine (4 percent) or in the sacrum (1 to 2 percent).[108, 110]

Metastases may be present in 10 percent of patients,[109] most commonly involving the skeleton and

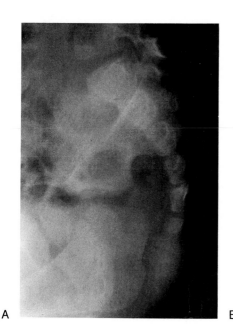

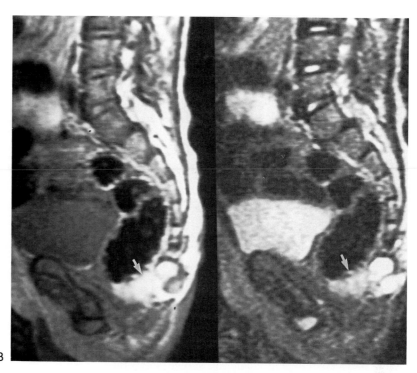

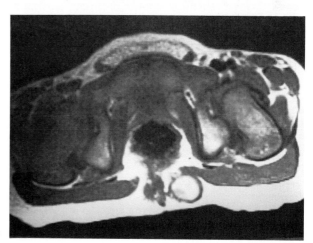

Figure 16–6. *Sacrococcygeal teratoma.* ***A,*** Lateral plain film of the sacrum in this 2-year-old boy reveals absence of the coccyx. ***B,*** Sagittal proton density and T2 weighted images (2000/30/80) show small well-defined, high-signal lesions inferior (*arrows*) to the sacrum. These lesions have signal intensity higher than that of fluid. ***C,*** Axial T1 weighted image (600/20) shows a well-defined rounded mass posterior to the rectum. The high signal may be due to fat. Adjacent intermediate soft-tissue-intensity tumor is less well defined.

lung (92 and 93 of 229 patients, respectively).[111] Bony metastases usually involve the skull or spine, accounting for the frequency of spinal cord compression in preterminal cases.[111] Other areas of metastasis include lymph nodes and soft tissues.[109]

Clinical Findings

Clinically, these lesions usually present with pain.[108,109,111] Initially the pain is an intermittent dull ache that, if untreated, becomes constant and severe.[109,111] Since the initial symptoms are nonspecific, significant delays in diagnosis can result. Focal tenderness with swelling and a palpable mass may also be seen.[111] There may be an associated low-grade fever and increased sedimentation rate.[109,111] Because of this, Ewing's sarcoma frequently is confused with inflammatory processes such as osteomyelitis.[108,109]

Pathology

Grossly, these tumors are soft, gray-white masses.[111] Histologically, they are composed of small, round cells that may arise from mesenchymal connective tissue.[111] These highly anaplastic lesions are very cellular, containing numerous cells with scant cytoplasm and little stroma.[107,111] There is still controversy regarding the cell of origin.[112] There may be areas of hemorrhage, necrosis, and cyst formation within these lesions.[111]

Imaging

Plain films show mottled lytic changes (88 of 107 patients) and an associated soft tissue mass (52 of 107).[48, 109, 111, 113] The "onion-peel" periosteal reaction (35 of 107 patients) is classic.[109] This laminated periosteum is reactive in nature and not secondary to actual bony proliferation by malignant cells.[58] Since the tumor quickly transgresses the bony margins, an adjacent soft tissue mass is often seen.[114]

The diagnosis is frequently uncertain from plain films since the "pathognomonic" findings often are not present. In a series of 26 patients, 16 (62 percent) showed only lytic areas and did not show the classic "onion-peel" reaction. Although plain films may show lytic bony changes, periosteal reaction, or an associated soft tissue mass, the associated soft tissue mass often is not well defined on plain films alone.[48, 109, 111, 113] In addition, plain films are unable to evaluate the extent of disease within the marrow cavity, information that is vital for adjusting radiation portals.[113, 114] Biopsy is needed to confirm the diagnosis regardless of the findings on imaging.

Because this tumor spreads rapidly through the medullary marrow over relatively long distances within bone, the ideal imaging technique should show the extent of involvement so that appropriate treatment may be devised. CT shows the soft tissue mass associated with the bony lesion; however, it is limited in its evaluation of the disease within the marrow cavity.[114] MRI successfully demonstrates marrow invasion. On MRI, Ewing's sarcoma is of decreased signal intensity on T1 weighted images and increased signal intensity on T2 weighted images. It can be differentiated from surrounding normal marrow. The tumor can be inhomogeneous secondary to hemorrhage, calcification, or necrosis. Soft tissue paraskeletal masses are readily evident.

Treatment

The prognosis depends on the location of the lesion. Overall, lesions in the extremities carry a better prognosis since they are more accessible to surgical amputation.[111] The 5-year survival rate for tumors in the extremities is 22 percent compared with 8 percent elsewhere.[111]

The primary treatment for Ewing's sarcoma, if amputation is not possible or is unsuccessful, is radiation therapy. This tumor is so sensitive to radiation that exposure to therapy before biopsy may cause problems with histologic recognition of this tumor.[109] Radiation therapy may also decrease symptoms such as pain and any associated soft tissue mass.[109]

Eosinophilic Granuloma

Eosinophilic granuloma (Langerhans Cell Histiocytosis) is a non-neoplastic condition, the cause of which is uncertain.[115] In one series of 28 patients, the disorder was most frequently seen in those 6 to 10 years old.[116] In another series of 46 patients, 38 percent were under 10 years of age and the youngest patient was 6 months old.[115] Overall, there is a male predilection.[115–118]

Clinical Findings

Symptoms are extremely variable, ranging from nonexistent to severe.[60, 115, 116, 118] The most common symptom is localized pain, especially when the skull and ribs are involved.[60, 115, 116, 118, 119] Tenderness can be seen with or without an associated soft tissue mass.[115, 117–119] Other symptoms include headache and fatigability.[115, 119] The duration of the symptoms may be days to months.[115] Signs include fever, weight loss, and increased sedimentation rate.[60, 115, 116]

These lesions may be single or multiple. In a study of 46 patients, 36 had solitary and 10 had multiple lesions.[115] Overall, the skull, pelvis, vertebrae, ribs, and long bones may be involved.[115, 116, 118] When the lesions are multiple, the ribs and vertebrae are more commonly involved, frequently at numerous levels.[115] With spinal lesions, collapse of the vertebral body may result in spinal cord compression, nerve root impingement, and deformity of the spine.[115, 118, 120] Lesions of the spine, skull, and ribs are more likely than lesions located elsewhere to be associated with soft tissue swelling.[115] There is one reported case of leptomeningeal spread of diffuse histiocytosis with cervical disease seen in the subarachnoid space.[121]

Pathology

Grossly, these lesions have cystic and hemorrhagic areas.[115, 119] The cysts may be 1 to 4 cm in size and are filled with lipid and blood, having a yellow to reddish-brown appearance.[60, 115, 122] As they evolve, intermittent lesions have increased amounts of lipid and finally heal with bone formation in the later stages.[115]

On a cellular basis there are initially a large number of eosinophils.[115, 123] Subsequently, in the intermediate phase, the number of eosinophils decreases and numerous large, vacuolated, foamy macrophages appear.[115, 123] Finally, in the healing stages, connective tissue is present, with bone formation occurring.[115, 123]

Imaging

Plain films show round or oval, sharply marginated, lytic, punched-out lesions with well-defined borders.[115, 118] These lesions may be solitary or multiple and there may or may not be an associated soft tissue mass.[115] When the vertebral body is involved, it is usually affected in its entirety.[60] This weakens the vertebral body and may result in collapse, with vertebra plana.[60] There may be unusual angulation to the spine and resultant deformity. Associated epidural hematoma may cause spinal cord compression.

CT shows findings similar to the plain films and better demonstrates any associated soft tissue mass (Figs. 16–7, 16–8).[124] MRI offers more information, especially regarding possible spinal cord compression. Lesions are usually of decreased signal intensity on T1

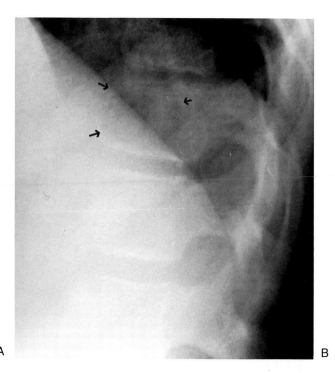

A

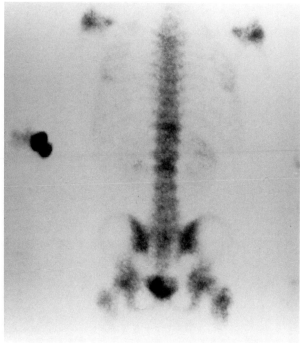

B

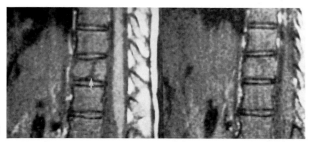

C

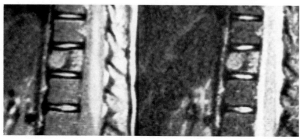

D

Figure 16–7. *Langerhans cell histiocytosis (eosinophilic granuloma).* ***A,*** Lateral plain film of the thoracolumbar region in this 10-year-old boy shows a lytic lesion (*arrows*) involving the anterior aspect of the T11 vertebral body. ***B,*** Bone scan (posterior image) shows increased activity in several vertebral bodies. ***C,*** Sagittal T1 weighted image (600/20) confirms the mild compression of the T11 vertebral body and discloses a lower signal cleft (*arrow*) representing the fracture through the midportion. ***D,*** Sagittal proton density and T2 weighted images (1800/30/80) show that the T11 vertebral body now has increased signal.

weighted images and increased signal intensity on T2 weighted images, unless hemorrhage is present; they are frequently indistinguishable in appearance from metastatic disease (Figs. 16–7 to 16–9).[125]

Osteosarcoma

Osteosarcoma occurs most commonly in the 10- to 20-year-old age group.[126] It is the most common primary malignant bone tumor in the pediatric population.[127] In the 1967 Mayo Clinic series of 600 cases of osteosarcoma, 285 cases occurred in patients 10 to 19 years old.[127] The youngest patient in this series was 4 years of age and several other children were between 4 and 5 years of age.[127] In another series of 552 patients, one-third were seen in the second decade of life; in this study, the median age at diagnosis was 26 years.[127, 128]

This tumor has a male predilection:[126, 129, 130] in the Mayo Clinic series, 373 cases were seen in males and 227 in females.[127]

Clinical Findings

The most common locations for this tumor are in the long bones; 50 percent are at the knee.[100, 128] Very rarely, this tumor originates in the spine; two out of 552 cases in the study from Memorial Sloan-Kettering Cancer Center and six out of 430 cases from the Mayo Clinic series involved the spine.[100, 129] There were only five reported cases of primary osteogenic sarcoma of the spine between the years 1925 and 1976.[131] Metastatic disease to the spine from osteogenic sarcoma arising elsewhere is very common, however.

Osteosarcomas may arise within bone that has been previously irradiated (16 of 600 patients in the Mayo Clinic series.[127, 128] There is usually a 5- to 25-year

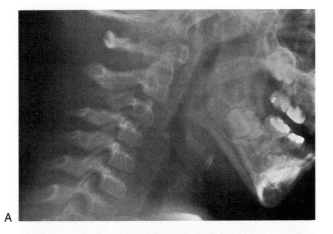

A

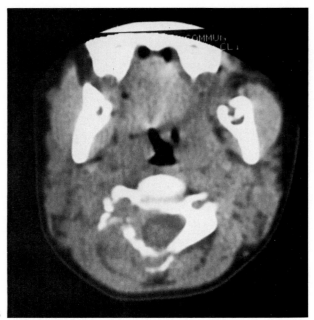

B

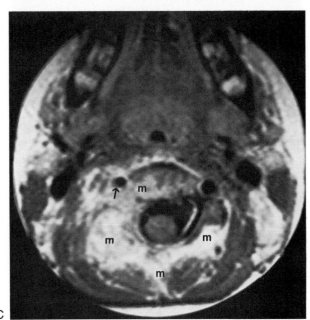

C

Figure 16–8. *Langerhans cell histiocytosis (eosinophilic granuloma) in a patient with a history of pain in the cervical spine.* **A,** Lateral radiograph shows destruction of the spinous process of the third cervical vertebra. **B,** CT scan shows a destructive lesion involving the posterior lateral and anterior parts of the third cervical vertebra. There is an adjacent soft tissue mass. **C,** Transverse T1 image (750/26) at the level of C3, obtained after intravenous gadolinium-DTPA injection, shows a mass lesion (m) hyperintense with soft tissue. There is invasion of the spinous process lamina, lateral mass, and part of the body of the C3 vertebra on both sides, with extension into the adjacent soft tissues. There is anterior displacement of the right vertebral artery (*arrow*). The spinal cord (C) appears normal. MRI shows more abnormality than CT.

latent period after the irradiation before the osteosarcoma develops.[127] Osteosarcomas may arise in osteochondromata, as in two of the 600 patients in the Mayo Clinic series.[127] Osteochondromas that become painful and show swelling should be regarded with suspicion.[129]

Pathology

Grossly, these lesions are calcified and firm. They are composed primarily of sarcomatous connective tissue that forms osteoid or bone, the amount of which may be extremely variable.[131] These tumors can be further subcategorized on the basis of their predominant histologic differentiation.[131] In the Mayo Clinic series involving osteosarcomas of all ages, 55 percent were osteoblastic, 23 percent fibroblastic, and 22 percent chondroblastic.[100]

Imaging

Plain film findings are nonspecific. CT may show osteoblastic or osteolytic bony changes. There may or may not be an associated soft tissue mass within either the epidural space or the paraspinal region.[132]

As with other invasive bone tumors, MRI is superior to CT in demonstrating the extent of osteosarcoma within the marrow space.[133] The degree of osteoid, bone, cartilage, or fibrotic tissue affects its appearance on MRI. MRI readily shows infiltration of low-signal tumor into the high-signal marrow cavity.[54, 126] In younger patients, normal marrow may appear of somewhat low intensity, since it is primarily hematopoietic and has a paucity of fat. In these patients, T2 weighted sequences, short T1 inversion recovery sequences, or gradient-echo sequences may provide additional information. With these sequences, normal marrow ap-

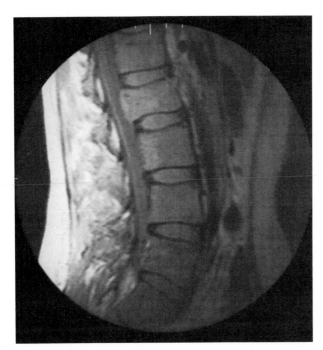

Figure 16–9. *Medulloblastoma bone metastasis.* Spin density image (1550/20) in the sagittal plane reveals areas of moderate increase in signal intensity at several levels, with partial collapse of L2 and encroachment into the spinal canal.

fibrotic or has sclerotic areas, such as seen in osteoblastic sarcoma.[54, 126] When the normal signal void of cortical bone is infiltrated by tumor, a mottled appearance results.[134] T1 weighted images after gadolinium-DTPA administration are not as useful as unenhanced T1 weighted images in showing the bony extent of the tumor, since the signal intensity of enhancing lesion may approach that of fatty marrow.[135, 136] Areas of periosteal reaction or of cortical thinning or cortical expansion may be shown on MRI as areas of low signal.[126, 133] Multiple imaging planes may also be employed to better document the extent of disease within the bone and the adjacent soft tissue.[54, 133]

MRI is also extremely sensitive for delineating tumor extension into the paraspinal soft tissue masses.[54, 131] Although the tumor may be hypointense or isointense with muscle, obliteration of normal fat planes may indicate extension of the neoplasm out of the vertebral bodies (Fig. 16–10).[126, 136] However, after administration of gadolinium-DTPA, these highly vascular malignancies often show immediate intense enhancement.[131, 135] The enhancing tumor now is readily separable on T1 weighted images from the lower signal intensity of muscle, which only minimally enhances.[135] Enhancing areas on T1 weighted images reflect the more vascular and probably the more "aggressive" viable areas of the tumor.[135] Biopsy is usually directed at these areas in order to best characterize the mass.[135] Associated necrotic or sclerotic areas either slowly enhance or fail to enhance.[135] These groups can be separated, since on T2 weighted images necrotic and cystic areas have increased signal, while sclerotic

pears of lower signal intensity and the lesions stand out as of higher intensity in comparison. However, occasionally the tumor may also be of very low signal intensity on some of these sequences if the lesion is primarily

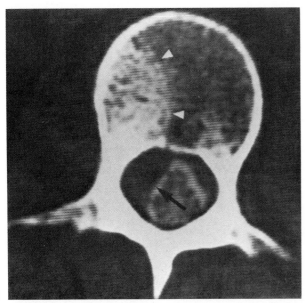

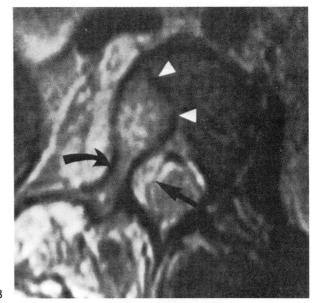

A   B

Figure 16–10. *Metastatic osteosarcoma to L2 with spinal canal invasion.* ***A, B,*** Axial metrizamide-enhanced CT scan and axial MR image (SE 1500/60). Both studies demonstrate greater than 25 percent involvement of the vertebral body (*arrowheads*); each also shows obliteration of the epidural fat by tumor and compression of the thecal sac (*straight arrows*). Only MRI demonstrates involvement of the right pedicle and transverse process (*curved arrow*). Note the extension of the tumor into the right paraspinal area on both images. (Beltran J, Noto AM, Chakeres DW, Christoforidis AJ. Tumors of the osseous spine: staging with MR imaging versus CT. Radiology 1987; 162:565–569.)

areas have decreased signal.[135] Finally, peritumoral edema may be seen on T2 weighted images.[133, 135] MRI is not as good as CT in showing associated calcification within the tumor or in defining the bony margins of the tumor.[133]

Treatment

Therapy for osteosarcoma in an extremity initially involves surgery, but when the spine is involved, generally only chemotherapy or radiation therapy is given, or both.

After radiation therapy there are histopathologic changes within the bone marrow of the spinal vertebrae. The cellular marrow within the vertebral body is eventually replaced by fatty marrow. This results in increased signal intensity within the vertebral body, most apparent on T1 weighted images.[137] This change may occur rapidly, as reported in one patient in whom the change was seen on T1 weighted images 9 days after 1 month of radiation therapy with 3,000 cGy.[11] As a result of the increased signal intensity on T1 weighted images, any recurrent or residual tumor is even more apparent owing to the greater contrast between the high signal intensity of fatty replaced vertebral body marrow and the low-signal-intensity tumor.

Chondrosarcoma

Chondrosarcomas account for 7 to 20 percent of all primary bone tumors.[138, 139] Overall, these are the third most common primary bone tumor after multiple myeloma and osteosarcoma.[139] There is a slight male predilection.[138, 140, 141] Peak incidence is in the third to sixth decade.[139–142] In a series of 493 cases of chondrosarcoma collected over a 54-year period at the Memorial Sloan-Kettering Cancer Center, only 79 (16 percent) occurred in patients under 21 years of age. In this group the age range was 5 years to 20 years, with an average of 16 years.[138]

Chondrosarcoma may arise as a primary de novo lesion or as a secondary lesion from a preexisting cartilaginous lesion,[143] especially osteochondromas or enchondromas. The incidence of malignant generation is 1 percent for a solitary osteochondroma and 5 to 25 percent for multiple hereditary exostosis.[141] In the 1987 Memorial Sloan-Kettering Cancer Center series, 71 percent of all chondrosarcomas were of the primary type in patients under 21 years of age, compared with 63 percent in adults.[138] Secondary chondrosarcomas occur slightly less often in children.[138, 141]

Chondrosarcoma rarely arises in the spine.[138, 140, 144–146] In the Sloan-Kettering study, only 3.8 percent of cases in children and 2.6 percent in adults involved the spine.[138] Camins and associates reviewed several series of patients with chondrosarcoma involving the spine and found a fairly equal distribution of cases throughout the spine.[146] Of 34 cases, eight were in the cervical region, six in the cervicothoracic junction, seven in the thoracic region, five in the lumbar region, and eight in the sacrum.[146]

Clinical Findings

The signs and symptoms are nonspecific. Pain is the most frequent symptom and frequently is mild, leading to a delay in evaluation.[140, 146] A palpable mass may be present.[140, 146] When the lesion involves the spine, there may be signs of spinal cord compression.[144, 146]

Imaging

These lesions are lytic, with sclerotic borders, and have a calcified matrix;[140, 146] the amount of calcification varies according to the differentiation of the tumor.[29, 143, 146] Frequently there is an associated soft tissue mass.

CT can often help distinguish between a malignant chondrosarcoma and a benign osteochondroma.[29] This distinction is critical, especially in multiple hereditary exostosis. Malignant lesions tend to have large soft tissue masses, irregular disorganized calcifications, destruction of bone, and growth into adjacent soft tissues.[146] The cortical margins may appear irregular and discontinuous with the parent bone. The thin cartilaginous cap typical of benign osteochondromas is usually not seen.

On MRI, the T1 signal intensity of chondrosarcomas may be increased as a result of their cartilaginous nature.[147] Focal areas of decreased signal intensity on T2 weighted images may be seen when the calcifications are very prominent.[147] Areas of hemorrage also contribute to the overall heterogeneity of this lesion. Again, MRI is excellent at defining an associated soft tissue mass.[136]

Leukemia

Leukemia is the most common malignancy in children, with an incidence of 42 cases per million in the United States.[148, 149] Each year, 4,000 new cases are diagnosed.[150] One-third of childhood neoplastic deaths are caused by leukemia.[151] There is a greater incidence of leukemia in Caucasian children. Acute lymphoblastic leukemia (ALL) represents 80 percent of all childhood leukemia; acute myelogenous leukemia accounts for 10 percent of the other cases.[148, 152, 153] The greatest incidence of ALL is in the 2- to 5-year-old age group, with a peak at 3 years.[153] There is a slight male predilection in ALL.[152–154]

Clinical Findings

Children with leukemia are systemically ill.[148] As leukemic cells proliferate, they replace normal bone marrow, resulting in abnormally low production of all cellular components.[152] Clinically, this manifests with increased susceptibility to infection, thrombocytopenia, anemia, pallor, and fatigue.[149, 152, 155] Splenomegaly and hepatomegaly are often noted.[154] Spinal involvement may cause local pain and swelling.[148,151,154] The pain may be migratory in nature and associated with swelling, thus mimicking juvenile rheumatoid arthritis.[154]

Imaging

Infiltration of the spine by leukemic cells results in osteoporosis, seen in 60 percent of cases.[148,151,155] There is also a decreased number of bony trabeculae within the vertebral bodies.[151,148] The infiltration and decreased number of trabeculae together can weaken the vertebral body and lead to compression fractures.[151] In addition, lucent bands may be seen in the spine;[148] this lucency does not represent actual tumoral deposit but rather impaired enchondral bone formation with abnormally small trabeculae.[151,154,155] Multiple focal lucencies of varying size may be seen within the marrow cavity, secondary to actual leukemic infiltrates.[151] Osteosclerotic areas secondary to increased trabecular formation may rarely be noted.[151,154]

MRI shows a homogeneous decreased signal on T1 weighted images secondary to replacement of the high-signal fatty marrow by low-signal leukemic cells (Fig. 16-11).[156-158] Young children, especially those under 7 years of age, may have a paucity of fat in the marrow. In these patients, leukemia infiltration may be more

difficult to detect. Enhancement with gadolinium-DTPA may be useful, since diffuse tumor infiltration enhances while normal marrow does not. Compression deformities of the vertebral bodies may be seen as a result of axial forces on the weakened vertebral body (Fig. 16-12). Foci of leukemic infiltration are of increased signal intensity on T2 weighted images.[158] Dense sclerotic foci may occur and yield low signal intensity on T1 and T2 weighted images.

Moore examined T1 relaxation times in 17 children with ALL: eight with new ALL, four with ALL in relapse, and five with ALL in remission.[158] In this study the authors found a significant increase in the T1 relaxation times of spine marrow in patients with newly diagnosed ALL or ALL in relapse over healthy children or patients with ALL in remission. Although iliac crest or bone biopsies are still necessary for the initial diagnosis and characterization of the tumor, MR relaxation times may be helpful in following the phases of this disease.[158] Specifically, MRI can help distinguish children with inactive disease or healthy children from children with active disease, eliminating the necessity of serial bone biopsies. T2 weighted images were not helpful in distinguishing the different stages of the disease.[158]

Most authors agree that bone involvement with leu-

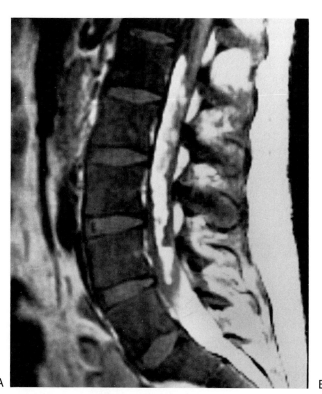
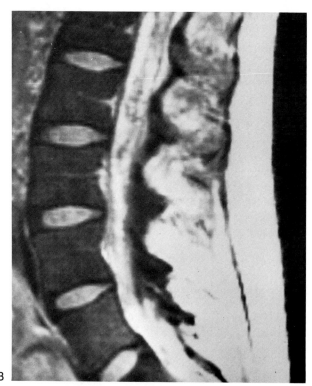

A   B

Figure 16-11. *Diffuse leukemic infiltration.* **A,** Sagittal T1 weighted image (800/20) shows diffuse low signal to the vertebral bodies, which are now of lower signal intensity than the adjacent intervertebral disc. Incidentally noted is blood in the subarachnoid space following lumbar puncture in this patient with a very low platelet count. **B,** Sagittal proton density (2000/35) image again shows the vertebral bodies to be of low signal intensity, and again blood in the subarachnoid space.

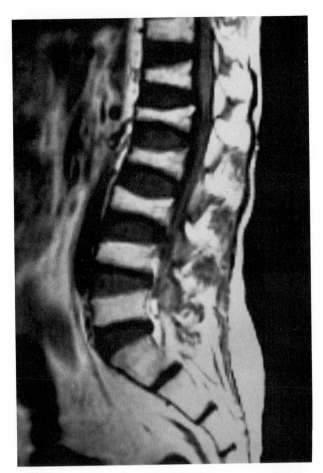

Figure 16–12. *Leukemia in remission.* Sagittal T1 weighted image (600/20) shows multiple vertebral body compression deformities in this 13-year-old boy with leukemia in remission. Radiation change is evidenced by increased signal intensity within the vertebral bodies.

kemic cells at the initial time of presentation does not influence the prognosis, although one study found a worse outcome in patients who had early osseous involvement.[159] Even if bony involvement is shown, treatment generally remains systemic chemotherapy. In selected patients bone marrow transplants may be performed.[160]

Non-Hodgkin's Lymphoma

Non-Hodgkin's lymphoma may involve bone primarily as an isolated lesion or secondarily as part of a systemic disease.[148] It occurs in approximately seven individuals per million population.[150] Each year 400 new cases of non-Hodgkin's lymphoma in children are diagnosed.[161]

Primary non-Hodgkin's lymphoma, previously referred to as reticulum cell sarcoma of bone, is more

frequently seen in older age groups, 93 percent of cases occurring in patients over 20 years of age.[148,162] Males are affected twice as commonly as females.[163] Primary non-Hodgkin's lymphoma usually occurs in long bones, although 13 of 94 cases reported in several series occurred in the spine.[162–165] These patients often have pain and swelling of the involved area but characteristically lack constitutional symptoms.[148,151,163,164] The tumor is grossly gray-pink in color and has frequent areas of necrosis.[164] It is highly cellular and has a very vascular stroma.[164]

Non-Hodgkin's lymphoma may also affect the spine in the form of metastatic disease. The peak incidence in the pediatric population is in children 5 to 9 years of age, with a second peak in the teenage years.[166–168] Greater involvement of the axial than of the appendicular skeleton is seen in secondary non-Hodgkin's lymphoma, with involvement of the facial bones, skull, ribs, and spine.[148]

This aggressive tumor grows rapidly; there are symptoms for a short time before diagnosis. These include bone pain, weakness, fatigue, abdominal pain, weight loss, cough, and symptoms referable to the central nervous system.[167] Signs include intestinal obstruction, lymphadenopathy, splenomegaly, anemia, leukocytosis, and thrombocytopenia.[169]

There is osseous involvement in 20 percent of children at the time of diagnosis; 25 percent eventually develop bony disease sometime during the illness.[148] Lesions of the spine are seen in 40 percent of cases with osseous involvement.[156]

Imaging

There is a wide spectrum of plain film radiographic manifestations of osseous non-Hodgkin's lymphoma, including changes ranging from a permeative moth-eaten appearance to a more lytic geographic area of bony destruction.[148,151,162,170] Pathologic fractures may be seen and are more common than in Hodgkin's disease.[151,171] Osteosclerotic lesions are uncommon and are characteristically less dense than those seen in Hodgkin's disease.[151] MR findings are described below with those of Hodgkin's disease.

Hodgkin's Disease

Hodgkin's disease has an incidence of six cases per million population in the United States.[150] This is, however, an unusual neoplasm in the pediatric age group.[172] The peak incidence is in the 20- to 30-year-old age group, with a second peak in the seventh decade.[173] About 10 percent of all cases of Hodgkin's disease occur in children under 10 years of age.[152] There is a male predominance of 1.5 to 1.[173]

The initial sign is palpable lymphadenopathy. Later, fever, abdominal pain, pallor, anemia, leukocytosis, and anorexia may be seen.[152] Only about 1 percent of patients show osseous involvement at the time of diagnosis, although 10 to 30 percent of children develop bony involvement at some time during the course of the disease.[148, 172] The vertebrae, especially the lower thoracic and lumbar spine, are the most frequently affected of the bones.[148, 151, 172] Bony involvement occurs either via direct spread from lymph nodes or by hematogenous dissemination.[172]

Imaging

On plain films overall, the lesions are usually mixed, osteolytic, and osteoblastic and frequently are multiple.[151] Vertebral lesions, however, tend to be mostly lytic, and therefore vertebral body collapse may be seen.[148, 151, 172] Scalloping of the vertebral body may result from contiguous para-aortic lymph node involvement.[151, 160] Generalized or localized bony sclerosis may occur, secondary to osseous involvement or myelofibrosis.[148, 151]

MRI OF NON-HODGKIN'S LYMPHOMA AND HODGKIN'S DISEASE. On MRI, both non-Hodgkin's lymphoma and Hodgkin's disease are typified by frequent vertebral body involvement. All these cellular lesions lead to infiltration of the normal high-signal-intensity fatty marrow of the vertebral bodies, and result in focal or diffuse areas of decreased signal intensity on T1 weighted images.[174] As the fatty marrow is replaced by cellular elements, the signal intensity decreases on T1 weighted images;[175-177] this is a sensitive but not a specific finding. On T2 weighted images, focal areas of tumor infiltrate have increased signal intensity.[175] Gadolinium-DTPA often is not helpful in delineating disease in the extradural compartment, since many extradural lesions may enhance and become isointense with the normal high signal intensity of fatty marrow, obscuring some of these lesions.[178, 179] However, gadolinium-DTPA may prove useful in particular cases. Specifically, enhancement may help characterize unusual lesions or direct biopsy.[179] In addition, studies after administration of gadolinium-DTPA may help document the response to therapy.[179]

INTRADURAL EXTRAMEDULLARY TUMORS

Neurofibroma

Neurinoma, neurofibroma, neurilemoma, and schwannoma are various names for tumors that arise from Schwann cells of nerve sheaths. Schwannoma, neuroma, and neurilemoma are synonyms, but schwannomas and neurofibromas are different entities.[180] Schwannomas do not envelop the adjacent nerve root, which is usually the dorsal sensory root; generally are solitary; and clinically are not associated with neurofibromatosis.[10, 181, 182] In contrast, neurofibromas envelop the dorsal sensory root, frequently are multiple, and are seen in neurofibromatosis.[180, 181, 183]

In the general population, neurofibromas are the most common intraspinal lesion, representing 16 to 30 percent of all intraspinal masses.[18, 62] These lesions most commonly present in the fourth decade of life.[182, 184]

Neurofibromas are less commonly seen in the pediatric population. Their incidence is probably less than 10 percent of all intraspinal lesions, although some authors report it to be as high as 29 percent.[6, 23] These tumors usually present in the teenage years.[6] The youngest patient reported was a 13-month-old female. In children, there is no sexual predilection. These tumors most commonly are intradural extramedullary in location (70 percent);[185] the remainder are purely extradural (14 percent), dumbbell-shaped with both an extradural and an intradural component (15 percent), and, rarely, intramedullary (1 percent).[6, 185] Harwood-Nash and Fitz reported 13 cases in children and found the most common location to be the cervical region, followed by the lumbar and thoracic regions.[6]

Neurofibromatosis is a phakomatosis that occurs spontaneously in 50 percent of patients and as an autosomal dominant condition in 50 percent. Skin manifestations consist of café au lait spots more than 15 mm in size; the presence of six or more spots is considered diagnostic. Patients with neurofibromatosis have a predisposition to other neoplasms in addition to neurofibromas, including intramedullary lesions such as astrocytomas, ependymomas, and hamartomas.[186]

Spinal findings in neurofibromatosis include posterior scalloping of the vertebral bodies, widening of the neural foramina, scoliosis, dural ectasia, and lateral meningoceles.[180, 186, 187] These last two lesions may look similar to neurofibromas on plain films. On CT, dural ectasia and lateral meningoceles may be difficult to differentiate from neurofibromas, since they both have low values on CT and present as paraspinal masses. However, on MRI this differentiation is readily made, since both dural ectasia and lateral meningoceles have signal intensities that parallel those of cerebrospinal fluid (CSF) on both T1 and T2 weighted images.[125, 186] In addition, after administration of gadolinium-DTPA, these two lesions do not enhance, whereas neurofibromas readily enhance. Lateral meningoceles can be shown to be in direct continuity with the thecal sac and do not result in displacement of the spinal cord.

Malignant degeneration is uncommon in neurofibromatosis, being seen in 2 to 12 percent of patients.[10, 22, 182, 188, 189] Malignant neoplasms arise either from neurofibromas or de novo from nerve sheaths. The varied terminology reflects controversy as to their origin; it includes malignant schwannoma, malignant neuroma, nerve sheath fibrocarcinoma, and neurofibrosarcoma. Developing neurofibrosarcoma probably has a latency period of 10 to 20 years.[188, 190] These malignant neural tumors are seen in the 15- to 39-year-old age group.[188] The 5-year survival rate is poor, between 15 and 30 percent.[188,190–192] Local recurrence and metastatic disease primarily to the lung, liver, and bone are common.[8] In patients with neurofibromatosis, therefore, it is important to make the distinction between large plexiform neurofibromas and neurofibrosarcoma.

Clinical Findings

The most frequent symptoms of neurofibromas are pain and radiculopathy, which are present for an average of 26 months before diagnosis.[183,184]

Pathology

Neurofibromas consist of mixtures of fibroblasts and proliferated Schwann cells between dispersed nerve fibers. The matrix of a neurofibroma contains acid mucopolysacharides and large amounts of tissue fluids with numerous fibrous strands. The matrix spreads apart the axons to produce the fusiform shape of the neurofibroma.

Imaging

On CT, neurofibromas are of decreased attenuation and present as paraspinal or intraspinal masses. Differentiation of the intraspinal portion of the neurofibromas from the adjacent spinal cord and thecal sac can be difficult without instillation of intrathecal contrast material.

Neurofibromas on MRI tend to have increased signal intensity compared with muscle on noncontrast T1 weighted images (in 11 of 12 patients).[186] The increased signal intensity on T1 weighted images may be secondary to shortening of the T1 by mucopolysaccharide molecules interacting with tissue water.[186] On T2 weighted images these lesions may have markedly increased signal intensity secondary to the high water content of these lesions.[186,193,194] Also frequently seen on T2 weighted images are central areas of decreased signal intensity (seven of 12 patients), which may represent more dense areas of collagen and Schwann cells as shown pathologically.[186] Decreased signal may result from the fact that fewer mobile protons are available within the fibrous matrix in the central portions of the lesions.[186] These lesions enhance intensely and fairly homogeneously,[195] and often are multiple. MRI demonstrates in superb detail the intraspinal portions of these tumors, especially on T1 weighted images after gadolinium-DTPA administration, and shows any displacement or compression of the spinal cord (Fig. 16–13).[194]

The most common spinal lesion in the differential diagnosis is a meningioma. Several criteria help to differentiate these two lesions. Neural tumors tend to be more anteriorly sited within the spinal cord, whereas spinal meningiomas have a posterolateral location except when they are in the cervical region, where they are more likely to be anterior.[196] Neurofibromas are often multiple whereas meningiomas tend to be solitary. Neurofibromas are not attached to the dura and therefore have more mobility than meningiomas.[183] Neurofibromas on T2 weighted images may have a central area of decreased attenuation not seen with meningiomas.

Imaging modalities can help differentiate plexiform neurofibromas from neurofibrosarcomas. On CT and MRI, both benign and malignant lesions show inhomogeneity,[186] but malignant schwannomas more often have irregular, infiltrative margins whereas benign lesions tend to have smooth margins.[190] Also, neurofibrosarcomas tend to lack the decreased central area of low signal intensity on T2 weighted images that is frequently noted in benign schwannomas.[186,190] Finally, neurofibrosarcomas tend to be larger than the benign lesions. Gallium scans may also be useful, since uptake is frequently seen in malignant tumors but not in their benign counterparts.[190]

Meningioma

Overall, meningiomas involving the CNS are rarely seen in the pediatric population. A review of 2,226 cases of CNS tumors involving children showed that only 19 were meningiomas.[9,197] In the younger age group, meningiomas are frequently associated with neurofibromatosis. Childhood meningiomas are usually intracranial lesions.[9,197] Meningiomas of the spinal canal are generally lesions of adults.[198] The average age of presentation is in the fifth and sixth decades, with 60 to 80 percent in females.[7,10,196,198] Roughly 3 to 6 percent of all spinal meningiomas occur in children. The thoracic region is involved in 82 to 90 percent of patients;[182,196] most of the remaining cases occur in the cervical region.[198]

Meningiomas in the spine tend to be encapsulated, are attached to the dura, do not invade the spinal cord but displace it, and usually are very small at presentation.[183] These lesions are usually posterolateral in location except those in the cervical region, which are more likely to be anterior. They are primarily intradural extramedullary (76 out of 84 cases) but may be both intradural and extradural (five out of 84) or, less likely, purely extradural (three out of 84).[198] When meningiomas are purely extradural, they tend to be malignant.[198] Rarely, spinal meningiomas may be multiple.[196]

Clinical Findings

The most common symptom is pain, either local or radicular.[196] Other findings include paresthesias, numbness, weakness, and bowel or bladder abnormalities.[196]

Pathology

Histologically, meningothelial, fibroblastic, psammomatous, and angiomatous types are seen,[10] and calcifications are noted in up to 72 percent of meningiomas.[198]

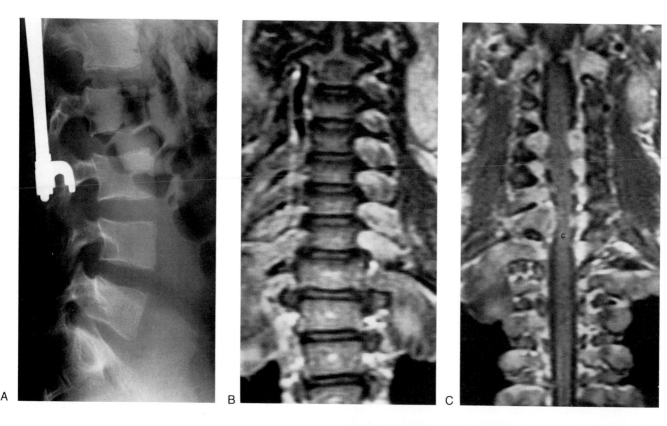

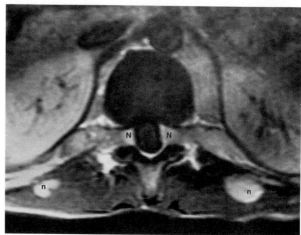

Figure 16–13. *Multiple neurofibromas with intraspinal extension.* ***A,*** Lateral plain film of the lumbar spine shows widening of all the neural foramina, erosion of the pedicles, and scalloping of the posterior portions of the L4 vertebral body. ***B, C,*** Coronal T1 weighted images (400/20) after gadolinium-DTPA administration show intraspinal extension of the neurofibromas in a "dumbbell" fashion with resultant compression of the spinal cord (C). ***D,*** Axial T1 weighted image (500/20) after gadolinium-DTPA shows bilateral neurofibromas (N) with intraspinal extension. Two enhancing neurofibromas (n) are seen in the posterior musculature.

Imaging

Meningiomas in the spine tend to be well circumscribed, are frequently located anterolateral or posterolateral to the spinal cord, and tend to displace it.[198] MRI shows bony abnormalities associated with these lesions, such as pedicle erosion and widening of the neural foramina, although these changes are more commonly seen with neurofibromas.[10] T1 weighted images show the lesions to be hypo- to isointense, and T2 weighted images to be slightly hyperintense, to the spinal cord.[199] In the intradural extramedullary location they are silhouetted against the high signal intensity of the CSF on T2 weighted images. These vascular tumors usually enhance immediately, intensely, and homogeneously after gadolinium-DTPA administration.[199, 200] There may be areas of signal void representing calcifications, especially in the psammomatous type.[198]

Spinal Subarachnoid Tumor

The most common cause of subarachnoid seeding is the primary intracranial neoplasm.[201, 202] In the pediatric population, the most common intracranial tumor to yield subarachnoid seeding is the medulloblastoma.[203] Eleven to 44 percent of patients have spinal leptomeningeal metastases at the time of initial diagnosis of the primary intracranial medulloblastoma.[203] The reason for this large discrepancy is unclear, but may be related to a multitude of factors, including the size of the original lesion at the time of diagnosis, variation in surgical techniques among institutions, and the temporal relationship of the myelogram to the initial surgery.[203]

Other primary CNS lesions in childhood that have been shown to metastasize to the leptomeninges of the spine include the more aggressive lesions, such as the primitive neuroectodermal tumors, ependymoma, oligodendroglioma, choroid plexus papilloma, and malignant glioma.[201,204] Rarely, even benign tumors may seed the subarachnoid space. In 42 cases of subarachnoid seeding in the general population, medulloblastoma was found to be the most common, representing 47.6 percent of cases.[6,204] Glioblastoma (grades III and IV) was next, occurring in 14.3 percent. Ependymoma was seen in 11.9 percent of cases, oligodendroglioma in 11.9 percent, astocytoma in 7.1 percent, retinoblastoma in 4.8 percent, and pinealoma in 2.4 percent.[204] Finally, in the pediatric population, choroid plexus papilloma may also show subarachnoid spread. The importance of establishing the presence of leptomeningeal disease with an intracranial lesion is paramount, since this information significantly alters the choice of therapy. If tumor is present within the spinal canal, spinal axis radiation is employed.[203]

Although the tumors that spread to the subarachnoid space in the pediatric population are usually primary intracranial neoplasms, tumors outside the CNS may also spread to the meninges.[205] There are many theories as to the mechanism by which systemic tumors spread to the leptomeninges, including direct extension into the subarachnoid space, peripheral lymphatic invasion, hematogenous dissemination, and seeding via the choroid.[205]

There are two age peaks for leptomeningeal carcinomatosis in the pediatric population, the first at roughly 6 years of age and the second at 14 to 15 years.[6] The second peak occurs in patients who have had spinal axis radiation and in whom there is either delayed spread of a primary tumor into the radiated spine, or secondary recurrence intracranially with later spread through the subarachnoid space into the spinal column.[6] Thirty-three percent of patients with intracranial recurrence of medulloblastoma show leptomeningeal spread into the spine at the time the recurrence is diagnosed.[203]

In the spine, leptomeningeal tumor most often spreads to the lumbosacral region (73 percent).[203] This probably reflects the effects of gravity, with most of the tumor cells settling in this area.[203] However, some lesions are seen in the cervical and thoracic region.[203] In one series, three of 26 patients with subarachnoid spread had lesions within the cervical region.[203] Lesions in the cervical and thoracic region tend to be dorsal in location.[203] Again, this distribution may reflect the natural flow of CSF, which travels from the brain dorsally to the cord and then returns to the brain ventrally to the cord.

Subarachnoid spread of tumor is often asymptomatic.[203,206] When symptoms are present, they may be attributed to the primary lesion within the posterior fossa. These problems are compounded by the fact that children frequently have difficulty in relaying symptoms accurately. Thus, preoperative imaging of the spinal axis is extremely important, since the therapy and the prognosis hinge on this information.

Imaging

Myelography has been shown to be sensitive in detecting subarachnoid tumor nodules,[206] and subarachnoid tumor has several appearances.[205] There may be parallel longitudinal filling defects due to thickened nerve roots within the contrast material, irregular filling defects with varying degrees of block resembling those of arachnoiditis, or multiple nodular defects.[6,202,205] Myelography is accurate, but it requires the use of general anesthesia in younger children, and also ionizing radiation. MRI with gadolinium-DTPA administration has been shown to be competitive with myelography in the detection of subarachnoid tumor, and is often the imaging modality of choice. Although myelography may be more sensitive in showing small, focal areas of leptomeningeal tumor, MRI is often more sensitive in documenting tumor coating the cord, causing subtle enlargement.

Noncontrast MRI has been found relatively insensitive for subarachnoid tumor.[193,202,207] In one series, myelography was shown to be much more sensitive than noncontrast MRI.[207] Of fifteen positive myelographic results for subarachnoid tumor, only four had positive findings on noncontrast MRI.[202] A large number of noncontrast MR images were equivocal or falsely negative (31 and 44 percent, respectively), since leptomeningeal tumor tends to blend with the adjacent CSF.[202]

In one study of leptomeningeal disease, on T1 weighted images, four of 12 patients showed normal results and five showed equivocal MR findings. The equivocal studies showed either less than optimal visualization of the conus medullaris or heterogeneity involving the intensity of the CSF signal.[208] Findings were similar on noncontrast T2 weighted images.

Tumor in the subarachnoid space may be difficult to visualize on noncontrast imaging for several reasons.[209] Since leptomeningeal disease and drop metastases are frequently associated with elevated protein in the CSF, shortening of the T1 and T2 relaxation times of the surrounding CSF compared with pure CSF results.[201,208] In addition, the tumor within the subarachnoid space, coating the nerve roots or spinal cord, has high water content, which results in prolongation of the T1 and T2 relaxation times with respect to more compact tumor.[208] Signal intensities may parallel those of the altered signal intensity of proteinaceous CSF.[201] Very little differentiation between the CSF and the subarachnoid tumor may be apparent on noncontrast imaging.[209] Small nodules may also be missed as a result of partial voluming.[208] Finally, movement artifact within the time frame that it takes to image the spinal canal may obscure lesions; artifacts may cause signal inhomogeneity within the CSF.[208]

After administration of gadolinium-DTPA, MRI is sensitive to the subarachnoid spread of tumor.[209] Enhancement of drop metastases may be prominent. On T1 weighted images, these high-signal enhancing lesions are easily seen against the low signal intensity of the CSF (Fig. 16–14).[209] The patterns of enhancement on contrast MRI should parallel those seen on myelography, i.e., thickened enhancing nerve roots, irregular areas of enhancement with varying degrees of block, or multiple enhancing nodules.[205, 208] Enhancing nodules as small as 2 to 3 mm have been identified on contrast MRI (Fig. 16–15).[208]

In evaluating patients for subarachnoid tumor, both noncontrast and contrast T1 weighted images in the sagittal plane should be obtained, as well as axial images through selected areas. The noncontrast T1 weighted images are needed for comparison.[208] The noncontrast T1 weighted images permit detection of subtle areas of enhancement when the two portions of the study are compared. Comparison between the noncontrast and contrast portions of the examination also allows for differentiation between epidural high-signal fat and areas of enhancement.[208] This is especially important, since there is a large amount of epidural fat in the lumbosacral region, the area where leptomeningeal disease is most commonly found.[207, 208] T2 weighted images do not appear to be necessary in evaluating the subarachnoid space for leptomeningeal tumor.

In the intradural extramedullary location, delayed imaging may show strandlike enhancement slightly greater than on the immediate postinjection images, but this increase is infrequent.[208] Furthermore, tumor nodules are generally best seen on immediate postcontrast scans. Therefore, delayed images have no positive effectiveness in the routine evaluation for leptomeningeal disease.[208]

INTRAMEDULLARY TUMORS

Astrocytoma

Although ependymomas may be more common in the adult population, there is an increased incidence of spinal astrocytomas in relation to ependymomas in children.[2, 185] Most series show that among primary pediatric spinal neoplasms, astrocytoma is slightly more common than neuroblastoma, neurofibroma, ependymoma, or ganglioneuroma.[2, 6, 23] Astrocytomas

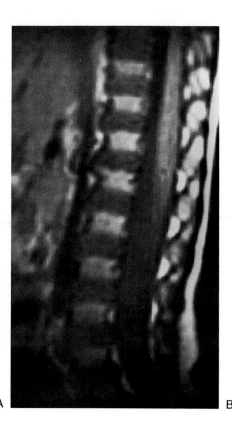
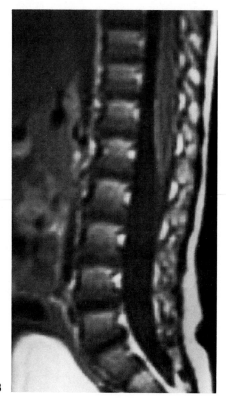

Figure 16–14. *Leptomeningeal metastases. **A,** Unenhanced sagittal T1 weighted image (600/20) in this 7-year-old boy with a pinealoblastoma is normal. **B,** Sagittal T1 weighted image (600/20) after gadolinium-DTPA administration shows a thin layer of tumor coating the conus medullaris. This is seen as a diffuse hazy enhancement. Leptomeningeal tumor was confirmed by CSF examination.*

A   B

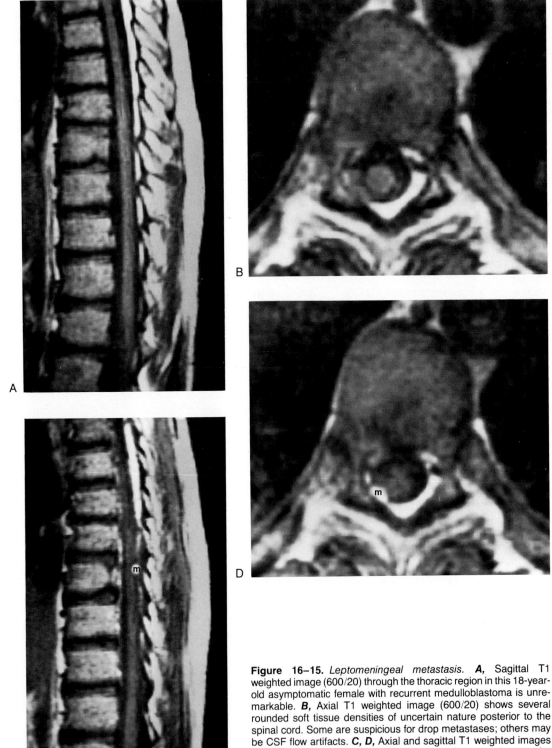

Figure 16–15. *Leptomeningeal metastasis.* **A,** Sagittal T1 weighted image (600/20) through the thoracic region in this 18-year-old asymptomatic female with recurrent medulloblastoma is unremarkable. **B,** Axial T1 weighted image (600/20) shows several rounded soft tissue densities of uncertain nature posterior to the spinal cord. Some are suspicious for drop metastases; others may be CSF flow artifacts. **C, D,** Axial and sagittal T1 weighted images (600/20) after gadolinium-DTPA administration now show an intensely enhancing, small, rounded mass (m) posterior and to the right of the spinal cord in the lower thoracic region. This appearance suggested leptomeningeal tumor, which was later proved by surgery.

represent over 50 percent of intramedullary mass lesions in children, while ependymoma constitutes approximately 38 percent.

Overall, the peak incidence of spinal astrocytomas is in the third and fourth decade. In patients under 20 years of age, however, the average age at diagnosis is 11.5 years. There is either no sexual predilection or a slight male predilection;[210] in a series of 11 patients with astrocytomas, nine were boys and two were girls.[9]

Astrocytomas are most often in the proximal spinal cord, with an increased incidence in the cervicomedullary and cervicothoracic junctions. Sloof and associates found that in patients of all ages, 41 of 86 astrocytomas were in the thoracic region, 11 in the cervicothoracic region, and 13 in the thoracolumbar area.[211] The prevalence of astrocytomas decreases in the lower thoracic and lumbar regions, unlike ependymomas, the prevalence of which increases in the caudal spinal canal.[2] In fact, it is rare for astrocytomas to be in the filum terminale, a common site for ependymomas. Only 7 percent of astrocytomas are seen in the filum. DeSousa and colleagues studied 11 children with spinal cord astrocytomas and found four cervicomedullary, one cervical, two cervicothoracic, three thoracic, and one lumbar in location.[9] Most astrocytomas are intramedullary, although rarely they may be exophytic and intradural extramedullary.[6]

Clinical Findings

The presenting symptoms are frequently nonspecific and ill defined, resulting in a delay in diagnosis.[210] Patients present with local or remote pain, gait disturbance, and genitourinary abnormalities such as incontinence or urgency.[10,210,211] On physical examination, motor and sensory changes, abnormal reflexes, or scoliosis may be seen.[210]

Pathology

These lesions usually result in fusiform expansion of the spinal cord.[182] Grossly, astrocytomas are gray-yellow to beefy red, depending on the degree of hemorrhage.[183,211] Cystic change is present 25 to 38 percent of the time in these potentially friable lesions.[183,185,210] These low-grade tumors do not have a clear line of demarcation from the normal spinal cord.[211] Frequently, they are eccentric in location, usually posteriorly sited by the posterior columns.[199,211] They often involve the spinal cord over multiple segments and can even involve the entire spinal cord.[6] Astrocytomas are composed of neoplastically transformed astrocytes, which vary from well differentiated to anaplastic. Seventy-five percent of astrocytomas are benign in adults (grades I and II); however, in younger individuals there is an increased tendency for astrocytomas to be of a higher histologic grade.[210]

Imaging

Imaging with myelography and postmyelography CT reveals an intramedullary mass. Based on the location and morphologic appearance, astrocytoma is usually considered, but the differential diagnosis may be more extensive.

Because of its superior ability to evaluate and characterize lesions of the spinal cord, MRI is the modality of choice in the evaluation of suspected intramedullary tumors.[212] MRI shows these lesions to be of low signal intensity on T1 weighted images.[213] Generally, there is spinal cord expansion.[199,212–214] On T2 weighted images, these lesions and the surrounding edema appear of high signal intensity.[213,214] On noncontrast MR imaging it may be difficult to distinguish the lesion from its surrounding edema. After contrast administration these lesions almost always enhance, but owing to the infiltrative nature of the tumor, without a capsule or cleavage plane between the lesion and the spinal cord, the margins of the lesion are often fuzzy and irregular.[199,214] The contrast enhancement may be inhomogeneous in nature and may reveal the tumor, which may not be evident in the noncontrast portion of the examination (Fig. 16–16).[199,209] Enhancement usually occurs immediately after the administration of contrast, although in necrotic tumors, delayed enhancement may be seen.[178]

MRI is also advantageous in its ability to show the tumor separate from associated cyst formation.[214] Cysts may be either caudal or rostral to the tumor, or within the tumor. Rostral and caudal cysts are usually reactive.[215] The reactive cysts may be formed by secretions from the tumor; they generally do not have tumorous elements within the wall, but are surrounded by gliosis and represent a "benign" type of cyst.[215] A second type of cyst is that formed by necrosis within the tumor.[215] The distinction between these two types of cysts is crucial, since a simple reactive cyst needs only to be drained, whereas a tumorous cyst may require surgical resection.[215] The distinction between these cysts can markedly affect the choice of surgery, since the extent of laminectomy may be limited when a reactive cyst is present.[215]

Both reactive and neoplastic cysts tend to have a decreased T1 signal intensity and an increased T2 signal intensity in relation to the tumor.[125] However, the signal intensity may become indistinguishable from the solid tumor on noncontrast MRI, especially when the cavity is caused by necrosis within the tumor.[215] Hemorrhage or increased protein within the cyst fluid may decrease T1 and T2 relaxation times, making the cyst isointense with the spinal cord and tumor.[214]

Complex benign syrinxes can resemble cystic astrocytomas. They have gliosis within their walls secondary to chronic CSF pulsations.[215] This tissue may have increased signal intensity on T2 weighted images and may be indistinguishable from tumor.[215] On noncontrast MRI, some characteristics may favor a simple syrinx cavity: these include cyst fluid, which is isointense with CSF; uniform signal intensity of the fluid; distinct margins to the cyst; and the presence of pulsations.[216] Factors on noncontrast MRI that may indicate a neoplastic cavity include indistinct margins, non-

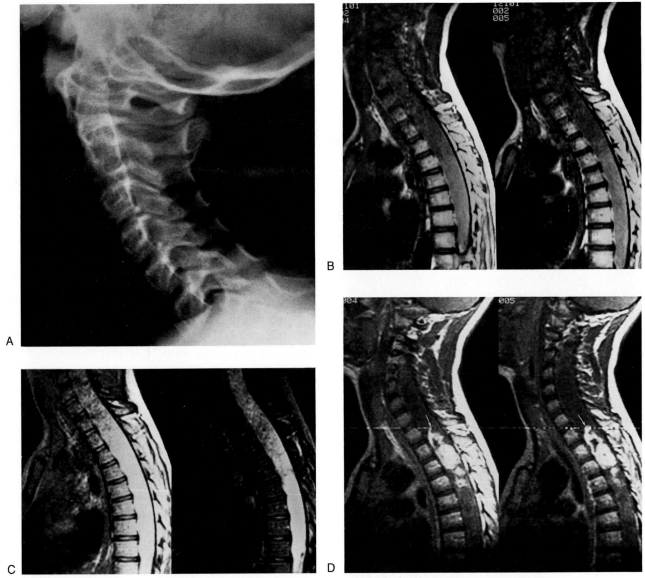

Figure 16–16. *Spinal cord astrocytoma with holocord syrinx in a 9-year-old boy.* **A,** Lateral plain film of the cervical spine shows an increased anteroposterior diameter to the spinal canal. **B,** Sagittal T1 weighted image (600/20) again demonstrates the abnormally increased anteroposterior diameter to the spinal canal as well as the thoracic region. There is inhomogeneous signal in the markedly expanded spinal cord. **C,** Sagittal proton density and T2 weighted images (2118/30/80) show inhomogeneity to the thecal sac-cord. **D,** Sagittal T1 weighted image (600/20) after gadolinium-DTPA administration discloses an irregular, intramedullary, enhancing mass lesion (*arrow*) from levels T1 to T4. There is associated expansion of the cord above and below this lesion with low-signal cysts, which extend from the medulla to the conus medullaris.

uniform signal intensity within the cyst, and a signal intensity of the fluid that does not parallel CSF.[216]

With gadolinium-DTPA, the vast majority of astrocytomas enhance.[199, 209] On T1 weighted images, cysts associated with tumor usually are easily separable from benign syrinxes, since tumorous components within the cyst wall generally enhance (Fig. 16–17);[199] However, there may be exceptions.

Ependymoma

Ependymomas are more commonly located intracranially than within the spine.[217] Barone and Elvidge reported on 74 ependymomas of patients of all ages; 47 of these were intracranial, and 27 were spinal.[218] In the pediatric population, ependymomas are second to astrocytomas in incidence.[217] These lesions usually occur

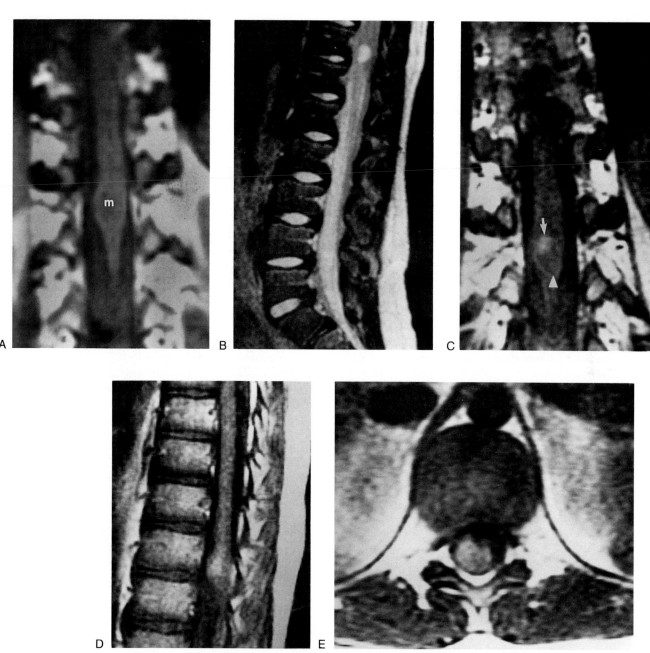

Figure 16–17. *Cord astrocytoma.* ***A,*** Coronal T1 weighted image (600/20) shows a lobular low-signal mass (m) expanding the conus medullaris. ***B,*** Sagittal T2 weighted image (2000/90) shows the conus mass to be of high signal intensity. ***C,*** Coronal T1 weighted image (600/20) after gadolinium-DTPA administration shows a nodular area of enhancement (*arrow*) with an inferior lower-signal necrotic or cystic area (*arrowhead*). ***D, E,*** Sagittal and axial T1 weighted images (600/20) after gadolinium-DTPA administration show the enhanced area anteriorly and the lower-signal cystic portion posteriorly.

after the age of 20 years.[2] Of all ependymomas involving the spinal canal, Sloof found that 10 percent occurred in the first two decades.[211] Similarly, in a series of 77 myxopapillary ependymomas from the Mayo Clinic, 19 percent presented in patients under 20 years old.[217] These tumors constitute between 5 and 13 per-

cent of mass lesions in the spinal canal of children.[4, 6] The average age in the pediatric population is 13.4 years; most patients are older than 8 years.[6] Although in all age groups combined there is a slight male predilection, there is probably a slight female predominance in the pediatric population.[2, 6, 10]

Ependymoma is the most common primary cord tumor of the lower spinal cord, conus medullaris, and filum terminale.[10,210] Ependymomas tend to be more common in the lower spinal cord. Of the 77 cases in the Mayo Clinic series involving patients of all ages, 65 percent were limited to the filum, 30 percent involved the filum and the conus medullaris, and only 5 percent were in the cervicothoracic spinal cord,[217] in contradistinction to astrocytomas, which are more common proximally and less prevalent in the distal spinal cord. Like intracranial ependymomas, spinal ependymomas may lead to leptomeningeal tumor spread.

Clinical Findings

Clinically these lesions have a presentation similar to that of astrocytomas. Pain, genitourinary abnormalities, and motor and sensory disturbances may be seen.

Pathology

Ependymal cells line the central spinal canal as well as the remainder of the internal surfaces of the central nervous system.[210] Thus, ependymomas often tend to be central in location and exhibit centrifugal growth.[199]

Grossly, ependymomas are cylindric elongated masses that cause localized fusiform expansion of the spinal cord.[199,183] They are brownish-red and blue in color, depending on their blood content. The most common histologic appearance is that of the cellular type.[199] However, the most common lesion of the filum terminale is the myxopapillary type, which is especially prone to hemorrhage and may present as an unexplained subarachnoid bleed.[6,199,217] Ependymomas are soft, friable lesions that frequently have a plane of cleavage between themselves and the spinal cord.[183,199] These tumors are invested by a delicate capsule; they may grow into the conus and adhere to the lumbar nerve roots.[217] Cyst formation is seen in 50 percent of cases, especially in the myxopapillary variety at the filum terminale.[10,214] Although ependymomas in the brain often calcify, calcification is extremely uncommon in spinal ependymomas.

Imaging

Plain films, CT, and myelography may be performed to localize the lesion and show its extent and the degree of spinal cord block. These modalities, however, are frequently nonspecific.

Noncontrast MRI demonstrates spinal cord widening. The lesion is isointense with the spinal cord on T1 weighted images and hyperintense on T2 weighted images.[219] These lesions may have a multinodular appearance on T2 weighted images.[219] Although the tumors have a pseudocapsule and may be fairly demarcated from the spinal cord pathologically, it is difficult to distinguish these tumors from astrocytomas by imaging criteria.

After the administration of gadolinium-DTPA, ependymomas tend to enhance intensely and homogeneously.[199,209] The lesions often have well-defined bor-

ders. Gadolinium-DTPA helps to show intratumoral and peritumoral cysts better, especially those that may be isointense with the lesion on the noncontrast MRI examination (Fig. 16–18).[209,215]

Treatment

Treatment is aimed at surgical removal. After complete removal of an encapsulated tumor, there is little chance of recurrence (10 percent).[217] Sometimes, however, the tumor is poorly encapsulated or cannot be removed entirely.[217] These tumors may metastasize via CSF dissemination or by distant metastases to the lung (up to 17 percent).[217]

Hemangioblastoma

Although hemangioblastomas are the most common primary posterior fossa tumor in the adult, they rarely involve the spinal cord. Hemangioblastomas account for 1.6 to 3.6 percent of all spinal cord tumors, but are uncommon in the pediatric population.[227–230] Overall, there is no sexual predilection. These lesions usually present in the fourth decade.[18]

Thirty percent of patients with spinal cord hemangioblastomas have von Hippel-Lindau syndrome.[231] This autosomal dominant disorder with almost 100 percent penetrance is typified by cerebellar hemangioblastomas (36 to 60 percent), retinal angiomatosis (more than 50 percent), renal cell carcinoma (25 to 38 percent), pheochromocytoma (more than 10 percent), or spinal hemangioblastomas (less than 5 percent).[220–223] However, the incidence of spinal cord hemangioblastomas in von Hippel-Lindau syndrome may be underestimated, since these lesions are frequently asymptomatic.[222,223] When patients with von Hippel-Lindau syndrome have retinal or cerebellar hemangioblastomas coexisting with spinal hemangioblastomas, they usually present with symptoms from the former lesions rather than from the spinal cord lesions.[221,222] If there is a positive family history for an asymptomatic patient, MRI is now recommended to evaluate for cerebellar or spinal cord lesions.

Hemangioblastomas involving the spinal cord tend to be single (79 percent), although multiple tumors in a single patient are not unusual. In spinal hemangioblastomas, the proximal spinal cord is the site most frequently involved.[220] Forty percent of lesions occur in the cervical cord and 50 percent in the thoracic cord.[221,223] There is a predilection for the cervicothoracic and thoracolumbar regions.[220] Most hemangioblastomas are intramedullary (60 percent); the remainder are either intradural extramedullary or purely extradural.

These vascular tumors are prone to hemorrhage, with associated cyst formation. These cysts may have high protein content as a result of the previous hemorrhage.[185] Overall, 43 percent of hemangioblastomas have cysts; however, when purely intramedullary he-

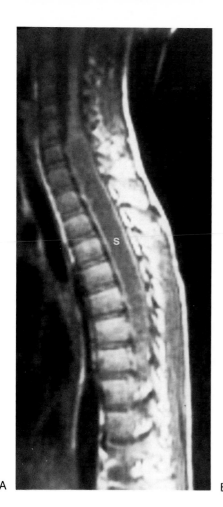

A

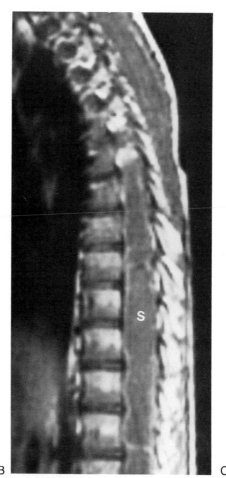

B

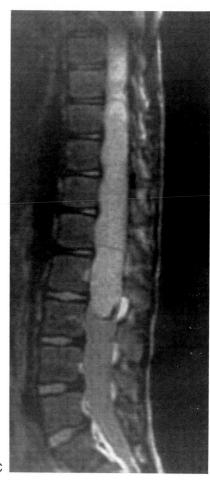

C

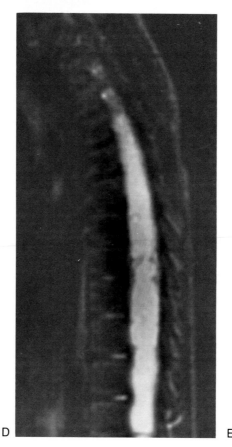

D

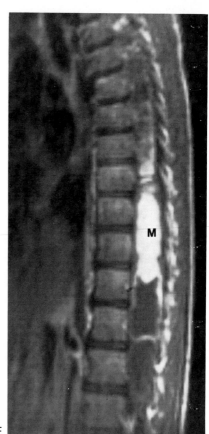

E

Figure 16–18. *Thoracic ependymoma in a 7-year-old boy with paraparesis and a neurogenic bladder.* **A, B,** Contiguous precontrast sagittal T1 weighted image (600/20) reveals syringomyelia (S) from C6 to L2, expanding the cord and spinal canal. Although several septations are present within the cyst, no tumor focus is identified. Note that the signal intensity of the cyst contents is slightly higher than that of the CSF, suggesting an elevated protein concentration. **C, D,** Precontrast spin density weighted (2000/30) (*C*) and T2 weighted (2000/80) (*D*) images demonstrate diffuse hyperintensity within the cyst cavity, obscuring the focal tumor. **E,** Gadolinium-enhanced T1 weighted image (600/20) shows a mass centered at levels T8 to T11, which expands the spinal canal. Surgical resection of the mass (M) revealed an ependymoma of the cord, with proteinaceous fluid within the peritumoral cyst. (Dillon WP, Norman D, Newton TH, Bolla K, Mark A. Intradural spinal cord lesions: gadolinium-DTPA enhanced MR imaging. Radiology 1989; 170: 229–237.)

mangioblastomas are considered, cyst formation is seen in up to 67 percent.[10,185,221,224] Polycythemia, reported in association with cerebellar hemangioblastomas, has never been seen with lesions involving the spinal cord.[221]

Pathology

Histologically, hemangioblastomas are composed of a mixture of endothelial cells intermixed with stromal cells containing fat and hemosiderin.[221] The origin of these endothelial and stromal cells remains controversial. Taking into account the common location of these lesions and a familial tendency, Browne states in his review of hemangioblastomas of the spinal cord that Lindau theorized that hemangioblastomas may arise from congenital rests.[221] The abnormality may occur in the second and third fetal months when the normal vascular structures are forming within the retina, fourth ventricle, and cerebellum.[221] The endothelial cells form the solid portions of the tumor and the vessels;[16] it is this portion of the tumor that makes up the actual growing mass.[221] Eventually the tumor consists of a compact collection of capillaries with small feeding arteries and dilated draining veins.[16,223] In three patients reported at autopsy, no tumor cells were seen in the wall of the cyst cavity associated with hemangioblastoma. This finding supports the theory that the cyst cavity may form secondary to secretions and is not due to necrosis within the tumor.[221]

Imaging

Myelography frequently shows expansion of the spinal cord as a result of cyst formation. In addition, serpiginous filling defects posterior to the spinal cord may be seen representing meningeal varicosities. CT scanning of spinal cord hemangioblastomas may show widening of the spinal cord with a hypodense tumor nidus that markedly enhances after contrast administration.[185] Spinal angiography shows equivalent findings, such as feeding arteries and draining veins and an intense blush of the tumor nidus.

Unenhanced MRI may show widening of the spinal cord.[224] Associated cyst formation may give the spinal cord an inhomogeneous appearance on noncontrast T1 weighted images.[199,224] There may be considerable edema within the adjacent cord, as shown by low signal on T1 and increased signal on T2 weighted images. The cyst itself may have signal characteristics that parallel those of CSF,[224] or may be of greater intensity as a result of increased protein content secondary to previous hemorrhage.[185] Because of this increased signal intensity, the cyst occasionally may be indistinguishable from the tumor nidus on noncontrast sequences.[223] Adjacent serpiginous areas of signal void may be seen;[223] these may represent large feeding arteries or, more commonly, draining meningeal varicosities associated with the very vascular tumor nidus.[10,185,221,223]

Enhanced MRI shows that the tumor nidus enhances markedly.[185,209] T1 weighted enhanced scans allow differentiation of the small enhancing tumor nidus from the adjacent edematous spinal cord and the cyst.[185] MRI therefore may accurately locate the tumor nidus and distinguish it from cyst or surrounding edema.[185] This helps to direct surgery toward accurate removal of the tumor nidus and decompression of the adjacent cyst. Complete surgical removal offers the only chance of cure at the present time.

Finally, intradural extramedullary and extradural spinal hemangioblastomas may present symptomatically with radicular pain and sensory loss as well as weakness of the lower extremities.[221] Again, treatment consists of surgical removal.[221]

REFERENCES

1. Miller J, Fishman LS. Spinal cord tumors. Imaging of pediatric oncology. Baltimore: Williams & Wilkins, 1985:101–105.
2. Farwell JR, Dohrman GJ. Intraspinal neoplasms in children. Paraplegia 1977; 15:262–273.
3. Parker BR, Castellino RA. Pediatric oncologic radiology. St Louis: CV Mosby, 1977:373–375.
4. Munk PL, Helms CA, Holt RG, et al. MR imaging of aneurysmal bone cysts. AJR 1989; 153:99–101.
5. Rand RW, Rand CW. Intraspinal tumors of childhood. Springfield, IL: Charles C Thomas, 1960:3–399.
6. Harwood-Nash DC, Fitz CR. Neuroradiology in infants and children. St Louis: CV Mosby, 1976:1167–1226.
7. Haft H, Ransohopf J, Carter S. Spinal cord tumors in children. Pediatrics 1959; 23:1152–1159.
8. Matson DD, Tachdjian MD. Intraspinal tumors in infants and children. Review of 115 cases. Postgrad Med 1963; 34:279–285.
9. DeSousa AL, Kalsbeck JE, Mealy J, et al. Intraspinal tumors in children. J. Neurosurg 1979; 51:437–445.
10. Dorwart RH, LaMasters DL, Watanabe TJ. Tumors. In: Newton TH, Potts DG, eds. Computed tomography of the spine and spinal cord. San Anselmo, CA: Clavadel Press, 1983:115–147.
11. Stowens D. Neuroblastoma and related tumors. Arch Pathol 1957; 63:451–459.
12. Siegel MJ, Jamroz GA, Glazer HS, Abramson CL. MR imaging of intraspinal extension of neuroblastoma. J Comput Assist Tomogr 1986; 10:593–595.
13. Dietrich RB, Kangarloo H, Lenarsky C, Feig SA. Neuroblastoma: the role of MR imaging. AJR 1987; 148:937–942.
14. Miller JH, Sato JK. Adrenal origin tumors. Imaging in pediatric oncology. Baltimore: Williams & Wilkins, 1985:305–339.
15. Dargeon HW. Neuroblastoma. Med Prog 1962; 61:456–471.
16. Reed JC, Hallet KK, Feign DS. Neural tumors of the thorax: subject review from the AFIP. Radiology 1978; 126:9–17.
17. Balakrishnan V, Rice M, Simpson D. Spinal neuroblastomas. Diagnosis, treatment and prognosis. J. Neurosurg. 1974; 40:631–637.
18. Bodian M. Neuroblastoma. Pediatric Clin North Am 1959; 6:449–472.
19. Koop CE, Hernandez JK. Neuroblastoma: experience with 100 cases in children. Surgery 1964; 56:726–733.
20. Punt J, Pritchard J, Pincott JR, Till K. Neuroblastoma: a review of 21 cases presenting with cord compression. Cancer 1980; 45:3095–3101.
21. Edeu K. The dumb-bell tumours of the spine. Br J Surg 1941; 28:549–569.
22. Kirks DR. Practical pediatric imaging. Boston: Little, Brown, 1984:159–177.
23. Resjo IM, Harwood-Nash D, Fitz CR, Chuang S. CT metrizamide myelography for intraspinal and paraspinal neoplasms in infants and children. AJR 1979; 132:367–372.
24. Adam A, Hochholzer L. Ganglioneuroblastoma of the posterior mediastinum: a clinicopathologic review of 80 cases. Cancer 1981; 47:373–381.

25. Inglis AE, Rubin RM, Lewis RJ, Villacin A. Osteochondroma of the cervical spine. Case report. Clin Orthop 1977; 126:127–129.
26. Ilgenfritz HC. Vertebral osteochondroma. Am J Surg 1951; 17:917–922.
27. Malat J, Virapongse C, Levine A. Solitary osteochondroma of the spine. Spine 1986; 11:625–628.
28. Gokay H, Bucy PC. Osteochondroma of the lumbar spine. Report of a case. J Neurosurg 1955; 12:72–78.
29. Kenney PJ, Gilula LA, Murphy WA. The use of computed tomography to distinguish osteochondroma and chondrosarcoma. Radiology 1981; 139:129–137.
30. Karian JM, DeFilipp G, Buchheit WA, et al. Vertebral osteochondroma causing spinal cord compression. Neurosurgery 1984; 14:483–484.
31. Twersky J, Kassner EG, Tenner MS, Camera A. Vertebral and costal osteochondromas causing spinal cord compression. AJR 1978; 124:124–128.
32. Novick GS, Pavlov H, Bullough PG. Osteochondroma of the cervical spine: report of two cases in preadolescent males. Skeletal Radiol 1982; 8:13–15.
33. Palmer FJ, Blum PW. Osteochondroma with spinal cord compression. Report of three cases. J Neurosurg 1980; 52: 842–845.
34. Cohn RS, Fielding JW. Osteochondroma of the cervical spine. J Pediatr Surg 1986; 21:997–999.
35. Kozlowski K, Beluffi G, Masel J, et al. Primary vertebral tumours in children. Report of 20 cases with brief review of the literature. Pediatr Radiol 1984; 14:129–139.
36. Glass RB, Poznanski AK, Fisher MR, et al. Case report: MR imaging of osteoid osteoma. J Comput Assist Tomogr 1986; 10:1065–1067.
37. Swee RG, McLeod RA, Beabout JW. Osteoid osteoma. Radiology 1979; 130:117–123.
38. Jackson RP, Reckling FW, Mantz FA. Osteoid osteoma and osteoblastoma. Clin Orthop 1977; 128:303–313.
39. Gamba JL, Martinez S, Apple J, et al. CT of axial skeletal osteoid osteomas. AJR 1984; 142:769–772.
40. Fountain E, Burgie C. Osteoid osteoma of the cervical spine. J Neurosurg 1950; 18:380.
41. Heiman ML, Cooley CJ, Bradford DS. Osteoid osteoma of a vertebral body: report of a case with extension across the intervertebral disk. Clin Orthop 1976; 118:159–163.
42. Mustard WT, Duval FL. Osteoid osteoma of the vertebrae. J Bone Joint Surg 1959; 41B:132–136.
43. MacLellan DI, Wilson FC. Osteoid osteoma of the spine. J Bone Joint Surg 1967; 49A:111–121.
44. Freiberger RH. Osteoid osteoma of the spine. Radiology 1960; 75:232–235.
45. Sherman MS. Osteoid osteoma. J Bone Joint Surg 1947; 29:918–930.
46. Omojola MF, Cockshott P, Beatty EG. Osteoid osteoma: an evaluation of diagnostic modalities. Clin Radiol 1981; 32:199–204.
47. Bell RS, O'Connor GD, Waddell JP. Importance of magnetic resonance imaging in osteoid osteoma: a case report. Can J Surg 1989; 32:276–278.
48. deSantos LA, Goldstein HM, Murray JA, Wallace S. Computed tomography in the evaluation of musculoskeletal neoplasms. Radiology 1978; 128:89–94.
49. Doran Y, Gruszkiewicz J, Gelli B, Deyser E. Benign osteoblastoma of vertebral column and skull. Surg Neurol 1977; 7:86–90.
50. Myles ST, MacRae ME. Benign osteoblastoma of the spine in childhood. J Neurosurg 1988; 68:884–888.
51. Lichtenstein L. Benign osteoblastoma. Cancer 1956; 9:1044–1052.
52. McCleod RA, Dahlin DC, Beabout JW. The spectrum of osteoblastoma. AJR 1976; 126:321–335.
53. Steiner GC. Ultrastructure of osteoblastoma. Cancer 1977; 39:2127–2136.
54. Jaffe H. Benign osteoblastoma. Bull Hosp JT Dis 1956; 17:141–151.
55. DeSouza L, Frost HM. Osteoblastoma of the spine. A review and report of 8 new cases. Clin Orthop 1973; 91:144–151.
56. Dias LD, Frost HM. Osteoblastoma of the spine: a review of eight cases. Clin Orthop 1973; 91:141–151.
57. Tonai M, Campbell CJ, Ahn GH, et al. Osteoblastoma: classification and report of 16 patients. Clin Orthop 1982; 167:222–235.
58. Bloom MH, Bryan RS. Benign osteoblastoma of the spine: case report. Clin Orthop 1969; 65:157–162.
59. Jackson RP, Reckling FW, Mantz FA. Osteoid osteoma and osteoblastoma. Clin Orthop 1977; 128:303–313.
60. Steiner GC. Ultrastructure of osteoblastoma. Cancer 1977; 39:2127–2136.
61. Omojola MJ, Fox AJ, Vinuela FV. Computed tomographic metrizamide myelography in the evaluation of thoracic spinal osteoblastoma. AJNR 1982; 3:670–673.
62. Tucker AS, Aramsri B, Hughes CR. Roentgenographic diagnosis of spinal tumors. AJR 1957; 78:54–65.
63. Seki T, Fukuda H, Ishii Y, et al. Malignant transformation of a benign osteoblastoma: a case report. J Bone Joint Surg 1975; 57A:424–427.
64. Krol G, Sundaresan N, Deck M. Computed tomography of axial chordomas. J Comput Assist Tomogr 1983; 7:286–289.
65. Heffelfinger MJ, Dahlin DC, McCarty CS, Beabout JW. Chordomas and cartilaginous tumors at the skull base. Cancer 1973; 32:410–420.
66. Beaugie JM, Mann CV, Butler CB. Sacrococcygeal chordoma. Br J Surg 1969; 56:586–588.
67. Sze G, Uichanco LS, Brant-Zawadzki M, et al. Chordomas: MR imaging. Radiology 1988; 166:187–191.
68. Higinbotham NL, Phillips RF, Farr HW, Hustu HO. Chordoma: thirty-five year study at Memorial Hospital. Cancer 1967; 20:1841–1850.
69. Firooznia H, Pinto RS, Lin JP, Zausner J. Chordoma: radiologic evaluation of 20 cases. AJR 1976; 127:797–805.
70. Cory DA, Fritsch SA, Cohen MD, et al. Aneurysmal bone cysts: imaging findings and embolotherapy. AJR 1989; 153:369–373.
71. Spjut HJ, Ayala AG. Skeletal tumors in childhood and adolescence. Pathology of neoplasia in children and adolescents. Philadelphia, WB Saunders, 1984.
72. Dahlin DC, McLeon RA. Aneurysmal bone cyst and other non-neoplastic conditions. Skeletal Radiol 1982; 8:243–250.
73. Biescker JL, Marcove RC, Huvos AG, Mike V. Aneurysmal bone cyst: a clinical pathologic study of 66 cases. Cancer 1970; 26:615–625.
74. Hay MC, Paterson D, Taylor TK. Aneurysmal bone cysts of the spine. J Bone Joint Surg 1978; 60B:406–411.
75. Gunterberg B, Kindblom LG, Laurin S. Giant cell tumor of bone and aneurysmal bone cyst. Skeletal Radiol 1977; 2:65–74.
76. Sherman RS, Soong KY. Aneurysmal bone cyst; its roentgen diagnosis. Radiology 1957; 68:54–64.
77. Tillman BP, Dahlin DC, Lipscomb PR, Stewart JR. Aneurysmal bone cyst: an analysis of 95 cases. Mayo Clin Proc 1968; 43:478–495.
78. Wang A, Lipson S, Hay Kal HA, et al. Computed tomography of aneurysmal bone cyst of the CT vertebral body. J Comput Assist Tomogr 1984; 8:1186–1189.
79. Banna M. Clinical radiology of spine and spinal cord. Rockville, MD: Aspen Publishers, 1985.
80. Beltran J, Simon D, Levy M, et al. Aneurysmal bone cysts: MR imaging at 1.5T. Radiology 1986; 158:689–690.
81. Zimmer WD, Berquist TH, Sim FH, et al. Magnetic resonance imaging of aneurysmal bone cyst. Mayo Clin Proc 1984; 59:633–636.
82. Lichtenstein L. Aneurysmal bone cyst. Further observations. Cancer 1953; 6:1228–1237.
83. Daffner RH, Linetsky L, Zabkar JH. Case Report 433. Skeletal Radiol 1987; 16:428–432.
84. Munk PL, Helms CA, Holt RG, et al. MR imaging of aneurysmal bone cysts. AJR 1989; 153:99–101.
85. Beltran J, Noto AM, Chakeres DW, Christoforidis AJ. Tumors

of the osseous spine staging with MR imaging versus CT. Radiology 1987; 162:565–569.

86. Hudson TM, Hamlin DJ, Fitzsimmons JR. Magnetic resonance of fluid levels in an aneurysmal bone cyst and in anticoagulated human blood. Skeletal Radiol 1985; 13:267–270.

87. Ross, JS, Masaryk TJ, Modic MT. Vertebral hemangiomas: MR imaging. Radiology 1987; 165:165–169.

88. McAllister VL, Kendall BE, Bull JW. Symptomatic vertebral hemangiomas. Brain 1975; 98:71–80.

89. Ghormley RK, Adson AW. Hemangioma of the vertebrae. Bone Joint Surg 1941; 23:887–895.

90. Laredo JD, Reizine D, Bard M, Merland JJ. Vertebral hemangiomas: radiologic evaluation. Radiology 1986; 161:183–189.

91. Krueger EG, Sobel GL, Weinstein C. Vertebral hemangioma with compression of the spinal cord. J. Neurosurg 1961; 18:331–338.

92. Fraumeni JF. Stature and malignant tumors of bone in childhood and adolescence. Cancer 1963; 20:967–973.

93. Robbins S, Cotran RS. Pathologic basis of disease. 2nd ed. Philadelphia: WB Saunders, 1979.

94. McInerney DP, Middlemiss JH. Giant cell tumor of bone. Skeletal Radiol 1978; 2:195–204.

95. Jacobs P. The diagnosis of osteoclastoma (giant cell tumours): a radiological and pathological correlation. Br J Radiol 1972; 45:121–136.

96. Goldenberg RR, Campbell CJ, Bonfiglio M. Giant cell tumor of bone, an analysis of 218 cases. J Bone Joint Surg 1970; 52A:619–664.

97. Williams RR, Dahlin DC, Ghormley RK. Giant cell tumor of bone. Cancer 1954; 7:764–773.

98. Brady TJ, Gebhardt MC, Pickett IL. NMR imaging of forearms in healthy volunteers and patients with giant cell tumor. Radiology 1982; 144:549–552.

99. Aisen AM, Martel W, Braunstein EM, et al. MRI and CT evaluation of primary bone and soft tissue tumors. AJR 1986; 146:749–756.

100. Coventry MB, Dahlin DC. Osteogenic sarcoma: a critical analysis of 430 cases. J Bone Joint Surg 1957; 39A:741–758.

101. Smith WL, Stokka C, Franken EA. Arteriography of sacrococcygeal teratomas. Radiology 1980; 137:653–655.

102. Williams AO, Lagundoye SB, Bankole MA. Sacrococcygeal teratoma in Nigerian children. Arch Dis Child 1975; 45:110–113.

103. Schey WL, Shkolnik A, White H. Clinical and radiographic considerations of sacrococcygeal teratomas: an analysis of 26 new cases and review of the literature. Radiology 1977; 125:189–195.

104. Moazam F, Talbert JL. Congenital anorectal malformations. Arch Surg 1985; 120:856–859.

105. Izant RJ, Filston HC. Sacrococcygeal teratomas. Analysis of forty-three cases. Am J Surg 1975; 130:617–620.

106. McDonald P. Malignant sacrococcygeal teratoma. Report of 4 cases. AJR 1973; 118:444–449.

107. Glass AG, Fraumeni JF. Epidemiology of bone cancer in children. J Natl Cancer Inst 1970; 44:187–190.

108. Wang CC, Shulz MD. Ewing's sarcoma: a study of fifty cases treated at Massachusetts General Hospital 1930–1952 inclusive. JAMA 1953; 248:571–576.

109. Bhansali SK, Desai PB. Ewing's sarcoma, observations of 107 cases. J Bone Joint Surg 1963; 45A:541–553.

110. Swenson PC. The roentgenologic aspects of Ewing's tumor of bone marrow. AJR 1943; 50:343–354.

111. Pritchard DJ, Dahlin DC, Dauphine RT, et al. Ewing's sarcoma: a clinopathological and statistical analysis of patients surviving five years or longer. J Bone Joint Surg 1975; 57A:10–16.

112. Dahlin DC, Coventry MB, Scanlon PW. Ewing's sarcoma: a critical analysis of 165 cases. J Bone Joint Surg 1961; 43A:185–193.

113. Berger PE, Kuhn JP. Computed tomography of tumors of the musculoskeletal system in children. Radiology 1978; 127:171–175.

114. Ginaldi S, deSantos LA. Computed tomography in the evaluation of small round cell tumors of bone. Radiology 1980; 134:441–446.

115. Dundon CC, Williams HA, Liapply TC. Eosinophilic granuloma of bone. Radiology 1946; 47:433–444.

116. McGavran MH, Spady HA. Eosinophilic granuloma of bone, a study of 28 cases. J Bone Joint Surg 1960; 42A:979–992.

117. Hamilton JB, Barner JL, Kennedy PC, McCort JJ. The osseous manifestations of eosinphilic granuloma: report of nine cases. Radiology 1945; 47:445–456.

118. Green WT, Farber S. "Eosinophilic or solitary granuloma" of bone. J Bone Joint Surg 1942; 24:499–526.

119. Childs DS, Kennedy RL. Reticulo-endotheliosis of children: treatment with roentgen rays. Radiology 1951; 57:653–660.

120. Oschsner SF. Eosinophilic granuloma of bone; experience with 20 cases. AJR 1966; 97:719–726.

121. Drolshagen LF, Kessler R, Partain CL. Cervical meningeal histiocytosis demonstrated by magnetic resonance imaging. Pediatr Radiol 1987; 17:63–64.

122. Lichtenstein L, Jaffe HL. Eosinophilic granuloma of bone. Am J Pathol 1940; 16:595–604.

123. Arcomano JP, Barnett JC, Wunderlich HO. Histiocytosis. AJR 1961; 85:663–679.

124. Norman P, Mills CM, Brant-Zawadzki M, et al. Magnetic resonance imaging of the spinal cord and canal: potentials and limitations. AJR 1983; 141:1147–1152.

125. Han JS, Kaufman B, Yousef SJ, et al. NMR imaging of the spine. AJR 1983; 141:1137–1145.

126. Redmond OM, Stack JP, Dervan PA, et al. Osteosarcoma: use of MR imaging and MR spectroscopy in clinical decision making. Radiology 1989; 172:811–815.

127. Dahlin DC, Coventry MB. Osteogenic sarcoma, a study of 600 cases. J Bone Joint Surg 1967; 49A:101–110.

128. Felson B, Wiot J. Osteogenic sarcoma: an update. Semin Roentgenol 1989; 24:143–200.

129. McKenna RJ, Schwinn CP, Soong KY, Higinbotham NL. Sarcoma of the osteogenic series (osteosarcoma, fibrosarcoma, chondrosarcoma, parosteal osteogenic sarcoma, and sarcomata arising in abnormal bone). J Bone Joint Surg 1966; 48A:1–26.

130. Marcour RC, Mike V, Hajek JV, et al. Osteogenic sarcoma under the age of twenty-one. J Bone Joint Surg 1970; 52A:411–423.

131. Fielding WJ, Fietti VG, Hughes JE, Gabriellian JC. Primary osteogenic sarcoma of the cervical spine. J Bone Joint Surg 1976; 58A:892–894.

132. Berger PE, Kuhn JP. Computed tomography of tumors of the musculoskeletal system in children. Radiology 1978; 127:171–175.

133. Zimmer WD, Berguist TH, McLeod RA, et al. Magnetic resonance imaging of osteosarcomas. Comparison with computed tomography. Clin Orthop 1986; 208:289–299.

134. Zimmer WD, Berguist TH, McLeod RA. Bone tumors: MR imaging versus CT. Radiology 1985; 155:709–718.

135. Erlemann R, Reiser MF, Peters PE, et al. Musculoskeletal neoplasms: static and dynamic Gd-DTPA-enhanced MR imaging. Radiology 1989; 171:767–773.

136. Sundaram M, McGuire MH, Herbold DR. Magnetic resonance imaging of osteosarcoma. Skeletal Radiol 1987; 16:23–29.

137. Ramsey RG, Zacharis CE. MR imaging of the spine after radiation therapy: easily recognizable effects. AJR 1985; 144:1131–1135.

138. Huvos AG, Marcove RC. Chondrosarcoma in the young. A clinicopathologic analysis of 79 patients younger than 21 years of age. Am J Surg Pathol 1987; 11:930–942.

139. Aprin H, Riseborough EJ, Hall JE. Chondrosarcoma in children and adolescents. Clin Orthop 1982; 166:226–232.

140. Barnes R, Catto M. Chondrosarcoma of bone. J Bone Joint Surg 1966; 48A:729–764.

141. Garrison RC, Unni KK, McCleod RA, et al. Chondrosarcoma arising in osteochondroma. Cancer 1982; 49:1890–1897.

142. Frassica FJ, Unni KK, Beabout JW, Sim FH. Dedifferentiated chondrosarcoma. J Bone Joint Surg 1986; 68A:1197–1205.
143. Blaylock RL, Kempe LG. Chondrosarcoma of the cervical spine. Case report. J Neurosurg 1976; 44:500–503.
144. Marcove RC. Chondrosarcoma: diagnosis and treatment. Orthop Clin North Am 1977; 8:811–820.
145. Wronski J, Bryc S, Kaminski J, Chibowski D. Chondrosarcoma of the cervical spine causing compression of the cord. J Neurosurg 1964; 21:419–421.
146. Camins MB, Duncan AW, Smith J, Marcove RC. Chondrosarcoma of the spine. Spine 1978; 3:202–209.
147. Pettersson H, Gillespy T, Hamlin D, et al. Primary musculoskeletal tumors: examination with MR imaging compared with conventional modalities. Radiology 1987; 164:237–241.
148. Parker BR, Marglin S, Castellino RA. Skeletal manifestations of leukemia, Hodgkin disease, and non-Hodgkin lymphoma. Semin Roentgenol 1980; 15:302–315.
149. Pinkel D. Treatment of acute leukemia. Pediatr Clin North Am 1976; 23:117–130.
150. Young JL, Miller RW. Incidence of malignant tumors in US children. J Pediatr 1975; 86:254–258.
151. Pear BL. Skeletal manifestations of the lymphomas and leukemias. Semin Roentgenol 1974; 9:229–240.
152. Murphy ML. Leukemia and lymphoma in children. Pediatr Clin North Am 1959; 6:611–638.
153. Pierce MI, Borges WH, Heyn R, et al. Epidemiological factors and survival experience in 1770 children with acute leukemia. Cancer 1969; 6:1296–1304.
154. Silverman FN. The skeletal lesions in leukemia. Clinical and roentgenographic observations in 103 infants and children with a review of the literature. AJR 1948; 59:819–843.
155. Baty JM, Vogt EC. Bone changes of leukemia in children. AJR 1935; 34:310–314.
156. Daffner RH, Lupetin AR, Dash N, et al. MRI in the detection of malignant infiltration of bone marrow. AJR 1986; 146:353–358.
157. Olson DO, Shields AF, Scheunch CJ, et al. Magnetic resonance imaging of the bone marrow in patients with leukemia, aplastic anemia and lymphoma. Invest Radiol 1986; 21:540–546.
158. Moore SG, Gooding CA, Brasch RC, et al. Bone marrow in children with acute lymphocytic leukemia; MR relaxation times. Radiology 1986; 160:237–240.
159. Masera G, Carnelli V, Ferrari M, et al. Prognostic significance of radiologic bone involvement in childhood acute lymphoblastic leukemia. Arch Dis Child 1977; 52:530–533.
160. Johnson FL. Marrow transplantation in the treatment of acute childhood leukemia. Am J Pediatr Hematol/Oncol 1981; 3:389–395.
161. Wollner N. Non-Hodgkin's lymphoma in children. Pediatr Clin North Am 1976; 23:371–378.
162. Dahlin DC. Reticulum cell sarcoma of bone. J Bone Joint Surg 1953; 35A:835–842.
163. Magnus HA, Wood LC. Primary reticulosarcoma of bone. J Bone Joint Surg 1956; 38B:258–278.
164. Wilson TW, Pugh DG. Primary reticulum cell sarcoma of bone, with emphasis on roentgen aspects. Radiology 1955; 65:343–351.
165. Sherman RS, Snyder RE. The roentgen appearance of primary reticulum cell sarcoma of bone. AJR 1947; 58:291–306.
166. Lanberg T, Garwicz S, Akerman M. A clinico-pathological study of non-Hodgkin's lymphomata in childhood. Br J Cancer 1975; 31:332–336.
167. Schey WL, White H, Conway JJ, Kidd JM. Lymphosarcoma in children. A roentgenologic and clinical evaluation of 60 children. AJR 1973; 117:59–72.
168. Pinkel D, Johnson W, Aur RJA. Non-Hodgkin's lymphoma in children. Br J Cancer 1975; 31:298–323.
169. Gall EA, Mallory TB. Malignant lymphoma. A clinico-pathologic survey of 618 cases. Am J Pathol 1942; 18:381–414.
170. Edwards J. Primary reticulum sarcoma of the spine. Report of a case with autopsy. J Bone Joint Surg 1953; 35A:835–843.
171. Valls J, Muscolo D, Schajowicz F. Reticulum cell sarcoma of bone. J Bone Joint Surg 1952; 34B:588–598.
172. Grossman H, Winchester PH, Bragg DG, et al. Roentgenographic changes in childhood Hodgkin's disease. AJR 1970; 108:354–364.
173. Baroni CD, Malchiodi F. Histology, age and sex distribution, and pathologic correlations of Hodgkin's disease. A study of 184 cases observed in Rome, Italy. Cancer 1980; 45:1549–1555.
174. Weaver GR, Sandler MP. Increased sensitivity of magnetic resonance imaging compared to radionuclide bone scintigraphy in the detection of lymphoma of the spine. Clin Nucl Med 1987; 12:333–334.
175. Walker HS, Dietrich RB, Flannigan BD, et al. Magnetic resonance imaging of the pediatric spine. Radiographics 1987; 7:1129–1152.
176. Cohen MD, Klatte EC, Baehner R, et al. Magnetic resonance of bone marrow disease in children. Radiology 1984; 151:715–718.
177. Kangarloo H, Dietrich RB, Taira RT, et al. MR imaging of bone marrow in children. J Comput Assist Tomogr 1986; 10:205–209.
178. Sze G, Bravo S, Krol G. Spinal lesions: quantitative and qualitative temporal evolution of gadopentate dimeglumine enhancement in MR imaging. Radiology 1989; 170:849–856.
179. Sze G, Krol G, Zimmerman R, Deck MDF. Malignant extradural spinal tumors: MR imaging with Gd-DTPA. Radiology 1988; 167:217–233.
180. Epstein B. The spine, a radiologic text and atlas. 4th ed. Philadelphia: Lea & Febiger, 1976.
181. Lewis TT, Kingsley DP. Magnetic resonance imaging of multiple spinal neurofibromata-neurofibromatosis. Neuroradiology 1987; 29:562–564.
182. Brasfield RD, Das Gupta TK. Von Recklinghausen's disease: a clinical pathologic study. Ann Surg 1972; 175:86–104.
183. Hughes JT. Pathology of the spinal cord. Tumors. London: Lloyd-Luke, 1966:160–180.
184. Gautier-Smith PC. Clinical aspects of spinal neurofibromatosis. Brain 1967; 90:359–393.
185. Zimmerman RA, Bilaniuk LT. Imaging of tumors of the spinal canal and cord. Radiol Clin North Am 1988; 26:65.
186. Burk DL, Brunberg JA, Kanal E, et al. Spinal and paraspinal neurofibromatosis: surface coil MR imaging at 1.5T. Radiology 1987; 162:797–801.
187. Laws JW, Dallis CP. Spinal deformities in neurofibromatosis. J Bone Joint Surg 1963; 45B:674–682.
188. Sordillo PP, Helson L, Hajdu SI, et al. Malignant schwannoma—clinical characteristics, survival and response to therapy. Cancer 1981; 10:2503–2509.
189. Wachstein M, Wolfe E. General neurofibromatosis (von Recklinghausen's disease) with local sarcomatous change and metastasis to regional lymph nodes. Arch Path Lab Med 1944; 37:331–333.
190. Levine E, Huntrakoon M, Wetzel LH. Malignant nerve-sheath neoplasms in neurofibromatosis: distinction from benign tumors by using imaging techniques. AJR 1987; 149:1059–1064.
191. Herrman J. Sarcomatous transformation in multiple neurofibromatosis (von Recklinghausen's disease). Ann Surg 1950; 131:206–217.
192. White HR. Survival in malignant schwannoma, an 18-year study. Cancer 1971; 3:720–729.
193. Davis PC, Hoffman JC, Ball TI, et al. Spinal abnormalities in pediatric patients: MR imaging findings compared with clinical, myelographic, and surgical findings. Radiology 1988; 166:679–685.
194. Scotti G, Scialfa G, Colombo N, Landoni, L. MR imaging of intradural extramedullary tumors of the cervical spine. J Comput Assist Tomogr 1985; 9:1037–1041.
195. Breger RK, Czernonke LF, Kass EG, et al. Truncation artifact in MR images of the intervertebral disk. AJNR 1988; 9:825–828.

196. Levy WJ, Bay J, Dohn D. Spinal cord meningioma. J Neurosurg 1982; 57:804–812.

197. Merten DF, Godding CA, Newton TH, Malamud N. Meningiomas of childhood and adolescence. Pediatrics 1974; 84:696–700.

198. Lombardi G, Passerini A. Spinal cord disease, a radiologic and myelographic analysis. Baltimore: Williams & Wilkins, 1964.

199. Parziel PM, Baleriaux D, Rodesch G, et al. Gd-DTPA enhanced MR imaging of spinal tumors. AJNR 1989; 10:249–258.

200. Bydder, GM, Kingsley PE, Brown J, et al. MR imaging of meningiomas including studies with and without gadolinium-DTPA. J Comput Assist Tomogr 1985; 9:690–697.

201. Barloon TJ, Yuh WT, Yang CJ, Schulz DH. Spinal subarachnoid tumor seeding from intracranial metastasis: MR findings. J Comput Assist Tomogr 1987; 11:242–244.

202. Krol G, Sze G, Malkin M, Walker R. MR of cranial and spinal meningeal carcinomatosis comparison with CT and myelography. AJNR 1988; 9:709–714.

203. Dorwart RH, Wara WM, Norman D, Levin VA. Complete myelographic evaluation of spinal metastases from medulloblastoma. Radiology 1981; 139:403–408.

204. Bryan P. CSF seeding of intracranial tumors: a study of 96 cases. Clin Radiol 1974; 25:355–360.

205. Kim KS, Ho SO, Weinberg PE, Lee C. Spinal leptomeningeal infiltration by systemic cancer: myelographic features. AJNR 1982; 3:233–237.

206. Deutsch M, Reigel DH. The value of myelography in the management of childhood medulloblastoma. Cancer 1980; 45:2194–2197.

207. Davis PC, Griedman NC, Fry SM, et al. Leptomeningeal metastasis: MR imaging. Radiology 1987; 163:449–454.

208. Sze G, Abramson A, Krol G, et al. Gadolinium-DTPA in the evaluation of intradural extramedullary disease. AJNR 1988; 9:153–163.

209. Dillon WP, Norman D, Newton TH, et al. Intradural spinal cord lesions: Gd-DTPA enhanced MR imaging. Radiology 1989; 170:229–237.

210. Reimer R, Onofrio BM. Astrocytomas of the spinal cord in children and adolescents. J Neurosurg 1985; 63:669–675.

211. Sloof JL, Kernohan JW, MacCarty CS. Primary intramedullary tumors of the spinal cord and filum terminale. Philadelphia: WB Saunders, 1969.

212. Packer RJ, Zimmerman RA, Bilaniuk LT, et al. Magnetic resonance imaging of lesions of the posterior fossa and upper cervical cord in childhood. Pediatrics 1985; 76:84–90.

213. Nokes SR, Murtagh FR, Jones D, et al. Childhood scoliosis: MR imaging. Radiology 1987; 164:791–797.

214. Goy AM, Pinto RS, Raghavenda BN, et al. Intramedullary spinal cord tumors: MR imaging with emphasis on associated cysts. Radiology 1986; 161:381–386.

215. Slasky BS, Bydder GM, Niendorf HP, Young IR. MR imaging with gadolinium-DTPA in the differentiation of tumor, syrinx and cysts of spinal cord. J Comput Assist Tomogr 1987; 11:845–850.

216. Williams AL, Haughton VM, Pojunas KW, et al. Differentiation of intramedullary neoplasms and cysts by MR. AJNR 1987; 8:527–532.

217. Sonneland PR, Scheithauer BW, Onofrio BM. Myxopapillary ependymoma, a clinicopathologic and immunocytochemical study of 77 cases. Cancer 1985; 56:883–893.

218. Barone BM, Elridge AR. Ependymomas, a clinical survey. J Neurosurg 1970; 33:428–438.

219. Kucharozyk W, Brant-Zawadzki M, Sobel D, et al. Central nervous system tumors in children: detection by magnetic resonance imaging. Radiology 1985; 155:131–136.

220. Kendall B, Russell J. Hemangioblastomas of the spinal cord. Br J Radiol 1966; 39:817–823.

221. Browne TR, Adams RD, Roberson GH. Hemangioblastoma of the spinal cord. Review and report of five cases. Arch Neurol 1976; 33:435–441.

222. Sato Y, Wazirim, Smith W, et al. Hippel-Lindau disease: MR imaging. Radiology 1988; 166:241–246.

223. Enomoto H, Shibata T, Ito A, et al. Multiple hemangioblastomas accompanied by syringomyelia in the cerebellum and the spinal cord. Surg Neurol 1984; 22:197–203.

224. Kaffenberger DA, Sah CP, Mortagh FR, et al. MR imaging of spinal cord hemangioblastoma associated with syringomyelia. J Comput Assist Tomogr 1988; 12:495–498.

Miscellaneous Disorders of the Spine

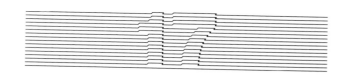

MARY K. EDWARDS, M.D.
TODD M. HARRIS, M.D.

Magnetic resonance imaging (MRI) of the normal pediatric spine reveals several distinct differences compared with the normal adult spine. From infancy through childhood the spine grows from a fetal or straight configuration to a more complex curve, reflecting the cervical and lumbar lordosis and thoracic kyphosis. The more straightened infant spine is more easily studied in the coronal and sagittal image planes in comparison with the adult spine. As children begin to hold their heads up, the cervical lordosis is seen. The lumbar lordosis develops as children begin walking. The intervertebral disc spaces are thicker and more rounded in infants (Fig. 17–1). As the child begins weight bearing, the disc spaces become more flattened and less spherical (Fig. 17–2). In newborns, the neural canal is quite capacious compared with the vertebral body size. Within the capacious canal there is a large amount of epidural fat that is most apparent in the lower lumbar and sacral regions. Within the spine of small children, the signal of the vertebral bodies is less bright on T1 weighted images than in older children and adults. The signal of the vertebral bodies is even less bright than that of the intervertebral disc spaces (Fig. 17–3). The decreased signal of the vertebral bodies on T1 weighted images in infants is due to the relative paucity of fat within the marrow compared with the abundant hematopoietic marrow.[1] In older children or adults, the marrow contains proportionately more fatty elements, causing normal vertebral bodies always to appear bright compared with the adjacent disc spaces (Fig. 17–4).

INTRADURAL LIPOMA AND LIPOMENINGOCELE

The exquisite sensitivity of MRI to fat on T1 weighted images has permitted the detection of many small intraspinal lipomas that were not apparent on computed tomography (CT) or other imaging modalities (see also the chapter on Spinal Dysraphism). In its most benign form, fat may be present at the conus medullaris and filum terminale in up to 5 percent of normal individuals.[2] Small lipomas present as incidental findings in other locations throughout the spinal canal (Figs. 17–5, 17–6). Lipomas should be differentiated from subacute hemorrhage, which is also bright on T1 weighted images. As opposed to subacute hemorrhage or methemoglobin, which is bright on both T1 and T2 weighted sequences, lipomas become less bright on T2 weighted sequences. Dysraphic spinal conditions remain the most common cause of intraspinal lipomas. Lipomas are frequently found in association with tethered cord or lipomyelomeningocele (Fig. 17–7).[3] Intraspinal lipomas may occur in association with mild forms of dysraphism, but without attachment of the distal cord to a neural placode. This finding indicates lipomeningocele, or intradural lipoma,

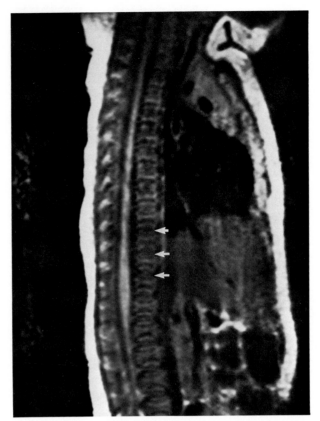

Figure 17–1. *Normal 7-month-old infant.* Sagittal proton-density image (2000/20) demonstrates rounded disc spaces (*arrows*), which are much larger compared with the vertebral bodies than in older children or adults. Note the straightened configuration of the infant spine.

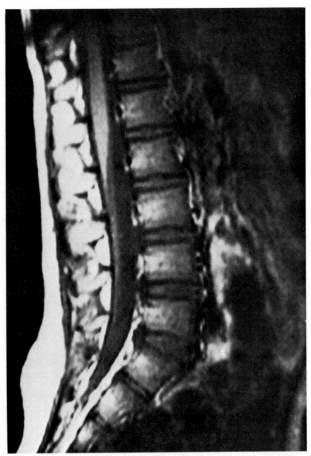

Figure 17–2. *Normal 7-year-old child.* Sagittal T1 weighted image (500/26) demonstrates normal lumbar lordosis of the older child as well as flattened disc spaces compared with the infant in Figure 17–1.

rather than Chiari malformation. Intracranial malformations such as hydrocephalus and tonsillar herniation do not commonly accompany lipomeningocele or intradural lipoma.

Other embryonal tumors also containing fatty elements may be found in the pediatric spine. These include epidermoid, dermoid, and teratomas, each with an MR appearance reflecting the components of the tissues within the tumor.[4] Epidermoids tend to be homogeneous in consistency, but may have signal characteristics on T1 weighted images ranging from fat to soft tissue density, reflecting the fat and squamous components of the tumor. Dermoids, arising from ectoderm and mesodermal rests, may have a more complex appearance. Teratomas, formed from all three germ layers, may have fat, solid keratin or cholesterol, fibrous tissue, muscle, or bone (Fig. 17–8).

SPINAL CORD CYSTS

Syringomyelia is a spinal cord disorder characterized by longitudinally oriented cavities containing cerebrospinal fluid (CSF), surrounded by a damaged or gliotic spinal cord. The term hydromyelia refers to dilatation of the central canal of the spinal cord; the term syringomyelia is used to describe cavities within the spinal cord parenchyma itself. In fact, it is impossible to differentiate hydromelia from syringomyelia, and when the central canal becomes dilated, rupture into the spinal cord parenchyma probably occurs quite early. For this reason, the terms syringomyelia and hydromyelia may be combined in the single diagnosis of syringohydromyelia. In this chapter the terms syringomyelia and syrinx refer to the entire disease process of spinal cord cyst, without consideration of etiology.

Intramedullary cystic cavities within the spinal cord have several potential etiologies that usually are not distinguishable by their clinical presentations.[5] MRI has proved helpful in differentiating among the several causes of intramedullary cavities, syringomyelia, tumor cyst, post-traumatic syrinx, and cord infarction. Tumor cysts may extend the length of the spinal cord and mimic syringomyelia, but are easily differentiated from benign spinal cord cysts by use of gadolinium-

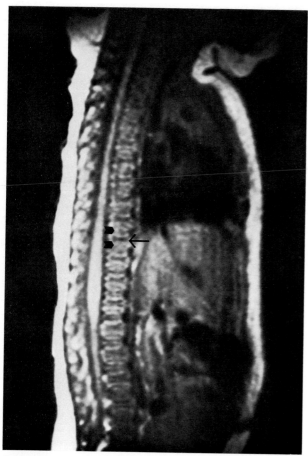

Figure 17–3. *Normal infant.* On sagittal T1 weighted sequence (500/26) the vertebral bodies appear slightly less bright (*arrow*) than the adjacent discs (*arrowheads*).

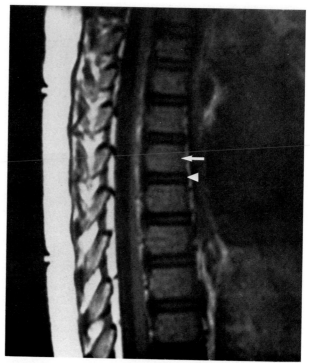

Figure 17–4. *Normal 7-year-old child.* Sagittal T1 weighted image (500/26) shows the marrow of the vertebral bodies (*arrow*) to be brighter than the adjacent discs (*arrowhead*).

DTPA enhancement.[6] Tumor cyst with enhancement is discussed more fully in the chapter on Tumors of the Spine.

Syringomyelia

The mechanism of development of syringomyelia is not clear. Many causes have been considered, including obstruction of the communication between the central canal of the spinal cord and the fourth ventricle at the obex. Although the exact cause of syringomyelia is not fully understood, there are well-recognized predisposing factors, including hydrocephalus, Chiari malformation, and other complex congenital malformations.[7] Syrinx cavities are common in both Chiari I and Chiari II malformations.

MR examination of cystic spinal cord lesions is undertaken whenever the clinical diagnosis of Chiari malformation, complex congenital malformation, spinal cord trauma, or spinal tumor is suspected. Syringomyelia may also occur as an isolated entity, usually appearing between the second and fourth decades.

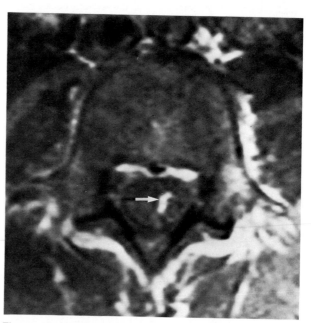

Figure 17–5. *Small filum lipoma.* Axial T1 weighted image (500/20) demonstrates an incidental lipoma of the filum terminale (*arrow*) appearing bright.

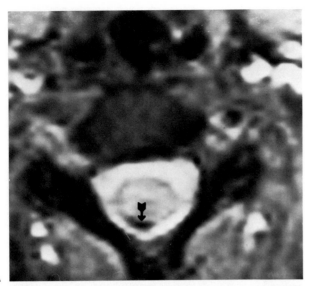
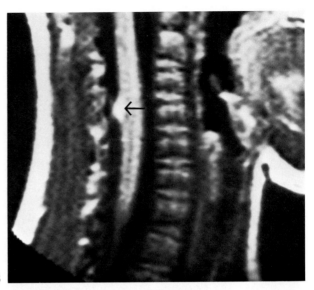

A

B

Figure 17–6. *Lipoma.* **A,** Axial T2 weighted sequence (2000/80) shows an asymptomatic cervical lipoma as an area of decreased signal and the posterior surface of the cervical spinal cord (*arrow*). **B,** Sagittal T1 weighted image (500/26) demonstrates increased signal corresponding to a small cervical lipoma (*arrow*).

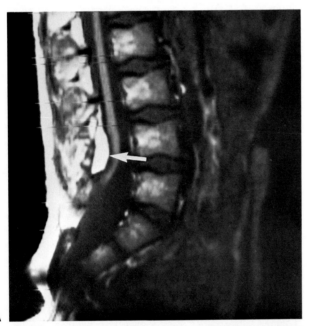
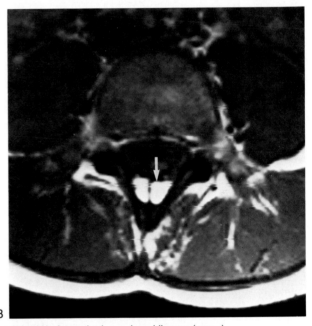

A

B

Figure 17–7. *Lipomyelomeningocele.* **A,** Sagittal T1 weighted image (500/26) shows the large dorsal lipoma (*arrow*) posterior to the tethered spinal cord just above the level of dysraphic posterior elements. **B,** Axial T1 weighted image (500/26) confirms the posterior location of the lumbar lipoma (*arrow*).

Children with syrinx commonly present with decreased pain and temperature sensation in the arms, with preservation of the sense of touch. Wasting of the intrinsic muscles of the hand may also be found. Severe pain may be the initial clinical presentation. Spastic weakness of the lower extremities and loss of bladder control are late findings in syringomyelia.

MRI has proved invaluable in the imaging of syringomyelia. Sagittal views are useful in providing an overview of cord morphology and in examining the craniocervical junction (Fig. 17–9). T1 weighted sequences are best for demonstrating cord morphology. Multiple septations are frequently demonstrated within the expanded syrinx cavity (Fig. 17–10). The

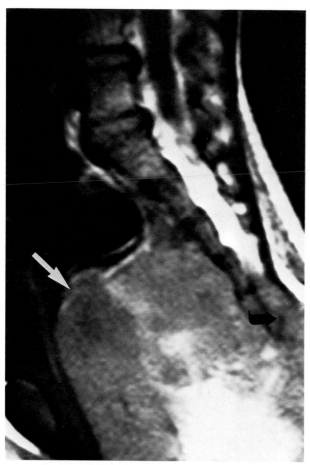

Figure 17–8. *Teratoma.* Sagittal T1 weighted image (500/26) demonstrates a huge anterior sacral teratoma (*arrow*) with mixed signal, and shows communication with the distal neural canal (*curved arrow*).

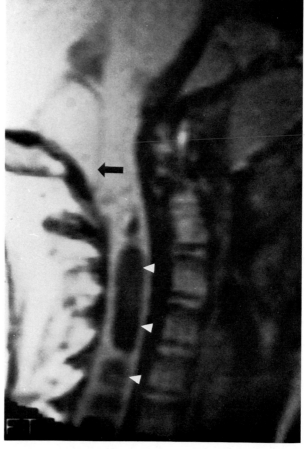

Figure 17–9. *Syrinx with Chiari II malformation.* Sagittal T1 weighted image (500/26) demonstrates low tonsils (*arrow*) with multiseptated syrinx in the cervical spinal cord (*arrowheads*).

thoracic spinal cord is a common location for syrinx cavities associated with Chiari malformation (Fig. 17–11). Pulsatile CSF motion within spinal cord cysts can be demonstrated with MRI, flow void being seen within the syrinx cavity. The observation of pulsations within a spinal cord cyst is indicative of a non-neoplastic cyst.[9] The decrease in pulsation after a shunt procedure may be a valuable indication of the success of surgery.[9] To maximize flow information, the T2 weighted images should be obtained with nonmotion compensated and nongated axial views. If fluid within a cyst is in motion, it will show low signal intensity on both first and second echoes of a multiecho T2 weighted sequence; the signal intensity is lowest on the second echo.

Post-traumatic Syrinx

Post-traumatic myelomalacia resulting in cystic destruction of the spinal cord may be indistinguishable from other causes of syrinx.[10,11] Post-traumatic spinal

cord cysts are usually diagnosed late, when the neurologic sequelae of the spinal cord trauma have not resolved. MRI is the most accurate method of demonstrating these cysts.[12] Post-traumatic syrinx cavities may present clinically within a few months or many years after trauma.[13] The traumatic event is usually severe enough to have caused paraplegia or tetraplegia. The syrinx should be suspected when spinal cord symptoms persist after injury, or when the deficits progress after being static for months or years following the injury.[13] Sagittal MR scans may demonstrate both the bony injury and the spinal cord injury after trauma (Fig. 17–12). Axial T1 weighted images may better define the location of the post-traumatic syrinx within the spinal cord (Fig. 17–13).

Spinal Subarachnoid Cysts

Arachnoid cysts do occur in the neural canal, although less commonly than in the head. Their cause is not clear, but they have been found in conjunction with

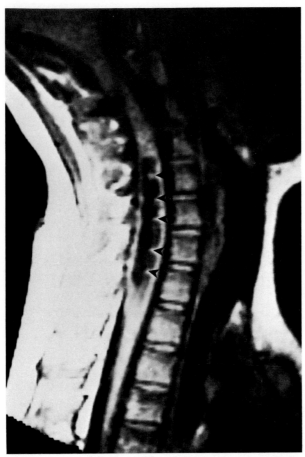

Figure 17-10. *Septations within a cervical syrinx.* Sagittal T1 weighted image (500/26) demonstrates multiple septations (*arrowheads*) within a syrinx cavity.

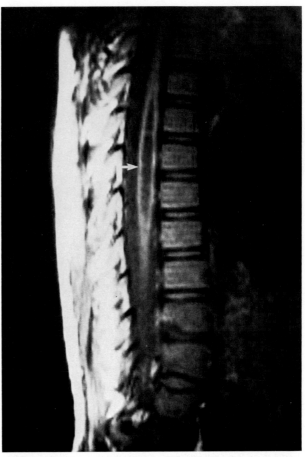

Figure 17-11. *Thoracic syrinx cavity.* Sagittal T1 image (500/26) shows focal expansion of the thoracic spinal cord (*arrow*) due to a localized syrinx cavity.

arachnoiditis and post-traumatic syrinx.[14] Arachnoid cysts may cause symptoms by compressing the spinal cord or nerve roots. Syringomyelia is commonly found in association with arachnoid cysts in the spine. It is important to identify arachnoid cysts, because failure of symptoms to improve after syrinx shunting may be the result of CSF trapping in an arachnoid cyst rather than failure of surgery.[14] T1 weighted axial MR sequences are the most accurate method for diagnosing arachnoid cysts (Fig. 17-14). Intrathecal contrast enhanced CT is limited in its ability to define arachnoid cysts, because the arachnoid adhesions prevent the normal flow of contrast within the subarachnoid space.

Root Sheath Cysts

Perineural cysts, also known as Tarlov's cysts, are common throughout the neural canal. They may reach a large size in the lumbosacral regions and present with pressure erosion of the surrounding bony canal (Fig.

17-15). Other cystic lesions in this region that may mimic perineural cysts and include meningeal diverticula or occult intrasacral meningocele.[15]

SCOLIOSIS

Scoliosis is usually idiopathic in young females, but should be pursued with MRI if any indication of underlying spinal abnormality is found. These indications include dextroscoliosis in any child, scoliosis in a boy, and scoliosis in association with dimple, hairy patch, or paraspinal abnormality. If the scoliosis progresses quickly, or if clubfoot is found in addition to scoliosis, MRI is helpful in defining a possible spinal abnormality. Vertebral body abnormalities, paravertebral masses, and segmentation anomalies can be well defined by MRI.[1] A common cause of scoliosis is dysraphic spine with tethered spinal cord, which may be occult (Fig. 17-16). In a child who has undergone previous repair of myelomeningocele, scoliosis com-

Text continues on page 508

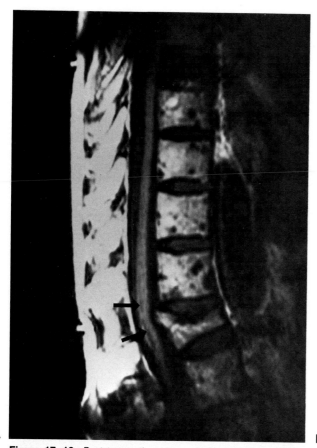

A

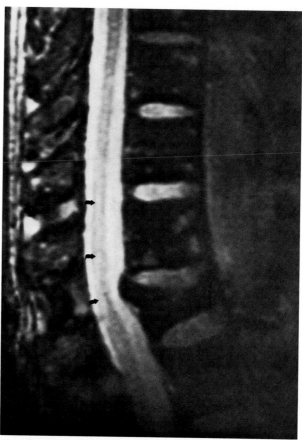

B

Figure 17–12. *Post traumatic syrinx.* ***A,*** Sagittal T1 weighted image shows pathologic fracture of a lower thoracic vertebra causing marked cord impingement. A focal post-traumatic syrinx is identified within the adjacent spinal cord (*arrows*). ***B,*** Sagittal gradient-echo image (500/18/20) shows faint but definite increased signal within the spinal cord related to the post-traumatic syrinx and myelomalacia (*arrows*).

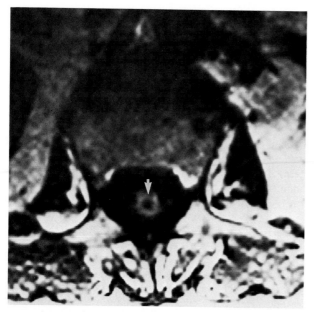

Figure 17–13. Post-traumatic syrinx is best defined in the axial T1 weighted sequence (500/26). The syrinx cavity is clearly defined as an area of low signal within the center of the cord (*arrow*).

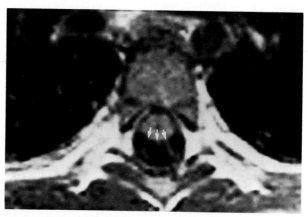

Figure 17–14. *Arachnoid cysts.* Axial T1 weighted image (500/26) demonstrates multiple arachnoid cysts separated by septations (*arrows*) posterior to the thoracic spinal cord.

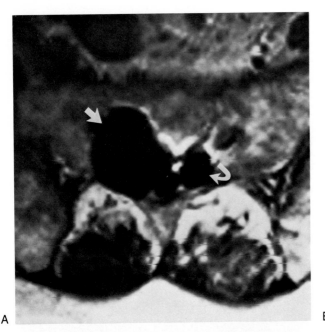

A

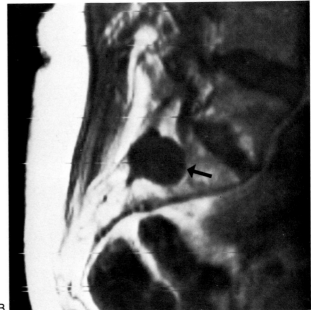

B

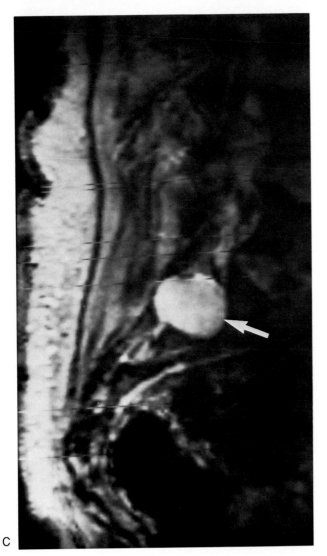

C

Figure 17–15. *Perineural cyst.*   **A,** Axial T1 weighted image of the sacrum shows a huge perineural cyst (*arrow*) on the right and a smaller perineural cyst (*curved arrow*) on the left. Bony erosion secondary to the large right cyst is evident. **B,** Sagittal T1 weighted image clearly defines the extent of bony erosion related to the large right perineural cyst (*arrow*). **C,** Sagittal T2 weighted image (2000/80) shows increased signal within the perineural cyst consistent with cerebrospinal fluid (CSF) (*arrow*).

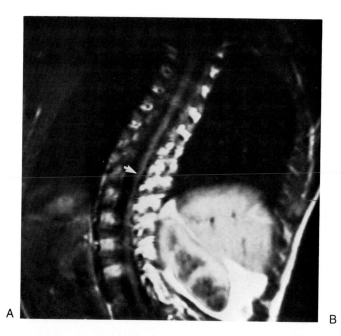

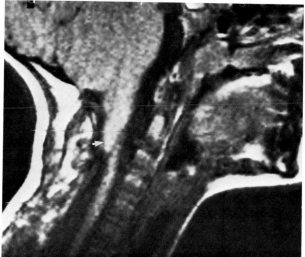

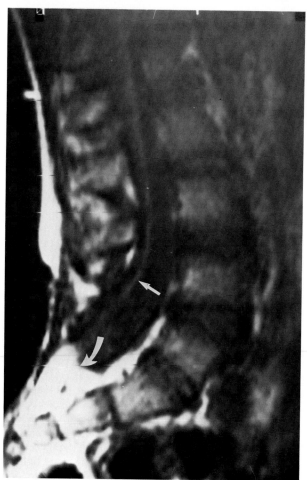

Figure 17–16. *Scoliosis secondary to Chiari malformation.* ***A,*** Coronal T1 weighted image (500/26) clearly defines the relationship of the spinal cord (*arrow*) to the scoliotic spine. ***B,*** Sagittal T1 weighted image (500/26) at the level of the foramen magnum shows the very low tonsils (*arrow*) related to the Chiari malformation. ***C,*** Sagittal T1 weighted image (500/26) at the lumbosacral region shows the tethered spinal cord (*arrow*) and intraspinal lipoma (*curved arrow*) at the level of the dysraphic spinal defect.

monly develops in adolescence during the growth spurt. When this occurs, the possibility of tethered spinal cord or syringomyelia should be considered.[16]

Fusion and segmental anomalies of the spine are commonly associated with childhood scoliosis.[17] The complex fusion anomalies of the spine are well studied by MRI, with excellent visualization of the spinal cord in relation to the bony anomaly. Plain film and CT scans better define the bony changes (Fig. 17–17), but MRI best defines the associated anomalies of the spinal cord. Hemivertebra and scoliosis are commonly associated with diastematomyelia. MRI is the best noninvasive method of diagnosing and defining the extent of diastematomyelia.[18] T1 weighted axial images clearly define both the bony spur and the divided cord characteristic of diastematomyelia (Fig. 17–18). In up to one-half of cases of diastematomyelia, only the divided cord can be found, with no associated bony spur. Occasionally, only a fibrotic or dural band is found separating the two halves of the spinal cord (see also the chapter on Spinal Dysraphism).[19]

CAUDAL REGRESSION

The incidence of caudal regression is approximately one in 3,000.[19] Caudal regression syndrome includes a spectrum of spine malformations with associated absence or regression of the sacrum. The most severe form, known as sirenomelia, is characterized by fusion of the lower extremities, with variable absence of the distal spine, anal atresia, and malformation of the external genitalia.[1] This degree of spinal agenesis is variable, and in the more benign forms, only the distal sacrum or coccyx may be missing. The clinical presentation reflects the severity of the spinal agenesis. Absent coccyx is usually asymptomatic. The most common form of sacral agenesis, occurring in approximately 50 percent of cases, is characterized by symmetric absence of the distal sacrum, usually with stable articulation of the proximal sacral alae with the ilia.[1] Sacral agenesis may be unilateral in up to one-third of cases.[19] The neural canal usually ends abruptly or is severely narrowed at the level of the bony agenesis, with severe constriction of the neural canal ending in fibrous bands or dural stenosis. The spinal cord either terminates or is dysplastic at the level of the spinal anomaly. Dysraphism, tethered cord, and dermal sinus tract may be seen with caudal agenesis, but occur infrequently.

Non-neurologic abnormalities are occasionally associated with caudal regression syndrome, including pulmonary hypoplasia and severe renal dysplasia or aplasia. There is a strong association with sacral agenesis and diabetic mothers. Mental retardation and cardiac malformations are found in up to one-third of patients with sacral agenesis.

MRI is the best method of evaluating the complex spinal and cord malformations of caudal agenesis. As-

sociated malformations may be detected and characterized by MRI. T1 weighted sagittal MR images clearly define the extent of the bony and neural anomaly (Fig. 17–19).

Absence of a portion of the vertebral body may be clearly defined by MRI. Absent pedicle may occur in the lumbar region (Fig. 17–20), and absence of one or both laminae is common in the cervical region. MRI is helpful in defining the extent of the congenital malformation and in demonstrating normal fat filling the bony void. This may help to exclude bone destruction from soft tissue mass as a cause of the absent bone (see also the chapter on Spinal Dysraphism).

SPINAL STENOSIS

Spinal stenosis is an uncommon problem in the pediatric population, usually presenting in the fifth or sixth decade. Achondroplasia is one cause of spinal stenosis. Children with achondroplasia may be spared the symptoms of spinal stenosis, but when the disease is advanced they may experience mild to moderate paraparesis and pain. Short, thick pedicles narrowing the spinal canal in the anteroposterior direction are the most important factors in the pathogenesis of congenital spinal stenosis. In achondroplasia there is narrowing and constriction at the level of the foramen magnum, as well as throughout the remainder of the neural canal (Fig. 17–21). MRI clearly defines the extent of spinal cord compression throughout the constricted neural canal. It also clearly reveals the posterior scalloping of the vertebral bodies. Early degenerative changes may accentuate the symptoms of cord compression (Fig. 17–22).

Other causes of spinal stenosis in children are uncommon and are frequently idiopathic. Bony dysplasias, Morquio's disease, and trauma are among the recognized causes of spinal stenosis. Presenting symptoms are usually radiculopathy; back, neck, or shoulder pain; and occasionally some degree of spasticity and weakness. Weakness and spasticity are usually due to involvement of the cortical spinal tracts, spinal thalamic tracts, or posterior columns.[20] MRI provides excellent detail of the degree of compression of the spinal cord. Sagittal T2 weighted or gradient-echo images have the benefit of defining the dark margin of cortical bone in contrast to CSF and spinal cord, to best define the extent of spinal stenosis (Fig. 17–23).

Spondyloepiphyseal dysplasia is an uncommon cause of spinal cord compression and scoliosis. Compression at the level of the foramen magnum is well demonstrated on sagittal images, and myelomalacia is more clearly demonstrated on axial T2 weighted sequences (Fig. 17–24). Coronal MR images are helpful in defining the bony deformity that results in scoliosis in patients with spondyloepiphyseal dysplasia (Fig. 17–25). As the disease progresses the vertebral body deformity may result in severe spondylosis, with spinal stenosis at an early age (Fig. 17–26).

Text continues on page 512

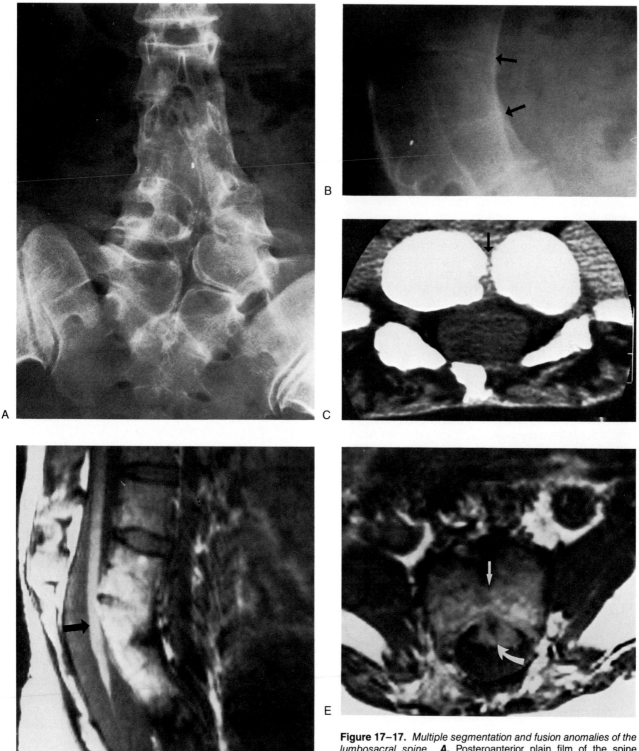

Figure 17–17. *Multiple segmentation and fusion anomalies of the lumbosacral spine.* ***A,*** Posteroanterior plain film of the spine shows multiple fusion and segmentation anomalies from L3 to S2. ***B,*** Lateral plain film of the spine confirms the fusion of L3 to L5 (*arrows*). ***C,*** Axial CT image shows a cleft in the L5 vertebral body (*arrow*). ***D,*** Sagittal T1 weighted image (500/26) defines the relationship of the tethered spinal cord (*arrow*) to the bony anomalies. ***E,*** Axial T1 weighted image (500/26) at L5 demonstrates not only the cleft vertebral body (*arrow*) but also the cleft of the tethered spinal cord (*curved arrow*).

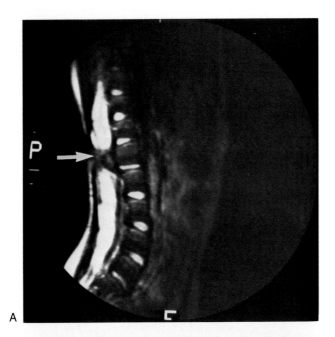

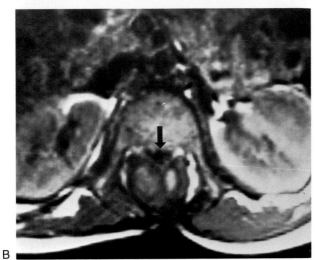

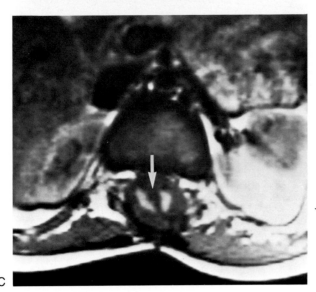

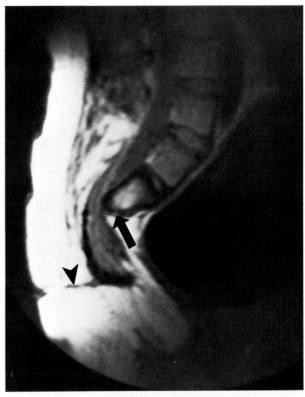

Figure 17–19. *Caudal regression.* Sagittal T1 weighted image (500/20) demonstrates the abrupt termination of the sacrum (*arrow*) and distal extension of the caudal sac to connect with a dermal sinus tract (*arrowhead*).

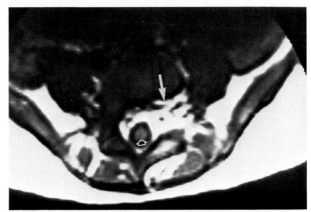

Figure 17–20. *Absent pedicle.* Axial T1 weighted image (500/26) clearly demonstrates not only the absence of the left pedicle at L5 (*long arrow*) but also a tethered spinal cord within the neural canal (*open arrow*).

◄ **Figure 17–18.** *Diastematomyelia.* **A,** Sagittal T2 weighted image (2000/80) shows a large bony spur arising from T12 and L1 (*arrow*) piercing the subarachnoid space. **B,** Axial T1 weighted image (500/26) shows the bony spur (*arrow*) bisecting the conus medullaris. **C,** Axial T1 weighted image (500/26) below the level of the diastematomyelia shows a persistent cleft in the distal conus medullaris (*arrow*).

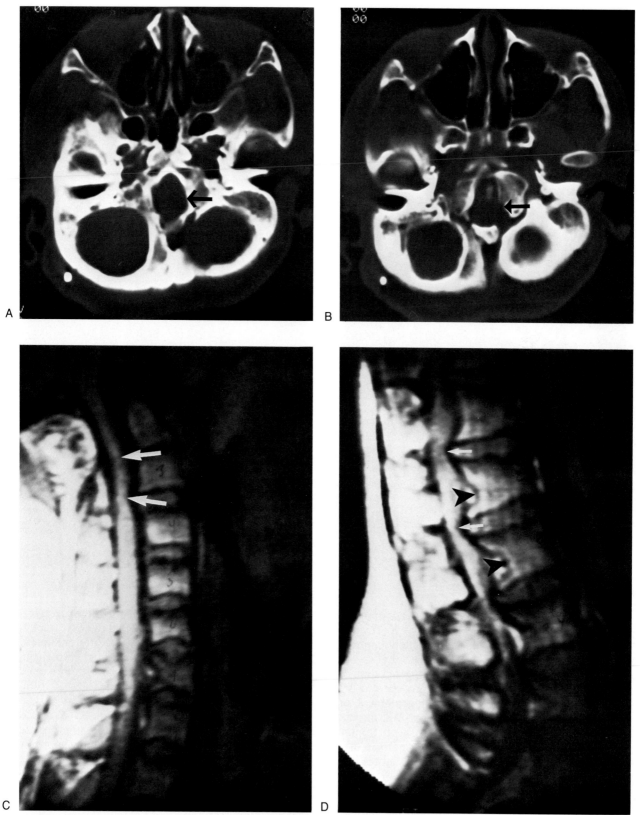

Figure 17–21. *Spinal stenosis.* *13-year-old patient with achondroplasia and gait disturbance.* ***A,*** Axial CT scan at the level of the foramen magnum clearly shows constriction of the bony foramen (*arrow*). ***B,*** Axial CT scan at C1 shows bony stenosis (*arrow*). ***C,*** Sagittal T1 weighted image (500/26) of the cervical spine shows marked cord narrowing at C2 and C3 (*arrows*). ***D,*** Sagittal T1 weighted image (500/26) at the lumbar region shows extensive spinal stenosis (*arrows*) with posterior scalloping of the vertebral bodies (*arrowheads*).

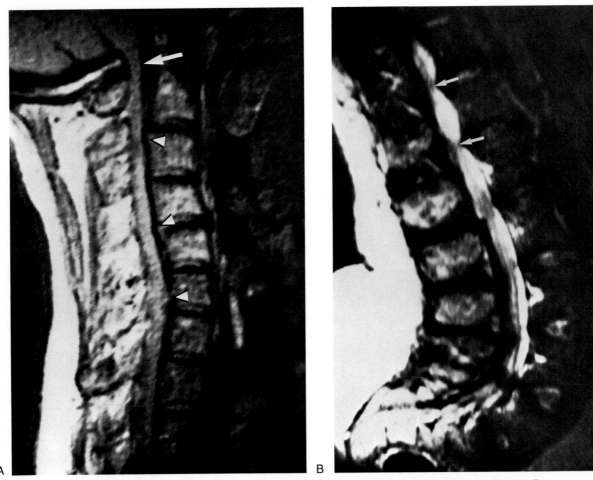

A   B

Figure 17–22. *17-year-old patient with achondroplasia and early degenerative spine changes.* ***A,*** Sagittal T1 weighted image (500/26) shows constriction at the level of the foramen magnum (*arrow*) as well as diffuse spinal stenosis throughout the cervical region, compounded by cervical spondylosis creating extensive cord compression (*arrowheads*). ***B,*** Sagittal gradient-echo image (550/18/20) shows extensive bony hypertrophy (*arrows*) accentuating the spinal stenosis.

DISC DEGENERATION

Disc disease and bony spondylosis, common in adults, are uncommon in children. Bony hypertrophy with spinal or foraminal stenosis is virtually nonexistent in childhood, unless accompanied by severe trauma or congenital bony dysplasia. Degeneration of the intervertebral disc, however, is a process that begins early in life and may present with acute neck or back pain in adolescence or teenage years. Disc herniation in children is commonly the result of acute trauma and is often accompanied by a history of sports injury. The nucleus pulposus in children is much more fluid than in adults. When herniation occurs in a young disc, large volumes of disc material may be extruded. The herniated disc material may appear viscous at surgery rather than cartilaginous as in adults. The herniated disc material may rupture through the posterior longitudinal ligament or be confined in the subligamentous location.

MRI is more sensitive to disc degeneration and disc herniation than CT or myelography.[22–24] Radiologists interpreting MRI must become familiar with its response to CSF flow and must understand flow compensation pulse sequences available from different manufacturers of MR equipment. Variable flip-angle, gradient-echo pulse sequences may provide more rapid imaging of the spine. Some authors suggest that gradient-echo scans should be performed in the cervical and thoracic region, but conventional T1 or T2 weighted spin-echo images are thought to be more appropriate in the lumbar region.[25,26] Surface coil imaging improves the resolution of both cervical and lumbar disc disease.

Sagittal MR images provide excellent detail and determine the alignment of the spine as well as the focal impingement on the neural canal caused by disc bulge or herniation. When the posterior longitudinal ligament is intact, herniated disc material is confined by the posterior longitudinal ligament to the immediate disc space or posterior vertebral body region (Fig.

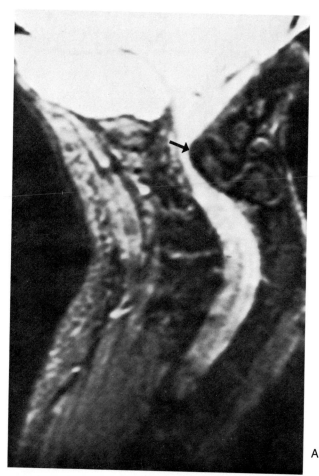

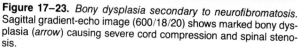

Figure 17–23. *Bony dysplasia secondary to neurofibromatosis.* Sagittal gradient-echo image (600/18/20) shows marked bony dysplasia (*arrow*) causing severe cord compression and spinal stenosis.

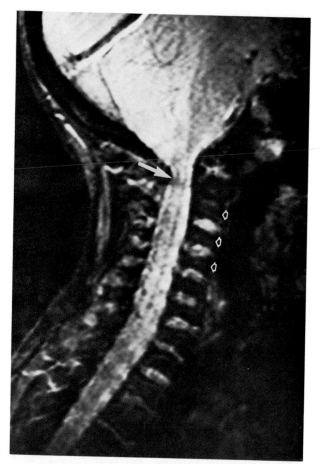

A

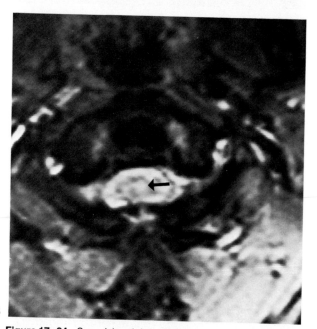

B

17–27). MRI provides better definition of the intact posterior longitudinal ligament than is possible on either CT or myelography. MRI is less helpful in determining whether a disc is bulging or herniated in the subligamentous dislocation (Fig. 17–28). When disc herniation has occurred with rupture of the nucleus pulposus through both the annulus fibrosus and the posterior longitudinal ligament, the term "free fragment" is used. Disc fragments commonly appear as areas of bright signal surrounded by a thin dark rim on gradient-echo images (Fig. 17–29).[27] When large disc fragments compromise the anteroposterior diameter of the neural canal in the cervical and thoracic regions, cord compression and myelomalacia may result. Myelomalacia appears on gradient-echo and T2 weighted images as abnormally bright signal within the cord parenchyma (Fig. 17–30).

MRI is generally more sensitive than other imaging modalities to lesions in the spine, possibly resulting in better detection of disc disease. Unfortunately, a lesion

Figure 17–24. *Spondyloepiphyseal dysplasia.* **A,** Sagittal gradient-echo image (550/18/20) shows flattening of the vertebral bodies (*open arrows*) and anteroposterior narrowing at C1 (*long arrow*). **B,** Axial gradient-echo image (550/18/20) better defines the myelomalacia of the upper cervical spinal cord (*arrow*) related to the bony stenosis.

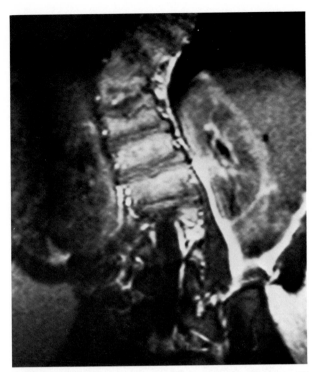

Figure 17–25. *Spondyloepiphyseal dysplasia.* Coronal T1 weighted image (500/26) shows severe scoliosis related to multiple vertebral body fractures.

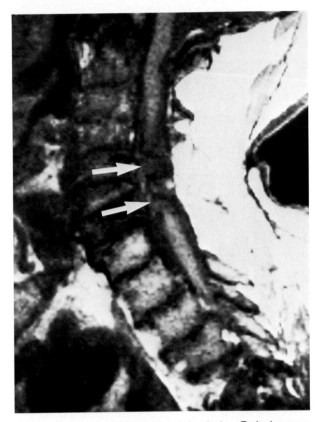

Figure 17–26. *Spondyloepiphyseal dysplasia.* Early degenerative changes cause marked cord compression (*arrows*) on this sagittal T1 weighted image (500/26).

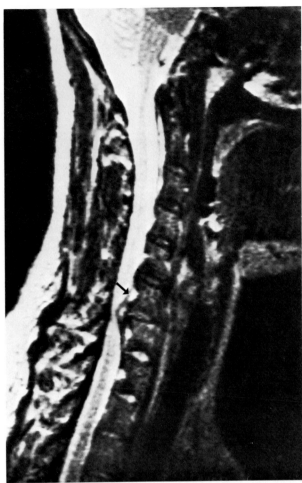

Figure 17–27. Sagittal T2 weighted image (2000/80) shows an intact posterior longitudinal ligament (*arrow*) being displaced by a huge, herniated cervical disc.

detected by MRI is not necessarily the cause of radicular or cord symptoms, and the MR findings must always be considered in conjunction with clinical history. MR images obtained in the supine position do not always reflect the appearance of the disc when the patient is weight bearing, at which time disc herniation or bulge may be accentuated.

Disc degeneration is associated with a loss of disc hydration and appears as a decrease in signal within the disc on all image sequences, although T2 weighted images best define the loss of hydration within the disc.[28] Lumbar disc herniation appears as an area of slightly increased signal in the neural canal, similar to the adjacent disc space, with obliteration of the normal fat planes in the neural canal and neural foramen (Fig. 17–31).

In both children and adults, signal changes are seen in the vertebral body end plate adjacent to disc disease. The vertebral body changes have been noted to take three main forms.[29] The earliest vertebral body change with disc disease, termed type 1 change, is that

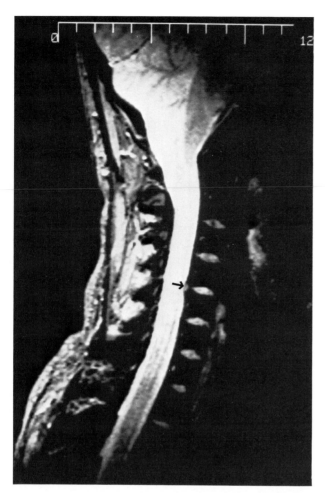

Figure 17-28. *Small disc herniation versus bulge in the cervical region.* Sagittal gradient-echo image (550/18/20) shows a focal soft tissue defect (*arrow*) at the C4–C5 location. MRI may not be able to differentiate among a small disc herniation and a subligamentous location and a disc bulge.

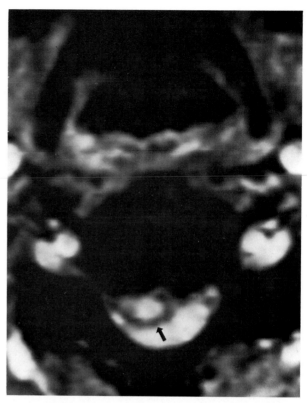

Figure 17-29. *Huge extruded disc fragment in the cervical region.* Axial gradient-echo image (550/18/20) shows the fragment (*arrow*) as an area of bright signal surrounded by a dark rim.

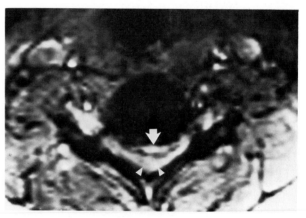

Figure 17-30. *Myelomalacia.* A huge cervical disc (*arrow*) results in spinal stenosis, cord compression, and abnormally bright signal within the cervical spinal cord (*arrowheads*).

of decreased signal on T1 weighted images, with a slight increase in signal on T2 weighted images, in the vertebral body adjacent to a degenerated disc. Type 2 changes appear as increased signal intensity in the vertebral body marrow on T1 weighted images and isointense or slightly hyperintense on T2 weighted images (Fig. 17-32). Patients with type 1 change have been observed to develop type 2 changes with time. The third type of vertebral body change is uncommon in children and appears to be related to severe bony sclerosis on plain radiographs. It appears as lack of signal, related to the absence of marrow in areas of advanced sclerosis.

SPONDYLOLISTHESIS

Spondylolisthesis is a condition in which a superior vertebral body is displaced in relation to the adjacent inferior vertebral body. In the lumbar region the supe-

rior vertebral body is prone to slip forward in relation to the inferior vertebral body because of the lumbar lordosis. Posterior slip of the superior vertebral body may occur, especially in the cervical region, and is termed retrolisthesis. Spondylolisthesis may occur either with or without an intact pars interarticularis. When spondylolisthesis occurs with an intact pars in-

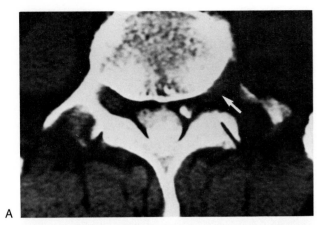

A

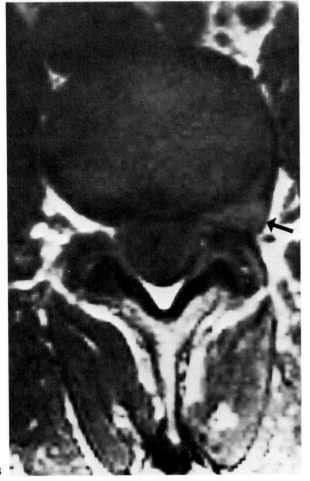

B

Figure 17–31. *A,* Axial CT image only poorly defines a focal lateral disc herniation (*arrow*). Axial T1 weighted image (500/26) shows the disc herniation to excellent advantage (*arrow*). *B,* Axial T1 weighted image (500/26) clearly defines the extent of the large lateral herniated disc (*arrow*).

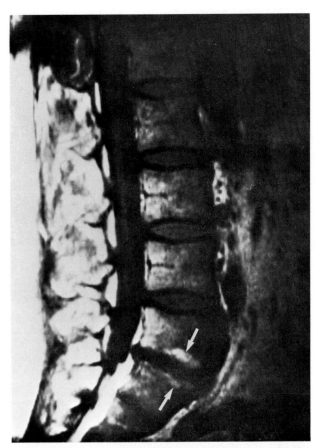

Figure 17–32. *Type 2 degenerative vertebral body change.* Focal bright signal is seen within the vertebral bodies adjacent to disc degeneration at the L5–S1 level (*arrows*) on this sagittal T1 weighted image (500/26).

terarticularis, the disc at the involved level is always degenerative and the degree of spondylolisthesis is always mild. In children, spondylolisthesis is far more likely to be the result of a defect of the pars interarticularis (spondylolysis). The degree of subluxation may be mild, moderate, or severe with spondylolysis. Spondylolysis is the result of traumatic fracture of the pars interarticularis, usually in susceptible individuals with a congenitally thin or weak pars interarticularis.[21]

Sagittal T1 weighted MR images provide the most accurate and noninvasive means of identifying the degree of spondylolisthesis as well as the relationship of the bony canal to the cauda equina (Fig. 17–33). Axial images may better define the bony defect in the pars interarticularis.

RHEUMATOID ARTHRITIS

Cervical cord compression may be the most significant clinical abnormality in patients with rheumatoid arthritis (see also the chapter on Miscellaneous Disorders of the Musculoskeletal System). Cord compres-

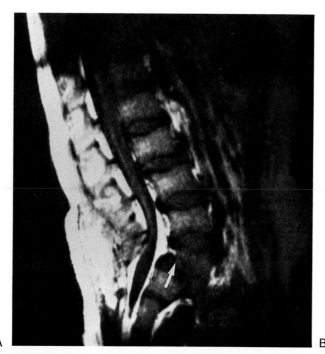
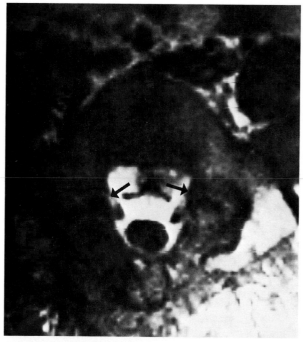

A

B

Figure 17–33. *Spondylolysis and spondylolisthesis.* **A,** Sagittal T1 weighted image (500/26) shows anterior subluxation of L5 on S1 (*arrow*). **B,** Axial T1 weighted image (500/26) best defines the pars defect (*arrows*).

sion results from dislocations within the cervical spine and can lead to paresis, paralysis, or even death. Subluxation of the spine in patients with rheumatoid arthritis is due in large part to the ligamentous laxity characteristic of the disease. Other factors may contribute to the cord compression, including erosion of the dens, basilar settling, ligamentous calcification, and osteophyte formation.[30–32] A large mass of pannus may also occur posterior to the dens, further compressing the cervical medullary spinal cord. In the atlantoaxial region subluxation is both common and significant in patients with rheumatoid arthritis. It may take many forms, including anterior atlantoaxial subluxation, basilar settling, lateral subluxation of C1 on C2, and posterior atlantoaxial subluxation.[33] Subluxation also occurs at other levels in the spine. Juvenile rheumatoid arthritis is similar to the adult form in the propensity of the spine to undergo subluxation, in pannus formation, and in atlantoaxial impaction. Juvenile rheumatoid arthritis differs from the adult form in the tendency to have extensive fusion of the posterior elements of the spine. This may result in thinning of the vertebral bodies.

MRI has proved helpful in evaluating patients with rheumatoid arthritis.[30] It is the best imaging tool for measuring the cervical medullary angle. Angles of less than 135 degrees in patients with rheumatoid arthritis have a high correlation with brain stem compression, myelopathy, or C2 nerve root pain.[30] The associated cord compression, subluxation, dens erosion, and pannus formation are clearly evaluated by MRI (Fig.

17–34). Bony fusion is also identified on sagittal MR images (Fig. 17–35). Pannus formation is commonly found posterior to the dens and is seen as an increased amount of soft tissue material adjacent to a sclerotic dens. Sagittal MRI consistently demonstrates the anatomic cause of brain stem symptoms in patients with rheumatoid arthritis.[30]

DEMYELINATING DISEASES OF THE SPINAL CORD

Multiple sclerosis (MS) is the most common and most typical of demyelinating diseases. Demyelinating, or myelinoclastic, diseases are those in which normally formed myelin is later destroyed. The causes of myelinoclastic diseases are related to infectious, postinfectious autoimmune, vascular, toxic, and idiopathic mechanisms. Although MS is poorly understood, there is a significant body of information that suggests a viral etiology in genetically susceptible individuals.[34]

Multiple Sclerosis

Although most patients with MS develop the first symptoms in early adulthood, 15 percent become ill before the age of 20 years.[34] The clinical presentation of spinal cord involvement with multiple sclerosis is weakness, numbness, tingling, and gait disturbance. Loss of sphincter control and paralysis may develop.

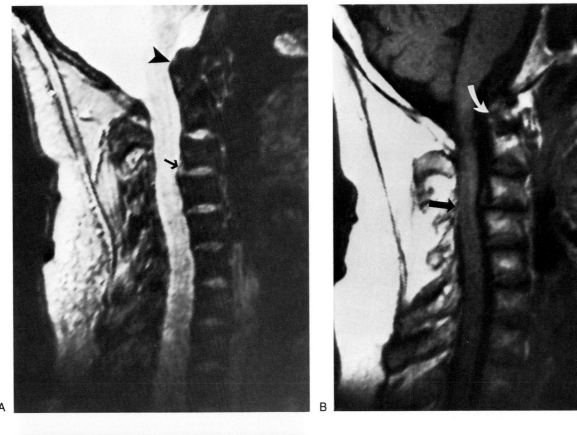

A

B

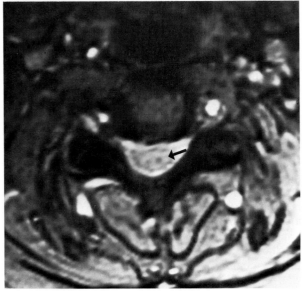

C

Figure 17–34. *Rheumatoid arthritis.* **A,** Sagittal gradient-echo image (550/18/20) shows pannus formation of the dens (*arrowhead*) and subluxation of C3 on C4 (*arrow*). **B,** Sagittal T1 weighted image (500/26) shows cord compression related to the subluxation at C3–C4 (*arrow*). Irregular signal at C1–C2 is due to pannus formation (*curved arrow*). **C,** Axial gradient-echo image (550/18/20) shows myelomalacia of the cervical cord (*arrow*).

Areas of demyelination occur within the white matter that is peripherally located in the spinal cord. Lesions may be focal, multifocal, or confluent and extensive throughout the spinal cord (Fig. 17–36). T2 weighted or gradient-echo images are most helpful in demonstrating the abnormal areas of demyelination, which appear bright and usually acentric within the spinal cord (Fig. 17–37). The role of spinal MRI in MS is not only to demonstrate the focal spinal cord abnormality, but to exclude other, treatable causes of focal neurologic deficit such as disc disease, tumor, or syrinx. MRI also may help stage the clinical severity of the disease by demonstrating multiple lesions that may not necessarily be symptomatic. The number and size of lesions

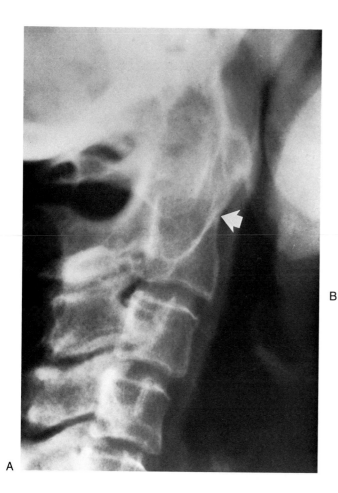

A

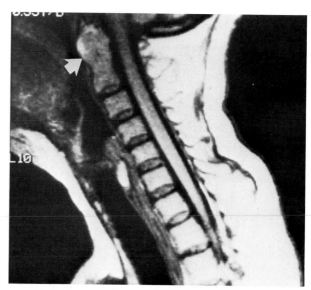

B

Figure 17–35. *Juvenile rheumatoid arthritis.* ***A,*** Plain film of the lateral cervical spine shows fusion of the dens and anterior arch of C1 (*arrow*). ***B,*** Sagittal T1 weighted image (500/40) confirms the bony fusion of C1 and the dens (*arrow*), with bright signal of marrow in a large bony mass. No cord compression or subluxation is seen.

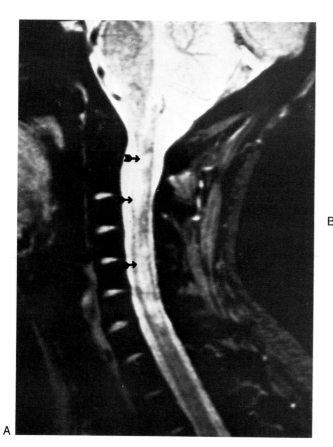

A

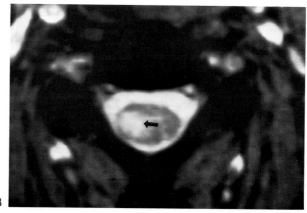

B

Figure 17–36. *Multiple sclerosis.* ***A,*** Sagittal T2 weighted image (2000/100) shows extensive areas of bright signal throughout the cervical spinal cord (*arrows*). ***B,*** Axial T2 weighted image (2000/100) shows an eccentric lesion in an area of demyelination in the right portion of the cervical spinal cord (*arrow*).

519

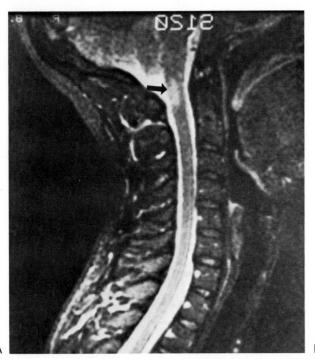
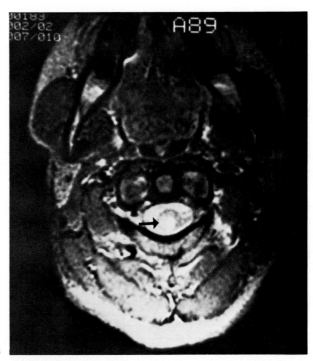

A   B

Figure 17–37. *Multiple sclerosis.* ***A,*** Sagittal gradient-echo image (550/18/20) shows a single focus of abnormal signal in the cervical spinal cord (*arrow*). ***B,*** Axial gradient-echo image (550/18/20) at the same location confirms the area of demyelination (*arrow*).

detected by MRI correlate well with the severity of disease.[35]

Postviral Immune-Mediated White Matter Diseases

Occasionally, after a viral illness, a patient develops an autoimmune response to white matter with variable and usually reversible demyelination. Guillain-Barré syndrome, Devic's syndrome, and acute disseminated encephalomyelitis (ADEM) are examples of virally induced, immune-mediated white matter diseases. Transverse myelitis is a nonspecific term used to refer to viral or postviral immune-mediated disease of the spinal cord. ADEM commonly presents within weeks after varicella or influenza infection or immunization. ADEM may involve only the brain but may present with spinal cord symptoms. Devic's syndrome is similar to ADEM but includes optic nerve and spinal cord involvement. On T2 weighted images, white matter lesions are seen within the spinal cord, appearing similar to multiple sclerosis plaques (Fig. 17–38).[36]

VASCULAR MALFORMATIONS

Spinal vascular malformations have been classified according to many criteria, including location, histology, angiographic pattern, and etiology.[37–39] It may be simplest to understand vascular malformations according to their location: extradural, intradural, subpial, and intramedullary. These vascular malformations may occur as isolated lesions but may also involve more than one layer at the same location.[40] Some of the difficulty in understanding the classification of spinal vascular malformations is due to their extreme rarity, lesions accounting for only 3 to 11 percent of spinal space-occupying lesions.[41] Vascular malformations tend to occur more commonly on the dorsal surface of the cord and in the more caudal aspect of the cord, because of the embryologic development of extensive arterial anastomoses on the dorsal surface of the cord between the third and sixth weeks. The ventral and cephalic portions of the spinal vasculature differentiate earlier than the dorsal and caudal portions. An insult to the fetus at around 6 weeks will lead to persistence of the thin-walled tortuous vessels, with abnormal arteriovenous connections characteristic of spinal vascular malformations.

Differentiation among the various morphologic and histologic types of vascular malformations is not possible with MRI. However, it is possible to assess the location of the malformations and observe their effect on the spinal cord. The location of the vascular malformations does carry some implication as to the degree of the shunting. The different layers that may be involved, in order, are vertebral, extradural, intradural, subpial, arachnoidal, and intramedullary. These vascular anomalies may occur in isolation or may span

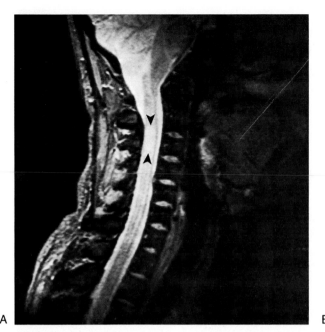 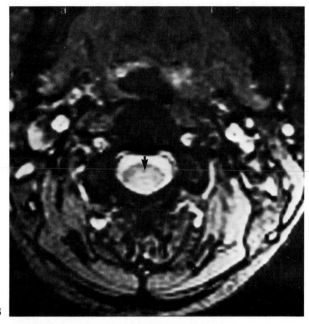

A   B

Figure 17–38. *Transverse myelitis.* **A,** Sagittal gradient-echo image (550/18/20) shows focal increased signal in the cervical spinal cord (*arrowheads*). **B,** Axial gradient-echo image (667/18/20) defines the location of the lesion in the midline posterior spinal cord (*arrow*).

different layers, even to include the skin. In up to 20 percent of cases, cutaneous vascular malformations are seen at the same level as vertebral vascular malformations.[38]

Vertebral angiomas, involving the vertebral bodies, are most common in the middle and thoracic spine. These malformations may extend into the extradural space. Extradural malformations are fairly common, accounting for 15 to 20 percent of all spinal vascular anomalies.[38] They are more common in older patients, usually those over 40 years of age, and are thought to be acquired rather than congenital.

A subpial site is the most frequent location of spinal vascular malformations. Many of these malformations may be confined to the cord surface, but increased pressure in the dilated draining veins may be manifest as dilatation of the intramedullary veins. Arterial and venous aneurysms are common and provide a source for subarachnoid hemorrhage. The juvenile form of vascular malformation is characterized by a vascular nidus lying within the cord, cord tissue being found within the interstices of the vascular mass.[42] Isolated intramedullary vascular malformations are uncommon. When confined to the spinal cord, the glomus type of vascular malformation is more common. In this form of malformation a nidus is seen, usually within the dorsal aspect of the spinal cord, with no cord tissue existing within the tangle of abnormal vessels. In both the subpial and intramedullary forms of vascular malformation, venous drainage is usually extensive, with dilated tortuous veins seen extending for long distances before emptying into the epidural venous plexus.

Many complications can result from spinal vascular malformations. Subarachnoid hemorrhage has been found in up to 30 percent.[38] There is a greater incidence of subarachnoid hemorrhage from vascular malformations with a large arteriovenous shunt than with the slower-flow malformations. Extradural and subdural hemorrhages are rare with vascular malformations, however. Hemorrhage within the spinal cord is a rather frequent complication of intramedullary vascular malformations and may be found in association with some degree of subarachnoid hemorrhage. It is not uncommon for the dilated veins of the vascular malformation to present as mass lesions with spinal cord and nerve root compression. Ischemia and infarction of the spinal cord occur as the result of a steal phenomenon. This may develop into chronic progressive radiculo-myelopathy (also known as Foix-Alajouanine syndrome) with progressive ascending weakness and anesthesia.

The MR findings in extradural and vertebral malformations are usually related to the dilated extradural veins (Fig. 17–39). The small nidus of the vascular malformation usually is not detected. The dilated veins present as large areas of signal void replacing the extradural fat.[43] Enlargement of the spinal cord at the level of the vascular malformation, commonly at the level of the conus, is thought to be due to venous congestion.

Subpial and intramedullary vascular malformations present on MRI with serpentine areas of signal void within the nidus of the vascular malformation as well as in larger dilated draining veins. When the malformation involves the spinal cord, the lesion appears ob-

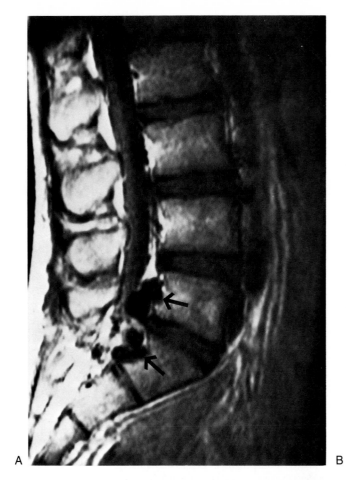

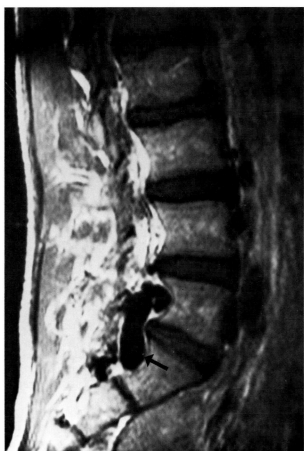

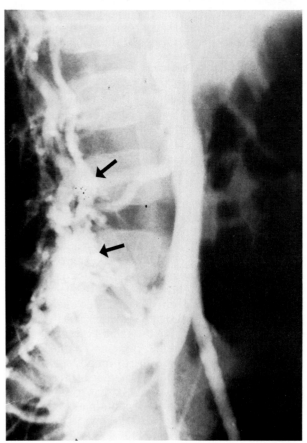

Figure 17–39. *Extradural vascular malformation.* **A,** Sagittal T1 weighted image (500/26) shows huge dilated extradural veins replacing extradural fat and causing bony erosion (*arrows*). **B,** Sagittal T1 weighted image (500/26) shows confluence of these large veins (*arrow*). **C,** Spinal angiogram confirms the extensive venous network draining the malformation (*arrows*).

vious on MRI. Subarachnoid veins may be more subtle on MRI, the dark signal void blending with CSF on T1 weighted images, and CSF pulsation creating confusing artifacts on T2 weighted images. MRI has been found superior to both CT and myelography in the detection of intraspinal lesions.[44] Cord edema and ischemia appear bright on gradient-echo or T2 weighted images (Fig. 17–40).[45] MRI may be of value in demonstrating thrombosis of a vascular malformation in which the signal void is replaced by increased signal on T1 and T2 weighted sequences. MRI provides excellent definition of the presence and extent of associated hemorrhage. Chronic hemorrhage may appear as superficial siderosis or dark hemosiderin staining of the margin of the spinal cord, seen best on T2 weighted or gradient-echo images. Subacute hemorrhage appears bright on both T1 and T2 weighted sequences (Fig. 17–41). The abnormal bright signal seen within the spinal cord on T2 weighted sequences may be caused by either edema or myelomalacia. MRI therefore may not be an accurate predictor of the prognosis after surgery.[45] Gadolinium-DTPA contrast enhancement is rarely helpful in spinal vascular malformations, but may occasionally enhance ischemic lesions secondary to the steal phenomenon.

INFECTION

Infection may involve the spine, epidural space, meninges, and cord.

Discitis

Infections involving the spinal column include osteomyelitis, referring to vertebral body infections, and discitis, referring to disc infections. It is rare to have infection of the vertebral body or the disc alone, and the more general term infectious spondylitis is probably more accurate. Many different names have been used to describe spinal infections including septic discitis, pyogenic vertebral osteomyelitis, spondyloarthritis, and nonspecific discitis. The inflammatory process causes destruction of the intervertebral disc and adjacent vertebral end plates. Diagnosis of discitis is difficult and often delayed owing to nonspecific symptoms and the late appearance of abnormalities on conventional radiographs. Plain radiographs, nuclear scintigraphy, CT, and MRI have been found useful in detecting discitis and its complications.

The clinical presentation of children with discitis is often nonspecific or misleading.[46] Symptoms and signs include back or hip pain, lumbar splinting, limp, refusal to stand or walk, radicular pain, meningeal irritation, abdominal pain, fever, and general irritability. There may be pain on straight-leg raising and local tenderness over the site of involvement. The clinical manifestations may be confused with those of meningitis, appendicitis, and septic arthritis. The erythrocyte sedimentation rate is elevated in most cases. White blood cell count may be elevated and blood cultures are frequently positive.

Hematogenous spread is the most common means of

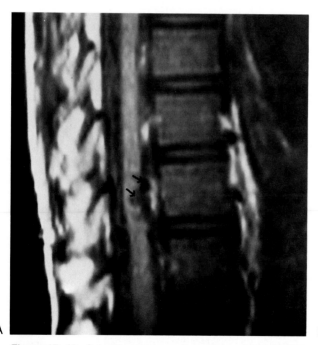
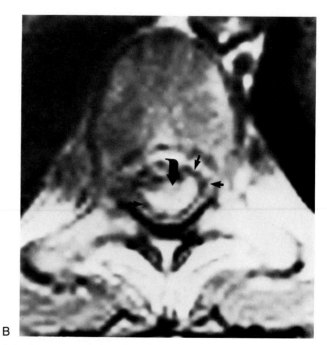

A   B

Figure 17–40. *Subpial vascular malformation.* ***A,*** Sagittal T1 weighted image (500/26) shows dilated veins in the subarachnoid space extending into the intramedullary location (*arrows*). ***B,*** Axial gradient-echo image (550/18/20) shows hemosiderin outlining the spinal cord (*arrows*), indicating previous hemorrhage. The spinal cord has increased signal (*curved arrow*) due to the steal phenomenon.

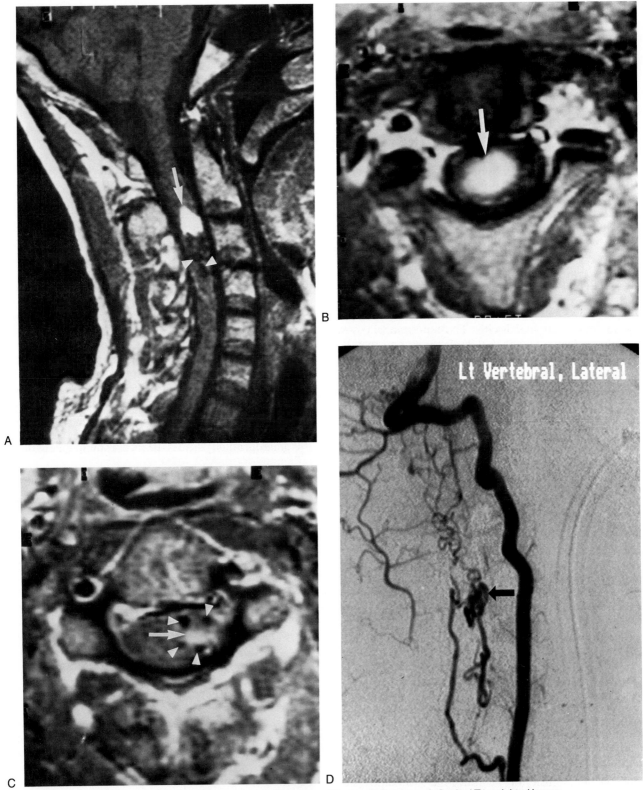

Figure 17–41. *Glomus-type intramedullary vascular malformation of the cervical spine.* **A,** Sagittal T1 weighted image (500/26) demonstrates subacute hemorrhage (*arrow*) above an area of flow void within the cord parenchyma (*arrowheads*). **B,** Axial T1 weighted image (500/26) at the level of cord hemorrhage demonstrates clearly the extent of hemorrhage within the spinal cord (*arrow*). **C,** Axial T1 weighted image (500/26) at a lower level shows a small residual hemorrhage (*arrow*) surrounded by abnormally dilated parenchymal vessels (*arrowheads*). **D,** Vertebral angiogram shows the abnormal intraparenchymal vascular nidus (*arrow*).

infection in childhood discitis. The intervertebral disc or adjacent vertebral end plate is the initial site of infection. In children, the disc space may be primarily infected owing to the persistence of direct arterial supply. By age 20 to 30 years, the disc space becomes avascular, and hematogenous infection must then begin in the vertebral end plate, with subsequent spread to the disc space.[47] The infecting organism is usually bacterial, and *Staphylococcus aureus* is the most common causative organism.[46,48] Viruses have been implicated in some cases, and fungal infections have been reported.[49,50] Discitis involves the lumbar, thoracic, and cervical regions in decreasing order of frequency.[51]

The patient with suspected discitis is initially evaluated on plain films. Unfortunately, spine films may not show an abnormality for 2 to 8 weeks after the onset of symptoms. Plain film findings include loss of disc height followed by end-plate erosion and sclerosis (Fig. 17–42A). Herniation of disc material into the vertebral body may occur.[52] A paravertebral soft tissue mass may also be visible.

Both Tc-99m bone scan and gallium scintigraphy are useful for detection of discitis. The bone scan will show uptake in two adjacent vertebral bodies and may be positive within 7 days of onset of symptoms. Gallium accumulates in the region of the abnormal disc as early as 2 weeks after the onset of symptoms.[49]

CT clearly demonstrates the findings of discitis in pediatric patients.[53] Bony end-plate destruction, paravertebral inflammation or abscess, and epidural abscess may be seen (Fig. 17–42B).

MRI has been shown to be useful in diagnosis of discitis.[54–57] Both T1 and T2 weighted images are obtained in the sagittal plane. Imaging parameters are not yet well established, but we have found the following parameters to be useful on a 1.5T MR unit. T1 weighted images are generated using TE of 26 milliseconds and TR of 500 milliseconds. T2 weighted images are generated using TE of 80 milliseconds and TR of 2000 milliseconds. In the normal spine, T1 weighted images show the disc and marrow space of the vertebral body to be of approximately equal signal intensity, separated by a narrow band of low signal representing the bony end plate. In the presence of inflammation, the disc space narrows and bony end plates are destroyed. There is increased water content in both the disc space and adjacent marrow. This is reflected in T1 weighted images as abnormally decreased signal intensity from the disc space, and particularly the adjacent marrow. The disc space is narrowed and the low-intensity signal of the end plate is lost, so that disc and marrow become confluent (Fig. 17–42C).[54]

T2 weighted images of the normal young spine show high signal intensity of the entire nucleus pulposus of the disc. This varies from the normal adult patient in whom a lower-signal intranuclear cleft is seen in the middle of the higher-signal nucleus pulposus.[58] The normal pediatric vertebral body marrow is of lower signal than the disc on T2 weighted images and is separated from the disc by low-signal vertebral end plates. In the presence of inflammation of the disc, T2 weighted images show no change or slightly decreased signal from the disc space.[55] Again, this differs from the findings in adult patients in whom the low-signal intranuclear cleft is lost and the disc signal increases. With involvement of adjacent vertebrae, there is abnormally increased signal in the adjacent marrow space (Fig. 17–42D). Paravertebral and epidural inflammatory masses or abscesses also show abnormally increased signal. Compression of the thecal sac and nerve roots may be seen. Follow-up MRI after treatment and resolution of inflammation may show residual disc narrowing and abnormally decreased signal from the disc space on T2 weighted images. No large studies of MR findings in pediatric discitis have been performed. Modic and colleagues, in a study of adult patients with suspected discitis, showed that MRI has a sensitivity, specificity, and accuracy of 96, 92, and 94 percent, respectively. This was compared with Tc-99m bone scan and gallium scintigraphy, which showed sensitivity, specificity, and accuracy of 90, 100, and 94 percent, respectively.[56]

MRI effectively discriminates between inflammatory, degenerative, and neoplastic diseases of the spine.[57] In degenerative disease, the disc space shows abnormally low signal on T2 weighted images. In neoplastic disease, the disc space is usually preserved in the presence of vertebral body destruction and signal alteration. Tuberculous spondylitis is an exception to this generalization; the disc space may be spared in this inflammatory disease process.

Use of gadolinium-DTPA may be helpful in the diagnosis of discitis. We have not yet studied discitis in pediatric patients with this agent, but several adult patients have been imaged. T1 weighted images enhanced with gadolinium-DTPA have shown increased signal from the disc space and adjacent end plates and marrow space of the involved vertebral bodies. Associated inflammatory masses may also be enhanced.

MRI is an attractive tool in pediatric patients because of the lack of ionizing radiation. Unfortunately, MRI is extremely sensitive to patient motion and requires more imaging time than other modalities. Sedation or general anesthesia is often required.

Epidural Abscesses

Epidural abscess may accompany vertebral body infection or may appear as an isolated finding. The source of the infectious organism may be a contiguous infected vertebral body, but hematogenous spread also occurs. In the cervical spine an abscess may result from spread of infectious tonsillitis or nasopharyngeal infections. Many organisms may cause epidural abscesses, but *Staphylococcus aureus* is the most common.[59–61] The MR findings in an epidural abscess may be less characteristic than those in discitis and osteomyelitis.[62]

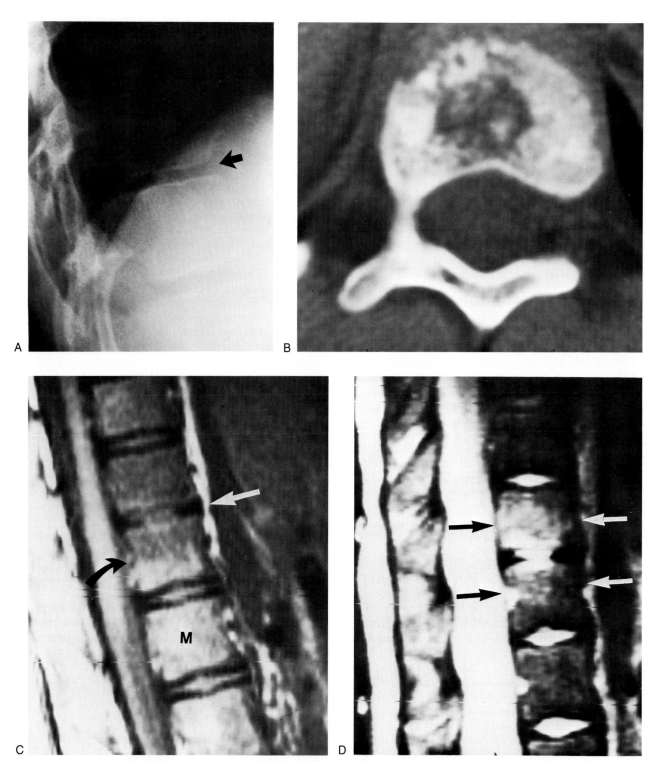

Figure 17–42. *Discitis in T11–T12*. This 9-year-old patient had a 10-week history of abdominal pain before 5 days of back pain. Blood cultures were positive for *Staphylococcus aureus*. The erythrocyte sedimentation rate was 50 mm per hour. *A,* Plain film demonstrates disc space narrowing at T11–T12 (*arrow*). *B,* CT scan shows end-plate destruction. *C,* T1 weighted MRI (500/26). There is poor definition of end plates at T11–T12 (*arrow*). Note the disc narrowing and abnormally decreased signal from the disc space and adjacent vertebral body marrow. There is an abrupt transition from abnormal to normal marrow (*curved arrow*). Note the normal high-signal marrow in the L1 vertebral body (M). *D,* T2 weighted MRI (2000/80). There is disc space narrowing with continued high signal intensity of the disc. Note the loss of low-signal end plates and the abnormally increased signal from adjacent vertebral bodies (*arrows*).

A variable appearance is reported. The signal intensity of epidural abscesses may be heterogeneous or high signal on T2 weighted sequences. When the infected area is large, obvious replacement of epidural fat is demonstrated (Fig. 17–43). When large, epidural abscesses are clearly identifiable masses that are isointense with the spinal cord on T1 weighted images and of high intensity on T2 weighted images. The extradural location of the abscess is usually apparent and easily distinguished from the adjacent compressed spinal cord and subarachnoid space. In some cases, however, the signal from the abscess may be similar to that of spinal fluid in the adjacent subarachnoid space and may be difficult to distinguish. CT following myelography may be helpful in these conditions.[62]

Epidural abscesses may span the spectrum between cellulitis and frank collections of pus. MRI does not distinguish between acute and more chronic infections.[62] Meningitis complicating epidural abscess or presenting as an isolated finding is not easily detected by MRI. Even in the brain, meningitis is imaged infrequently.

Cord Infections

Infections and abscesses of the spinal cord are rare.[63] The blood supply to the spinal cord is limited, accounting for the infrequent hematogenous spread of infection to the spinal cord. When infection does occur, however, the effects are devastating, and rapid diagnosis and treatment are imperative. The MR findings in spinal cord infection include mass effect, low or isointense signal on T1 weighted images, and enhancement with contrast material (Fig. 17–44). Patients with AIDS have a predisposition to the development of spinal cord abscesses.

TRAUMA AND HEMORRHAGE

Pediatric spine injury differs in several significant ways from adult spine injury. As many as 20 percent of children with spinal cord trauma show no plain film evidence of bone injury.[64] In the cervical spine the upper cervical spinal cord is damaged more frequently

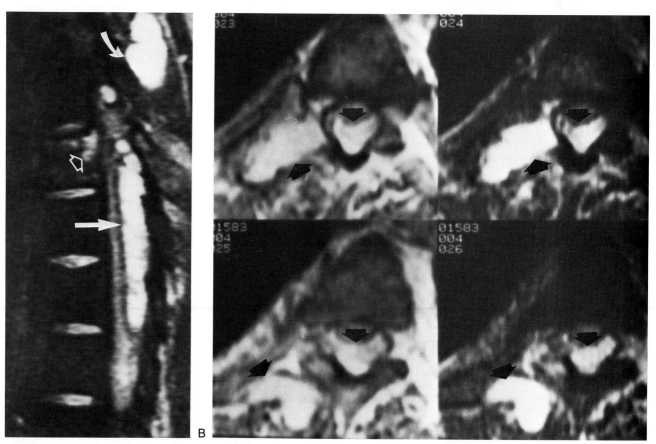

Figure 17–43. *Epidural abscess.* **A,** Sagittal gradient-echo image (600/18/15) demonstrates a large septated area of abnormally bright signal within the neural canal (*arrow*) with involvement of the adjacent vertebral body (*open arrow*) and paraspinal space (*curved arrow*). **B,** Serial axial gradient-echo images (600/18/15) show extensive paraspinal and epidural infection (*arrows*).

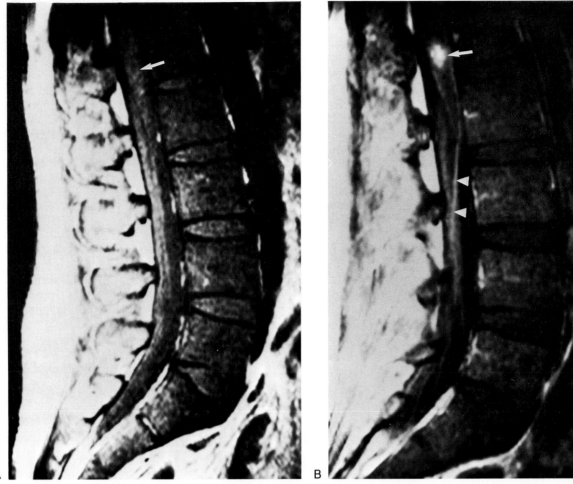

A   B

Figure 17–44. *Abscess of the conus.* ***A,*** Nonenhanced sagittal T1 weighted image (500/26) shows slight enlargement of the conus medullaris (*arrow*). ***B,*** Sagittal T1 weighted image (500/26) with gadolinium-DTPA enhancement shows marked enhancement of the conus medullaris (*arrow*). Enhancement of the cauda equina is also seen (*arrowheads*). Toxoplasmosis was cultured from the spinal cord biopsy.

in children under 8 years of age, whereas lower cervical cord injury occurs more commonly after age 8. The propensity for upper cervical cord injury in younger children is due to the greater laxity in their ligamentous structures, allowing increased motion of the bony elements. Delayed onset of symptoms is common in children with spinal cord injury.[65]

Assessment of the stability of the spine after injury is a significant consideration. Specifically, in children, evidence of ligament injury should be recognized because of the possibility of subluxation and further spinal cord injury. Plain film assessment of instability is made from measurements of subluxation or angulation. MRI provides additional information by directly imaging the ligaments.

The signs and symptoms of injury directly reflect the pattern of cord involvement. Transection of the spinal cord, for example, results in complete anesthesia and paralysis below the level of cord injury. Brown-Séquard syndrome, in which one-half of the cord is injured, results in contralateral loss of pain and temperature sensation and ipsilateral loss of motor function. Central cord syndrome, usually the result of vascular compromise, presents with a variable degree of quadriparesis, generally with greater involvement of the upper extremity than of the lower extremity. Sensory deficits usually are not complete. The anterior cord syndrome, generally the result of direct mechanical injury, presents with quadriparesis, usually more severe in the lower than in the upper extremities.

MRI is sensitive to the presence of vertebral dislocation, ligament injury, and hemorrhage. Hemorrhage may be found in epidural, subdural, or intramedullary locations. Spinal cord edema and contusion without hemorrhage also appear clearly on MRI. The greatest advantage of MRI is its ability to image spinal cord damage directly.[66]

The most subtle sign of spinal cord injury is that of increased signal within the cord parenchyma on T2 weighted images (Fig. 17–45). This finding represents a nonhemorrhagic spinal cord injury with edema.[67] This injury may extend for several segments and usually returns to a normal appearance on MRI within 3 weeks of injury.[68] Clinical symptoms generally also resolve quickly.

Evidence of hemorrhage within the spinal cord has much more serious prognostic implications.[68] Acutely, hemorrhage appears with a decreased signal in the spinal cord on T2 weighted or gradient-echo se-

quences, reflecting the presence of deoxyhemoglobin in acute injury (Fig. 17–46). The hemorrhage is commonly seen at the gray and white matter junction.[68] The increased capillary network at the gray and white junction is proposed as the reason for the propensity for hemorrhage in this location.[68] In the subacute phase, hemorrhage may appear as a mixture of bright and dark signal on T2 weighted sequences, reflecting a mixture of deoxyhemoglobin and methemoglobin (Fig. 17–47). As the injury evolves, the signal characteristics may reflect methemoglobin entirely with bright signal on T1 weighted sequences (Fig. 17–48). Even small amounts of hemorrhage may be detected, and one small hemorrhage does not necessarily represent a serious injury with permanent sequelae. Cord transection usually results from penetrating injury or massive subluxation. In a small child with great ligament laxity, severe stretching injury of the spine may result in cord transection (Fig. 17–49). The relationship of spinal fracture and dislocation to the level of cord injury is best assessed on sagittal images (Fig. 17–50). Compression fractures are more common in the thoracic and lumbar vertebra, presenting as wedge-shaped deformities (Fig. 17–51).

Epidural hematomas may occur spontaneously or as the result of trauma.[69] Rapid accumulation of an epidural mass may cause compression of the spinal cord or cauda equina (Fig. 17–52).[69] Rapid surgical decompression is necessary to prevent the development of permanent sequelae and progression of the hematoma. Subdural hematomas may extend for a consider-

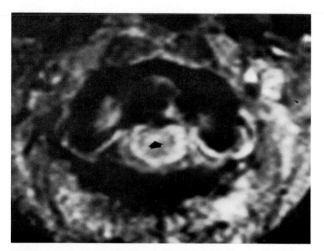

Figure 17–45. *Cord contusion without hemorrhage.* Increased signal within the spinal cord parenchyma (*arrow*) is clearly defined on this axial T2 weighted image (2000/80).

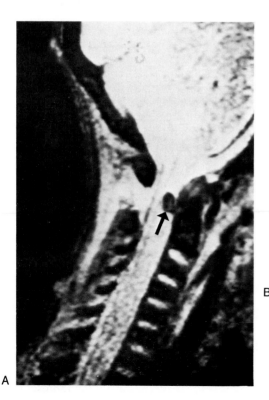

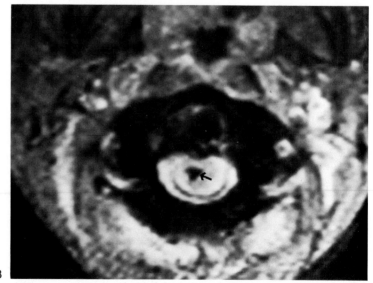

Figure 17–46. *Acute hemorrhagic cord injury.* **A,** Sagittal T1 weighted image (2000/80) shows an area of decreased signal consistent with deoxyhemoglobin (*arrow*). **B,** Axial gradient-echo image (550/18/20) clearly defines the location of the acute hemorrhage within the spinal cord parenchyma (*arrow*).

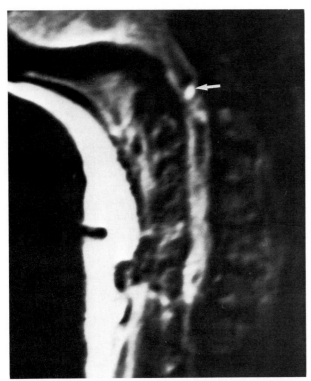

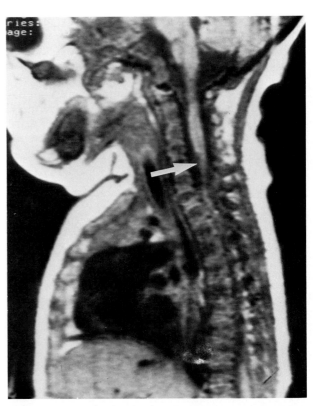

Figure 17–47. *Subacute spinal cord hemorrhage.* Sagittal T2 weighted image (2000/100) shows a mixture of bright and dark signal within the upper cervical spinal cord (*arrow*), reflecting a mixture of deoxyhemoglobin and methemoglobin.

Figure 17–49. *Cord transection.* Sagittal T1 weighted image (500/26) shows abrupt termination of the cervical spinal cord (*arrow*) after an acute flexion injury.

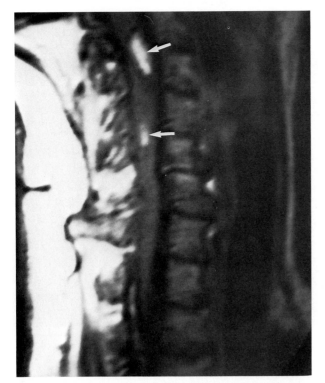

Figure 17–48. *Subacute spinal cord hemorrhage.* Sagittal T1 weighted image (500/26) shows two areas of methemoglobin within the cervical spinal cord (*arrows*) appearing as areas of bright signal.

able distance throughout the neural canal. In the subacute phase, these appear as bright signal on T1 weighted sequences (Fig. 17–53).

Late sequelae of spinal cord injury include myelomalacia and spinal cord cyst.[70] MRI provides the best definition of the extent of spinal cord injury. T1 weighted sequences demonstrate intramedullary cysts extending for a variable distance (Fig. 17–54). Myelomalacia may appear as of signal intensity similar to that of CSF on T2 weighted sequences.[70] Thinning of the cord may be seen with a variable degree of cord destruction on T1 weighted sequences (Fig. 17–55).

IATROGENIC COMPLICATIONS

Postoperative complications in the spinal column are clearly assessed on MRI.[71] Pseudomeningocele may be the result of dural leak and appears as a cystic collection isointense to CSF on both T1 and T2 weighted sequences (Fig. 17–56).

Gadolinium-DTPA enhancement has been found to be of great value in detecting postoperative scar.[72] Scar formation generally shows some degree of enhancement on T1 weighted images with gadolinium-DTPA (Fig. 17–57). The enhancement is usually homogeneous, but heterogeneous enhancement may be noted.

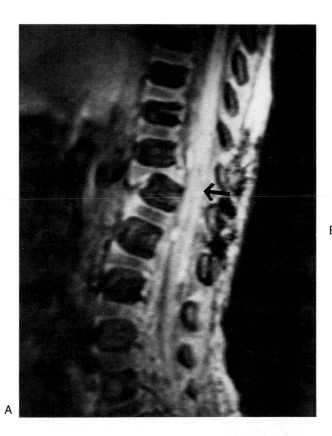

A

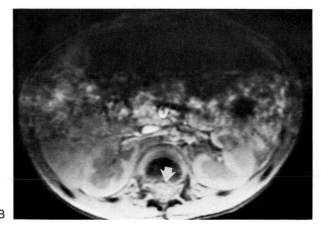

B

Figure 17–50. *Thoracic cord subluxation.* ***A,*** Sagittal gradient-echo image (550/18/20) in a small infant shows severe anterior subluxation in the midthoracic region (*arrow*). ***B,*** Axial gradient-echo image (550/18/20) shows abnormally bright signal within the spinal cord at this level (*arrow*).

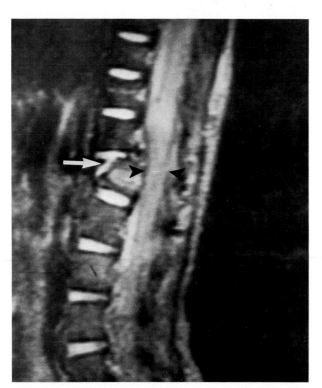

Figure 17–51. *Fracture subluxation of the lower thoracic region.* Sagittal gradient-echo image (550/18/20) shows anterior wedging and fracture of a lower thoracic vertebra (*arrow*) and anteroposterior narrowing of the neural canal related to the fracture (*arrowheads*).

Arachnoiditis occurs in 6 to 16 percent of patients after spinal injury, and may be the cause of prolonged pain and disability.[73] The diagnosis of arachnoiditis has traditionally been made by myelography and CT following myelography. Arachnoiditis appears as clumped nerve roots in the cauda equina with streaky subarachnoid filling defects and blunting of the root sleeves. On MRI, arachnoiditis may appear as a soft tissue mass within the thecal sac caused by fibrosis and adhesions (Fig. 17–58). The subarachnoid space may appear obliterated. Both sagittal and axial images may be helpful in defining the conglomerations of clumped nerve roots, whether peripherally or centrally. Both T1 and T2 weighted sequences may define the abnormality. The more subtle signs of arachnoiditis, with blunting of root sheaths, are better visualized on myelography.

Postoperative injury to the spinal column in children may result in growth disturbance and accentuated spinal curvature (Fig. 17–59). MRI clearly defines the extent of spinal curvature and its relationship to the spinal cord.

After radiation, characteristic vertebral body changes can be seen (see also the chapter on Primary Disorders of Bone Marrow). Increased signal on T1 weighted images is typically found within the vertebral body marrow after radiation injury (Fig. 17–60). The increased signal on T1 weighted sequences is due to

Text continues on page 535

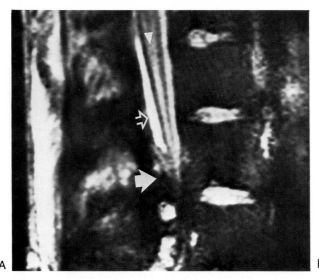

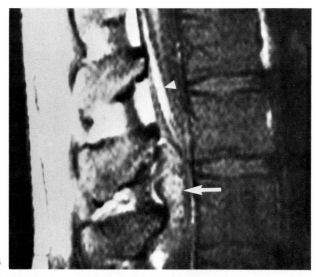

A

B

Figure 17–52. *Spontaneous epidural hematoma in a 14-year-old boy with low platelet count, recent pain, and neurogenic bladder.* **A,** Sagittal T2 weighted sequence shows hematoma (*arrow*) with mixed bright and dark signal causing severe compression of the conus medullaris, which has abnormally bright signal consistent with edema (*arrowhead*). Subdural hematoma, superior to the epidural hematoma (*open arrow*), appears bright. **B,** Sagittal T1 weighted image (500/26) confirms both the acute epidural hematoma (*arrow*) and the subacute subdural hematoma (*arrowhead*).

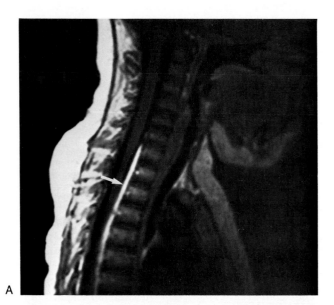

A

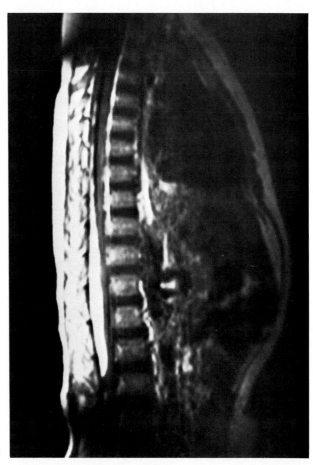

B

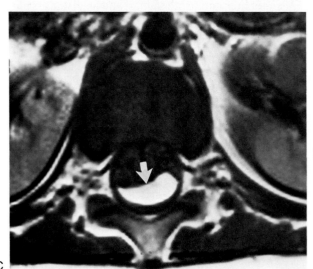

C

Figure 17–53. *Large subdural hematoma presenting with neck stiffness 5 days after lumbar puncture.* **A,** Sagittal T1 weighted image (500/20) in the thoracolumbar region shows a huge posterior subacute hematoma (*arrow*). **B,** Sagittal T1 weighted image (500/20) in the cervical region shows anterior extension of the hematoma in the upper thoracic and cervical regions. **C,** Axial T1 weighted image (650/20) at the level of the conus confirms the subdural location of the hematoma (*arrow*).

532

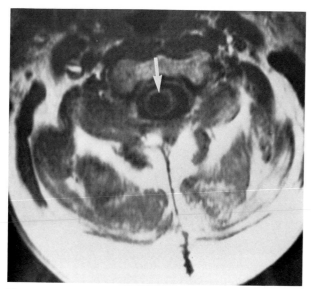

Figure 17–54. *Post-traumatic intramedullary cyst.* Axial T1 weighted image (550/26) shows a large CSF-containing cyst (*arrow*) occupying most of the spinal cord.

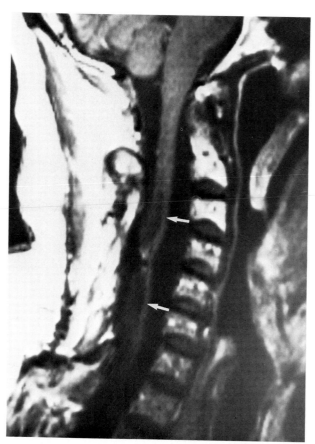

Figure 17–55. *Postsurgical myelomalacia.* Sagittal T1 weighted image (550/26) shows extensive myelomalacia in the cervical spinal cord manifest as marked thinning of the spinal cord (*arrows*), with associated myelomalacia appearing as dark signal posterior to the thinned spinal cord remnant.

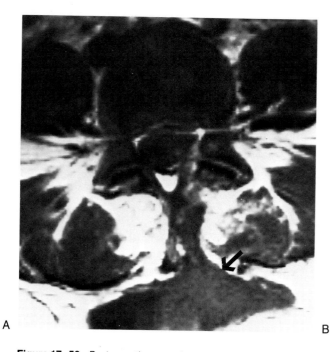

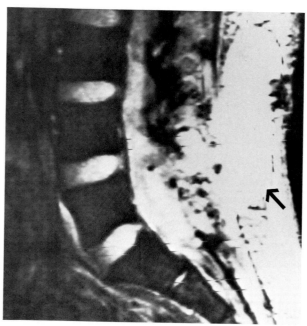

A   B

Figure 17–56. *Postoperative pseudomeningocele.* **A,** Axial T1 weighted image (550/26) shows a large posterior cystic collection with dark signal similar to CSF (*arrow*). **B,** Sagittal T2 weighted sequence (2000/80) confirms the spinal fluid characteristics of the cystic mass appearing as bright signal (*arrow*).

533

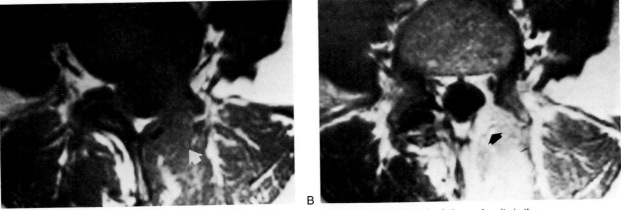

Figure 17–57. *Postoperative scar.* **A,** T1 weighted axial image (550/26) shows a large area of soft tissue density in the region of previous surgery (*arrow*). **B,** Axial T1 weighted image (550/26) with gadolinium-DTPA enhancement shows the same area with marked enhancement, indicating an extensive scar (*arrow*).

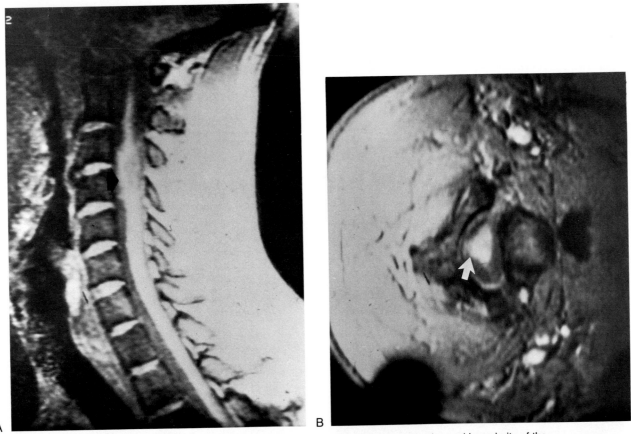

Figure 17–58. *Arachnoiditis.* **A,** T1 weighted sagittal image (550/26) demonstrates thickening and irregularity of the upper cervical spinal cord (*arrow*). **B,** Axial T1 weighted image (550/26) shows irregularity and increased size of the cervical spinal cord (*arrow*).

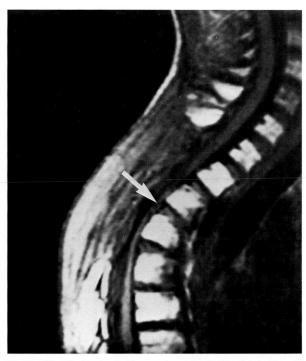

Figure 17–59. *Postoperative and postradiation kyphosis.* T1 weighted sagittal image (500/20) demonstrates marked kyphosis (*arrow*) secondary to growth disturbance after treatment of Ewing's sarcoma of the posterior elements.

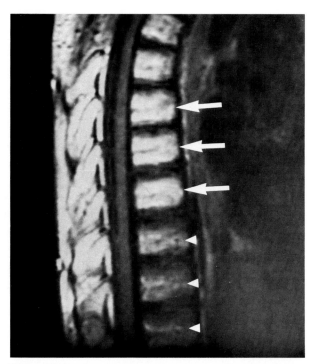

Figure 17–60. *Fatty replacement of marrow after radiation therapy to the spine.* T1 weighted sagittal image shows increased signal in the affected vertebral bodies (*arrows*). Note the sharp demarcation with normal vertebral bodies outside the radiation ports (*arrowheads*).

fatty replacement of normal marrow following radiation.

CONCLUSION

MRI provides the first method of directly imaging the spinal cord. It has proved invaluable in determining the severity of spinal cord injury in the myriad conditions that affect the spinal column. Because of the sensitivity of MRI, a better understanding is now possible of many primary spinal cord inflammatory and demyelinating lesions. With improved MR imaging techniques and pulse sequences, the possibility of expanding our understanding of spinal disease is bright.

REFERENCES

1. Flannigan-Sprague BD, Modic MT. The pediatric spine: normal anatomy and spinal dysraphism. In: Modic MT, Masaryk TJ, eds. Magnetic resonance imaging of the spine. Chicago: Year Book, 1989:240–256.
2. Masaryk TJ. Spine tumors. In: Modic MT, Masaryk TJ, eds. Magnetic resonance imaging of the spine. Chicago: Year Book, 1989:183–213.
3. Barnes PD, Lester PD, Yamanashi WS, et al. Magnetic resonance imaging in infants and children with spinal dysraphism. AJNR 1986; 7:465–472.
4. Davidson HD, Ouchi T, Steiner RE. NMR imaging of congenital intracranial germ layer neoplasms. Neuroradiology 1985; 27:301–303.
5. Lee BCP, Zimmerman RD, Manning JJ, Deck MDF. MR imaging of syringomyelia and hydromyelia. AJR 1985; 144: 1149–1156.
6. Slasky BS, Bydder GM, Niendorf HP, Young IR. MR imaging with gadolinium-DTPA in the differentiation of tumor, syrinx, and cyst of the spinal cord. J Comput Assist Tomogr 1987; 11:845–850.
7. Kokmen E, Marsh WR, Baker HL Jr. Magnetic resonance imaging in syringomyelia. Neurosurgery 1985; 17:267–270.
8. Yeates A, Brant-Zawadzki M, Norman D, et al. Nuclear magnetic resonance imaging of syringomyelia. ANJR 1983; 4: 234–237.
9. Enzmann ER, O'Donohue J, Rubin JB, et al. CSF pulsations within nonneoplastic spinal cord cysts. AJR 1987; 149:149–157.
10. Pojunas K, Williams AL, Daniels DL, Haughton VM. Syringomyelia and hydromyelia: magnetic resonance evaluation. Radiology 1984; 153:679–683.
11. Sherman JL, Barkovich AJ, Citrin CM. The MR appearance of syringomyelia: new observations. AJNR 1986; 7:985–995.
12. Gabriel KR, Crawford AH. Identification of acute post-traumatic spinal cord cyst by magnetic resonance imaging: a case report and review of the literature. J Pediatr Orthop 1988; 8:710–714.
13. Enzmann DR. Syringomyelia. In: Enzmann DR, DeLaPaz RL, Rubin JB, eds. Magnetic resonance of the spine. St Louis: CV Mosby, 1990:341–364.
14. Andrews BT, Weinstein PH, Rosenblum ML, et al. Intradural arachnoid cysts of the spinal canal associated with intramedullary cysts. J Neurosurg 1988; 68:544–548.
15. DeLaPaz RL. Congenital anomalies of the spine and spinal cord. In: Enzmann DR, DeLaPaz RL, Rubin JB, eds. Magnetic resonance of the spine. St Louis: CV Mosby, 1990:176–236.
16. Samuelsson L, Bergstrom K, Thomas KA, et al. MR imaging of syringomyelia and Chiari malformations in myelomeningocele patients with scoliosis. AJNR 1987; 8:539–546.
17. Nokes SR, Murtagh FR, Jones JD III, et al. Childhood scoliosis: MR imaging. Radiology 1987; 164:791–797.
18. Han JS, Benson JE, Kaufman B, et al. Demonstration of di-

astematomyelia and associated abnormalities with MR imaging. AJNR 1985; 6:215–219.

19. Thron A, Schroth G. Magnetic resonance imaging (MRI) of diastematomyelia. Neuroradiology 1986; 28:371–372.

20. Shellinger D, Wener L, Ragsdale BD. Facet joint disorders and their role in the production of back pain and sciatica. Radiographics 1987; 7:923–944.

21. Modic MT. Degenerative disorders of the spine. In: Modic MT, Masaryk TJ, Ross JS, eds. Magnetic resonance imaging of the spine. Chicago: Year Book, 1989:75–119.

22. McAfee PC, Bohlman HH, Han JS, Salvagno RT. Comparison of nuclear magnetic resonance imaging and computed tomography in the diagnosis of upper cervical spinal cord compression. Spine 1986; 11:295–304.

23. Ross JS, Perez-Reyes N, Masaryk TJ, et al. Thoracic disk herniation: MR imaging. Radiology 1987; 165:511–515.

24. Modic MT, Masaryk T, Coumphrey F, et al. Lumbar herniated disk disease and canal stenosis: prospective evaluation by surface coil MR, CT, and myelography. AJR 1986; 147:757–765.

25. Enzmann DR. Degenerative disk disease. In: Enzmann DR, DeLaPaz RL, Rubin JB, eds. Magnetic resonance of the spine. St Louis: CV Mosby, 1990:437–509.

26. Enzmann DR, Rubin JB. The cervical spine: MR imaging with partial flip angle, gradient-refocused pulse sequence. Part 1. General considerations and disk disease. Radiology 1988; 166:467–472.

27. Hedberg MC, Drayer BP, Flom RA, et al. Gradient-echo (GRASS) MR imaging in cervical radiculopathy. AJR 1988; 150:683–689.

28. Modic MT, Pavicek W, Weinstein MA, et al. Magnetic resonance imaging of intervertebral disk disease: clinical and pulse sequence considerations. Radiology 1984; 152:103–111.

29. Modic MT, Steinberg PM, Ross JS, et al. Degenerative disk disease: assessment of changes in vertebral body marrow with MR imaging. Radiology 1988; 166:193–199.

30. Bundschuh C, Modic MT, Kearney F, et al. Rheumatoid arthritis of the cervical spine: surface-coil MR imaging. AJR 1988; 151:181–187.

31. Aisen AM, Maetel W, Ellis JH, McCune WJ. Cervical spine involvement in rheumatoid arthritis: MR imaging. Radiology 1987; 165:159–163.

32. Breedveld FC, Algra PR, Vielvoye CJ, Katz A. Magnetic resonance imaging in the evaluation of patients with rheumatoid arthritis and subluxations of the cervical spine. Arthr Rheum 1987; 30:624–629.

33. Ross JS. Inflammatory disease. In: Modic MT, Masaryk TJ, Ross JS, eds. Magnetic resonance imaging of the spine. Chicago: Year Book, 1989:167–182.

34. Edwards MK, Smith RR. White matter diseases. Topic Magn Reson Imaging 1989; 2:41–48.

35. Edwards MK, Farlow MR, Stevens JC. Multiple sclerosis: MRI in clinical correlation. AJR 1986; 147:571–574.

36. Merine D, Wang H, Kumar AJ, et al. CT myelography and MR imaging of acute transverse myelitis. J Comput Assist Tomogr 1987; 11:606–608.

37. Rubinstein LJ. Tumors and malformation of blood vessels. In: Firminger HI, ed. Tumors of the central nervous system. Washington DC: Air Force Institute of Pathology, 1985:235–256.

38. Jellinger K. Pathology of spinal vascular malformations and vascular tumors. In: Pia HW, Djin Djian R, eds. Spinal angiomas: advances in diagnosis and therapy. New York: Springer-Verlag, 1978:18–44.

39. Masaryk TJ. Miscellaneous topics. In: Modic MT, Masaryk TJ, Ross JS, eds. Magnetic resonance imaging of the spine. Chicago: Year Book 1989:257–273.

40. Aminoff MJ, Barnard RO, Valentine L. The pathophysiology of spinal vascular malformations. J Neurol Sci 1974; 23:255–263.

41. Masaryk TJ, Ross JS, Modic MT, et al. Radiculomeningeal vascular malformations of the spine: MR imaging. Radiology 1987; 164:845–849.

42. Rosenblum B, Oldfield EH, Doppman JL, et al. Spinal arteriovenous malformations: a comparison of dural arteriovenous fistulas and intradural AVM's in 81 patients. J Neurosurg 1987; 67:795–802.

43. Ross JS, Masaryk TJ, Modic MT, et al. Vertebral hemangiomas: MR imaging. Radiology 1987; 165:165–169.

44. Fontaine S, Melanson D, Cosgrove R, Bertrand G. Cavernous hemangiomas of the spinal cord: MR imaging. Radiology 1988; 166:839–841.

45. Minami S, Sagoh T, Nishimur K, et al. Spinal arteriovenous malformation: MR imaging. Radiology 1988; 169:109–115.

46. Rocco HD, Eyring EJ. Intervertebral disk infections in children. Am J Dis Child 1972; 123:448–451.

47. Resnick D, Niwayama G. Osteomyelitis, septic arthritis, and soft tissue infection: the axial skeleton. In: Resnick D, Niwayama G, eds. Diagnosis of bone and joint disorders. 2nd ed. Philadelphia: WB Saunders, 1988:224–248.

48. Wenger DR, Bobechko WP, Gilday DL. The spectrum of intervertebral disc-space infection in children. J Bone Joint Surg 1978; 60A:100–108.

49. Fischer GW, Popich GA, Sullivan DE, et al. Diskitis: a prospective diagnostic analysis. Pediatrics 1978; 62:543–548.

50. Holmes PF, Osterman DW, Tullos HS. Aspergillus discitis. Clin Orthop 1988; 226:240–246.

51. Menelaus MB. Discitis: an inflammation affecting the intervertebral discs in children. J Bone Joint Surg 1964; 46B:16–23.

52. Smith RF, Taylor TKF. Inflammatory lesions of intervertebral discs in children. J Bone Joint Surg 1967; 49A:1508–1520.

53. Sartorius DJ, Moskowitz PS, Kaufman RA, et al. Childhood diskitis: computed tomographic findings. Radiology 1983; 149:701–707.

54. Forster A, Pothmann R, Winter K, Baumann-Rath CA. Magnetic resonance imaging in non-specific discitis. Pediatr Radiol 1987; 17:162–163.

55. Szalay EA, Green NE, Heller RM, et al. Magnetic resonance imaging in the diagnosis of childhood discitis. J Pediatr Orthop 1987; 7:164–167.

56. Modic MT, Feiglin DH, Piraino DW, et al. Vertebral osteomyelitis: assessment using MR. Radiology 1985; 157:157–166.

57. Ross JS. Inflammatory disease. In: Modic MT, Masaryk TJ, Ross JS, eds. Magnetic resonance imaging of the spine. Chicago: Year Book, 1989:000–000.

58. Aguila LA, Piraino DW, Modic MT, et al. The intranuclear cleft of the intervertebral disk: magnetic resonance imaging. Radiology 1985; 155:155–158.

59. Whelan MA, Schonfeld S, Post JD, et al. Computed tomography of nontuberculous spinal infection. J Comput Assist Tomogr 1983; 7:25–29.

60. Mickhael MA, Ciric IS, Tarkington JA. MR imaging in spinal echinococcosis. J Comput Assist Tomogr 1985; 9:398–400.

61. de Roos A, van Persijn van Meerten EL, et al. MRI of tuberculous spondylitis. AJR 1986; 146:79–82.

62. Post MJD, Quencer RM, Montalvo BM, et al. Spinal infection: evaluation with MR imaging and intraoperative US. Radiology 1988; 169:765–771.

63. Enzmann DR. Infection and inflammation. In: Enzmann DR, DeLaPaz RL, Rubin JB, eds. Magnetic resonance of the spine. St Louis: CV Mosby, 1990:260–300.

64. Hadley MN, Sabramski JM, Browner CM, et al. Pediatric spinal trauma: review of 122 cases of spinal cord and vertebral column injuries. J Neurosurg 1988; 68:18–25.

65. Enzmann DR, DeLaPaz RL. Trauma. In: Enzmann DR, DeLaPaz RL, Rubin JB, eds. Magnetic resonance of the spine. St Louis: CV Mosby, 1990:237–259.

66. Hackney DB, Asato D, Joseph PM, et al. Hemorrhage and edema in acute spinal cord compression: demonstration by MR imaging. Radiology 1986; 161:387–390.

67. Beers GJ, Raque GH, Wagner GG, et al. MR imaging in acute cervical spine trauma. J Comput Assist Tomogr 1988; 12:755–761.

68. Kulkarni MV, McArdle CB, Kopanicky D, et al. Acute spinal cord injury: MR imaging at 1.5T. Radiology 1987; 164:837–843.

69. Rothfus WE, Chedid MK, Deeb ZL, et al. MR imaging in the

diagnosis of spontaneous spinal epidural hematomas. J Comput Assist Tomogr 1987; 11:851–854.

70. Quencer RM, Sheldon JJ, Post MJD, et al. MRI of the chronically injured cervical spinal cord. AJR 1986; 147:125–132.

71. Ross JS, Masaryk TJ, Modic MT. Postoperative cervical spine: MR assessment. J Comput Assist Tomogr 1987; 11:955–962.

72. Hueftle MG, Modic MT, Ross JS, et al. Lumbar spine: postoperative MR imaging with Gd-DTPA. Radiology 1988; 167:817–824.

73. Burton CV, Kirkaldy-Willis WH, Yong-Hing K, et al. Causes of failure of surgery on the lumbar spine. Clin Orthop 1981; 157:191–199.

SECTION

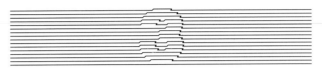

BODY IMAGING

Cardiovascular System

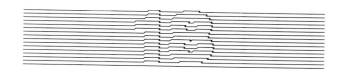

GEORGE S. BISSET III, M.D.

In the era of modern cardiology, many imaging modalities (including both invasive and noninvasive techniques) have become part of the diagnostic armamentarium and have been utilized to characterize cardiovascular anatomy, function, and metabolism. Although there is some overlap of information gained from the techniques, each plays an important role in cardiac diagnosis and research.

In recent years there has been a trend toward evaluation of better noninvasive techniques in an attempt to obviate the need for more invasive workups. This will spare risk and discomforts for the patient, which become an even greater problem in the pediatric population, in which small size may limit contrast material and catheter size.

Early experience with magnetic resonance imaging (MRI) has been remarkably fruitful.[1-5] In the cardiovascular system, MRI provides the most accurate anatomic detail available. The inherent natural contrast between flowing blood and myocardial or vessel wall permits diagnosis without the use of intravenous or intra-arterial contrast material. In addition, the ability to acquire multiplanar images provides for three-dimensional information, which is particularly useful for the surgeon in planning operative intervention. Another advantage of MRI in the pediatric population is the lack of ionizing radiation. This is particularly important in children who require cardiac catheterization or multiple radiographic examinations.

The major focus of cardiovascular MRI has been on an anatomic definition of pathologic states. With the advent of gradient refocused image acquisition, attention is now turning toward assessment of cardiac function. Also, newer areas of research are exploring the role of MR spectroscopy in the evaluation of myocardial metabolism.

The final role of MR in cardiac imaging has yet to be determined. Early studies indicated excellent accuracy for MRI in defining cardiac anomalies. For example, Didier, in a review of 72 patients with congenital heart lesions, categorized MRI as excellent or diagnostic in 96 percent of cases.[1] Boxer and colleagues found that, in 34 of 36 children with congenital heart disease, the anatomic detail provided by MRI was sufficient to make a diagnosis.[6] Great strides have been made in imaging techniques since these two manuscripts appeared. Jacobson, writing for the Council on Scientific Affairs, stated that at the present time no unequivocal recommendations can be made for the use of MRI and that further studies critically comparing MRI with ultrasonography are needed.[7] However, this committee felt that the role of MRI in the evaluation of congenital heart disease was extremely promising. Areas in which MRI will have a major early impact are in the evaluation of disorders of the great vessels in the thorax, abnormalities of the main pulmonary artery and its branches, abnormalities of venous return to the heart, and evaluation of postoperative palliative shunts and corrective procedures for congenital heart lesions.[4, 7-9]

TECHNIQUES

The ability to complete a cardiac MR examination successfully depends largely on patient cooperation. In the pediatric population, painstaking efforts must sometimes be made to ensure that nonperiodic motion artifact is suppressed. In infants and young children, maintaining a relatively motion-free state for up to 1 hour requires sedation. Techniques for sedation and monitoring are discussed elsewhere.[10, 11]

The cyclic motion of the heart creates blurred images on a standard nongated spin-echo acquisition. An averaged image of the heart results from information being recorded in systole and diastole. Therefore, to acquire accurate anatomic information, one must be able to "freeze-frame" the heart. This is accomplished by gating the image acquisition to the patient's electrocardiogram (ECG).

The most common MR method to view anatomy is the multislice technique. One must bear in mind that this ECG-gated technique will acquire multiple slices at different anatomic locations, as well as at different phases of the cardiac cycle. Because the major goal is to enhance contrast between flowing blood and myocardium, the information acquisition should be relatively closely confined to systole (when blood flow is rapid). As the information is acquired closer to the diastolic phase of the cardiac cycle, there is a resultant increase in flow-related artifact within the cardiac chambers and great vessels.

Patient preparation involves the placement of three specially designed electrodes on the patient's back. This posterior placement minimizes the motion of lead wires in a supine patient, thus creating fewer artifacts and optimal triggering. If the signal amplitude of the ECG tracing is unsatisfactory, an anterior precordial lead placement may be used. In children weighing less than 15 kg the examinations are performed with the patient positioned in the head coil; larger children are examined in the body coil. Newer coils matched to body size should provide even better signal-to-noise ratios (SNR) in cardiac imaging.

The ECG-gated imaging sequence begins with the R wave of the telemetrically transmitted ECG (Fig. 18–1). The R-R interval of the ECG determines the "effective" repetition time (TR). This number is a fixed value even though the actual R-R interval varies slightly from beat to beat, hence the term "effective." The actual acquisition begins shortly after the onset of the R wave. This "lag time" is related to a short hardware delay. An additional operator programmable delay is added to ensure that imaging begins after isovolumetric contraction. All MR images in this chapter have been obtained utilizing a TR that varies between 380 and 1,000 msec.

A short echo time (TE) is generally used in most cardiac imaging to optimize SNR and maximize the number of slice locations (TE $\leq$20 msec). Occasionally, longer TE and TR intervals (gated to every other or every third beat) are used to evaluate the signal characteristics of cardiac tumors or paracardiac masses. A 256 $\times$ 128 matrix size is generally sufficient for most cardiac imaging.

An important new technique to decrease intracardiac and vascular flow motion artifacts uses spatial slab presaturation pulses.[12] The application of these pulses, followed by spoiler gradients, saturates nuclei outside the imaging slice. Therefore, flowing blood (moving spins) entering the imaging plane between successive excitations is saturated and unable to generate signal. In this instance, decreased signal equates with decreased artifact. New software also creates the potential to eliminate aliasing in the phase and frequency encoding directions, thus reducing wraparound artifacts.

Slice thicknesses in the pediatric cardiovascular system are generally 5 mm, with 0.5- to 1-mm interslice gaps. In small children, thicker slices (>5 mm) result in a loss of anatomic information because of partial volume averaging. Thinner slices (<5 mm) significantly

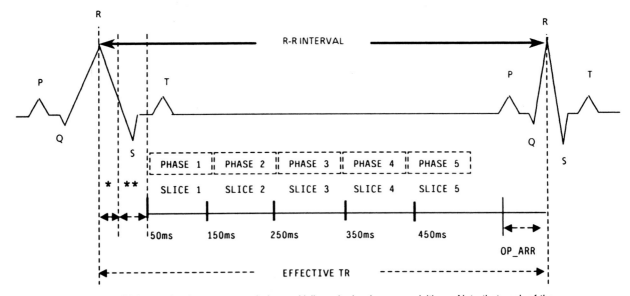

Figure 18–1. *Typical ECG gated pulse sequence during multislice, single-phase acquisition.* Note that each of the multiple slices is obtained at a different point in the systolic phase. * denotes a hardware delay; ** denotes the programmable delay following the R-wave trigger. This delay is important to ensure that imaging takes place after isovolumetric contraction. (Courtesy of General Electric Corporation.)

decrease the SNR and usually do not provide enough volume coverage. Occasionally, however, thin (3-mm) slices are used to obtain better spatial resolution of a small anatomic structure. In most cases, two to four excitations provide enough sampling information to construct adequate images.

The ability to obtain multiplanar orthogonal and oblique images has created some difficulty in adhering to prescribed cardiovascular MR protocols.[13, 14] Standard sagittal, coronal, and axial planes suffice in most cases in which anatomic information is sought. However, in patients in whom specific questions are asked (e.g., regarding patency and size of pulmonary arteries, presence of coarctation), oblique images are invaluable. Information concerning chamber diameters, thicknesses, or function is better delineated with imaging planes parallel to the long and short axes.[2] In planning the cardiac MR examination, the cardiac imaging planes are best tailored to each patient and the specific questions asked.

Another spin-echo imaging technique used to evaluate ventricular mechanics is rotated, gated image acquisition.[15] With this technique, several anatomic slices are imaged at successive phases in the cardiac cycle. The ventricles are then assessable in systole and diastole, providing important information about ventricular function.[16] In pediatric patients, myocardial dynamics are readily assessed with other modalities, resulting in a limited use of this technique.

Cine MRI has been developed recently to create dynamic cardiac images.[17–19] Short TE and TR values are combined with a narrow flip angle (15 to 30 degrees) and a gradient reversal to acquire multiple (16 to 45) frames of a single cardiac slice during an averaged cardiac cycle. Each of the multiple images corresponds to a different temporal location. These images are sequentially displayed to produce a cine-type movie. Between each excitation, fully magnetized blood enters the imaging volume, resulting in high signal intensity of normally flowing blood. Abnormally turbulent high velocity flow, as through a stenotic valve, results in signal loss. The rapid acquisition of this relatively large volume of images and the cine format make this an ideal technique for evaluation of valve motion, flow characteristics, and ventricular dynamics.[16, 17] The major focus currently is on the evaluation of regurgitant or stenotic valvular lesions, but newer applications are being described. Although this cine technique has been used to evaluate cardiac function, it currently is not as practical as other techniques for rapid noninvasive assessment. This is primarily related to the high cost of the MR examination.

The future of cardiovascular MRI appears bright. Early experience with three-dimensional image reconstruction has resulted in improved operative planning.[20] High-speed imaging techniques such as echo-planar imaging, ultrafast (short TR) imaging, and newer short acquisition window protocols have reduced image acquisition times to 40 to 100 msec.[21–23] Although these techniques currently have shortcom-

ings in the form of poor spatial resolution, decreased SNR, and other technical limitations, this advanced technology may result in great strides in the near future.

MR spectroscopy is now being investigated as a biochemical probe.[24, 25] This technology has long been used for in vitro laboratory work. Recently, techniques have been developed to obtain in vivo spectroscopic information from the beating heart. The potential to evaluate myocardial metabolism (particularly high energy phosphate metabolism) has been a particular focus of scientific research attention. When MR spectroscopy time constraints are better addressed, and spectral resolution and field-of-view problems are solved, this technique should prove very useful in the assessment of cardiac muscle disease and cardiac response to therapy. At the present time, MR spectroscopy represents a purely investigational tool.

CONTRAINDICATIONS

MR scanning may be performed with relative impunity in most cardiac patients. The only absolute contraindications to MRI have been in patients with cardiac pacemakers, cerebral aneurysm clips, and ferromagnetic foreign bodies around the eyes. In patients with pacemakers, radiofrequency (RF) pulses have been shown to affect pacemaker activity.[26] Currents induced in pacemaker leads may lead to incorrect sensing by the pacemaker, resulting in suppression of output. At the other extreme, atrial triggering rates of up to 800 per minute have been reported in dual chamber pacemakers.[27] RF pulses may also reprogram or damage electronic circuitry within the pacemaker, causing malfunction. A final problem relates to actual torquing of the pacemaker generator or lead wires.[28] This is not a significant concern, because these are usually well anchored. The presence of a cardiac pacemaker is still an absolute contraindication to cardiac MRI.

Cerebral aneurysm clips may torque as a result of the magnetic fields, subjecting the patient to the risk of vessel rupture.[29] New and colleagues demonstrated the effect of the magnetic field on several vascular clips used in aneurysm surgery.[30] Because of this torque effect, these patients should be excluded from the MRI suite. Abdominal clips, sternal wires, and other intrathoracic clips are generally surrounded by perilesional fibrosis and therefore should be relatively stable in most clinical magnetic field strengths.[31]

Ferromagnetic foreign bodies around the orbit also contraindicate the use of MRI. The danger of migration resulting in damage to the globe or retina militates against this technique. If there is clinical concern about a possible foreign body, a Waters view of the orbits may be used to screen for metallic objects.

With regard to prosthetic valves, MRI is generally a safe imaging technique under most circumstances. Soulen and colleagues demonstrated that the extrinsic forces placed on the prosthetic valve secondary to cardiac motion and flow effects create more torque than generated by magnetic fields used in clinical imaging.[32] Before patients with prosthetic valves are imaged, two precautions should be taken. First, one should ensure by fluoroscopy that the prosthesis is not dehiscent. Second, reference should be made to the article by Shellock, which compiles all available literature on the ferromagnetic properties of each of the prosthetic valves.[33] In addition, when these patients are imaged, cognizance of the ferromagnetic artifact created by the local distortion of the magnetic field will result in fewer image interpretive errors (Fig. 18–2).

NORMAL ANATOMY

Cardiovascular pathology may be appropriately evaluated only when there is an awareness of normal anatomy and morphology. It is difficult to demonstrate all the anatomy in every obliquity, but a basic atlas of the relationships in the standard orthogonal planes (axial, sagittal, and coronal) is essential to an understanding of pathologic alterations. The sets of images in Figures 18–3 to 18–5 were obtained in normal children aged from 4 to 16 years. All used a TE of 20 msec and a TR adjusted to the patient's ECG R-R interval (380 to 1,000 msec). Imaging was performed on a 1.5 Tesla system.

MRI provides accurate anatomic information with excellent spatial resolution. Cardiac chambers, atrial and ventricular septa, great vessels, hila, and pericardium are well visualized. Frequently, atrioventricular valves are demonstrated. Although the spin-echo tech-

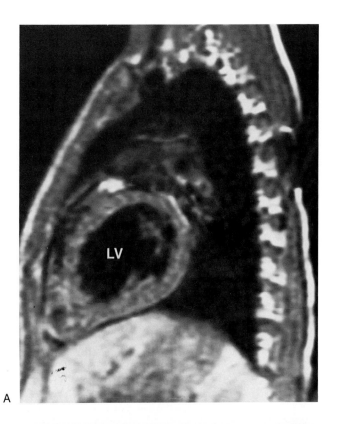

A

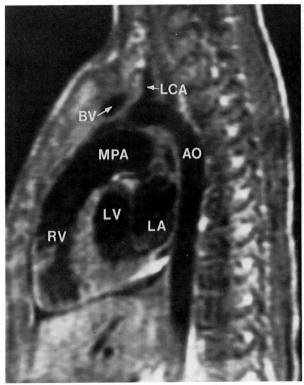

B

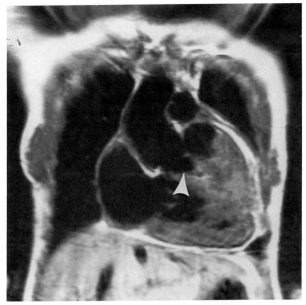

Figure 18–2. *Artifact from a prosthetic aortic valve.* Coronal image through the aortic root in a patient with a Starr-Edwards prosthetic valve in the aortic position. The arrowhead denotes a ferromagnetic signal void artifact that may simulate a ventricular septal defect.

Figure 18–3. *Normal cardiac anatomy.* Sagittal images obtained in a normal volunteer extending from *A,* most leftward scan, through the body of the left ventricle through *E,* the most rightward scan, through the right atrium. AA, Aortic arch; AO, aorta; Ap, right atrial appendage; AzV, azygos vein; BV brachiocephalic vein; HV, hepatic veins; IVC, inferior vena cava; LA, left atrium; LV, left ventricle; MPA,

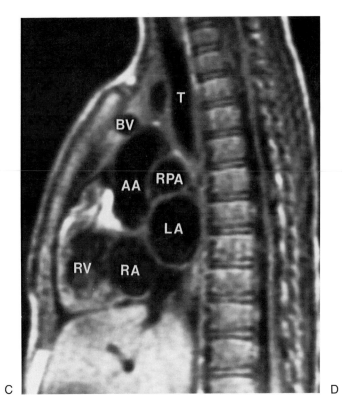

C

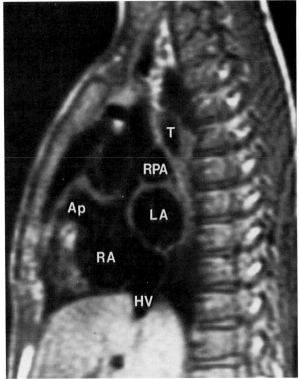

D

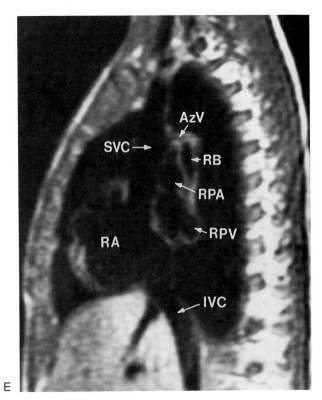

E

Figure 18–3. *Continued.*
main pulmonary artery; RA, right atrium; RB, right mainstem bronchus; RPA, right pulmonary artery; RPV, right pulmonary veins; RV, right ventricle; SVC, superior vena cava; T, trachea. (Figures 18–3 through 18–16 from Bisset GS III. Cardiac and great vessel anatomy. In: El-Khoury GY, Bergman RA, Montgomery WJ. Sectional anatomy by MRI/CT. New York: Churchill Livingstone, 1990:219–243.)

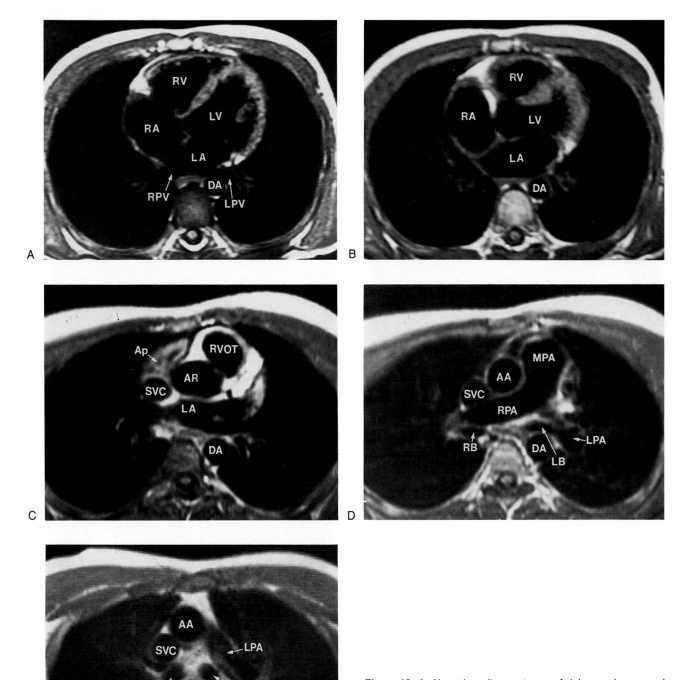

Figure 18–4. *Normal cardiac anatomy.* Axial scans in a normal volunteer extending from *A,* the inferior aspect of the heart to *E,* the most superior aspect of the left pulmonary artery. DA, Descending aorta; LB, left mainstem bronchus; LPA, left pulmonary artery; LPV, left pulmonary veins; see previous figures for other abbreviations. (Several figures from Bisset GS III. Cardiac and great vessel anatomy. In: El-Khoury GY, Bergman RA, Montgomery WJ. Sectional anatomy by MRI/CT. New York: Churchill Livingstone, 1990:219–243.)

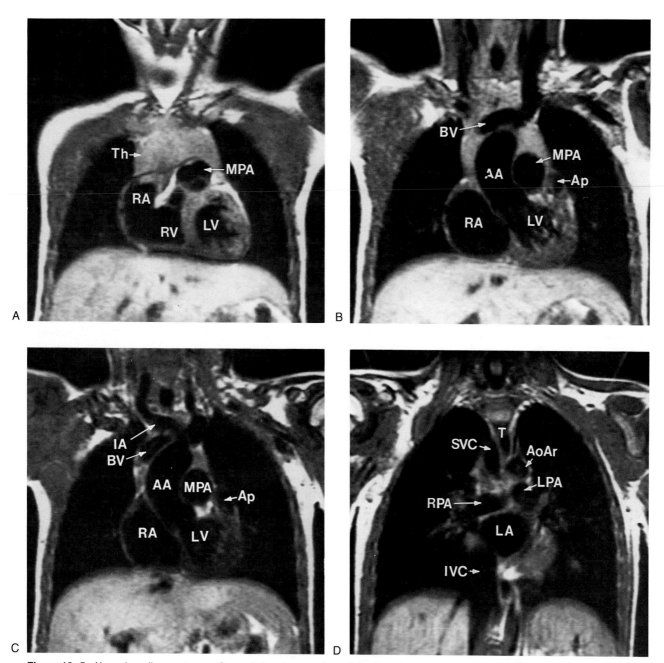

Figure 18–5. *Normal cardiac anatomy.* Coronal plane images through the heart in a normal child. *A,* the most anterior scan, which extends through the right ventricular outflow tract. *D,* the most posterior section extends through the aortic arch. AoAr, Aortic arch; Ap, left atrial appendage; IA, innominate artery; Th, thymus; see previous figures for other abbreviations. (Several figures from Bisset GS III. Cardiac and great vessel anatomy. In: El-Khoury GY, Bergman RA, Montgomery WJ. Sectional anatomy by MRI/CT. New York: Churchill Livingstone, 1990:219–243.)

nique is suboptimal for visualizing rapidly moving semilunar valves, the cine technique permits relatively detailed investigation.

CONGENITAL DISORDERS

Echocardiography has been the primary noninvasive imaging modality for the evaluation of congenital heart disease, and when coupled with Doppler is a

powerful tool for assessing real-time anatomy. Also, the portability, noninvasiveness, and low cost of echocardiography make this an ideal screening technique. Occasional obstacles arise in its technical performance. Shortcomings include (1) air or excessive fat between the transducer and region of interest, (2) sternotomy wires, (3) prosthetic valves, (4) small acoustic windows, and (5) the limitations of a "pie-slice" type of view. In these instances, and in patients in whom it is important to assess global anatomy, MRI may contribute additional information. Table 18–1 compares MRI and echocardiography with regard to the advantages and disadvantages of each technique.

Overview of Embryology

The embryology of the heart is extremely complex. A detailed knowledge of cardiac embryology is not absolutely essential for image interpretation, but some basic understanding of the development of the heart is necessary in order to assess congenital heart disease comprehensively.

A simplistic view of the embryonic tubular heart indicates the presence of five primitive chambers. These include the:

1. Sinus venosus.
2. Atrium.
3. Ventricle.
4. Bulbus cordis.
5. Truncus arteriosus.

The sinus venosus does not persist as a separate structure and eventually is incorporated into the wall of the right atrium. The importance of this structure is that maldevelopment at this level may result in a relatively uncommon atrial septal defect (sinus venosus ASD), which lies close to the entry of the superior vena cava into the right atrium.

The primitive atrium is partitioned into the right atrium and left atrium by two septa. Initially a septum primum forms, which grows cephalad from the posterosuperior aspect of the primitive atrium, dividing the chamber into left and right atria. As it develops, a gap between its lower free edge and the endocardial cushion remains patent: this is the foramen primum. As this foramen closes, a secondary foramen develops as a collection of coalescing perforations, more cephalad in the septum primum: this is the foramen secundum. Failure of the foramen primum to close results in an ostium primum atrial septal defect.

A second septum, the septum secundum, develops later and to the right side of the septum primum. If it fails to cover the foramen secundum, the resulting defect is a secundum type of atrial septal defect. After birth the rim of the septum secundum fuses with the septum primum to obliterate the potential communication (foramen ovale) between the two atria.

The primitive ventricular chamber is also divided by a septum into a right and left ventricle. This septum

forms only the inferior, muscular portion of the final ventricular septum. The remainder of the ventricular septum arises from the bulbus cordis and the truncus arteriosus.

The primitive bulbus cordis is divided by the membranous septum into right and left sides. Partitioning of this structure forms both right and left ventricular outflow tracts, and also contributes to the aortic and pulmonary valves. With further development, there is resorption of most of the left ventricular outflow tract. This results in the aortic valve lying in continuity with the mitral valve. On the right side the bulbus cordis outflow tract persists as the right ventricular outflow tract. This results in separation of the pulmonary and tricuspid valves and also the persistent anterior position of the pulmonary artery relative to the aorta.

The primitive truncus arteriosus also becomes divided by a septum. This septum forms a spiral and divides the truncus arteriosus into an anterior pulmonary artery and a posterior proximal aorta. Abnormalities of development of the truncal septum result in several common congenital malformations. If the septum completely fails to develop, one is left with a truncus arteriosus. It should be noted that, as the truncal septum does contribute to the final ventricular septum, a ventricular septal defect is always present in patients with a persistent truncus arteriosus. A hole or defect in the truncal septum results in the formation of an aorticopulmonary window. If the truncal septum forms in a straight single plane (without spiraling), transposition of the great vessels results, with the aorta lying anteriorly and the pulmonary artery posteriorly. If the truncal septum does not form in the middle of the primitive truncus arteriosus, the resulting defect is tetralogy of Fallot. In this condition the truncal septum forms in an eccentric position with a resultant small pulmonary artery, large proximal aorta, and overriding of the ventricular septum.

The lungs normally develop as buds from the gut. The pulmonary veins therefore initially connect to the gut by the cardinal and umbilical vitelline veins. Normally they lose these connections and join an outpouching from the left atrium. Defects in this anastomotic process result in anomalous venous return from the lungs to the right heart.

Early in development there is a ventral and a dorsal aorta on each side, connected by six branchial arches. The left ventral aorta becomes the ascending aorta and the left dorsal aorta becomes the descending aorta. The left fourth arch becomes the aortic arch. The ventral part of each sixth arch becomes the pulmonary artery on each side. The dorsal segment of the left sixth arch becomes the ductus arteriosus. An understanding of the development of the aortic arches clarifies the nature of double aortic arch anomalies.

The heart initially develops as a tube within the pericardium. Early in this development the tube becomes too long for the available space and bends to form a loop, which is almost always to the right and is therefore a dextro or D loop. This results in the right

Table 18–1. COMPARISON OF THE ADVANTAGES OF MRI AND ECHOCARDIOGRAPHY

MRI	Echocardiography
Excellent global anatomy	Portability
No body habitus limitations	Low cost
No bone or air penetration limitations	Real-time imaging (functional assessment)
Excellent contrast resolution	Easier patient monitoring

ventricle coming to lie to the right of the left ventricle and the ascending aorta lying to the right of the proximal pulmonary artery. Left or L looping results in ventricular inversion and corrected transposition of the great vessels (the aorta lying to the left of the pulmonary artery).

Left-to-Right Shunt Lesions

Left-to-right shunt lesions represent the most common congenital heart defects. These include the more common atrial septal defects, ventricular septal defects, atrioventricular canal defects, and patent ductus arteriosus. The more unusual left-to-right shunts are the total and partial anomalies of pulmonary venous return, aorticopulmonary windows, aberrant origins of the left coronary artery, and peripheral arteriovenous fistulas. Although in many of these lesions MRI may clearly identify the presence and exact site of the defect, this may be superfluous information. Most of these anomalies are well evaluated by echocardiography. Only rarely are we asked to perform MRI on patients with uncomplicated atrial or ventricular septal defects. However, it is still important to be able to recognize and categorize these defects, since they may be detected on MRI performed for other reasons or may be noted as part of a more complex cardiac anomaly.

Atrial Septal Defects

Atrial septal defects (ASDs) are relatively common congenital heart defects. They are most frequently recognized in childhood, but occasionally escape detection until later in life.

There are four types of atrial septal defect. The most common is the secundum defect. Ostium primum and sinus venosus defects are the less common types of atrial level shunts. A fourth type represents a complete failure of septal development, resulting in a common atrium (Fig. 18–6). In each case the net physiologic effect of the atrial level left-to-right shunt is right ventricular volume overload, manifested by dilatation of the right atrium and right ventricle. The left atrium and left ventricle remain of normal size, or may be slightly smaller than normal.

The ideal MR plane for diagnosis of atrial septal defect has not been completely defined. Long axis oblique views through the left ventricle and standard orthogonal axial views have both demonstrated high sensitivity and specificity for detection of defects.[34,35] In a study of 31 patients with atrial septal defects, MRI was able to identify 97 percent of the malformations and identified their location with an accuracy of over 96 percent.[35] Our experience has also indicated that the axial view is very accurate for detection of atrial level shunts (Fig. 18–7). The primary findings are related to the actual defect, and the secondary findings to the physiologic effect of the shunt. Each of the defects is demonstrated as an interruption of the atrial septum at

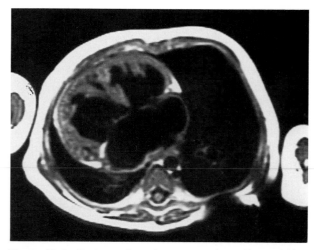

Figure 18–6. *Dextrocardia and common atrium.* Transaxial image through the heart. Note the complete lack of formation of the atrial septum.

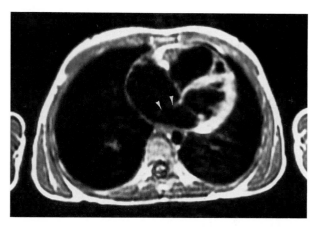

Figure 18–7. *Secundum atrial septal defect.* Transaxial image through the midportion of the atrial septum. The arrowheads denote the blunt edges at the periphery of the defect.

the affected location. The size of the defect can be fairly well characterized. The secondary findings are those of right atrial and right ventricular dilatation. An additional finding, particularly in patients with sinus venosus defects, may be partial anomalous pulmonary venous return. The pulmonary venous structures are well characterized by MRI, which may be at least as accurate as two-dimensional echocardiography and angiography for the evaluation of abnormal pulmonary venous connections.

An occasional pitfall with MRI is the interpretation of normal thinning at the level of the fossa ovalis as a secundum type of defect.[16] Blunt edges must be demonstrated at the periphery of the true defect, rather than subtle tapering at the fossa ovalis. In patients who have previously undergone operative repair of an atrial defect, the low signal intensity patch may be demonstrated, surrounded by higher signal intensity neointima (Fig. 18–8).

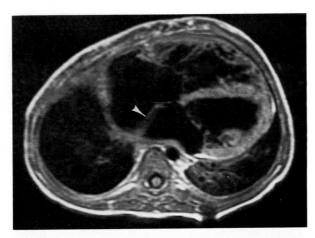

Figure 18–8. *Repaired atrial septal defect.* Transaxial image. The patch (*arrowhead*) is demonstrated as a low signal intensity structure surrounded by higher signal intensity neointima. Note the lack of normal convexity of the atrial septum at the patch site, and the residual right atrial and right ventricular enlargement.

Although MRI is useful in evaluating defects in the atrial septum, it is seldom used for this purpose. Because of its sensitivity and specificity, echocardiography, coupled with the Doppler technique, has proved to be a reliable noninvasive method for evaluating these defects.[36]

Ventricular Septal Defects

Ventricular septal defects (VSDs) are the most commonly recognized congenital heart defects. Although they are usually isolated anomalies, they are often associated with other cardiac abnormalities. As with atrial level shunts, there are multiple types of defects. There are numerous nosologic descriptions of these anomalies, but the most practical classification divides the ventricular septal defects according to their position in the septum: (1) inlet septal defects (atrioventricular canal), (2) trabecular defects (muscular), (3) infracristal defects (subaortic or perimembranous), and (4) supracristal defects (subpulmonic). The infracristal defects are the most common (80 percent).

The net physiologic effect of each of these defects is left ventricular volume overload. The extra volume of blood recirculated into the pulmonary circuit through the defect increases the return volume to the left atrium and left ventricle, resulting in dilatation of these two chambers. If the pulmonary resistance rises, as noted in some of the larger defects, the right ventricle will enlarge as a result of pressure overload. Frequently the main pulmonary artery is also dilated as a result of the increased pulmonary arterial flow. In patients with atrioventricular canal defects, the mitral or tricuspid valve clefts may result in additional right atrial and right ventricular dilatation, resulting from left ventricle–to–right atrium shunting.

In patients with ventricular septal defects, the development of pulmonary vascular disease (Eisenmenger's syndrome) results in thickening of the right ventricle

and marked dilatation of the proximal pulmonary arteries. As the pressures in the right and left ventricles equilibrate, the left-to-right shunt decreases and the left-sided volume overload features resolve. In these patients, an abnormal MR signal may be found in the pulmonary arteries during systole, suggesting diminished flow.[37, 38]

The optimal MR plane for visualizing ventricular defects is variable, depending on the exact location of the defect.[39, 40] The ventricular septum, rather than being a planar structure, has a complex curvature, with the major trabecular portion convex toward the right ventricle. This complex curve may vary, depending on the attendant pathology. Right and left ventricular volume overloads affect the septum in different ways. Most of the inlet, trabecular, and infracristal defects are best visualized in the transaxial plane (Fig. 18–9). Planes through the long axis of the left ventricle are also accurate in demonstrating the defects. Supracristal defects may best be detected on transaxial imaging, but visualization in the coronal plane may also be necessary. Sagittal images may be useful when the defect is complicated by right ventricular enlargement (Fig. 18–10). As this chamber dilates, the septum aligns more parallel with the coronal plane. Therefore, sagittal imaging provides more of a cross-sectional view through the ventricular septum than can be obtained on a coronal view.

The cine MR technique has demonstrated an ability to demonstrate left-to-right shunting across ventricular septal defects[41] and may also be useful in quantification of shunt volume. In each of the uncomplicated ventricular septal defects the major finding is an abrupt edge, with dropout of signal, at the defect. One would also expect to see left atrial and left ventricular enlargement. Occasionally, a septal aneurysm may be demonstrated at the site of the defect. The detection rate of these defects depends on the size, larger defects being more obvious; small defects, particularly in the muscu-

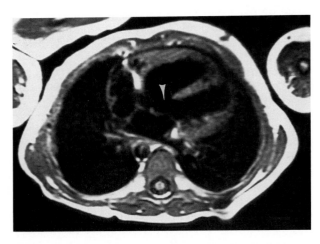

Figure 18–9. *Ventricular septal defect.* Transaxial plane image through the subaortic region in a patient with tetralogy of Fallot and a typical subaortic ventricular septal defect (*arrowhead*).

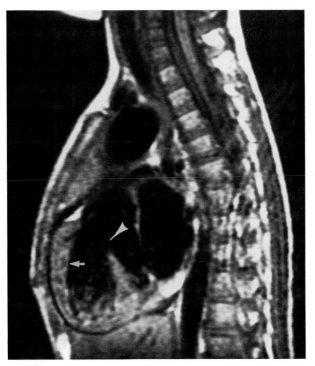

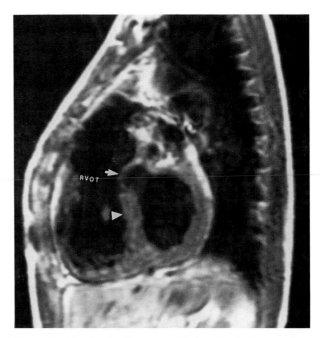

Figure 18–11. *Repaired tetralogy of Fallot.* Sagittal plane image. The right ventricular outflow tract (RVOT) is markedly widened following extensive resection. Note the ventricular septal defect patch (*arrow*) immediately cephalad to the native septum (*arrowhead*).

Figure 18–10. *Subaortic ventricular septal defect.* Sagittal plane section in a patient with tetralogy of Fallot demonstrates a large subaortic ventricular septal defect (*arrowhead*). Note the thickening of the anterior wall of the right ventricle (*arrow*).

lar septum, frequently go undetected. In postoperative repair patients, the septal patch may be demonstrated (Fig. 18–11).

As noted with atrial septal defects, cardiac MR scans are not often performed to diagnose ventricular septal defects, since these lesions are easily demonstrated by two-dimensional echocardiography. When echocardiography is coupled with Doppler, even small defects may be shown, or inferred from Doppler findings.[42] Ventricular level defects, however, are occasionally noted on MRI performed to evaluate more complex congenital heart disease. Information as to the type and size of the defect may be invaluable for the surgeon planning operative repair.

Atrioventricular Canal Defects

In this defect (endocardial cushion defect) there is a combination of a primum type of atrial septal defect, a high posterior inlet ventricular septal defect, and a common atrioventricular valve ring. The disease presents as a spectrum of abnormalities, the most complete form having all of the above malformations. The simplest form is an isolated primum type of atrial septal defect without any ventricular level shunt. One study of nine patients with atrioventricular canal defects reported that MRI was able to identify the abnormality in each patient.[43] The defects were well recognized in the transaxial plane. Three patients with partial defects were accurately distinguished from six individuals

with complete atrioventricular canals. In patients with a partial defect, MRI identifies a dense fibromuscular bridge of tissue that courses from the atrioventricular valve to the crest of the ventricular septum, obliterating the interventricular communication.

Patent Ductus Arteriosus

The ductus arteriosus is an embryonal vascular structure that permits the fetal right heart output to bypass the high-resistance (and functionally inert) lungs. This vessel connects the origin of the left pulmonary artery to the descending aorta at the level of the aortic isthmus. Normally this vessel closes at birth as a response to high oxygen tensions related to respiration. In some individuals the vessel wall does not constrict normally and the ductus arteriosus remains patent. This patent vessel varies considerably in size and configuration. The net physiologic effect of this maintained patency is a left-to-right shunt from the higher pressure aorta into the lower pressure pulmonary arteries. This extra volume of blood entering the pulmonary circuit results in the left atrium and left ventricle receiving larger volumes. These two chambers dilate as a response to the overload.

The optimal plane in which to image a patent ductus arteriosus (PDA) is transaxial (Fig. 18–12A). They are also demonstrated in the right anterior oblique equivalent view, which profiles the condition (Fig. 18–12B). The primary finding is a small tubular structure with signal void, connecting the aortic isthmus with the distal main or proximal left pulmonary artery. Second-

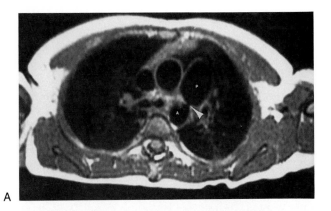

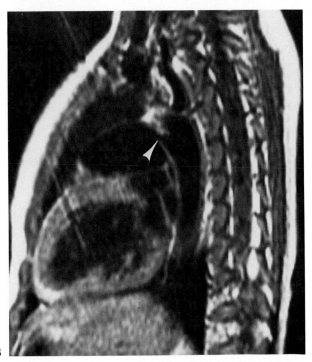

Figure 18–12. *Patient ductus arteriosus.* ***A,*** Axial scan through the superior aspect of the main pulmonary artery. The arrowhead denotes a small patent ductus arteriosus that connects the proximal portion of the descending aorta (A) to the main pulmonary artery (P). Note the slight dilatation of the main pulmonary artery. ***B,*** Sagittal oblique image obtained in a plane directly paralleling the patent ductus arteriosus on the transaxial view. The arrowhead denotes the small patent ductus arteriosus.

ary findings include dilatation of the left atrium and left ventricle.

MR scans are infrequently requested to evaluate a patent ductus arteriosus. As with the aforementioned left-to-right shunt lesions, duplex Doppler echocardiography is sensitive and accurate for the diagnosis of this condition. Occasionally, MRI may be useful for differentiating a patent ductus arteriosus from an aorticopulmonary window; both behave in a clinically similar fashion. In some instances the echocardiogram may not be able to distinguish between the two lesions.

Miscellaneous

Little experience has been acquired in MRI of the more unusual left-to-right shunts. Experience with imaging lesions such as aorticopulmonary windows, aberrant origins of the coronary arteries, and non–central nervous system (CNS) arteriovenous fistulas (Fig. 18–13) has been limited to isolated case reports.[44] The ability to acquire cine-type MR displays has demonstrated early promise for mapping of arteriovenous fistulas before attempted embolization. We have also used this technique to follow the progress of embolization therapy.

Obstructive Lesions

Right Heart Outflow Obstruction

Most obstructive lesions of the right heart are typified by cyanosis and are addressed in the section on cyanotic disease. The only significant acyanotic obstructive right heart lesions consist of isolated infundibular stenosis (rare), pulmonary valve stenosis, and pulmonary artery coarctation. Although pulmonary hypertension frequently presents as a cyanotic form of right heart outflow obstruction (because of associated congenital heart disease), these patients may have acyanotic etiologies. In each case the pathophysiology is related to pressure overload of the right ventricle, resulting in right ventricular hypertrophy.

The main, proximal right, and proximal left pulmonary arteries are ideally suited for MRI.[45, 46] Transaxial or axial oblique images, paralleling the identified axis of the main pulmonary artery in the sagittal plane, are best for visualizing the right and left pulmonary arteries (Fig. 18–14). The direct sagittal plane may be more appropriate for imaging the main pulmonary artery and subvalvar area (infundibulum). In these planes, focal areas of narrowed vessel or infundibulum are identified. In the case of valvar pulmonic stenosis the thickened, domed valve is occasionally identified, but more often the abnormal valve is not seen with conventional spin-echo imaging. Cine MR has proved beneficial in imaging the thickened valve and its motion, and in demonstrating the abnormal flow pattern in the proximal pulmonary arteries. Frequently, post-stenotic dilatation of the main pulmonary artery is visualized on the sagittal images.

In the case of peripheral pulmonic stenosis areas of narrowing may be demonstrated, if present proximal to the hila (Figs. 18–15, 18–16). Distal areas of narrowing are difficult to visualize because of an inability to separate vessel flow void from lung parenchyma.

In patients with severe pulmonary hypertension, although pulmonary artery pressures are significantly elevated, flow velocity may be diminished. Rather than visualizing signal void in the pulmonary arteries, the slow flow may result in an increased intraluminal signal (Fig. 18–17). Didier and Higgins demonstrated signal in the pulmonary arteries on systolic images in ten

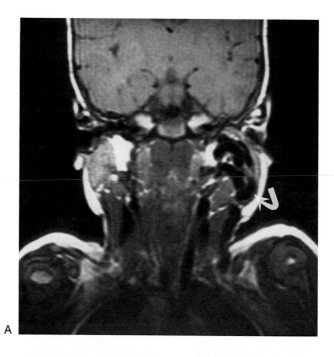

A

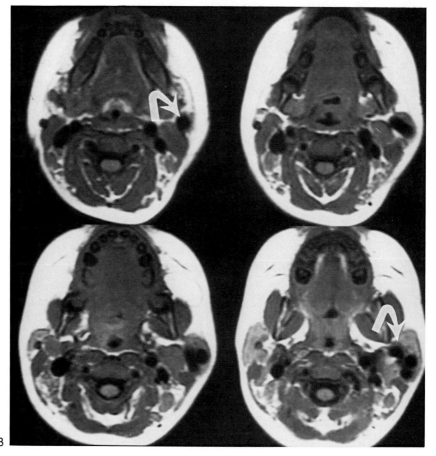

Figure 18–13. *Arteriovenous malformation.* **A,** Coronal image through the neck of a 7-month-old child with clinical findings of a moderate left-to-right shunt. The curved arrow indicates a prominent arteriovenous malformation extending from the carotid artery to the external jugular vein. **B,** Transaxial images in the same patient, extending from cranial to caudal locations, demonstrate the prominent low signal intensity vessels (*curved arrow*) just medial to the sternocleidomastoid muscle.

B

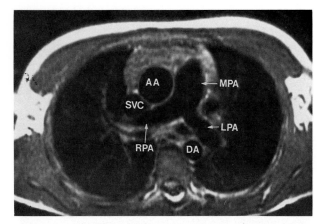

Figure 18–14. *Normal pulmonary artery.* Transaxial image through the axis of the main pulmonary artery demonstrating a normal bifurcation of the main pulmonary artery trunk. AA, Ascending aorta; DA, descending aorta; LPA, left pulmonary artery; MPA, main pulmonary artery; RPA, right pulmonary artery; SVC, superior vena cava.

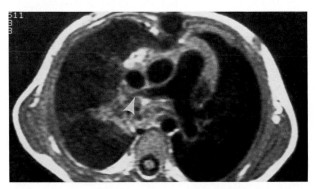

Figure 18–15. *Peripheral pulmonary stenosis.* Transaxial image through the axis of the main pulmonary artery demonstrating marked tapering (*arrowhead*) of the proximal right pulmonary artery. This narrowing was documented at cardiac catheterization. This patient also had marked right pulmonary vein stenosis.

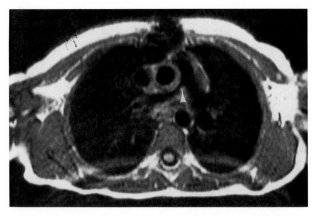

Figure 18–16. *Peripheral pulmonary stenosis.* Transaxial image through the axis of the main pulmonary artery in a patient after operative placement of a right ventricular outflow tract conduit. There is moderately severe stenosis of the proximal right pulmonary artery (*arrowhead*).

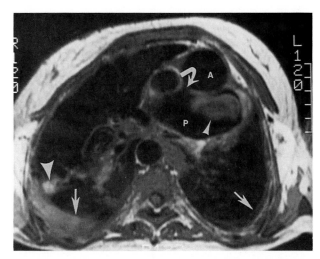

Figure 18–17. *Pulmonary hypertension.* Transaxial image in a patient with tetralogy of Fallot and a Waterston shunt (*curved arrow*) from the ascending aorta (A) to the right pulmonary artery (P). This patient has catheterization-proved absence of the left pulmonary artery and severe pulmonary hypertension. Within the right pulmonary artery there is a focal area of increased signal intensity (systolic image) indicating slow flow (*small arrowhead*). In addition, the patient has a focal area of intrapulmonary hemorrhage in the right lower lobe (*large arrowhead*). There are also small bilateral pleural effusions (*arrows*). (From Bisset GS III. Magnetic resonance imaging in pediatrics. Clear Images 1987; 1:6–17.)

patients with Eisenmenger's syndrome.[47] In these patients there was a direct linear relationship between pulmonary artery signal intensity and pulmonary vascular resistance. Associated findings may include areas of intrapulmonary hemorrhage, dilatation of the main pulmonary artery, and right ventricular hypertrophy (Fig. 18–17).

Left Heart Inflow Obstruction

Left heart obstructive lesions include inflow and outflow abnormalities. The inflow obstructive lesions include pulmonary vein stenosis, cor triatriatum, supravalvar stenosing mitral ring, and mitral stenosis. In each the physiology is characterized by pulmonary venous congestion and signs of right ventricular pressure overload (thickened, dilated right ventricle and dilated pulmonary arteries). The direct findings include visualization of narrowed or obliterated pulmonary veins (Fig. 18–18), an intra-atrial membrane or ring (Fig. 18–19), and (in the case of mitral stenosis) a markedly dilated left atrium. Occasionally, a thickened mitral valve is demonstrated.

In patients with cor triatriatum, MRI may play a particularly important role.[48] This is a rare congenital anomaly in which a fibromuscular membrane divides the left atrium into an accessory posterior chamber, which receives pulmonary venous return, and an anteroinferior chamber, which communicates with the left ventricle. In this lesion, M-mode and two-dimensional echocardiography may occasionally lead to false-negative results. If the intra-atrial membrane is not imaged

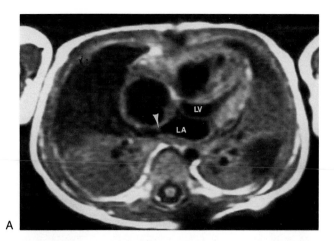

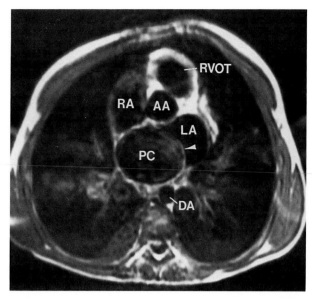

Figure 18–19. *Cor triatriatum.* Transaxial view through the left atrium. The arrowhead denotes the intra-atrial membrane, which separates the posterior chamber (receiving pulmonary venous inflow) from the portion of the left atrium (including the left atrial appendage), which communicates with the left ventricle by way of the mitral valve. AA, Ascending aorta; DA, descending aorta; LA, anterior portion of the left atrium; PC, posterior chamber; RA, right atrium; RVOT, right ventricular outflow tract. (From Bisset GS III, Kirks DR, Strife JL, Schwartz DC. Cor triatriatum: diagnosis by magnetic resonance imaging. AJR 1987; 149:567–568.)

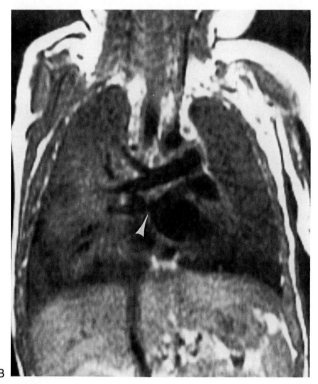

Figure 18–18. *Pulmonary vein stenosis.* ***A,*** Transaxial view through the right pulmonary veins. The arrowhead denotes a membrane obstructing the inflow from the right upper pulmonary vein. The left pulmonary veins had similar obstructive lesions, resulting in the diffuse pulmonary edema. Note the small size of the left atrium (LA) and left ventricle (LV). ***B,*** Coronal image through the right upper pulmonary vein in the same patient, demonstrating the discrete stenosis at the junction of the right upper pulmonary veins with the left atrium (*arrowhead*). Again, note the pulmonary edema.

in an optimal plane, it may go undetected. Angiography, as well as being potentially harmful in these patients, may also lead to false-negative results. If the membrane is parallel to the imaging plane, detection is difficult. MRI, because of its multiplanar capabilities, provides excellent delineation of the membrane (Fig. 18–19).

Optimal imaging planes for these lesions are variable. Thin (3-mm) coronal and axial images are best suited to visualizing small pulmonary venous structures and intra-atrial membranes or rings. An oblique plane parallel to the longitudinal axis of the left ventricle may be best for demonstrating the mitral valve. In these obstructive lesions, one may see higher signal intensity within the pulmonary veins or left atrium as a result of partially obstructed slow blood flow (Fig. 18–19).

Although the mitral valve is best visualized by echocardiography, intra-atrial membranes or rings and pulmonary venous structures may be better visualized by MRI.[48, 49] In patients with pulmonary venous hypertension in whom no obvious cause is demonstrated by echocardiography, MRI has been invaluable as a problem-solving tool.[48]

Left Heart Outflow Obstruction

Left heart outflow obstructive lesions include hypoplastic left heart, subvalvar discrete aortic stenosis, hypertrophic cardiomyopathy (idiopathic hypertrophic subaortic stenosis, IHSS), valvar aortic stenosis, supravalvar aortic stenosis, and coarctation of the thoracic aorta. In each of these lesions the net physiologic effect of obstruction is left ventricular hypertrophy (except hypoplastic left heart). Each of the intracardiac lesions is best evaluated by echocardiography.

Supravalvar aortic stenosis (Fig. 18–20) and coarctation of the thoracic aorta, however, are difficult to evaluate with this modality because of superimposed lung tissue.

Coarctation of the Aorta

MRI is ideally suited for imaging the thoracic aorta.[50–54] The ability to perform sagittal oblique imaging allows visualization of the entire arch on a single series acquisition. Thoracic coarctation may be classified into two types: discrete juxtaductal and diffuse hypoplastic. If the coarctation is proximal to the insertion of the ductus arteriosus, the lower half of the body will be supplied by the patent ductus arteriosus in the neonatal period. When the ductus arteriosus closes in response to physiologic stimuli, the infant becomes acidotic and hypoperfused. With juxtaductal coarctation the only pathway for blood to reach the lower half of the body is via the narrowed aorta and prominent collateral vessels.

In the evaluation of coarctation of the aorta it is important to define the location and severity of the coarctation (Figs. 18–21 to 18–23), the length of the coarctation, the presence or absence of collateral vessels (Fig. 18–24), the presence or absence of an associated bicuspid aortic valve, and the degree of left ventricular hypertrophy. The left subclavian artery must also be delineated; this vessel may be used in the

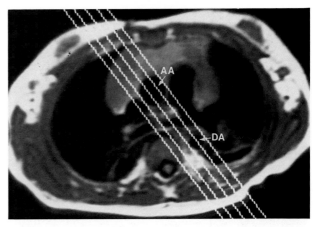

Figure 18–21. *Normal aorta.* Oblique imaging technique for acquiring direct sagittal images of the aorta. After transaxial images are obtained through the ascending and descending aorta, electronic angling is used to establish a plane through the ascending aorta (AA) and descending aorta (DA).

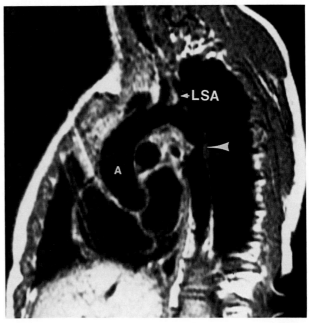

Figure 18–22. *Coarctation of the aorta.* In the sagittal oblique plane a discrete coarctation of the aorta is identified in a typical juxtaductal location (*arrowhead*). The relationship of the coarctation to the left subclavian artery (LSA) is readily established. Post-stenotic dilatation of the ascending aorta (A) is secondary to aortic valve stenosis.

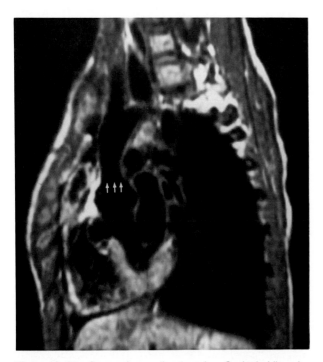

Figure 18–20. *Supravalvar aortic stenosis.* Sagittal oblique image through the ascending aorta in a patient with Williams' syndrome. Note the focal narrowing (*arrows*) of the ascending aorta just distal to the sinuses of Valsalva. This is a typical form of supravalvar aortic stenosis.

operative repair of the coarctation (Fig. 18–22). Pseudocoarctation, characterized by tortuosity and kinking of the aortic arch, may be distinguished from true coarctation by means of MRI (Fig. 18–25). In all but complicated cases, MRI has supplanted cardiac catheterization and cineangiography in the preoperative assessment of aortic coarctation.

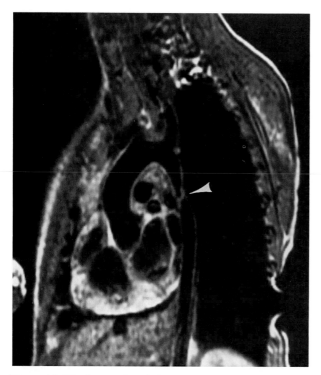

Figure 18–23. *Coarctation of the aorta.* Sagittal oblique image through aortic arch in a child with Williams' syndrome. A severe discrete coarctation is identified in a juxtaductal position (*arrowhead*).

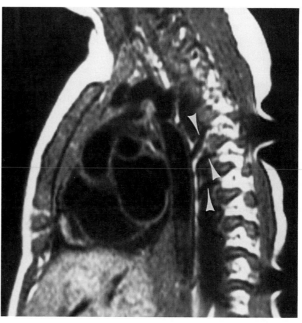

Figure 18–24. *Coarctation of the aorta.* Sagittal oblique image through the aortic arch demonstrating a discrete juxtaductal coarctation of the thoracic aorta, as well as several prominent collateral vessels (*arrowheads*).

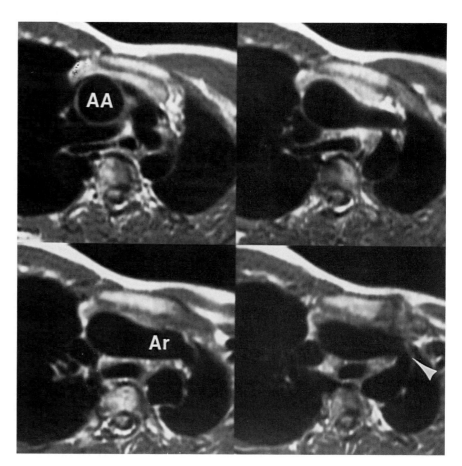

Figure 18–25. *Pseudo coarctation.* Series of axial oblique scans through the aortic arch extending in a caudal to cranial direction. Note the buckling and marked tortuosity (*arrowhead*) of the aortic arch in this patient with a proved pseudocoarctation anomaly. AA, Ascending aorta; Ar, aortic arch.

Right-to-Left Shunt Lesions (Cyanotic Disease)

The major cyanotic lesions include tetralogy of Fallot, D-transposition of the great vessels, truncus arteriosus, total anomalous pulmonary venous return, and tricuspid atresia. More unusual defects, such as double outlet right ventricle and single ventricle, generally combine a ventricular septal defect with pulmonary stenosis. As in many of the left-to-right shunt lesions, most cyanotic defects are well characterized by echocardiography. On occasion, however, MRI may provide a unique capability, not readily available with any other noninvasive or invasive imaging tool.

Tetralogy of Fallot

The lesions associated with the classic tetrad described by Fallot include ventricular septal defect, right ventricular hypertrophy, pulmonic stenosis (infundibular, valvar, supravalvar, or a combination), and aortic override of the ventricular septum. The physiologic effect of a ventricular septal defect combined with pulmonic stenosis results in shunting of unoxygenated blood from right to left into the aorta. The right ventricle hypertrophies as a result of the increased pressure overload, and the aorta dilates as a consequence of markedly increased aortic flow. A right aortic arch is commonly present.

The key role of MRI in this lesion is in delineation of the main right and left pulmonary arteries and in assessment of bronchial collateral flow. Echocardiography and, on occasion, angiography often cannot identify a distinct pulmonary confluence, particularly with small right and left branches. This information is of vital importance to the surgeon planning operative repair. MRI may also be used to follow the growth of small pulmonary arteries after a shunt procedure.

The transaxial or axial oblique planes (parallel to the main pulmonary artery, identified on sagittal localizer) are best for evaluating the pulmonary outflow tract (Figs. 18–26, 18–27).[46] Bronchial collateral flow arising from the descending aorta is best imaged in the coronal plane (Fig. 18–28). Although the large subaortic ventricular septal defect may be visualized with MRI (Fig. 18–29), this information is generally obtainable by echocardiography.

Treatment of tetralogy consists of complete surgical repair in childhood. If there is severe pulmonary obstruction, a palliative shunt (Blalock-Taussig or Waterston) may be performed during infancy.

D-Transposition of Great Vessels

This is the most common of the cyanotic congenital heart lesions, usually presenting in the newborn period with profound hypoxemia. D-transposed great vessels (D-TGV) result when the aorta and pulmonary artery are reversed in position so that the aorta arises anteriorly from the right ventricle, and the main pulmonary artery posteriorly from the left ventricle. The proximal aorta lies to the right of the pulmonary artery. This physiology results in parallel circulatory systems, rather than the normal situation of series-type flow. These patients must have a natural or artificially created shunt to survive. The diagnosis is usually established by echocardiography in the neonatal period. Therefore, although reports have documented the efficacy of MRI in defining this condition, MRI may not provide any unique information.[1,3] This defect should be recognizable, however, because of its frequent association with more complex congenital disease. In this anomaly and in L-transposed great vessels, the transaxial views through the level of the pulmonary artery bifurcation demonstrate the aforementioned anterior

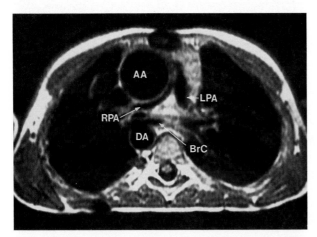

Figure 18–26. *Tetralogy of Fallot.* Transaxial image through the pulmonary outflow tract. Note the small right pulmonary artery (RPA) and the slightly larger, but still diminutive, left pulmonary artery (LPA). The slightly larger left pulmonary artery results from a previous left Blalock-Taussig shunt. Note the right-sided aortic arch and the prominent bronchial collateral (BrC) vessel arising from the anterior aspect of the descending aorta (DA). AA, Ascending aorta.

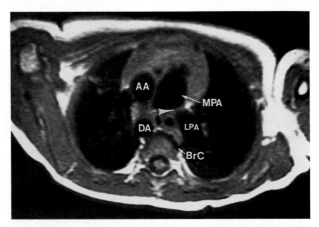

Figure 18–27. *Tetralogy of Fallot.* Transaxial image through the main pulmonary artery. Note the discontinuity (*arrowhead*) between the main (MPA) and left (LPA) pulmonary arteries. Also note the bronchial collateral (BrC) vessel anterior to the vertebral body. A right aortic arch (AA) is also demonstrated. This patient had a predominant left-to-right shunt at this age because of relatively mild infundibular pulmonic stenosis. This factor is responsible for the slightly enlarged main pulmonary artery. DA, Descending aorta.

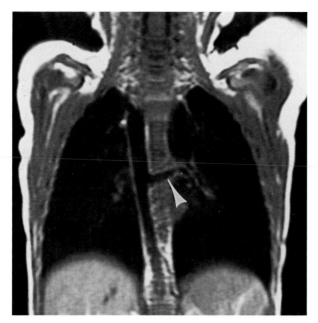

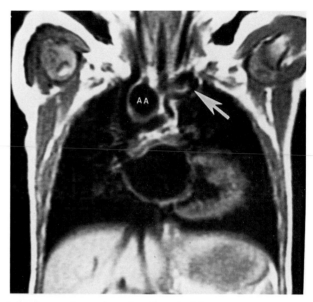

Figure 18–28. *Tetralogy of Fallot.* Sequential coronal images through the descending aorta and aortic arch. A large bronchial collateral vessel (*arrowhead*) supplies blood to the left lung. A Blalock-Taussig shunt (*arrow*) supplies blood to the right pulmonary artery. The aortic arch (AA) is to the right of the trachea.

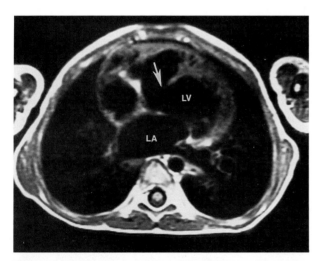

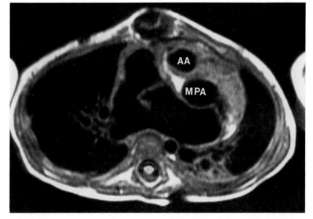

Figure 18–30. *D-transposition after Senning procedure.* Transaxial image through the origins of the great vessels. Note the anterior and rightward position of the ascending aorta (AA) relative to the main pulmonary artery (MPA). (From Bisset GS III. Pediatric thoracic applications of MRI. J Thorac Imaging 1989; 4(2):51–57.)

Figure 18–29. *Tetralogy of Fallot.* Transaxial image through the ventricular septum. Note the large subaortic ventricular septal defect (*arrow*). The left atrium (LA) and left ventricle (LV) are moderately dilated in this patient secondary to an artificially created aorticopulmonary shunt.

position of the aorta (Figs. 18–30, 18–31). The sagittal localizer views also show the aorta arising from the right ventricle in the retrosternal space.

Truncus Arteriosus

Truncus arteriosus occurs when there is inadequate conotruncal septation. This embryologic insult results in a single large truncal vessel arising from the base of the heart (overriding a large VSD), which gives rise to an aorta and pulmonary arteries.

Classification of the varying types of truncus arteriosus was initially based on the origin of the pulmonary arteries. More recently, Van Praagh modified the classification as follows:[55]

Type I: Incomplete formation of the aorticopulmonary septum, resulting in a partially separate main pulmonary artery.

Type II: Absent aorticopulmonary septum resulting in both pulmonary arteries arising directly from the truncus.

Type III: One pulmonary artery branch is absent.

Type IV: Preductal hypoplasia, coarctation, atresia, or interruption.

The classification is important in planning the surgical approach and predicting the outcome. Each type may be readily defined by means of MRI.

As with D-transposition of the great vessels, MRI plays a small role in the initial diagnosis, but may be used to evaluate small pulmonary arteries or postoperative problems. Transaxial views generally provide all the necessary information (Fig. 18–32).

Total Anomalous Pulmonary Venous Return

Total anomalous pulmonary venous return (TAPVR) is characterized by the entire pulmonary venous drainage emptying into the right atrium. Three types include supracardiac, cardiac, and infracardiac level return. In the supracardiac type the pulmonary veins join together behind the left atrium and then drain via a persistent cardinal vein into the left innominate vein. Occasionally, drainage may be directly into a left or right superior vena cava. In the cardiac type of abnormality the anomalous venous return is either directly into the coronary sinus or to the right atrium. Infradiaphragmatic return of anomalous pulmonary veins is usually to the portal veins. Each of these may have slightly different clinical manifestations, but the net effect is that oxygenated blood returning from the lungs to the heart enters the right atrium and may reach the left atrium only through an atrial septal defect. This results in marked right-sided enlargement with relatively small left-sided chambers. As with the other cyanotic defects, the diagnosis is usually established in early infancy by echocardiography. MRI may have a role in identifying anomalous pulmonary veins in patients being evaluated for more complex disease (Figs. 18–33, 18–34).

Transaxial and thin (3-mm) coronal sections have been best for identifying the origins of the pulmonary veins.

Tricuspid Atresia

Tricuspid atresia arises as a result of failure of the right-sided atrioventricular connection to develop. There generally is hypoplasia or absence of the right ventricle and defective development of the ventricular septum. Pulmonary stenosis or atresia is frequently present. Patients with this anomaly are diagnosed in the first 3 months of life because of persistent cyanosis. Because the right ventricle contains no significant inlet and is hypoplastic, the left ventricle dilates to accommodate the overload. Once again, the diagnosis is generally made by two-dimensional echocardiography. Occasionally, however, MRI may provide useful infor-

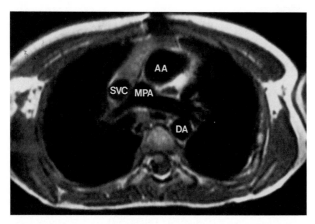

Figure 18–31. *L-transposition.* Transaxial image through the pulmonary artery. The ascending aorta (AA) is positioned anterior and to the left of the main pulmonary artery (MPA). DA, Descending aorta; SVC, superior vena cava.

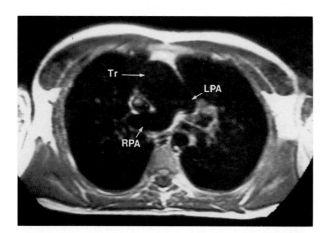

Figure 18–32. *Truncus arteriosus: type II.* Transaxial image through the great vessels. Note the origins of the pulmonary arteries (RPA, LPA) from the posterior aspect of the truncus (Tr). (Courtesy of Dr. Kerry Link, Winston-Salem, NC.)

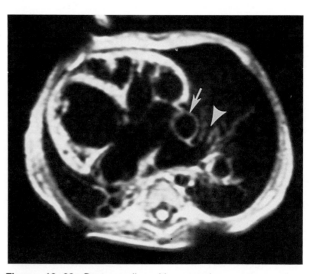

Figure 18–33. *Dextrocardia with anomalous venous return.* Transaxial image through the pulmonary veins. Note the pulmonary vein (*arrowhead*) draining into the left side of the common atrium behind a left-sided superior vena cava (*arrow*).

mation about small pulmonary arteries or the status of the atrial septum.[56]

MRI is best performed in the transaxial plane and usually shows an atretic tricuspid plate, associated with a diminutive right ventricle and a large left ventricle (Fig. 18–35). In the classic form of tricuspid atresia the atrioventricular valve is absent and the muscular floor of the right atrium is separated from the ventricular mass by fat in the atrioventricular sulcus, in the region where the valve would be expected to be. This fat appears of bright signal intensity on T1 and T2 weighted pulse sequences.[57] This finding is not present

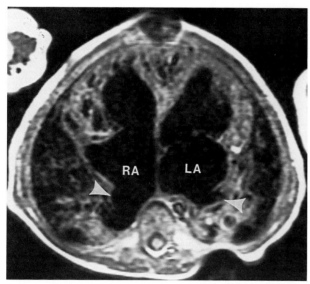

Figure 18–34. *Anomalous venous return.* Transaxial view through the middle heart in a patient with complex congenital heart disease. Note the pulmonary venous structures (*arrowheads*) draining into the posterior aspects of the right (RA) and left (LA) atrium.

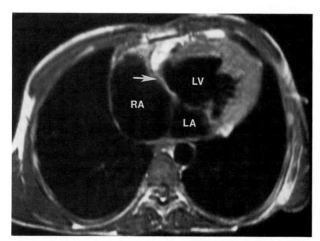

Figure 18–35. *Tricuspid atresia.* Transaxial plane through the left ventricle. Note the atretic tricuspid plate (*arrow*) and the moderately dilated right atrium (RA). The right ventricle is markedly hypoplastic. LA, Left atrium; LV, left ventricle.

in patients with a rare form of imperforate tricuspid valve, which helps to differentiate this condition from classic tricuspid atresia.[57] The size of the pulmonary arteries is directly related to pulmonary blood flow.

Intrathoracic Arterial and Systemic Venous Anomalies

Vascular rings result from an abnormal development of the aortic arch system in which derivatives of the arch encircle the trachea and esophagus. The various components of the vascular rings represent segments of the six primitive aortic arches that have persisted abnormally.

Anomalies of the aortic arch complex include (1) the "classic" vascular rings: the double aortic arch, and right aortic arch with left ligamentum arteriosus and anomalous left subclavian artery (Figs. 18–36, 18–37); (2) the cervical aortic arch (Fig. 18–38); and (3) the left aortic arch with an aberrant right subclavian artery (Fig. 18–39). Each of these lesions may be associated with esophageal or tracheal compression. The pulmonary sling is another anomaly that may result in tracheal compression (Fig. 18–40). In this aberrancy the left pulmonary artery arises from the right pulmonary artery and passes between the trachea and esophagus to cross to the left.

Although most of these arch anomalies may be diagnosed by plain films and barium esophagography, the precise anatomy must frequently be inferred rather than precisely visualized. Ninety percent of these lesions are best approached through a left thoracotomy.[58] In the remaining 10 percent a right-sided thoracotomy is indicated. The condition in these patients may not always be predicted by standard imaging techniques, and there are outspoken proponents of angiography for evaluation of these anomalies. Noninvasive MRI provides accurate anatomic information in these patients.[59]

A study of a large series of 18 patients with congenital arch anomalies concluded that MRI is extremely accurate in evaluation of arch anomalies and that it can be used as a substitute for other techniques, including esophagram and angiography.[60] MRI can identify the position of the aortic arch and, with right arch, the presence or absence of mirror image branching. This is important, because a high percentage of children with mirror image branching have associated severe cardiac defects. MRI can also be used to demonstrate these defects.

In each of the arch anomalies and in the pulmonary sling, the transaxial plane provides optimal information. Coronal images may better demonstrate origins of the "strap" vessels but are not absolutely necessary to establish the diagnosis. The excellent soft tissue contrast provided by MRI permits visualization of the encircled (and usually compressed) trachea and esophagus.

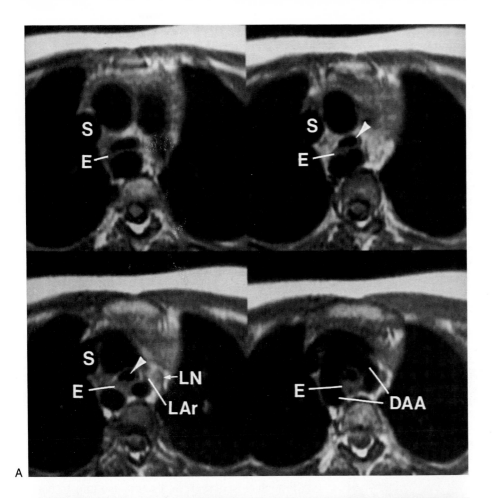

A

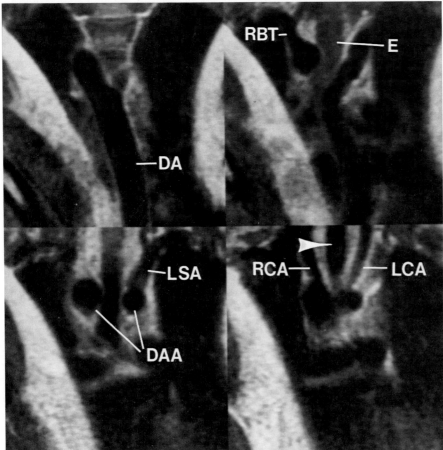

B

Figure 18–36. *Double aortic arch (DAA).* **A,** Serial transaxial images through the upper thorax. (DAA). Sections progress from caudal to cranial. **B,** Sequential coronal images in the same patient. *Arrowhead,* Trachea; DA, descending aorta; E, esophagus; LAr, ligamentum arteriosum; LN, lymph node; LCA, left common carotid artery; LSA, left subclavian artery; RBT, right brachiocephalic trunk; RCA, right common carotid artery; S, superior vena cava. (From Bisset GS III, Strife JL, Kirks DR, Bailey WW. Vascular rings: MR imaging. AJR 1987; 149:251–256.)

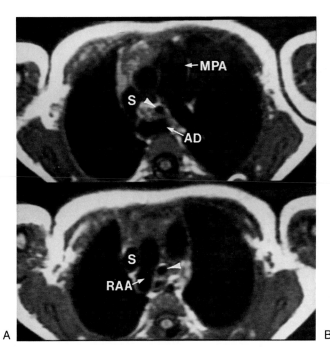
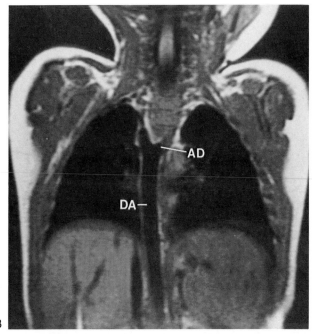

Figure 18–37. *Right aortic arch (RAA) and aberrant left subclavian artery.* ***A,*** Serial transaxial images through the upper thorax. This aberrant vessel arises from an aortic diverticulum (AD). Note the encirclement of the trachea (*arrowhead*). ***B,*** Coronal scan through the descending aorta (DA) shows the origin of the aortic diverticulum. MPA, Main pulmonary artery; S, superior vena cava. (From Bisset GS III, Strife JL, Kirks DR, Bailey WW. Vascular rings: MR imaging. AJR 1987; 149:251–256.)

Systemic venous anomalies of the thorax include infrahepatic interruption of the inferior vena cava with azygos continuation (Fig. 18–41), persistent left superior vena cava (Fig. 18–42), and congenital forms of ectasia (Fig. 18–43). In one study, MRI was excellent in identifying venous anomalies in nine patients;[61] in this study, three patients had persistent left superior vena cava. This was best shown in the transaxial images as a round signal void structure lying lateral to the aortic arch and main pulmonary artery and anterior to the left hilum. In patients with interruption of the inferior vena cava, the inferior vena cava is found to end in the abdomen, venous return is through the azygous venous system, and the azygous vein is significantly distended. This structure can be differentiated from a normal inferior vena cava in that it lies behind the right crus of the diaphragm. Occasionally the continuation may occur on the left side with drainage into the hemiazygous vein (e.g., in patients with polysplenia). With azygous continuation of the inferior vena cava the suprahepatic segment of the latter may still be patent. This segment may receive hepatic venous flow. As with the major arch anomalies, anatomy on MRI is generally best defined in the transaxial plane, although coronal planes may permit the abnormal vessel to be seen in its entirety. Information concerning aberrant systemic venous anatomy may be particularly important for planning surgical strategy in patients with more complicated associated forms of congenital heart disease.

Miscellaneous Congenital Lesions

The ability of MRI to display multiplanar anatomy makes it particularly useful for the evaluation of complex congenital heart lesions (Figs. 18–44, 18–45). Entities such as double outlet right ventricle, Ebstein's anomaly, single ventricle, dextrocardia, crisscross heart, polysplenia, and asplenia are sometimes difficult to evaluate completely with echocardiography and cineangiography.[64, 65] MRI may highlight key anatomic relationships that are vital to successful surgical palliation or correction.

Double Outlet Right Ventricle

Double outlet right ventricle is another conotruncal abnormality. Both the aorta and pulmonary artery arise completely or almost completely from the right ventricle. Surgical planning depends on accurate definition of the relationship of the ventricular septal defect to the great vessels. Aortic commitment of this defect allows internal repair by an intraventricular baffle. It is suggested that because of the multiplanar imaging capability, MRI may have a role to play in accurately defining the relationship of the great vessels to the ventricular septal defect.[62]

Ebstein's Anomaly

Ebstein's is a rare congenital anomaly of the tricuspid valve, characterized by varying degrees of downward displacement and dysplasia of the tricuspid

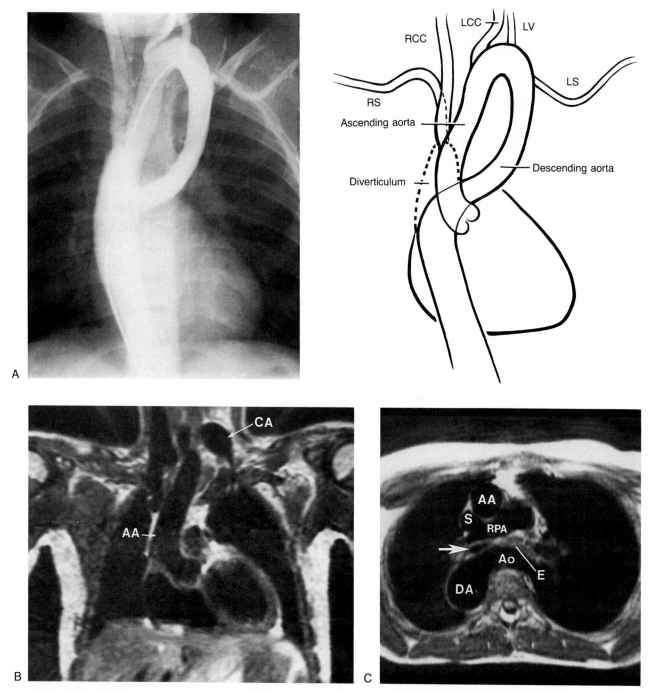

Figure 18–38. *Cervical aortic arch.* **A,** Aortic angiogram and diagrammatic representation of the anatomy in a patient with a cervical aortic arch; right common carotid artery (RCC), left common carotid artery (LCC), left subclavian artery (LS), right subclavian artery (RS), left vertebral artery (LV). **B,** Coronal image demonstrates elongation of the ascending aorta (AA). The cervical arch (CA) is identified in the left neck. **C,** Transaxial image through the retroesophageal component (Ao) of the descending aorta (DA). E, Esophagus; RPA, right pulmonary artery; S, superior vena cava; arrow, right mainstem bronchus. (From Bisset GS III, Strife JL, Kirks DR, Bailey WW. Vascular rings: MR imaging. AJR 1987; 149:251–256.)

valve, with resultant atrialization of a portion of the right ventricle and decreased pumping ability of the remainder of the right ventricle. The anterior leaflet of the tricuspid valve remains medially connected to the atrioventricular groove, while the lateral edge of this cusp is attached variably to the right ventricular wall.

The posterior and septal leaflets are attached to the right ventricular wall below the atrioventricular junction. In four patients with Ebstein's anomaly, MRI was able to identify accurately the markedly dilated right atrium, the thin-walled atrialized part of the right ventricle, and dilatation of the right ventricular infun-

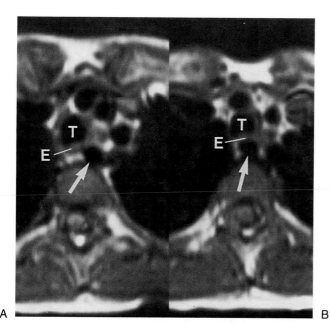

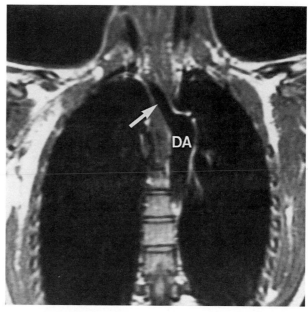

A   B

Figure 18–39. *Left aortic arch and aberrant right subclavian artery.* ***A,*** Sequential transaxial images through the upper thorax. Note the passage of the aberrant vessel (*arrow*) behind the esophagus (E) and trachea (T). ***B,*** Coronal image through the proximal descending aorta (DA). Note the origin of the aberrant right subclavian artery (*arrow*) and its retroesophageal passage. (From Bisset GS III. Pediatric thoracic applications of MRI. J Thorac Imaging 1989; 4(2):51–57.)

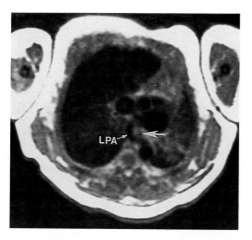

Figure 18–40. *Aberrant left pulmonary artery.* Transaxial image through the main pulmonary artery in a newborn with a pulmonary sling. Note the origin of the left pulmonary artery (LPA) passing posterior to the trachea (*large arrow*), resulting in severe tracheal compression. Also demonstrated is marked hyperinflation of the right lung and atelectasis of the left lung.

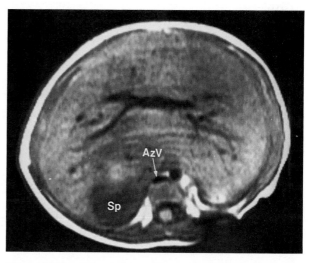

Figure 18–41. *Polysplenia syndrome.* Transaxial image through the liver in an infant with polysplenia and infrahepatic interruption of the inferior vena cava with azygos continuation. Note the midline position of the liver and the right-sided spleen (Sp). The azygos vein (AzV) is demonstrated as a focal area of signal void in the retrocrural region. (From Bissett GS III. Pediatric thoracic applications of MRI. J Thorac Imaging 1989; 4(2):51–57.)

dibulum.[63] The posterior and septal leaflets are generally dysplastic and not well visualized.

Pericardial Defects

Partial or complete absence of the pericardium is a rare congenital defect that may manifest clinically with angina-like pain. Although standard chest radiography may be diagnostic (shift of the heart into the left hemi-

thorax and prominence of the pulmonary artery shadow), further workup is indicated if surgical treatment is warranted. Diagnostic pneumothorax and cineangiography provide invasively acquired information. Generally, the pericardium is easily delineated as a low signal intensity "line" surrounding the heart (Fig. 18–46). High signal intensity epicardial fat or

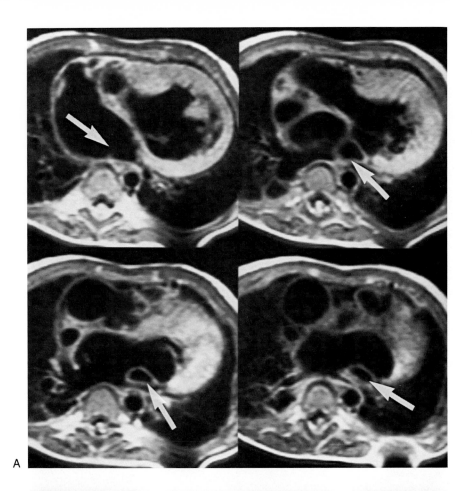

A

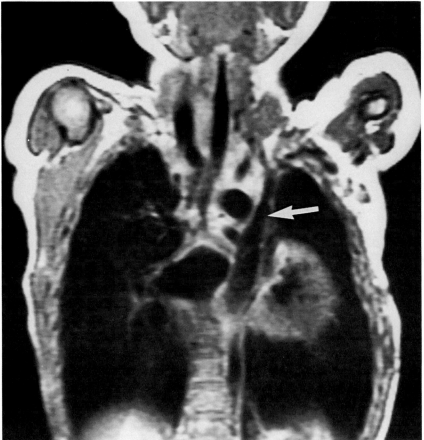

B

Figure 18–42. *Persistent left superior vena cava.* ***A,*** Sequential transaxial scans. The superior vena cava (*arrows*) joins the coronary sinus on the most inferior axial (first) scan. ***B,*** Coronal image in the same patient demonstrates the major portion of the persistent left superior vena cava (*arrow*). (From Bisset GS III. Pediatric thoracic applications of MRI. J Thorac Imaging 1989; 4(2):51–57.)

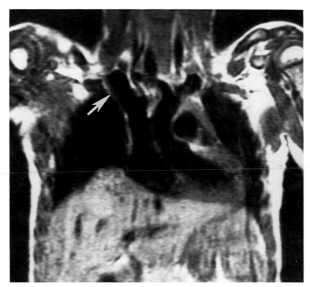

Figure 18–43. *Venous dilatation.* Coronal image through the superior vena cava in a child with a connective tissue disorder. There is moderate ectasia of the right upper superior vena cava (*arrow*). The dilatation extended into the right external jugular vein.

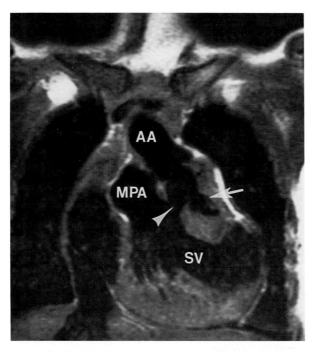

Figure 18–44. *Single ventricle and L-transposed great vessels.* Coronal image through the outflow tract. Note the communication (*arrowhead*) between the single ventricle (SV) and the rudimentary outflow tract chamber (*arrow*). AA, Ascending aorta; MPA, main pulmonary artery.

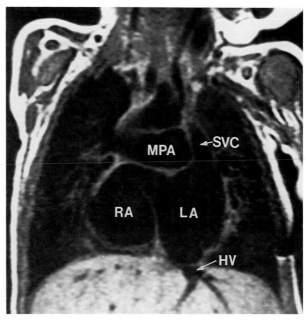

Figure 18–45. *Abnormal venous connections.* Coronal image in a patient with complex congenital heart disease. MRI was used to evaluate the systemic and pulmonary venous return patterns. The superior vena cava (SVC) returns to the left-sided atrium (LA). The inferior vena cava was absent, but the hepatic veins (HV) also emptied into the left-sided atrium. A large superior atrial septal defect is also noted. MPA, Main pulmonary artery; RA, right atrium.

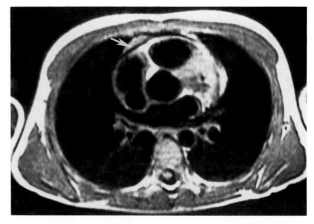

Figure 18–46. *Normal aortic root.* Transaxial image through the aortic root in a normal volunteer. The arrow indicates the normal low signal intensity pericardium, surrounded by epicardial fat centrally and mediastinal fat peripherally.

Postoperative Complications

MRI is particularly well suited for evaluation of the postoperative cardiac patient.[67] Metallic sternotomy wires, fibrosis around the sternotomy site, altered bony anatomy, and prosthetic valves and conduits may limit acoustic windows through which echocardiography may be performed. Although the sternotomy wires and prosthetic valves may create small ferromag-

intermediate signal intensity myocardium is demonstrated along the inner aspect of the pericardium, with mediastinal fat exterior to the pericardium. A focal disappearance of this "line" suggests partial pericardial absence (Figs. 18–47, 18–48).[66]

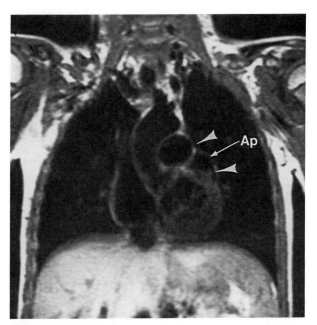

Figure 18–47. *Partial absence of left pericardium.* Coronal image through the left atrial appendage (Ap). Note the discontinuation of the normal low signal intensity pericardium (*arrowheads*) at the level of the left atrial appendage. In this patient with recurrent chest pain, operative intervention confirmed the diagnosis. (Figures 18–47 through 18–49 from Ross RD, Bissett GS III, Meyer RA, et al. Magnetic resonance imaging for diagnosis of pulmonary vein stenosis after "correction" of total anomalous pulmonary venous connection. Am J Cardiol 1987; 60:1199–1201.)

netic artifacts on MR images, they tend to be relatively unobtrusive. In many patients who have undergone previous surgery, the imaging questions relate to specific anatomic structures. MRI may provide the answers, obviating more invasive procedures.

Table 18–2 lists postoperative entities and frequent problems that are well evaluated by MRI. In each case the MR examination must be tailored to the questions asked. Evaluation of the aorta is best accomplished with visualization in the sagittal oblique plane. The pulmonary arteries, pulmonary veins, and pericardial space are best visualized in the transaxial plane. Occasionally, the coronal plane may be ideal for evaluation of extracardiac shunts or complicated intracardiac lesions (Figs. 18–49 to 18–56).

MRI has been fairly widely used for the evaluation of shunts in the thorax. Even at an early stage in technologic development, a report demonstrated shunts in 11 of 17 patients.[70]

Some fairly large studies have reported the use of MRI to evaluate patients after thoracic cardiovascular palliative surgery. In patients who have undergone Fontan procedures, MRI was able to assess the size of the right atrium and of the pulmonary arteries.[71] In patients in whom a conduit had been placed between the right atrium and the right pulmonary artery, MRI identified the entire conduit and was able to demonstrate thrombosis, if present, within it. Ultrasound penetrates the conduit wall poorly.

In patients who have undergone previous Rastelli procedures, the conduit from the right ventricle to the pulmonary artery lies behind the sternum and is also poorly assessed by echocardiography. MRI can identify fibrin deposition and any decrease in caliber of the conduit.[71] There are some difficulties with MR evaluation of surgically created vascular shunts.[72] In a series of 27 patients it was found that MRI was 100 percent accurate in differentiating patency from occlusion, but less accurate in identifying stenosis, particularly in

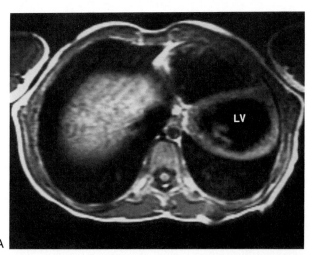

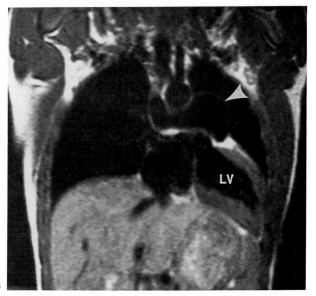

Figure 18–48. *Absent left pericardium.* ***A,*** Transaxial image. The heart is to the left of the normal position. No identifiable pericardial line is demonstrated around the left ventricle (LV). ***B,*** Coronal image in the same patient demonstrates a prominent pulmonary artery (*arrowhead*) and a left ventricular apex positioned at the left costophrenic sulcus. No pericardium is identified around the left ventricle or main pulmonary artery.

Table 18-2. POSTOPERATIVE COMPLICATIONS

Postoperative Conditions	Possible Problems
Coarctation (Figs. 18-60, 18-61)[67-69]	Residual stenosis? Aneurysm formation?
Blalock-Taussig shunt (subclavian artery–pulmonary artery) or Waterston shunt (ascending aorta–right pulmonary artery) (Fig. 18-62)[70]	Patency? Growth of pulmonary arteries? Size of anastomosis?
Pulmonary artery banding (Fig. 18-63)	Migration of band? Too tight?
Senning or Mustard procedure for D-TGV (Fig. 18-64)[67]	Pulmonary venous or systemic venous baffle obstruction? Patch disruption?
Rastelli conduit (right ventricle–pulmonary artery)	Anastomosis? Thrombus?
Glenn shunt (superior vena cava–pulmonary artery)	Anastomosis? Thrombus?
Fontan procedure (right atrium–pulmonary artery)	Flow? Thrombus?
TAPVR (Fig. 18-65)[49]	Pulmonary venous occlusive disease?
Prosthetic valve placement (Figs. 18-2, 18-66)[32]	Aneurysm or dissection? Stenosis?
Nonspecific (Fig. 18-67)	Pericardial effusion? Postoperative status?

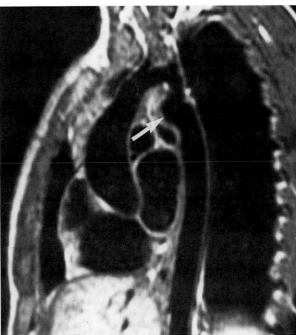

Figure 18-50. *Coarctation: post angioplasty.* Sagittal oblique image through the aortic arch in a patient who had previous balloon angioplasty of a discrete juxtaductal aortic coarctation. Note the aneurysmal dilatation at the angioplasty site (*arrow*). Also demonstrated is post-stenotic dilatation of the ascending aorta, secondary to valvar aortic stenosis. (From Bisset GS III. Pediatric thoracic applications of MRI. J Thorac Imaging, 1989; 4(2):51–57.)

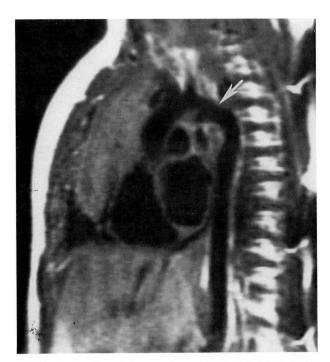

Figure 18-49. *Coarctation: post repair.* Sagittal oblique image through the aortic arch in a 1-year-old infant who had undergone subclavian flap aortoplasty for aortic coarctation. There is no residual stenosis at the repair site (*arrow*).

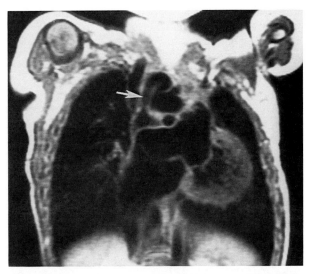

Figure 18-51. *Tricuspid atresia: patent shunt.* Coronal image. An intact Blalock-Taussig shunt (*arrow*) is identified between the right subclavian artery and right pulmonary artery. The presence of signal void indicates normal velocity flow.

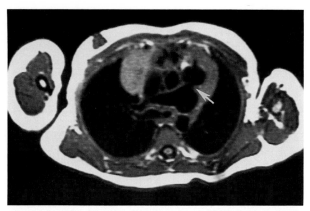

Figure 18–52. *Pulmonary artery band.* Transaxial image through the main pulmonary artery in an infant. Note the constriction (*arrow*) in the midportion of the main pulmonary artery at the site of the band.

small vessels. These authors caution that not all signal in the vessel represents occlusion or thrombus, but that bright signal may be noted with slow flow, even echo rephasing and diastole.[72]

MRI has been extensively evaluated for its ability to assess patients after corrective surgery for transposition of the great vessels. Two surgical procedures are used, both of which achieve physiologic correction. In the Mustard procedure a baffle is constructed from a trouser-shaped patch of pericardium, sewn into the atrial cavity after resection of the atrial septum. Within the lumen of the baffle, blood flows from the superior and inferior venae cavae through the mitral valve into the left ventricle. Pulmonary venous blood flows around the baffle, through the tricuspid valve, into the right ventricle. In the Senning procedure a similar type of redirection of blood flow is achieved by utilizing the atrial septum and part of the right atrial wall to form the baffle, rather than a pericardial patch. In one study of 15 patients, complete obstruction in two individuals was easily identified by MRI.[73] Direct visualization of partial narrowing was more difficult; secondary signs strongly suggestive of narrowing included an increase in the diameter of the superior vena cava and the azygos vein.[73] In another study of eight patients all under the age of 8 years who underwent Mustard procedures, MRI identified complete obstruction at the junction of the superior vena cava and right atrium in three children.[74] There was also an increase in size of the azygos vein in these patients. These findings were confirmed by angiography or surgery. This study utilized cine MRI and was able to identify atrioventricular valve regurgitation in five of the eight patients.[74] The ventricular outflow tracts and pulmonary veins were normal in all eight. Ejection fraction measured by the

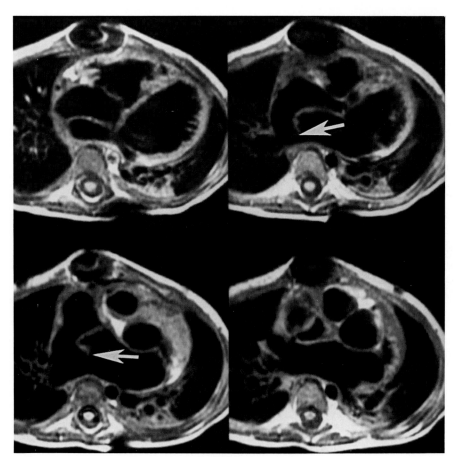

Figure 18–53. *D-transposition: post Senning procedure.* Serial transaxial images in a patient who underwent a Senning procedure for D-transposed great vessels. The more cephalad scans are on the bottom row. There is disruption of the intra-atrial baffle (*arrows*).

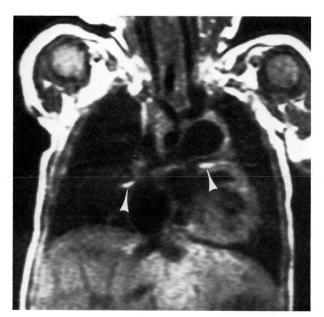

Figure 18–54. *Pulmonary vein stenosis.* Coronal image through the pulmonary veins in a patient who underwent repair of total anomalous pulmonary venous return. The presence of focal linear high signal intensity areas (*arrowheads*) suggests acquired pulmonary veno-occlusive disease. These high signal intensity areas represent small pulmonary veins with markedly diminished flow velocity. (From Ross RD, Bisset GS III, Meyer RA, et al. Magnetic resonance imaging for diagnosis of pulmonary vein stenosis after "correction" of total anomalous pulmonary venous connection. Am J Cardiol 1987; 60:1199–1201.)

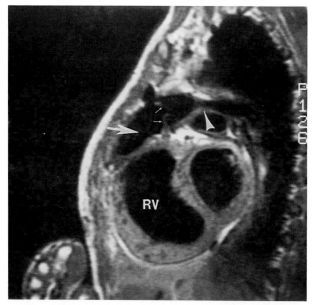

Figure 18–55. *Conduit with stenosed anastomosis.* Sagittal image through the right ventricular outflow tract in a child who underwent repair of tetralogy of Fallot. A porcine valved conduit (*large arrow*) is noted arising from the markedly thickened right ventricle (RV). Note the narrowing at the junction of the conduit with the left pulmonary artery (*arrowhead*). Thickened valve cusps (*small arrows*) are identified within the conduit.

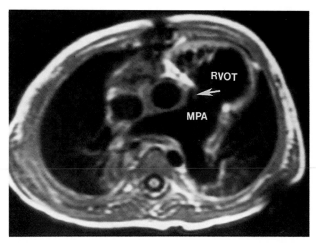

Figure 18–56. *Pulmonary valvectomy.* Transaxial image through the pulmonary outflow tract in an infant. Note the small nubbin of residual pulmonary valve tissue (*arrow*). There is marked dilatation of the right ventricular outflow tract (RVOT) and the proximal pulmonary arteries, secondary to gross pulmonary insufficiency. MPA, Main pulmonary artery.

cine MRI technique in four patients correlated well with measurements obtained at angiography.

Seventeen adult patients were studied 9 to 20 years after Mustard procedures with MRI, echocardiography, nuclear studies, and angiography.[75] Ejection fraction values with MRI were found to be higher than those obtained with nuclear studies. Long-term complications of the Mustard procedure are mainly those related to right heart failure and tricuspid regurgitation. In the evaluation of patients following Senning or Mustard procedures, it seems that a combination of MRI and echocardiography offers the best information.[73] In evaluating patients following the Mustard procedure, the sagittal plane is best for demonstrating pulmonary venous return, whereas the coronal plane is best for showing the superior venous channel and Mustard baffle.[71] The axial plane is best for defining the baffle in Senning procedure patients.

ACQUIRED DISORDERS

Acquired heart disease in the pediatric population represents a relatively small proportion of the cardiac disease spectrum. Unlike adults, children rarely experience "classic" ischemic disease related to arteriosclerotic disease, or cardiomyopathy related to drugs or alcohol. However, MRI may play a role in the evaluation of a select group of acquired pediatric cardiac diseases.

Valvar Insufficiency

Angiography and Doppler echocardiography are the modalities of choice for demonstration of valvular incompetence. Recently developed gradient-echo techniques, however, permit the demonstration of incompetence by MRI. With these techniques, normal blood in the cardiac chambers appears of bright signal intensity. In two series of adult patients, MRI was able to demonstrate valvular regurgitation in 49 in whom it was identified by either echocardiography or angiography.[76, 77] The regurgitation is identified as an area of low signal "jetting" back across the valve. Unfortunately, false-positive findings with MRI were as high as 25 percent, probably as a result of normal turbulence.[76]

Infectious and Inflammatory Diseases

In the infectious forms of pericarditis, myocarditis, and endocarditis, MRI is of limited benefit. In these acquired lesions, clinical examination is directed toward assessing the amount of pericardial fluid, the quality of myocardial function, and the presence and size of valvular vegetations. Echocardiography is an ideal means of acquiring the necessary data.

Some inflammatory circumstances may support a role for MRI. If there is a clinical suspicion of loculated effusion, MRI may provide accurate localization (Fig. 18–57).[78] The regions of pericardium adjacent to the lungs are often difficult to evaluate with echocardiography. Additionally, MRI may be able to separate high signal intensity blood from nonhemorrhagic effusions. In chronic constrictive pericardial disease, MRI may provide ancillary information. The demonstration of a thickened and low signal intensity pericardium, small ventricular chambers, prominent atria, and the appropriate clinical picture confirms the diagnosis.

In the absence of cine MRI, myocardial function and valvular lesions are difficult to evaluate. The spatial resolution limitations and valve motion currently do not permit identification of valvular vegetations.

One inflammatory condition in which MRI may play an increasing role is Kawasaki's disease.[79] This multisystem inflammatory process characteristically affects infants and young children. The major morbidity and mortality in this disease is related to the formation of coronary artery aneurysms. Although two-dimensional echocardiography is the primary screening modality for detection of aneurysms, MRI may provide information in patients in whom echocardiography is not technically feasible or not diagnostic. MRI may also detect other intrathoracic aneurysms not suspected by echocardiography (Fig. 18–58). In this disease and in other lesions involving the coronary arteries, maximal MR information has been obtained in the axial, coronal, and axial oblique (through the short axis of the left ventricular outflow tract) planes, using 3-mm thick slices with 0.5-mm interslice gaps (Figs. 18–59 to 18–61).

Cardiomyopathy

Cardiomyopathies include disorders affecting primarily the cardiac muscle. The disorder may be idiopathic, infectious, ischemic (e.g., anomalous origin of the left coronary artery), or metabolic (e.g., glycogen storage disease type II) in origin. Evaluation of cardiomyopathy in children focuses on excluding such correctable conditions as anomalous left coronary artery, hypoxemia, and anemia. Also, myocardial functional assessment is important in determining therapy and prognosis. Although this evaluation may be accomplished by echocardiography, MRI may play a role in selected cases. In patients with congestive or dilated cardiomyopathy, MRI may be used for cine assessment of myocardial function.

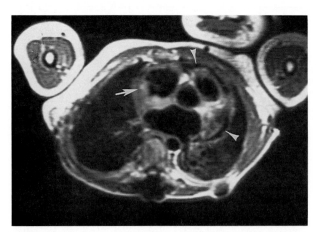

Figure 18–57. *Pericardial effusion.* Transaxial image through the heart in a patient with a small pericardial effusion (*arrowheads*). A thrombus extends from the tip of a central venous catheter positioned in the superior vena cava (*arrow*).

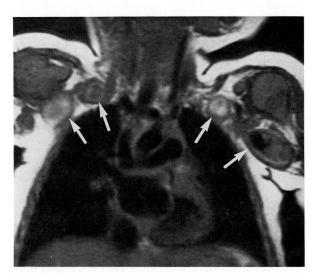

Figure 18–58. *Kawasaki's disease.* Coronal image through the upper thorax in a 6-month-old infant. Note the multiple axillary and subclavian artery aneurysms (*arrows*). (From Bisset GS III. Pediatric thoracic applications of MRI. J Thorac Imaging 1989; 4(2):51–57.)

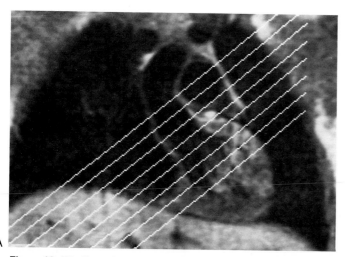

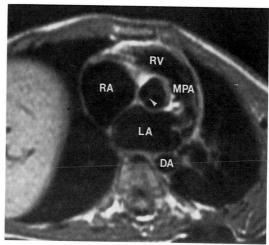

Figure 18–59. *Normal oblique imaging.* **A,** Technique for obtaining axial oblique scans. After initial coronal images are taken, electronically angled scans are obtained perpendicular to the axis of the left ventricular outflow tract. **B,** Corresponding axial oblique image demonstrating normal anatomy. Aortic valve cusps (*arrowhead*); DA, descending aorta; LA, left atrium; MPA, main pulmonary artery; RA, right atrium; RV, right ventricle.

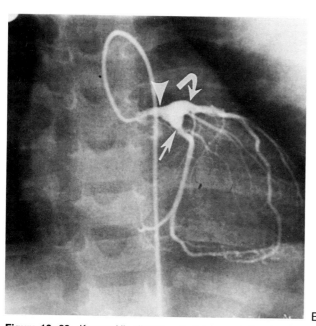

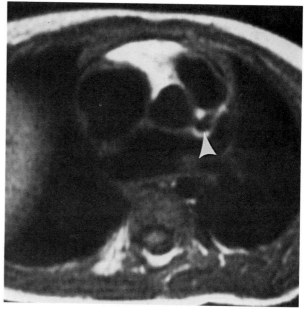

Figure 18–60. *Kawasaki's diease.* **A,** Anteroposterior view of left coronary artery angiogram. An aneurysm is seen extending from just distal to the origin of the left main coronary artery (*arrowhead*) to the origins of the left anterior descending branch (*curved arrow*) and circumflex branch (*straight arrow*). **B,** Axial oblique image through the aortic root shows an aneurysm of the proximal left coronary artery and proximal left anterior descending branch (*arrowhead*). (From Bisset GS III, Strife JL, McCloskey J. Magnetic resonance imaging of coronary artery aneurysms in children with Kawasaki's disease. AJR 1989; 152:805–807.)

Hypertrophic Cardiomyopathy

Patients with hypertrophic cardiomyopathy are also readily assessed by echocardiography. The thickened ventricular wall and septal hypertrophy are well demonstrated. MRI may be useful, however, when there is diagnostic confusion or when quantitative information concerning myocardial function is sought. Cine MRI has been of particular benefit in this role, demonstrat-

ing complete systolic obliteration of the left ventricular cavity in some cases (Fig. 18–62).

Restrictive Cardiomyopathy

MRI may provide unique information in patients with restrictive cardiomyopathy. In this particular entity, ventricular compliance is decreased, resulting in dilatation of the atria (Fig. 18–63). Unfortunately, it

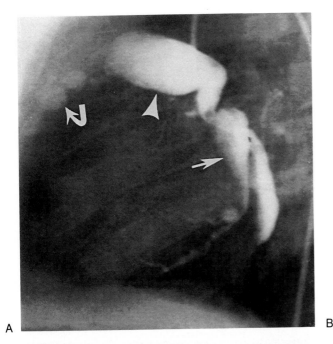

A

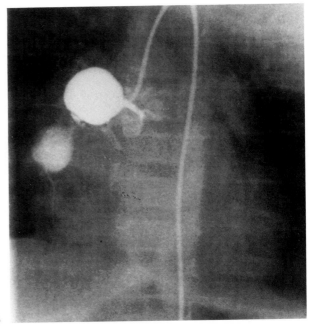

B

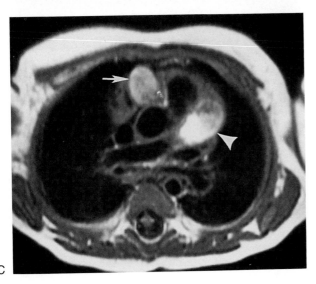

C

Figure 18–61. *Kawasaki's disease.* **A,** Lateral view of a left coronary artery angiogram in a 7-month-old infant shows large aneurysms in the left main coronary artery (*arrowhead*), left anterior descending branch (*curved arrow*), and circumflex branch (*straight arrow*). **B,** Anteroposterior view of a right coronary artery angiogram demonstrates giant aneurysms of the proximal right coronary artery. **C,** Axial scan through the aortic root performed 3 weeks after the angiogram demonstrates thrombus and/or slow flow in the proximal left (*arrowhead*) and right (*arrow*) aneurysms. (From Bisset GS III, Strife JL, McCloskey J. Magnetic resonance imaging of coronary artery aneurysms in children with Kawasaki's disease. AJR 1989; 152:805–807.)

may be extremely difficult to differentiate between restrictive myocardial disease and constrictive pericardial disease;[80] in both lesions there is ventricular inflow obstruction. MRI has been very useful in distinguishing between the two entities. As noted earlier, the thickened, low signal intensity pericardium in constrictive pericarditis may be distinguished from a normal (<3 mm thickness) pericardial sac. This may be the only clue in differentiating between the two diseases, which behave clinically and angiographically in identical fashions. Even pressure data acquired by catheterization may not be diagnostic. As with other myocardial or pericardial diseases, transaxial scans provide

maximal information. Cine-acquired short and long axis views of the ventricles may be used to evaluate function.

Metabolic Disorders

Glycogen storage disease type II results in the accumulation of glycogen in the myocardium. There is marked ventricular hypertrophy, which may cause outflow tract obstruction. The ventricular septum is also enlarged. MRI in one patient demonstrated diffuse ventricular hypertrophy with a resultant decrease in ventricular lumen size.[81] The signal intensity from the myocardium was very irregular and nonhomogeneous.

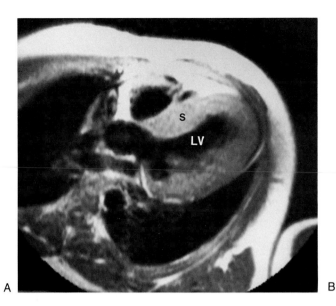

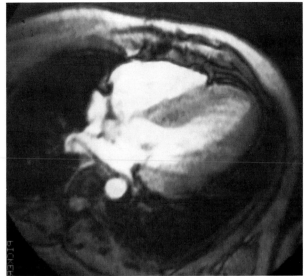

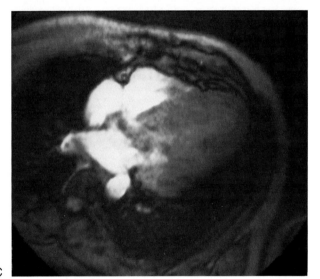

Figure 18–62. *Hypertrophic cardiomyopathy.* ***A,*** Spin-echo long axis oblique view through the left ventricle (LV). Note the markedly thickened left ventricular free wall and septum (S). ***B,*** End-diastolic gradient-echo acquisition image in the same patient demonstrates high signal intensity blood flow within the left ventricular cavity. ***C,*** During systole, there is complete obliteration of the left ventricular cavity, typical of hypertrophic cardiomyopathy. (Courtesy of Dr. Kerry Link, Winston-Salem, NC)

Intracardiac and Paracardiac Masses

Intracardiac and paracardiac masses in the pediatric population include thrombus (Fig. 18–64), pericardial cyst, bronchopulmonary foregut malformation (Fig. 18–65), atrial myxoma, rhabdomyoma (Fig. 18–66), fibroma (Fig. 18–67), lymphoma (Fig. 18–68), teratoma, and metastatic foci. Echocardiography is generally used as the primary screening tool in patients with suspected masses. If a mass is suggested, MRI may be crucial in characterizing its location and extent, as well as in defining the relationship of the paracardiac mass to the pericardium, myocardium, and adjacent mediastinal vessels.[82] This information may be of vital importance in operative planning.

MRI may provide tissue characterization in some cases, although it is often difficult to distinguish benign from malignant disease. Lipomas, thrombi, and mucinous cysts may show typical high signal intensity on T1 weighted sequences. Intermediate signal intensity lymph nodes may not change on T2 weighted sequences, while cystic masses become high in signal intensity.

Tumors in or around the heart are relatively rare. Primary tumors include rhabdomyoma, rhabdomyosarcoma, and angiosarcoma. Direct cardiac invasion may occur from adjacent mediastinal tumors, particularly lymphoma.[83] Patients with tuberous sclerosis show an increased incidence of cardiac rhabdomyomas. Both MRI and ultrasonography are effective means of demonstrating these cardiac tumors. In one

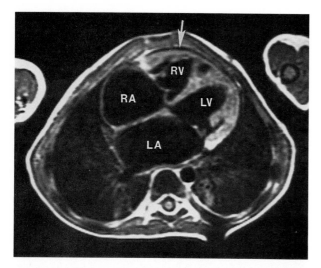

Figure 18–63. *Restrictive cardiomyopathy.* Transaxial image. Note the normal size of the right (RV) and left (LV) ventricular chambers. There is marked dilatation of the right (RA) and left (LA) atria. The normal thickness of the pericardium (*arrow*) differentiates this lesion from constrictive pericardial disease.

series of 14 patients with tumors, MRI was found to be particularly helpful in patients in whom the echocardiographic study was equivocal.[83] Ultrasonography appears superior to MRI in defining the mobility of a tumor mass lying within a cardiac chamber. Patients with tuberous sclerosis and cardiac rhabdomyomas may present initially with cardiac arrhythmia. In these patients, diagnosis of the tumor is sometimes delayed. It is possible that in the future MRI may have a definite role in early diagnosis of these lesions. With regard to signal characteristics, tumors generally become brighter on T2 weighted sequences (Fig. 18–66), but, as noted earlier, a specific histologic picture may not be predicted.

VASCULAR DISORDERS

The inherent natural contrast between flowing blood and vessel walls makes MRI an ideal modality for evaluation of the vascular system. With conventional

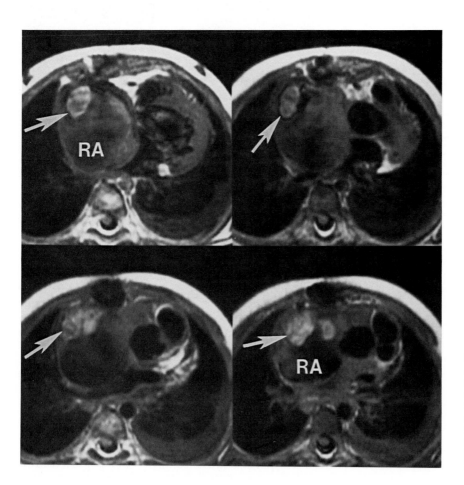

Figure 18–64. *Tricuspid atresia: post Fontan procedure.* Sequential transaxial images. In this procedure the right atrium (RA) is anastomosed directly to the main pulmonary artery. Two months after surgery the patient developed a thrombus (*arrow*) along the anterior wall of the right atrium. Slow blood flow is identified as diffusely increased signal intensity within the right atrium.

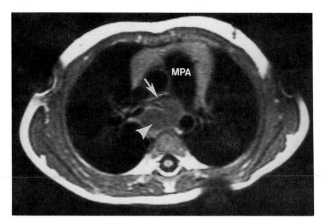

Figure 18–65. *Bronchogenic cyst.* Transaxial scan through the main pulmonary artery (MPA) in an infant. The cyst (*arrowhead*) causes moderate compression of the right pulmonary artery (*arrow*).

spin-echo imaging, rapidly moving blood creates signal void. As the flow diminishes in velocity, the signal intensity increases in a nonlinear fashion. Stationary blood (thrombus) is usually relatively high in signal intensity because of increased proton density and relatively high concentrations of free methemoglobin (Fig. 18–64).

With the advent of gradient-recalled echo techniques (fast scanning), flowing blood is depicted with bright signal, producing an "angiographic effect." The vast array of blood flow phenomena and their inherent complexities are beyond the scope of this chapter and are discussed in the chapters on Basic Physics.

MRI should provide a noninvasive imaging tool that will be extremely useful in imaging the vascular system. The potential to avoid the need for angiography in many patients has already become apparent.

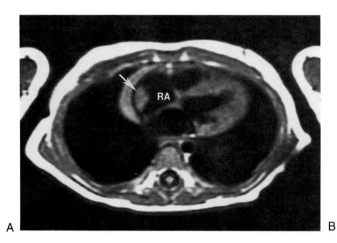

A

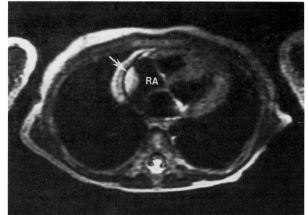

B

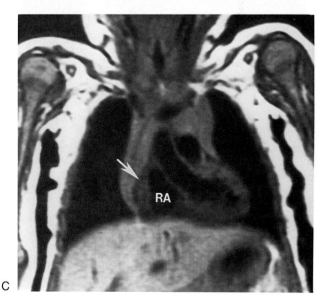

C

Figure 18–66. *Tuberous sclerosis.* **A,** Transaxial image through the heart in a newborn. An intracardiac rhabdomyoma (*arrow*) is identified along the lateral wall of the right atrium (RA). **B,** On a T2 weighted axial scan (SE 1800/80) the tumor (*arrow*) demonstrates high signal intensity. **C,** A coronal scan through the right atrium demonstrates the "layering" of the tumor (*arrow*) along the lateral wall of the right atrium.

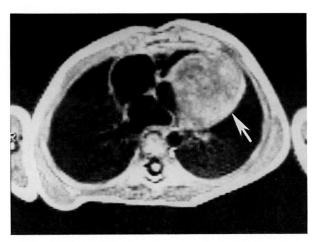

Figure 18–67. *Cardiac fibroma.* Transaxial image from a child with a large fibroma (*arrow*) arising from the outflow tract septum. The tumor almost completely obliterates the outflow tract. (From Higgins CB. The heart: congenital disease. In Higgins CB, Hvicak H, eds. Magnetic resonance imaging of the body. New York: Raven Press, 1987:267–294.)

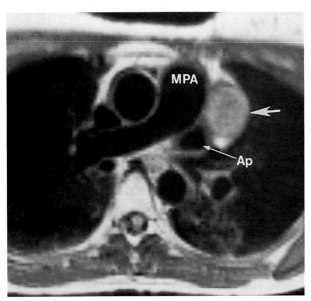

Figure 18–68. *Lymphoma.* Transaxial image through the main pulmonary artery (MPA) in a patient with a lymphomatous mass (*arrow*). The mass abuts, but does not invade, the main pulmonary artery or left atrial appendage (Ap). (Courtesy of Dr. Charles Gooding, San Francisco, CA.)

MR examination of the vascular system, just as in the heart, must be tailored to each patient. Intrathoracic vessels are best evaluated with ECG gating, using a TE of 20 msec. In the extremities and abdomen, larger areas may be covered with fewer attendant artifacts using a TR of 600 msec and a TE of 20 msec. As in the thorax, spatial slab presaturation pulses are used to diminish flow-related artifacts in the imaging plane. If questions arise concerning differentiation of slow blood flow from thrombus, gradient-recalled echo images are obtained using a TE of 12 msec, a TR of 22 msec, and a flip angle of 30 degrees. In the abdomen and pelvis, these images are obtained during breath holding. Thrombus results in low signal intensity on this pulse sequence. An alternative technique for distinguishing between slow flow and thrombus involves obtaining first and second echoes at evenly spaced time periods (i.e., TEs of 30 and 60 msec). Slow flow is subject to the phenomenon of even-echo rephasing, resulting in increased signal in the vessel containing any flow.[84, 85]

MRI has multiple applications in the vascular system, several of which have already been discussed. In general, the transaxial plane provides optimal information, resulting in the fewest artifacts, least partial volume averaging, and most accurate cross-sectional vessel lumen diameters. In the thoracic aorta, electronic angling of the imaging plane may be used to achieve sagittal oblique images of the aortic arch. This is an ideal view for evaluating thoracic aortic aneurysms or dissections. Occasionally, direct sagittal and coronal views may be used to follow the course of a large intrathoracic or intra-abdominal vessel.

Marfan's Syndrome

Marfan's syndrome affects many different areas of the body. Involvement of the cardiovascular system (in particular, aneurysmal dilatation of the aortic root) is the most important factor causing death in these patients. Early surgical intervention may improve long-term survival. It is for this reason that patients with Marfan's syndrome need long-term follow-up evaluation of the aortic root.[86] Echocardiography has been used to evaluate and follow the aortic root size. Limitations may arise, however, because of small acoustic windows (in patients with pectus excavatum or pectus carinatum) and because of an inability to evaluate the remainder of the aorta for aneurysm or dissection. MRI performed in the transaxial and sagittal oblique planes through the aortic root and arch, respectively, provides accurate measurements of the aorta and allows assessment for aneurysmal dilatation or intimal flaps (Fig. 18–69). Sequential studies may be used to follow the thoracic aortic diameter in patients at risk.

Measurements of the transverse diameter of the aortic root, obtained with MRI, correlate extremely well with those obtained with either echocardiography or computed tomography (CT).[86, 87] The pattern of dilatation of the aortic root in Marfan's syndrome differs from that seen when aortic dilatation is caused by other disorders. If the ratio of the transverse diameter of the aorta measured at the sinus of Valsalva and 2 cm proximal to the midaortic arch is greater than 1.4:1, the diagnosis of Marfan's syndrome is virtually assured.[88]

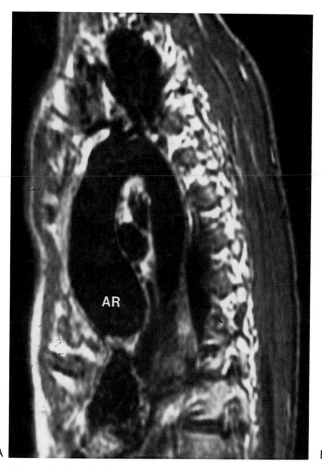

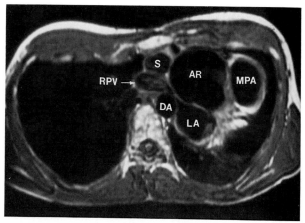

A B

Figure 18–69. *Marfan's syndrome.* ***A,*** Sagittal oblique image through the aortic arch in an adolescent. There is moderate dilatation of the aortic root and the patient has a pectus excavatum. ***B,*** Transaxial image through the aortic root in another patient with Marfan's syndrome. Again noted is marked dilatation of the aorta at the level of the sinuses of Valsalva, associated with a moderately severe pectus excavatum. The heart is displaced into the left hemithorax because of the chest wall deformity. AR, Aortic root; DA, descending aorta; LA, left atrium; MPA, main pulmonary artery; RPV, right pulmonary vein; S, superior vena cava. (From Bissett GS III. Pediatric thoracic applications of MRI. J Thorac Imaging 1989; 4(2):51–57.)

Aortic Aneurysm and Dissection

The greatest potential for MRI in vascular disease may be in evaluating the thoracic aorta for aneurysms or dissections.[89] In the pediatric population these entities are relatively rare, but certain disease states may predispose to the development of aortic disease, including Marfan's syndrome, cystic medial necrosis, Ehlers-Danlos syndrome, relapsing polychondritis, connective tissue disease, coarctation of the aorta, and post-traumatic conditions.

Angiography has been considered the "gold standard" for evaluation of aortic dissection, but it has several limitations. During angiographic evaluation, only the patent lumen (true or false) containing blood flow is visualized with contrast material.[12] Sometimes the intimal flap is visualized. MRI, unlike angiography, does not suffer from the necessity to have flow

present in order to demonstrate a lumen. Therefore, the extent of the intimal flap, flow in the true or false lumen, the relationship of the flap to the strap vessels, and the effect of the dissection on adjacent structures may be assessed. With the use of two perpendicular planes (transaxial and sagittal oblique), the origin and extent of the intimal flap may be accurately evaluated, thus permitting important decisions in patient management (Figs. 18–70, 18–71).

One of the pitfalls in the assessment of aortic dissections results from basing diagnostic decisions solely on signal intensity changes within the aortic lumen. Focal areas of increased signal intensity do not necessarily implicate slow flow or thrombus (Fig. 18–72). With the use of cardiac gating, such phenomena as entry slice enhancement, imaging point in time during the cardiac cycle, and direction of flow play complex roles in determining signal intensity. A second pitfall may result

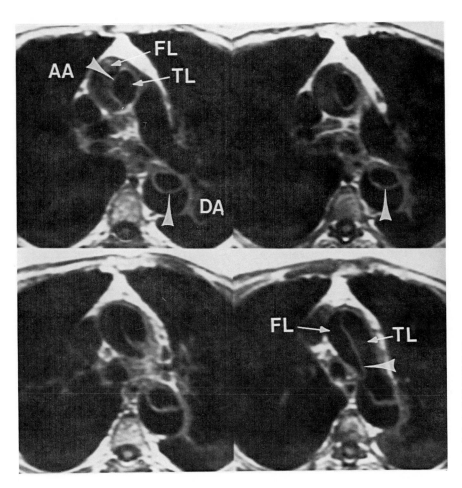

Figure 18–70. *Dissecting aortic aneurysm.* Sequential transaxial images through the aortic arch in a patient with a DeBakey type I aortic dissection. The intimal flap (*arrowheads*) originates in the ascending aorta (AA) and is seen well into the descending aorta (DA). At the level of the aortic arch, there is relatively normal velocity flow in both the true (TL) and false (FL) lumen. (Courtesy of Dr. Jon Moulton, Cincinnati.)

from incorrect interpretation of the superior pericardial recess (which contains signal void) as a false lumen at the level of the aortic root. This results in misdiagnosing a DeBakey I or II type dissection.

Sinus of Valsalva aneurysms represent focal dilatations of the right or posterior aortic root sinuses. These may be associated with Marfan's syndrome or may be isolated anomalies. Prolapse and progressive dilatation of the sinus and possible development of aortic insufficiency may result from diminished aortic valve support in patients with subpulmonic ventricular septal defects. In each of these entities, the finding of aneurysmal dilatation of the sinus of Valsalva is best demonstrated on transaxial views (Fig. 18–73). Ectasia of the ascending aorta (which may also be associated with this lesion) is best seen on sagittal oblique (left anterior oblique equivalent) scans. Occasionally, these may be difficult to distinguish from para-aortic abscesses by MRI (Fig. 18–74), but the clinical presentations are vastly different.[90]

Abdominal Aortic Disease

The abdominal aorta also is quite amenable to MR imaging. In the pediatric population, dissections in this vessel are extremely rare, but areas of focal or diffuse narrowing associated with Williams' syndrome or neurofibromatosis may be imaged. In these patients, sagittal localizing scans are obtained (ECG gating is not required), followed by electronically angled images in the coronal oblique plane. The entire abdominal aorta may be imaged on two or three 3-mm slices. As with other vascular applications, spatial slab presaturation pulses are used to diminish flow-related artifacts.

Although experience is limited at this time, MRI may be a useful technique for mapping peripheral arteriovenous malformations (Fig. 18–13). Although angiography is necessary to assess the detailed anatomic relationships and for embolization therapy, MRI may be used to follow the response of the malformation to therapy.

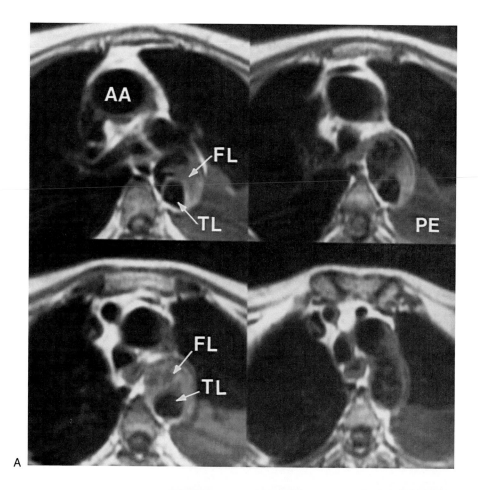

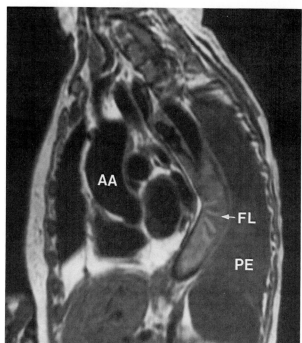

Figure 18–71. *Dissecting aortic aneurysm.* **A,** Sequential transaxial images through the aortic arch in a patient with DeBakey type III dissection. Note the signal void within the true lumen, indicating normal velocity flow (TL). The false lumen (FL) demonstrates higher signal intensity, indicating slow flow or thrombus. Note the normal ascending aorta (AA), indicating that the dissection has not extended into this portion of the aorta. **B,** Sagittal oblique lumen in the same patient showing the slightly dilated but otherwise normal ascending aorta, and the extensive thrombus in the false lumen of the aortic dissection. Incidental note is made of a large left pleural effusion (PE). (Courtesy of Dr. Jon Moulton, Cincinnati.)

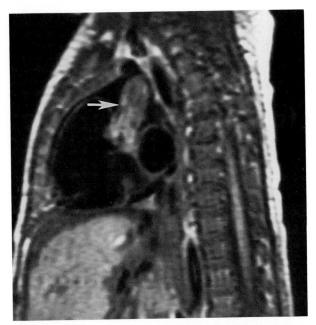

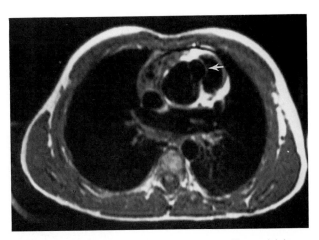

Figure 18–73. *Sinus of Valsalva aneurysm. Transaxial image through the aortic root.* The aneurysm (*arrow*) bulges into the right ventricular outflow tract.

Figure 18–72. *Normal aorta.* Sagittal view through the ascending aorta in a patient with a normal ascending aorta. This image was obtained 25 msec after the onset of the R wave of the ECG. Because flow has not had time to accelerate in the ascending aorta, there is abnormal signal intensity (*arrow*), which may mimic aortic slow flow or thrombus.

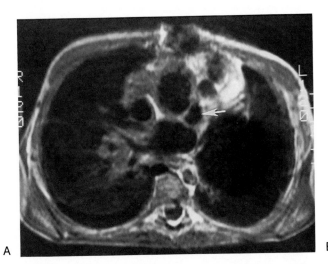

A

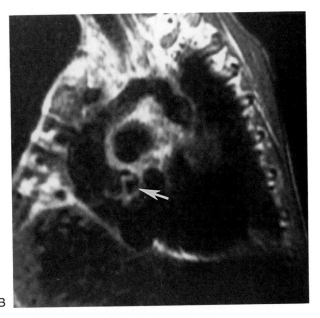

B

Figure 18–74. *Infected prosthetic valve.* **A,** Transaxial image through the aortic root in a patient with a bioprosthetic aortic valve. The arrow denotes a para-aortic abscess. **B,** Sagittal oblique view through the aortic arch. The arrow again shows the small para-aortic abscess adjacent to the bioprostheic valve. On both views this lesion may simulate a sinus of Valsalva aneurysm, but this patient was extremely ill. The large signal void in the left posterior paracardiac region originates from embolization coils in an apico-aortic conduit.

REFERENCES

1. Didier D, Higgins CB, Fisher MR, et al. Gated magnetic resonance imaging in congenital heart disease: experience in initial 72 patients. Radiology 1986; 158:227–235.
2. Miller SW, Brady TJ, Dinsmore RE, et al. Cardiac magnetic resonance imaging: the Massachusetts General Hospital experience. Radiol Clin North Am 1985; 23:745–764.
3. Fletcher BD, Jacobstein MD, Nelson AD, et al. Gated magnetic resonance imaging of congenital cardiac malformations. Radiology 1984; 150:137–140.
4. Higgins CB. Overview of MR of the heart—1986. AJR 1986; 146:907–918.
5. Higgins CB, Byrd BF II, McNamara MT, et al. Magnetic resonance imaging of the heart: a review of the experience in 172 subjects. Radiology 1985; 155:671–679.
6. Boxer RA, Singh S, LaCorte MA, et al. Cardiac magnetic resonance imaging in children with congenital heart disease. J Pediatr 1986; 109:460–464.
7. Council on Scientific Affairs, Report of the Magnetic Resonance Imaging Panel. Magnetic resonance imaging of the cardiovascular system. Present state of the art and future potential. JAMA 1988; 259:253–259.
8. Bank ER, Hernandez RJ. CT and MR of congenital heart disease. Radiol Clin North Am 1988; 26:241–260.
9. Reed JD, Soulen RL. Cardiovascular MRI: current role in patient management. Radiol Clin North Am 1988; 26:589–604.
10. Bisset GS III. Magnetic resonance imaging in pediatrics. Clear Images 1987; 1:6–17.
11. Strain JD, Campbell JB, Harvey LA, Foley LC. IV Nembutal: safe sedation for children undergoing CT. AJNR 1988; 9: 955–959.
12. Felmlee JP, Ehman RL. Spatial presaturation: a method for suppressing flow artifacts and improving depiction of vascular anatomy in MR imaging. Radiology 1987; 164:559–564.
13. Murphy WA, Gutierrez FR, Levitt RG, et al. Oblique views of the heart by magnetic resonance imaging. Radiology 1985; 154:225–226.
14. Dinsmore RE, Wismer GL, Levine RA, et al. Magnetic resonance imaging of the heart: positioning and gradient angle selection for optimal imaging planes. AJR 1984; 143:1135–1142.
15. Fisher MR, von Schulthess GK, Higgins CB. Multiphasic gated magnetic resonance imaging: normal regional left ventricular wall thickening. AJR 1985; 145:27–40.
16. Higgins CB. The heart: congenital disease. In: Higgins CB, Hricak H, eds. Magnetic resonance imaging of the body. New York: Raven Press, 1987:267–294.
17. Sechtem U, Pflugfelder PW, White RD, et al. Cine MR imaging: potential for the evaluation of cardiovascular function. AJR 1987; 148:239–246.
18. Utz JA, Herfkens RJ, Heinsimer JA, et al. Cine MR determination of left ventricular ejection fractionating the interventricular communication. AJR 1987; 148:839–843.
19. Edelman RR, Thompson R, Kantor H, et al. Cardiac function: evaluation with fast-echo MR imaging. Radiology 1987; 162:611–615.
20. Laschinger JC, Vannier MW, Gronemeyer S, et al. Noninvasive three-dimensional reconstruction of the heart and great vessels by ECG-gated magnetic resonance imaging: a new diagnostic modality. Ann Thorac Surg 1988; 45:505–514.
21. Rzedzian RR, Pykett IL. Instant images of the human heart using a new, whole-body MR imaging system. AJR 1987; 149:245–250.
22. Stehling MK, Ordidge RJ, Coxon R, et al. Cinematic imaging in a single heart cycle with echo planar imaging: technique and application. Radiology 1988; 169:377.
23. Atkinson DJ, Edelman RR. Ultrafast MR imaging of the heart. Radiology 1988; 169:37.
24. Bottomley PA. Noninvasive study of high energy phosphate metabolism in human heart by depth-resolved P-31 NMR spectroscopy. Science 1985; 229:769–772.
25. Bottomley PA, Herfkens RJ, Smith LS, Bushore TM. Altered phosphate metabolism in myocardial infarction: P-31 MR spectorscopy. Radiology 1987; 165:703–707.
26. Pavlicek W, Geisinger M, Castle L, et al. The effects of nuclear magnetic resonance on patients with cardiac pacemakers. Radiology 1983; 147:149–153.
27. Erlebacher JA, Cahill PT, Pannizzo F, Knowles RJ. Effect of magnetic resonance imaging on DDD pacemakers. Am J Cardiol 1986; 57:437–440.
28. Fetter J, Aram G, Holmes DR Jr, et al. The effects of nuclear magnetic resonance imagers on external and implantable pulse generators. PACE 1984; 7:720–727.
29. Dujovny M, Kossovsky N, Kossowsky R, et al. Aneurysm clip motion during magnetic resonance imaging: in vivo experimental study with metallurgical factor analysis. Neurosurgery 1985; 17:543–548.
30. New PFJ, Rosen BR, Brady TJ, et al. Potential hazards and artifacts of ferromagnetic and nonferromagnetic surgical and dental devices in nuclear magnetic resonance imaging. Radiology 1983; 147:139–148.
31. Barrafato D, Henkelman RM. Magnetic resonance imaging and surgical clips. Can J Surg 1984; 27:509–512.
32. Soulen RL, Budinger TF, Higgins CB. Magnetic resonance imaging of prosthetic heart valves. Radiology 1985; 154:705–707.
33. Shellock FG. MR imaging of metallic implants and materials: a compilation of the literature. AJR 1988; 151:811–814.
34. Dinsmore RE, Wismer GL, Guyer D, et al. Magnetic resonance imaging of the interatrial septum and atrial septal defects. AJR 1985; 145:697–703.
35. Diethelm L, Dery R, Lipton MJ, Higgins CB. Atrial-level shunts: sensitivity and specificity of MR in diagnosis. Radiology 1987; 162:181–186.
36. Hatle L, Angelsen B. Doppler ultrasound in cardiology, 2nd ed. Philadelphia: Lea & Febiger, 1985.
37. von Schulthess GK, Fisher MR, Higgins CB. Pathologic blood flow in pulmonary vascular disease as shown by gated magnetic resonance imaging. Ann Intern Med 1985; 103:317–323.
38. Bouchard A, Higgins CB, Byrd BF III, et al. Magnetic resonance imaging in pulmonary arterial hypertension. Am J Cardiol 1985; 103:317–323.
39. Didier D, Higgins CB. Identification and localization of ventricular septal defects by gated magnetic resonance imaging. Am J Cardiol 1986; 57:1363–1368.
40. Lowell DG, Turner DH, Smith SM, et al. The detection of atrial and ventricular septal defects with ECG synchronized magnetic resonance imaging. Circulation 1986; 73:89–94.
41. Sechtem U, Pflugfelder P, Cassidy MC, et al. Ventricular septal defect: visualization of shunt flow and determination of shunt size by cine MR imaging. AJR 1987; 149:689–692.
42. Stevenson JG, Kawabori I, Dooley T, et al. Diagnosis of ventricular septal defect by pulsed Doppler echocardiography—sensitivity, specificity, and limitations. Circulation 1978; 58: 322–326.
43. Jacobstein M, Fletcher B, Goldstein S, Riemenschneider T. Evaluation of atrioventricular septal defect by magnetic resonance imaging. Am J Cardiol 1985; 55:1158–1161.
44. Cohen JM, Weinreb JC, Redman GC. Arteriovenous malformations of the extremities: MR imaging. Radiology 1986; 158: 475–479.
45. Fletcher BD, Jacobstein MD. MRI of congenital abnormalities of the great arteries. AJR 1986; 146:941–948.
46. Formanek AG, Witcofski RL, D'Souza VJ, et al. MR imaging of the central pulmonary arterial tree in conotruncal malformation. AJR 1986; 147:1127–1131.
47. Didier D, Higgins CB. Estimation of pulmonary vascular resistance by MRI in patients with congenital cardiovascular lesions. AJR 1986; 146:919–924.
48. Bisset GS III, Kirks DR, Strife JL, Schwartz DC. Cor triatriatum: diagnosis by magnetic resonance imaging. AJR 1987; 149:567–568.

49. Ross RD, Bisset GS III, Meyer RA, et al. Magnetic resonance imaging for diagnosis of pulmonary vein stenosis after "correction" of total anomalous pulmonary venous connection. Am J Cardiol 1987; 60:1199–1201.

50. von Schulthess GK, Higashino SM, Higgins SS, et al. Coarctation of the aorta: MR imaging. Radiology 1986; 158:469–474.

51. Amparo EG, Higgins CB, Shafton EG. Demonstration of coarctation of the aorta by magnetic resonance imaging. AJR 1984; 143:1192–1194.

52. Bank ER, Aisen AM, Rocchini AP, Hernandez RJ. Coarctation of the aorta in children undergoing angioplasty: pretreatment and posttreatment MR imaging. Radiology 1987; 162:235–240.

53. Soulen RL, Kan J, Mitchell S, White RI. Evaluation of balloon angioplasty of coarctation restenosis by magnetic resonance imaging. Am J Cardiol 1987; 60:343–345.

54. Simpson IA, Chung KJ, Glass RF, et al. Cine magnetic resonance imaging for evaluation of anatomy and flow relations in infants and children with coarctation of the aorta. Circulation 1988; 78:142–148.

55. Van Praagh R. Classification of truncus arteriosus communis (TAC). Am Heart J 1976; 92:129–132.

56. Jacobstein MD, Fletcher BD, Goldstein S, Riemenschneider TA. Magnetic resonance imaging in patients with hypoplastic right heart syndrome. Am Heart J 1985; 110:154–158.

57. Fletcher BD, Jacobstein MD, Abramowsky CR, Anderson RH. Right atrioventricular valve atresia: anatomic evaluation with MR imaging. AJR 1987; 148:671–674.

58. McFaul R, Millard P, Nowicki E. Vascular rings necessitating right thoracotomy. J Thorac Cardiovasc Surg 1981; 82:306–309.

59. Bisset GS III, Strife JL, Kirks DR, Bailey WW. Vascular rings: MR imaging. AJR 1987; 149:251–256.

60. Kersting-Sommerhoff BA, Sechtem UP, Fisher MR, Higgins CB. MR imaging of congenital anomalies of the aortic arch. AJR 1987; 149:9–13.

61. Fisher MR, Hricak H, Higgins CB. Magnetic resonance imaging of developmental venous anomalies. AJR 1985; 145:705–709.

62. Akins EW, Martin TD, Alexander JA, et al. MR imaging of double-outlet right ventricle. AJR 1989; 152:128–130.

63. Link KM, Herrera MA, D'Souza VJ, Formanek AG. MR imaging of Ebstein anomaly: results in four cases. AJR 1988; 150:363–367.

64. Peshock RM, Parrish M, Fixler D, Parkey RW. Magnetic resonance imaging of single ventricle. Circulation 1985; 72(Suppl III):III-29.

65. Link KM, Weesner KM, Formanek AG. MR imaging of the criss-cross heart. AJR 1989; 152:809–812.

66. Schiavone WA, O'Donnell JK. Congenital absence of the left portion of parietal pericardium demonstrated by nuclear magnetic resonance imaging. Am J Cardiol 1985; 55:1439–1440.

67. Soulen RL, Donner RM, Capitanio M. Postoperative evaluation of complex congenital heart disease by magnetic resonance imaging. RadioGraphics 1987; 7:975–1000.

68. Bisset GS III, Strife JL, Kirks DR, et al. Magnetic resonance imaging of the aorta following coarctation repair. Radiology 1987; 165(P):247.

69. Boxer RA, LaCorte MA, Singh S, et al. Nuclear magnetic resonance imaging in evaluation and follow-up of children treated for coarctation of the aorta. J Am Coll Cardiol 1986; 7:1095–1098.

70. Jacobstein MD, Fletcher BD, Nelson AD, et al. Magnetic resonance imaging: evaluation of palliative systemic pulmonary artery shunts. Circulation 1984; 70:650–656.

71. Soulen RL, Donner RM. Magnetic resonance imaging of rerouted pulmonary blood flow. Radiol Clin North Am 1985; 23:737–744.

72. Katz ME, Glazer HS, Siegel MJ, et al. Mediastinal vessels: postoperative evaluation with MR imaging. Radiology 1986; 161:647–651.

73. Campbell RM, Moreau GA, Johns JA, et al. Detection of caval obstruction by magnetic resonance imaging after intraatrial repair of transposition of the great arteries. Am J Cardiol 1987; 60:688–691.

74. Kyung JC, Simpson IA, Glass RF, et al. Cine magnetic resonance imaging after surgical repair in patients with transposition of the great arteries. Circulation 1988; 77:104–109.

75. Rees S, Somerville J, Warnes C, et al. Comparison of magnetic resonance imaging with echocardiography and radionuclide angiography in assessing cardiac function and anatomy following Mustard's operation for transposition of the great arteries. Am J Cardiol 1988; 61:1316–1322.

76. Utz JA, Herfkens RJ, Heinsimer JA, et al. Valvular regurgitation: dynamic MR imaging. Radiology 1988; 168:91–94.

77. Sechtem U, Pflugfelder PW, Cassidy MM, et al. Mitral or aortic regurgitation: quantification of regurgitant volumes with cine MR imaging. Radiology 1988; 167:425–430.

78. Stark DD, Higgins CB, Lanzer P, et al. Magnetic resonance imaging of the pericardium: normal and pathologic findings. Radiology 1984; 150:469–474.

79. Bisset GS III, Strife JL, McCloskey J. Magnetic resonance imaging of coronary artery aneurysms in children with Kawasaki disease. AJR 1989; 152:805–807.

80. Soulen RL, Stark DD, Higgins CB. Magnetic resonance imaging of constrictive pericardial disease. Am J Cardiol 1985; 55:480–484.

81. Boxer RA, Fishman M, LaCorte MA, et al. Cardiac MR imaging in Pompe disease. J Comput Assist Tomogr 1986; 10:857–859.

82. Amparo EG, Higgins CB, Farmer D, et al. Gated MRI of cardiac and paracardiac masses: initial experiment. AJR 1984; 143:1151–1156.

83. Gomes AS, Lois JF, Child JS, et al. Cardiac tumors and thrombus: evaluation with MR imaging. AJR 1987; 149:895–899.

84. Bradley WG, Waluch V. Blood flow: magnetic resonance imaging. Radiology 1985; 154:443–450.

85. Bradley WG, Waluch V. NMR even echo rephasing in slow laminar flow. J Comput Assist Tomogr 1984; 8:594–598.

86. Soulen RL, Fishman EK, Pyeritz RE, et al. Marfan syndrome: evaluation with MR imaging versus CT. Radiology 1987; 165:697–701.

87. Schaefer S, Peshock RM, Malloy CR, et al. J Am Coll Cardiol 1987; 9:70–74.

88. Kersting-Sommerhoff BA, Sechtem UP, Schiller NB, et al. MR imaging of the thoracic aorta in Marfan patients. J Comput Assist Tomogr 1987; 11:633–639.

89. Amparo EG, Higgins CB, Hricak H, Sollitto R. Aortic dissection: magnetic resonance imaging. Radiology 1985; 155:399–406.

90. Winkler ML, Higgins CB. MRI of perivalvular infectious pseudoaneurysms. AJR 1986; 147:253–256.

Respiratory System

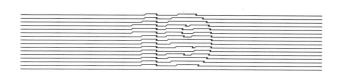

MARILYN J. SIEGEL, M.D.
PAUL L. MOLINA, M.D.

PEDIATRIC THORAX

Magnetic resonance imaging (MRI) has become recognized as an excellent method for evaluating thoracic anatomy and disease. In comparison with computed tomography (CT), MRI has several distinct advantages as a thoracic imaging technique, including direct multiplanar imaging capability, superior contrast resolution, and sensitivity to blood flow. Because MRI has no associated ionizing radiation and does not require administration of intravenous contrast material, it is particularly attractive for use in children. The disadvantages of MRI include poorer spatial resolution and longer acquisition times than for CT, thus increasing the potential for motion degradation of the image. Nevertheless, valuable diagnostic information can be gained from MRI of the chest in children.[1]

TECHNIQUES

Patient Preparation

Children under the age of 5 years often require sedation to prevent motion artifacts during scanning. The administration of pentobarbital (Nembutal), 5 mg per kilogram (up to a maximal dose of 100 mg) intramuscularly 20 to 30 minutes before the procedure, provides adequate sedation in most cases. For children over 5 years of age, explanation and reassurance are usually all that is necessary.

Imaging Techniques

Pulse Sequences

For most studies of the chest, both T1 and T2 weighted spin-echo pulse sequences are helpful.[1-5] T1 weighted images are obtained using a short repetition time (TR = 500 msec) and a short echo delay (TE = 15 to 30 msec). Such pulse sequences provide the best contrast between abnormal soft tissue masses (low signal intensity) and normal mediastinal fat (higher signal intensity), making masses easier to detect. On balanced images (long TR, short TE), relative signal intensities are increased, improving the signal-to-noise ratio (SNR) and image quality. This is helpful in demonstrating parenchymal and pleural disease, but the contrast between normal fat and tumor decreases, which makes delineation of mass lesions more difficult. T2 weighted sequences are obtained with a longer repetition time (TR = 2500 msec) and echo delay (TE = 60 to 90 msec). A pulse sequence that is more T2 weighted is advantageous in the delineation of tissues with longer T2 relaxation times, such as fluid. On T2 weighted sequences the cystic components of masses and pleural fluid have intense signals and are more easily seen. The contrast between tumor, of high signal, and muscle, of relatively low signal, is also improved. However, the contrast between mediastinal fat and most tumors is decreased on T2 weighted images because of overlap in their T2 values. In general, the resolution of bronchi and mediastinal vascular structures improves with longer TR values.

Cardiac Gating

Cardiac gating reduces blurring and motion artifact by acquiring data at specific phases in the cardiac cycle. This is routinely accomplished by "triggering" the MR imaging sequence with the R wave of the electrocardiogram (ECG), or at some preselected time after the R-wave signal has been received.[6,7] Cardiac gating can significantly increase the resolution of the heart and great vessels, and structures immediately adjacent to them (i.e., pulmonary hila, paracardiac mediastinal masses),[8–10] but it has several disadvantages. These include a longer setup time, since ECG electrodes and leads must be applied, and slightly prolonged imaging time. Moreover, the TR interval is relatively fixed, being determined by the R-to-R interval on the ECG. Images with a longer TR can be obtained by triggering MR data acquisition to alternate heart beats; this may be particularly useful in newborns and young infants who normally have a very fast heart rate. Cardiac gating cannot be successfully performed in patients with cardiac arrhythmias.

Reduction of Respiratory Motion

MR images of the chest are subject to degradation by respiratory motion, which causes spatial blurring and increased image noise from "ghost" artifacts.[11] To minimize image degradation, several techniques have been developed that acquire MR data during selected phases of the respiratory cycle. These include various modes of respiratory gating,[12,13] as well as the technique of respiratory ordered phase encoding (ROPE). Although ROPE reduces ghost artifacts, it does not correct spatial blurring.[11,14] Respiratory gating reduces both spatial blurring and ghost artifacts, but prolongs imaging time by a factor of 2 to 3, making its routine clinical use impractical. More recently, the technique of first moment nulling has been used to reduce respiratory motion artifacts. However, in our experience, the simplest method of reducing respiratory motion-related artifacts in children is to shorten imaging time by the use of fast spin-echo or gradient-echo sequences.

Planes of Section

MR imaging of the mediastinum and lungs in children is performed in the transverse imaging plane. Transaxial images obtained at 1-cm intervals with scan thickness of 5 mm or 1 cm are sufficient in most cases. Sagittal and coronal sections are used in selected patients, such as in imaging of the aorta and great vessels, evaluation of the aortopulmonary window, and defining the relationship of a mass to the spinal canal.[15–19] Although oblique imaging is particularly applicable to the heart and aorta, it generally is not required in imaging the mediastinum and lungs. Most MR studies are tailored to a particular clinical problem, and the whole thorax often is not imaged. The average study requires 45 to 60 minutes to accomplish.

NORMAL ANATOMY

The anatomy of the thorax on MR images is illustrated through a series of characteristic sections, including levels through the (1) aortic arch, (2) pulmonary arteries, (3) left atrium, and (4) cardiac ventricles (Figs. 19–1, 19–2).

Specific Anatomic Structures

Mediastinal Vessels

In normal children the mediastinal vascular structures seen on CT are visible on MRI. The lumina of the aorta and superior vena cava and their branches have no significant signal intensity because of the rapidly flowing blood they contain.[20,21] Hence, they are easily distinguished from both the surrounding mediastinal fat, which displays high signal intensity on T1 and T2 weighted images, and adjacent muscle, which usually has an intermediate signal intensity on most sequences. Increased signal within the aorta and superior vena cava can be seen occasionally in normal patients as a result of flow-related enhancement effect, or during diastole.[20]

Thymus

The appearance of the thymus changes dramatically with age. Awareness of the variations in the morphology of the thymus is essential lest it be mistaken as a mass lesion. The normal thymus is a bilobed structure, each lobe having a separate fibrous capsule. In neonates and infants, the thymus consists primarily of dense aggregates of lymphocytes separated by fibrous septa. Beginning at puberty, the lymphocytes gradually involute and are replaced by fat. The thymus is largest with respect to patient age in neonates and young infants (average weight 20 g). Maximal thymic weight (average 30 g) is reached at puberty.

The thymus is visible on MRI in all patients in the first two decades of life. In patients under 5 years of age, the thymus lies in the anterior mediastinum between the horizontal portion of the left brachiocephalic vein superiorly and the horizontal portion of the right pulmonary artery inferiorly. The largest portion is between the aortic arch and the main pulmonary artery. In these younger patients, the thymus generally has a quadrilateral shape with convex lateral contours (Figs. 19–3, 19–4).[22] With increasing age the appearance of the thymus changes, assuming a triangular or bilobed configuration with straight outer borders (Fig. 19–5). By the age of 15 years the triangular appearance should be present in all patients. The left lobe of the thymus parallels the aortic arch, and usually is slightly larger and extends more caudal than the right lobe.[22,23]

In prepubescent patients the signal intensity of the normal thymus is slightly greater than that of muscle on T1 weighted images, and slightly less than or equal to that of fat on T2 weighted images. After puberty the

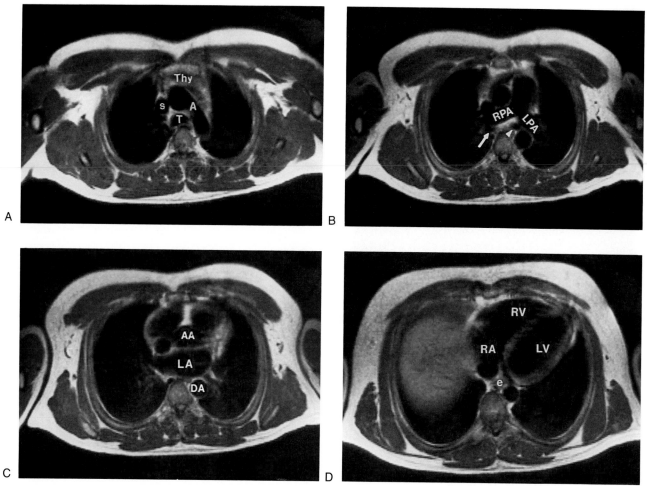

Figure 19–1. *Normal mediastinal and lung anatomy.* Sequential axial scans through the following levels in caudad order: *A,* aortic arch; *B,* pulmonary arteries; *C,* left atrium; *D,* cardiac ventricles. s, superior vena cava; T, trachea; e, esophagus; A, aortic arch; Thy, thymus; LPA, left pulmonary artery; RPA, right pulmonary artery; LA, left atrium; AA, ascending aorta; DA, descending aorta; RA, right atrium; LV, left ventricle; RV, right ventricle; arrow, right mainstem bronchus; arrowhead, left mainstem bronchus.

T1 value of the thymus decreases, reflecting fatty infiltration. The T2 relaxation times of the thymus overlap with those of fat and generally do not change with age. Because of its long T1 relaxation time in comparison to fat, the normal thymus is more easily delineated on T1 weighted MR images. It may be difficult to identify the thymus on T2 weighted images because of the similar signal intensities of thymic parenchyma and fat, as well as the poor anatomic resolution compared with T1 weighted images.[22, 23]

Although generally not required for identification of an abnormality, the most reliable measurement of the thymus is its thickness. Before the age of 15 years the normal average thickness on MRI is 1.50 cm (1 S.D. = 0.3 cm).[22] Measurements of the thickness of the thymic soft tissues are slightly larger on MRI than on CT, and are believed to be related to the lower lung volumes on MR images.[23] MRI is performed during quiet respira-

tion, whereas CT generally is performed in suspended or full inspiration.

Rarely, the thymus may extend either superiorly above the brachiocephalic vessels or into the posterior mediastinum. The abnormally positioned thymus can be recognized on MRI by its direct continuity with the anterior mediastinal thymic tissue, a signal intensity similar to that of normal thymic tissue, and the absence of compression of the adjacent mediastinal vessels or tracheobronchial tree (Fig. 19–6).[24]

Mediastinal Lymph Nodes

Lymph nodes in the mediastinum are rarely seen in children under 15 years of age. Occasionally, normal lymph nodes are seen in older adolescents. When normal nodes are identified, they are less than 1 cm in size and have a signal intensity between that of muscle and fat on both T1 and T2 weighted MR images. At times

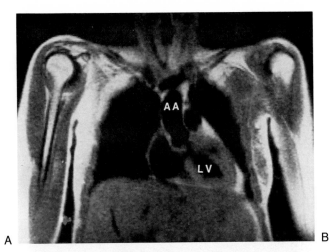

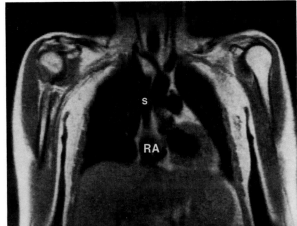

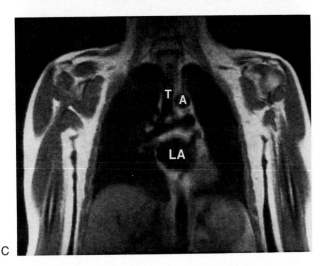

Figure 19–2. *Normal mediastinal and lung anatomy.* **A** to **C,** Coronal images (500/30) from anterior to posterior. (See Figure 19–1 for abbreviations.)

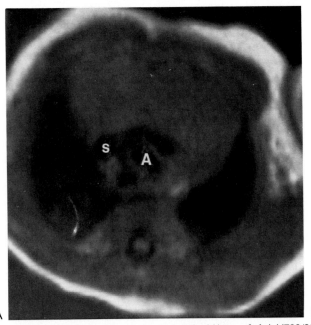

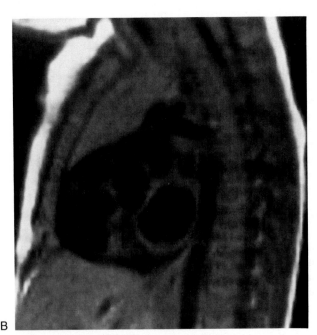

Figure 19–3. *Normal thymus in a 4-month-old boy.* **A,** Axial (700/30) and **B,** sagittal (900/30) MR images demonstrate a quadrilateral thymus with slightly convex lateral borders and a broad retrosternal component. Signal intensity is homogeneous and slightly greater than chest wall musculature. A, Aorta; s, superior vena cava.

588

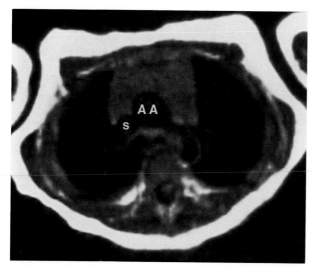

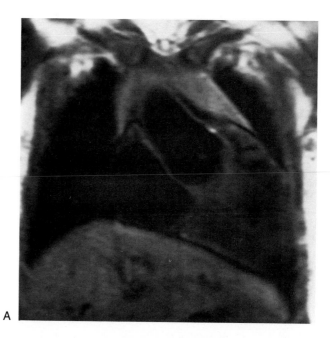

Figure 19–4. *Normal thymus in a 4-year-old boy.* Axial T1 weighted (600/30) image shows a smaller quadrilateral thymus with relatively straight margins and a signal intensity slightly greater than muscle. AA, ascending aorta; s, superior vena cava.

A

on MRI a closely clustered group of normal-sized lymph nodes may appear as a conglomerate mass rather than as discrete nodal structures, because of the inferior spatial resolution of MRI compared with CT.[1, 5, 25]

Pulmonary Hilum

The normal pulmonary hilum is composed of the mainstem bronchi, pulmonary arteries and veins, hilar lymph nodes, and nerve plexuses, all of which are enclosed by connective tissue. The right and left main bronchi, lobar bronchi, and main pulmonary artery branches are seen frequently on MRI. Most segmental bronchi, as well as peripheral arterial branches and small pulmonary vessels, are not seen or are poorly visualized.[26, 27] Likewise, hilar lymph nodes are seen infrequently in children. Rarely, normal collections of soft tissue, representing both fat and small lymph nodes, may be large enough to be confused with abnormally enlarged hilar lymph nodes. Typically, this confusion arises in three sites: at the level of the bifurcation of the right pulmonary artery, at the origin of the middle lobe bronchus, and at the level of the left upper lobe bronchus.[28]

Other Structures

The trachea generally can be well visualized by MRI and appears as an area of signal void. The esophagus usually is collapsed, appearing as an area of intermediate signal intensity.[29] On occasion a collapsed esophagus may be mistaken for an enlarged retrotracheal lymph node mass on a single MR image, but review of sequential images usually permits correct identification of the structure as the esophagus.[3]

The pulmonary parenchyma, pleura, fissures, and ligaments are not as well delineated by MRI as by CT.

B

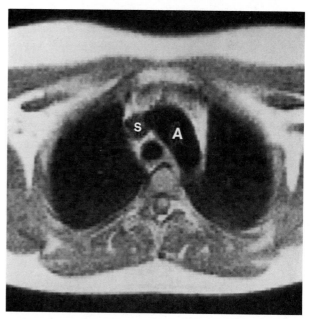

Figure 19–5. *Normal thymus.* **A,** Coronal T1 weighted image (500/30) in a child and **B,** T1 weighted axial image in an adolescent show a bilobed thymus. The left lobe is more prominent than the right. A, Aortic arch; s, superior vena cava.

The normal pulmonary parenchyma has a low signal intensity on T1 and T2 weighted images because of the very low hydrogen concentration in the alveoli, air in the bronchi, and flow in the vessels. Fissures are not seen because they are too thin to be resolved. Inadequate identification of pulmonary fissures is an important limitation because the fissures serve as major landmarks, allowing for accurate localization of disease within the pulmonary parenchyma. The normal pericardium generally can be seen by MRI, particularly

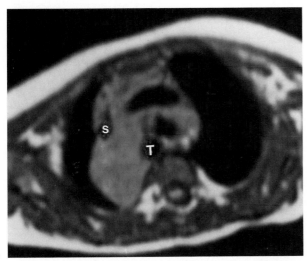 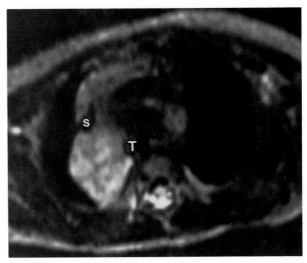

Figure 19–6. *Posterior mediastinal thymus.* ***A,*** T1 weighted axial image (700/20) demonstrates normal homogeneous thymic tissue in the anterior mediastinum. Posteriorly, the thymus extends between the superior vena cava (s) and trachea (T) to reach the chest wall. The signal intensity of the thymus is intermediate between muscle and fat. ***B,*** On a T2 weighted axial image (3200/80) the thymus has a signal intensity slightly greater than fat.

with ECG gating.[30] On ECG-gated MRI the pericardium is seen as a thin curvilinear area of low signal intensity between the higher-intensity pericardial fat and the medium-intensity myocardium or high-intensity epicardial fat.[30, 31]

MEDIASTINUM AND HILUM

Indications for MR Imaging

MR imaging of the mediastinum in childhood is used most often to further evaluate the nature and extent of a mediastinal mass seen on CT scanning. In most patients the anatomic information provided by MRI is comparable with that from CT.[1] However, in patients in whom there is a contraindication to the administration of intravenous contrast material, or in cases in which the CT findings are equivocal, MRI may give clinically relevant data. MRI appears particularly useful for the evaluation of posterior mediastinal masses, which have a propensity for spinal invasion. Because of its superior contrast resolution, MRI can allow confident identification of intraspinal extension without the use of intrathecal contrast material.

Further assessment of an enlarged or questionably abnormal pulmonary hilum noted on plain chest radiography is usually performed with CT. On CT the diagnosis of a hilar mass or lymphadenopathy is based on separation of normal vessel from soft tissue mass. This often requires a bolus injection of contrast medium to produce vascular opacification. Because rapidly flowing blood produces little MR signal, the hilar vessels are easy to detect on MRI. In patients whose CT examinations are equivocal, MRI can be a helpful supplement in confirming the diagnosis of a hilar mass

or lymph node enlargement.[28] It can assume a more primary role if there is a known contraindication to, or an inability to use, intravenous contrast material. When contrast material is used with CT, the accuracy of MRI and CT is comparable.[1]

Congenital Abnormalities

Mediastinal Cysts

Most mediastinal cysts are congenital in origin and classified as bronchogenic, enteric, or neurenteric, depending on their histologic picture. In children, most cysts produce clinical symptoms because they compress the airway or esophagus, causing dyspnea and dysphagia. Occasionally, mediastinal cysts are discovered as incidental findings on plain chest radiographs.

The CT appearance of a mediastinal cyst is usually that of a well-circumscribed near-water-density mass that does not enhance. In some cases the density may be equal to soft tissue, usually because of viscid contents. Most mediastinal cysts have long T1 and T2 relaxation times, reflecting their serous contents (Fig. 19–7). On T1 weighted images these fluid-filled cysts have a low signal intensity similar to that of muscle. On T2 weighted sequences the cyst contents are more intense relative to adjacent soft tissues.[32, 33] On occasion the signal intensities may be higher than those of simple cysts on T1 weighted images, because the cyst contents are proteinaceous or hemorrhagic rather than serous.[32] Cysts with short T1 values may be indistinguishable from necrotic soft tissue neoplasms, although their location may be a clue to the correct diagnosis.

Bronchogenic cysts are lined by respiratory epithelium and result from anomalous budding of the tra-

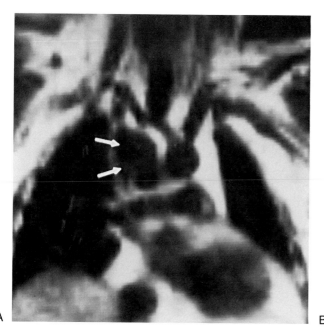
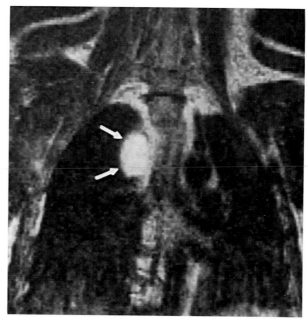

A   B

Figure 19–7. *Duplication cyst.* **A,** T1 weighted (300/15) coronal MR image shows a well-circumscribed low signal intensity mass (*arrows*) in the right paratracheal region. **B,** On a T2 weighted (2100/90) image the mass (*arrows*) is higher in signal intensity and as bright as fat. The long T1 and T2 relaxation values are consistent with a cystic lesion containing pure fluid. At surgery a duplication cyst was confirmed.

cheobronchial tree. The subcarinal and right paratracheal areas are the most common locations of these cysts, although they may be found in the posterior mediastinum and within the lung parenchyma. Their contents can range from serous material to mucoid material, with variable viscosities.[34]

Enteric cysts, also known as esophageal duplications, are lined by gastrointestinal mucosa and arise either as a diverticulum from the dorsal bud of the primitive foregut or from aberrant recanalization of the gut. Those cysts that contain gastric mucosa may produce pain from peptic ulceration or hemoptysis from erosion into the tracheobronchial tree. Enteric cysts are usually located in the posterior mediastinum adjacent to the esophagus, or within the esophageal wall.

Neurenteric cysts arise from incomplete separation of the primitive foregut from the notochord during early embryonic life and are usually connected to the meninges through a midline defect in one or more vertebral bodies. Histologically, the cyst wall contains both gastrointestinal and neural elements, while the lining is composed of GI epithelium. Like the enteric cysts, neurenteric cysts tend to occur in the posterior mediastinum. They may be distinguished by their location, as well as by their association with spinal anomalies.

Cystic hygromas are lymphogenous cysts that occur in the superior mediastinum. Almost all the lesions are inferior extensions of cervical hygromas. On CT they appear as multiloculated masses with an attenuation value near water.[35] On MRI they have a signal intensity

equal to or slightly less than that of muscle on T1 weighted images, and greater than that of fat on T2 weighted images (Fig. 19–8). This appearance correlates with the preponderance of fluid-filled cystic spaces. Rarely, the signal intensity may be equal to that of fat on T1 weighted images, reflecting the presence of blood or increased amounts of fat. Septations are present in nearly all patients and appear as low signal intensity structures.[36] Lymphangiomas may be distinguished from other mediastinal cysts by their usual association with a cervical component.

Occasionally, soft tissue neoplasms have fluid-filled areas secondary to necrosis, radiation, chemotherapy, or previous hemorrhage, and thus may mimic mediastinal cysts. This appearance can be seen with thymomas, teratomas, and Hodgkin's disease. An MR diagnosis of a cystic neoplasm should be possible on the basis of demonstration of a cystic mass with thick walls in conjunction with other findings such as lymph node enlargement or pleuro-pericardial disease. In other cases, tissue sampling is required for definitive diagnosis. Currently, MRI appears to have no diagnostic advantage over CT in the evaluation of mediastinal cysts.

Diaphragmatic Hernia

Diaphragmatic hernias usually are easily identified by plain radiography or CT scanning. In children, most diaphragmatic hernias are congenital, occur through the posterior foramen of Bochdalek, and are found on the left, because the liver protects the right hemidiaphragm. Anterior diaphragmatic hernias through

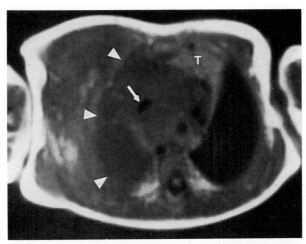
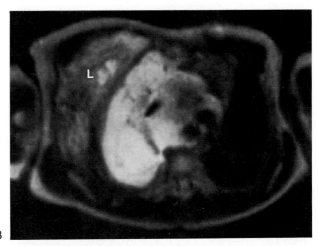

Figure 19–8. *Mediastinal lymphangioma.* ***A,*** T1 weighted axial MR image (500/30) in a 2-month-old girl demonstrates a low signal intensity mass (*arrowheads*) in the superior mediastinum displacing the superior vena cava (*arrow*) anteriorly. T, Normal left lobe of the thymus. ***B,*** On the T2 weighted image (1800/120) the mass is much brighter than all surrounding tissues, reflecting its fluid nature. Margins of the lesion are seen better on the T2 weighted sequence. Also note lymphangioma (L) in the right chest wall.

the foramen of Morgagni are less frequent. The internal contents of the herniation determine the signal intensity. If the hernia contains fatty omental tissue, the signal intensity may be the same as that of subcutaneous fat. Coronal MR sections are particularly valuable in showing the relationship of the thoracic mass to the diaphragm.

Tumor

The mediastinum is the most common site of primary thoracic masses in childhood. There is an almost equal frequency of mass lesions in the three mediastinal compartments, approximately 30 percent of lesions occurring in the anterior, 30 percent in the middle, and 40 percent in the posterior mediastinum. The most common mass lesions are neurogenic tumors, lymphoma, teratomas, and cysts of foregut origin.[37] Aneurysms and excessive fat deposition are rare causes of mediastinal widening in childhood.

Germ Cell Neoplasm

Germ cell tumors, which can be benign or malignant, are derived from one or more of the three embryonic germ cell layers. Dermoid cysts (containing only ectodermal elements) and benign teratomas (containing more than one germinal layer) are the most common mediastinal germ cell tumors. When located in the chest, they are frequently found within the thymus. Rarely, teratomas can be in the posterior mediastinum or along the base of the heart. In younger children, germ cell neoplasms often produce dyspnea, wheezing, and rarely superior vena cava obstruction; in older patients, they usually are asymptomatic and discovered incidentally on chest radiographs.

The diagnosis of a germ cell neoplasm can be made with certainty by CT if calcifications, fat, and soft tissue components are demonstrated within an anterior mediastinal mass with a well-defined thick wall.[38] On MRI the internal contents of dermoids and teratomas demonstrate some inhomogeneity because of the variable admixture of components. The signal intensities depend on the relative amounts of fluid and fat within the lesion. Predominantly cystic lesions have signal intensities slightly greater than that of muscle on T1 weighted images. On T2 weighted sequences the relative signal intensity usually markedly increases (Fig. 19–9). The appearance of germ cell neoplasm is nonspecific and cannot be distinguished from thymomas with cystic or necrotic areas. For practical purposes, MRI offers no advantage in patients with benign teratomas over CT, which can detect calcification more readily.

A malignant germ cell tumor appears on CT or MRI as a poorly defined mass that infiltrates mediastinal fat and encases or invades mediastinal vessels or airways.[39] Besides malignant teratoma, other rare malignant germ cell tumors that invade locally are seminoma, embryonal cell carcinoma, choriocarcinoma, and endodermal sinus tumor. The appearance on MRI of malignant germ cell tumors is indistinguishable from that of lymphoma or an invasive thymoma. However, by demonstrating their full extent, MRI can be valuable in treatment planning and follow-up evaluation of these tumors.

Lymphoma

Lymphoma frequently involves the thorax, especially the mediastinum. At clinical presentation, approximately two-thirds of patients with Hodgkin's lymphoma have intrathoracic disease, and in 90 percent of

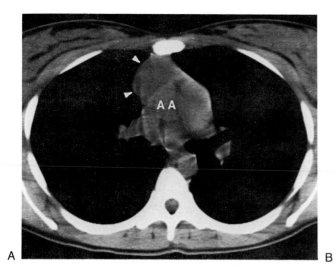

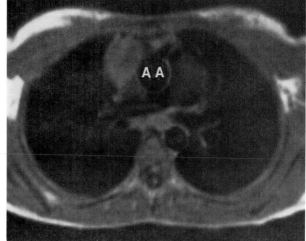

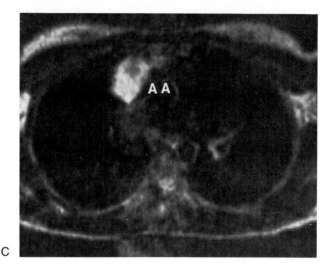

Figure 19–9. *Benign cystic teratoma.* **A,** CT scan through the superior mediastinum shows a well-defined homogeneous mass (*arrowheads*), anterior to the ascending aorta (AA), arising from the right lobe of the thymus in an 18-year-old girl. The lesion is composed mainly of water. At a higher level, faint calcifications were seen. **B,** T1 weighted MR image (750/15) at a comparable level demonstrates a low signal intensity mass equal to that of muscle. **C,** On a T2 weighted image (2400/90) the signal intensity of the mass is equal to that of fat. The areas of calcification, noted on CT, were not seen on MRI.

these there is mediastinal involvement.[40–42] In contrast, about 40 percent of patients with non-Hodgkin's lymphoma have intrathoracic disease, and about 50 percent of these have mediastinal involvement.[41, 42] Lymphoma most often involves the anterior mediastinum and may appear as a mediastinal mass, reflecting infiltration and enlargement of the thymus, or as discrete lymphadenopathy.

CT has been the examination of choice to evaluate the extent of disease in patients with Hodgkin's disease and non-Hodgkin's lymphoma. On CT, lymphoma produces massive infiltration of both lobes of the thymus; the outer margins of the thymus are convex and lobulated.[43] Concomitant lymphadenopathy elsewhere in the thorax, displacement of vascular structures and airways, and direct invasion of the anterior chest wall are frequently present. Accurate assessment of the extent of disease is especially important when radiation therapy is planned.

The appearance on MRI is similar to that seen on CT. Lymphoma may involve one lobe of the thymus or

produce diffuse enlargement of the gland (Fig. 19–10).[22] The infiltrated thymus often has a quadrilateral shape with convex lateral borders and is inhomogeneous. The inhomogeneity of the thymus is attributed to underlying necrosis, cystic degeneration, or fibrosis (Fig. 19–11). The signal intensity of the infiltrated thymus is slightly greater than muscle on T1 weighted sequences and close to that of fat on T2 weighted images. Difficulty may arise in distinguishing lymphomatous infiltration of the thymus from an invasive thymoma. The presence on MRI of lymph node disease elsewhere in the mediastinum suggests lymphoma, whereas multiple pleural implants at distant sites favor a thymoma.

The manifestations of lymphadenopathy on MR, as on CT, consist mainly of nodal enlargement (Figs. 19–12, 19–13). However, whether such enlargement is caused by tumor or inflammation usually cannot be ascertained by MRI or CT alone. There is no size criterion that allows both high sensitivity and high specificity for predicting nodal enlargement. In infants

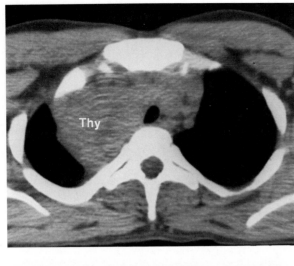

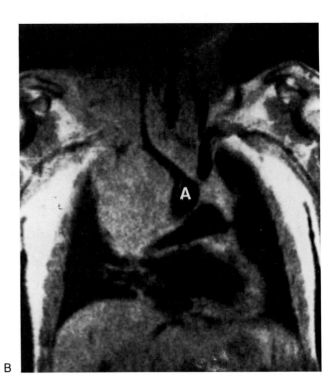

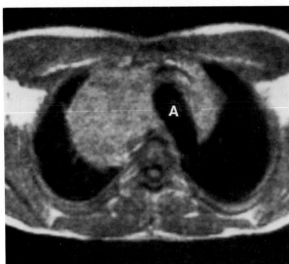

Figure 19–10. *Thymic Hodgkin's disease, nodular sclerosing type.* ***A,*** CT scan through the superior mediastinum shows massive infiltration of the right lobe of the thymus (Thy). ***B,*** T1 weighted (500/20) coronal and ***C,*** axial images demonstrate similar findings. A markedly enlarged thymus (thickness = 7.5 cm) with convex lateral margins is present. The signal intensity is intermediate between muscle and fat and mildly heterogeneous. The superior vena cava is not visualized secondary to compression by the enlarged thymus. A, Aortic arch.

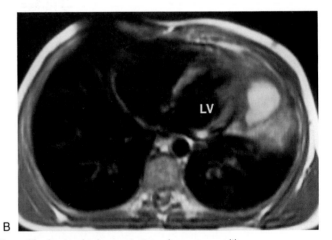

Figure 19–11. *Cystic lymphoma.* ***A,*** CT image in a 14-year-old boy with chest pain demonstrates a large mass with central necrosis in the area of the left lobe of the thymus. ***B,*** T1 weighted (700/30) MR image shows an intermediate signal intensity mass with a high signal intensity center adjacent to the left ventricle (LV). Multiple enlarged nodes were present on other images. Hodgkin's disease was confirmed by lymph node biopsy.

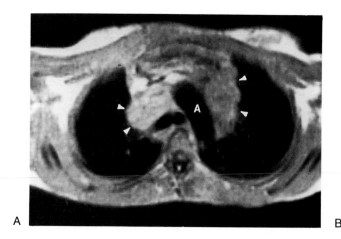

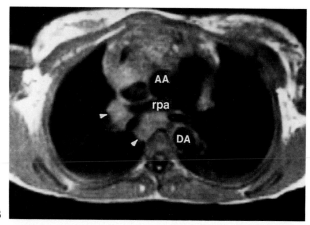

Figure 19–12. *Lymph node enlargement in various mediastinal regions.* Multiple enlarged nodes (*arrowheads*) secondary to Hodgkin's disease are seen on T1 weighted images (700/15). *A,* Enlarged pretracheal and lateral aortic nodes. *B,* Right hilar and posterior subcarinal lymphadenopathy. *C,* Superior diaphragmatic (pericardial) lymphadenopathy. On T1 weighted images the lymph nodes have an intermediate signal intensity, between that of muscle and fat. A, Aortic arch; AA, ascending aorta; DA, descending aorta; rpa, right pulmonary artery.

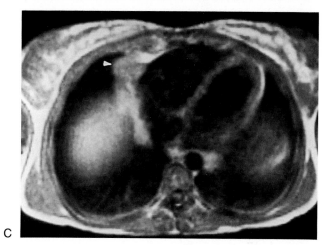

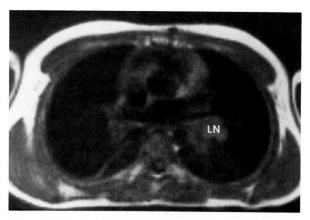

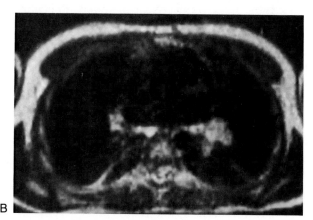

Figure 19–13. Hilar lymph node enlargement on *A,* T1 weighted (500/15) and *B,* T2 weighted (2100/90) images in a patient with Hodgkin's disease. Lymph nodes are of intermediate signal intensity on T1 weighted images and increased signal intensity on T2 weighted images. LN, Lymph node.

and younger children, lymph nodes normally are not seen and their presence should be considered abnormal. In adolescents, any lymph node exceeding 1 cm in diameter is believed to be pathologic. MRI also can be used to evaluate airway compression. MRI and CT are equivalent in assessing tracheal compression by adenopathy, but MRI is not as good as CT in evaluating bronchial narrowing (Fig. 19–14).

MRI imaging appears to be helpful in the follow-up evaluation of patients with lymphoma who have under-

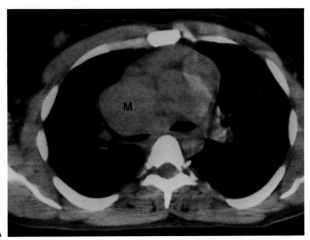

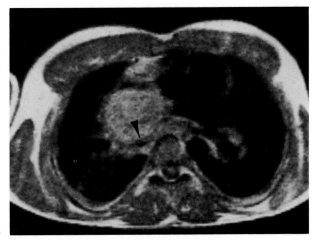

A   B

Figure 19–14. *Hodgkin's disease with bronchial compression.*   **A,** CT scan in a 16-year-old boy shows a mediastinal mass (M) anterior to and compressing the right mainstem bronchus. **B,** T1 weighted MR image (500/30) demonstrates the mediastinal mass and extensive narrowing of the right mainstem bronchus (*arrowhead*). The signal intensity of the mass is nonspecific and between that of muscle and fat. Note that the degree of bronchial compression is more severe on MR than on CT. The patient, however, was asymptomatic, and the narrowing on MR was believed to be overestimated, owing to partial volume averaging and respiratory motion.

gone radiation therapy and have a residual mass.[44] In some cases, MRI may be able to distinguish residual or recurrent tumor from post-treatment fibrosis. On both T1 and T2 weighted pulse sequences, radiation fibrosis usually has a low signal intensity similar to that of muscle.[45] Tumor has a slightly greater signal intensity than muscle on T1 weighted images. On T2 weighted images, however, tumor demonstrates strong signal intensity, reflecting its longer T2 value. Unfortunately, the presence of relatively high signal intensity on T2 weighted images is not necessarily specific for recurrent tumor. Acute radiation pneumonitis, infection, hemorrhage, and sometimes even regions of radiation fibrosis may have a signal intensity similar to that of neoplasm, and thus may be confused with recurrent disease. In these cases, serial MR examinations or biopsy are necessary for diagnosis.

Thymoma

Thymomas are exceedingly rare in patients 20 years old and younger, representing less than 5 percent of all mediastinal tumors in childhood.[37] These tumors, which can be benign or malignant, occur in association with myasthenia gravis or (rarely) other conditions such as red cell aplasia or hypogammaglobulinemia. They may also occur sporadically.

On CT a benign thymoma appears as a soft tissue density mass that is round, oval, or lobulated and well delineated.[46] A similar appearance is noted on MRI. The signal intensity of a thymoma is similar to that of muscle on short TR and TE spin-echo pulse sequences. On longer TR and TE sequences, the relative signal intensity increases and is greater than that of muscle, but less than that of fat.[47] Thymomas that contain calcification or necrosis show heterogeneous signal intensity on T1 and T2 weighted images (Fig. 19–15).[48]

The signal characteristics of thymomas with necrotic degeneration are indistinguishable from those of other cystic lesions such as dermoids or teratomas.

Approximately 10 to 15 percent of thymomas are invasive (i.e., malignant). The presence of neoplastic growth through the capsule determines whether the tumor is invasive. Experience with CT suggests that an invasive thymoma should be suspected when, in addition to an anterior mediastinal mass in the location of the thymus, there are pleural or pericardial implants, most commonly on only one side of the thoracic cavity.[49, 50] Although we have had no experience with malignant thymomas on MRI, presumably a malignant or invasive thymoma would appear as an anterior mediastinal mass in the location of the thymus, associated with local invasion and pleura- or pericardium-based metastatic implants.

Thymic Cyst

Thymic cysts are rare lesions that can be easily distinguished from solid lesions by their long T1 and T2 relaxation times. On T1 weighted images, thymic cysts have a low signal intensity and generally are homogeneous in appearance. If the cyst contains blood or mucoid contents, the signal intensity may be higher (Fig. 19–16). T2 weighted images typically show an increase in signal intensity of the cyst contents. Differentiation of thymic cysts from teratomas or necrotic thymomas may be difficult, although in general the latter tumors have thicker walls.

Thymic cysts may also occur in association with Hodgkin's disease. They are believed to be related to initial involvement of the thymus with disease, rather than being the result of chemotherapy or radiation therapy.[51] The presence of diffuse thymic enlargement and associated lymphadenopathy and pleuropa-

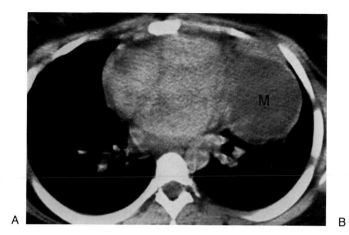

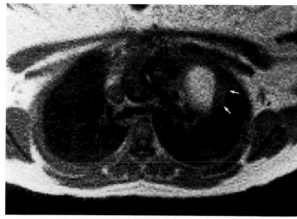

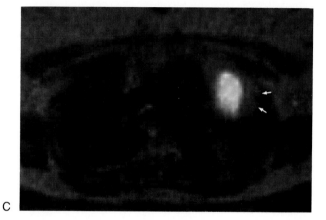

Figure 19–15. *Cystic thymoma.* ***A,*** CT scan through the superior mediastinum demonstrates an 8-cm mass (M) in the area of the left lobe of the thymus in a 15-year-old girl. The central portion of the lesion has a low attenuation value consistent with necrosis. ***B,*** T1 weighted (700/17) and ***C,*** T2 weighted (2500/90) images demonstrate a large mass involving the left lobe of the thymus. The more solid component of the mass (*arrows*) is lower in signal intensity than the central cystic component. A thymoma of the left lobe with central necrosis and hemorrhage was confirmed pathologically.

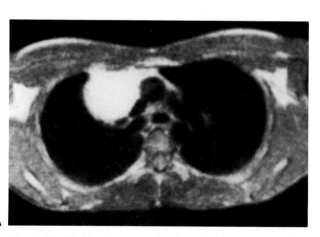

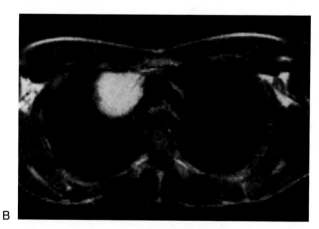

Figure 19–16. *Thymic cyst in a 22-year-old man with right pleuritic chest pain.*   A CT scan had demonstrated a large, near-water-density anterior mediastinal mass. ***A,*** T1 weighted (500/30) and ***B,*** T2 weighted (2500/90) MR images show a homogeneously high signal intensity mass in the right lobe of the thymus, suggesting the diagnosis of a hemorrhagic cyst. At surgery, a benign thymic cyst containing old hemorrhage was confirmed. (From Sagel SS, Glazer HS. Mediastinum. In: Lee KTL, Sagel SS, Stanley RJ. Computed body tomography with MRI correlation. New York: Raven Press, 1989:283.)

renchymal disease suggests lymphoma rather than an uncomplicated thymic cyst. Such cysts may present or enlarge following treatment, despite regression of other disease.

Neurogenic Tumor

Posterior mediastinal tumors are of neurogenic origin in approximately 95 percent of cases and may originate from sympathetic ganglion cells or from nerve roots. The former include neuroblastomas, ganglioneuroblastomas, and ganglioneuromas; the latter include neurofibromas and schwannomas. Nerve root tumors are rarely malignant, whereas ganglion cell tumors have variable degrees of malignancy. Other rare causes of posterior mediastinal masses in children are diaphragmatic or esophageal hiatal hernias; paraspinal abscess, usually secondary to tuberculosis; and lymphoma.

Most patients with neurogenic tumors are evaluated initially by CT. The tumors usually are paraspinal in location and spherical or fusiform in shape in a cephalocaudad direction. Benign lesions typically are sharply marginated, while malignant tumors tend to have poorly defined borders.[52] Typically, neural tumors are of soft tissue density, although they may be lower in attenuation value if they contain high amounts of lipid within the neural tissue. Calcifications frequently are identified on CT, especially within the neuroblastomas. CT scanning with metrizamide myelography can be used to depict intraspinal tumor extension.[53]

MRI is superb for determining the extent of neurogenic tumors, especially malignant ones. The multiplanar imaging capabilities and the excellent soft tissue contrast allow evaluation of intraspinal extension without myelography.[54] Neurogenic tumors may have low signal intensity on T1 weighted images and relatively higher signal intensity on T2 weighted images, similar to other solid tumors (Figs. 19–17, 19–18). In these instances, the location in the posterior mediastinum should suggest the diagnosis. Occasionally, neurogenic tumors show high intensity on T1 and T2 weighted images, possibly owing to their high lipid content.[32]

The disadvantage of MRI is its inability to detect calcifications, which are present in up to 40 percent of mediastinal neuroblastomas. The recognition of these calcifications is important for diagnosis. However, the ability of MRI to diagnose infiltration of surrounding mediastinal tissues and intraspinal extension without the use of contrast medium is an important enough factor to outweigh the disadvantages (Fig. 19–19). Presently, MRI imaging appears to be the method of choice to evaluate a posterior mediastinal mass suspected on plain chest radiography.

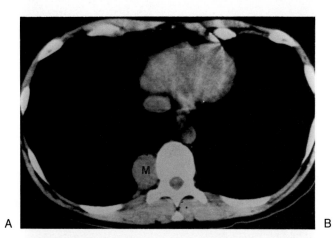

A

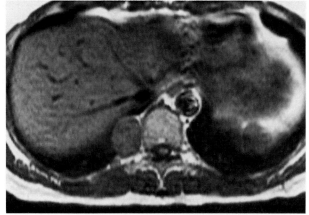

B

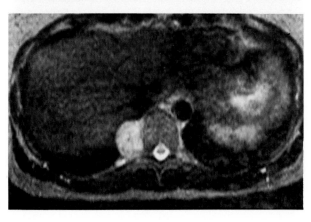

C

Figure 19–17. *Ganglioneuroma.* **A,** CT scans shows a soft tissue mass (M) in the right paravertebral area. **B,** Axial T1 weighted (500/30) MR image shows a well-defined mass with a signal intensity slightly above muscle. **C,** On a T2 weighted (2800/90) image the signal intensity of the mass approaches that of fat.

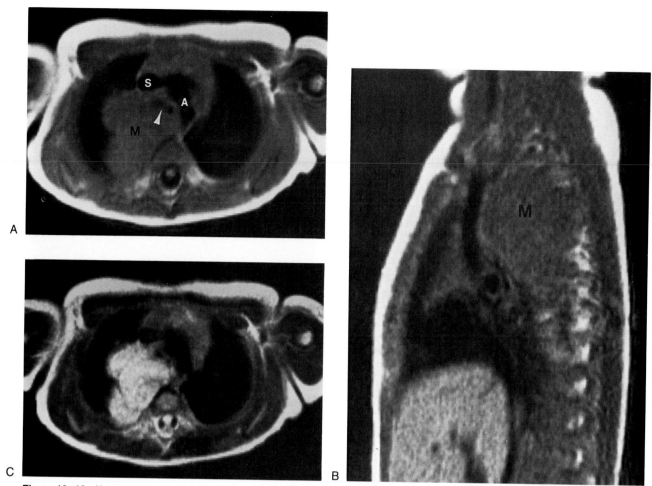

Figure 19–18. *Neuroblastoma.* *A,* Axial and *B,* sagittal T1 weighted images (500/15) demonstrate a posterior mediastinal mass (M) with a signal intensity equal to muscle. The mass compresses and displaces the trachea (*arrowhead*) to the left. *C,* On an axial T2-weighted image (2100/90) the neoplasm is much brighter than muscle and slightly lower in intensity than fat. There is no evidence of intraspinal extension. S, Superior vena cava; A, aortic arch.

Infection and Inflammation

Lymphadenopathy

The main causes of lymph node enlargement in children are granulomatous disease and lymphoma. An MR diagnosis of lymphadenopathy is based on identification of nodal enlargement, rather than on any characteristic signal intensity. Lymph node enlargement may appear as discrete round soft tissue densities or as a single solid mass. Abnormal lymph nodes usually have a homogeneous appearance on MR images but may appear inhomogeneous if they contain areas of calcification or necrosis.

On T1 weighted images, involved lymph nodes have signal intensities slightly greater than that of muscle. On T2 weighted images, nodal signal intensity increases, and thus the contrast between lymph nodes and muscle increases while that between nodes and fat decreases. At the present time, MRI cannot reliably distinguish benign from malignant adenopathy. Some investigators have suggested that the T1 and T2 relaxation times of neoplastic nodes are longer than those of inflamed or reactive nodes. However, other workers have noted a wide overlap in these values.

MRI has no proved advantage over contrast-enhanced CT in depicting mediastinal lymphadenopathy. Both examinations are nonspecific for distinguishing between benign and malignant lymphadenopathy. CT, however, has the ability to reveal calcification, which can be a considerable advantage. Calcification within mediastinal or hilar lymph nodes generally connotes old granulomatous disease.

Fibrosing Mediastinitis

Mediastinal lymph nodes involved by granulomatous diseases, particularly histoplasmosis, may heal with extensive fibrosis, leading to compression and sometimes occlusion of the superior vena cava or tracheobronchial tree. This result has been labeled "fibrosing mediastinitis." On T1 and T2 weighted MR

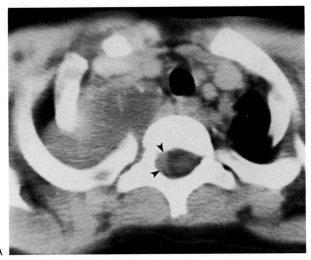

A

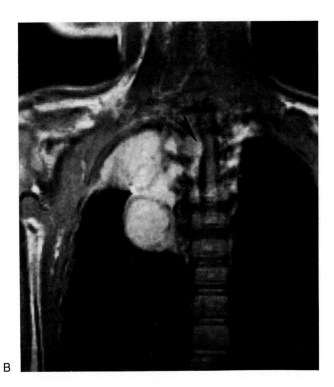

Figure 19–19. *Neuroblastoma with spinal invasion.* **A,** CT scan through the superior mediastinum in a 7-year-old boy shows a large soft mass in the right apex. Increased density is noted in the right side of the spinal canal (*arrowheads*). **B,** Balanced coronal MR image (2100/30) shows a high signal intensity paraspinal mass (*arrowhead*) displacing the spinal cord to the left. (From Siegel MJ, Nadel SN, Glazer HS, Sagel SS. Mediastinal lesions in children: Comparison of CT and MR. Radiology 1986; 160:241–244.)

B

images, adenopathy associated with fibrosing mediastinitis is of relatively low signal intensity with respect to muscle (Fig. 19–20).[55] MRI is equivalent to CT in defining the extent of adenopathy, but CT is superior at detecting calcifications and the effects of the fibrotic process on the bronchi. MRI, however, offers complementary information, particularly in evaluating vascular patency without the need for intravenous contrast medium.[55, 56]

Miscellaneous

Thymic Hyperplasia

True thymic hyperplasia, characterized by the presence of numerous, active, lymphoid germinal centers in both the medulla and cortex, can occur with red cell aplasia, with hyperthyroidism, or after chemotherapy.[57] On MRI, as on CT, the hyperplastic thymus may be of normal size or diffusely enlarged, especially in thickness. When enlarged, it is usually homogeneous, has a normal signal intensity for age, and retains its normal triangular or bilobed configuration (Fig. 19–21).

Rebound hyperplasia following chemotherapy may simulate recurrent or residual disease, especially in patients being treated for lymphoma. In general, if the patient is doing well clinically and shows no evidence of disease in the chest or elsewhere, the presumed diagnosis is rebound thymic overgrowth. Since this is a transient and benign phenomenon, our policy is to follow the size of the thymus with serial CT or MR

imaging. A gradual reduction in size of the thymus supports the diagnosis of hyperplasia as the cause of enlargement.

LUNG

Although MRI has proved useful in evaluating a number of mediastinal abnormalities, it has not been extensively used for the evaluation of pulmonary parenchymal disease. As previously noted, the major reasons are its poor spatial resolution compared with CT, and degradation by respiratory motion. The normal lungs have very little signal intensity since they contain only a small amount of solid tissue. On occasion, more intense linear structures corresponding to segments of vessels or bronchi can be seen in the lung parenchyma. Because there is so little signal in the lung parenchyma, abnormalities are easily recognized. However, since pulmonary fissures and segmental bronchi and vessels cannot be demonstrated in detail, it is often difficult on MRI to localize disease precisely.

Congenital Lung Lesions

Congenital lobar emphysema, cystic adenomatoid malformation, sequestration, and vascular malformations are lung anomalies resulting from abnormal bronchial or vascular development that can be demonstrated by MRI.

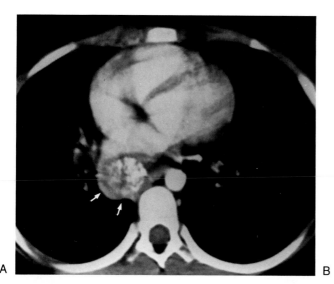

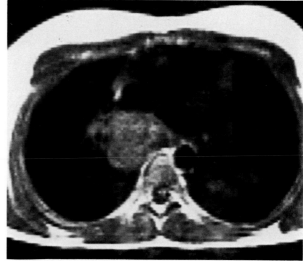

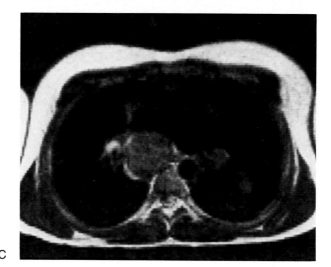

Figure 19–20. *Fibrosing mediastinitis due to histoplasmosis.* ***A,*** Postcontrast CT image in an 11-year-old boy demonstrates densely calcified subcarinal lymph nodes (*arrows*). ***B,*** On a T1 weighted (500/35) MR image the subcarinal nodal mass has a signal intensity slightly greater than that of muscle, but less than that of fat. Calcifications present on CT are not well appreciated on MRI. ***C,*** The subcarinal lymphadenopathy maintains an intermediate signal intensity on the T2 weighted (1500/90) image.

Congenital Lobar Emphysema

Congenital lobar emphysema is a condition characterized by hyperinflation of a lobe, or rarely several lobes. The etiology is unknown, but postulated causes of obstruction include localized deficiency, dysplasia or immaturity of cartilage, mucosal folds or webs, bronchial stenosis, extrinsic vascular compression, and extrinsic mass compression. Most patients with congenital lobar emphysema are symptomatic in the neonatal period, presenting with respiratory distress. Chest radiography typically shows hyperinflation of the lobe and mediastinal shift. The left upper lobe is involved in 43 percent of cases, the right middle lobe in 32 percent, the right upper lobe in 20 percent, and two lobes in 5 percent. The MR appearance is similar to that of conventional radiography, showing a hyperinflated lobe with attenuated vascularity and compression of adjacent lung (Fig. 19–22).

Cystic Adenomatoid Malformation

Congenital cystic adenomatoid malformation of the lung is a rare abnormality that is usually discovered shortly after birth because of respiratory distress. Its cause is unknown, but it is thought to result from failure of the respiratory portion of the lung to canalize and join with the bronchial portion. On pathologic section, the affected lobe is overdistended and composed of a cystic lesion, with an overgrowth of the terminal portion of the bronchial tree. Some bronchial communication is usually present and the blood supply is from the pulmonary circulation. Histologically, three types of cystic adenomatoid malformation have been described. Type I involves the presence of single and multiple large cysts, type II contains multiple small cysts, and type III is a large noncystic lesion. The lesion occurs with equal frequency in both lungs, and there is a tendency to upper lobe predominance. Chest radio-

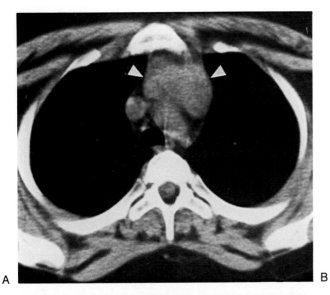

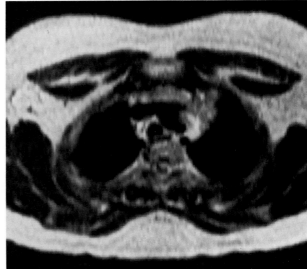

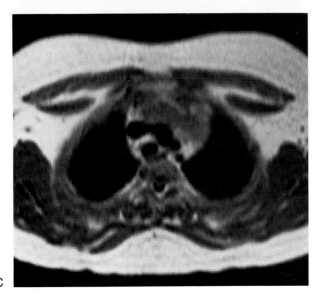

Figure 19–21. *Rebound thymic hyperplasia.* ***A,*** A 15-year-old boy treated 6 months previously with chemotherapy for osteosarcoma, now clinically well, has symmetric enlargement of both lobes of the thymus (*arrowheads*) on CT. (A previous CT of the mediastinum was normal.) ***B,*** T1 weighted (700/17) and ***C,*** T2 weighted (1800/90) images confirm enlargement of the thymus, which maintains its normal shape. The thickness of both lobes was 3.2 cm. On T1 and T2 weighted sequences the thymus is homogeneous and has a signal intensity greater than muscle but less than fat. The CT and MR findings in the clinical context were believed to be the result of rebound hyperplasia, and biopsy was not performed. A follow-up CT study 6 months later showed slight reduction in the size of the thymus and no other evidence of disease.

graphic examination of affected neonates typically shows the multilocular cystic mass causing mediastinal shift. On CT or MR imaging, cystic adenomatoid malformation appears as an intrapulmonary mass containing variable amounts of solid and cystic components (Fig. 19–23).

Sequestration

Pulmonary sequestration is a congenital mass of aberrant pulmonary tissue that has no normal connection with the tracheobronchial tree and is supplied by an anomalous artery, usually arising from the descending aorta in about 70 percent of cases and from the aortic arch, abdominal aorta, intercostal arteries, or bronchial arteries in the remaining 30 percent. The sequestered lung is termed "intralobar" when it lies within the visceral pleura and has pulmonary venous drainage. When it is outside the visceral pleura and has systemic or portal venous drainage, it is termed "extralobar." Sequestrations usually are located in the lower lobes, particularly the left lower lobe, but may arise in an upper lobe, interlobar fissure, mediastinum, abdomen, or pericardium. Rarely, bilateral sequestrations have been reported.

Sequestrations in children are usually detected because of superimposed infection of the sequestered segment. Chest radiography frequently shows a homogeneously dense mass or infiltrate in the medial and posterior portion of the lower lobe. If a communication with the bronchus develops secondary to collateral air drift through the pores of Kohn or from infection, the sequestration may appear cystic or may have an air fluid level. CT or MRI can provide a definite diagnosis of sequestration by demonstrating the anomalous ves-

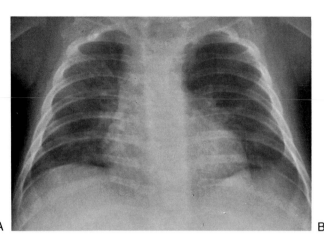

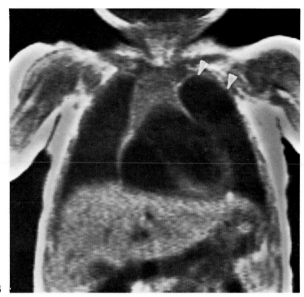

A   B

Figure 19–22. *Congenital lobar emphysema.* **A,** Posteroanterior chest radiograph shows a hyperlucent left upper lobe with attenuated vascularity. **B,** T1 weighted coronal MR image (500/26) demonstrates an emphysematous left upper lobe (*arrowheads*) with mild compression of adjacent parenchyma.

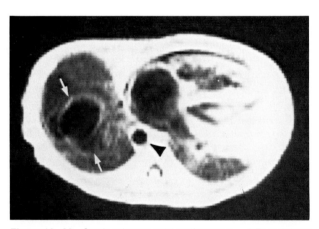

Figure 19–23. *Cystic adenomatoid malformation.* A T1 weighted axial MR image at the level of the heart shows a multilocular low signal intensity mass (*arrows*) in the right lung. The mass was high in signal intensity on T2 weighted images. Arrowhead, descending aorta (the patient also had a right aortic arch).

sel feeding the abnormal lung. The CT diagnosis of systemic blood flow is based on enhancement of the sequestration immediately after enhancement of the thoracic or abdominal aorta. On MRI the feeding vessels and draining veins appear as areas of signal void. The appearance of the parenchymal portion of the sequestration on CT and MRI depends on the presence or absence of aeration. When the sequestered segment communicates with the remainder of the lung, usually after being infected, it appears as an aerated lesion. When the sequestration does not communicate, it appears as a homogeneous density on CT and as an area of intermediate or high signal intensity on MRI.

Although MR imaging can detect sequestration, it usually is not required for the diagnosis. However, it can be useful in determining the extent of abnormality or in defining the anatomy of pulmonary arteries and veins and their relationships to the cardiac chambers. Thus, it can avoid the need for more invasive studies, such as angiography.[58]

Vascular Anomalies

Abnormalities of the pulmonary vessels are rare and more likely to be congenital than acquired. The most common abnormality is the pulmonary arteriovenous fistula (hemangioma), which represents an abnormal vascular connection between a pulmonary artery and vein as a result of abnormal capillary development. The abnormal communication is usually supplied by a single artery and drained by a single vein, but occasionally more complex fistulas with many feeding arteries and veins may be present. The typical radiographic appearance is that of a well-defined, somewhat lobulated mass, usually in the inner third of the lung, with linear branching shadows in close proximity. Confirmation of the vascular nature of the lesion can be obtained by dynamic CT or by MR imaging. However, if surgery or embolization is planned, arteriography is required, because multiple tiny lesions and the precise vascular anatomy of complex fistulas may not be visible on CT scans or MR images.

Tumor

Pulmonary Nodules

MRI can detect large parenchymal nodules, although it is less sensitive than CT in detecting nodules less than 1 cm in diameter because of its poorer spatial resolution.[59] In a study comparing CT and MR imaging for the detection of lung nodules, CT was more sensitive in detecting nodules near the diaphragm or chest wall. On the other hand, some pulmonary nodules situated close to blood vessels were better displayed by MR imaging.[59] Although MRI can demonstrate large pulmonary nodules, it is inferior to CT in defining their borders or the presence or absence of calcification. The presence of calcium in a nodule can be important in distinguishing a benign granuloma from a metastasis. CT remains the current method of choice for detecting pulmonary nodules.

Infection and Inflammation

Parenchymal Infiltrates

Although MRI cannot diagnose parenchymal disease as well as can CT, it can detect processes that fill alveoli or interstitial structures.[60-64] In patients with pulmonary consolidation or pneumonia, fluid replaces air within the alveoli. On T2 weighted images, the areas of pneumonic consolidation are high in signal intensity, presumably reflecting the high water content of the exudative process (Fig. 19–24). In general, the differences in signal intensity are not specific enough to permit confident diagnosis as to etiology, although pulmonary alveolar proteinosis may produce a relatively low signal intensity on T2 weighted images, presumably because the intraalveolar material contains high levels of protein and lipid rather than water.[63] Unfortunately, this appearance is not always present, and alveolar proteinosis can at times result in MR findings similar to those of other parenchymal diseases, limiting the usefulness of MRI in diagnosis.

A wide variety of disorders cause diffuse interstitial infiltrates, including cystic fibrosis, inflammatory disorders (viral pneumonia, tuberculosis, pneumocystis infection), hemorrhage, congenital lymphangiectasia, pulmonary edema, allergic reactions, and idiopathic disorders (histiocytosis). MRI can identify abnormality in these conditions, although it cannot provide a specific diagnosis. In some instances, the distribution of disease and the intensity with different pulse sequences may be helpful in differentiation.

In patients with cystic fibrosis, MRI is capable of demonstrating areas of peribronchial inflammation and mucoid impaction, both of which appear as branching tubular structures of high signal intensity. Associated atelectasis, bronchiectasis, hilar adenopathy, and enlarged central pulmonary vessels may also be depicted by MRI.[61, 62] Some disorders, such as pulmonary edema and histiocystosis (Fig. 19–25), have a uniform intensity on MRI. Pulmonary edema also has a perihilar distribution. By contrast, lymphangiectasia appears as coarse, irregular, streaky areas of increased signal intensity.

Pulmonary Abscesses

Lung abscesses in children result from the aspiration of material infected with anaerobic organisms, as a complication of bacterial pneumonia, or from superinfection of a chronic abscess cavity. Conventional radiography is an excellent means of diagnosing a lung abscess. However, CT or MRI is indicated when routine radiographs are equivocal and cavitation cannot be excluded, or to define the extent of the mass before drainage. A lung abscess is defined as a localized area of suppuration with destruction of underlying pulmonary parenchyma. On MRI the abscess appears as a round, thick-walled cavity with a nodular inner margin and an irregular wall that is often poorly separated from the adjacent consolidated parenchyma (Fig. 19–26). Because of its prolonged T1 and T2 relaxation times, the lesion is low in signal intensity on T1 weighted images and high on T2 weighted images.

Miscellaneous

Pulmonary Collapse

In most patients, MRI provides information similar to that obtainable from CT with respect to detecting lobar collapse and assessing the underlying medi-

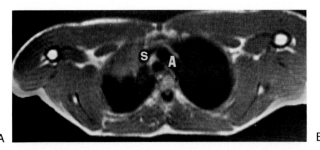
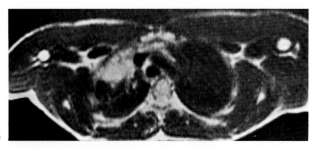

A   B

Figure 19–24. *Right upper lobe pneumonia.* ***A,*** T1 weighted MR image (500/26) shows a right upper lobe anterior segment infiltrate with signal intensity equal to that of muscle. ***B,*** On the T2 weighted image (2000/60) the pneumonic infiltrate is high in signal intensity, reflecting the underlying exudative process. s, Superior vena cava; A, aortic arch.

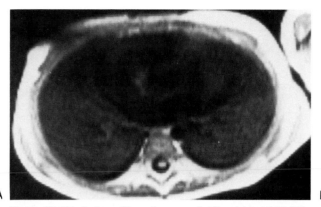

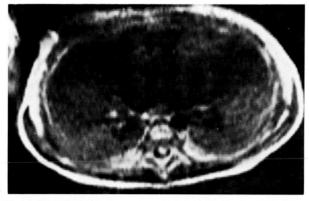

A | B

Figure 19–25. *Letterer-Siwe disease.* **A,** T1 weighted (500/30) and T2 weighted (2000/60) images show diffuse lung disease causing a homogeneous increase in the signal intensity of the lung fields. Instead of being low, the signal intensity in the lung fields is intermediate.

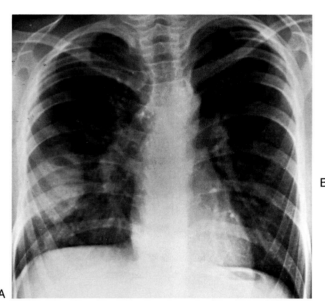

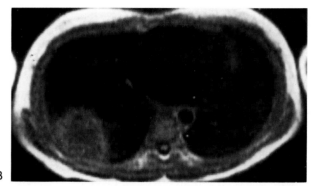

B

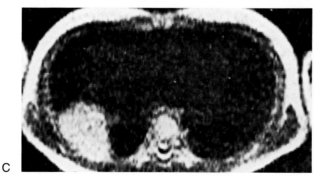

A

Figure 19–26. *Lung abscess.* **A,** Posteroanterior chest radiograph shows a cavitary lesion in the right lung. **B,** T1 weighted MR image (500/20) demonstrates a round, low signal intensity mass with irregular margins and acutely angled interfaces with the chest wall. **C,** On a relatively T2 weighted image (1000/60) the lung abscess is high in signal intensity.

C

astinum (Fig. 19–27). T2 weighted pulse sequences are best for distinguishing between mediastinal tumor and distal collapsed lung.[65] Collapsed lung usually has a higher signal intensity than that of the more proximal tumor, presumably because of the higher water content of atelectatic lung. Unfortunately, the water content of tumors and collapsed lung is variable, and differentiation may not always be possible by MRI.

Because of its better spatial resolution, the patency of the bronchi is usually evaluated better with CT than with MRI. On the latter, bronchial narrowing or ob-

struction may be overestimated because of the degradation of image quality by respiratory motion and poor spatial resolution. Moreover, in some patients, MRI may suggest bronchial narrowing when the bronchial lumen is essentially normal.[1, 28]

Radiation-induced Pulmonary Injury

Radiation-induced pulmonary changes seen on chest radiography, CT, or MRI vary depending on radiation dose, radiation portals, and the time elapsed since treatment. Acute changes usually are seen on

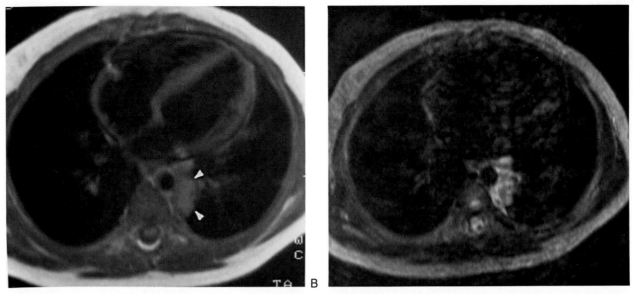

A   B

Figure 19–27. *Left lower lobe atelectasis.* **A,** On a T1 weighted (680/30) image the segment of collapsed lung (*arrowheads*) is of medium signal intensity. **B,** On a T2 weighted (2600/90) MR image the atelectatic lung increases in signal intensity, reflecting the higher water content of collapsed lung.

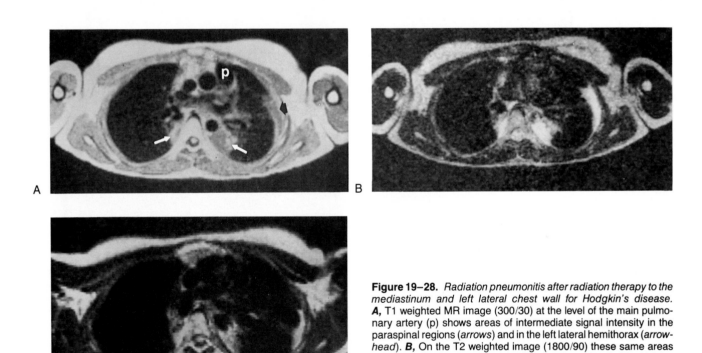

A   B

C

Figure 19–28. *Radiation pneumonitis after radiation therapy to the mediastinum and left lateral chest wall for Hodgkin's disease.* **A,** T1 weighted MR image (300/30) at the level of the main pulmonary artery (p) shows areas of intermediate signal intensity in the paraspinal regions (*arrows*) and in the left lateral hemithorax (*arrowhead*). **B,** On the T2 weighted image (1800/90) these same areas are high in signal intensity, approximating that of fat. **C,** T2 weighted image obtained 12 months later demonstrates little change in the relatively high signal intensity paraspinal areas. The patient was asymptomatic and showed no other clinical evidence of disease; the MR findings were presumed to be related to radiation pneumonitis.

plain chest radiographs 6 to 8 weeks after completion of therapy. These changes gradually become fibrotic and stabilize by 9 to 12 months after therapy is ended. Post-treatment changes can be seen somewhat earlier on CT, occasionally as early as 3 to 4 weeks after

treatment.[66] The earliest changes are patchy areas of consolidation conforming to the radiation ports. Gradually the margins of the infiltrates become more sharply demarcated, reflecting the development of fibrosis. Bronchiectasis and volume loss may be additional findings. On MRI, acute radiation changes may have a high signal intensity on T2 weighted images, reflecting a high water content. With time, the signal intensity decreases, reflecting fibrosis.[45]

The significant problem after radiation therapy is distinguishing fibrosis from residual or recurrent tumor. On CT, parenchymal changes inside the radiation ports suggest fibrosis, whereas abnormalities outside the radiation ports are considered suspicious for tumor. In the lung parenchyma, as in the mediastinum, MRI may be more helpful than CT in differentiating between post-treatment radiation fibrosis and residual or recurrent tumor. Radiation fibrosis has a low signal intensity on both T1 and T2 weighted images, whereas tumor demonstrates increased signal intensity on T2 weighted images. However, high signal intensity is a

nonspecific finding and can be seen with recurrent tumor, infection, and even radiation change, probably reflecting persistent inflammation (Fig. 19–28).[45]

PLEURA AND CHEST WALL

The normal pleural space is not seen by MRI, although subpleural fat within the chest wall can be easily visualized. MRI can be used to confirm the presence of a pleural lesion and its extent, but usually is not required, since in most cases CT can provide the necessary information. In addition, CT can be used to assess the pulmonary parenchyma. In some patients, MRI can be helpful in distinguishing between a parenchymal process and a pleural or extrapleural process. On MRI the features of parenchymal lesions are a rounded or oval shape, acute or abrupt angles at the interface with the chest wall, and poorly defined margins with the adjacent lung (Fig. 19–26). The MR features of pleural disease are a lenticular or crescentic shape, obtuse or tapering angles at the interface with the chest wall, and well-defined margins with adjacent lung, bone, and soft tissues (Fig. 19–29). Extrapleural lesions are lenticular in shape, have poorly defined margins, and have obtuse or tapering angles at the interface with the pleura.

MRI can be valuable in displaying the individual components of the chest wall, specifically muscular and fatty structures, including lymph nodes, vessels, and nerves. T1 weighted sequences are preferable for separating soft tissue from fat; T2 weighted sequences are better for distinguishing between tumor and muscle (Fig. 19–30). The chest wall is best evaluated by techniques that suppress respiratory motion. Surface coils can be used to improve resolution in superficial areas such as the neck, shoulder, and brachial plexus.

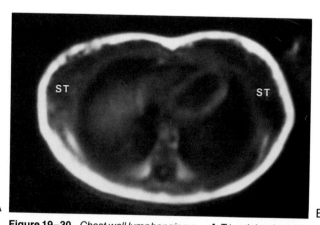

Figure 19–29. *Empyema.* T2 weighted MR image (2000/60) demonstrates a crescentic, high signal intensity right pleural fluid collection with well-defined margins. An area of signal void (*arrowhead*) within the pleural space represents air associated with the empyema.

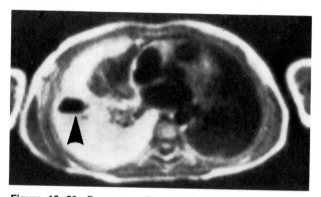

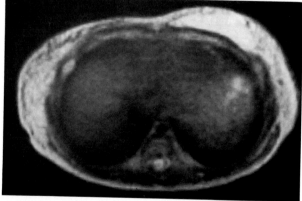

A   B

Figure 19–30. *Chest wall lymphangioma.* ***A,*** T1 weighted axial MR image (500/15) of the lower chest in a 1-year-old boy shows inhomogeneous thickening of the soft tissues (ST) of the anterior and lateral chest walls. Signal intensity of the infiltrated tissue is equal to that of paraspinal muscle. ***B,*** On the T2 weighted image (2100/90) the lymphangioma has a very bright signal intensity (greater than paraspinal muscle) because of increased water content, and contains internal septations.

REFERENCES

1. Siegel MJ, Nadel SN, Glazer HS, Sagel SS. Mediastinal lesions in children: comparison of CT and MR. Radiology 1986; 160:241–244.
2. Gamsu G, Webb WR, Sheldon P, et al. Nuclear magnetic resonance imaging of the thorax. Radiology 1983; 147:473–480.
3. Levitt RG, Glazer HS, Roper CL, et al. Magnetic resonance imaging of mediastinal and hilar masses: comparison with CT. AJR 1985; 145:9–14.
4. Webb WR, Gamsu G, Stark DD, et al. Evaluation of magnetic resonance sequences in imaging mediastinal tumors. AJR 1984; 143:723–727.
5. Webb WR, Moore EH. Differentiation of volume averaging and mass on magnetic resonance images of the mediastinum. Radiology 1985; 155:413–416.
6. Crooks LE, Barker B, Chang H, et al. Magnetic resonance imaging strategies for heart studies. Radiology 1984; 153:459–465.
7. Lanzer P, Barta C, Botvinick EH, et al. ECG-synchronized cardiac MR imaging: method and evaluation. Radiology 1985; 155:681–686.
8. Amparo EG, Higgins CB, Farmer D, et al. Gated MRI of cardiac and paracardiac masses: initial experience. AJR 1984; 143:1151–1156.
9. Lanzer P, Botvinick EH, Schiller NB, et al. Cardiac imaging using gated magnetic resonance. Radiology 1984; 150:121–127.
10. Lieberman JM, Alfidi RJ, Nelson AD, et al. Gated magnetic resonance imaging of the normal and diseased heart. Radiology 1984; 152:465–470.
11. Lewis CE, Prato FS, Drost DJ, Nicholson RL. Comparison of respiratory triggering and gating techniques for the removal of respiratory artifacts in MR imaging. Radiology 1986; 160:803–810.
12. Ehman RL, McNamara MT, Pallack M, et al. Magnetic resonance imaging with respiratory gating: techniques and advantages. AJR 1984; 143:1175–1182.
13. Runge VM, Clanton JA, Partain CL, James AE. Respiratory gating in magnetic resonance imaging at 0.5 Tesla. Radiology 1984; 151:521–523.
14. Bailes DR, Gilderdale DJ, Bydder GM, et al. Respiratory ordered phase encoding (ROPE): a method for reducing respiratory motion artifacts in MR imaging. J Comput Assist Tomogr 1985; 9:835–838.
15. Higgins CB, Stark D, McNamara M, et al. Multiplane magnetic resonance imaging of the heart and major vessels. Studies in normal volunteers. AJR 1984; 142:661–667.
16. O'Donovan PB, Ross JS, Sivak ED, et al. Magnetic resonance imaging of the thorax. The advantages of coronal and sagittal planes. AJR 1984; 143:1183–1188.
17. Ross JS, O'Donovan BP, Paushter DM. Tracheobronchial tree and pulmonary arteries: MR imaging using electronic axial rotation. Radiology 1986; 160:839–841.
18. Webb WR, Gamsu G, Crooks LE. Multisection sagittal and coronal magnetic resonance imaging of the mediastinum and hila. Radiology 1984; 150:475–478.
19. Webb WR, Jensen BG, Gamsu G, et al. Coronal magnetic resonance imaging of the chest. Normal and abnormal. Radiology 1984; 153:729–735.
20. Bradley WG, Waluch V. Blood flow: magnetic resonance imaging. Radiology 1985; 154:443–450.
21. McMurdo KK, deGeer G, Webb WR, Gamsu G. Normal and occluded mediastinal veins: MR imaging. Radiology 1986; 159:33–38.
22. Siegel MJ, Glazer HS, Wiener JI, Molina PL. Normal and abnormal thymus in childhood: MR imaging. Radiology 1989; 172:367–371.
23. deGeer G, Webb WR, Gamsu G. Normal thymus. Assessment with MR and CT. Radiology 1986; 158:313–317.
24. Rollins NK, Currarino G. MR imaging of posterior mediastinal thymus. J Comput Assist Tomogr 1988; 12:518–520.
25. Aronberg DJ, Glazer HS, Sagel SS. MRI and CT of the mediastinum: comparisons, controversies and pitfalls. Radiol Clin North Am 1985; 23:439–448.
26. Brasch RC, Gooding CA, Lallemand DP, Wesbey GE. Magnetic resonance imaging of the thorax in childhood. Radiology 1984; 150:463–467.
27. Fletcher BD, Dearborn DG, Mulopulos GP. MR imaging in infants with airway obstruction. Preliminary observations. Radiology 1986; 160:245–249.
28. Webb WR, Gamsu G, Stark DD, Moore EH. Magnetic resonance imaging of the normal and abnormal pulmonary hila. Radiology 1984; 152:89–94.
29. Quint LE, Glazer GM, Orringer MB. Esophageal imaging by MR and CT: study of normal anatomy and neoplasms. Radiology 1985; 156:727–731.
30. Sechtem U, Tscholakoff D, Higgins CB. MRI of the normal pericardium. AJR 1986; 147:239–244.
31. Stark DD, Higgins CB, Lanzer P, et al. Magnetic resonance imaging of the pericardium: normal and pathologic findings. Radiology 1984; 150:469–474.
32. Naidich DP, Rumancik WM, Ettenger NA, et al. Congenital anomalies of the lungs in adults. MR diagnosis. AJR 1988; 151:13–19.
33. von Schulthess GK, McMurdo K, Tscholakoff D, et al. Mediastinal masses: MR imaging. Radiology 1986; 158:289–296.
34. Nakata H, Sato Y, Nakayama T, et al. Bronchogenic cyst with high CT numbers. Analysis of contents. J Comput Assist Tomogr 1986; 10:360–362.
35. Pilla TJ, Wolverson MK, Sundaram M, et al. CT evaluation of cystic lymphangiomas of the mediastinum. Radiology 1982; 144:841–842.
36. Siegel MJ, Glazer HS, St. Amour TE, Rosenthal DD. Lymphangiomas in children. MR imaging. Radiology 1989; 170:467–470.
37. Bower RJ, Kiesewetter WB. Mediastinal masses in infants and children. Arch Surg 1977; 112:1003–1009.
38. Suzuki M, Takashima T, Itoh H, et al. Computed tomography of mediastinal teratomas. J Comput Assist Tomogr 1983; 7:74–76.
39. Levitt RG, Husband JE, Glazer HS. CT of primary germ-cell tumors of the mediastinum. AJR 1984; 142:73–78.
40. Castellino RA. Hodgkin disease: practical concepts for the diagnostic radiologist. Radiology 1986; 159:305–310.
41. Khan A, Herman PG. Intrathoracic manifestations of lymphoma. Seminars US, CT, MR 1986; 7:18–42.
42. Neuman CH, Parker BR, Castellino RA. Hodgkin's disease and the non-Hodgkin lymphomas. In: Bragg DG, Rubin P, Youker JE, eds. Oncologic Imaging. New York: Pergamon Press, 1984: 477–500.
43. St. Amour TE, Siegel MJ, Glazer HS, Nadel SN. CT appearances of the normal and abnormal thymus in childhood. J Comput Assist Tomogr 1987; 11:645–650.
44. Nyman RS, Rehn SM, Glimelius BLG, et al. Residual mediastinal masses in Hodgkin disease: prediction of size with MR imaging. Radiology 1989; 170:435–440.
45. Glazer HS, Lee JKT, Levitt RG, et al. Radiation fibrosis: differentiation from recurrent tumor by MR imaging. Radiology 1985; 156:721–726.
46. Brown LR, Muhm JR, Sheedy PF II, et al. The value of computed tomography in myasthenia gravis. AJR 1983; 140:31–35.
47. Batra P, Hermann C Jr, Mulder D. Mediastinal imaging in myasthenia gravis: correlation of chest radiography, CT, MR, and surgical findings. AJR 1987; 148:515–519.
48. Gamsu G, Stark DD, Webb WR, et al. Magnetic resonance imaging of benign mediastinal masses. Radiology 1984; 151:709–713.
49. Scatarige JC, Fishman EK, Zerhouni EA, Siegelman SS. Transdiaphragmatic extension of invasive thymoma. AJR 1985; 144:31–35.
50. Zerhouni EA, Scott WW Jr, Baker RR, et al. Invasive thymomas: diagnosis and evaluation by computed tomography. J Comput Assist Tomogr 1982; 6:92–100.
51. Lindfors KK, Meyer JE, Dedrick CG, et al. Thymic cysts in mediastinal Hodgkin disease. Radiology 1985; 156:37–41.

52. Kumar AJ, Kuhajda FP, Martinez CR, et al. CT of extracranial nerve sheath tumors. J Comput Assist Tomogr 1983; 7:857–865.

53. Resjo IM, Harwood-Nash DC, Fitz CR, Chung S. CT metrizamide myelography for intraspinal and paraspinal neoplasms in infants and children. AJR 1979; 132:367–372.

54. Siegel MJ, Jamroz GA, Glazer HS, Abramson CL. MR imaging of intraspinal extension of neuroblastoma. J Comput Assist Tomogr 1986; 10:593–595.

55. Rholl KS, Levitt RG, Glazer HS. Magnetic resonance imaging of fibrosing mediastinitis. AJR 1985; 145:255–259.

56. Farmer DW, Moore E, Amparo E, et al. Calcific fibrosing mediastinitis: demonstration of pulmonary vascular obstruction by magnetic resonance imaging. AJR 1984; 143:1189–1191.

57. Choyke PL, Zeman RK, Gootenberg JE, et al. Thymic atrophy and growth in response to chemotherapy: CT evaluation. AJR 1987; 149:269–272.

58. Pessar ML, Soulen RL, Kan JS, et al. MRI demonstration of pulmonary sequestration. Pediatr Radiol 1988; 18:229–231.

59. Muller NL, Gamsu G, Webb WR. Pulmonary nodules: detection using magnetic resonance and computed tomography. Radiology 1985; 155:687–690.

60. Cohen MD, Eigen H, Scott PH, et al. Magnetic resonance imaging of inflammatory lung disorders: preliminary studies in children. Pediatr Pulmonol 1986; 2:211–217.

61. Fiel SB, Friedman AC, Caroline DF, et al. Magnetic resonance imaging in young adults with cystic fibrosis. Chest 1987; 91:181–184.

62. Gooding CA, Lallemand DP, Brasch RC. Nuclear magnetic resonance imaging of cystic fibrosis. J Pediatr 1984; 105:384–388.

63. Moore EH, Webb WR, Muller N, Sollitto R. MRI of pulmonary airspace disease. Experimental model and preliminary clinical results. AJR 1986; 146:1123–1128.

64. Schmidt HC, Tsay DG, Higgins CB. Pulmonary edema: an MR study of permeability and hydrostatic types in animals. Radiology 1986; 158:297–302.

65. Tobler J, Levitt RG, Glazer HS, et al. Differentiation of proximal bronchogenic carcinoma from postobstructive lobar collapse by magnetic resonance imaging. Comparison with computed tomography. Invest Radiol 1987; 22:538–543.

66. Libshitz HI, Shuman LS. Radiation-induced pulmonary change: CT findings. J Comput Assist Tomogr 1984; 8:15–19.

Gastrointestinal System

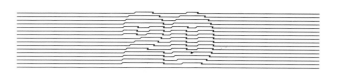

MERVYN D. COHEN, M.B., Ch.B.

NORMAL ANATOMY

With magnetic resonance imaging, all the organs of the abdomen can be seen. The clarity and extent of the visualization vary from patient to patient. The liver and the spleen are well seen in virtually every patient; the pancreas is less well seen and the bowel loops are visualized to a variable extent. The shape and contour of the various organs are not distorted and the organs appear as one would expect from gross anatomic and other imaging studies. One difference between MRI and other imaging modalities is the ability of the former to display the abdominal organs in any imaging plane. We are accustomed to the appearance of the various abdominal organs on CT and ultrasonography and need to learn their normal appearance when different imaging planes are used with magnetic resonance. As mentioned above, we are accustomed to the size, shape, and contour of the abdominal organs on non-MR imaging. We are also accustomed to a predictable appearance of the internal structures of each of the organs on CT, ultrasound, or barium studies. With non-MR imaging this appearance is fairly predictable and constant. With MRI the normal appearance of each of the organs varies, depending on the pulse sequence used. For the intestine the appearance also varies greatly, depending on the physical and chemical nature of the contents of the bowel lumen. The signal intensity obtained from the abdominal organs depends on their T1 and T2 relaxation times. Of all the abdominal organs, the liver normally has the shortest T1 and T2 relaxation times. The pancreas, spleen, renal cortex, and renal medulla, in that order, tend to have increasing T1 and T2 relaxation times. On most pulse sequences a long T1 relaxation time results in low signal intensity on T1 weighted images, and a long T2 relaxation time results in high signal intensity on T2 weighted images.

611

Liver

There is good contrast differentiation between liver and adjacent tissues so that, except where motion degrades image quality, the liver is well visualized by MRI in all children (Figs. 20–1 to 20–3). The liver parenchyma has relatively short T1 and T2 relaxation times, and therefore appears of greater intensity than the spleen on T1 weighted images and lower intensity than the spleen on T2 weighted images (Figs. 20–1, 20–2).[1] The overall texture of the liver appears relatively homogeneous. Intrahepatic vessels (Fig. 20–4) are usually well identified, appearing with a very low or absent signal on most spin-echo pulse sequences. The main portal vein and its right and left branches and the right, middle, and left hepatic veins can be traced along their course through the liver. On some field-echo pulse sequences, and in certain other situations, the vessels appear of very bright signal.[2] The intrahepatic bile ducts usually are not seen, and the falciform ligament usually is not visible.[2]

Gallbladder

The gallbladder is well seen (Fig. 20–5). The appearance of normal bile in the gallbladder changes, depending on whether the bile is fresh or not. With fast-

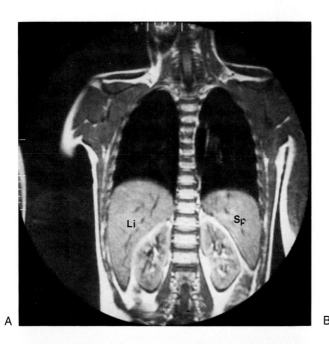

A

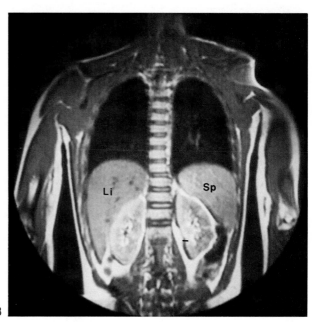

B

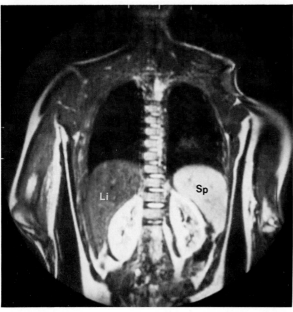

C

Figure 20–1. *Normal liver and spleen: effect of alteration of pulse sequence. Series of coronal abdominal images all obtained at 1.5T.* ***A,*** *800/260. The liver intensity is similar to that of spleen. Both organs are very well identified.* ***B,*** *1500/20. On this slightly more spin-density weighted image the spleen is of a little greater intensity than the liver.* ***C,*** *1500/70. On this T2 weighted image the spleen is of much greater signal intensity than the liver. Normal spleen has a longer T1 and longer T2 relaxation time than normal liver. Li, Liver; Sp, spleen.*

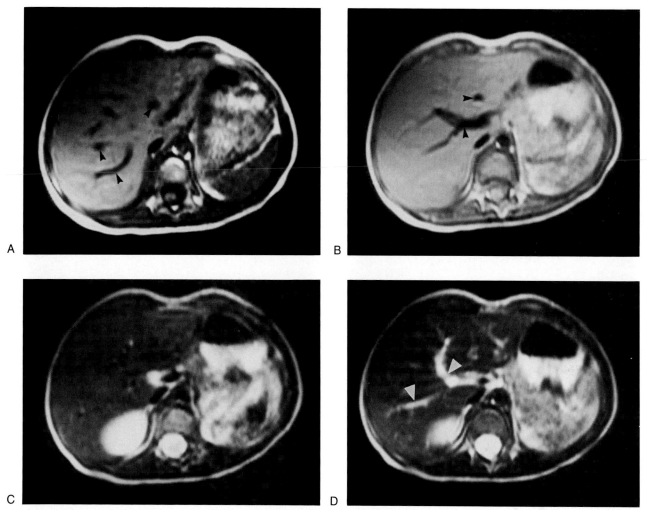

Figure 20–2. *Normal liver: effect of alterations of imaging pulse sequence. All images are transverse hepatic images obtained at 1.5T.* ***A,*** *T1 weighted image (500/16). The liver is of homogeneous intensity. Liver vessels (arrowheads) are seen as areas of low signal intensity owing to flow void.* ***B,*** *2000/20. Once again the liver appears of homogeneous intensity with vessels (arrowheads) appearing as regions of low signal.* ***C,*** *T2 weighted image (2000/80). The liver is of lower intensity than on the T1 and spin-density weighted images. It is also slightly less homogeneous in appearance. Blood vessels (arrowheads) again appear of low intensity owing to flow void.* ***D,*** *T2 weighted image with motion suppression (MAST) technique (2000/80). On this T2 weighted image the liver is of low intensity. This particular MAST technique causes the vessels (arrowheads) to appear of high signal intensity. The major vessels are clearly identified as vessels. Smaller branches of the vessels, particularly when seen end on, would be very difficult to differentiate from lesions such as inflammation or tumor.*

ing, bile becomes concentrated, as water is removed from it. The normal gallbladder absorbs 90 percent of the water content of the bile within 4 hours after the gallbladder is filled. Fresh bile has a long T1 relaxation time and appears of low signal intensity on T1 weighted images, whereas concentrated bile has a short T1 relaxation time and appears of high signal intensity on T1 and T2 weighted images, because of water binding by macromolecules.[3] In gallbladder disease bile is not concentrated, so even with fasting a low signal is obtained from the bile on T1 weighted images. The extrahepatic bile ducts may be visualized but are not seen in all patients. The best visualization of the extrahepatic

bile ducts is obtained using T2 pulse sequences in the transverse imaging plane.[4]

Spleen

As with the liver, the spleen is usually well visualized by MRI in all patients, unless there are motion artifacts. The spleen outline is smooth. The internal signal intensity is moderately homogeneous. The T1 and T2 relaxation times of the spleen show some variation[5] but are generally between 40 and 60 percent longer than those obtained from the liver.[6] This means that on T1

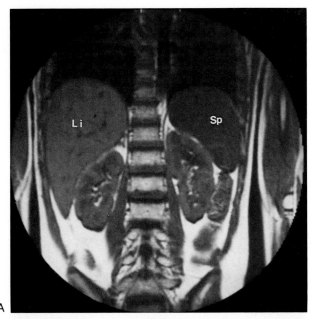
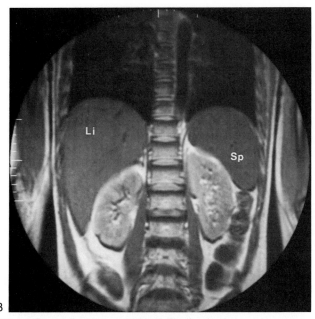

A   B

Figure 20–3. *Normal liver and spleen. Coronal images obtained at 1.5T.* ***A,*** T1 weighted image (500/16). The liver is of stronger signal intensity than the spleen. ***B,*** Spin-density image (2000/20). The liver and spleen are of similar intensity. Li, Liver; Sp, spleen.

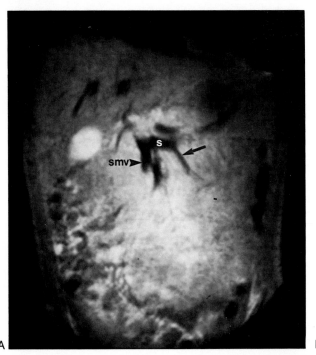
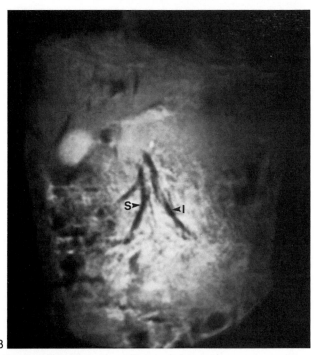

A   B

Figure 20–4. *Normal portal and mesenteric vessels.* ***A,*** Coronal MR image (2000/20). The splenic vein (s) and its confluence with the superior mesenteric vein (smv) are clearly identified. The inferior mesenteric vein (*arrow*) is also nicely identified. ***B,*** Coronal image (2000/20). This image is obtained immediately anterior to ***A.*** It shows the superior mesenteric vein (S) and the inferior mesenteric vein (I).

weighted images the spleen is of lower signal intensity than the liver, and on T2 weighted images is of higher signal intensity than the liver (Fig. 20–1). In some normal patients, the T2 relaxation time of the spleen may be so long that on strongly T2 weighted images the signal intensity from the spleen is similar to that of adjacent fat, and this may partly obscure the contour of the spleen. The splenic vein and its internal branches within the spleen are usually well visualized in almost all patients.

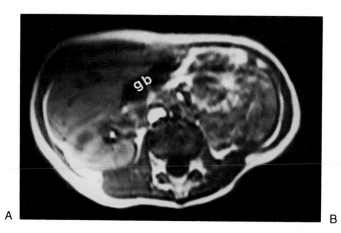

A

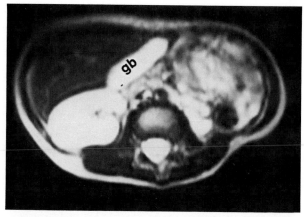

B

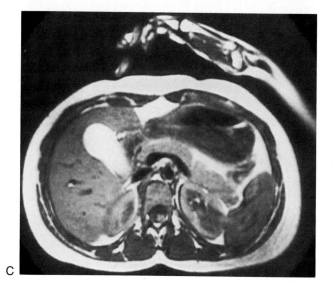

C

Figure 20–5. *Normal gallbladder.* **A,** Transverse T1 weighted MR image through the gallbladder in a nonfasting patient (500/16). The gallbladder (gb) appears of very low signal intensity. **B,** T2 weighted MR image obtained at the same level as **A** (200/80). The gallbladder now appears of very high signal intensity. **C,** Transverse T1 image (600/30) in a fasting patient. The gallbladder is of strong signal intensity.

Pancreas

The signal intensity obtained from normal pancreas tends to be between that of liver and spleen on both T1 and T2 weighted pulse sequences, but there is a definite variation between patients (Figs. 20–6, 20–7). At 0.35T Tscholakoff and colleagues found little signal difference between normal pancreas and liver.[7] At 1.5T Piccirillo and colleagues found signal intensity of pancreas to be greater than that of liver but less than that of spleen in most patients on T2 pulse sequences (Fig. 20–7).[8]

The transverse plane is best for imaging the pancreas. The pancreas is much less readily identified than the liver or spleen. The major factors compromising pancreatic visualization are the difficulty in separating the pancreas from adjacent loops of bowel, and motion artifact.[8] Also, in some patients the signal intensity from the pancreas on T2 weighted images is similar to that of adjacent fat, obscuring definition of the margins of the pancreas. The pancreatic duct usually is not identifiable. Because the pancreas is often so difficult to see, we must use several excellent landmarks to help us localize it. The second part of the duodenum, the common bile duct, the portal vein, and the gastroduodenal artery are landmarks for the head of the pancreas. The splenic vein is the landmark for the body and tail of the pancreas, with the vein lying posterior to the pancreas (Fig. 20–6).

Bowel

Visualization of the stomach, duodenum, and small and large bowel is extremely variable. In many patients the walls of individual loops of bowel cannot be identified at all. Poor visualization of the bowel is due to motion artifact from respiration and peristalsis, and also to the fact that the bowel contents may be of similar T1 and T2 relaxation times to adjacent tissues (Fig. 20–8). If air is present, the lumen of the air-filled loops of bowel is well defined (Figs. 20–9, 20–10). The retroperitoneal segments of the bowel are better visualized than intraperitoneal segments. This is because they are farther away from artifacts produced by anterior abdominal wall motion, and also because retro-

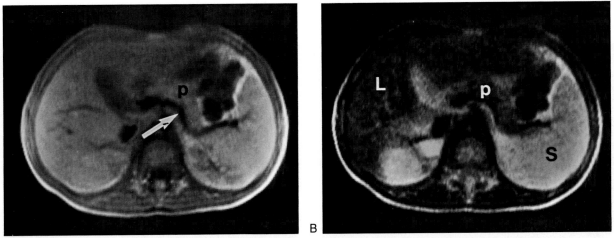

Figure 20–6. *Normal pancreas. In this patient, scanned at 0.15T, the pancreas is of similar intensity to liver on both T1 and T2 weighted images.* ***A,*** Transverse MR T1 weighted image (500/30). The pancreas (p) is seen anterior to the splenic vein (*arrow*). ***B,*** Transverse T2 weighted MR image (1500/60). The pancreas (p) is of similar intensity to liver (L). Note that both the liver and the pancreas are of much lower intensity than the spleen (S).

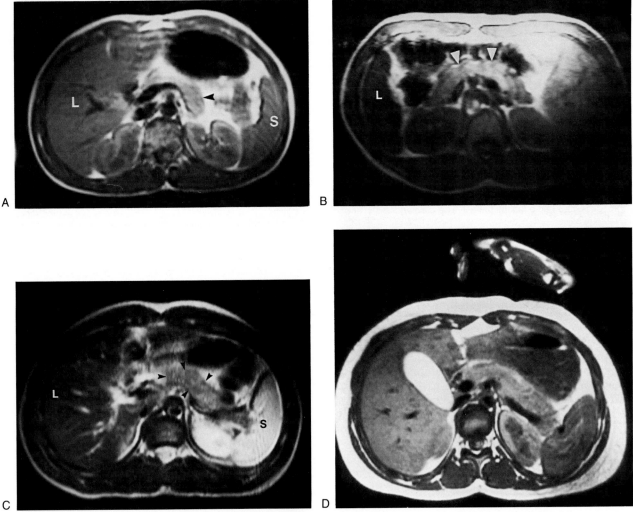

Figure 20–7. *Normal pancreas in different patients with different imaging techniques at 1.5T.* ***A,*** Transverse image (600/20). The tail of the pancreas (*arrowhead*) is of fairly homogeneous intensity, slightly greater than that of either liver (L) or spleen (S). ***B,*** 500/16. This image was obtained using a surface coil. Most of the pancreas (*arrowheads*) is well visualized. It is of moderately homogeneous appearance and of signal intensity slightly higher than that of liver (L). ***C,*** Transverse MR image (2000/80). On this strongly T2 weighted image the pancreas (*arrowheads*) has a slightly nonhomogeneous granular appearance. The signal intensity is less than that of fat and spleen (S) but greater than that of liver (L). ***D,*** Transverse T1 MR image (700/30). The pancreas is well seen. It is of slightly higher signal than that of liver, spleen, or fluid in the stomach.

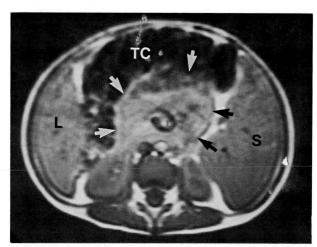

Figure 20–8. *Normal bowel mimics retroperitoneal lymphadenopathy.* T1 weighted transverse abdominal MR image (450/26). The liver (L), spleen (S), and transverse colon (TC) are all well seen. There is an ill-defined region of moderate intensity (*arrows*) seen in the midabdomen anterior to the spine and great vessels. These are in fact normal fluid-filled loops of bowel with strong signal intensity, presumably the result of ingestion of food containing either fat or paramagnetic ions that have shortened T1 relaxation time. They cannot be differentiated from diffuse retroperitoneal lymphadenopathy.

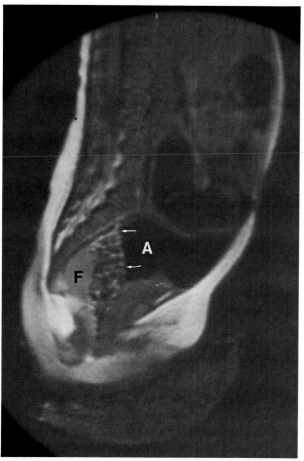

Figure 20–10. *Normal rectal feces.* Sagittal midline image with the patient supine (800/26). On this T1 weighted image three distinct substances are seen within the rectum, separated from each other by sharply defined horizontal lines. The anterior substance is of very low intensity and represents air (A). It is separated by an air fluid level (*arrows*) from bubbly fecal material of mixed low and high signal intensity. Behind this is more homogeneous fecal material of intermediate signal intensity, probably representing semisolid feces (F), not mixed with any air.

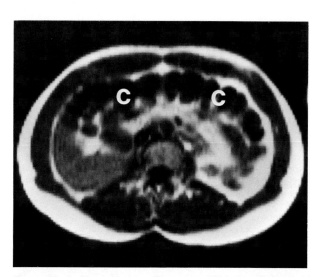

Figure 20–9. *Normal colon.* Transverse MR image (500/30). Visualization of the bowel on MR images varies considerably. When the bowel lumen contains air, and when there is fat surrounding the bowel, as in this patient, the bowel can be beautifully seen. The transverse colon (C) in this patient is very well identified.

peritoneal fat helps outline the contour of the bowel loops (Fig. 20–11). Signal intensity from bowel content is incredibly variable (Figs. 20–11 to 20–14). Air produces a very low signal on all pulse sequences. Simple fluid is of low signal on T1 and high signal on T2 pulse sequences. Fecal material has an extremely varied appearance that is completely unpredictable (Figs. 20–10, 20–12, 20–14). Foods contain many natural

contrast agents that also affect signal intensity from the bowel contents. For example, milk that contains a relative high content of fat causes strong signal from the bowel lumen on both T1 and T2 pulse sequences. Many other food substances contain iron, which exerts a paramagnetic effect, reducing T1 and T2 relaxation times (Fig. 20–12). The content of protein, water, and many other minerals affects signal intensity. The bowel contents range from homogeneous to very nonhomogeneous in appearance.

The anatomy of the anal canal and distal rectum is exquisitely demonstrated by MRI. In normal patients the bowel lies symmetrically in the midline, passing through the levator ani muscle. The levator muscle blends with the muscles of the internal sphincter, and these muscles appear of relatively low intensity on T1 pulse sequences.

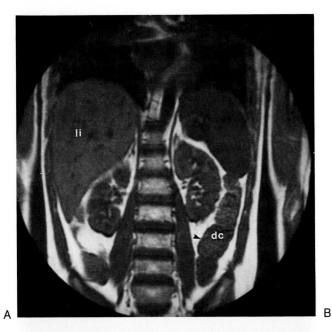

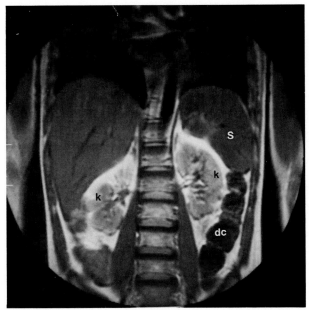

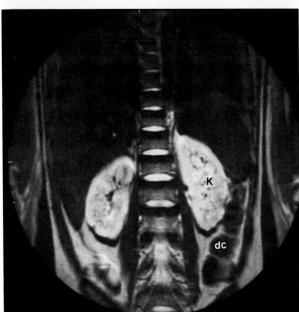

Figure 20–11. *Normal appearance of bowel loops. These three images show the descending colon, which is very well outlined by retroperitoneal fat.* **A,** Coronal T1 image (500/16). The descending colon (dc) is of heterogeneous appearance with predominant signal intensity slightly greater than that of liver (li). Very low-intensity areas probably represent air, which is mixed with feces. The vertical lucency (*arrowhead*) to the left of the bowel content is not the bowel wall, but a chemical shift artifact. **B,** Image obtained in the same plane as A (2000/20). On this spin-density image the signal intensity from the fecal material in the descending colon (dc) is of lower intensity than on A. This probably indicates the solid or semisolid nature of the material, rather than the presence of fluid feces. k, Kidney; S, spleen. **C,** Strongly T2 weighted image (2000/70). The appearance of the fecal material in the descending colon (dc) is now of even lower signal intensity than on the previous images. K, kidney. It must be emphasized that the appearance of the content of the bowel is extremely variable.

Major Abdominal Blood Vessels

Without the need for any injection of contrast agents, most major abdominal arteries and veins are well seen on MR images (Fig. 20–15). They appear of low signal intensity on most, but not all, pulse sequences (see the discussion of flow in the chapter on Modifying and Interpreting the MRI) (Figs. 20–4, 20–16).

CONGENITAL DISORDERS

Duplication Cysts

Duplication cysts can occur at any site in the bowel. They are most common in the small bowel; the esophagus is the second most common site (Fig. 20–17). These cysts usually do not communicate with the adjacent bowel lumen, although they may do so. The cysts

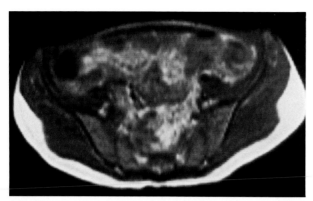

Figure 20–12. *Normal feces.* Transverse T1 MR image (500/30). This T1 weighted image shows high signal intensity from the bowel contents in the distal loops of small bowel. This high signal must be due to the presence of paramagnetic substances within ingested food. The appearance of bowel is extremely variable on MR images.

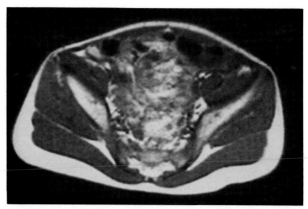

Figure 20–13. Normal variation in the appearance of bowel. Distal loops of small bowel are seen in the pelvis. The signal is very mixed, but predominantly strong. The wall of the individual loops of bowel cannot be clearly defined, giving an overall very heterogeneous appearance. This appearance should not be confused with tumor, inflammation, or hemangioma.

may contain ectopic gastric or pancreatic tissue, and because of this, bleeding ulceration or perforation may occur. The cysts can be multiple. Occasionally, duplication cysts arise as a result of poor separation of bowel from the primitive neurenteric canal. These particular cysts commonly occur in the chest and are associated with vertebral anomalies. Duplication cysts may be diagnosed as an incidental finding or may produce symptoms from mass effect or ectopic bowel mucosa (bleeding or pain). Clinically a mass may be detected.

Plain film and barium studies show a mass with indentation and displacement of adjacent segments of bowel. Ultrasonography shows a cystic mass, but the precise tissue of origin cannot be defined; this modality, for example, cannot differentiate a duplication cyst from a mesenteric cyst. CT usually provides little additional information to that provided by ultrasonography.[9, 10] On MRI the cysts are well seen.[9, 10] The cyst wall appears of low intensity,[9] but if infected may appear of high signal intensity on T2 images.[10] The cyst fluid

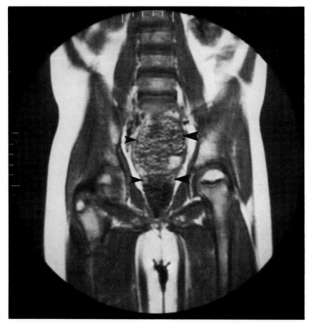

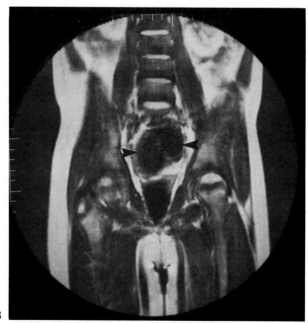

A   B

Figure 20–14. *Normal feces.* ***A,*** Coronal T1 weighted image (800/26). Fecal material (*arrowheads*) is seen in the rectum, of mottled mixed low and high density. ***B,*** Coronal T2 weighted image (1700/90) obtained at the same level as ***A.*** Most of the fecal material (*arrowheads*) now appears of low intensity. Its appearance is therefore consistent with relatively short T1 and also short T2 relaxation times.

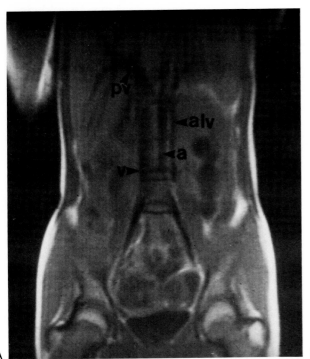

A

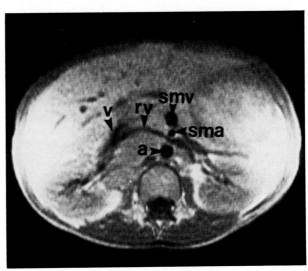

B

Figure 20–15. *Normal abdominal vessels.*   Without the need for any intravenous contrast agent, MRI identifies the major abdominal vessels with great clarity. *A,* Coronal MR image (550/30) demonstrating the inferior vena cava (v), the abdominal aorta (a), the main portal vein (pv) with its main branches, and the ascending lumbar vein on the left side (alv). *B,* Transverse MR image (500/30) demonstrating the aorta (a), superior mesenteric artery (sma), superior mesenteric vein (smv), left renal vein (rv), and inferior vena cava (v). Note that the left renal vein passes between the aorta and the superior mesenteric artery. The inferior vena cava has been displaced by a tumor.

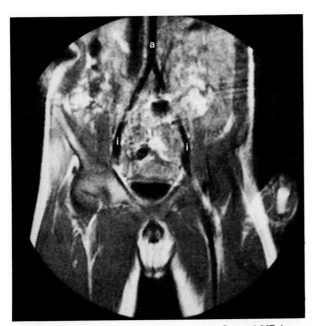

Figure 20–16. *Normal abdominal vessels.* Coronal MR image (700/26). Without any requirement for injection of contrast agents, MRI demonstrates normal abdominal vessels extremely well. This image shows the inferior part of the abdominal aorta (a) and its bifurcation into the right and left common iliac arteries (i).

appears of very high signal intensity on T2 weighted images. On T1 weighted images the appearance of the fluid varies. Simple fluid is of very low signal, infection causes a slightly higher signal, and hemorrhage may cause a strong signal. Inflammatory debris may cause the appearance of a fluid-fluid level within the cyst.[10] Continuity of the cyst with the adjacent bowel wall may be demonstrated on MRI (Fig. 20–17).[10] In this regard the ability of MRI to image in multiple planes is a definite advantage.

For the demonstration of ectopic gastric mucosa within the wall of a duplication cyst, nuclear scanning with technetium pertechnetate is the modality of choice. MRI probably has no role in this.

Treatment of symptomatic or large duplication cysts consists of simple surgical excision.

Choledochal Cysts

Choledochal cysts (Fig. 20–18) are focal areas of dilatation of the biliary duct system. The most common type is a tubular dilatation of the common bile duct. It may extend proximally to involve the origin of the right and left hepatic duct. Occasionally the cyst is a diverticulum arising from the common bile duct. The etiology of choledochal cysts is believed to be an anatomic abnormality of the lower end of the common bile duct, which permits reflux of pancreatic juices into the duct. Clinical symptoms include pain, jaundice, and an abdominal mass. MRI reveals a right upper quadrant mass lesion. The diagnosis of a choledochal cyst on MRI is suggested by an elongated or oval shape to the cyst, by a location in the expected site of the biliary ducts,[3] and by a finding that the signal intensity from the bile in the cyst is the same as that from bile in the gallbladder on all pulse sequences.[11] The diagnosis can be confidently confirmed by demonstrating continuity of the cyst with adjacent normal bile ducts.[3]

Plain film radiographs are of little help in making the diagnosis. Ultrasonography identifies a right upper quadrant cystic mass. If continuity with adjacent bile ducts can be identified, the diagnosis is confirmed. If not, the diagnosis can be readily made and confirmed by nuclear medicine studies with technetium-labeled DISIDA; provided the liver is functioning, the radioisotope will be seen to accumulate both within normal ducts and within the choledochal cyst. An occasional choledochal cyst occurs with biliary atresia, and in these patients the radioisotope cannot reach the cyst. MRI probably has little role to play in routine evaluation of patients with suspected choledochal cyst. However, the cyst may be found incidentally on MRI of the abdomen for other reasons, and its appearance should therefore be recognized.

Treatment of choledochal cyst consists of surgical excision.

Congenital Diaphragmatic Hernia

Morgagni hernia (Fig. 20–20) is a result of failure of the anterior aspect of the diaphragm to fuse to the chest wall. Bochdalek hernia occurs posterolaterally and represents failure of fusion of the pleural peritoneal canal. Bochdalek hernias usually present very early in life and are more common on the left side than on the right. Morgagni hernias may present at any age and are frequently an incidental finding in older persons. Bowel loops, liver, spleen, or omentum may herniate through the diaphragm defect into the chest. Plain film radiographs suggest the diagnosis and are often fairly diagnostic, particularly with Bochdalek hernia in newborns and when loops of bowel are in the hernia. When required, the diagnosis usually is readily made using gastrointestinal contrast material to confirm the presence of herniated bowel loops. Herniated liver is most readily identified with ultrasonography but can be accurately defined using technetium sulfur colloid nuclear medicine scan. The spleen can be similarly defined. Neither contrast studies nor nuclear medicine studies demonstrate herniated omentum. MRI can identify the herniation of abdominal material through the diaphragm, although the actual defect in the diaphragm may not be defined. One advantage of

MRI is that, because of multiplanar scanning, it can demonstrate continuity of the herniated and intra-abdominal segments of the involved tissue,[12] which is absolute evidence of a diaphragmatic hernia (Figs. 20–19, 20–20). A major disadvantage of CT in evaluation of diaphragmatic hernia is the restriction to the transverse imaging plane, which is probably the least favorable plane for evaluation.

Treatment of diaphragmatic hernia consists of surgical reduction of the hernia and repair of the diaphragm defect.

Anal Atresia

Anal atresia[13–16] is a not uncommon congenital anomaly diagnosed in newborns. To fully understand this abnormality a detailed knowledge of the anatomy of the muscles of this area is essential (Figs. 20–21, 20–22). Normal bowel wall has an outer longitudinal and an inner circular layer of smooth muscle. In the anal canal the circular smooth muscle is enlarged to form the internal anal sphincter. The outer longitudinal smooth muscle is prominent. Close to the distal anus, fibers from this muscle turn inward to blend with the internal sphincter and outward to blend with the overlying external sphincter. This outer longitudinal smooth muscle is sometimes called the conjoined longitudinal muscle. The next layer of muscle that surrounds the rectum is striated muscle; this is called the external anal sphincter. This muscle is divided into three segments. Inferiorly (superficially), there is the subcutaneous external sphincter. As one moves farther away from the skin surface, one encounters the superficial external sphincter and then the deep external sphincter. The deep external sphincter blends imperceptibly with fibers of the levator ani muscle: this is a very important point to remember. The outer wall of the external anal sphincter forms the medial boundary of the ischiorectal fossa, which is itself filled with fat. The levator ani muscle lies in the plane between the pubis symphysis and the coccyx. Three segments of this muscle are called respectively the pubococcygeal muscle, the puborectalis muscle, and the iliococcygeal muscle; these blend with each other.

The abnormality in anal atresia may be classified as high, intermediate, or low. High abnormality stops above the level of the levator muscles; intermediate stops at the muscle; and low lesions have the anus patent through the levator with just a superficial covering at the skin margin. Other associated congenital anomalies are very common, being present in over 50 percent of patients with high abnormality.

Conventional imaging is not greatly used in evaluation of anal atresia. The disorder is diagnosed clinically, and the old inverted lateral plain film to determine the level of atresia is no longer popular. Renal ultrasonography and cystography are usually performed to detect associated urinary tract anomalies.

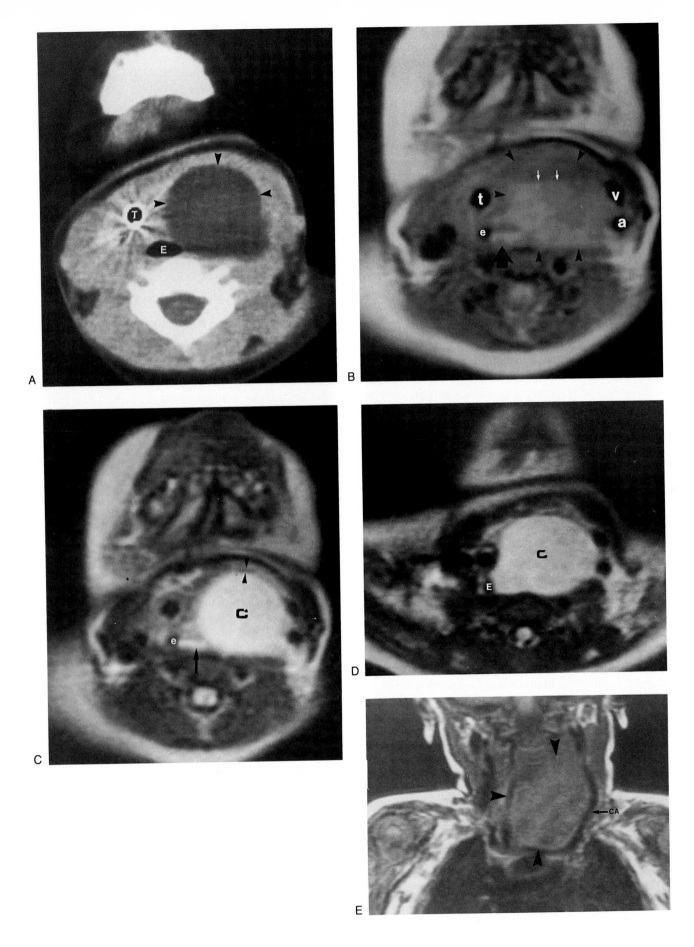

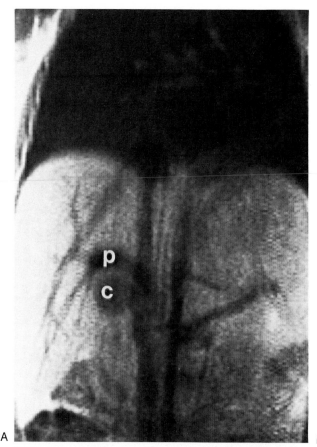 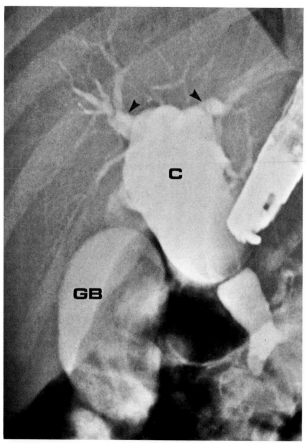

A   B

Figure 20–18. *Choledochal cyst.* **A,** Coronal T1 weighted MR image (500/30). A well-defined, low-intensity choledochal cyst (c) is seen just inferior to the portal vein (p). **B,** ERCP. This clearly identifies the choledochal cyst (C) with the right and left hepatic ducts (*arrowheads*) draining into it. The gallbladder (GB) has also filled with contrast material.

CT is not routinely used in the workup of these patients.

Magnetic resonance has an important role in both the preoperative and postoperative evaluation of patients with anal atresia. From a technical point of view, one is interested only in anatomic image quality, and T2 images are not required. T1 or spin-density images should be performed with adequate repetition times to provide excellent anatomic resolution. All three imaging planes should be used. In the transverse plane there are some useful anatomic landmarks. The plane through the symphysis pubis and coccyx corresponds to the pubococcygeal plane, which was previously identified on inverted conventional radiographs. At this level the rectum lies just behind the prostate or cervix and is surrounded by the puborectalis part of the levator ani muscle. Also at this level the gluteus muscles approximate each other in the midline over the

Figure 20–17. *Cervical esophageal duplication cyst in a 9-month-old female with a 5-day history of poor feeding and swelling of the left side of the neck.* **A,** Transverse CT scan. There is displacement of a mildly dilated esophagus (E) and trachea (T) by a low-density cystic mass (*arrowheads*). **B,** Transverse T1 weighted MR image (500/20). The cyst (*arrowheads*) is of moderate intensity with relatively poorly defined margins. A fluid fluid level (*small arrows*) is identified within the cyst. At surgery the cyst contained turbid infected material and the MR image shows layering out of some of the sediment in the fluid. Note the bridge (*large arrow*) between the cyst and the esophagus (e). The common carotid artery (a), internal jugular vein (v), and trachea (t) are also identified. **C,** Transverse T2 weighted image (2000/70). The cyst (C) is much better defined. The fluid is of more uniform intensity with high signal. A band of tissue (*arrow*) joins the cyst through the esophagus (e). This is of the same signal intensity as the fluid in the cyst. This appeared to correspond to the level of communication that was noted intraoperatively. Note that part of the cyst wall (*arrowheads*) demonstrates relatively low signal intensity similar to that of muscle. **D,** Transverse T2 weighted image (2000/70) at a more caudad level than **C.** The continuity of the cyst (C) with the esophagus (E) is well demonstrated. **E,** Coronal T1 weighted image (500/20). This shows nicely the cephalocaudal extent of the cyst (*arrowheads*). The marked lateral displacement of the left common carotid artery (CA) is well shown. (Rhee RS, Ray CG, Kravetz MH, et al. Cervical esophageal duplication cyst: MR imaging. J Comput Assist Tomogr 1988; 12:693–695.)

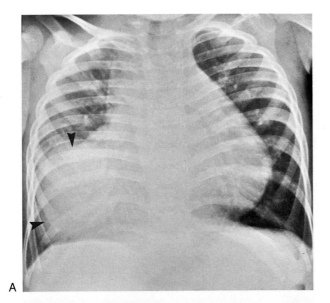

A

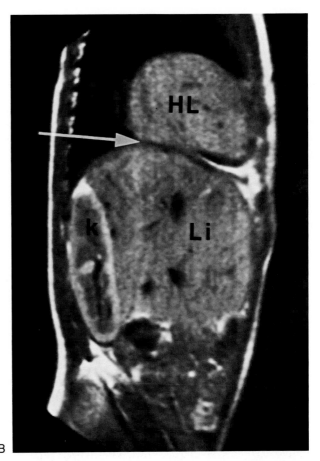

B

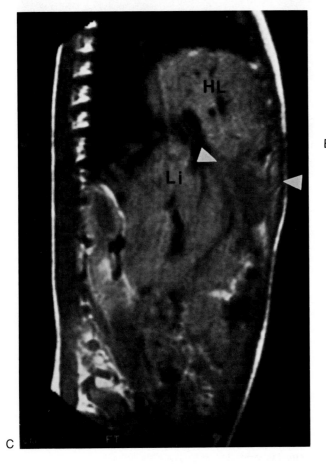

C

Figure 20–19. *Morgagni hernia in a 2-year-old child with imperforate anus. There is an incidental finding of density in the right lower lung field on chest radiography.* **A,** Chest x-ray. There is a well-defined homogenous soft tissue density (*arrowheads*) in the right lower hemithorax, obscuring the right heart border. The right and left hemidiaphragms are still both visualized. **B,** Sagittal MR image (700/26). This image is obtained to the right of the midline at the level of the right kidney (K). Liver (Li) is identified anterior to the kidney. A homogeneous soft tissue mass of herniated liver (HL) is seen above the right hemidiaphragm (*arrow*), in the thorax. It is of similar intensity to the liver below the diaphragm. **C,** Sagittal MR image (700/26) obtained closer to the midline than **B.** It clearly shows anterior continuity between liver (Li) below the diaphragm and herniated liver (HL) above the diaphragm. The herniation is occurring through an anterior defect (*arrowheads*) and is therefore a Morgagni hernia.

coccyx. The other important transverse plane is that through the ischial rami and ischial tuberosity. At this level the image passes through the external anal sphincter. The sphincter and the anus are slightly oval, with the long axis lying in the sagittal plane. Also at this level the superficial transverse perineal muscles are identified running transversely from the central point

of the perineum (just anterior to the external anal sphincter) to the ischial tuberosity.

In the preoperative period, MRI can exquisitely demonstrate the levator ani muscle and the residual external sphincter muscle mass (Fig. 20–23). In patients with associated anomalies of the sacrum, the external sphincter mass may be in an eccentric posi-

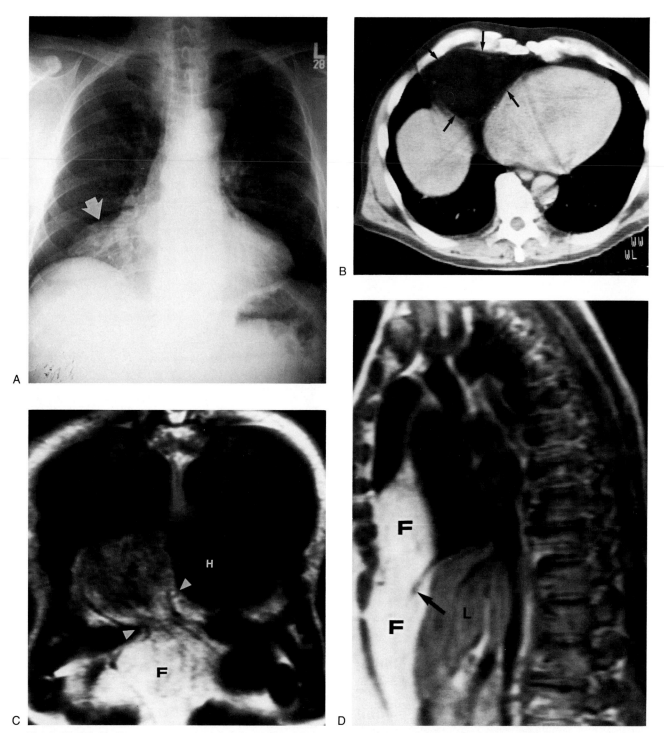

Figure 20–20. *Morgagni hernia: herniation of omental fat.*   ***A,*** Chest radiograph shows a mass lesion (*arrow*) in the right cardiophrenic angle. ***B,*** Transverse CT scan shows that the paracardiac mass (*arrows*) is fatty in origin. ***C,*** Coronal MR image (600/20). Omental fat (F) is identified below and above the diaphragm. It is constricted as it passes through the diaphragm defect (*arrowheads*). There is clear continuity between the thoracic and abdominal components. H, Heart. ***D,*** Sagittal MR image (600/20), which also demonstrates the omental fat (F) herniating into the chest. The herniation is occurring through an anterior defect in the diaphragm. The free edge of the diaphragm is well identified (*arrow*). L, Liver. (Yeager BA, Guglielmi GE, Scheibler ML, Gefter WB. Magnetic resonance imaging of Morgagni hernia. Gastrointest Radiol 1987; 12:296–298.)

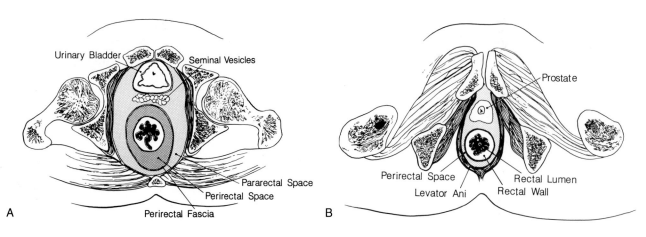

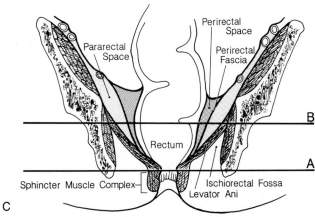

Figure 20–21. *Normal perirectal anatomy.* ***A,*** Transverse diagram through the pelvis, superior to the level of the levator ani. ***B,*** Transverse diagram of the pelvis at the level of the levator ani muscle. ***C,*** Coronal image through the plane of the rectum; ***A,*** junction of the rectum and the anus, ***B,*** junction of the rectum and the sigmoid. (Courtesy of Dr. A. Vade, Chicago.)

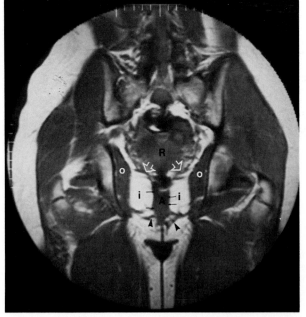

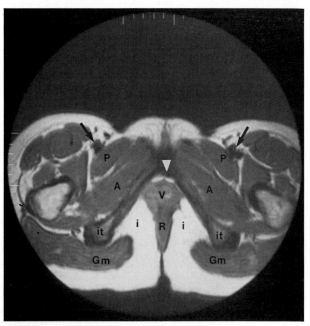

Figure 20–22. *Normal perineal anatomy.* ***A,*** Coronal image through the rectum (1500/20). The rectum (R) and anal canal (A) are well identified. The anal canal lies between the ischiorectal fossae (i). Just lateral to the ischiorectal fossae are the obturator internus muscles (o). The superficial fibers of the external sphincter (*arrowheads*) are seen surrounded in fat. The deeper external sphincter and the internal sphincter (*arrows*) cannot be differentiated from each other. The levator ani muscle on each side is well identified (*open arrows*). ***B,*** Transverse MR image (1500/20), demonstrating the vagina (V), rectum (R), ischiorectal fossa (i), ischial tuberosity (it), and gluteus maximus muscle (Gm). Note the femoral vessels (*arrows*) lying off the pectineus muscle (P). Deep to the pectineus are the adductor muscles (A). The urethra is seen as a small round lucency (*arrowhead*).

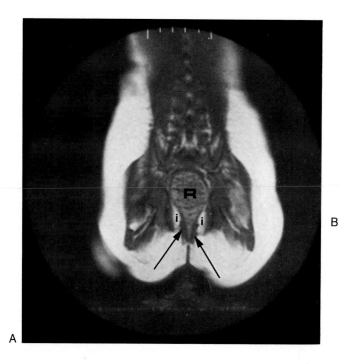

A

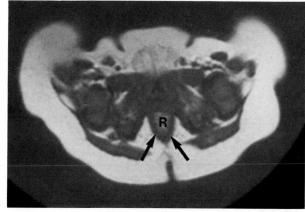

B

Figure 20–23. *Low anal atresia: normal muscles. A 3¹/₂-month-old female who presented with rectocutaneous fistula at birth. This was incised. MR study confirms the normal location of the rectum within the sphincter muscle.* **A,** *Coronal image (800/26). The rectum (R) is seen well located within the external sphincter (arrows). Note the ischiorectal fossae filled with fat (i) and the well-defined external sphincter.* **B,** *Transverse MR image (800/26), showing the rectum (R) with well-developed external sphincter muscles (arrows).*

tion, and its preoperative location is essential for guiding the pull-through surgical procedure. MR identification of the external sphincter mass is crucial. Originally, surgery for anal atresia involved pulling the rectum through the levator ani muscle, and it was believed that these patients lacked an external sphincter. Modern surgery still involves pulling the rectum down through the levator muscle sling. In addition, however, present-day surgery involves splitting the residual existing external anal sphincter muscles with electrostimulation to guide the dissection. The bowel is then placed within the external sphincter muscle mass. MRI also defines many of the associated congenital abnormalities in the pelvis such as fistula, sacral malformation, and tethered cord.

Before surgery, MRI can thus determine the level of the anal atresia (Figs. 20–23, 20–24), demonstrate the size and position of the levator sling and of the external sphincter muscle mass (Figs. 20–24, 20–25), and reveal associated anomalies (Fig. 20–26). In addition, MRI can accurately identify the degree of distention of the distal rectum, so that the surgeon knows whether rectal tapering needs to be included in the surgical procedure.

MRI also has a vital role in the postoperative evaluation of these patients (Figs. 20–27, 20–28). This is particularly true in patients troubled with incontinence. MRI provides information to indicate whether a repeat surgical procedure offers a potential for ameliorating fecal incontinence. In some patients, MRI demonstrates an appropriately placed rectum but with very small hypoplastic muscles and sphincters; in this situation, no further surgical revision will be helpful. In many other patients, however, MRI identifies complications of the surgery, many of which are potentially correctable by surgical revision. The rectum may be inappropriately placed (Figs. 20–29, 20–30). There are two common locations for this malplacement. First, the rectum may be placed outside the levator sling and external sphincter muscle mass. This is easily identified in all imaging planes. The rectum is usually seen lying adjacent to the appropriate muscles and not contained within them as it should normally be. The second malposition that is not uncommonly seen is anterior malplacement of the rectum within the external sphincter muscle mass. Another problem identified on MRI is the inclusion of mesenteric fat within the sphincter ring. In this situation, mesenteric fat is pulled down with the rectum as it is being surgically relocated. The mesenteric fat causes problems with incontinence because it interferes with normal sphincter muscle contraction.

MRI provides unique information compared with other imaging modalities. Contrast studies are still indicated for optimal visualization of fistulas from the rectum to the bladder, vagina, or urethra. For demonstration of the level of atresia, the integrity of the levator ani and sphincter muscles, and postoperative complications, MRI should be the tool of choice.

Treatment of high or intermediate anal atresia consists of initial decompression colostomy, with definitive pull-through corrective surgery at age 1 to 2 years.

Text continues on page 630.

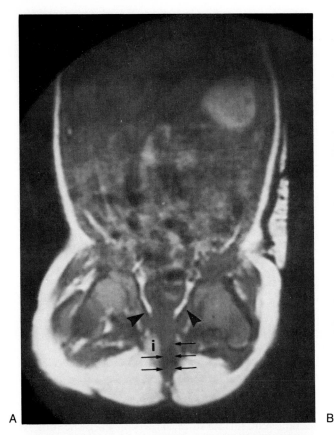

A

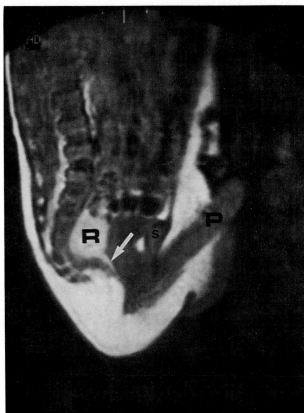

B

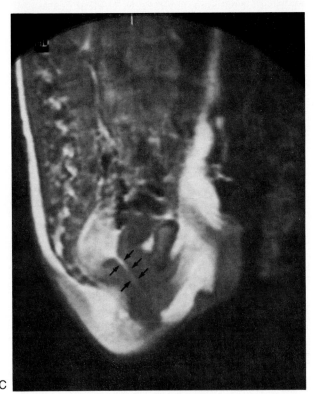

C

Figure 20–24. *High anal atresia and fistula: preoperative study in a 3-week-old male.* ***A,*** Coronal T1 weighted image (700/26). The levator ani muscles appear present and reasonably well developed (*arrowheads*). The external sphincter muscle mass (*arrows*) also appears to be present and of reasonable size. There is decrease in size of the ischiorectal fossa (i) with almost complete absence on the left side. ***B,*** Midline sagittal image (700/26). The rectum (R) is blind ending and has a curved inferior margin. The level of the inferior aspect of the rectum lies above the lower sacrum. From the anteroinferior aspect of the rectum a fistula (*arrow*) leads anteriorly and inferiorly. P, Penis; S, symphysis pubis. ***C,*** Sagittal MR image (700/26), showing the full extent of the fistula (*arrows*), which is extending forward to the region of the prostatic urethra. The urethra itself is not precisely visualized. Note that the MR images also demonstrated normal lumbar spine and sacrum. The strong signal from the rectum is believed to be due to mucoid fluid within it.

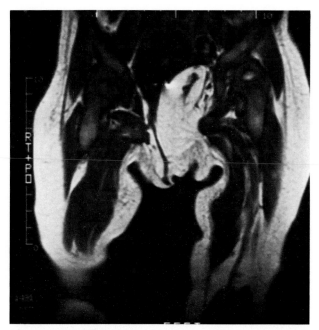

Figure 20–25. *Anal atresia: preoperative study.* Coronal T1 image (933/20). There is little normal perineal muscle, and diffuse infiltration of the perineum by fat.

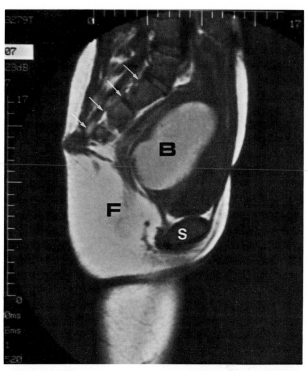

Figure 20–26. *Anal atresia.* Midline sagittal image (900/26), showing two anomalies associated with anal atresia. The sacrum (*arrows*) is very dysplastic, pointing backward with no normal curvature and reduction in the number of sacral segments present. There is a large increase in the amount of perineal fat (F), which extends well into the pelvis. S, Symphysis pubis, B, bladder.

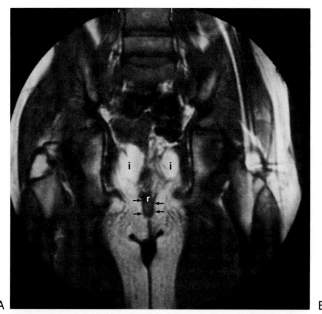

A

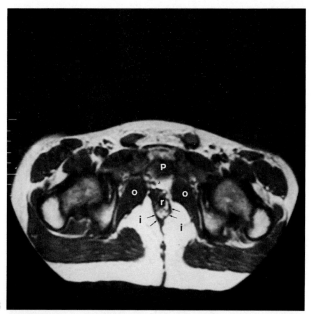

B

Figure 20–27. *Anal atresia: normal postoperative appearance in a 10-year-old child.* ***A,*** Coronal T1 weighted image (850/26). The rectum (R) lies in normal position. Fibers of the external sphincter (*arrows*) can be identified surrounding the rectum. Note that there is some distortion in size and contour of the ischiorectal (i) fossae. ***B,*** Transverse T1 weighted image (850/26). The rectum (R) is well visualized, lying contained within the fibers of the levator ani muscle (*arrows*). The ischiorectal fossae (i) are well identified. Note also the obturator internus muscles (O). The prostate (P) lies anterior to the rectum.

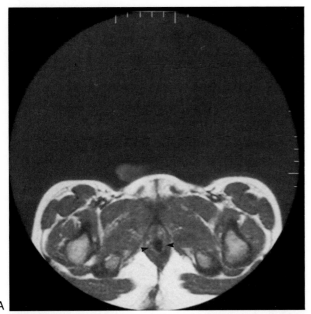
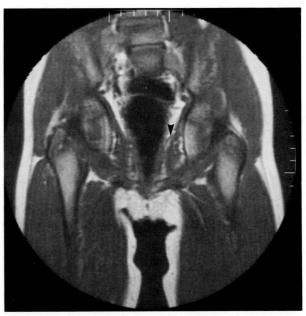

A   B

Figure 20–28. *Anal atresia: excellent result after pull-through surgical procedure in a 7-year-old male.* **A,** Transverse MR image (800/26). The rectum is normally located and the external and internal sphincter muscles (*arrowheads*) are well developed. **B,** Coronal MR image (800/26). This also shows normal rectal position. The levator ani muscle is seen, particularly well on the left side (*arrowhead*).

Duodenal and Small Bowel Atresia

There are no reports of MR imaging in these disorders. Plain film radiographs, with or without contrast studies, are excellent, and I do not consider that MRI can add any further information.

Other Congenital Disorders

There are many other congenital bowel disorders (e.g., asplenia, malrotation, situs), for which the role of MRI can only be further evaluated with time. MRI will almost certainly reveal many of these abnormal-

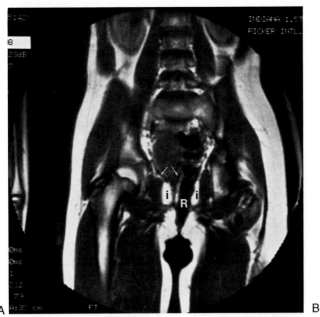
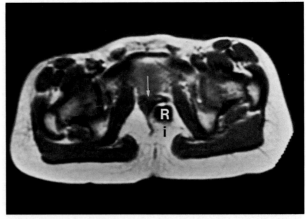

A   B

Figure 20–29. *Repaired anal atresia: malposition of the rectum.* **A,** Coronal MR image (800/30). The air-filled rectum (R) lies to the left of the midline. Fibers of the levator ani muscle are seen as low-intensity oblique bands (*arrows*). The rectum lies to the left of the left levator ani muscle. The ischiorectal fossae (i) are well seen; the rectum passes through the fat of the left fossa. **B,** Transverse image (2000/30). The rectum (R) is seen to lie within the fat of the left ischiorectal fossa. It lies outside the levator sling and sphincter muscle complex (*arrow*).

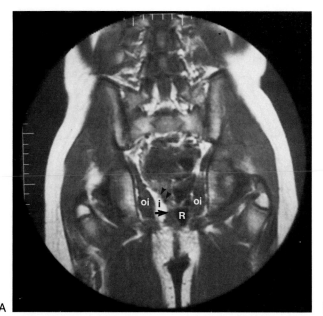

A

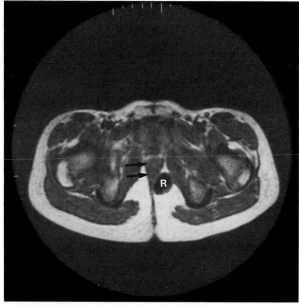

B

Figure 20–30. *Anal atresia: incorrect placement of the rectum in a 10-year-old boy with incontinence.* ***A,*** Coronal T1 weighted image (700/26). The rectum (R) lies to the left of the midline and to the left of the external sphincter muscle mass (*arrow*). Some fibers of the right levator ani are seen (*arrowheads*). The left levator muscle is not clearly identified. Note fat in the ischiorectal fossa (i) and also the obturator internus muscles (oi). ***B,*** Transverse T1 weighted image (700/26). The rectum (R) lies to the left of the external sphincter muscle mass (*arrow*) and seems to pass through the left ischiorectal fossa.

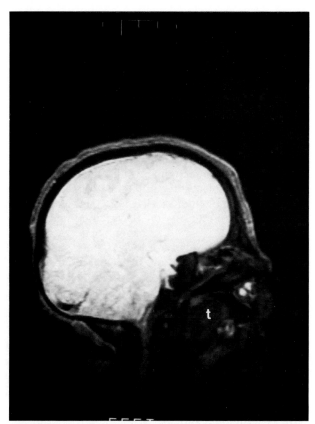

Figure 20–31. *Pierre Robin syndrome: demonstration of tongue position (2500/80).* The mandible is hypoplastic. The tongue (t) lies in the posterior part of the mouth, almost occluding the airway.

ities (Fig. 20–31), but its value and role are yet to be determined.

INFECTION AND INFLAMMATION

Ulcerative Colitis and Crohn's Disease

Both of these inflammatory disorders of the bowel occur in children, although less commonly than in adults (Fig. 20–32). Crohn's disease is more common than ulcerative colitis. Both have an unknown etiology. Ulcerative colitis pathologically is predominantly a superficial mucosal ulceration, always affecting the distal large bowel and a variable extent of the proximal colon. Crohn's disease is a more aggressive inflammation involving the entire bowel wall; it is most commonly seen in the distal ileum but can occur at any site in the bowel.

There are a few isolated reports demonstrating MR findings in these disorders, but no large series indicating any specific role for MRI has yet been published. In the few published cases the MR findings appear relatively nonspecific, with identification of swelling of the bowel wall due to inflammation, and signal intensity consistent with prolonged T1 and T2 relaxation times. At this time it seems unlikely that MRI will be used routinely to evaluate these disorders.

Possible uses for MRI may include seeking complications such as an abscess, or differentiating inactive fibrous strictures from narrowed segments of bowel with active Crohn's disease.

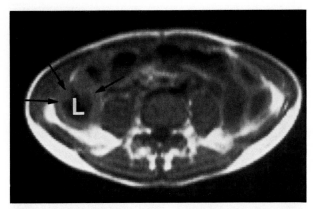

Figure 20–32. *Ulcerative colitis.* Transverse T1 MR image through the abdomen. The wall of the ascending, and to a lesser extent the descending, colon is markedly thickened. This finding is nonspecific and could be seen with tumor, inflammation from other causes, or edema. Arrow, Bowel wall; L, bowel lumen.

Abscess

Abscesses (Figs. 20–33 to 20–38) can occur at any site within the peritoneal cavity or within any of the abdominal organs. Organisms may reach the abscess site either by perforation of the bowel or by blood spread. There may or may not be a history of trauma or surgery. Clinical signs are as expected, with fever, elevated white blood cell count, and variable abdominal pain that may or may not be localized. The appearance of abscess is variable on MR images. It is seen as a poorly or well-defined lesion of low signal intensity on T1 images (Fig. 20–35). Fluid within the abscess cavity has a high signal intensity on T2 images (Fig. 20–36). An inflamed abscess wall also has a high signal on T2 images. With healing and fibrosis, signal intensity from the abscess wall decreases (Figs. 20–33, 20–37). Variable amounts of adjacent edema and inflammation are also identified as areas of high signal intensity on T2 weighted images (Fig. 20–36). Air fluid levels may be identified within the abscess, and their presence strongly suggests the correct diagnosis (Fig. 20–33). The accuracy of MRI in identifying abdominal abscesses is not known at this time. Because of the sensitivity of MRI to inflammation, with time it may prove a sensitive screening test for an abdominal abscess. However, the findings on MRI are not specific (Fig. 20–34). Differential diagnosis includes fluid-filled loops of bowel, other fluid collections, and necrotic tumors.[17] Recent experimental work in animals suggests that gadolinium-DTPA contrast enhancement may prove helpful in abscess evaluation. Gadolinium-DTPA was found to improve visualization of the abscess by improving lesion to background contrast. It was also found that the enhancement pattern varied with abscess evolution, so that it may be possible to predict the age or activity of an abscess. Abscesses a few days old showed a ring-enhancement pattern, whereas abscesses a few weeks old had a more homogeneous enhancing pattern.[18]

Ultrasound, CT, and gadolinium-DTPA scanning remain the primary methods of evaluation of an abdominal abscess. The role of MRI remains to be clearly defined.

Hepatitis

Almost nothing has been published on the clinical use of MRI in the evaluation of hepatitis. In experimental animals, hepatitis can be identified within 12 hours of its onset, indicating great sensitivity for MRI.[19] There has been no evidence to suggest that MRI can distinguish various types of hepatitis, or differentiate neonatal hepatitis from biliary atresia.

Pancreatitis

Pancreatitis, which is uncommon in children, can be detected by MRI. It is seen as a patchy or diffuse area of increased signal intensity on T2 images and decreased signal intensity on T1 images.[20] The margins of the pancreas may often be blurred, and extension of the inflammation into adjacent tissues can be identified. The appearance of the pancreatitis is somewhat nonspecific, and it may not be possible on the MR image to differentiate focal inflammation from disorders such as tumor.[7]

Compared with CT, MRI has not been found to offer any specific advantages, and its routine use for evaluation of pancreatitis is not yet recommended.[7]

Cholecystitis

Although biliary tract disease is not especially common in children, infection and gallstones do occur. In patients with cholecystitis, inflammatory edema in the wall of the gallbladder can be identified as a rim of increased signal intensity on T2 weighted images and decreased intensity on T1 images.[21] The gallbladder may also be increased in size. An inflamed gallbladder cannot concentrate bile, and the signal intensity from bile is low on T1 and high on T2 weighted images irrespective of whether the patient is fasting. Gallstones behave as solids and are not easily detectable, since they mainly produce a very weak MR signal.[22] They are seen as areas of low signal against a background of high-signal bile on T2 images.

Necrotizing Enterocolitis

In experimental animals, MRI can detect abnormal signal from affected bowel within hours of onset of this necrotizing enterocolitis. In infants, MRI should be

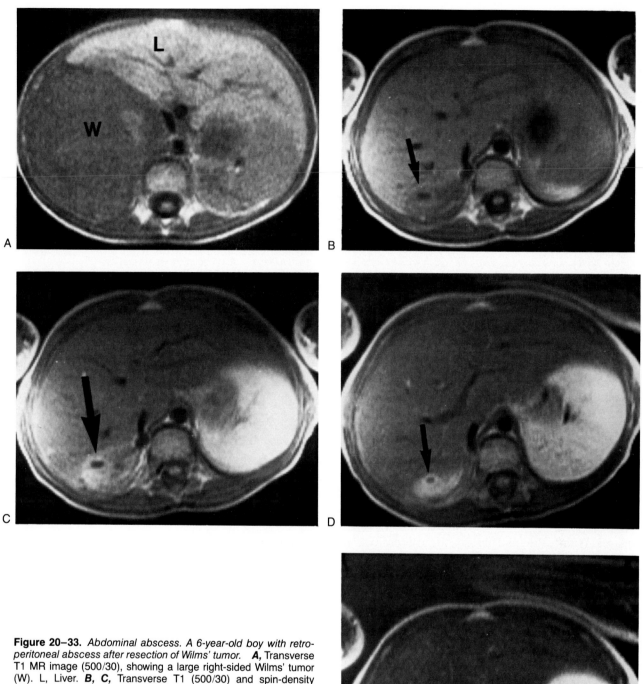

Figure 20–33. *Abdominal abscess. A 6-year-old boy with retro-peritoneal abscess after resection of Wilms' tumor.* ***A,*** Transverse T1 MR image (500/30), showing a large right-sided Wilms' tumor (W). L, Liver. ***B, C,*** Transverse T1 (500/30) and spin-density (1000/30) images show an abscess (*arrow*) in the region of the right renal fossa. The abscess is composed of a very thick wall with a small cavity containing air. The signal intensity of the wall is below that of liver on the T1 image and increases to that above liver on the spin-density image. ***D, E,*** Transverse spin-density (1000/30) and T2 (1000/60) weighted images, obtained 10 days after the previous pair of images. They show marked reduction in the size of the abscess (*arrow*). The signal intensity from the wall to the abscess is still very strong on the T2 weighted image, indicating the presence of inflammatory activity. The diagnosis in this patient is made by the clinical history of pain and fever following abdominal surgery, and is confirmed by the MR findings.

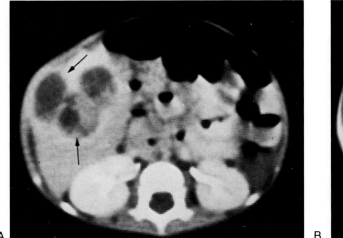

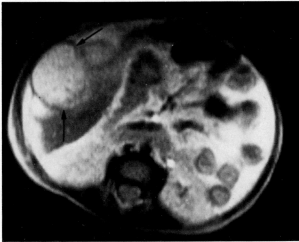

Figure 20–34. *Liver abscess in a 1-year-old infant with right upper quadrant fullness.* **A,** CT scan shows several low-intensity areas in the inferior aspect of the right lobe of the liver (*arrows*). **B,** T2 MR image (1000/60). The lesions (*arrows*) on the CT scan are identified on the MR scan. They appear of very high intensity against a background of liver of lower intensity. MRI is sensitive for the detection of the mass lesion. The appearance in this case is nonspecific, and differential diagnosis would include vascular malformation and tumor.

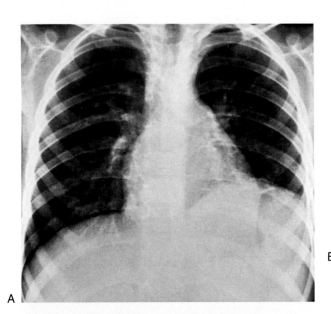

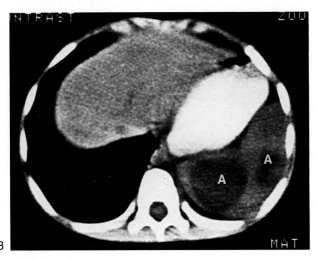

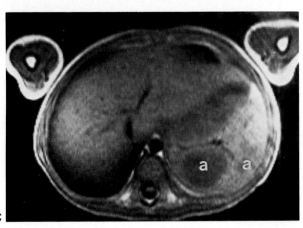

Figure 20–35. *Splenic abscess in a 5-year-old child who presented with unexplained fever and abdominal pain.* **A,** Chest radiograph shows elevation of the left hemidiaphragm due to a subdiaphragmatic fluid collection. **B,** CT scan shows two low-intensity areas (A) in the spleen. **C,** T1 weighted transverse MR image (500/30). The two abscesses (a) in the spleen are seen as moderately well defined lesions of signal intensity lower than that of normal spleen on this T1 weighted image. The very low signal intensity suggests the presence of fluid. A tumor or cyst might have a similar appearance.

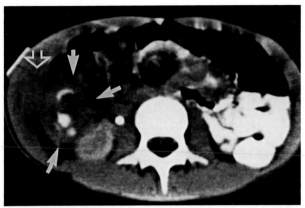 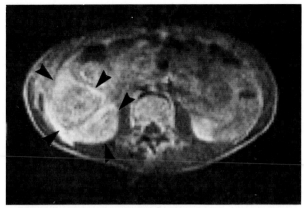

A   B

Figure 20–36. *Abdominal abscess in a 12-year-old girl with right lower quadrant pain and fever.* **A,** Transverse CT scan. A small amount of contrast material is seen in the ascending colon. A moderate-sized soft tissue mass (*arrows*) surrounds the ascending colon. At surgery this was found to be an abscess. Note also the marked thickening of the muscle layers of the abdominal wall (*open arrow*), just lateral to the abscess. **B,** Transverse T2 weighted image (1000/60). The appearance of the abscess (*arrowheads*) corresponds fairly well to the CT scan. The abdominal wall is thickened. The abscess is seen as a lesion with a wall of very strong intensity and central area of slightly lower intensity. The appearance is not absolutely diagnostic of abscess; other lesions, including tumor or Crohn's disease, might look somewhat similar.

able to identify strong signal on T2 images in affected bowel. The sensitivity, specificity, and clinical utility all remain to be determined.

Gastroenteritis

There are no reports of MR imaging in gastroenteritis. No advantages in the use of MR are anticipated.

Histoplasmosis

The spleen is commonly involved with histoplasmosis. Lesions may have T1 and T2 relaxation times similar to normal spleen and thus be difficult to visualize (Fig. 20–39).

Hydatid Cyst

Hydatid cysts in the liver are easily and well defined. The characteristic daughter cysts can also be well demonstrated by MRI (Fig. 20–40).

TUMORS

Tumors of the intestine, pancreas, and spleen are all rare. The liver is the most common site of tumor involving the gastrointestinal tract.

Pancreatic Tumors

Pancreatic tumors are rare in children. Hormone-producing tumors tend to be small and there are few reports of their identification by MRI. One report of an

insulinoma indicated that the tumor had a fairly nonspecific appearance, with signal intensity lower than normal pancreas on T1 images and higher than normal pancreas on T2 images.[18] The appearance of most pancreatic tumor lesions is relatively nonspecific, and MRI cannot accurately differentiate benign from malignant lesions.[7]

Lymphoma may involve the pancreas, and this involvement may be diffuse (Fig. 20–41) or focal. Signal intensity may be different from that of normal pancreas, but in some patients may be very similar to that of normal pancreas on both T1 and T2 pulse sequences.[7] In this situation the only abnormality identified is enlargement of the gland.

Pancreatic carcinoma (Fig. 20–42) presents as a solid mass lesion with no specific features. Pancreatic cyst adenocarcinoma has mixed solid and cystic components.

Currently, it is not known whether MRI has advantages over ultrasonography or CT in the evaluation of pancreatic tumors. The sensitivity of MRI in detecting small hormone-producing tumors of the pancreas is also not known.

Hemangioma of the Liver

Hemangiomas are very common benign liver tumors (Figs. 20–43 to 20–47). Pathologically they are endothelium-lined, cystic, blood-filled spaces.[23] There is some overlap in the pathologic description of cavernous hemangiomas and hemangioendotheliomas. The term "cavernous hemangioma" is usually applied only to focal, fairly well defined lesions, whereas "hemangioendothelioma" is generally used to describe more diffuse lesions, particularly in newborns. Focal hemangioendotheliomas should probably be consid-

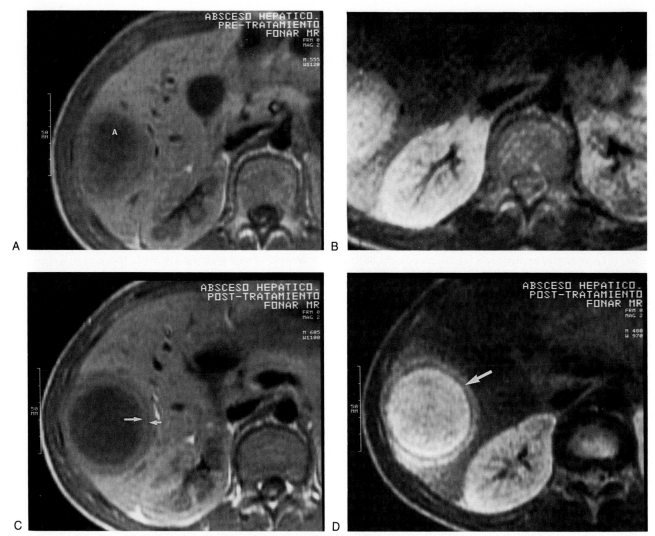

Figure 20–37. *Amebic liver abscess before and after drug therapy.* **A, B,** These are transverse images through the liver with T1 (500/28) and T2 (2000/84) weighting. The T1 weighted image shows a sharply circumscribed, fairly heterogeneous low-signal-intensity abscess mass (A) in the right lobe of the liver. The T2 weighted image shows hyperintensity in the area of the abscess mass. The abscess is surrounded by a larger region of hyperintensity corresponding to edematous liver tissue. **C, D,** The same abscess after 10 days of drug therapy. On the T1 weighted image (C) the cavity is now of homogeneous low intensity. It is bordered by an inner ring (*large arrow*) of moderate intensity believed to be inflamed granulation tissue, and an outer ring (*small arrow*) of low intensity believed to be collagen. The T2 weighted image (**D**) shows that the size of the overall abscess abnormality is the same as that in **C,** indicating that the perifocal edema has largely resolved. The outer intense rim (*arrow*) represents residual focal liver edema. (Elizondo G, Weissleder R, Stark DD, et al. Amebic liver abscess: diagnosis and treatment evaluation with MR imaging. Radiology 1987; 165:795–800.)

ered the same as cavernous hemangiomas without trying to differentiate these lesions. When these lesions are large, they may show internal areas of fibrosis or thrombosis; this greatly affects the MR image.[24]

Clinically, small cavernous hemangiomas are usually asymptomatic and are often incidental findings on imaging studies performed for other reasons, or at post mortem. Hemangioendotheliomas, particularly when large, may present in newborns. In this situation, shunting of blood through the lesion is so extensive as to cause congestive cardiac failure. In these patients the large shunt of blood causes marked enlargement of

the hepatic artery, and there is an abrupt decrease in caliber of the aorta at the level of the origin of the celiac artery. The flow of blood through the enlarged vascular spaces is usually fairly slow. In patients with large lesions, thrombocytopenia is common.

Plain film radiographs are normal, or may show enlargement of the liver and occasionally calcification. On ultrasonography the lesions may be large or small and poorly or well defined, and consist of mixed areas of increased and decreased echoes. With large shunts a large hepatic artery is also clearly identified, as is the decreased caliber of the aorta below the celiac artery.

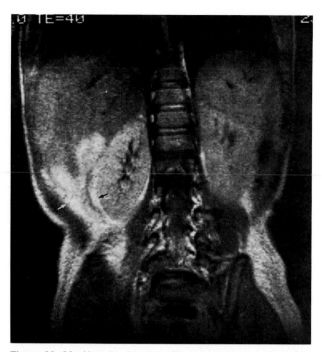

Figure 20–38. *Hepatic abscess.* T2 weighted image. There is a high-intensity lesion in the inferior aspect of the right lobe of the liver. The appearance of this lesion is relatively nonspecific. High-intensity signal is also seen from the adjacent soft tissues (*white arrow*), consistent with extension of the inflammatory process. This involves the renal fascia as well (*black arrow*). (Riddlesberger MM. Evaluation of the gastrointestinal tract in the child: CT, MRI and isotopic studies. Pediatr Clin North Am 1988; 35:281–310.)

On CT scan, with dynamic imaging following bolus injection of contrast material, there is a fairly characteristic appearance: low intensity of the lesion before contrast injection is followed by a fairly early peripheral vascular blush with slow filling in of the center of the lesion over a period of 2 to 20 minutes. Large areas of necrosis or hemorrhage show no contrast enhancement. MRI shows the presence of one or more mass lesions within the liver. With large shunts, vessel enlargement is easily appreciated. The lesions are usually of lower signal intensity than liver on strongly T1 weighted images, variable intensity on moderately T1 weighted images, and increased signal intensity on T2 weighted images. The large hemangioendotheliomas tend to be nonhomogeneous in appearance, probably in part owing to central areas of fibrosis, thrombosis, or mucoid change (Fig. 20–44).

Specific characterization of these lesions varies from patient to patient. The classic MR appearance of a small cavernous hemangioma is of a well-defined lobulated lesion with sharp margins, with low signal intensity on strongly T1 weighted images and very high signal on strong T2 images (Fig. 20–43).[24, 25] In these patients the diagnosis may strongly be suspected, but very vascular metastases in the liver or simple liver cysts occasionally may have a similar appearance.[25] Some lesions, however, are atypical, with nonhomogeneous irregular contours and an irregular, moderately enhancing signal on T2 images.[25, 26] Gross patho-

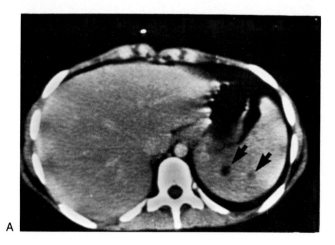

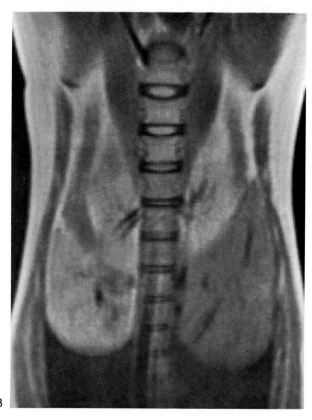

Figure 20–39. *Splenic histoplasmosis: false-negative MR study.* ***A,*** Transverse CT scan shows two low-intensity lesions in the spleen (*arrows*). ***B,*** Coronal MR image (200/30) obtained at 0.15T. The spleen appears normal. The spleen normally has relatively long T1 and T2 relaxation times, seen also in many pathologic conditions. Because of this, it may sometimes be difficult to identify focal lesions within the spleen. In this patient, CT scan identified two lesions. At surgery, hundreds of smaller lesions were also found.

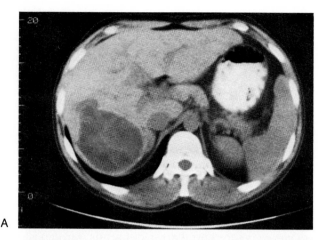

A

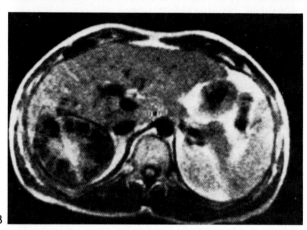

B

Figure 20–40. *Hydatid cyst.* Transverse CT (*A*) and MR (*B*) (800/40) images of the abdomen show a large cystic abnormality in the posterior aspect of the right lobe of the liver. The cyst is well defined. A very characteristic finding strongly suggesting the correct diagnosis is the appearance of the sharply defined multiple daughter cysts lying within the larger cysts. (Morris DL, Buckley J, Gregson R, et al. Magnetic resonance imaging in hyatid disease. Clin Radiol 1987; 38:141–144.)

logic examination of specimens in these patients reveals that the inhomogeneity is due to areas of fibrosis, thrombosis, and calcification (Figs. 20–44, 20–46).[26] In difficult cases, several things can be done to assist the differential diagnosis. On CT the enhancing pattern starting from the periphery and moving inward is suggestive of hemangioma. Nuclear medicine studies are even more specific. Using technetium-labeled red blood cells, the demonstration of increased activity within the lesion on a 2-hour image is markedly characteristic of a hemangioma. This appearance is seen even in hemangiomas that are atypical on MRI.[27] The enhancement pattern following injection of gadolinium-DTPA may also be helpful. The changes are similar to those seen following contrast injection in CT scanning. In five of seven patients with cavernous hemangiomas, it was shown that dynamic imaging using very short scan times showed early peripheral enhancement of the lesion immediately following gad-

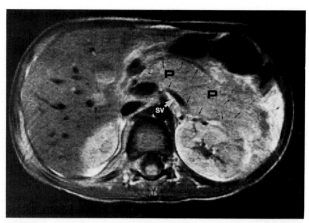

Figure 20–41. *Burkitt's lymphoma of the pancreas.* Transverse T2 weighted image of the abdomen at the level of the pancreas. There is diffuse uniform enlargement of the pancreas (P), which has signal of moderate intensity. The splenic vein (SV) is seen posterior to the pancreas. The uniform intensity and the absence of abnormality in the adjacent soft tissues favor tumor rather than pancreatitis. (Riddlesberger MM. Evaluation of the gastrointestinal tract in the child: CT, MRI and isotopic studies. Pediatr Clin North Am 1988; 35:281–310.)

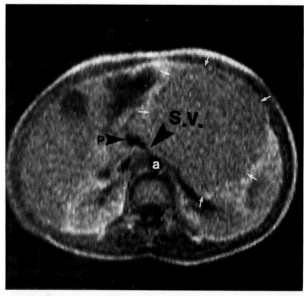

Figure 20–42. *Pancreatic carcinoma in a 12-year-old boy.* Transverse MR image (1000/30). There is a large tumor mass (*small arrows*), which is homogeneous and of similar intensity to liver. The mass lies immediately anterior to the splenic vein (SV). This close association of the tumor with the splenic vein strongly suggests a pancreatic origin. A neuroblastoma would be expected to cause downward displacement of the kidney. In this patient the tumor lies predominantly anterior to the kidney. Note also that the aorta (a) lies in normal position. With a neuroblastoma of this size, one would expect some displacement or encasement of the aorta. P, Portal vein.

olinium-DTPA injection, with enhancement of the entire lesion seen 5 minutes after contrast injection (Fig. 20–45).[28] This pattern of enhancement was not seen with other abnormalities.

MRI is very sensitive for detection of liver hemangiomas and has been able to demonstrate more lesions than either CT or ultrasonography.[29] MRI can characterize many of these lesions (Fig. 20–43) and can be used to follow the involution of these lesions in newborns.

Many hemangiomas require no therapy and resolve spontaneously (Fig. 20–43). In newborns with large hemangioendotheliomas, severe congestive cardiac failure may occur. In these patients, focal lesions can be resected (Fig. 20–44). Diffuse lesions can be treated with steroids, hepatic artery ligation, or embolization.

Lymphoma

Lymphoma (Figs. 20–48, 20–49) involving the liver, spleen, and intestine is discussed in detail in Chapter 22. MRI is very good at demonstrating diseased lymph nodes (Fig. 20–50) and can identify disease in other locations (Figs. 20–51, 20–52).

Hepatocellular Carcinoma and Hepatoblastoma

These two tumors account for two-thirds of all pediatric liver tumors (Figs. 20–53 to 20–57). They are less common than either neuroblastoma or Wilms' tumor. Hepatoblastoma is usually a single well-defined mass with a tendency to invade portal and hepatic veins and metastasize to lungs. Histologically, hepatoblastomas are classified into fetal and embryonal types; they are more common in the right lobe of the liver; and this may produce hormones causing unusual clinical signs and symptoms such as osteoporosis, virilization, precocious puberty, and hypercalcemia. Nearly all patients with hepatoblastoma have elevated serum levels of alpha-fetoprotein. This finding can be used both for diagnosis and in monitoring therapy. Hepatoblastoma is usually seen in children under the age of 3 years. Hepatocellular carcinoma is uncommon before the age of 5 years; this tumor occurs equally in either lobe of the liver. There is an increased incidence of hepato-

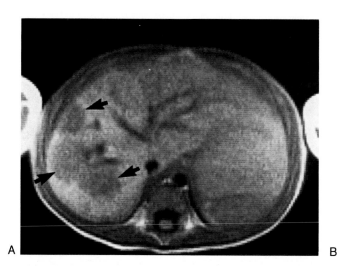

A

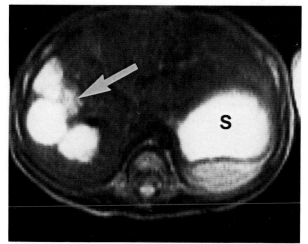

B

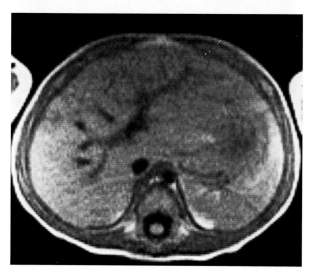

C

Figure 20–43. *Cavernous hemangioma of the liver in a 9-month-old infant.* ***A,*** Transverse MR image (500/30) shows a moderately well defined, trilobed, low-intensity lesion (*arrows*) in the right lobe of the liver. ***B,*** On the T2 weighted image (1500/60) there is a marked increase in signal intensity from the lesion (*arrow*). It is well defined and lobulated. The appearance is fairly characteristic of cavernous hemangioma. The strong signal from the stomach (S) is due to milk. ***C,*** Transverse T1 weighted image (500/30) obtained 3 months later shows almost complete spontaneous involution of the hemangioma. This is not uncommon.

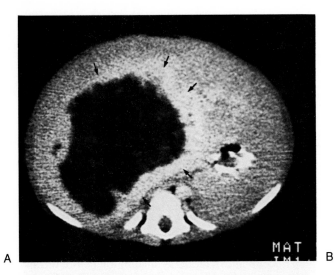

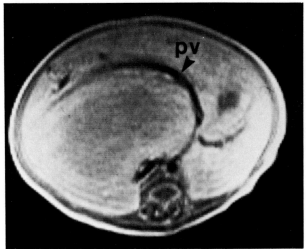

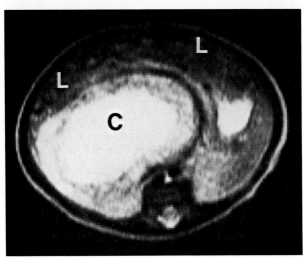

Figure 20–44. *Hemangioendothelioma in a newborn with clinical presentation of an abdominal mass. There was no bruit, no skin hemangiomas, and no evidence of congestive cardiac failure. The tumor was surgically resected.* **A,** CT scan taken immediately after bolus injection of contrast material shows a large lesion in the right lobe of the liver. The center of the lesion is of low intensity. There is an irregular rim of moderate enhancement (*arrows*), just over 1 cm wide and surrounding the low-intensity center of the lesion. **B,** Transverse MR image (1000/30). The lesion in the right lobe of the liver is well seen. It is elevating the portal vein (pv). The appearance of the lesion corresponds fairly well to the CT scan, with a low-intensity center and a slightly higher-intensity rim. **C,** Strongly T2 weighted image (1000/240). The center (C) of the lesion, because of its fluid nature, has become of very strong signal intensity. The rim of the lesion is of moderate intensity, less than the center, but much more than the normal liver (L), which is of very low intensity on this image.

blastoma in patients with biliary atresia and metabolic disorders involving the liver, such as cystinosis and Wilson's disease.

The clinical presentation of primary liver tumors is varied and includes incidental findings such as an abdominal mass, pain, or secondary syndromes from hormone production.

Plain film findings in these liver tumors are those of a right upper quadrant abdominal mass. Calcification may be seen in between 25 and 50 percent of patients. Ultrasonography usually identifies a focal mass lesion within the liver. The margins of the lesion sometimes are not as well seen on ultrasonography as on CT or MRI. Ultrasonography shows mixed areas of increased and decreased echogenicity, and is probably the best modality for identifying the hepatic veins. The left hepatic vein separates the medial and lateral segments of the left lobe of the liver, the middle hepatic vein separates the right and left lobes of the liver, and the right hepatic vein separates the anterior and posterior segments of the right lobe of the liver. Demonstration

of the hepatic veins is crucial for segmental localization of the tumor, on which successful surgical resection depends. CT identifies liver lesions well. They are usually well defined and of lower intensity than normal liver before intravenous contrast is given. With bolus injection of contrast, there is usually early enhancement of the tumor mass. Areas of hemorrhage and necrosis in the tumor do not enhance. Hepatic veins may be seen but are less well seen than on either MRI or ultrasonography. In one study of 60 patients, MRI was found to be better than CT for the detection of pseudocapsule around these tumors, and for the identification of internal trabeculae and also vessel involvement.[30] MRI has also been shown to be better than CT in identifying the recurrence of these tumors in the liver (Fig. 20–58).[24] Sulfur colloid liver-spleen scans in patients with primary liver malignancy show a focal mass lesion within the liver but do not add information. Angiography has traditionally been used to aid in demonstration of vascular anatomy before surgery. In almost all cases angiography should no longer be neces-

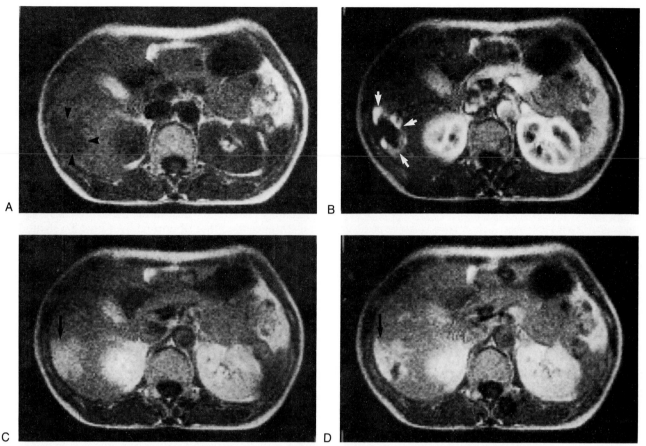

Figure 20–45. *Cavernous hemangioma of the liver: effect of bolus injection of gadolinium-DTPA. Rapid scan technique was utilized, the acquisition of time for each image being 26 seconds. The pulse sequence was 100/15 or 100/20.* **A,** *Transverse MR image of the liver obtained before administration of contrast media. The cavernous hemangioma (arrowheads) appears of low intensity compared with normal liver.* **B,** *Image obtained immediately after administration of contrast. There is peripheral enhancement (arrows) of the lesion.* **C, D,** *Images obtained 2 and 5 minutes after contrast administration show that the lesion (arrows) is of fairly uniform high intensity. This pattern of enhancement corresponds fairly well to that which would be seen on CT scan. (Ohtomo K, Itai Y, Yoshikawa K, et al. Hepatic tumors: dynamic MR imaging. Radiology 1987; 163:27–31.)*

sary, because of excellent vessel visualization on MRI (Fig. 20–57) and ultrasonography (Fig. 20–59).

These liver tumors are well identified on MRI, being seen as mass lesions with signal intensity consistent with increase in T1 and T2 relaxation time, compared with normal liver (Figs. 20–55, 20–56). The internal structure of the lesions is variable, ranging from fairly homogeneous to very irregular (Figs. 20–54, 20–55). Calcification is usually speckled and not well seen on the MR images. MRI can show compression, displacement, or tumor invasion of vessels. In most patients, segmental localization of the tumor can be accurately defined because of the excellent visualization of the hepatic veins (Fig. 20–54). The overall MR appearance is relatively nonspecific,[24] and many other pathologic conditions may have a similar appearance, including metastases, lymphomas, granulomas, and hamartomas.[2]

Intravenous injection of gadolinium-DTPA shows immediate enhancement of signal intensity on T1 im-

ages (Fig. 20–54). The location of this enhancement is variable, involving the center or rim of the tumor, and it may be patchy or diffuse. Imaging 5 minutes after gadolinium-DTPA injection shows no enhancement of the tumor in 75 percent of patients. Forty percent show a halo of enhancement in the capsule of the tumor.[28]

There is an unusual type of hepatocellular carcinoma that has a characteristic appearance on MRI (Fig. 20–60): the fibrolamellar carcinoma.[31] This tumor occurs in the later teenage years. It is more benign than the classic hepatocellular carcinoma, and patients have normal serum levels of alpha-fetoprotein. The tumor has a central stellate scar seen as an area of low signal in the middle of the tumor on both T1 and T2 weighted pulse sequences.

Liver malignancies may metastasize to many sites, including lung and bone (Fig. 20–61).

The mainstay of therapy for primary liver tumors in children is surgery. Unless the tumor is completely resected, the chance of survival is almost nil. MRI is

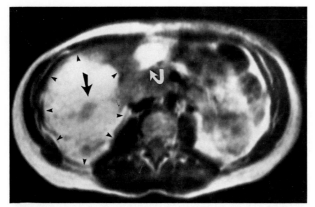

Figure 20–46. *Hemangioma of the right lobe of the liver.* T2 weighted transverse MR image. A loop of bowel is seen as of strong signal intensity in the midabdomen (*curved arrow*). The hemangioma (*arrowheads*) is identified in the right lobe of the liver, and has a characteristic, well-defined, lobulated shape. However, the appearance is not homogeneous and there is a central area of decreased signal (*black arrow*). This corresponded pathologically to a nodular fibrosis. Many large hemangiomas are not homogeneous on T2 weighted images, and this finding should not exclude the diagnosis. Nonhomogeneity is due to fibrosis, as in this case, or thrombus formation. (Ros PR, Lubbers PR, Olmsted WW, Morillo G. Hemangioma of the liver: heterogenous appearance of T2-weighted images. AJR 1987; 149:1167–1170.)

extremely valuable in predicting resectability. In patients whose tumors are initially unresectable, MRI can be used effectively to monitor tumor response to chemotherapy and predict the best time for delayed surgical resection (Figs. 20–53, 20–54).

Hepatic Metastases

Many kinds of tumors may metastasize to the liver. In children, neuroblastoma is probably the most common of these disorders (Fig. 20–62). Wilms' tumor also metastasizes to liver, as do many other less common tumors. The appearance of metastases in the liver is extremely varied.[32, 33] Most of the metastasis has a signal stronger than that of normal liver on T2 weighted pulse sequences. On T1 pulse sequences the intensity varies and can be either less than, equal to, or greater than that of normal liver. Metastases may be focal or diffuse; neuroblastoma, particularly in young infants, often tends to be diffuse (Fig. 20–62). These metastases have a very strong signal intensity on T2 pulse sequences. Differential diagnosis for metastasis includes hemangioma, abscess, hematoma, and hamartoma. There is much controversy in the literature re-

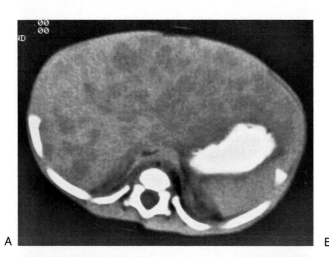

A

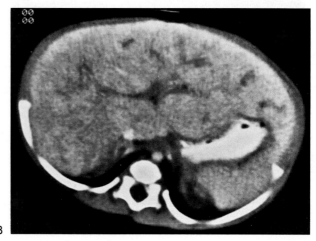

B

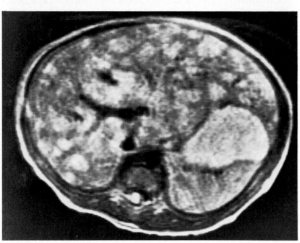

C

Figure 20–47. *Hemangioendothelioma of the liver in a 1-month-old boy.* **A,** Non-contrast-enhanced CT scan. There are multiple low attenuation masses distributed throughout the liver. **B,** CT scan after contrast administration shows marked enhancement of the nodules. **C,** Transverse T2 weighted image (1500/56). There is very high signal intensity from the lesions seen scattered throughout the liver. (Boechat MI, Kangarloo H, Ortega J, et al. Primary liver tumors in children: comparison of CT and MR imaging. Radiology 1988; 169:727–732.)

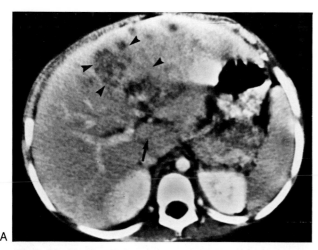
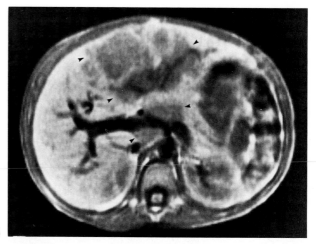

A

B

Figure 20–48. *Hepatic lymphoma in an 8-year-old girl.* ***A,*** Postcontrast CT scan. There is a mass (*arrowheads*) in the central part of the liver. It has a very heterogenous appearance and seems to invade the portal vein (*arrow*). ***B,*** Transverse MR image (500/28). The portal vein is compressed and encased by lymphadenopathy at the porta hepatis, but is not invaded by tumor. The tumor is outlined by arrowheads. (Boechat MI, Kangarloo H, Ortega J, et al. Primary liver tumors in children: comparison of CT and MR imaging. Radiology 1988; 169:727–732.)

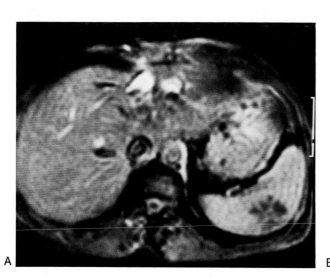
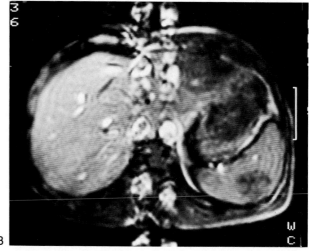

A

B

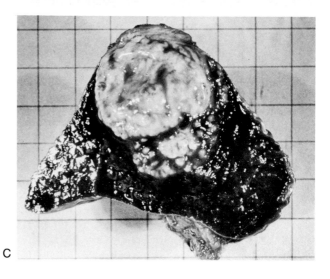

Figure 20–49. *Splenic lymphoma.* ***A,*** Transverse MR image (field echo 80/16), 30-degree flip angle. There is an area of low intensity in the spleen, due to focal involvement with lymphoma. ***B,*** Transverse MR image (field echo 80/16), 60-degree flip angle. The lesion remains of lower intensity than that of normal spleen on this slightly more T1 weighted image. ***C,*** Gross specimen showing the macroscopic lymphoma, which corresponds well to the abnormalities seen on the MR images. (Hess CF, Griebel J, Schmiedl U, et al. Focal lesions of the spleen: preliminary results with fast MR imaging at 1.5T. J Comput Assist Tomogr 1988; 12:569–574.)

C

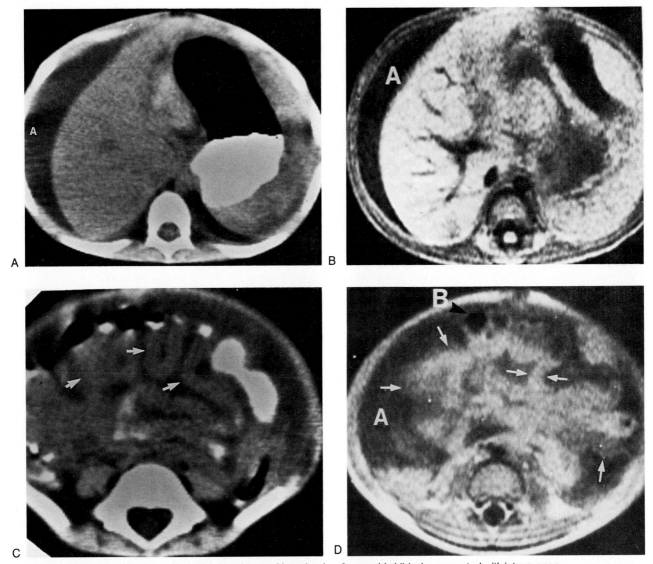

Figure 20–50. *Mesenteric non-Hodgkin's lymphoma with ascites in a 6-year-old child who presented with intussusception.* ***A,*** CT scan showing a large amount of ascitic fluid (A). ***B,*** Transverse MR image (500/30). The ascites (A) is easily identified. The MR image corresponds well to the CT scan. ***C,*** CT image shows diffuse thickening of the bowel mesentery (*arrows*) consistent with widespread lymphadenopathy. ***D,*** Transverse MR image (500/30). The thickened mesentery (*arrows*) is identified by the moderately strong signal. Air-filled loops of bowel (B) are seen anteriorly. The low intensity in the flanks represents ascites (A).

garding the use of MRI to evaluate hepatic metastasis. The dispute involves both the role of MRI and the pulse sequences that should be used. The information provided by the literature is somewhat confusing and conflicting.[34] Some radiologists favor utilizing strongly T1 weighted pulse sequences such as the STIR pulse sequence for screening the liver; others prefer T2 weighted pulse sequences.[35–38] The optimal pulse sequence will vary with magnetic field strength. There is also conflicting evidence regarding the sensitivity and specificity of MRI compared with other modalities such as CT and ultrasonography. There are reports in which MRI has demonstrated metastases not seen by other imaging tools.[2, 39] MRI may also exclude metas-

tases suspected from other imaging studies (Fig. 20–63).

In summary, MRI has proved sensitive in identifying liver metastases, especially in adults. New motion suppression methods and new contrast agents will only improve MR imaging of the liver. MRI should play a major role in screening the liver for metastases in children.

Angiomyolipoma

Angiomyolipoma is an unusual tumor that may involve the liver.[40] The lesion is well defined. A characteristic finding is increased signal intensity on both T1

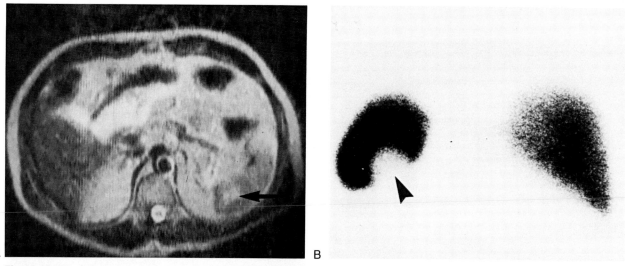

Figure 20–51. *Splenic lymphoma.* ***A,*** Transverse T2 weighted MR image (2350/120). There is a small focal lesion (*arrow*) lying within the spleen. It has greater signal intensity than the surrounding spleen. ***B,*** Posterior scintiscan shows a photogenic defect (*arrowhead*) larger than the lesion seen on the MR image.

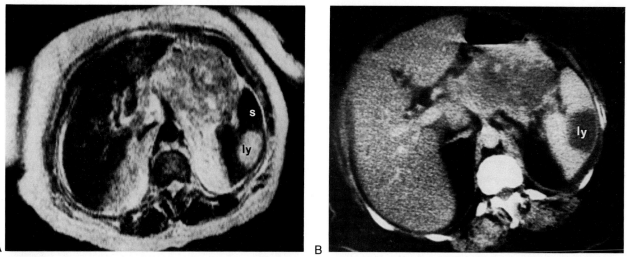

Figure 20–52. *Splenic lymphoma.* ***A,*** Transverse T2 weighted image (1620/120). There is a lymphoma (ly) lesion that is hyperintense relative to the surrounding spleen (S). ***B,*** Contrast-enhanced transverse CT scan correlates well with the MR image. The tumor (ly) fails to enhance with intravenous contrast administration. (Hahn PF, Wiessleder R, Stark DD, et al. MR imaging of focal splenic tumors. AJR 1988; 150:823.)

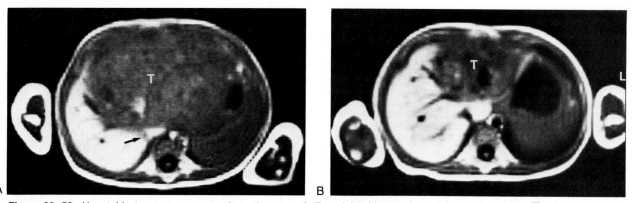

Figure 20–53. *Hepatoblastoma: response to chemotherapy.* ***A,*** T1 weighted image shows a large tumor mass (T). ***B,*** Repeat MRI after five cycles of chemotherapy shows marked interval tumor (T) shrinkage. The tumor is in the left lobe of the liver. It was resected. (Rollins NK. MRI of the pediatric patient. Curr Concepts MRI 1988; 2:5–18.)

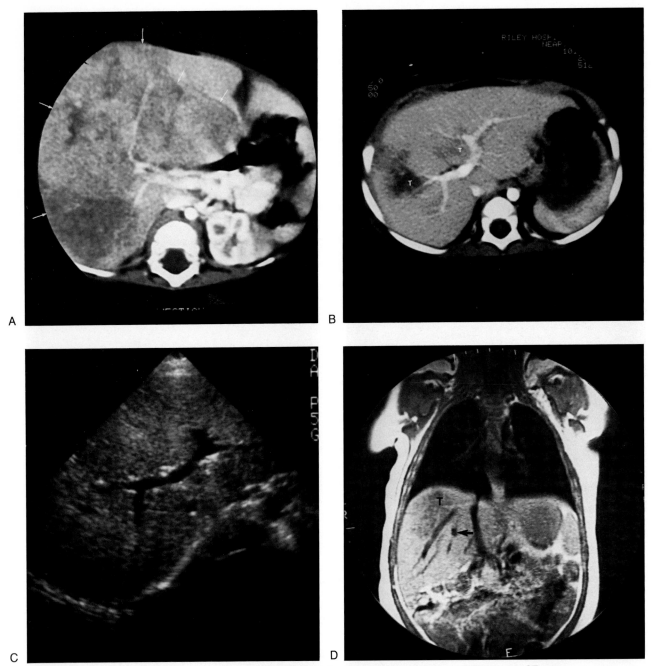

Figure 20–54. *Hepatoblastoma: preoperative MR evaluation after 3 months of chemotherapy.* **A,** Transverse CT scan at the time of presentation demonstrates a gigantic mass (*arrows*) involving most of the liver. **B,** CT scan obtained 3 months later. There is marked reduction in the size of the tumor (T), which extends up to the left branch of the portal vein and therefore involves the right and quadrate lobes of the liver. **C,** Comparative ultrasound study. The tumor is of increased ethogenicity. Note that it is more difficult to identify the tumor margins on the ultrasound image than on the CT scan. **D,** Coronal MR image (900/26), demonstrating complete patency of the right and left hepatic veins. The middle hepatic vein (*arrow*) is less well seen. T, Tumor. **E,** Transverse T1 (900/26) weighted image. This again corresponds well to the CT scan. The portal vein is well seen. Tumor is seen as a low-intensity abnormality. **F, G,** Transverse MR images (900/26) obtained just superior to the portal vein before and after administration of gadolinium-DTPA. Before administration the tumor is of patchy, very low intensity; after administration there is marked enhancement of the rim of the tumor. The enhancement is somewhat patchy. At surgery the central area of the tumor was found to be hemorrhagic and fibrotic. Hemosiderin was present. **H,** Transverse T2 weighted image (2000/80) obtained with motion suppression technique. Even on this T2 weighted image, tumor is of mainly low intensity with some higher-intensity background. The low intensity is consistent with T2 shortening from the hemosiderin and fibrosis. Note that the motion suppression technique turns the portal veins (*arrow*) white, and the appearance corresponds fairly well to that seen on the CT scan. There is good correlation between the three modalities; MRI and CT are superior to ultrasound. MRI was extremely good at characterizing the pathologic nature of the tumor.

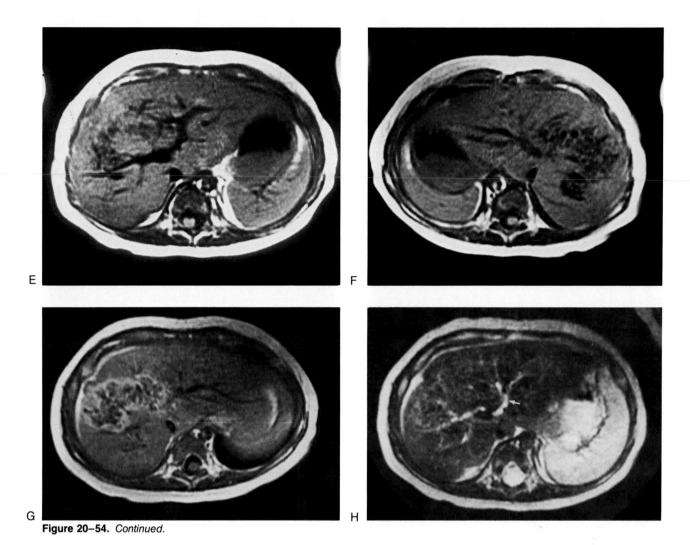

E

F

G

H

Figure 20–54. *Continued.*

and T2 pulse sequences due to areas of fat within the tumor. However, the appearance is not absolutely specific, because similar findings can be noted in other tumors containing regions of hemorrhage.

Liver Cysts

Simple liver cysts are not uncommon. Unless very large, they will produce no symptoms. They are well defined and round, with smooth margins. They are easily diagnosed by ultrasonography or CT. MRI of liver cysts identifies single, sharply defined lesions with very low signal intensity on T1 and very high signal on T2 images. Cavernous hemangiomas may have a similar appearance.

Mesenchymal Hamartoma

Mesenchymal hamartoma is a benign, well-defined liver tumor, usually presenting in infancy. It should be

well seen on MR images, but no cases have yet been reported.

Miscellaneous Tumors

Many abdominal and retroperitoneal tumors arise from organs other than those of the gastrointestinal tract. They do, however, need to be recognized and distinguished. Examples of such tumors include retroperitoneal teratomas (Fig. 20–64), lipomas (Fig. 20–65), yolk sac tumors (Fig. 20–66), and retroperitoneal neurofibromas (Fig. 20–67).

TRAUMA

There are virtually no reports of the use of MRI to evaluate acute abdominal trauma. This is probably due to the difficulty in getting acutely traumatized patients to remain still for the prolonged period required to

Text continues on page 652.

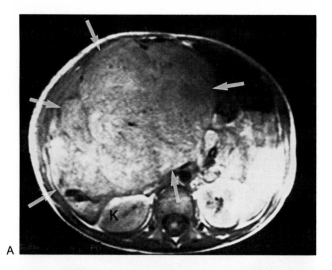

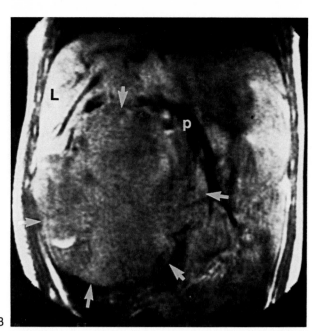

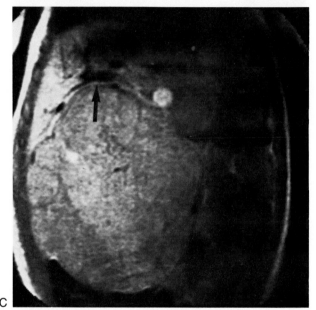

Figure 20–55. *Hepatoblastoma in a 2-year-old boy with an abdominal mass.* **A,** Transverse T2 weighted MR image (1500/60). There is a very large mass lesion (*arrows*) seen in the right upper abdomen, of mixed moderate and high intensity. The high-intensity areas correspond to regions of hemorrhage and/or necrosis. The mass lies anterior to the right kidney (K). **B, C,** Coronal T1 (600/30) and T2 (1500/60) weighted MR images. Both show the mass lesion well (*arrows*) and clearly demonstrate that the tumor is arising from the liver (L). It is situated in the inferior aspect of the right lobe of the liver. The tumor extends superiorly, close to the portal vein (p), which is patent and not invaded by tumor. The T2 image shows a thin rim of normal tissue (*arrow*) between the tumor and the portal vein. This was confirmed at surgery.

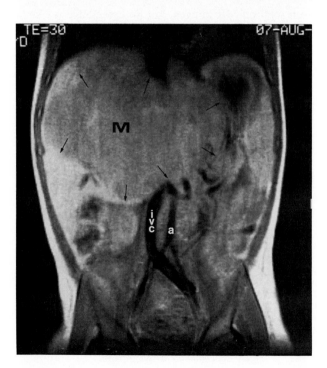

Figure 20–56. *Hepatoblastoma.* T1 weighted image. There is a very large mass (M) of homogeneous intensity occupying most of the posterior aspect of the right lobe of the liver (arrows indicate tumor margin). The tumor mass is causing compression and partial obstruction of the inferior vena cava (ivc). Below the level of the mass the inferior vena cava is distended. The aorta (a) is of normal caliber. (Riddlesberger MM. Evaluation of the gastrointestinal tract in the child: CT, MRI and isotopic studies. Pediatr Clin North Am 1988; 35:281–310.)

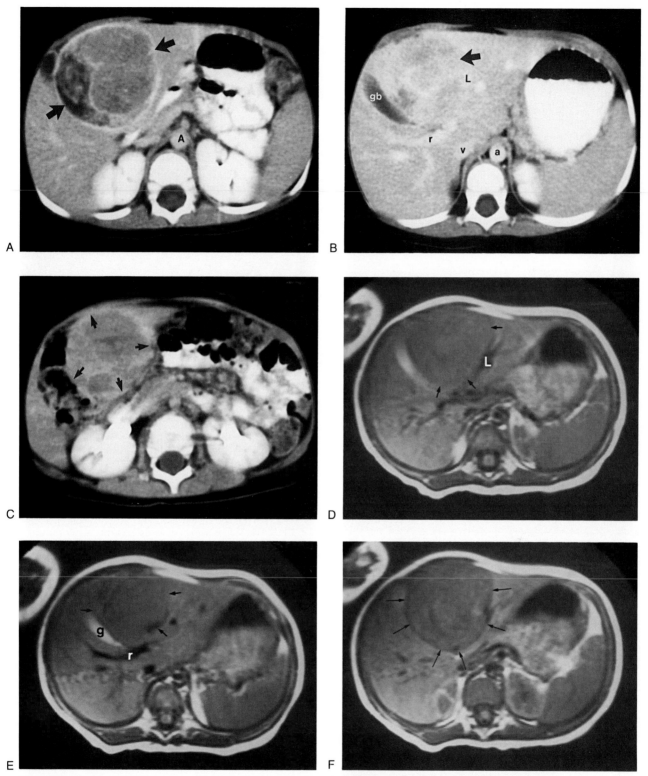

Figure 20–57. *Hepatoblastoma in an 18-month-old boy who presented with abdominal mass.* **A** to **C,** Transverse CT images taken at three levels through the liver (L), after administration of intravenous contrast material. There is a well-defined mass lesion (*arrows*) lying medial to the gallbladder (gb). The aorta (a), inferior vena cava (v), and right (r) and left (l) branches of the portal vein can be seen. The tumor appears to lie in the quadrate lobe and to hang down off the inferior surface of the liver. **D** to **F,** Transverse T1 weighted MR images taken at three levels through the liver (550/26). The mass lesion is well seen (*arrows*). It is of slightly lower intensity than that of normal liver and lies medial to the gallbladder (g). The right (r) and left (l) portal vein branches are well seen. The tumor is confined to the quadrate lobe. **G,** Sagittal T1 image through the plane of the right kidney (K) (550/26). This shows that the tumor (*arrows*) is well defined, and is composed of one large segment and a smaller posterior second lobule. **H,** T2 weighted sagittal image (2000/80). There is an increase in signal intensity from the well-defined tumor (T). It appears of much higher intensity than that of normal liver (L). **I,** Transverse field-echo T2 weighted MR image with 20-degree flip angle (400/14) shows a moderately strong signal from the tumor (*arrows*). Note that field-echo pulse sequences are more sensitive to motion and that there is significant blurring artifact in this image (compare with **D, E,** and **F,** which were obtained with spin-echo technique). The field echo takes less time to perform.

Figure continues on following page.

649

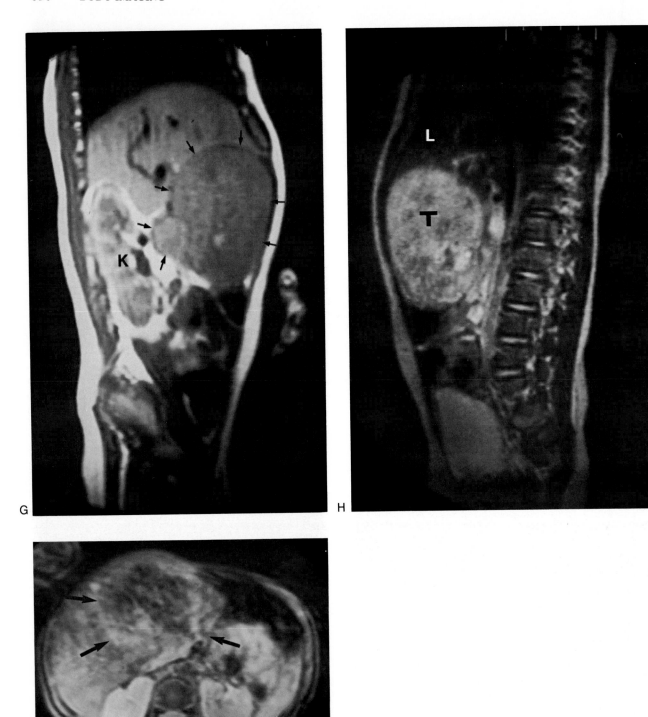

Figure 20–57. *Continued.*

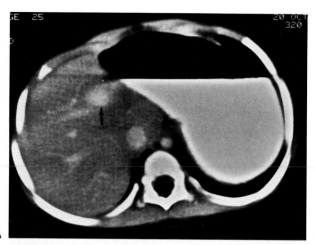

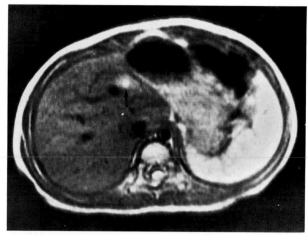

A B

Figure 20–58. *Recurrent hepatoblastoma in a 2-year-old girl 3 months after left hepatectomy.* **A,** Transverse CT image after bolus injection of intravenous contrast material. There is an area of enhancement close to the margin of the liver (*arrow*). On the CT image it is difficult to differentiate an enhancing blood vessels from tumor. **B,** Transverse T2 image (1500/56). The area of abnormality is hyperintense (*arrow*) on the MR image. Blood vessels are of low intensity. The appearance is strongly suggestive of tumor recurrence, which was confirmed at surgery. (Boechat MI, Kangarloo H, Ortega J, et al. Primary liver tumors in children: comparison of CT and MR imaging. Radiology 1988; 169:727–732.)

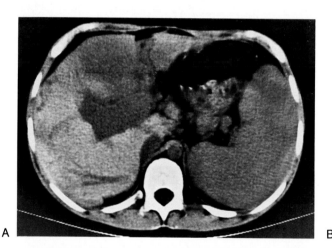

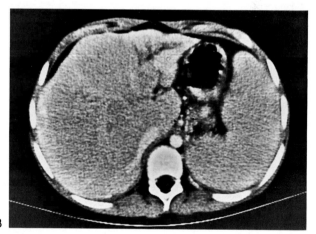

A B

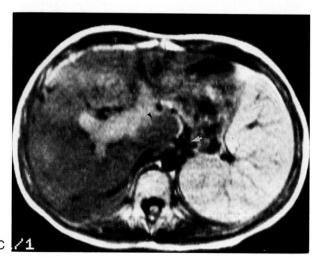

C /1

Figure 20–59. *Hepatocellular carcinoma with invasion of the portal vein in a 14-year-old boy.* **A,** Non–contrast-enhanced CT scan. There is a large low-attenuation mass in the liver. Note the splenomegaly. **B,** CT scan after intravenous contrast injection. The tumor is now isointense with liver parenchyma. The lack of enhancement of the portal vein and the presence of gastric varices (*arrows*) and splenomegaly suggest tumor infiltration of the portal vein, causing hypertension. **C,** Transverse T2 weighted image (1500/56) demonstrates a mass with low signal intensity invading the portal vein (*arrowhead*). Note the multiple dilated collateral vessels (*arrow*) and the splenomegaly. (Boechat MI, Kangarloo H, Ortega J, et al. Primary liver tumors in children: comparison of CT and MR imaging. Radiology 1988; 169:727–732.)

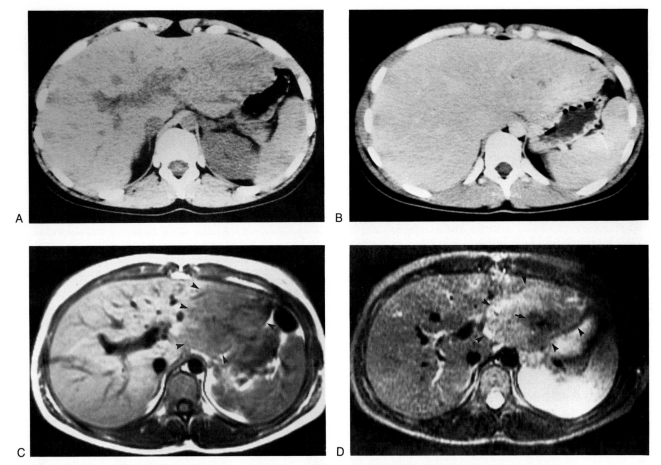

Figure 20–60. *Fibrolamellar hepatocellular carcinoma.* **A,** Enhanced CT scan shows a slightly hypodense mass in the lateral segment of the left lobe. **B,** CT scan after intravenous contrast injection. The mass is almost completely hypointense compared with normal liver. **C,** Transverse T1 weighted MR image (400/20). There is a hypointense mass in the lateral segment of the left lobe of the liver (*arrowheads*). **D,** T2 weighted MR image (2500/80). Most of the mass (*arrowheads*) is of heterogeneous high signal. The central area is of low signal intensity (*arrow*). (Teitelbaum DS, Hatabu H, Schiebler ML, et al. Fibrolamellar hepatocellular carcinoma: MR appearance. J Comput Assist Tomogr 1988; 12:588–591.)

obtain MR images. However, there is no reason why, with the newer, rapid pulse sequences, one should not attempt to use MR in evaluating these patients. CT is excellent for evaluating acute abdominal trauma, and it may be why there has been little enthusiasm for attempting the use of MRI for this purpose. MRI does offer the potential of partially characterizing tissues and fluids, and this could be helpful, for example, in differentiating blood in the peritoneal space from chylous ascites due to a ruptured gallbladder (Fig. 20–68).[41] Hematomas in the liver, for example, show low signal intensity on T1 pulse sequences early in their evolution. Within a day or two the signal intensity from the hematoma becomes strong.[33] Because MRI can characterize blood, it may have a role in the identification of hematomas in difficult or unusual locations in the abdomen. For example, the presence of a hematoma in the duodenal wall can be inferred from indentations in the barium column. On CT the diagnosis of a mass lesion may be easy to make, but accurate charac-

terization of the blood cannot be confident. MRI may prove more accurate in identifying duodenal hematomas (Fig. 20–69).

Pancreatic pseudocysts (Fig. 20–70) are easily identified on MRI, as well-defined lesions closely related to the pancreas. These have low signal (unless they contain blood) on T1 weighted images and high signal on T2 weighted images. It is not known whether MRI offers any advantages over CT or ultrasonography.

MRI has identified traumatic diaphragmatic rupture with herniation of bowel into the thorax (Fig. 20–71).

Mechanical Disorders

Mechanical lesions of the bowel are common and include bowel obstruction, volvulus, intussusception, and inguinal hernia. These disorders are usually well evaluated by conventional imaging techniques, and there appears to be no rush to use MRI to study them.

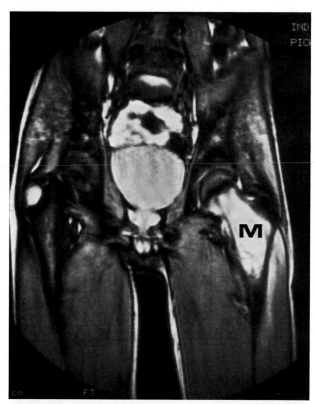

Figure 20–61. *Bone metastasis from hepatocellular carcinoma.* Coronal MR image (2000/30) shows high-intensity signal in the neck of the femur on the left side. The appearance is nonspecific, but in this patient was due to a hemorrhagic metastasis (M).

One possible area of research interest may be evaluation of bowel ischemia in children with volvulus.

Other mechanical disorders may be seen incidentally on MR images. An example is paralyzed diaphragm (Fig. 20–72).

VASCULAR DISORDERS

Splenic Infarction

Splenic infarction (Fig. 20–73) may be an incidental finding or may occur as a complication in disorders such as sickle cell anemia. An area of acute infarction in an otherwise normal-appearing spleen will have increased T1 and T2 relaxation times and may be difficult to differentiate from normal spleen, which has relatively long T1 and T2 relaxation times, compared with liver or muscle. In many patients with splenic infarction, however, there is associated iron overload from transfusions for hemolytic anemia.[5, 42] In these situations the spleen appears of very low intensity on T1 weighted images. Areas of infarction appear as round focal regions of signal intensity greater than that of muscle on T2 weighted pulse sequences (Fig. 20–73).[5] Using fast field-echo pulse sequences with varying flip

angles, it was found that old healed infarcts were indistinguishable from other disorders such as lymphoma and sarcoid. Recent infarcts less than 3 weeks old were seen as regions of high signal intensity with pulse sequences of 30-degree and 60-degree flip angles.[42]

Portal Vein Occlusion

MRI can be used to confirm or exclude the presence of portal vein thrombus (Figs. 20–74, 20–75). Thrombus formation in the portal vein can be identified on MRI. No large series comparing MRI with CT and ultrasonography have been reported. Criteria for the diagnosis of portal vein thrombosis include the presence of a persistent signal in the portal vein (Fig. 20–75) or failure to show the portal vein and the demonstration of enlarged collateral vascular channels (cavernous transformation of the portal vein).[43, 44] The signal intensity from the portal vein thrombus varies, depending both on the age of the thrombus and on the magnetic field strength.[43] The thrombus is of high signal on T2 images. At 0.5T, thrombi less than 5 weeks old were found to have only mild signal on T1 pulse sequences.[43] The differential diagnosis of intraluminal thrombus includes compression of the vessel, e.g., from enlarged lymph nodes, or intraluminal signal from entry slice phenomena (even echo rephasing) or slow or stagnant blood.[43] The presence of clot is strongly suggested if the abnormality is seen to be persistent on multiple pulse sequences,[43] if it persists on different imaging planes, and if the presence of an extrinsic mass is excluded on the T2 pulse sequence.

Cavernous transformation represents the development of enlarged collateral vessels in the chronic stage after portal vein thrombosis. These vessels are seen as linear regions of low signal intensity (due to flow) on most conventional spin-echo pulse sequences (Figs. 20–76, 20–77).[44] A varying number of these collateral vessels are identified in the region of the porta hepatis; no normal portal vein is seen. The hepatic veins may be enlarged.

Portal Hypertension

In children the most common cause of portal hypertension is idiopathic thrombosis of the portal vein. This usually occurs early in life and may be associated with previous use of umbilical venous catheters or previous episodes of abdominal infection. Collateral vessel channels develop in the porta hepatis, bypassing the occluded portal vein. These give the condition its other name of "cavernous transformation of the portal vein." Less commonly, in children, portal hypertension is due to liver cirrhosis (Fig. 20–78) from, for example, previous infection, biliary atresia, and metabolic disorders such as Wilson's disease and alpha$_1$-antitrypsin deficiency. Hepatic vein occlusion is rare in children.

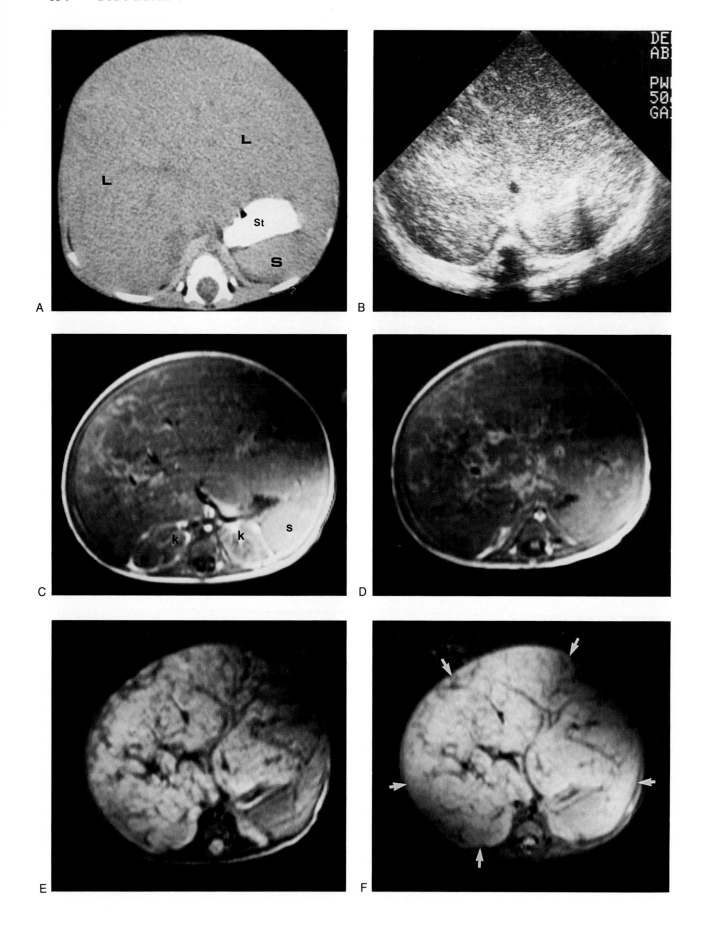

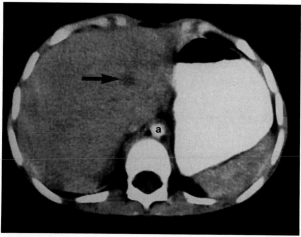
A

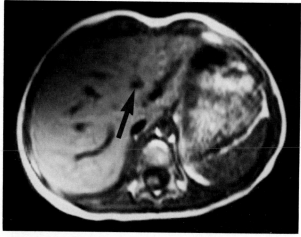
B

Figure 20–63. *False diagnosis of liver metastasis on CT scan.* **A,** Transverse CT image obtained immediately after bolus injection of contrast material. A low-intensity lesion (*arrow*) is seen in the left lobe of the liver. This was originally thought to be a metastasis in a patient with known Wilms' tumor. **B,** Transverse MR image (500/26) shows that the abnormality seen on the CT scan appears to be a normal branch of the portal vein (*arrow*), with low signal intensity due to flow. The correct diagnosis was of a normal vessel. On the CT scan a bolus of contrast material is clearly identified in the aorta, (a), but the contrast, at the time of the image acquisition, had not yet had time to circulate through the liver and opacify the portal vein.

MRI is rapidly becoming the imaging modality of choice for evaluating these children. It may well make angiography unnecessary in many patients. The only thing that MRI cannot do is measure the direction of flow, which is easily done by Doppler ultrasonography. MRI shows a normal liver in patients with cavernous transformation of the portal vein (Fig. 20–77). In cirrhosis the liver is abnormal but the appearance is extremely varied, depending to some extent on the underlying etiology. Patency or thrombosis of the portal vein can be identified. With cavernous transformation, multiple patent collateral channels are seen as of low signal intensity on all pulse sequences in the region of the porta hepatis. The patency and size of the splenic vein can be determined. This is particularly important in patients in whom splenorenal shunt is to be performed. Variceal dilatation of veins at various sites can be well identified (Fig. 20–77). This includes dilatation of the left gastric (coronary) vein, the short gastric

veins, the superior mesenteric veins, and the veins of the anterior abdominal wall. The spleen is enlarged in almost all patients with portal hypertension. Signal intensity from the spleen remains more or less normal. After a surgical shunt procedure, MRI can also be used to evaluate the patency and size of the shunt.

METABOLIC DISORDERS

Fatty Infiltration of the Pancreas

This is a common finding in patients with cystic fibrosis (Fig. 20–79). The pancreas is diffusely infiltrated with fat. It appears of fairly normal size and shape. The fat in the pancreas causes it to be of very high signal intensity on both T1 and T2 pulse sequences.

Text continues on page 658.

◀ **Figure 20–62.** *Stage IV-S neuroblastoma: hepatic involvement in a 3-month-old infant who presented with an abdominal mass, due to hepatomegaly.* **A,** CT scan shows massive hepatomegaly. The liver (L) is fairly homogeneous. Tumor cannot be differentiated from normal liver. S, Spleen; St, stomach. **B,** Transverse abdominal ultrasound image shows marked hepatomegaly. There is some ill-defined increase in echogenicity. The cause of the hepatomegaly cannot be determined from this image. **C, D,** Transverse T1 weighted images obtained at two levels in the liver (550/16), which fills almost the entire image. There is an irregular reticulated network of moderate signal intensity representing residual normal liver. The rest of the liver appears of lowish signal intensity owing to tumor infiltration. s, Spleen; k, kidney. **E,** Transverse T2 weighted image (2000/80). Normal liver at this pulse sequence should appear of very low signal intensity. Virtually the entire liver is replaced by neuroblastoma, which appears of strong signal intensity and has a lobulated nodular appearance. Note also the marked distortion of the hepatic and portal veins (the tubular low-intensity structures) by the infiltrating tumor. **F,** Transverse STIR image through the liver (*arrows*) (TE 200/TI 150). On this pulse sequence, almost no signal is obtained from subcutaneous fat. Tumor within the liver appears of strong signal intensity. Visualization of the tumor is very similar to that in **E.** MRI demonstrates the tumor infiltration throughout the liver and the distortion of the intrahepatic vessels much better than does either CT or ultrasonography.

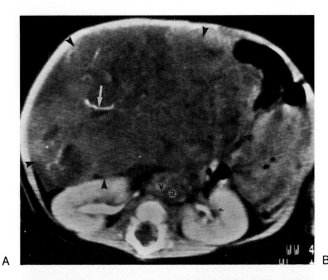

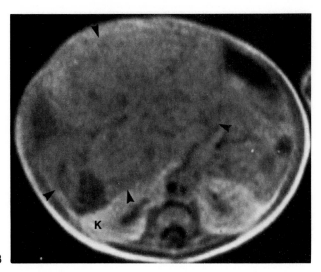

A

B

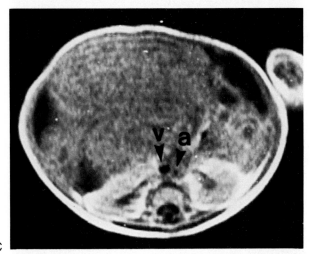

C

Figure 20–64. *Retroperitoneal teratoma in a 6-week-old infant.* ***A,*** CT scan shows a large abdominal mass (*arrowheads*) separate from the kidneys. A small amount of calcium (*arrow*) is seen within the mass. The aorta (a) and inferior vena cava (v) are displaced but not encased by the tumor mass. ***B,*** Transverse MR image (500/30). The size, shape, and outline of the mass (*arrowheads*) are similar to those seen on the CT scan. Once again, the mass is noted to be clearly separate from the kidney. There is some squashing of the right kidney (K). The aorta and inferior vena cava are slightly compressed by the mass. The absence of any large lymph nodes encasing the aorta and inferior vena cava is very much against the diagnosis of neuroblastoma. ***C,*** Transverse T2 image (1000/60). The signal intensity from the mass is increased. Note again the compression of the inferior vena cava (v) and aorta (a). The calcium seen on the CT scan cannot be identified on the MR images.

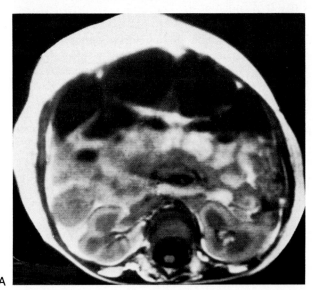

A

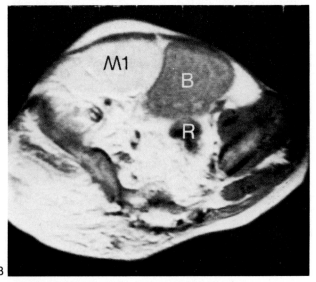

B

Figure 20–65. *Proteus syndrome. This disorder is characterized by hemihypertrophy with diffuse lipomas and lymphangiomas.* ***A,*** Transverse abdominal MR image (600/27). There is diffuse increase in the thickness of the subcutaneous fat owing to widespread lipomatosis. ***B,*** Transverse MR image through the pelvis. There is diffuse infiltration of the pelvis by fatty tissue. A better-defined fatty mass (M1) displaces the bladder (B) and also the rectum (R) to the left. (Cremin BJ, Viljoen DL, Wynchank S, et al. The proteus syndrome: the magnetic resonance and radiological features. Pediatr Radiol 1987; 17:486–488.)

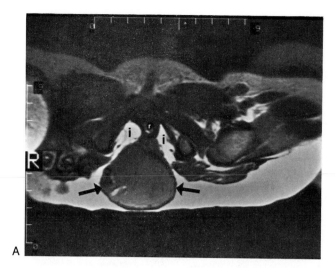

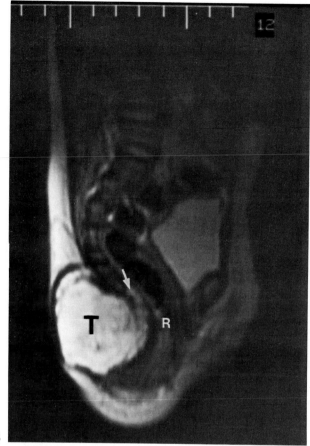

Figure 20–66. *Yolk sac tumor and teratoma in a 9-month-old infant with a perineal mass.* **A,** Transverse T1 weighted image (680/26). There is a large, well-defined soft tissue mass (*arrows*) lying posteriorly in the perineum. The rectum (r) is displaced forward and to the left by the mass. Both ischiorectal fossae (i) are compressed and distorted by the mass. **B,** Sagittal T2 weighted midline image (2000/80). The tumor (T) is well defined and appears of very strong intensity. The tumor extends anteriorly (*arrow*) around the coccyx to displace the rectum (R) forward.

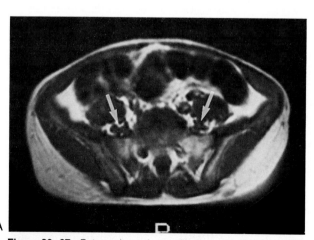

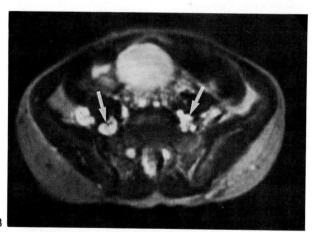

Figure 20–67. *Retroperitoneal neurofibromas. T1 (800/30).* (**A**) and T2 (1500/90) (**B**) weighted images show multiple retroperitoneal nodules (*arrows*). These are difficult to differentiate from muscle on the T1 images but appear of very strong signal intensity on the T2 weighted images. Apart from their location, it is very difficult to differentiate these lesions from high-intensity signal in loops of bowel.

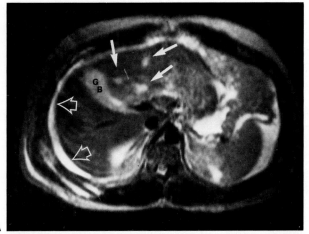

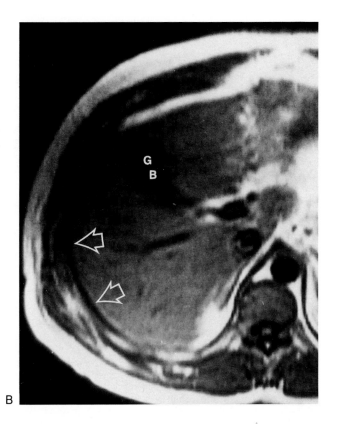

Figure 20–68. *Traumatic gallbladder rupture.* ***A,*** Transverse MR image (210/100) obtained through the level of the gallbladder (GB) demonstrates small foci of hyperintensity (*arrows*) in the medial segment of the left lobe of the liver. Intraperitoneal fluid (*open arrows*) is seen around the right liver margin and is of very strong signal intensity. ***B,*** T1 weighted image (683/26). The lesion in the left lobe of the liver is nearly isointense with normal liver. The intraperitoneal fluid along the right liver edge is of markedly decreased intensity (*open arrows*). The images were obtained 7 days after injury. At this stage one would expect traumatic ascites containing blood to be of strong signal intensity on the T1 weighted image. The fact that it is of low signal raises the possibility that the fluid is not blood. At surgery it proved to be bile, and a tear in the gallbladder was identified. (Baumgartner FJ, Barnett MJ, Velez M, Chiu LC. Traumatic disruption of the gallbladder evaluated by computerized tomography and magnetic resonance imaging. Br J Surg 1988; 75:386–387.)

Iron Storage Disorders

Hemochromatosis is rare. It represents abnormal accumulation of ferritin in the parenchymal liver cells[45] and is due to abnormal absorption of iron from the intestinal tract. The parenchymal cells are damaged, finally causing cirrhosis.

Hemosiderosis is far more common. It is due to the accumulation of abnormal amounts of hemosiderin within the cells of the reticuloendothelial system, and involves the liver, spleen, bone marrow, and other sites.[45] The deposited hemosiderin in the reticuloendothelial cells has little direct toxic effect.[46] The cause of the hemosiderin deposition is almost always iron overload in children, requiring chronic blood transfusions either for hemolytic anemia or for chronic renal failure.

The hemosiderin contains iron in a ferric state. This exerts a paramagnetic effect that alters the signal intensity from the tissues in which the hemosiderin is deposited. Using an in vitro experimental method, Brasch and colleagues demonstrated that the hemosiderin causes a reduction in both T1 and T2 relaxation times. The effect in decreasing T1 relaxation time is maximal at low concentrations of hemosiderin. Higher concentrations of hemosiderin exert a proportionately larger

effect in decreasing T2 relaxation time.[46] The effect of the reduction in T1 relaxation time is to cause an increase in signal intensity on T1 weighted images. The effect of the reduction in T2 relaxation time is to reduce markedly the signal intensity in T2 and T1 weighted images (Figs. 20–73, 20–80). The effect of signal reduction in T2 images is easily explained by the reduction in T2 relaxation time. The cause of the low signal on the T1 images is the effect of T2 shortening overwhelming the T1 shortening. Detection of signal stops when T2 relaxation is complete. If T2 is so short that there is inadequate time for signal to be detected, the signal intensity, even on T1 images, is very low, irrespective of the T1 relaxation time.[45, 46]

The MR findings in patients with hemosiderosis and hemochromatosis are exactly what one would predict from the above discussion. In two patients, one with hemosiderosis and one with hemochromatosis, very low signal was seen in the liver on both T1 and T2 pulse sequences.[45] In 18 children with transfusion-induced hemosiderosis for renal failure, the subjective liver intensity and the ratio of liver intensity to muscle intensity was low on T1 weighted images in all 18.[47] In 15 children with sickle cell disease and transfusion-induced hemosiderosis, liver signal intensity was low on T1 images in all 15.[48] This reduction in signal intensity

Text continues on page 662.

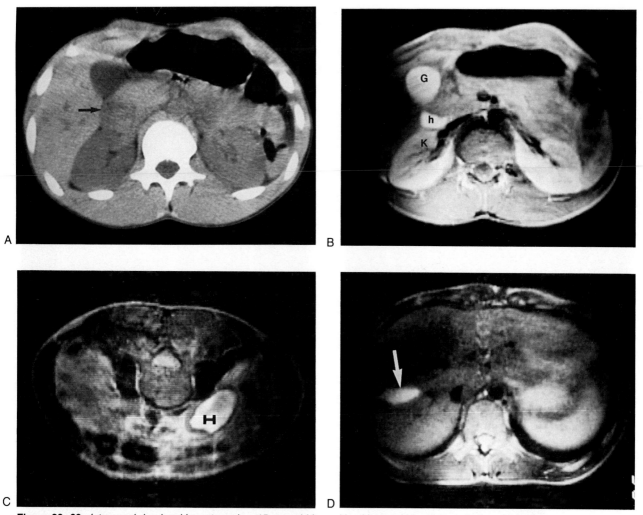

Figure 20–69. *Intramural duodenal hematoma in a 15-year-old boy with a history of blunt trauma to the midabdomen followed by pain and vomiting.* ***A,*** CT scan shows a very poorly defined soft tissue mass (*arrow*) anterior to the right kidney. ***B,*** Transverse spin-density image (2000/30). There is a crescentic area of high signal intensity anterior to the right kidney, which represents the hematoma (h). G, Gallbladder; K, kidney. This image was obtained at the same level as ***A.*** ***C,*** T2 weighted image (2000/75) 5 cm caudal to ***B.*** There is a large hematoma (H) of strong signal intensity at the junction of the second and third portions of the duodenum. ***D,*** Image obtained through the liver, showing an associated hematoma (*arrow*) lying within the liver, due to a partial laceration. The MR images were obtained 16 days after the trauma. The strong signal intensity is consistent with hematoma. Note that there is much more contrast between the hematoma and adjacent soft tissues on the MR compared with the CT scan. (Martin B, Mulopulos AP, Butler ME. MR imaging of intranural duodenal hematoma. J Comput Assist Tomogr 1986; 10:1042–1043.)

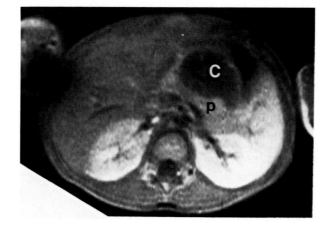

Figure 20–70. *Pancreatic pseudocyst in a 6-year-old child with a history of abdominal trauma.* Transverse MR image (500/30) showing a well-defined cyst (C). Normal pancreatic tissue is seen immediately posterior to the cyst. This close association suggests that the cyst has a pancreatic origin. Other cystic pathology such as a bowel duplication cyst would be included in the differential diagnosis. The low-intensity signal on this T1 weighted image is consistent with the presence of fluid. p, Pancreas.

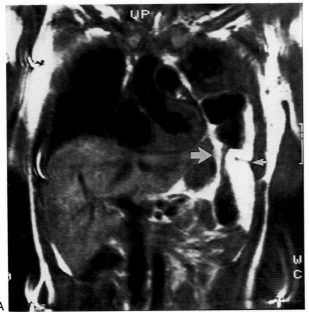

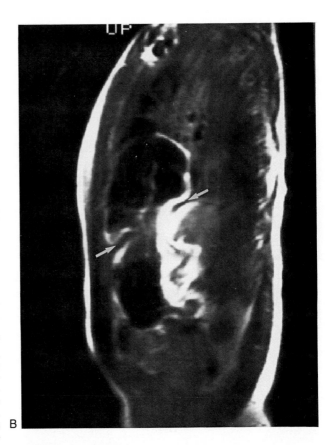

A

B

Figure 20–71. *Traumatic diaphragmatic rupture with herniation of the colon into the chest.* ***A,*** Coronal MR image (510/17). There is a defect in the left hemidiaphragm with herniation of the colon through the defect (*arrows*). Increased signal surrounding the colon represents fat. ***B,*** Sagittal T1 weighted image (510/17) that also demonstrates the ruptured diaphragm with herniation of the colon. The colon is constricted as it crosses the tear in the diaphragm (*arrows*). (Mirvis SE, Veramat B, Buckman R, et al. MR imaging of traumatic diaphragmatic rupture. J Comput Assist Tomogr 1988; 12:147–149.)

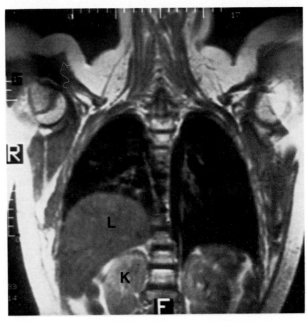

Figure 20–72. *Paralyzed right hemidiaphragm in a child with Hodgkin's lymphoma of the mediastinum. Coronal spin-density image (2000/20).* There is marked elevation of the right hemidiaphragm. The liver and right kidney are also elevated, which suggests the correct diagnosis of paralyzed diaphragm rather than hernia or eventration. Note the normal smooth contour of the diaphragm. L, Liver; K, kidney.

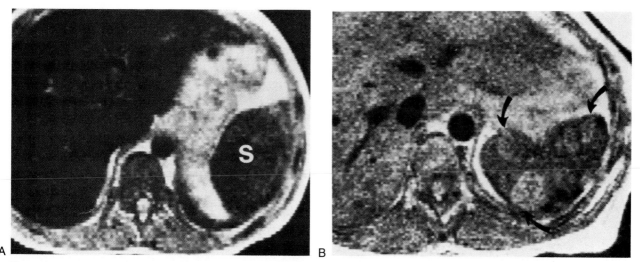

Figure 20–73. *Sickle cell anemia: secondary splenic infarction and hemosiderosis.* ***A,*** Transverse image (2000/28). There is low signal intensity from the spleen (S) and the liver due to shortening of T1 and T2 relaxation times from deposited hemosiderin. ***B,*** Transverse MR image (2000/28) in another patient. This shows multiple hyperintense splenic lesions (*arrows*) consistent with multiple infarcts. (Adler DD, Glazer GM, Aisen AM. MRI of the spleen: normal appearance and findings in sickle-cell anemia. AJR 1986; 147:843–845.)

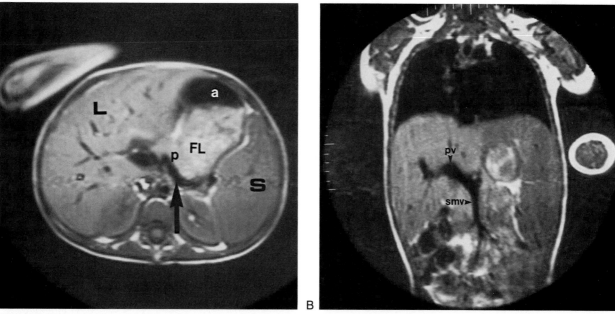

Figure 20–74. *Idiopathic splenomegaly in a 5-year-old girl with splenomegaly suspected to be the result of Henoch-Schönlein purpura. The MR study was performed to exclude portal vein obstruction as a cause of hypertension and splenomegaly.* ***A,*** Transverse T1 weighted image (450/26). The liver (L) and spleen (S) are well seen. In the stomach there is an air-fluid level with air (a) seen anteriorly and fluid (FL) with strong signal seen posteriorly. The strong signal is presumably due to ingestion of milk containing fat. It is difficult to differentiate the stomach from the pancreas (p). However, the splenic vein (*arrow*) is beautifully demonstrated and is patent. No enlarged collateral vessels or varices can be identified. ***B,*** Coronal MR image (250/26) that reveals a normal patent portal vein (pv). The superior mesenteric vein is also well identified (smv). Note that the liver appears of normal size with normal signal.

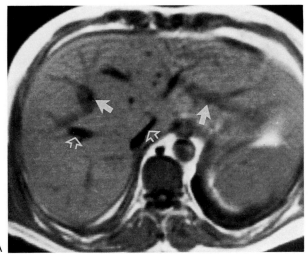

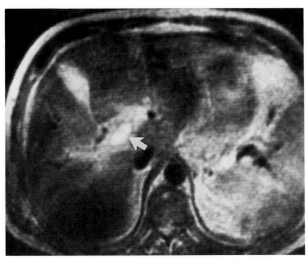

A   B

Figure 20–75. *Portal vein thrombosis.* **A,** Transverse T1 weighted image. Some signal is seen in the lumen of the right and left branches of the portal vein (*solid arrows*). The hepatic veins (*open arrows*) are void of signal. **B,** T2 weighted image shows a very bright signal (*arrow*) from the thrombus at the bifurcation of the portal vein. It is important to note that the signal intensity from the thrombus will vary, depending on the age of the clot and also on the magnetic field strength utilized. The above images were obtained at 0.5T. (Levy HM, Newhouse JH. MR imaging of portal vein thrombosis. AJR 1988; 151: 283–286.)

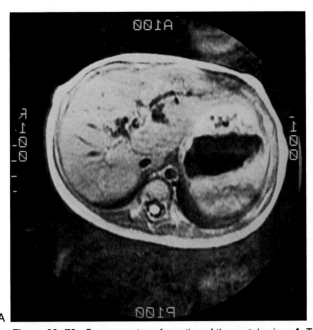

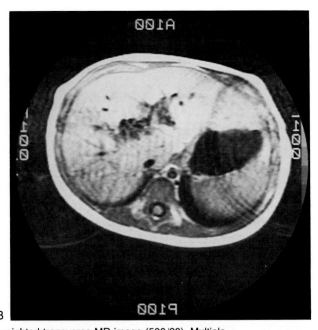

A   B

Figure 20–76. *Cavernous transformation of the portal vein.* **A,** T1 weighted transverse MR image (500/20). Multiple serpiginous, tubular, low-intensity areas are seen at the hilum of the liver. **B,** T2 weighted image (2500/40). The tubular serpiginous structures remain of low intensity, indicating the presence of flowing blood. They represent multiple enlarged collateral vessels secondary to thrombosis of the portal vein. (Courtesy of Dr. C. Weidenmeier, Jacksonville, FL.)

in the liver in hemosiderosis is also seen when field-echo pulse sequences are utilized.[42] In another study of 13 patients with sickle cell disease, low signal intensity was seen in the liver and spleen on T1 and T2 pulse sequences in all 13.[5] In three other patients with transfusion-induced hemosiderosis, signal intensity on all pulse sequences was low in the liver, spleen, and marrow but was increased compared with normal in kidney and muscle. This was explained as being due to only mild accumulation of hemosiderin in the kidneys and muscle (Fig. 20–81).

MRI is thus very sensitive for the identification of

change in tissues after accumulation of stored iron. It does not appear, however, that MRI can be used to give an accurate quantitative estimation of the amount of iron present. For example, Querfeld and associates found that the serum ferritin did not correlate with measured T1 relaxation times in the liver,[47] and Hernandez and associates noted no correlation between measured T1 and T2 relaxation times with either serum ferritin concentrations or liver iron concentrations measured by liver biopsy.[48] It was thought by these researchers that these findings were due to intrinsic difficulties in accurate measurements of T1 and T2 relaxation times. Two other studies have found lower measurements of T1 relaxation times in patients with liver iron storage,[5,49] but these studies did not correlate the amount of iron storage with the amount of T1 reduction. Hernandez and associates compared liver muscle intensity ratios with iron concentrations measured by liver biopsy (Fig. 20–82). They found that MRI could accurately differentiate between iron concentrations below 100 μg per milligram of liver and those above 100 μg per milligram. The intensity ratio changed with increasing iron concentration up to 100 μg per milligram. With iron concentrations of 100 to 400 μg per milligram, there was no further change in the intensity ratio.[48]

In summary, MRI seems to provide a very sensitive method for detection of iron overload, but gives only a very rough estimate of the amount of iron deposited in the tissue.

Fatty Infiltration of the Liver

MRI is relatively insensitive to changes in liver metabolism.[1] Diffuse fatty infiltration of the liver causes little or no change in the appearance of the liver, and may be difficult to detect on conventional spin-echo pulse imaging.[1] Focal deposits of fat may be more concentrated and are seen as areas of increased intensity on T1 weighted spin-echo pulse sequence images.[50]

Wilson's Disease

MR imaging has not proved to be a sensitive method for looking at the liver in Wilson's disease. In one study of 12 patients, nodular irregularities were identified in only two; the other ten appeared normal.[51]

IATROGENIC DISORDERS

Drug-induced Disorders

Little has been published on the MR appearance of iatrogenic disorders of the gastrointestinal tract. MRI has been used in an attempt to screen the liver for methotrexate-induced toxicity. In 51 patients, measurements of T1 relaxation time showed no correlation with liver biopsy findings.[52]

Radiation

In the acute stage after radiation therapy, MRI can detect hepatic abnormality, seen as a sharply demarcated area corresponding to the radiation port. The irradiated area of the liver shows signal changes consistent with edema and prolongation of T1 and T2 relaxation times. Compared with normal liver, there is low signal intensity on T1 weighted and high signal intensity on T2 weighted images.[53]

MISCELLANEOUS DISORDERS

Liver Transplantation

The preoperative evaluation of patients for liver transplantation (Figs. 20–83 to 20–86) requires careful demonstration of venous anatomy.[54] Ultrasonography is the primary screening procedure for evaluation of these structures. However, many potential recipients have distorted abdominal anatomy because of congenital anomalies, portal hypertension, tumor masses, or surgical change. In these difficult patients in whom sonography is inconclusive, MRI may prove useful.[54] In a study of nine pediatric liver transplant candidates, MRI was used to define venous anatomy. MRI was able to demonstrate portal vein patency in three patients (Fig. 20–83) in whom it was not seen on angiography, and in one patient in whom it was not well seen on ultrasonography. In two patients with either very slow flow or thrombosis, MRI was inferior to angiography or ultrasonography (Fig. 20–85).[54] MRI was excellent in identifying azygous continuation of the inferior vena cava in one patient (Fig. 20–86).[54] MRI can also permit accurate measurement of portal vein diameter; a minimum of 3 to 4 mm is required to perform transplantation (Fig. 20–84).

CONTRAST AGENTS

A major problem in MR imaging of the abdomen is that it is frequently difficult to identify normal loops of bowel. Because of this and the unpredictability of signal from the bowel, there is great difficulty in differentiating bowel content from lesions inside or outside the bowel. Because there is such limited natural contrast between the bowel and contiguous tissues, a wide variety of orally administered contrast agents have been used in an attempt to improve bowel visualization, either by making the bowel contents produce a strong signal or by creating a negative signal from the bowel lumen.

Text continues on page 666.

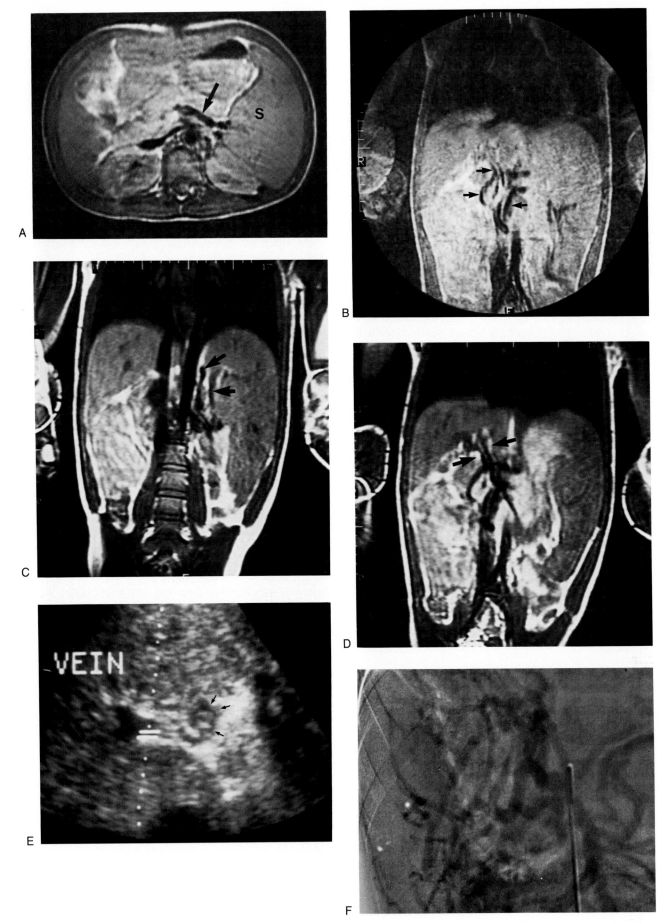

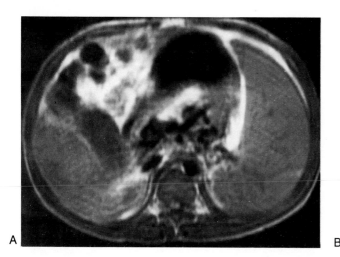

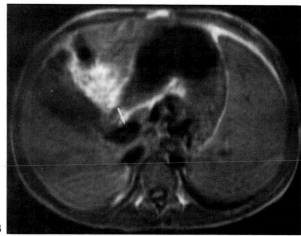

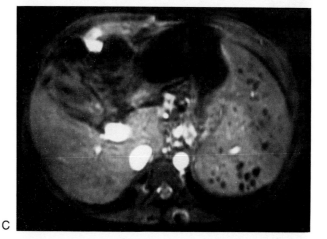

Figure 20–78. *Cirrhosis with portal hypertension in a 12-year-old boy.* ***A,*** Transverse T1 weighted image (600/20) showing multiple varices in the region of the gastric fundus. These are seen as serpiginous low-intensity regions. The spleen is enlarged. ***B,*** Transverse T1 image (600/20) through the porta hepatis. The portal vein (*arrow*) is enlarged. Multiple varices are again identified. ***C,*** Transverse field-echo image (21/12) in which multiple intrasplenic dilated sinusoids are seen as areas of low signal intensity owing to very slow flow. (Courtesy of Dr. George Bisset, Cincinnati.)

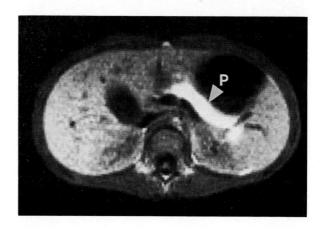

Figure 20–79. *Fatty infiltration of the pancreas in cystic fibrosis in a 12-year-old girl. Transverse T1 image (500/30).* There is a very strong signal from the entire pancreas (P) owing to diffuse fatty infiltration of this organ.

◄ **Figure 20–77.** *Cavernous transformation of the portal vein with varices in a 10-year-old child in whom the diagnosis has been known for 5 years. Preoperative study to evaluate vessel size and anatomy.* ***A,*** Transverse MR image (2017/20). The splenic vein (*arrow*) is patent and measures at least 5 mm in diameter, which is adequate for surgery. The spleen (S) is markedly enlarged. ***B,*** Coronal spin-density image (2017/20) showing variceal dilatation of mesenteric veins. Multiple enlarged veins (*arrows*) are identified along the path of the mesenteric veins. ***C,*** Coronal T1 image (433/26). Multiple esophageal varices are identified (*arrows*). ***D,*** Coronal T1 weighted image (433/26) demonstrating cavernous transformation of the portal vein with multiple collateral vessels (*arrows*) seen in the region of the porta hepatis. ***E,*** Ultrasound image. This also shows multiple enlarged vessels in the region of the porta hepatis (*arrows*). ***F,*** Angiogram obtained 5 years previously shows multiple serpiginous vessels in the region of the porta hepatis.

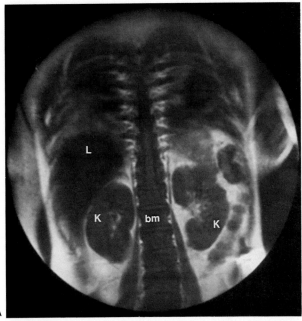

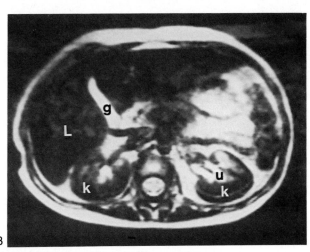

A

B

Figure 20–80. *Hemosiderosis in a 15-year-old boy due to multiple blood transfusions. The patient has autoimmune hemolytic anemia.* **A,** Coronal MR image (577/26). This T1 weighted image shows reduction in signal intensity from the liver (L), kidneys (K), and bone marrow (bm). Although T1 relaxation time is shortened by the deposited hemosiderin, this effect is overwhelmed by the very marked shortening of T2 relaxation time, resulting in the low signal. **B,** T2 weighted transverse MR image (1300/100). There is very low signal from the liver (L) and kidney parenchyma (k). This is due to T2 shortening from the hemosiderin. Note the strong signal from bile in the gallbladder (g) and urine in the collecting systems (u).

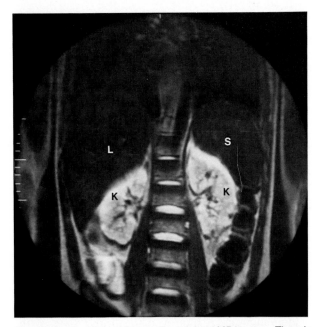

Figure 20–81. *Hemosiderosis. T1 weighted MR image.* There is marked reduction in signal from the liver (L) and spleen (S). The kidneys (K) are much less severely affected and still have a strong signal intensity owing to shortening of T1 relaxation time, which is not overwhelmed by marked T2 relaxation time shortening.

Potential contrast agents for MRI of the bowel may be divided into those producing positive and those producing negative signal from the bowel lumen compared with the signal from the native luminal contents. Positive agents increase luminal signal intensity and act through T1 shortening. Negative contrast agents act in one of two ways: they may produce no signal because they contain no hydrogen, or they may act by producing extreme shortening of T2 relaxation time so that, irrespective of which pulse sequence is used, there is inadequate time for a detectable signal to be generated.

Positive Intestinal Contrast Agents

These agents have the advantage of producing a very strong signal from the lumen of the bowel. The disadvantages of positive contrast agents are as follows:

1. About 50 percent of the noise in an MR image of the upper abdomen is caused by ghost artifacts from moving structures. Moving structures with very low signal, no matter how much they move, contribute little to this noise. Conversely, high-signal structures such as subcutaneous fat and positive contrast agents produce the majority of ghost artifacts in the upper

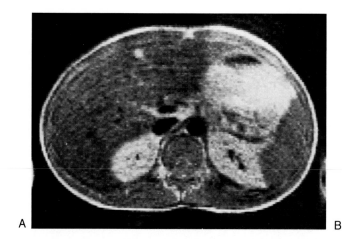

A

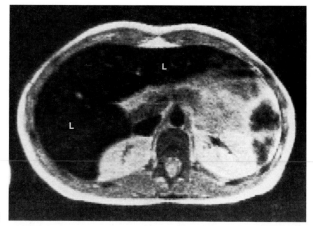

B

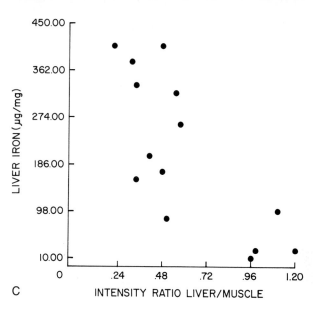

C

Figure 20–82. *Hemosiderosis: correlation of signal intensity with liver iron content.* ***A,*** Transverse MR image of the liver (2000/28). There is mild decrease in signal intensity from the liver. This patient had a liver iron concentration of 96 μg per milligram dry weight. ***B,*** Transverse MR image in another patient (2000/28). There is marked reduction in signal intensity from the liver (L). The liver iron concentration was 404 μg per milligram dry weight. ***C,*** Scatter plot of liver iron (dry weight) versus the intensity ratio of liver to muscle obtained from T1 weighted images (500/28), at 0.35T magnetic field strength. This diagram represents 15 patients with chronic blood transfusions. In all the patients the intensity ratio of liver to muscle is low. The normal value obtained at this field strength with this particular imager was 1.66 ± 0.33. Note that patients with iron levels less than 100 μg per milligram had higher intensity ratios than those with iron levels greater than 100 μg per milligram. This difference was statistically significant. (Hernandez RJ, Sarnaik SA, Lande I, et al. MR evaluation of liver iron overload. J Comput Assist Tomogr 1988; 12:91–94.)

abdomen. This occurs irrespective of whether the motion is produced by respiration, pulsation, or bowel peristalsis.

2. The signal intensity from positive contrast agents is unpredictable. In the correct concentration with the correct pulse sequence, they produce a positive strong signal. However, if the concentration of the agent is either too low or too high, the agent produces a negative rather than a positive effect. Because of this unreliability in response, clinical interpretation of images using positive contrast may prove difficult. Even if a standardized oral dose of the contrast agent is given, the effect in different segments of the bowel will vary considerably because the agent becomes diluted to an unpredictable extent by the natural bowel secretions.

3. The high signal produced from these contrast agents may make it difficult to differentiate bowel from adjacent fat.

Many different substances have been used as positive gastrointestinal contrast agents. Most authors report at least some improvement in visualization of the bowel and, because of this, improved visualization of adjacent structures, particularly the pancreas. Agents that have been tried are discussed below.

GADOLINIUM-DTPA. This agent (Fig. 20–87) has the advantage of being tasteless but the disadvantage of being very expensive. In one study in 20 human volunteers, it was found that best visualization of the bowel was obtained using a gadolinium-DTPA concentration of 1 millimolar given in a dose of 10 ml per kilogram body weight. The addition of mannitol to the gadolinium-DTPA improved the transit time of the mixture through the bowel and improved its mixing with bowel contents. This in turn improved bowel visualization. A disadvantage of the mannitol was the diarrhea induced in four of 15 patients.[55] In another study

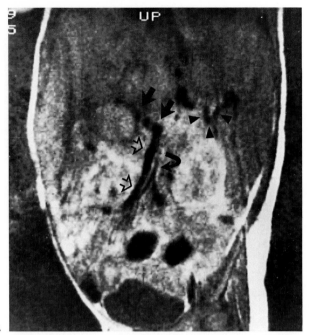

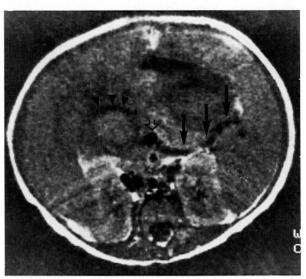

A   B

Figure 20–83. *Preoperative evaluation for liver transplantation: adequate portal vein caliber in a 34-month-old girl with extrahepatic biliary atresia.* **A,** Coronal MR image (500/30). Portions of the splenic vein (*arrowheads*), inferior vena cava (*curved arrow*), superior mesenteric vein (*open arrows*), and portal vein (*solid straight arrows*) are all demonstrated to be patent. The caliber of the portal vein is 4 mm, which is adequate for transplantation. The portal vein is displaced superiorly by cystic dilatation of bile ducts in the porta hepatis. **B,** Transverse MR image (300/35). The splenic vein (*solid arrows*), the superior mesenteric vein (*open arrow*), and a portion of the portal vein (*arrowheads*) are all well seen and are patent. (Day DL, Letourneau JG, Allan BT, et al. MR evaluation of the portal vein in pediatric liver transplant candidates. AJR 1986; 147:1027–1030.)

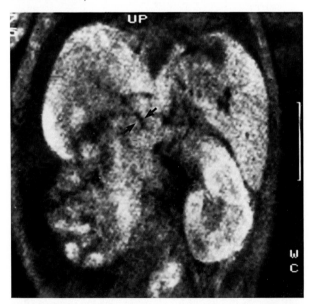

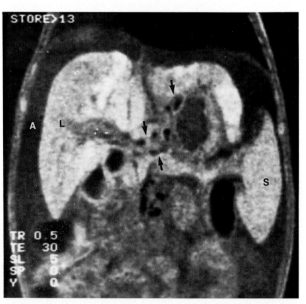

Figure 20–84. *Small portal vein in an 8-month-old infant with extrahepatic biliary atresia: prehepatic transplant evaluation.* Coronal MR image (500/30) showing a tiny portal vein (*arrows*) in the porta hepatis. This is a contraindication for hepatic transplantation. (Day DL, Letourneau JG, Allan BT, et al. MR evaluation of the portal vein in pediatric liver transplant candidates. AJR 1986; 147:1027–1030.)

Figure 20–85. *Nonvisualization of portal vein by MRI in a 10-month-old girl with extrahepatic biliary atresia: preoperative evaluation for liver transplantation.* Coronal MR image (500/30) of the upper abdomen. Multiple gastric and periportal venous collateral vessels are identified (*arrows*). The portal vein is not clearly identified as a separate structure and was believed to be thrombosed. Splenoportography, however, showed a 3-mm-caliber patent portal vein. Note also the ascites (A) seen as a low intensity around the liver (L). The liver parenchyma is inhomogeneous, probably due to cirrhosis. S, Spleen. (Day DL, Letourneau JG, Allan BT, et al. MR evaluation of the portal vein in pediatric liver transplant candidates. AJR 1986; 147:1027–1030.)

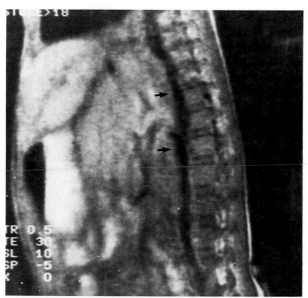

Figure 20–86. *Azygous continuation of the inferior vena cava (arrows): preoperative evaluation for hepatic transplantation.* Sagittal MR image (500/30). (Day DL, Letourneau JG, Allan BT, et al. MR evaluation of the portal vein in pediatric liver transplant candidates. AJR 1986; 147:1027–1030.)

of 41 patients, visualization of the pancreas was improved in 80 percent when a 10 millimolar gadolinium-DTPA solution was utilized in the bowel.[56]

MANGANESE. This substance[57] is too toxic for routine clinical use, but in rabbits it has been demonstrated that manganese can be used effectively as a combined gastrointestinal and liver contrast agent. This is because manganese is absorbed from the bowel and concentrated in the liver. Varying concentrations of manganese showed the predictable transition from a negative to a positive contrast agent. This effect is seen in both the bowel and the liver.

FOOD AGENTS. Many foods contain materials that exert a paramagnetic effect producing a positive contrast in the bowel (Figs. 20–88, 20–89). The advantage of these food materials is that they are readily available, cheap, safe, and palatable. The disadvantage is that the paramagnetic effect is produced by a variety of materials within the food product, and when they are used routinely it may be difficult to control the local concentration of these agents and therefore predict the contrast response. Agents within the food that produce contrast include minerals such as iron (Fig. 20–90) and manganese, protein, and fat.[58] Fat does not exert a paramagnetic effect but is a positive contrast agent because it produces strong signal on both T1 and T2 spin-echo pulse sequences. One study tried a number of food products including milk, ice cream, and Similac as contrast agents.[59] It was found that Similac with iron produced a better effect than Similac alone. In four normal volunteers the Similac with iron produced excellent delineation of stomach and duodenum, but less predictable improved visualization of the distal small bowel.

Negative Intestinal Contrast Agents

These have the advantage of producing a predictable effect that is not dependent on pulse sequence and does not vary depending on local concentrations of the agent. They also cause no motion ghost artifacts. Examples of these agents are listed below.

FERRITE AND MAGNETITE. These agents[60, 61] produce negative intraluminal contrast from strong reduc-

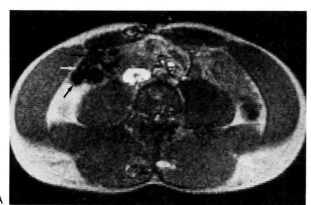

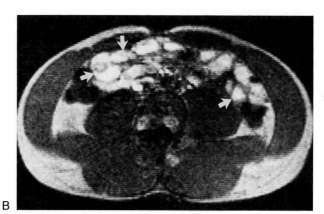

A   B

Figure 20–87. *Normal bowel loops. Use of gadolinium-DTPA as a contrast agent.* **A,** Precontrast image of the abdomen (flash technique 40/60, 40-degree flip angle). A few bowel loops are seen in the right anterior abdomen (*arrows*) as low-intensity areas. **B,** Transverse MR image obtained with the same pulse sequence and at the same level after administration of 10 ml per kilogram of a solution containing 1 millimolar gadolinium-DTPA and 15 g of mannitol per liter. This image shows much improved visualization of the bowel loops (*arrows*), which appear as regions of strong signal intensity. (Laniado M, Kornmesser W, Hamm B, et al. MR imaging of the gastrointestinal tract: value of Gd-DTPA. AJR 1988; 150:817–821.)

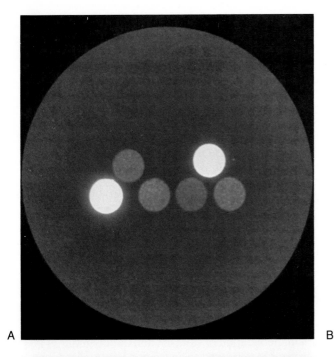

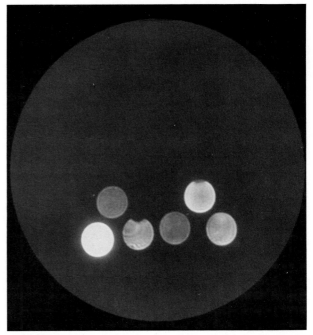

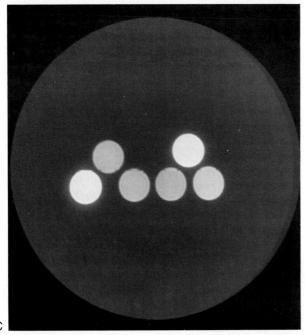

Figure 20–88. *Appearance of different food liquids at different pulse sequences.* Top row, left to right, 50 percent lemonade, 50 percent apple juice. Bottom row, left to right, undiluted apple juice, undiluted lemonade, 50 percent orange juice, undiluted orange juice. ***A,*** Inversion recovery (700/200). ***B,*** T1 weighted spin echo (800/40). ***C,*** T2 weighted spin echo (2000/90). The different fluids presumably appear differently because of varying concentrations of paramagnetic substances and protein.

tion in T2 relaxation time. They are ferromagnetic substances, some of which have the advantage of mixing freely with the bowel content and of not being absorbed.[62] In animal experiments and work with human volunteers, they have been found to improve the identification of bowel contour. Potential disadvantages of this group of agents are that they may be irritant to gastric mucosa,[60] and may cause image distortion and blurring at high concentrations.[60, 61] An-

other potential problem is that gastric acid may release ferric iron from these compounds. The ferric iron is absorbable and toxic. Therefore, an appropriate compound that is stable in acid must be chosen.

KAOLIN. This substance acts by reduction of T2 relaxation time. It thus produces a negative contrast effect. In volunteers a solution of kaolin in Kaopectate was found to improve bowel visualization (Fig. 20–91).[63]

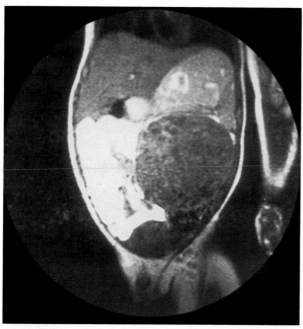

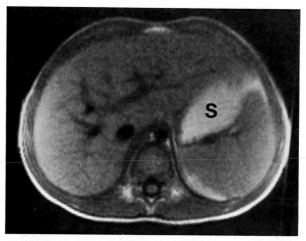

Figure 20–90. *Gastrointestinal contrast agent (iron).* Transverse MR image (500/30). The patient has been given oral Geritol, the iron in which has caused marked shortening of T1 relaxation time, so that the fluid in the stomach (S) appears of very strong intensity.

Figure 20–89. *Contrast agents, apple juice.* T1 weighted image (800/26) about 1 hour after ingestion of undiluted apple juice. Small bowel loops on the right side of the abdomen are well seen and appear of strong signal intensity.

BARIUM SULFATE. This agent may be used alone or in combination with deuterium oxide.[60] It contains no hydrogen and therefore produces negative contrast wherever it is present in the bowel. It is safe, cheap, and palatable. The deuterium is absorbed from the bowel. In human volunteers the agent was found to improve bowel visualization (Fig. 20–92).

AIR. Air contains an extremely low concentration of hydrogen and therefore acts as a negative contrast. It is cheap and can be administered in the form of gas-releasing tablets. The disadvantages of air are that it does not mix with the bowel contents, and that its transit and distribution through the bowel are extremely unpredictable and uncontrollable.

PERFLUOROCARBONS. These are organic compounds in which hydrogen is replaced by fluorine. Because they contain no hydrogen, they act as negative contrast agents and produce no signal. They are tasteless and odorless and have a rapid transit through the bowel. They do not mix with water.[64] In animals and human volunteers, these agents also improve bowel identification.

As can be seen from the above, there are many different agents that offer potential for improving bowel visualization. They may be used alone or with the addition of a bowel-paralyzing agent such as glucagon or Buscopan. At the present time, no ideal contrast agent has been developed. The ideal for which one strives is an agent that is cheap, palatable, and easily prepared; has no side effects; produces a desir-

able and predictable effect; and mixes well with bowel contents. No clinical trials have been reported using contrast agents to increase detection of pathology.

Liver Contrast Agents

The use of contrast agents[35] may be advantageous in a number of ways. They may improve visualization of an abnormality, which may then allow reduction in scan time by reducing the number of required repetitions or by reducing the number of pulse sequences used. Contrast agents may also help in characterization of pathologic tissues. Two different groups of contrast agents have been used in the liver: gadolinium-DTPA, which is available for routine clinical use, and ferrite, an experimental agent.

GADOLINIUM-DTPA. After intravenous injection of gadolinium-DTPA, it is distributed throughout the body in a manner similar to that of iodinated contrast agents, which are used for radiography. Gadolinium-DTPA is used in relatively low doses at which the T1 effect is maximal. These increase signal intensity and therefore visualization of a wide range of pathologic processes in the liver. On T1 weighted pulse sequences when gadolinium-DTPA is used, it is important that early dynamic images are acquired. This means the use of rapid pulse sequences with either a field-echo or a spin-echo pulse sequence with very short TE and TR relaxation times.

FERRITE. This is a super paramagnetic agent that exerts a powerful selective effect, decreasing the T2 relaxation time. After intravenous injection the agent is selectively taken up by phagocytic cells of the reticuloendothelial system. The marked decrease in T2 relaxation time caused by the ferrite produces a low-

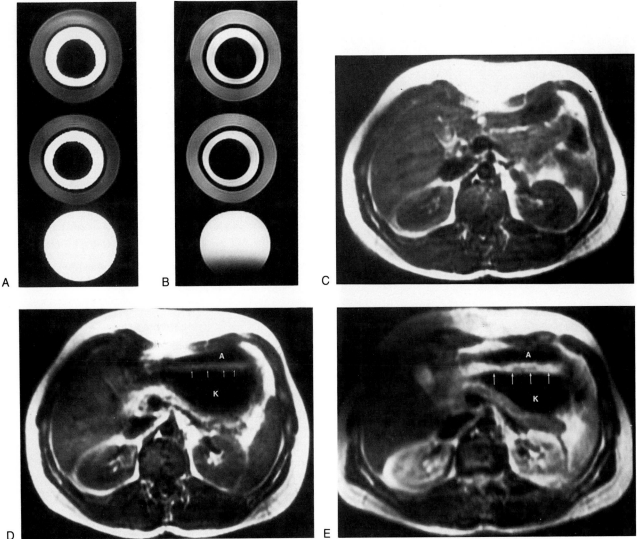

Figure 20–91. *Gastrointestinal contrast agents: use of clay minerals kaolin and bentonite.* T1 (400/25) (**A**) and T2 (200/80) (**B**) images of phantoms. The signal void in the center of the top phantom of each image is produced by Kaopectate, while the signal void in the center of the middle phantom is produced by a 5 percent solution of bentonite. A high-signal-intensity ring surrounding each signal void is due to a nickel acetate reference solution; the outer rings of lower signal intensity are from deionized water. The lowermost phantom is a solution of the nickel acetate reference fluid. **C,** Transverse image of the abdomen (800/25), obtained before contrast administration. **D, E,** Transverse images with pulse sequences (2000/30 and 2000/60), obtained after administration of Kaopectate (K), which is seen in the posterior aspect of the stomach and produces no signal. The pancreas (P) is seen behind it. Air (A) is present in the anterior part of the stomach. Fluid (*arrows*), between the air and the Kaopectate, is producing the horizontal high signal intensity between the air and the Kaopectate. (Litinsky JJ, Bryant RG. Gastrointestinal contrast agents: a diamagnetic approach. Mag Reson Med 1988; 8:285–292.)

intensity signal on both T1 and T2 pulse sequences. This means that the normal liver appears of very low signal intensity. The visualization of pathology is improved, since these diseased cells are not affected by the contrast agent and appear of strong signal against the dark background of normal liver.

MOTION SUPPRESSION IN MR GASTROINTESTINAL IMAGING

In the abdomen, motion artifacts (Figs. 20–93 to 20–95) are induced by vessel pulsation, bowel peristalsis, and respiratory motion.[65] Of these, respiratory

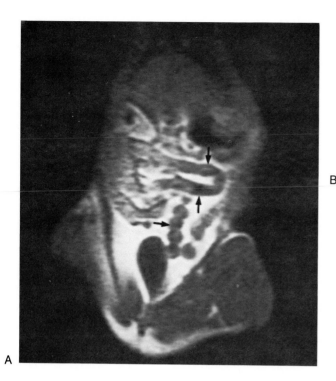

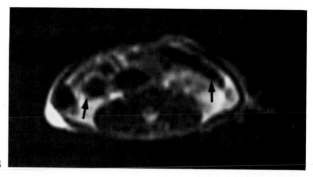

Figure 20–92. *Normal animal bowel demonstrating the effective use of barium sulfate and deuterium oxide mixture as a negative gastrointestinal contrast agent.* **A,** T1 weighted image obtained 80 minutes after administration of barium sulfate and deuterium oxide. Bowel loops (*arrows*) appear as low-intensity-areas owing to the presence of the contrast agent. **B,** T2 weighted image obtained just over 1 hour after contrast administration also demonstrates low-intensity signal from bowel loops containing the contrast agent. Barium sulfate is a negative contrast agent that contains neither hydrogen atoms nor paramagnetic substances. (Courtesy of Dr. A. Parikh, New Brunswick, NJ.)

motion is the most important. Movement causes two types of artifacts: (1) blurring of the image due to change in position of structures during motion and (2) ghost artifacts. These latter are ghostlike replicas of moving structures that superimpose on or obscure other structures. Ghosts obscure underlying structures and alter the true signal intensity of these structures. The maximal amount of ghosting is produced by structures with high signal intensity (e.g., fat) and by the number of pixels across which the tissue is moved (this means that for any given amplitude of motion, the use of a larger pixel size reduces ghosting).

RESPIRATORY GATING. This is seldom used now, first because it is not completely effective in eliminating the effects of motion, and second because it significantly increases the amount of time needed to image a patient.

BREATH HOLDING. It is now possible to use certain pulse sequences and obtain an image in 20 seconds or less. In cooperative patients the use of these fast gradient-echo pulse sequences together with breath holding eliminates the effects of respiratory motion.

SIGNAL AVERAGING. Instead of collecting a single set of data, two, four, or more sets of data can be collected from a single region of interest in the body. These signals can then be averaged, and this results in some improvement of the blurring artifacts caused by motion. This is a simple technique but it results in a proportional increase in imaging time. Doubling the number of acquisitions doubles imaging time. In general terms the averaging of two or even four sets of data produces a significant improvement in image quality.

Collection of more data sets than this results in little further elimination of motion artifacts. Signal averaging is best used with short TE, short TR pulse sequences.

SPECIALIZED INVERSION RECOVERY PULSE SEQUENCES. If an inversion recovery sequence is chosen with a very short time to inversion, tissues such as fat, which have a relatively short T1 relaxation time and which usually produce a strong signal on T1 weighted images, can be made to produce a very low signal. The strong signal from moving fat in the abdominal wall is a major contributor to the ghosting artifacts seen on abdominal images. By eliminating the signal from fat, the ghosting artifacts are significantly improved. The penalty that is paid with this pulse sequence is that the images are somewhat noisier than with other pulse sequences.

ALTERATION OF THE PHASING CODING AXIS IN ABDOMINAL IMAGING. In MRI, structures are spatially located in the abdomen by coding along the X- and Y-axes. Gradient fields (frequency) are used to code along one axis and signal phase along the other. Motion in any direction causes ghosts that are displayed in the phase encoding direction. One needs to choose the phase encoding direction to display the ghosts away from the organs of clinical interest.

SHORT TE, TR PULSE SEQUENCES. The effect of motion is proportional to the time taken to acquire the image. By using spin-echo pulse sequences with short TE and short TR relaxation times, image quality can be improved (Figs. 20–93, 20–94). The TE ideally should be less than 20 msec and the TR less than 400

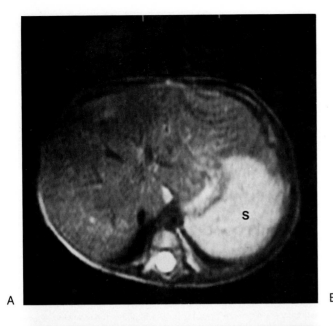

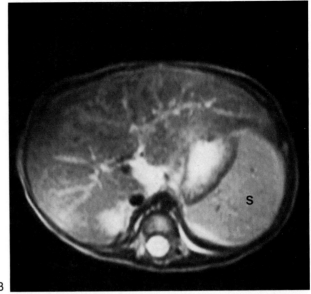

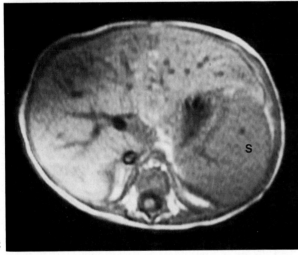

Figure 20–93. *Motion suppression techniques for liver imaging. All are transverse liver images obtained at 1.5T.* **A,** T2 weighted image (2000/80), showing visualization of the liver, and to a lesser extent the spleen (S), is significantly degraded by motion artifact. **B,** MAST technique. This is also known as first moment nulling and utilizes nonlinear gradient (2000/80). There is significant improvement of the motion artifacts compared with **A.** Note that with this technique the hepatic vessels appear of strong, rather than low, signal intensity. S, Spleen. **C,** Shortening of TE and TR (500/16). The use of shorter TE and TR times has also resulted in significant suppression of motion artifact and improvement of the image quality compared with **A.** S, Spleen.

msec. The advantage of this pulse sequence is that it takes a short time. One therefore has the luxury of also doing multiple data acquisitions and averaging the results. The disadvantage of these pulse sequences is that if the TR is too short, the overall signal strength falls, resulting in noisier images. In addition, these short TE, TR images are T1 weighted, and much pathology is best shown on T2 weighted images; also, the short TR limits the number of slices that can be obtained.

RESPIRATORY ORDERED PHASE ENCODING. This method of motion suppression monitors respiration and, instead of sequentially recording data, collects the data, depending on the phase of the respiratory cycle. In simple terms, the computer, by knowing at which stage during the respiratory cycle data were collected, can locate its position and compensate for the motion. This technique does improve image quality, but it requires very complex computer manipulations and at

the present time can only be used effectively for single-slice imaging. It therefore may not be practical for routine use.

NONLINEAR MAGNETIC FIELD GRADIENTS. An example is MAST (this technique is also called first moment nulling) (Fig. 20–93). As mentioned before, gradient magnetic fields are used to locate the position of a structure in an image slice. When a structure moves, the computer loses track of its precise location. This technique, instead of using linear gradients, continually changes the gradient wave forms to compensate for movement. An advantage is that good images can be obtained with only a single signal average per view. A disadvantage is that the technique requires long TE and TR relaxation times and therefore is best used for T2 imaging. Another disadvantage is that the blood vessels appear white and are often not as easily or well seen as when they are displayed as areas of

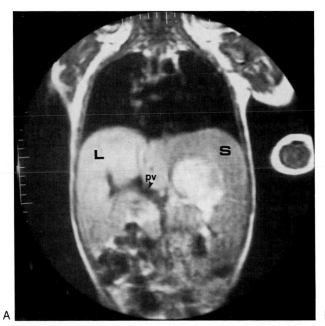

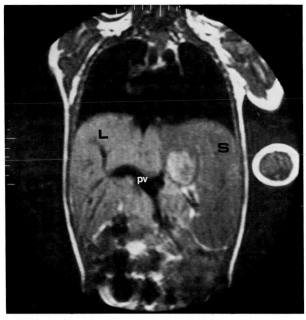

Figure 20–94. *Motion suppression using reduction of TR.* ***A,*** *Coronal MR image at the level of the portal vein (500/26). The liver (L), spleen (S), and portal vein (pv) can all be well seen, but there is slight blurring.* ***B,*** *Same image as* ***A*** *with reduced TR (250/26). The liver, spleen, and portal vein are again well visualized. Note the significant reduction in the blurring from motion artifact in this image with the shorter TR. This is a very effective method of suppressing motion artifact.*

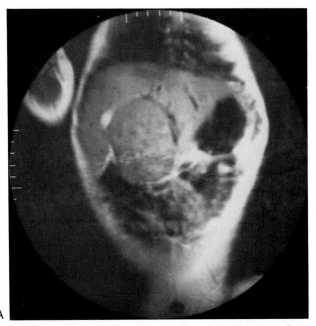

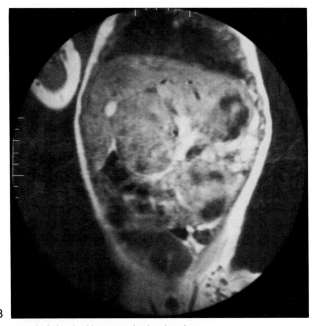

Figure 20–95. *Imaging technique: effect of slice thickness. Both are coronal abdominal images obtained at the same level. The pulse sequence is 550/26.* ***A,*** *10-mm-thick slice. This image has the best signal-to-noise ratio (SNR) but has slight blurriness.* ***B,*** *5-mm-thick slice. There is less blurring effect. However, the image is grainier because of poor SNR.*

signal void. This is a very promising technique that may become widely employed.

FIELD-ECHO IMAGING (GRADIENT-ECHO IMAGING). This also is a new technique that should become widely used very quickly. The physics is relatively com-plicated. The major difference from conventional spin-echo imaging is that no 180-degree of refocusing radio-wave pulse is used to generate a signal. Instead, the gradient fields are rapidly reversed to alter the rotation direction of the hydrogen atoms and produce a signal.

Another difference from spin-echo imaging is that, instead of a 90-degree tip angle, other angles can be used. With short tip angles and very short TE and TR relaxation times, images can be acquired rapidly, in as little as 20 seconds, and therefore can be used with breath holding to acquire or image. These field-echo images have more noise than spin-echo images, but because of their rapid acquisition and the significant improvement in motion artifact, they often are extremely good. However, if motion is still present, it greatly degrades the image.

For routine clinical use, the most effective and practical methods of reducing motion artifact are, for T1 images, to utilize short TE, short TR pulse sequences with a large number of signal averages. For T2 weighted images, one should try both nonlinear magnetic fields with spin echo, and the field-echo pulse sequences with short tip angles.

PERSPECTIVES IN ABDOMINAL IMAGING

MRI has the widely reported virtues of being safe and noninvasive. It has the potential for achieving some degree of tissue characterization, it has the ability to create images in any plane, it has outstanding soft tissue contrast resolution, and it makes possible excellent vessel visualization without the need for contrast material injection.[1] With all these attributes, MRI surely has a role to play in abdominal imaging. Abdominal MRI has lagged behind MRI in the central nervous and musculoskeletal systems. Problems with MRI include motion artifacts, poor visualization of calcium, and poor visualization of the bowel. The problems of motion artifacts are now largely being overcome and we are on the threshold of having an acceptable oral contrast agent that will permit accurate identification of loops of bowel. Many abnormalities are detected incidentally on abdominal MR images, and it is important to be aware of the MR features of the full range of abdominal pathology. What unique role MRI will play is yet to be determined. I would predict that an early impact will be on the visualization, localization, and characterization of focal lesions in the liver and to a lesser extent in the spleen. MRI will also become important in the evaluation of focal mass lesions elsewhere in the abdomen. MRI could become important in screening for disorders such as abdominal abscess. Its role in abdominal trauma is not known. MRI may prove sensitive in evaluating the effects of certain metabolic disorders on abdominal structures.

The plain film abdominal radiograph will still remain the foundation of abdominal imaging. It is cheap, simple, and quick to perform. It screens virtually all the different abdominal tissues and organs, and in many patients a final diagnosis can be obtained with a single technique. Sometimes treated with scorn, compared with its more expensive brothers, the abdominal radiograph is often viewed too rapidly. Often, when other imaging techniques have been used, one returns to the abdominal radiograph to find that if one had only looked carefully enough, the answer was already apparent.

Contrast bowel studies will remain the method of choice for evaluation of many lesions. Indications for performing these studies will include the evaluation of children with vomiting, gastroesophageal reflux, bowel stenosis or atresia, malrotation, Hirschsprung's disease, meconium ileus, and intussusception.

Nuclear medicine studies are widely used. Major areas of interest are gastrointestinal reflux, gastric emptying, congenital anomalies and function of the biliary system, liver scanning in patients with tumor, and the search for ectopic gastric mucosa.

Ultrasonography will probably remain the initial modality of choice after plain film in many abdominal disorders. It suffers from a limited field of view and from the fact that areas of the abdomen are always obscured by overlying bowel gas.

CT remains an excellent choice for abdominal imaging. It is widely available, accurate, and excellent for evaluation of solid mass lesion and screening for abdominal abscess. It does require the administration of oral and intravenous contrast agents, and accuracy depends on selecting the proper time of imaging after contrast injection. Spatial resolution is still superior to MRI, but soft tissue contrast resolution is inferior.

The indications for abdominal angiography in children are rapidly decreasing. Angiography is now rarely used in patients with tumors, and even in preoperative evaluation of patients for resection of liver tumors, ultrasonography and MRI together can usually provide excellent and adequate anatomic mapping of the blood vessels.

REFERENCES

1. Council on Scientific Affairs. Magnetic resonance imaging of the abdomen and pelvis. JAMA 1989; 261:420–433.
2. Weinreb JC, Cohen JM, Armstrong E, Smith T. Imaging the pediatric liver: MRI and CT. AJR 1986; 147:785–790.
3. Cohen MD. MRI of the gastrointestinal and musculoskeletal systems in children. Appl Radiol 1987; 16:50–53.
4. Spritzer C, Kressel HY, Mitchell D, Axel L. MR imaging of normal extrehepatic bile ducts. J Comput Assist Tomogr 1987; 11:248–252.
5. Adler DD, Glazer GM, Aisen AM. MRI of the spleen: normal appearance and findings in sickle-cell anemia. AJR 1986; 147:843–845.
6. Hahn PF, Weissleder R, Stark DD, et al. MR imaging of focal splenic tumors. AJR 1988; 150:823–827.
7. Tscholakoff D, Hricak H, Thoeni R, et al. MR imaging in the diagnosis of pancreatic disease. AJR 1987; 148:703–709.
8. Piccirillo M, McCarthy S, Rapoport S. High field strength MRI of the normal pancreas. Presented at the Society of Magnetic Resonance Imaging, San Francisco, CA, August, 1988.
9. Lupetin AR, Dash N. MRI appearance of esophageal duplication cyst. Gastrointest Radiol 1987; 12:7–9.
10. Rhee RS, Ray CG, Kravetz MH, et al. Cervical esophageal duplication cyst: MR imaging. J Comput Assist Tomogr 1988; 12:693–695.

11. Alexander MC, Haaga JR. MR imaging of a choledochal cyst. J Comput Assist Tomogr 1985; 92:357–359.
12. Yeager BA, Guglielmi GE, Schiebler ML, Gefter WB. Magnetic resonance imaging of Morgagni hernia. Gastrointest Radiol 1987; 12:296–298.
13. Sato, Y, Pringle KC, Bergman RA, et al. Congenital anorectal anomalies: MR imaging. Radiology 1988; 168:157–162.
14. deVries PA, Cox KL. Surgery of anorectal anomalies. Surg Clin North Am 1985; 65:1139–1169.
15. Mesacapo PM, Price AP, Haller JO, et al. MR and CT demonstration of levator sling in congenital anorectal anomalies. J Comput Assist Tomogr 1987; 11:273–275.
16. Pringle KC, Sato Y, Soper RT. Magnetic resonance imaging as an adjunct to planning an anorectal pull-through. J Pediatr Surg 1987; 22:571–574.
17. Wall SD, Fisher MR, Amparo EG, et al. Magnetic resonance imaging in the evaluation of abscesses. AJR 1985; 144:1217–1221.
18. Schmiedl U, Paajanen H, Arakawa M, et al. MR imaging of liver abscesses; application of Gd-DTPA. Magn Reson Imaging 1988; 6:9–16.
19. Stark DD, Bass NM, Moss AA, et al. Nuclear magnetic resonance imaging of experimentally induced liver disease. Radiology 1983; 148:743–751.
20. Stark DD, Moss AA, Goldberg HI, et al. Magnetic resonance and CT of the normal and diseased pancreas: a comparative study. Radiology 1984; 150:153–162.
21. Smith FW. Two years' clinical experience with NMR imaging. Appl Radiol 1983; 12:29–42.
22. Moon KL, Hricak H, Margulis AR, et al. Nuclear magnetic resonance imaging characteristics of gallstones in vitro. Radiology 1983; 148:753–756.
23. Ohtomo K, Itai Y, Yoshikawa K, et al. Hepatocellular carcinoma and cavernous hemangioma: differentiation with MR imaging. Radiology 1988; 168:621–623.
24. Boechat MI, Kangarloo H, Ortega J, et al. Primary liver tumors in children: comparison of CT and MR imaging. Radiology 1988; 169:727–732.
25. Li KC, Glazer GM, Quint LE, et al. Distinction of hepatic cavernous hemangioma from hepatic metastases with MR imaging. Radiology 1988; 169:409–415.
26. Ros PR, Lubbers PR, Olmsted WW, Morillo G. Hemangioma of the liver: heterogeneous appearance on T2-weighted images. AJR 1987; 149:1167–1170.
27. Brown RKJ, Gomes A, King W, et al. Hepatic hemangiomas: evaluation by magnetic resonance imaging and technetium-99m red blood cell scintigraphy. J Nucl Med 1987; 28:1683–1687.
28. Ohtomo K, Itai Y, Yoshikawa K, et al. Hepatic tumors: dynamic MR imaging. Radiology 1987; 163:27–31.
29. Itai Y, Ohtomo K, Furui S, et al. Noninvasive diagnosis of small cavernous hemangioma of the liver: advantage of MRI. AJR 1985; 145:1195–1199.
30. Itoh K, Nishimura K, Togashi K, et al. Hepatocellular carcinoma: MR imaging. Radiology 1987; 164:21–25.
31. Titelbaum DS, Hatabu H, Schiebler ML, et al. Fibrolamellar hepatocellular carcinoma: MR appearance. J Comput Assist Tomogr 1988; 12:588–591.
32. Wittenberg J, Stark DD, Forman BH, et al. Differentiation of hepatic metastases from hepatic hemangiomas and cysts by using MR imaging. AJR 1988; 151:79–84.
33. Kressel HY. Strategies for magnetic resonance imaging of focal liver disease. Radiol Clin North Am 1988; 26:607–615.
34. Bernardino ME. Variety of MRI methods useful in liver imaging. Diagn Imaging 1987; July:96–99.
35. Ferrucci JT. MR imaging of the liver. AJR 1986; 147:1103–1116.
36. Reinig JW, Dwyer AJ, Miller DL, et al. Liver metastases: detection with MR imaging at 0.5 and 1.5 T. Radiology 1989; 170:149–153.
37. Stark DD. MR imaging of focal liver masses. Radiology 1988; 168:323–328.
38. Stark DD, Wittenberg J, Rutch RJ, Ferrucci JT. Hepatic metastases: randomized, controlled comparison of detection with MR imaging and CT. Radiology 1987; 165:399–406.
39. Curati WL, Halevy A, Gibson RN, et al. Ultrasound, CT, and MRI comparison in primary and secondary tumors of the liver. Gastrointest Radiol 1988; 13:123–128.
40. Fobbe F, Hamm B, Schwarting R. Angiomyolipoma of the liver: CT, MR, and ultrasound imaging. J Comput Assist Tomogr 1988; 12:658–659.
41. Baumgartner FJ, Barnett MJ, Velez M, Chiu LC. Traumatic disruption of the gallbladder evaluated by computerized tomography and magnetic resonance imaging. Br J Surg 1988; 75:386–387.
42. Hess CF, Griebel J, Schmiedl U, et al. Focal lesions of the spleen: preliminary results with fast MR imaging at 1.5 T. J Comput Assist Tomogr 1988; 12:569–574.
43. Levy HM, Newhouse JH. MR imaging of portal vein thrombosis. AJR 1988; 151:283–286.
44. Ros PR, Viamonte M, Soila K, et al. Demonstration of cavernomatous transformation of the portal vein by magnetic resonance imaging. Gastrointest Radiol 1986; 11:90–92.
45. Leung AWL, Steiner RE, Young IR. NMR imaging of the liver in two cases of iron overload. J Comput Assist Tomogr 1984; 8:446–449.
46. Brasch RC, Wesbey GE, Gooding CA, Koerper MA. Magnetic resonance imaging of transfusional hemosiderosis complicating thalassemia major. Radiology 1984; 150:767–771.
47. Querfeld U, Dietrich R, Taira RK, et al. Magnetic resonance imaging of iron overload in children treated with peritoneal dialysis. Nephron 1988; 50:220–224.
48. Hernandez RJ, Sarnaik SA, Lande I, et al. MR evaluation of liver iron overload. J Comput Assist Tomogr 1988; 12:91–94.
49. Runge VM, Clanton JA, Smith FW, et al. Nuclear magnetic resonance of iron and copper disease states. AJR 1983; 141:943–948.
50. Wenker JC, Baker MK, Ellis JH, Glant MD. Focal fatty infiltration of the liver: demonstration by magnetic resonance imaging. AJR 1984; 143:573–574.
51. Lawler GA, Pennock JM, Steiner RE, et al. Nuclear magnetic resonance (NMR) imaging in Wilson disease. J Comput Assist Tomogr 1983; 7:1–8.
52. Rademaker M, Webb JAW, Lowe DG, et al. Magnetic resonance imaging as a screening procedure for methotrexate induced liver damage. Br J Dermatol 1987; 117:311–316.
53. Unger EC, Cohen MS, Gatenby RA, et al. Single breath-holding scans of the abdomen using FISP and FLASH at 1.5 T. J Comput Assist Tomogr 1988; 12:575–583.
54. Day DL, Letourneau JG, Allan BT, et al. MR evaluation of the portal vein in pediatric liver transplant candidates. AJR 1986; 147:1027–1030.
55. Laniado M, Kornmesser W, Hamm B, et al. MR imaging of the gastrointestinal tract: value of Gd-DTPA. AJR 1988; 150:817–821.
56. Tiling R, Fink U, Bauer WM, et al. Oral contrast medium. A valuable improvement in the diagnosis of pancreatic disorders. Presented at the Society of Magnetic Resonance Imaging, San Francisco, CA, August, 1988.
57. Cory DA, Schwartzentruber DJ, Mock BH. Ingested manganese chloride as a contrast agent for magnetic resonance imaging. Magn Reson Imaging 1987; 5:65–70.
58. Chen B, Gore JC, Zhong JH, et al. Gastrointestinal MRI contrast enhancement by liquid food. Presented at the Society of Magnetic Resonance Imaging, San Francisco, CA, August, 1988.
59. Bisset GS. Evaluation of potential practical oral contrast agents for pediatric magnetic resonance imaging: preliminary observations. Presented at the Society for Pediatric Radiology, Coronado, CA, April, 1988.
60. Parikh AM, Mezrich RS. Deuterated barium sulphate as an oral MRI contrast agent. Presented at the Society of Magnetic Resonance Imaging, San Francisco, CA, August, 1988.
61. Lonnemark M, Carlsten HJ, Ericsson A, et al. Superparamag-

netic particles as an MRI contrast agent for the gastrointestinal tract. Acta Radiol 1988; 29:599–602.

62. Hahn PF, Stark DD, Saini S, et al. Ferrite particles for bowel contrast in MR imaging. Design issues and feasibility studies. Radiology 1987; 164:37–41.

63. Listinsky JJ, Bryant RG. Gastrointestinal contrast agents: a diamagnetic approach. Magn Reson Med 1988; 8:285–292.

64. Mattrey RF, Hajek PC, Gylys-Morin VM, et al. Perfluorochemicals as gastrointestinal contrast agents for MR imaging: preliminary studies in rats and humans. AJR 1987; 148:1259–1263.

65. Wood ML, Runge VM, Henkelman RM. Overcoming motion in abdominal MR imaging. AJR 1988; 150:513–522.

Genitourinary System

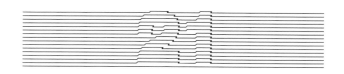

ROSALIND B. DIETRICH, M.B., Ch.B.

Although magnetic resonance (MR) rapidly gained acceptance as a useful imaging modality in the evaluation of the pediatric central nervous system, determination and implementation of its role in the evaluation of the pediatric genitourinary tract have been slow to become established.

Excretory urography was previously the predominant radiologic examination used in the evaluation of the pediatric genitourinary system. More recently it has been largely replaced by a combination of ultrasonography, giving structural information, and radionuclide scintigraphy, giving functional information.

These modalities are often excellent at demonstrating pathologic conditions but they have limitations. Excretory urography often reveals pathology indirectly by showing how an abnormality distorts the adjacent kidney, ureter, or bladder. Ultrasonography has the advantages of being relatively inexpensive and easy to perform, and it can directly image both normal structures and pathology. Unfortunately, the ultrasonographic field of view is limited by beam shape and it may be difficult to obtain an overall view of large lesions with this imaging modality. In addition, bowel gas and bone obscure underlying structures.

Newer technologies such as computed x-ray tomography (x-ray CT) and duplex ultrasonography have been added to the imaging armamentarium. The newest of these, MRI, has many characteristics that make it a potentially advantageous method of evaluating the pediatric genitourinary system. MRI is able to obtain direct multiplanar images of the abdomen and pelvis without the use of ionizing radiation. Its inherently excellent tissue contrast differentiation aids greatly in the differentiation of normal and abnormal structures. Its complementary role in the evaluation of this system is at last becoming established.

NORMAL ANATOMY

Kidney

Because the kidneys are positioned in the retroperitoneum, surrounded by perinephric fat, they are easily detected by MRI.[1–5] They are seen as structures of predominantly medium signal intensity well outlined by the high-signal-intensity fat. On spin-echo T1 weighted images of the normal kidney, the cortex demonstrates higher signal intensity than the adjacent medulla, and therefore the two can be clearly differentiated (Fig. 21–1).[1–5] On these sequences the renal pyramids appear even more prominent in neonates and young children than in older children and adults.[4]

The renal artery and vein usually demonstrate low signal intensity owing to the presence of rapidly flowing blood within them.[1–3] At times, however, an intraluminal signal may be identified within normal renal vessels. This signal may be due to slow flow of blood within the vessel or, when images are obtained demonstrating the cross section of a vessel, to flow-related enhancement.[6] The urine within the pelvocaliceal system and ureter also demonstrates low signal intensity on images obtained with this pulse sequence, because of its long T1 value.[1,2,4] The high signal intensity seen

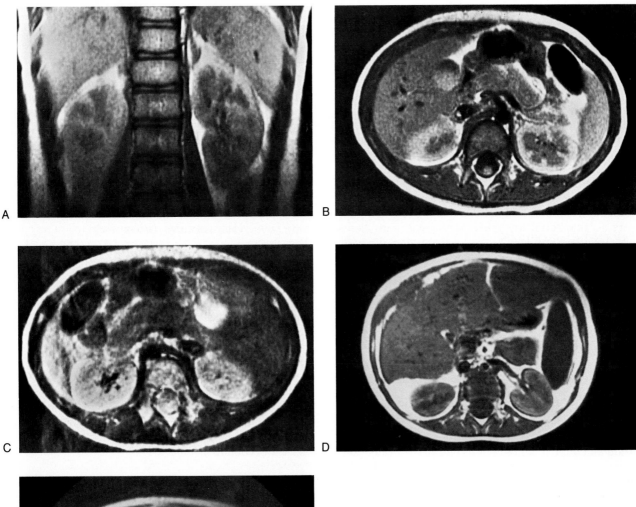

Figure 21–1. *Normal pediatric kidney.* **A,** Coronal (SE 500/30). This T1 weighted sequence demonstrates good corticomedullary differentiation. There is an absence of the high signal intensity seen in the renal hilum of adult kidneys, owing to the presence of adipose tissue. **B,** Axial (SE 500/30). Good corticomedullary differentiation is also seen on this T1 weighted image. The cortex is of higher signal than the medulla. **C,** Axial (SE 2000/85). On T2 weighted images both the cortex and medulla demonstrate high signal intensity with subsequent loss of corticomedullary differentiation. **D,** Axial image (800/60) shows good corticomedullary differentiation with higher signal in the cortex than in the medulla and almost no signal from the urine in the renal pelvis. **E,** Axial image with the same pulse sequence as **D** obtained approximately 15 minutes after intravenous administration of gadolinium-DTPA shows increase in signal intensity from the medulla with loss of corticomedullary differentiation. There is high signal intensity from the urine owing to shortening of the T1 relaxation time.

in the hilar region of adult kidneys, which is due to the presence of adipose tissue, is not visible in young children. In older children the signal intensity of the renal hilum progressively increases with age, and by puberty the kidney has a similar appearance to that in adults.[4] When there is a duplex collecting system, a lower-signal-intensity band, isointense with the cortex, crosses and separates the renal hilum.

On images obtained with T2 weighted sequences, both the normal cortex and medulla have high signal intensity, and corticomedullary differentiation is less well identified (Fig. 21–1).[4,5] Corticomedullary differentiation may be even more apparent on T1 weighted images obtained using inversion recovery pulse sequences than on those using spin-echo pulse sequences.[1,3] However, if too much T1 weighting is present, corticomedullary differentiation may again become less apparent, since both the cortex and medulla have low signal intensity.[7]

At times a chemical shift misregistration artifact may be identified at the interface between the kidney and the adjacent perinephric fat.[8] This appears as a low-signal-intensity line along one side of the kidney with a symmetric high-signal-intensity line along the opposite side. It is more pronounced on T2 weighted images and images obtained with magnets of higher field strength. Care must be taken not to attribute the low-signal-intensity band incorrectly to a rim of calcification.

In normal healthy volunteers,[9] intravenous injection of gadolinium-DTPA produces characteristic changes in the kidneys. The findings of Kikinis and colleagues were obtained utilizing rapid scanning with a gradient-echo technique and a 10-second acquisition time per image.[9] With spin-echo imaging and longer acquisition times, the findings are less pronounced. On T1 weighted images the renal cortex shows an increase in signal intensity after injection of the contrast agent; this is presumed to be due to shortening of T1 relaxation time. In the renal medulla there is a marked decrease in signal intensity approximately 1 minute after injection, followed by a gradual increase in intensity (Fig. 21–1D, E). The decrease in signal intensity in the medulla is believed to be due to overwhelming T2 shortening caused by very high concentrations of gadolinium that occur as a result of normal renal function. The urine in the renal pelvis shows similar but less dramatic effect than in the renal medulla.

Bladder

The bladder is easily identified by MRI, positioned on the anterior portion of the pelvic floor and separated from the symphysis pubis by the fat in the space of Retzius (Fig. 21–2).[1, 10, 11] On MR images, visualization of the bladder wall depends on the relative contrast between it, the urine within the bladder, and the adjacent perinephric fat.[1] It must be remembered that the wall thickness of the normal bladder varies, depending on the relative distention of the organ. On T1 weighted sequences the bladder wall and urine frequently are difficult to distinguish, because both demonstrate low signal intensity owing to their relatively long T1 values.[11–13] Therefore, images with longer TR and TE values are better for demonstration of the contour of the bladder wall and evaluation of its thickness. On images obtained with T2 weighted sequences the bladder wall has lower signal intensity than the adjacent high-signal-intensity urine and intermediate-signal-intensity perivesical fat.[11–13] On proton-density or only mildly T1 weighted images the bladder wall has a signal intensity intermediate between that of urine (low) and perivesical fat (high), and such sequences are preferred by some authors for bladder evaluation.[14] Air or rubber catheters in the bladder are of low signal on all pulse sequences (Fig. 21–3).

Prostate, Seminal Vesicles, and Penis

In older children the regional anatomy of the prostate, as described in adults, can be identified on proton-density and T2 weighted images.[15–18] On such images the central and transitional zones demonstrate lower signal intensity than the high-signal-intensity peripheral zone. In younger children it is not always possible to define these regions, and in such patients the prostate has a homogeneous appearance on MR images demonstrating medium signal intensity (similar to that of skeletal muscle) on T1 weighted images and higher signal intensity (slightly less than that of fat) on T2 weighted images (Fig. 21–2).

Seminal vesicles can also be clearly seen by MRI as discrete bilateral structures with medium to low signal intensity on T1 weighted images and high signal intensity on T2 weighted images owing to their high water content (Fig. 21–2).[16]

The anatomy of the penis can also be defined by MRI.[19] The corpora cavernosa, corpus spongiosum, and bulb of the penis demonstrate medium signal intensity on T1 weighted images and high signal intensity on T2 weighted images. They are clearly separated on both sequences by the low-signal-intensity tunica albuginea and Buck's fascia (Figs. 21–2, 21–4). The arteries of the corpora cavernosa, the deep dorsal vein, the dorsal artery, and the urethra can also be identified and have relatively low signal intensity compared with the corpora.

Uterus, Cervix, and Vagina

The normal uterus, cervix, and vagina can be identified on good quality MR images in children of all ages (Fig. 21–5),[10, 13, 20–22] and images obtained in the sagittal and axial planes are best for the identification of these midline structures.[23] The appearance of these organs varies, depending on their hormonal status.[24–26] Because of maternal hormonal stimulation, the newborn uterus has an appearance and relative proportions similar to those of the postpubertal adolescent uterus,[13, 20, 27] but of course its overall size is smaller (Fig. 21–5). At this time the high-signal-intensity, hormonally stimulated endometrium can be easily distinguished from the low-signal-intensity junctional line and medium-signal-intensity myometrium. These findings are seen especially well on T2 weighted sequences.

After the immediate postnatal period, when maternal hormonal stimulation is lost, the body of the prepubertal uterus has approximately the same size as the adjacent cervix (Fig. 21–5), and differentiation of the endometrium, junctional line, and myometrium is less distinct even on T2 weighted images.[22]

By puberty, the uterus has attained its adult size and configuration, and again clear differentiation of the different layers may be obtained by MRI (Fig. 21–5).

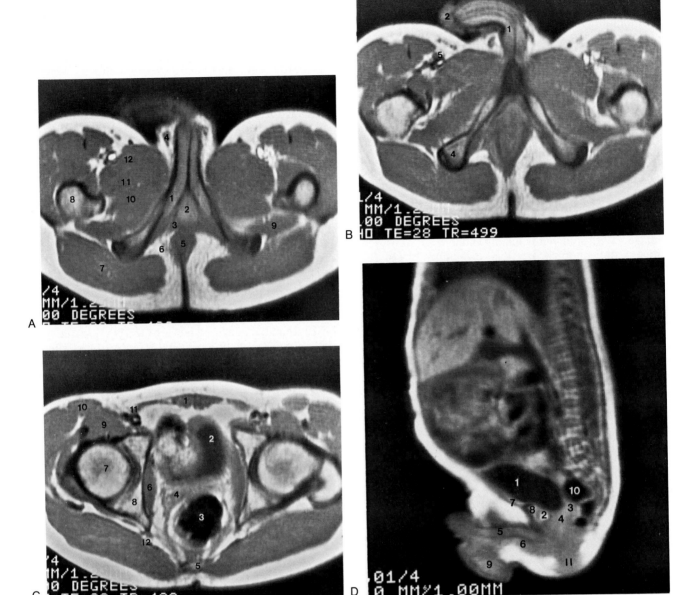

Figure 21–2. *Normal pediatric male pelvis.* **A,** Transverse plane; perineum (SE 500/28). 1, Crus of penis; 2, bulb of penis; 3, bulbocavernous m.; 4, pampiniform plexus and spermatic cord; 5, rectum; 6, ischiorectal fossa; 7, gluteus maximus m.; 8, femur; 9, quadratus femoris m.; 10, adductor magnus m.; 11, adductor brevis m.; 12, adductor longus m. **B,** Transverse plane; low pelvis (SE 500/28). 1, Corpus cavernosus; 2, glans penis; 3, prostate; 4, ischial tuberosity; 5, femoral a. and v. **C,** Transverse plane; middle pelvis (SE 500/28). 1, Rectus abdominis; 2, bladder; 3, rectum; 4, seminal vesicle; 5, coccyx; 6, obturator internus m.; 7, femur; 8, ischium; 9, iliopsoas m.; 10, sartorius m.; 11, femoral a. and v.; 12, inferior gluteal a. and v. **D,** Sagittal plane (SE 500/28); newborn. 1, Bladder; 2, retropubic space; 3, seminal vesicle; 4, prostate; 5, corpus cavernosum; 6, corpus spongiosum; 7, rectus abdominis m.; 8, pubis; 9, testis; 10, rectum; 11, external

After menarche, changes in the appearance of the uterus occur in different phases of the menstrual cycle. The central high-signal-intensity endometrial zone is thinnest immediately after menstruation and thickest at midcycle.[24–27] The signal intensity of the myometrium also changes cyclically and is highest during the secretory phase (Fig. 21–6).

The postpubertal cervix demonstrates two distinct layers on T2 weighted sequences. The inner layer has high signal intensity and is thought to represent cervical epithelium and mucus.[20, 27] The outer layer has homogeneous low signal intensity.

The anatomy of the vagina is best seen in the axial plane, and differentiation of the upper, middle, and

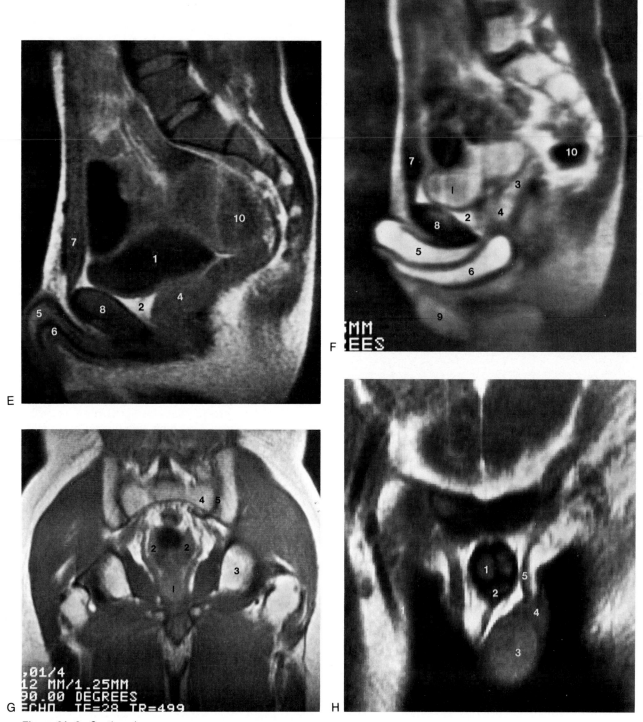

Figure 21–2. *Continued.*
anal sphincter. *E, F,* Sagittal plane; midline (SE 500/28) and (SE 200/84). 1, Bladder; 2, retropubic space; 3, seminal vesicles; 4, prostate; 5, corpus cavernosum; 6, corpus spongiosum; 7, rectus abdominis m.; 8, pubis; 9, testis; 10, rectum. *G,* Coronal plane (SE 500/28). 1, prostate; 2, seminal vesicles; 3, ischium; 4, sacrum; 5, sacroiliac joint. *H,* Coronal plane; scrotum (SE 500/28). 1, Corpus cavernosum; 2, corpus spongiosum; 3, testis, 4, epididymis; 5, spermatic cord. (From Dietrich RB, Kangarloo H. Pediatric body imaging. In: Stark DD, Bradley WG Jr., eds. Magnetic resonance imaging. St. Louis: CV Mosby, 1988:1434–1452.)

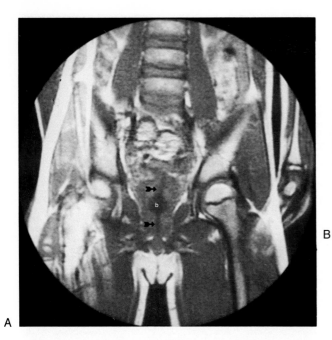

A

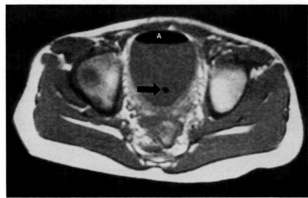

B

Figure 21–3. *Normal appearance of Foley catheter and air in the bladder.* **A,** Coronal image (700/26) shows a Foley catheter (*arrows*) in the bladder. The balloon (B) is inflated. Note that the rubber of the catheter and the air in the balloon are all of low signal intensity. **B,** Transverse image (700/26) shows the tip of the catheter (*arrow*) to be of low signal intensity. Air (A) in the anterior aspect of the bladder produces no signal.

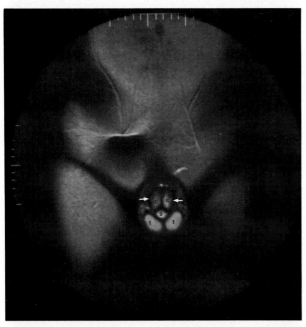

Figure 21–4. *Normal penis on coronal image.* On T2 weighted images (2000/80) the corpora cavernosa and corpus spongiosum appear of high signal intensity. They are surrounded by low-signal-intensity tunica albuginea (*arrows*). c, Corpus cavernosum; s, corpus spongiosum; t, testis.

lower thirds is possible by identification of its changing shape and of adjacent structures.[28] In its upper third the vaginal fornices can be seen laterally. The middle third of the vagina is seen at the level of the base of the bladder, and the lower third at the level of the urethra. As in the uterus and cervix, cyclic variation in the appearance of the vagina may be seen on T2 weighted images in postpubertal girls.[28]

Because the ovaries are bilateral structures, they are best identified in the axial or coronal planes.[13, 20, 21, 29] Since they demonstrate medium signal intensity on T1 weighted sequences and high signal intensity on T2 weighted sequences, they may be difficult to distinguish from adjacent bowel loops and fat (Fig. 21–5).[13, 21] It is important, therefore, to use the adjacent anatomic landmarks when trying to identify normal ovaries. The normally positioned ovaries lie on the muscles that compose the pelvic side wall, i.e., the obturator internus, iliopsoas, or pubococcygeus, and are seen directly adjacent to the internal iliac vessels.[30]

CONGENITAL DISORDERS

Kidney Malposition

Abnormal location of the kidneys, whether high (intrathoracic kidney) or low (pelvic kidney) (Fig. 21–7), as well as fusion anomalies, such as crossed-fused ectopia (Fig. 21–8) and horseshoe kidney (Fig. 21–9), are well seen by MRI.[4, 31] Although most of these anomalies can be accurately evaluated by ultrasonography, at times it is difficult to differentiate between renal agenesis and abnormal location of the kidney, especially if air-containing bowel loops are present in the region being scanned. Since visualization of abdominal and pelvic organs by MRI is not limited by bone or bowel gas, it provides an overall view of the area; it allows easy differentiation between renal agenesis (Fig. 21–10) and ectopia and demonstrates possible

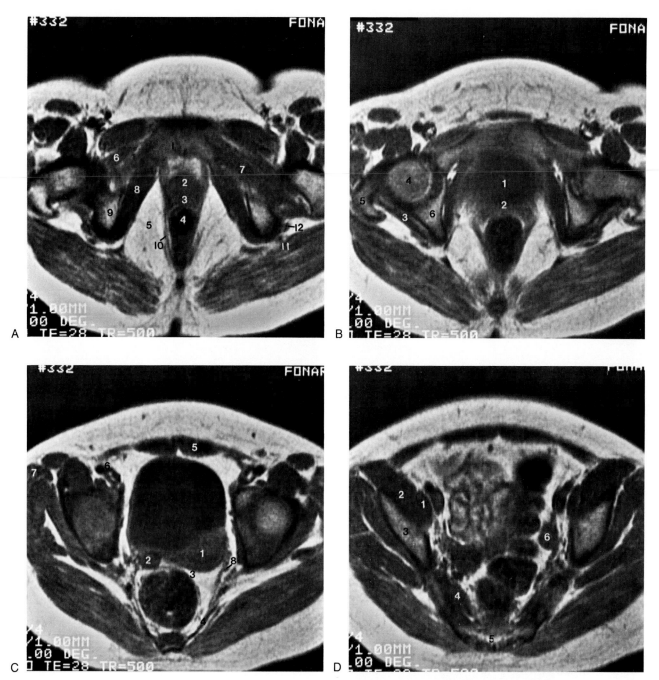

Figure 21–5. *Normal female pelvis.* **A,** Axial plane; perineum (SE 500/28). 1, Pubis; 2, base of bladder; 3, vagina; 4, rectum; 5, ischiorectal fossa; 6, pectineus m.; 7, obturator externus m.; 8, obturator internus m.; 9, ischial tuberosity; 10, levator ani m.; 11, inferior gluteal a. and v.; 12, sciatic n. **B,** Axial plane; lower pelvis (SE 500/28). 1, Bladder; 2, vagina; 3, inferior gemellus m.; 4, femoral head; 5, greater trochanter; 6, ischium. **C,** Axial plane; middle pelvis (SE 500/28). 1. Uterus; 2, ovary; 3, rectouterine space; 4, coccygeus m.; 5, rectus abdominis m.; 6, external iliac a. and v.; 7, tensor fasciae latae; 8, ureter. **D,** Axial plane; upper pelvis (SE 500/28). 1, Psoas m.; 2, iliacus m.; 3, ilium; 4, piriformis m.; 5, sacrum; 6, ovary.

Figure continues on following page.

complications: ectopic kidneys are more prone to injury or the development of obstruction.

Most congenital anomalies are best evaluated by T1 weighted images obtained in the coronal plane, which give good anatomic detail. In children with crossed-

fused ectopia, such images demonstrate the abnormally positioned fused kidney on one side and absence of renal tissue on the contralateral side (Fig. 21–9). Horseshoe kidneys are an exception and are easier to diagnose on transverse T1 weighted images

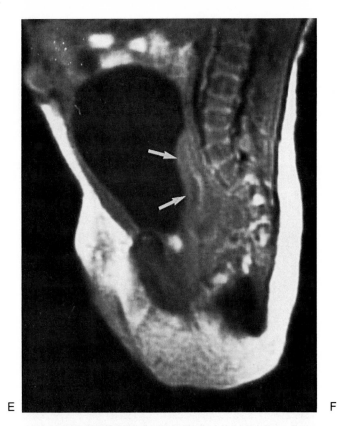

E

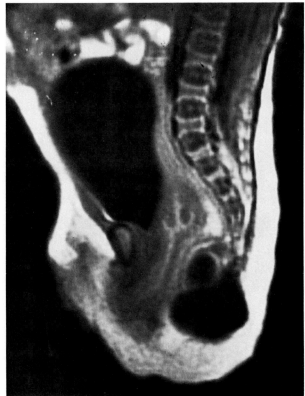

F

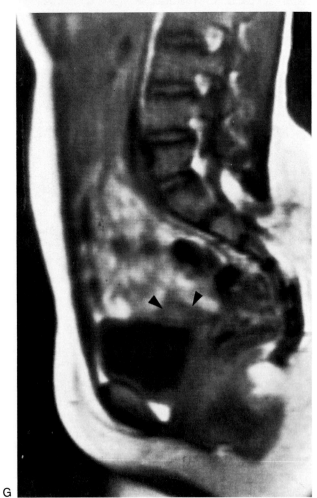

G

Figure 21–5. *Continued.*
E, F, Sagittal plane; maternal estrogen stimulation of the uterus in the newborn (SE 500/18). The uterus (*arrows*) has a postpubertal configuration, and clear differentiation of the endometrium, junctional line, and myometrium is seen. *G,* Sagittal plane; prepubertal uterus (SE 500/28). The uterine body (*arrowheads*) and cervix are of similar size and there is poor differentiation of endometrium and myometrium.

Figure continues on following page.

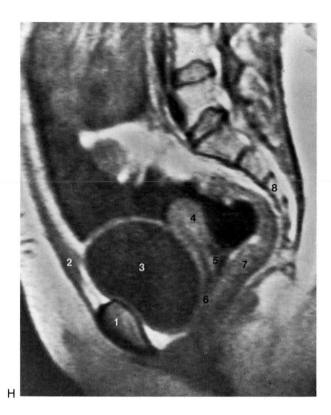

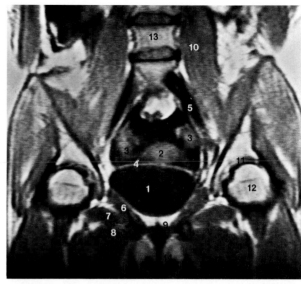

Figure 21–5. *Continued.*
H, Sagittal plane; postpubertal uterus (SE 500/28). The uterine body is larger than the cervix. The endometrium, junctional line, and myometrium can be identified even on this relatively T1 weighted image. ***I,*** Coronal plane; child with ascites (SE 500/28). 1, Bladder; 2, uterus; 3, ovary; 4, fallopian tube; 5, iliac a. and v.; 6, obturator internus m.; 7, obturator externus m.; 8, adductor brevis m.; 9, levator ani m.; 10, psoas m.; 11, acetabulum, 12, femur; 13, vertebra; 14, labium majus.

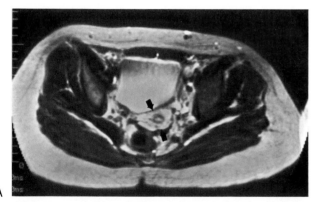

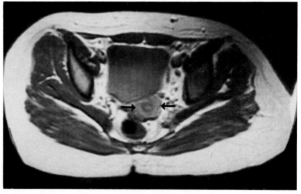

Figure 21–6. *Normal postpubertal uterus in secretory phase of cycle in a 15-year-old girl.* ***A,*** Transverse T2 image (2000/70). The uterus is outlined by arrows. The thick high-intensity outer rim is the myometrium. The thin low-intensity junctional zone represents the inner layer of the myometrium. The high-signal central area represents the endometrium. ***B,*** Spin-density image at the same level (1200/20) again shows the three layers of the uterus. Note that the contrast differentiation between these layers is less on this more T1 weighted image.

(Fig. 21–8). On posterior coronal cuts the axes of the kidneys appear normal, and only on more anteriorly positioned cuts can the lower pole fusion be visualized. Because the axes of the kidneys may be angled quite steeply, often only a small portion of renal tissue is identified on each slice, and the fusion of the lower poles across the midline can thus be easily missed on coronal images.

In children with agenesis of a kidney, the ipsilateral adrenal gland does not develop its characteristic inverted-V shape but instead has a discoid configuration. Discoid adrenal glands can be seen as elongated linear structures on coronal MR images (Fig. 21–10). Unilateral renal agenesis may also be associated with other abnormalities of the genitourinary tract. In females there may be anomalies of the uterus or vagina (dis-

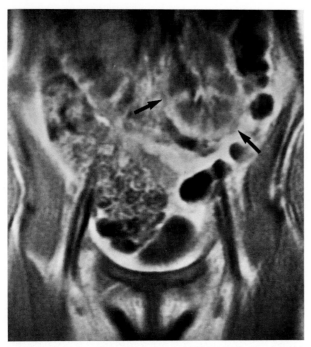

Figure 21–7. *Renal ectopia.* Coronal SE (500/28). The left kidney (*arrows*) is ectopically positioned inferiorly.

cussed later). In males there may be an associated cyst of the seminal vesicle (Figs. 21–11, 21–12).

Renal Cystic Diseases

The classifications of renal cystic disease are often confusing, and many are neither directly applicable nor helpful to the radiologist. Although early classifications were based on pathologic findings,[32] ones more directly related to imaging findings have recently been established.[33, 34] Cystic renal disorders include the polycystic diseases (infantile, juvenile, and adult), multicystic disease, and solitary cysts. Cysts may be confined to the medulla (medullary sponge kidney and juvenile nephrophthisis) or may be predominantly cortical in distribution (as seen in several of the multiple malformation syndromes and the trisomies).

Although all the renal cystic diseases can be well demonstrated by MRI,[4] ultrasonography is the primary modality used for their evaluation in most cases.[34] Thus, the role of MRI in this group of diseases is to clarify confusing cases and demonstrate complications that may occur, such as hemorrhage into the cysts.

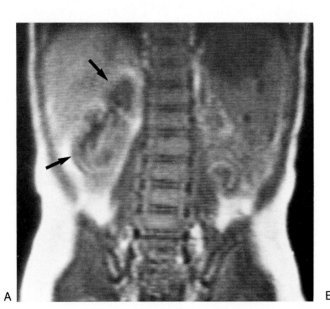

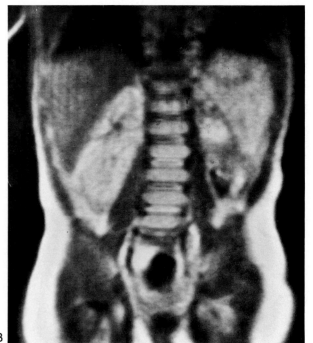

A

B

Figure 21–8. *Crossed-fused ectopia.* **A,** Coronal (SE 500/28). Both kidneys are fused and positioned in the right renal fossa (*arrows*). **B,** Coronal (SE 1500/56). Fused kidneys demonstrate high signal intensity on this T2 weighted image. (From Dietrich RB, Kangarloo H. Kidneys in infants and children: evaluation with MR. Radiology 1986; 159:215–221.)

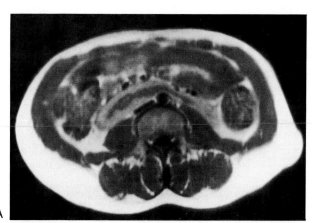

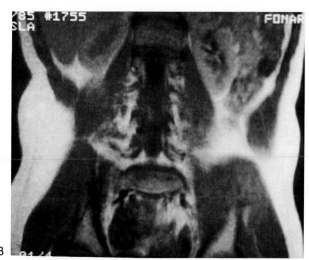

A   B

Figure 21–9. *Horseshoe kidney.* **A,** Axial SE (500/28). Fusion of lower poles of the kidney across the midline, anterior to the aorta. **B,** Coronal SE (500/28). Axes of kidneys appear normal on this image obtained through the posterior aspect of the kidneys. (From Dietrich RB, Kangarloo H. Pediatric body imaging. In: Stark DD, Bradley WG Jr., eds. Magnetic resonance imaging. St. Louis: CV Mosby, 1988:1434–1452.)

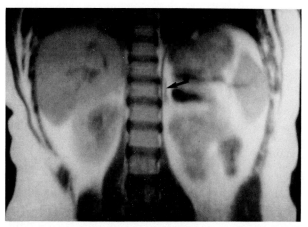

Figure 21–10. *Renal agenesis, discoid adrenal, and compensatory hyperplasia.* Coronal SE (500/28) showing discoid adrenal (*arrow*) lateral to the crus of the diaphragm and absent left kidney.

On MR images simple cysts appear as homogeneous, well-defined masses with clearly defined thin walls. If the fluid within the cyst is relatively pure, it will demonstrate low signal intensity on spin-echo and inversion recovery T1 weighted sequences.[1–4,55] On spin-echo T2 weighted sequences, the signal intensity of cyst fluid ranges from medium to high with progressive T2 weighting.[1,2,4,5] On images obtained using these pulse sequences, the cyst wall and the fluid within the cyst may not be easily distinguishable. Small amounts of calcification in the wall of the cyst are not readily identified by MRI, but larger amounts may be seen as a rim of signal void.

When the fluid within a cyst has a high protein content or contains subacute hemorrhage, the cyst may demonstrate inhomogeneous high signal intensity on both T1 and T2 weighted sequences.[1–3,32–40] However, there is a wide range of variability in the MR appearances of hemorrhagic cysts, even within the same kidney. Unfortunately it is not always possible to differentiate between hemorrhagic cysts, infected cysts, or neoplasms using the imaging sequences currently available[5,40] or even using T1 and T2 measurements.[40] Some authors have suggested that the presence of a fluid-iron level within a cyst correlates with a diagnosis of benign hemorrhage.[41]

Autosomal Recessive Polycystic Disease

Also frequently referred to as infantile polycystic disease, autosomal recessive polycystic disease is a congenital abnormality affecting both kidneys. Patients may present at varying ages and demonstrate a spectrum of pathology.[42] Associated liver disease ranges from proliferation and dilatation of the biliary radicles (biliary atresia) to severe periportal fibrosis,[43] and the severity of the renal cystic disease and hepatic fibrosis varies inversely.[44]

In infants presenting with polycystic disease, the kidneys are greatly enlarged in size bilaterally. Transection of the kidney shows multiple fusiform cysts, formed from dilated tubules.[45] In this group, liver pathology is rarely a problem.

Polycystic disease presenting in later childhood tends to have more severe liver involvement and less severe renal involvement. Patients frequently develop portal hypertension and gastrointestinal bleeding from varices. The renal cysts in these children may have a fusiform appearance similar to those of infants or may have a more rounded contour.[42]

MR images show the massively enlarged kidneys and the fusiform cysts contained within them (Fig. 21–13).[4]

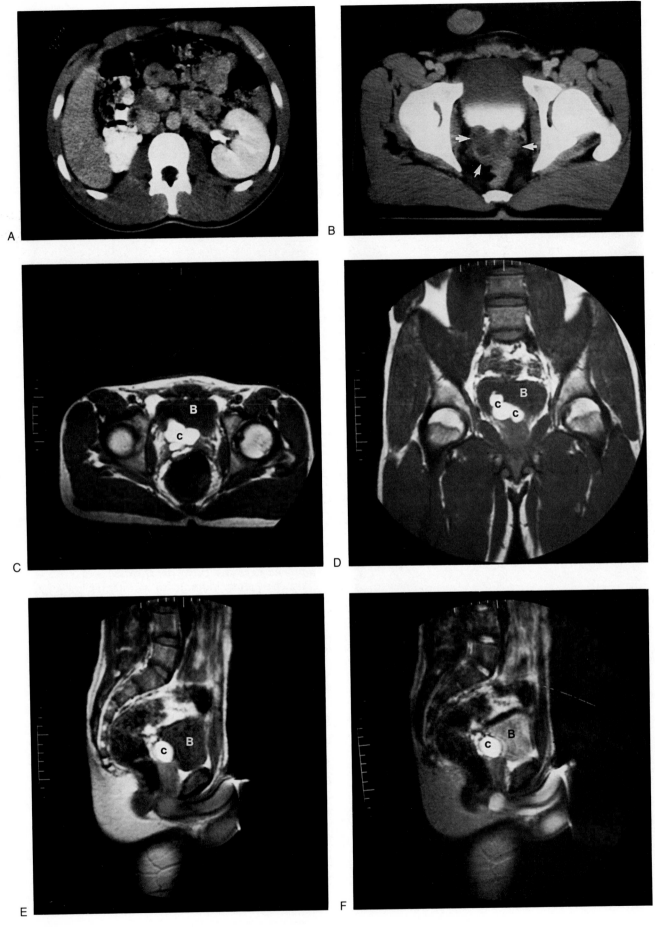

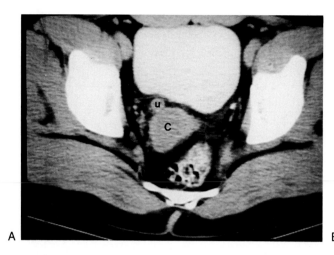

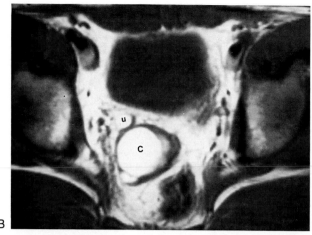

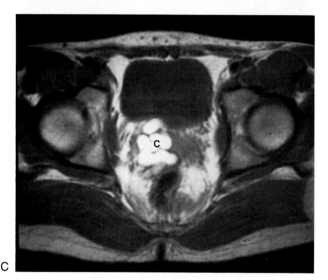

Figure 21–12. *Congenital seminal vesicle cyst in a 26-year-old male with a history of perirectal pain aggravated by ejaculation. The right kidney was absent. There was a blind-ending distal right ureter with insertion into the ejaculatory duct.* ***A,*** CT scan showing the dilated ureter (u) and a complex cystic mass (C) in the region of the seminal vesicle. ***B, C,*** Transverse MR images (2000/20). These also show the complex seminal vesicle cyst (C) and the dilated distal right ureteric stump (u). (Courtesy of B. King, Rochester, MN.)

On spin-echo T1 weighted images, areas of high signal intensity due to subacute hemorrhage present within the cysts may be seen (Fig. 21–13).[4]

Adult Polycystic Disease Presenting in Infancy

Adult autosomal dominant polycystic disease may present in childhood (Fig. 21–14). In neonates it may be difficult to distinguish from infantile polycystic disease, because the kidneys appear large and contain multiple small cysts.[46] As children become older, the cysts become larger in size and the more characteristic adult type appearance develops with multiple, asymmetrically positioned cysts involving both kidneys.[45]

MRI demonstrates both the simple cysts and those containing hemorrhage.[3, 41]

Multicystic Dysplastic Kidney

Multicystic dysplasia is the most common form of renal cystic disease in infants.[47] Both the classic and hydronephrotic forms are caused by obstruction of the ureter in early intrauterine life.[48, 49] By comparison, obstruction occurring after the formation of the functional kidneys results in the development of hydronephrosis.[48] Although usually unilateral, multicystic kidney disease may involve both kidneys and when it does so is, of course, incompatible with life. Neonates

◄ **Figure 21–11.** *Congenital seminal vesicle cyst in association with congenital renal agenesis in a 16-year-old boy with a history of recurrent genitourinary infections.* ***A,*** CT scan shows absence of the right kidney. ***B,*** CT scan of the pelvis shows a moderately poorly defined, irregular, mixed low and soft tissue density lesion (*arrows*) lying behind the bladder. ***C, D,*** Transverse and coronal T1 weighted images (800/26) showing a well-defined, high-intensity seminal vesicle cyst (c) indenting the posteroinferior aspect of the bladder (B). The high signal intensity from the fluid in the cyst is due to the presence of blood. ***E, F,*** Sagittal spin density (1700/20) and T2 weighted (1700/70) images again show the hemorrhagic seminal vesicle cyst (c) indenting the bladder (B).

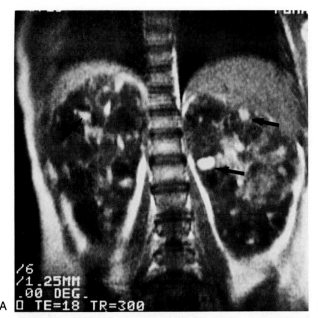
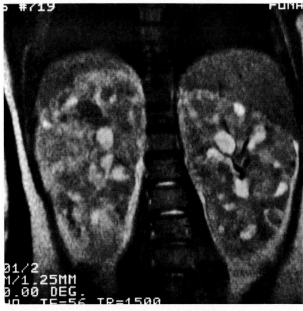

A B

Figure 21–13. *Juvenile onset autosomal recessive kidney disease.* **A,** Coronal (SE 300/18). The kidneys are greatly enlarged bilaterally and contain multiple low-signal-intensity cysts. Areas of high signal intensity (*arrows*) represent hemorrhage within the cysts. **B,** Coronal (SE 1500/56). Both hemorrhagic and nonhemorrhagic cysts have high signal intensity on this T2 weighted image. (From Dietrich RB, Kangarloo H. Pediatric body imaging. In: Stark DD, Bradley WG Jr., eds. Magnetic resonance imaging. St. Louis: CV Mosby, 1988:1434–1452.)

with bilateral involvement demonstrate the classic features of Potter's syndrome. With multicystic dysplastic kidney the proximal ureter is frequently atretic. The vascular pedicle may or may not be atretic. Contralateral urinary anomalies are found in up to 30 percent of patients. A common anomaly of the opposite side is uteropelvic junction obstruction.

The most common clinical presentation of multicystic dysplastic kidney is an asymptomatic abdominal mass found on routine examination.

MR images demonstrate multiple cysts that may vary greatly in size and are separated by a small amount of dysplastic renal tissue (Fig. 21–15).[4] The classic and hydronephrotic types of multicystic kidney can be distinguished by MRI. In the hydronephrotic type, smaller peripheral cysts can be seen surrounding a larger central cyst.

Simple Cysts

Although simple renal cysts are an uncommon autopsy finding in childhood,[50] the advent of ultrasonography demonstrated that they occur more frequently than previously thought.[51, 52] The incidence of simple renal cysts increases with age, and they are found in more than half of adults over 50 years of age.[53] Affected individuals are usually asymptomatic, and the presence of cysts is often an incidental finding on ultrasound studies performed for other reasons. Pathologically the cysts have a fibrous wall with a single layer of epithelium.

On MRI they are seen as single, well-defined masses of low homogeneous signal intensity on T1 weighted images and medium to high signal intensity on T2 weighted images (Fig. 21–16). When simple cysts are demonstrated in children, it is important to exclude the possibility of a Wilms' tumor or multilocular cyst.

Multilocular Cysts

Multilocular cyst is a benign tumor that contains multiple, noncommunicating cysts and causes displacement and compression of the adjacent normal renal tissue.[54] There are as yet no reports in the literature describing the MR appearance of this entity.

Medullary Cysts

Medullary cysts are seen during childhood in patients with juvenile nephronophthisis and medullary sponge kidney. The kidneys of children with juvenile nephronophthisis are normal or small in size and have small numbers of cysts in the medulla or corticomedullary region. These children usually present with azotemia.[55]

Children with medullary sponge kidney have cystic dilatation of the renal collecting ducts.[56] Although the disease occurs uncommonly in children, those affected usually present with hematuria or complications of the tubular ectasia such as development of stones or infection. Renal function remains normal.

There are no reports in the literature of the MR appearances of these diseases. However, as MRI is able to demonstrate the presence of small cysts in other

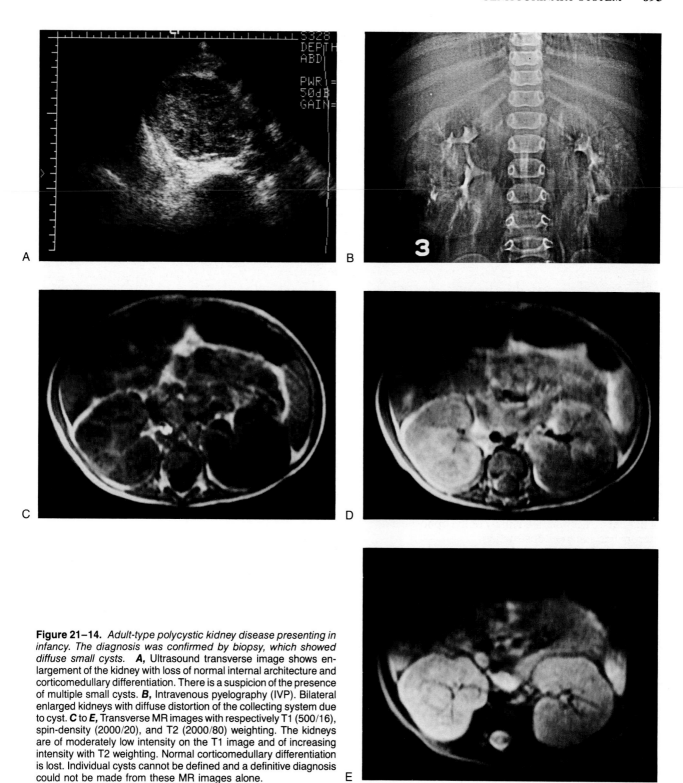

Figure 21–14. *Adult-type polycystic kidney disease presenting in infancy. The diagnosis was confirmed by biopsy, which showed diffuse small cysts.* **A,** Ultrasound transverse image shows enlargement of the kidney with loss of normal internal architecture and corticomedullary differentiation. There is a suspicion of the presence of multiple small cysts. **B,** Intravenous pyelography (IVP). Bilateral enlarged kidneys with diffuse distortion of the collecting system due to cyst. **C** to **E,** Transverse MR images with respectively T1 (500/16), spin-density (2000/20), and T2 (2000/80) weighting. The kidneys are of moderately low intensity on the T1 image and of increasing intensity with T2 weighting. Normal corticomedullary differentiation is lost. Individual cysts cannot be defined and a definitive diagnosis could not be made from these MR images alone.

renal cystic diseases, it is probable that it would reveal the cysts in the kidneys of children with juvenile nephronophthisis provided they are of sufficient size. It is unlikely, however, that MRI would show any abnormalities in children with medullary sponge kidneys.

The small stones and nephrocalcinosis occasionally seen by ultrasonography in the region of the pyramids in this entity[56] are unlikely to be seen by MR, because small amounts of calcium are not easily seen by the latter.

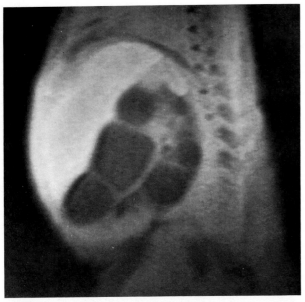

Figure 21–15. *Multicystic dysplastic kidney in a child with Potter's syndrome.* Sagittal (SE 500/28). Multiple low-signal-intensity cysts replace the parenchyma of the right kidney.

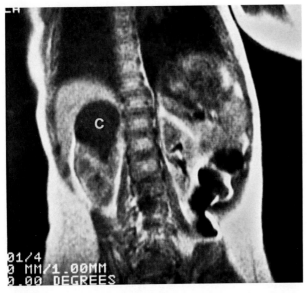

Figure 21–16. *Simple cyst.* Coronal (SE 500/28). A single cyst (C) containing homogeneous low-signal-intensity fluid and a thin, well-defined wall is present in the upper pole of the right kidney.

Cortical Cysts

Cortical cysts may be seen in several of the malformation syndromes, including tuberous sclerosis, von Hippel-Lindau disease, Jeune's asphyxiating dystrophy, Zellweger's cerebrohepatorenal syndrome, and the orofaciodigital syndrome. Microcystic changes are described in cases of trisomy D, trisomy E, Down's syndrome, and Turner's syndrome.[43] MRI can demon-

strate the cysts developing in these entities as long as they are of sufficient size.[57,58]

In addition to renal cysts, the kidneys of children with tuberous sclerosis may contain angiomyolipomas (Fig. 21–17).[57] On T1 weighted images, angiomyolipomas may demonstrate homogeneous medium signal intensity, but most also contain areas of high signal intensity owing to the presence of lipomatous tissue.[7] On T1 weighted images, it may not be possible to distinguish this fatty tissue from hemorrhagic cysts, but on images obtained with long enough TR and TE values, the lipomatous tissue will show lower signal intensity than the adjacent cysts. Phase contrast imaging may also aid in the differentiation of the two types of lesions.

Lower Urinary Tract

Multiplanar T1 weighted images are frequently the only sequences needed to evaluate congenital abnormalities of the lower urinary tract in children, since they demonstrate excellent anatomic resolution and clear depiction of fatty planes.[22] Since both large- and small-capacity bladders can be seen and bladder wall thickness can be demonstrated, MRI can be useful in the evaluation of children with neurogenic bladders. The same MR study of the pelvis used to image the bladder can also evaluate the lumbosacral spine for possible dysraphic abnormalities or spinal cord tumors that may be the cause of a neurogenic bladder (Fig. 21–18).[59]

Bladder Exstrophy

Abnormal location of the bladder with eversion of its posterior wall, separation of the pubic bones, absence of the rectus abdominis muscles, and anterior displacement of the anus can be seen by MRI in children with bladder exstrophy (Fig. 21–19). Other associated anomalies may be seen, such as a bifid clitoris and anterior tilting of the vagina in girls and bilateral inguinal hernias in boys.[60] Although these children have normal upper urinary tracts at birth, vesicoureteric reflux usually occurs after surgical closure of the bladder. Abnormalities of the upper tract may therefore be seen in older children with previously repaired exstrophy. Epispadias may also be seen in association with exstrophy of the bladder or as an isolated abnormality. In this entity, coronal images obtained at the level of the symphysis pubis demonstrate separation of the corpora cavernosa and displacement of the corpus spongiosum cephalad.[19]

Prune-Belly Syndrome

In children with the prune-belly syndrome, absence of abdominal musculature is seen in conjunction with urinary tract anomalies. Affected children are almost always male and two separate groups are identified. In one group an obstructing lesion of the urethra leads to

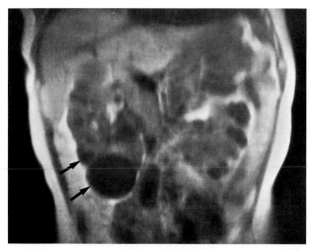 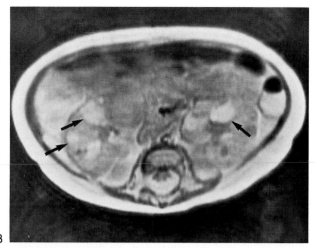

A   B

Figure 21–17. *Tuberous sclerosis.* ***A,*** Coronal (SE 500/28). Multiple low-signal-intensity cysts of varying sizes are seen within the right kidney (*arrows*). The high-signal-intensity areas most likely represent areas of fatty tissue within angiomyolipomas. ***B,*** Axial (SE 1500/56). Fluid within cysts (*arrow*) demonstrates higher signal intensity than the adjacent renal parenchyma.

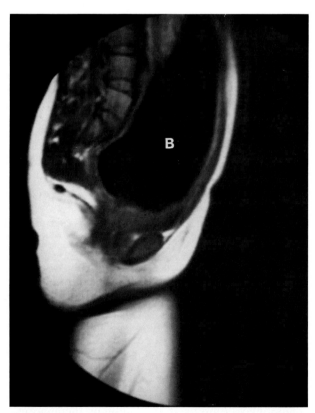

Figure 21–18. *Urogenic bladder due to partial sacral agenesis in a 7-year-old girl.* Midline sagittal image (700/26) shows absence of most of the sacrum. The bladder (B) is massively distended owing to flaccid urogenic paralysis.

the development of a hypertrophied bladder. By contrast, in the second group a functional abnormality of bladder emptying is present and the bladder is large and floppy.[61] Severe hydronephrosis and bilateral hydroureter may occur in both groups, and the dilatation of the ureters is frequently disproportionally severe compared with that of the renal pelvis and calyces.[62] A urachal remnant may be identified extending from the bladder to the umbilicus; part of this remnant may form a focal cyst. T1 weighted MR images are able to demonstrate the entire spectrum of anomalies in children with this disorder (Fig. 21–20).

MRI can also demonstrate many other abnormalities, such as ectopic ureterocele causing hydroureter and hydronephrosis (Fig. 21–21). Many or most of these abnormalities are well demonstrated by cheaper imaging modalities and MRI has no specific role to play in their evaluation. They may, however, be found incidentally on MR images taken for other reasons, and therefore their appearance should be recognized.

MRI can also demonstrate abnormal anatomy in less frequently seen lower urinary tract anomalies; a single report in the literature describes the MR findings in a patient with partial duplication of the bladder and incomplete diphallus.[19]

Genital Tract

MRI is an ideal modality for the evaluation of congenital anomalies of the genital tract. Before its introduction, diagnostic laparoscopy was often necessary to fully define the abnormal anatomy in patients with such anomalies.[63]

Congenital anomalies of the genital tract in children can be divided into several major groups: (1) disorders

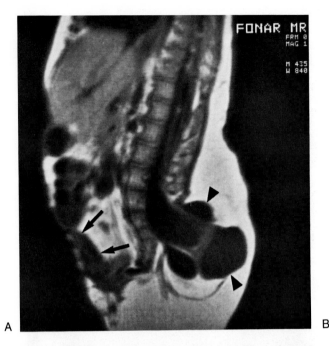

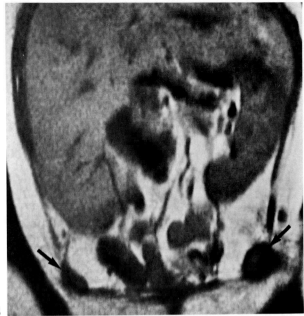

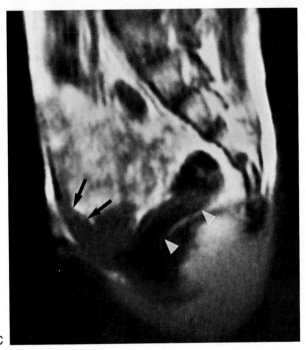

Figure 21–19. *Bladder extrophy.* **A,** Sagittal image (SE 500/28) shows bladder exstrophy (*arrows*). Absence of rectus abdominis muscles and myelomeningocele (*arrowheads*) are also seen. **B,** Coronal (SE 500/28). The pubic bones are separated and displaced laterally (*arrows*). **C,** Sagittal (SE 500/28). Midline cut demonstrates absence of the rectus abdominis muscles, and an anteriorly positioned bladder (*arrows*). The uterus, rectum (*arrowheads*), and anus are also displaced anteriorly. (From Dietrich RB, Kangarloo H. Pelvic abnormalities in children: assessment with MR imaging. Radiology 1987; 163:367–372.)

of sexual differentiation, (2) müllerian duct anomalies, (3) hydrometrocolpos-hematometrocolpos, and (4) undescended testis.

Disorders of Sexual Differentiation

MR images can clearly show the absence or abnormal location of pelvic organs in children with ambiguous genitalia or genetic abnormalities. Images obtained in the sagittal plane best demonstrate the uterine and cervical anatomy; axial images are best to show the vagina and gonads. Both T1 and T2 weighted images may be useful in fully defining the abnormal anatomy in these patients.

Turner's syndrome is a genetic disorder resulting from complete or partial monosomy of the short arm of the X chromosome. Complete monosomy (45,X) is the most frequent abnormality; (46,XXX) and (45,X) mosaics occur less often.[64] In these children the uterus, cervix, and vagina are always present but are usually hypoplastic, thus demonstrating an infantile configura-

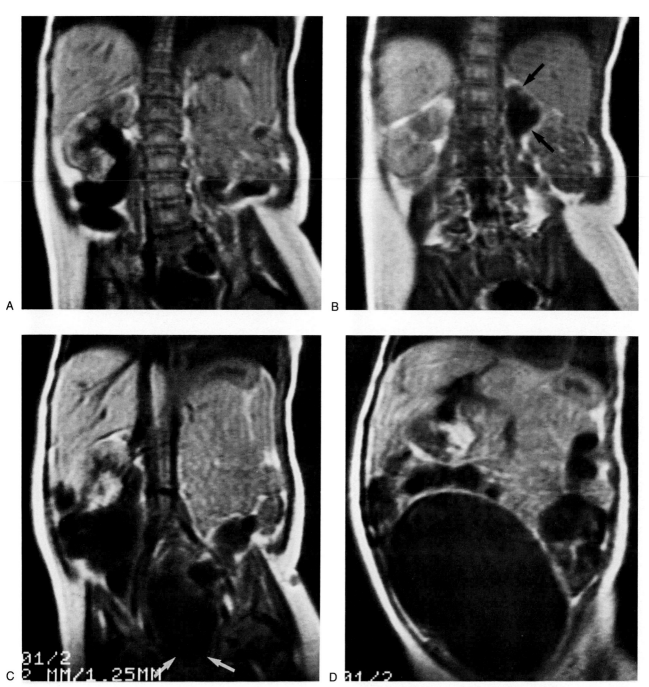

Figure 21–20. *Prune-belly syndrome.* **A,** Coronal (SE 500/28). Marked dilation and toruosity of the right ureter and to a lesser extent the pelvis and calices of the right kidney. **B,** Coronal (SE 500/28). Dysplastic left kidney (*arrows*). **C,** Coronal (SE 500/28). The bladder neck is clearly seen (*arrows*). There is no evidence of a dilated posterior urethra. **D,** Coronal (SE 500/28). Distended bladder and bulging of the abdominal wall. (From Dietrich RB, Kangarloo H. Kidneys in infants and children: evaluation with MR. Radiology 1986; 159:215–221; Dietrich RB, Kangarloo H. Pediatric body imaging. In: Stark DD, Bradley WG Jr., eds. Magnetic resonance imaging. St. Louis: CV Mosby, 1988:1434–1452.)

tion. Ovarian anatomy may range from single or (rarely) bilateral normal-appearing ovaries seen in a small number of patients who menstruate, to bilateral streak ovaries. Both ultrasonography and MRI can clearly define these abnormalities (Fig. 21–22).[65,66] On MRI, streak ovaries are seen as low-signal-intensity streaks on both T1 and T2 weighted images. Approximately 4 percent of patients with Turner's syndrome have (45,X/46,XY) mosaicism, and this group of children is at special risk. They have a propensity to develop gonadal neoplasia, particularly gonadoblastoma or dysgerminoma.[64] Because of this possibility, which

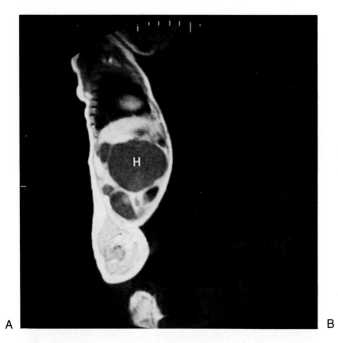

A

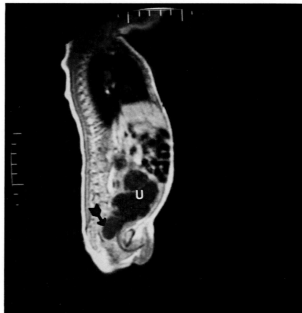

B

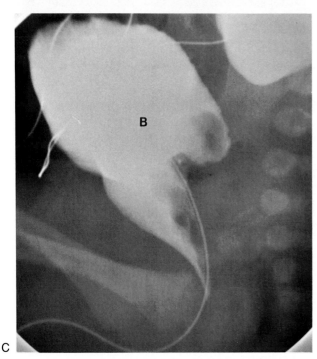

C

Figure 21–21. *Ectopic ureterocele with hydroureter and hydronephrosis in a 1-day-old infant.* ***A, B,*** Sagittal MR images (800/30) show hydronephrosis (H) with dilatation of the ureter (U) and a ureterocele (black arrow). ***C,*** Cystogram shows an irregular filling defect in the posteroinferior aspect of the bladder (B) due to the ureterocele.

has an incidence of 50 percent in this subgroup of children, thorough screening of these patients by ultrasonography and/or MRI is essential. On MRI, gonadoblastoma appears as an adnexal mass with medium signal intensity on T1 weighted images and high signal intensity on T2 weighted images, and thus has a markedly different appearance from that of streak ovaries (Fig. 21–23).[22, 66] The T2 weighted images are particularly important to help define the abnormal tissue and its extent. Associated renal anomalies in children

with Turner's syndrome include agenesis, ureteropelvic junction obstruction, ectopia, rotational abnormalities, double collecting systems, and horseshoe kidney.[67]

Children with testicular feminization have end-organ insensitivity to testosterone.[68] Although they have a male chromosome pattern of (46,XY), they are phenotypically female. Sagittal MR images show absence of the uterus and cervix; axial images show primitive gonads either in the adnexal region or in ectopic posi-

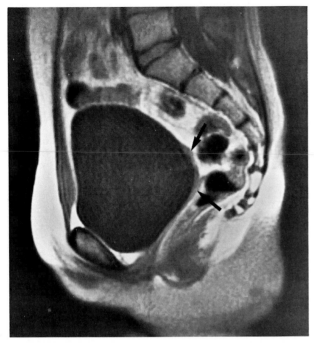

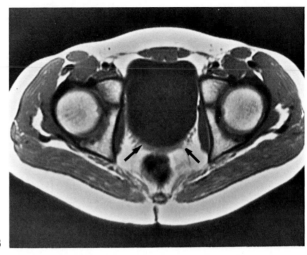

A

B

Figure 21–22. *Turner's syndrome.*   ***A,*** Sagittal (SE 500/30). A hypoplastic uterus and cervix (*arrows*) are present. ***B,*** Axial (SE 700/30). Small streak ovaries are present bilaterally (*arrows*).

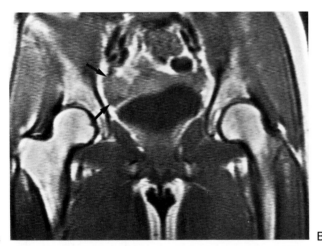

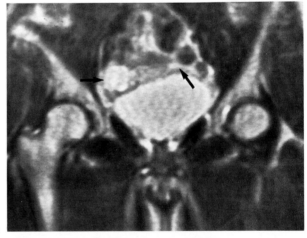

A

B

Figure 21–23. *Turner's syndrome with gonadoblastoma.*   ***A,*** Coronal (SE 500/28). A medium-signal-intensity right adnexal mass is present (*arrows*). ***B,*** Coronal (SE 2000/84). Regions of high signal intensity are seen in the right adnexal mass and also in the left streak ovary (*arrows*). This tissue was found to represent gonadoblastoma at surgery. (From Dietrich RB, Kangarloo H. Pelvic abnormalities in children: assessment with MR imaging. Radiology 1987; 163:367–372; Dietrich RB, Kangarloo H. Pediatric body imaging. In: Stark DD, Bradley WG Jr., eds. Magnetic resonance imaging. St. Louis: CV Mosby, 1988:1434–1452.)

tion within the inguinal canal (Fig. 21–24). In these patients the vagina ends in a blind pouch.

In children with hermaphroditism, both ovarian and testicular tissues are present. A uterus is present but may be hypoplastic or unicornate, and the appearance of the external genitalia ranges from feminine with slight clitoral prominence to fully masculine.[68] MR images obtained in multiple planes can help demon-strate the varied and complex anatomy in these children.

Pseudohermaphroditism occurs when there is a disturbance in the endocrinologic environment of the fetus. Exposure to excessive amounts of androgen leads to varying degrees of masculinization of the external genitalia in children who are genetically female and have normal female internal genitalia.[68]

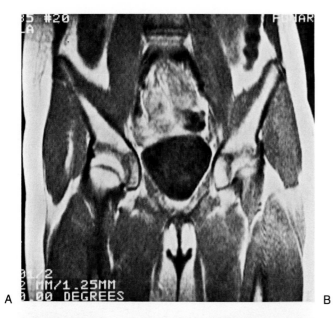

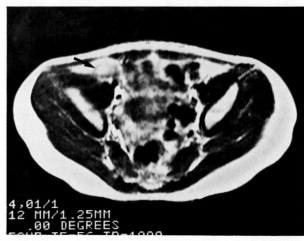

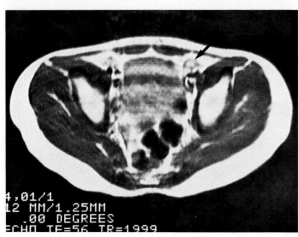

Figure 21–24. *Testicular feminization.* **A,** Coronal (SE 500/28). No uterus is identified. **B,** Axial (SE 2000/56). High-signal-intensity gonad with low-signal-intensity surrounding rim is seen adjacent to the right iliopsoas muscle (*arrow*). **C,** Axial (SE 2000/56). The left gonad is also identified (*arrow*). (From Dietrich RB, Kangarloo H. Pelvic abnormalities in children: assessment with MR imaging. Radiology 1987; 163:367–372.)

Male pseudohermaphrodites, by contrast, have testes, but the external genitalia are not fully masculinized owing to a deficiency of testicular secretions or a failure of target tissues to respond to the secretions elaborated.[68]

Müllerian Duct Anomalies

The fallopian tubes, uterus, cervix, and proximal vagina develop from the müllerian ducts. The distal two-thirds of the vagina develops from the urogenital sinus.[69]

FUSION DEFECTS. Abnormalities caused by incomplete fusion of the müllerian ducts are numerous (Fig. 21–25).[70] Complete failure of fusion results in the formation of two uteri, two cervices, and two vaginas (uterus didelphys) (Fig. 21–26). Incomplete fusion leads to the development of such lesions as bicornuate uterus (single vagina and cervix with two uteri) and uterus septus (single vagina, cervix, and uterus with a

uterine septum). Occasionally in children with a double vagina, one half is imperforate (Fig. 21–27).

These uterine abnormalities can frequently be diagnosed and differentiated by MRI, thus obviating the need for more invasive diagnostic procedures.[63, 71] MRI can differentiate bicornuate and septate uteri in postpubertal girls. This is extremely important clinically because the two anomalies require different surgical management. On axial T2 weighted images, patients with bicornate uteri show a medium-signal-intensity strip of myometrium separating the two low-signal-intensity junctional zones that is not seen in children with septate uteri. Müllerian duct anomalies are also associated with a wide spectrum of genitourinary anomalies such as agenesis or malposition of the kidney.[72]

ATRESIA DEFECT. This causes aplasia and atresia of the vagina and uterus. It is an uncommon abnormality with an incidence of approximately one in 5,000.[73]

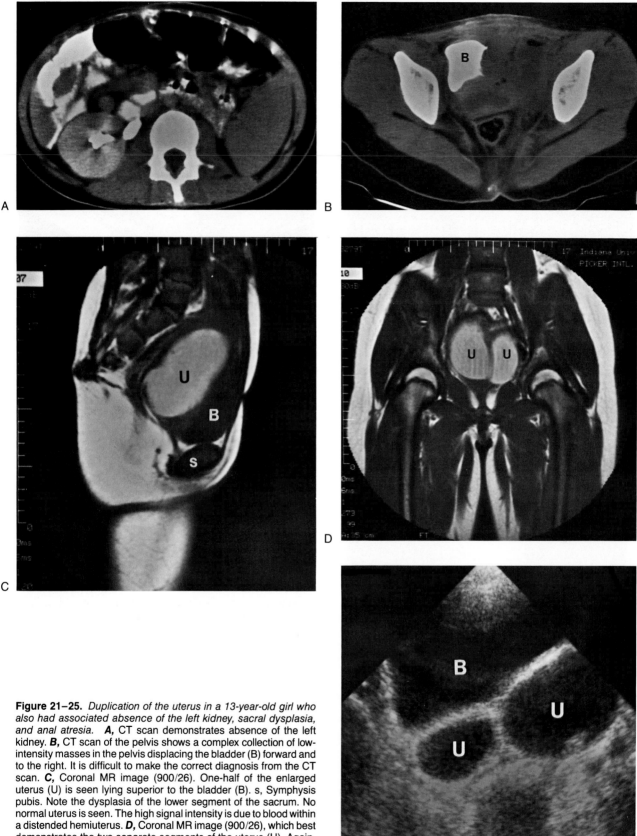

Figure 21–25. *Duplication of the uterus in a 13-year-old girl who also had associated absence of the left kidney, sacral dysplasia, and anal atresia.* ***A,*** CT scan demonstrates absence of the left kidney. ***B,*** CT scan of the pelvis shows a complex collection of low-intensity masses in the pelvis displacing the bladder (B) forward and to the right. It is difficult to make the correct diagnosis from the CT scan. ***C,*** Coronal MR image (900/26). One-half of the enlarged uterus (U) is seen lying superior to the bladder (B). s, Symphysis pubis. Note the dysplasia of the lower segment of the sacrum. No normal uterus is seen. The high signal intensity is due to blood within a distended hemiuterus. ***D,*** Coronal MR image (900/26), which best demonstrates the two separate segments of the uterus (U). Again, the high signal intensity is due to blood. ***E,*** Ultrasound also shows the two segments of the uterus (U) quite well. B, Bladder.

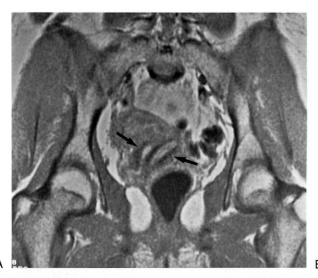
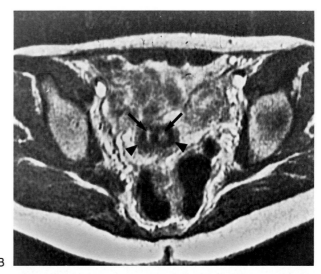

Figure 21–26. *Uterus didelphys.* **A,** Coronal (SE 500/18). A double uterine cavity is identified (*arrows*). **B,** Axial (SE 2000/85). Two separate high-signal-intensity endometrial linings are present (*arrows*). Two low-signal-intensity junctional lines are also identified (*arrowheads*) with medium-signal-intensity myometrium separating them.

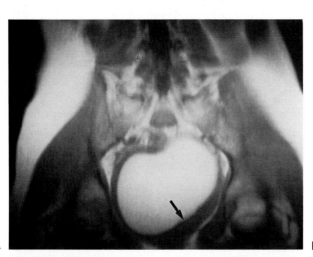
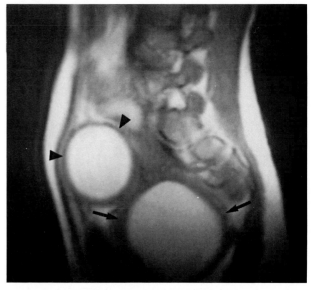

Figure 21–27. *Bicornuate uterus with obstruction of the right cavity.* **A,** Coronal (SE 500/28). A high-signal-intensity blood collection is seen distending the right uterine cavity. The medium-signal-intensity compressed left uterine cavity is seen adjacent to it (*arrows*). **B,** Parasagittal (SE 500/28). The high-signal-intensity blood collection distends the uterine cavity (*arrows*) and also the adjacent right fallopian tube (*arrowheads*).

The chromosomes, ovaries, and secondary sexual characteristics are usually normal. The range of abnormality is from simple partial agenesis of the vagina with a normal cervix and uterus to complete absence of these organs.

In patients with the Mayer-Rokitansky-Küster-Hauser syndrome, both the uterus and vagina are usually absent. Approximately one-third of patients have associated renal anomalies such as unilateral agenesis, uni- or bilateral ectopia, horseshoe kidney, abnormalities of the collecting system, or malrotation; vertebral anomalies may also be present.[73–76] Because MRI is able to demonstrate clearly both normal and abnormal vaginal anatomy noninvasively, it is the modality of choice for the evaluation of patients with this abnormality (Fig. 21–28).[28, 69]

Vaginal agenesis may be diagnosed early in life, but diagnosis is often delayed until teenage years. Patients may present with primary amenorrhea. In girls in whom a cervix and uterus are present, pain and an abdominal mass develop after the menarche.

MRI has a unique role to play in the evaluation of these patients. Because of the ability to image in multiple planes, MRI is the best modality for demonstrating

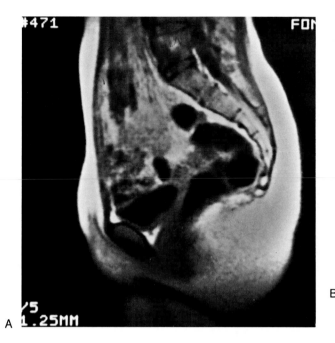

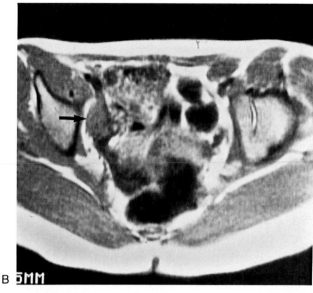

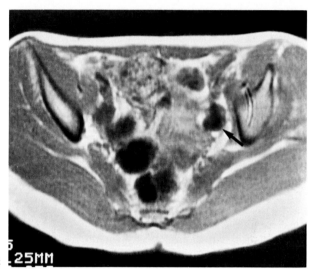

Figure 21–28. *Mayer-Rokitansky-Küster-Hauser syndrome.* **A,** Sagittal (SE 500/28). No uterus or vagina is identified between the bladder and rectum. **B,** Axial (SE 500/28). Normal right ovary is seen (*arrow*). **C,** Axial (SE 500/28). Normal left ovary is seen (*arrow*).

the extent of the abnormality. This information is critical for accurate planning of surgical reconstruction. In patients who have both a cervix and a uterus, the vaginal reconstruction must connect with these organs. In patients with only a uterus but no cervix, a blind-ending vagina is reconstructed and the uterus is removed.

MÜLLERIAN DUCT CYSTS. This is a very rare isolated congenital abnormality that arises from the caudal end of the fused müllerian duct.[77] It is a cyst of the prostatic utricle in males. It is usually diagnosed in adults but can be diagnosed in children. Symptoms result from hemorrhage into the cyst, infection, and mass effect on adjacent organs. The cyst can vary in size from small to large.

MRI shows a midline lesion arising from the prostate and bulging at the level of the verumontanum. Signal intensity is high on T2 weighted images; it may be low

on T1 weighted images, or high if the cyst contains hemorrhage or mucus. The midline location of the cyst differentiates it from a seminal vesicle cyst.[77]

Hydrometrocolpos-Hematometrocolpos

This involves the presence of fluid and/or blood in the vagina and/or uterus. There are many causes of this accumulation, including an imperforate hymen, a vaginal diaphragm, atresia of the vagina or cervix, or a persistent urogenital sinus or cloaca. In children with hematometrocolpos, a high-signal-intensity blood collection is seen within a markedly dilated upper vagina and uterine cavity on both T1 and T2 weighted images (Fig. 21–29).[22, 69] The dilated structures cause compression of the adjacent bladder and rectum. The sagittal plane best identifies the location of the fluid collection within the upper vagina and uterine cavity.[23] In some instances the fluid collection may extend into the

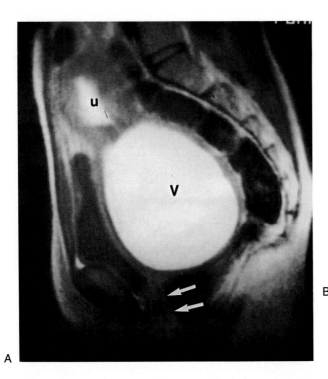

A

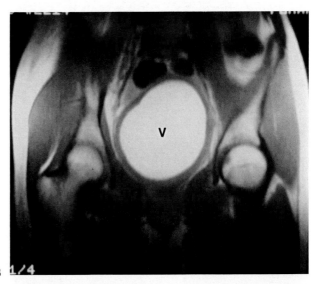

B

Figure 21–29. *Hematometrocolpos.* **A,** Sagittal (SE 500/28). A high-signal-intensity blood collection distends the upper vagina (V) and uterine cavity (u). The lower vagina appears normal (*arrows*). **B,** Coronal (SE 500/28). A high-signal-intensity fluid collection distends the upper vagina (V).

adjoining fallopian tube, and the tortuous and dilated fluid-filled fallopian tube can be seen extending into the abdomen. In the sagittal plane the nondistended lower portion of the vagina may also be identified (Fig. 21–29). In children with one abnormal müllerian duct, hematometrocolpos may involve only a portion of the uterine cavity (Fig. 21–27).[78]

Undescended Testis

Evaluation of male infants is frequently required for localization of an undescended testis before surgery. Ultrasonography is performed initially, and if this is unsuccessful in locating the gonad, MRI may be performed.[36,79] The undescended gonad most commonly lies within the inguinal canal. If, however, it is positioned within the abdomen or pelvis, it may be located adjacent to the lateral bladder wall, the psoas muscle, or the iliac vessels; in the retroperitoneum; or in the superficial inguinal pouch. In rare instances the gonad may be prepenile or perineal in position.[37] On T1 weighted images the ectopic gonad has medium signal intensity and can frequently be identified as it is outlined by the high-signal-intensity fat surrounding it (Fig. 21–30). In the search for ectopic gonads, a T2 weighted sequence may add useful information, since on such images gonads appear as high-signal-intensity structures with a surrounding rim of medium signal intensity, and are thus easily distinguished from muscles and lymphadenopathy (Fig. 21–30). This low-signal-intensity rim may be more difficult to see on images obtained at high field strength, because chemical shift misregistration is more apparent and may mask the

rim. A more detailed discussion of undescended testis is presented in the chapter on the Reticuloendothial and Endocrine Systems.

INFECTION AND INFLAMMATION

Infection

In children with a proven urinary tract infection or with symptoms suggestive of it, the workup consists of a combination of ultrasonography, excretory urography, and nuclear scintigraphy.[80–86] In this group of patients, evaluation by MRI does not routinely add any information. In more problematic cases or in patients who develop complications, MRI may be useful.

In the evaluation of acute pyelonephritis, the radiologic findings are frequently minimal and nonspecific irrespective of the modality used. On MR images the affected kidney may appear enlarged, and on T1 weighted images the increased water content may cause lower signal intensity and loss of corticomedullary differentiation. Visualization of thickening of the perirenal fascia by MRI has also been described.[7] If the infection affects only part or parts of the kidney, as in acute lobar nephronia, the affected areas may demonstrate lower signal intensity on T1 weighted images than the adjacent normal areas (Fig. 21–31). On T2 weighted images, both the normal and abnormal areas demonstrate similar signal intensity, although infected areas may show higher signal intensity than the adja-

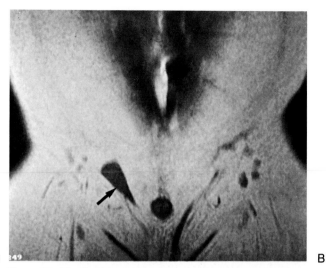
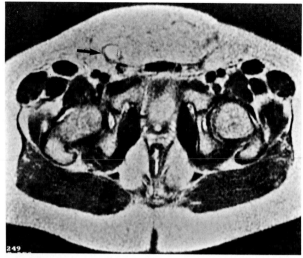

A   B

Figure 21–30. *Undescended testis.* **A,** Coronal (SE 300/18). A medium-signal-intensity gonad is present in the inguinal canal (*arrow*). **B,** Axial (SE 1500/60). On this T2 weighted image the gonad demonstrates high signal intensity with a medium-signal-intensity rim surrounding it (*arrow*).

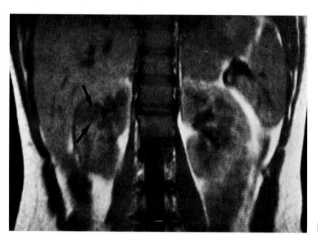
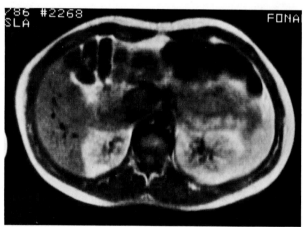

A   B

Figure 21–31. *Focal nephronia.* **A,** Coronal (SE 500/28). A low-signal-intensity region extends to the surface of the right kidney (*arrows*). **B,** Axial (SE 2000/84). The same area demonstrates slightly higher signal intensity than the adjacent renal parenchyma on this T2 weighted image.

cent normal parenchyma if the TR value is sufficiently long. Remember that kidneys normally have very long T1 and T2 relaxation times.

Renal abscesses and carbuncles occur less frequently in children than in adults. On MRI they demonstrate low to medium signal intensity on T1 weighted images and high signal intensity on T2 weighted images. In children with duplication of the renal collecting system, infection may develop in an obstructed upper moiety. When this occurs the MR signal intensity of the urine in the obstructed system may vary on T1 weighted images, depending on the protein content of the fluid. A fluid-fluid level may also be seen within the fluid collection on images obtained in an appropriate plane (Fig. 21–32). Perinephric abscesses may occur

secondary to severe pyelonephritis or as a consequence of carbuncle rupture. They usually have a similar appearance to that of infected fluid collections elsewhere in the body.[87]

Pelvic abscesses usually occur in association with an inflammatory process such as appendicitis or inflammatory bowel disease. As with other abscesses, the MR appearances of those occurring in the pelvis are equally nonspecific, and their signal intensity characteristics may vary depending on their content. It usually is not possible to distinguish them from other noninfected fluid collections, or from necrotic tumors arising or involving the soft tissues, either by their MR appearance alone or by evaluation of their T1 and T2 values.[87, 89]

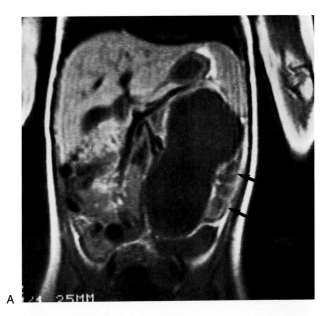

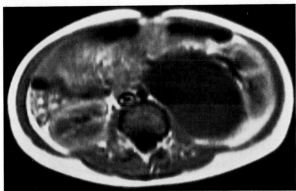

Figure 21-32. *Duplex renal collecting system with an infected, obstructed upper pole.* **A,** Coronal (SE 500-28). A low-signal-intensity fluid-filled upper pole displaces the lower pole of the kidney laterally and inferiorly (*arrows*). **B,** Axial (SE 500/28). Axial image obtained with the patient dependent demonstrates a fluid-fluid level within the infected upper pole. (From Dietrich RB, Kangarloo H. Pediatric body imaging. In: Stark DD, Bradley WG Jr., eds. Magnetic resonance imaging. St. Louis: CV Mosby, 1988:1434–1452.)

Glomerulonephritis and Other Causes of Acute Renal Failure

The most frequent causes of acute renal failure in children are different from those in the adult population. In the pediatric population, renal failure may have either a glomerular or a tubular etiology. Glomerular causes include glomerulonephritis, the nephrotic syndrome, inherited renal disease such as Alport's disease or sickle cell disease, and the hemolytic-uremic syndrome. Tubular causes are much rarer and include renal tubular acidosis, hypercalcemic syndromes, juvenile nephronophthisis, and Fanconi's syndrome.[90] In neonates, acute renal failure frequently is secondary to a vascular insult (see the section on vascular disorders below).

In acute renal failure, although MRI is able to detect abnormality within the kidney, the findings are nonspecific. Not only is MRI unable to differentiate the varying diseases causing acute renal failure from each other, but it also cannot distinguish them from such other entities as dehydration, transplant rejection, pyelonephritis, and infiltrative tumor on the MR appearance alone.[4, 31] In all these entities, T1 weighted MR images may demonstrate loss of corticomedullary differentiation in kidneys that are of normal size or slightly enlarged (Fig. 21–33). Although loss of corticomedullary differentiation is thus a nonspecific finding, it has been shown to be a sensitive indicator of renal disease.[91] The role of MRI in this group of patients lies therefore not in the diagnosis of the disease process, but in the demonstration of complications such as hemorrhage following renal biopsy (see the section on vascular disorders).

In children with chronic renal failure, the kidneys may be very small and are often difficult to visualize by ultrasonography owing to obscuration by adjacent bowel gas. MRI can easily show the small, shrunken kidneys that also demonstrate loss of corticomedullary differentiation (Fig. 21–34). These children, who have frequently been receiving long-term peritoneal dialysis, may develop multiple renal cysts or even renal carcinoma as a complication of their treatment.[92] MRI can be extremely useful in the identification and follow-up of such lesions (Fig. 21–34).[92] On T1 weighted images, cysts due to chronic dialysis appear as well-defined, low-signal-intensity areas as seen in other renal cystic diseases, and renal carcinoma appears as a medium-signal-intensity mass. On T2 weighted images, both types of lesions demonstrate high signal intensity.

TUMOR

The renal neoplasms that occur commonly in children include the various forms of leukemia, lymphoma, and Wilms' tumor. Less often, renal cell carcinoma, teratoma, and primary sarcomas such as rhabdomyosarcoma may be seen in the pediatric age group.

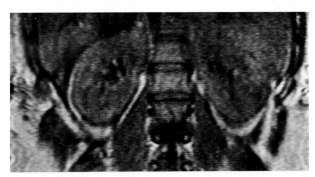

Figure 21–33. *Acute glomerulonephritis.* Coronal (SE 500/28). The kidneys are slightly enlarged and there is loss of corticomedullary differentiation.

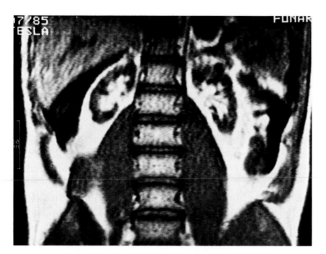

Figure 21–34. *Chronic renal failure.* Coronal (SE 500/28). There are small kidneys bilaterally with loss of corticomedullary differentiation. Multiple small cysts are present bilaterally.

Wilms' Tumor

Wilms' tumor is the most common primary renal neoplasm in children, making up 95 percent of cancers affecting the kidney, ureter, and bladder in children under 16 years of age.[93] Of these, 90 percent occur in children under 7 years of age, and there is a peak incidence between the ages of 1 and 3 years.[94] It is very rare in newborns. There is also an increased incidence of Wilms' tumor in children with aniridia, hemihypertrophy, genitourinary anomalies, and Beckwith-Wiedemann syndrome.[95, 96] Bilateral tumor involvement occurs in approximately 5 to 10 percent of cases of Wilms' tumor.

Pathologically, Wilms' tumors are usually large at the time of presentation and frequently contain areas of hemorrhage and/or necrosis. They are usually well defined, having a pseudocapsule of compressed tissue. Metastatic spread of Wilms' tumor depends on the histology. Over 90 percent of Wilms' tumors have a so-called classic or favorable histology. These spread by invasion of local tissues, including the renal veins and inferior vena cava, and also via the bloodstream to the liver and lungs. Regional lymph node metastasis can also occur. The remaining 10 percent of Wilms' tumors have a different histology (unfavorable histology). Several subtypes are recognized, including a rhabdoid tumor that classically metastasizes to brain, and an aplastic clear cell sarcoma that typically spreads to bone.

Children with Wilms' tumor most frequently present with a unilateral abdominal mass. Less commonly, children present with vague abdominal pain or hematuria.[97]

The initial diagnosis is usually made by ultrasonography, which demonstrates a solid mass arising from the kidney. MRI, however, has been shown to be superior to both ultrasonography and x-ray CT in diagnosing and defining the extent of Wilms' tumor.[23, 98, 99] Coronal T1 weighted images are excellent for defining the organ of origin of the lesions, and thus differentiating renal lesions from those arising in the adjacent liver and adrenal gland (Figs. 21–35 to 21–37). Both T1 and T2 weighted images, used in conjunction, define the full extent of the lesion, its possible invasion of adjacent organs, and the presence of associated lymphadenopathy (Fig. 21–35). MRI has not yet been shown to be any better than other imaging modalities at demonstrating capsule invasion and penetration by Wilms' tumor. At the present time this can be accurately determined only by a histologic evaluation of the resected tumor.

The internal structure of Wilms' tumors is varied on MR images. Most are not homogeneous. On T1 weighted images, tumor tissue appears of relatively low

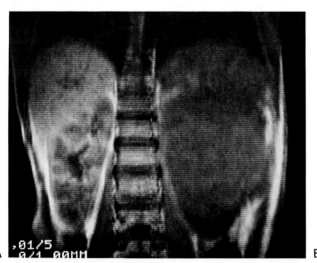
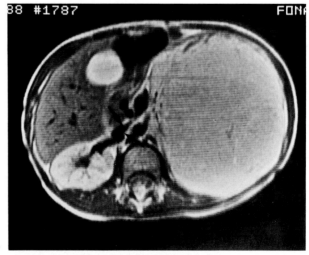

Figure 21–35. *Wilms' tumor.* **A,** Coronal (SE 500/28). There is a large medium-signal-intensity mass replacing the left kidney. **B,** Axial (SE 500/28). Tumor demonstrates high signal intensity on this T2 weighted image, enabling its exact borders to be identified. The distal left renal vein and inferior vein demonstrate a flow void with no evidence of tumor thrombus within them (*arrows*).

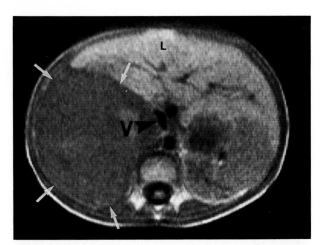

Figure 21–36. *Wilms' tumor.* Transverse T1 weighted image (500/30). There is a very large right upper quadrant mass (*arrows*) of low intensity, less than that of liver (L). The inferior vena cava (V) is displaced by the tumor but not encased. No tumor is seen within the lumen of the cava. Note that the tumor is clearly differentiated from the liver.

intensity. It may be lower than that of normal kidney, or of similar intensity. Necrotic regions in the tumor are of lower intensity than viable tumor in many cases. Focal areas of hemorrhage may be seen as regions of high signal intensity on T1 weighted images. On T2 weighted images there is a marked increase in signal intensity of the tumor tissue. Areas of necrosis (Fig. 21–38) usually increase in signal intensity even more than the primary tumor. Hemorrhage appears of varied signal intensity on T2 weighted images (Figs. 21–36, 21–37).

Although the MR contrast agent gadolinium-DTPA is not yet approved by the Federal Drug Administration for use in evaluation of the pediatric body, it is already being used experimentally at several sites. It shows early promise in helping to demonstrate the exact margins of lesions and in identifying associated adenopathy, especially in vascular tumors that demonstrate enhancement on T1 weighted images after contrast administration.

Because MRI so clearly defines patent vascular structures, owing to the low signal intensity of rapidly flowing blood within them, it is extremely useful in demonstrating the presence of tumor thrombus within the renal veins or inferior vena cava (Figs. 21–39, 21–40).[99, 100] Wilms' tumors usually displace, rather than encase, the abdominal aorta or inferior vena cava. The direction of displacement and the position of the displaced vessels can be well identified on MRI (Fig. 21–37) and this is helpful in planning surgical resection of the tumors. Lung metastases from Wilms' tumor can be seen on MR images, appearing as focal regions of very high signal intensity well seen against the background of normal low-signal-intensity lung (Fig. 21–41). There are no reports comparing MRI and CT for the detection of lung metastases in Wilms' tumor. CT is

exquisitely sensitive, and it is not thought that MRI is as accurate as CT for detection of very tiny metastases. MRI is also useful in evaluating children for residual or recurrent disease after chemotherapy or surgical resection of tumor.

The precise role of MRI in the evaluation of children with Wilms' tumor is still under debate. Ultrasonography and CT are very good. The main advantage of MRI is its potential for replacing all the other modalities for imaging children with suspected Wilms' tumor, its excellent visualization of blood vessels, and its ability potentially to better visualize direct spread of the tumor by imaging in multiple planes. MRI is limited only by motion artifacts, which vary from patient to patient.

Nephroblastomatosis

In newborn infants, small rests of primitive metanephric epithelium, nephrogenic blastema, are often present within the kidney. These rests, which usually regress by 4 months of age, are thought to be the precursor of Wilms' tumor. In a small number of patients, however, regression does not occur and the rests develop into Wilms' tumor. Both kidneys are usually affected and children frequently present with bilateral renal masses.[101] On gross inspection the kidneys are enlarged and lobulated. Enlargement of the kidneys, together with marked distortion and elongation of the pelvocaliceal system, is well seen by x-ray CT.[102] The same findings described on CT can be seen by MRI. It may thus be possible to differentiate between classic Wilms' tumor, which may obliterate the collecting system, and Wilms' tumor arising from nodular nephroblastomatosis, in which the collecting system is distorted but preserved (Fig. 21–42). In patients with nodular nephroblastomatosis presenting as a unilateral mass, the contralateral kidney should always be very carefully examined.

Leukemia and Lymphoma

Both leukemia and lymphoma may involve the kidney through infiltration of its interstitium by tumor cells. In acute leukemia, involvement is usually diffuse, causing generalized enlargement of the kidneys.[103] In lymphoma, although involvement may be diffuse, it may also be more focal, appearing as multiple nodules or even a solitary mass within the kidney.[104] MRI can demonstrate the enlarged kidneys and identify diffuse or focal disease in both these entities (Figs. 21–43 to 21–45). Focal disease appears as one or more masses that are isointense or slightly hypointense compared with the renal parenchyma on spin-echo T1 weighted sequences. Loss of corticomedullary differentiation can also be seen in the involved areas on spin-echo T1 weighted images. On T2 weighted sequences the masses are usually of lower signal intensity than the

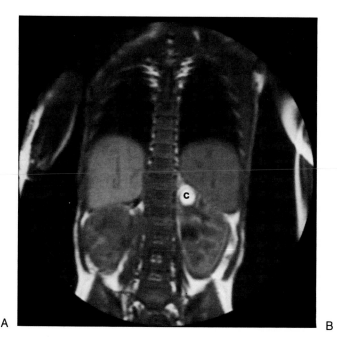

A

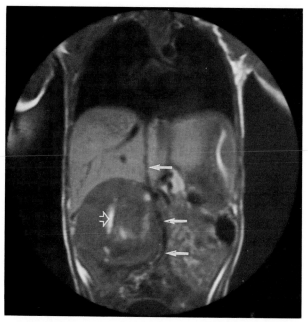

B

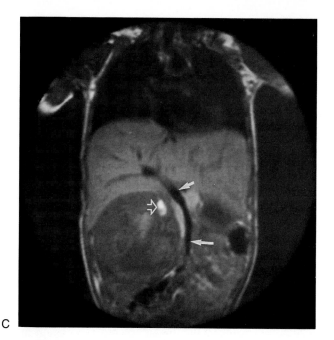

C

Figure 21–37. *Wilms' tumor with hemorrhage. Three coronal T1 images (500/16) at the level of the spine, vena cava, and portal vein, respectively.* **A,** This posterior image shows a mass lesion in the region of the right kidney. It is of lower intensity than liver, from which it is clearly separate. A well-defined high-intensity focus in the upper pole of the left kidney represents a small hemorrhagic cyst (C). **B,** A patent inferior vena cava (*arrows*) is displaced to the left by the tumor mass. Areas of high signal intensity (*open arrow*) in the tumor are due to hemorrhage. **C,** This more anterior image shows displacement of the portal vein (*arrows*), by the tumor mass. Areas of hemorrhage in the tumor (*open arrow*) are seen as focal high-intensity regions. The tumor is well separated from the liver.

adjacent high-signal-intensity renal tissue. Involvement of the adjacent vertebral or pelvic bone marrow also is often identified, thus helping to differentiate lymphoma from Wilms' tumor, which rarely metastasizes to bone marrow.

Rhabdomyosarcoma

Rhabdomyosarcoma is the most common tumor of the lower urinary tract in children and may arise from the bladder, urethra, or prostate.[93] It occurs more commonly in boys than in girls, and has peak incidences under 4 years of age and between 15 and 19 years of age.[105] Children with rhabdomyosarcoma present with urinary retention or, less commonly, hematuria. Bladder lesions most frequently arise in the submucosa of the trigone or bladder neck and then infiltrate the bladder wall. In girls, invasion of the vagina and uterus may occur.[106] Prostatic rhabdomyosarcoma tends to infiltrate the bladder neck, posterior urethra, and perirectal tissues early in its course, and tumor arising in this organ is more likely to metastasize distally.

Text continues on page 713.

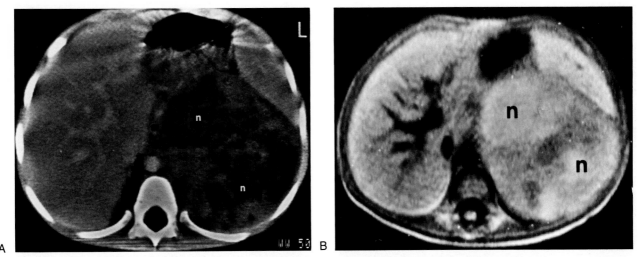

Figure 21–38. *Large left necrotic Wilms' tumor.* **A,** CT scan shows the large tumor mass. Most of the tumor is of very low intensity, consistent with necrosis. **B,** MR image (1000/60). The tumor mass is well seen. The areas of necrosis on the CT scan are seen as areas of very high intensity on the MR image. These necrotic areas are of greater intensity than the soft tissue components of the tumor. n, Necrosis.

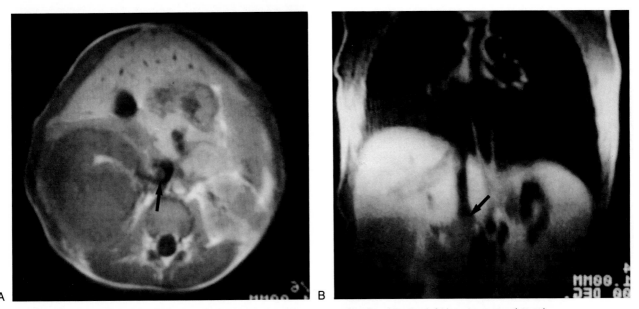

Figure 21–39. *Wilms' tumor of the right kidney with tumor thrombus extending into the inferior vena cava (arrow).* **A,** Axial (SE 500/28). **B,** Coronal (SE 500/28). The superior extent of the tumor thrombus within the inferior vena cava is seen in this plane (*arrow*).

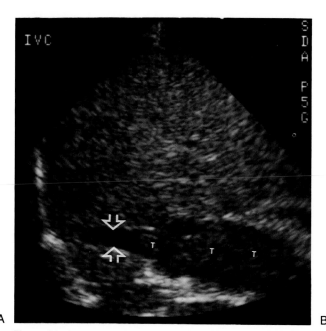

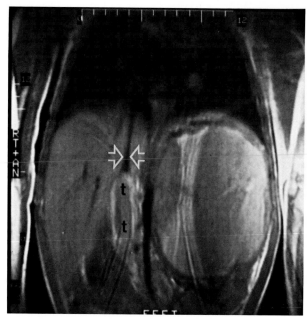

A   B

Figure 21–40. *Intracaval tumor. Good correlation between MRI and ultrasound.* ***A,*** Longitudinal ultrasound shows a large tumor (T) mass in the inferior vena cava. ***B,*** Coronal MRI (833/20) also shows the mass. The normal patent inferior vena cava above the tumor is indicated by arrows.

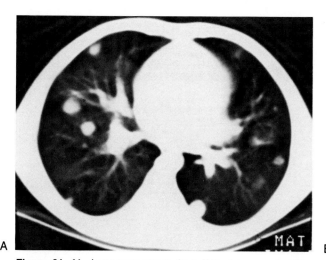

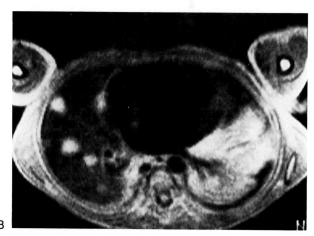

A   B

Figure 21–41. *Lung metastases from Wilms' tumor.* ***A,*** CT scan shows multiple metastases in both lung fields. ***B,*** Transverse spin-density image (2000/30). This is at a slightly different level from ***A.*** Multiple lung metastases are seen as well-defined high-intensity nodules against the background of low-intensity normal lung.

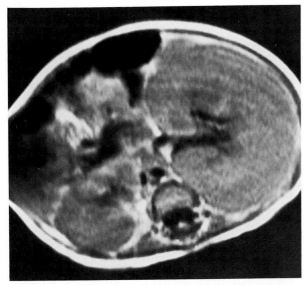

Figure 21–42. *Bilateral nephroblastomatosis.* Axial image (SE 500/28) shows loss of corticomedullary differentiation bilaterally. Although the left kidney is markedly enlarged, its collecting system is preserved.

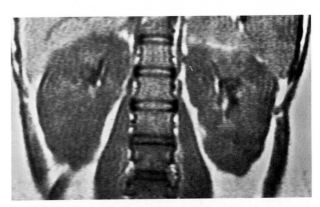

Figure 21–43. *Acute lymphoblastic leukemia.* Coronal (SE 500/28). The kidneys appear enlarged and lobular bilaterally with loss of corticomedullary differentiation. (From Dietrich RB, Kangarloo H. Kidneys in infants and children: evaluation with MR. Radiology 1986; 159:215–221; Dietrich RB, Kangarloo H. Pediatric body imaging. In: Stark DD, Bradley WG Jr., eds. Magnetic resonance imaging. St. Louis: CV Mosby, 1988:1434–1452.)

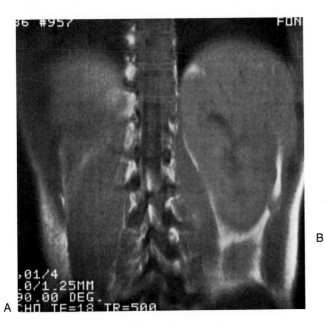

A

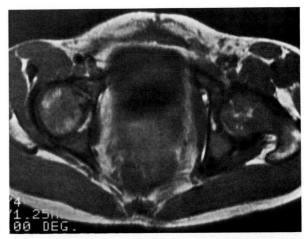

B

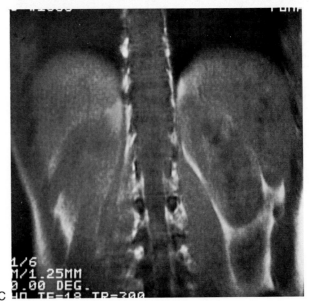

C

Figure 21–44. *Burkitt's lymphoma before and after chemotherapy.* **A,** Coronal (SE 500/18). Multiple masses are present within the left kidney, which also demonstrates loss of corticomedullary differentiation. **B,** Axial (SE 500/18). There is patchy replacement of the high-signal-intensity bone marrow by low-signal-intensity tumor cells. **C,** Coronal (SE 300/18). After chemotherapy the masses are reduced in size but corticomedullary differentiation is still absent.

The multiplanar capabilities of MRI are extremely useful in the evaluation of children with rhabdomyosarcoma (Figs. 21–46, 21–47). MRI can clearly demonstrate thickening of the bladder wall in patients with bladder neoplasms,[107–110] and use of the sagittal and coronal planes is particularly helpful for evaluation of the bladder base and demonstration of inferior, lateral, or posterior extension of tumors arising in this region. As with most neoplasms, the MR appearance of the lesion is nonspecific apart from the demonstration of a solid mass with medium signal intensity on T1 weighted images and high signal intensity on T2 weighted images (Fig. 21–48).[23] The signal intensity of pelvic rhabdomyosarcomas increases markedly on T1 weighted images after administration of intravenous gadolinium-DTPA (Fig. 21–47*B*).

The precise role of MRI as compared with CT has not yet been fully evaluated. MRI can identify the presence of a capsule surrounding a prostatic rhabdomyosarcoma and can also identify spread to local lymph nodes (Fig. 21–49). The multiplanar capabilities of MRI may make it useful for determining the full extent of a tumor mass and its relationship to adjacent structures. MRI may also prove useful in following the response of tumors to chemotherapy (Fig. 21–47*E,F*).

TRAUMA AND MECHANICAL DISORDERS

Hydronephrosis

In the pediatric age group, hydronephrosis may have many causes. It may be due to mechanical obstruction, secondary to reflux, or may be associated with a urinary tract infection. Frequent sites of obstruction include the ureteropelvic junction (usually from intrinsic causes) (Fig. 21–50), the lower ureter and ureterovesical junction (due to tumors, retrocaval ureters, intrinsic causes, megaureters, or ureteroceles), and the posterior urethra (due to valves and the prune-belly syndrome).

Dilatation of the collecting system is readily demonstrated by MRI in all patients with hydronephrosis.[111, 112] Once this has been seen, evaluation of T1 weighted coronal images will readily show the level of the obstruction, because on these sequences the signal intensity from the urine is low, and the dilated collecting system or ureter can easily be differentiated from adjacent structures (Fig. 21–51).

MRI can also demonstrate adjacent masses or aberrant vessels in patients in whom hydronephrosis occurs secondary to extrinsic compression. In cases of chronic obstruction, loss of corticomedullary differentiation and parenchymal atrophy are seen in the kidney proximal to the obstruction.[111]

Text continues on page 716.

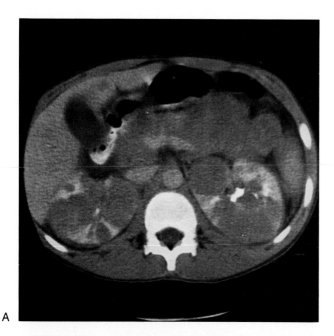

A

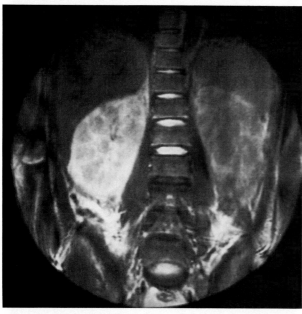

B

Figure 21–45. *Burkitt's lymphoma with extensive renal involvement in a 14-year-old patient.* ***A,*** CT scan, transverse image obtained after administration of intravenous contrast material. There is normal enhancement of residual functioning kidney tissue, but over 80 percent of the kidney remains of low intensity because of the presence of tumor. ***B,*** Coronal MR image (2000/70). There is loss of normal renal architecture and of corticomedullary differentiation. Residual normal kidney tissue shows very high signal intensity. The diffuse nodular tumor is of lower intensity. The margins between normal kidney and tumor are not as sharply defined as on the CT scan.

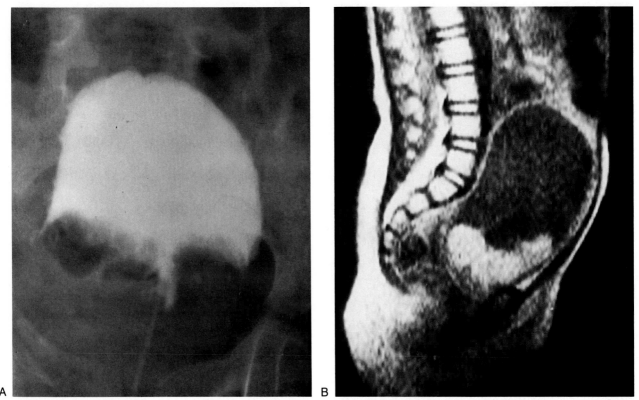

Figure 21–46. *Rhabdomyosarcoma.* ***A,*** Cystogram shows multiple irregular indentations of the bladder (B) base. The presence of a tumor can be inferred but its extent cannot be evaluated. ***B,*** Midline sagittal MR image (1000/60). The bladder (B) is distended. The large rhabdomyosarcoma (R) appears of strong intensity. It indents the bladder base. The entire extent of the tumor is well defined.

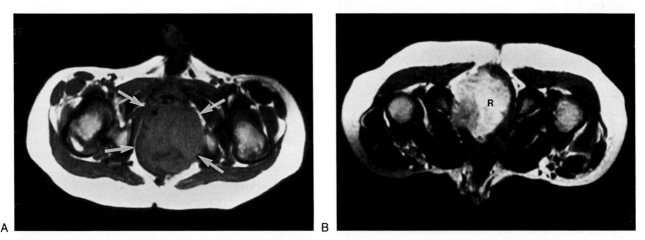

Figure 21–47. *Pelvic rhabdomyosarcoma in a 2-year-old boy who presented with a large perineal mass. The origin of the tumor is most likely in the prostate gland.* ***A, B,*** Transverse MR images (800/26). ***A*** shows a very large mass lesion (*arrows*) occupying most of the pelvic cavity. The mass is of slightly higher intensity than muscle. ***B*** is taken after injection of intravenous gadolinium-DTPA. Note the marked, slightly patchy enhancement of the rhabdomyosarcoma (R).

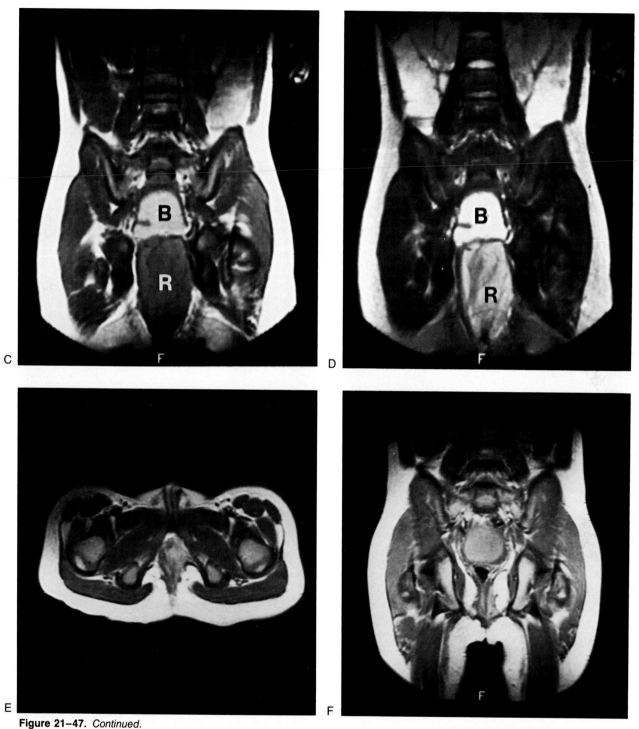

Figure 21–47. *Continued.*
C, D, Spin-density (2000/20) and T2 (2000/80) weighted images show the large, tubular-shaped rhabdomyosarcoma (R) lying inferior to the bladder (B). The base of the bladder is elevated by the tumor. *E, F,* Transverse T1 (900/26) and coronal spin-density (2050/30) weighted images obtained after 10 weeks of chemotherapy show almost complete resolution of the giant soft tissue tumor. A small amount of residual tumor is still identified, particularly on the left side (*arrow*).

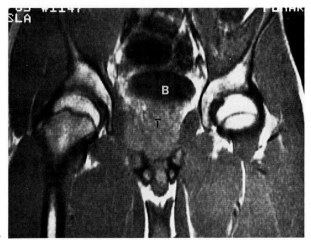

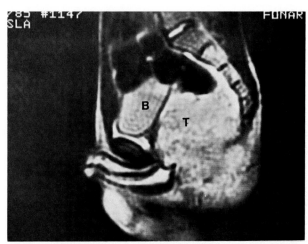

Figure 21–48. *Prostatic rhabdomyosarcoma.* ***A,*** Coronal (SE 500/28). A medium-signal-intensity tumor (T) elevates the bladder (B) and infiltrates the pelvic side wall. ***B,*** Sagittal (SE 2000/84). On T2 weighted sequence the tumor has high signal intensity and does not invade the bladder wall.

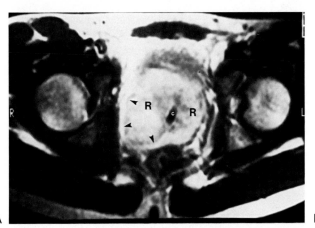

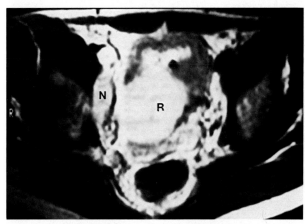

Figure 21–49. *Prostatic rhabdomyosarcoma with lymph node metastases in a 15-year-old boy.* ***A, B,*** Transverse T2 weighted images (1650/50). Most of the prostate is replaced by a large rhabdomyosarcoma (R). The central lucency is due to a catheter (c). The cavity tumor is encapsulated. The peripheral area of the prostate (*arrowheads*) is compressed but not involved with tumor. An enlarged metastatic lymph node (N) is well identified on the right side.

Renal Calculi

One of the limitations of MRI as an imaging modality of the genitourinary system is its frequent inability to demonstrate renal calculi. Fortunately, this is less of a problem in patients in the pediatric age group in whom the incidence of renal calculi is much lower than in adults.[113] Despite the introduction of many new techniques, excretory urography still remains the imaging modality of choice for the evaluation of stones. When renal calculi are seen by MRI, they appear as localized areas of signal void on both T1 and T2 weighted images. Since the urine within a dilated collecting system also demonstrates low signal intensity on T1 weighted images, calculi are particularly difficult to see on images obtained using these pulse sequences

(Fig. 21–52). On T2 weighted images, the presence of calculi may become more obvious if the low-signal-intensity stone is outlined by relatively higher-signal-intensity urine.

Renal Trauma

Blunt trauma to the abdomen and pelvis is a common problem in the pediatric age group, and in younger children the possibility of child abuse must always be considered. At the present time, x-ray CT is the tool of choice for evaluating children with suspected abdominal or pelvic trauma. It is able to demonstrate bony fractures, to show soft tissue injury, and to make a

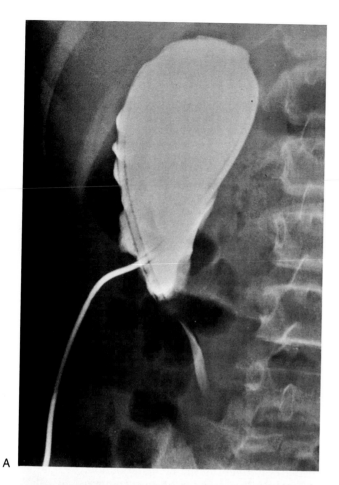

A

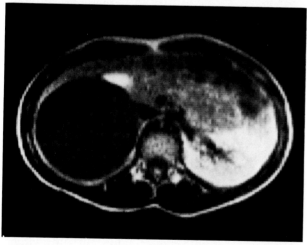

B

Figure 21–50. *Ureteropelvic junction obstruction.* ***A,*** Nephrosto-gram. There is marked dilatation of the renal pelvis (P). The ureter (*arrow*) is of normal caliber. The obstruction is at the level of the ureteropelvic junction. ***B,*** Transverse MR image (1000/60). The dilated renal pelvis (P) is seen as a large cystic mass. The calices are not well seen because they have been effaced by the pelvic distention. Note that a specific diagnosis cannot be made from the MR image.

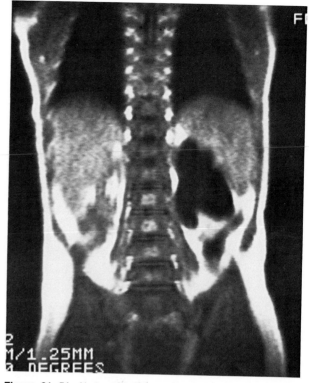

Figure 21–51. *Hydronephrosis: ureteropelvic junction obstruc-tion.* Coronal image (SE 500/28) shows dilatation of the left collect-ing system to the level of the proximal ureter.

specific diagnosis of acute hemorrhage if present.[114] At the same time, it can also evaluate renal function. In one series evaluating pediatric trauma, 12 percent of all intra-abdominal injuries involved the kidney.[115]

MRI is able to demonstrate some abnormalities due to trauma. In the perinephric region, hematoma may occur after trauma, surgery, percutaneous biopsy, or radiologic invasive procedures. Hematomas in the perirenal or pelvic areas, like those elsewhere in the body, frequently have characteristic appearances on MRI and can sometimes be easily differentiated from other fluid collections.[116–118] As a hematoma evolves over time, its MR appearance changes. Acute hema-tomas are isointense with muscle on T1 weighted se-quences, and clinically significant lesions may there-fore be missed on MR studies obtained immediately after surgery or trauma. By the end of the first week after development of a hematoma, inhomogeneous streaks may be present within it, or a fluid-fluid level may be identified if the supernatant fluid contained within it has a higher protein content, and thus shorter T1 and T2 values, than the dependent fluid. Subacute hematomas often demonstrate characteristically high signal intensity (Fig. 21–53) and may have an even more specific appearance, that of a concentric ring that may develop as early as 3 weeks after hemorrhage.[116] This sign is described on T1 weighted images and con-

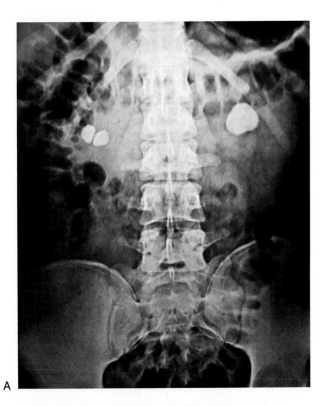

A

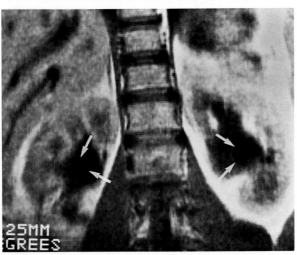

B

Figure 21–52. *Renal calculi.* **A,** Abdominal radiograph showing three renal calculi. **B,** Coronal (SE 500/28). The renal calculi (*arrows*) are extremely difficult to identify owing to obscuration by adjacent low-signal-intensity urine.

sists of two concentric rings surrounding a central core of intermediate signal intensity. The inner ring is bright and the outer rim dark on all pulse sequences. The paramagnetic susceptibility effects from insoluble hemosiderin digested by the phagocytic cells surrounding the hematoma are thought to account for the short T2 of the dark rim.[118]

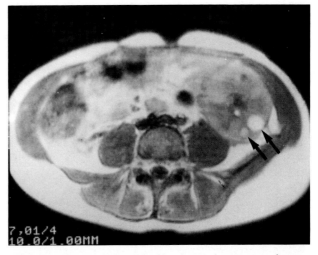

Figure 21–53. *Renal allograft with subacute hematomas after percutaneous biopsy.* Axial image (SE 500/28) shows two high-signal-intensity subacute hematomas (*arrows*) within the renal allograft.

VASCULAR DISORDERS

Renal Vein Thrombosis and Renal Infarction

Both renal artery occlusion and renal vein thrombosis may occur in the pediatric population and are particularly frequent in the neonatal period.[119–121] Renal vein thrombosis is by far the most common and usually results from hemoconcentration due to dehydration.[119] Other predisposing factors include hypercoagulable states and infants born to diabetic mothers.

Renal artery occlusion occurs less commonly but it too is often seen in conjunction with hemoconcentration. It may also occur secondarily to the development of thrombi around umbilical artery catheters.[121]

The MR appearances of the kidneys after experimental ligation of the renal arteries and veins of animals have been reported.[112, 122, 123] Although there is some conflict in the results presented by these authors, they do agree on the finding of prolongation of the T1 and T2 values of the cortex and outer medulla in both renal artery and renal vein ligation. In renal vein ligation the kidneys are described as appearing enlarged in size initially. No urine is seen in the collecting systems of the kidneys in both entities, consistent with nonfunction. After renal infarction, the kidneys become shrunken, and loss of corticomedullary differentiation is seen (Fig. 21–54).

Since rapidly flowing blood emits little or no signal, the blood vessels of children can be easily differentiated from the adjacent high-signal-intensity fat and medium-signal-intensity muscles, and appear as tubular structures with absent signal intensity.[5, 100] Signal within vessels may be due to the presence of thrombus

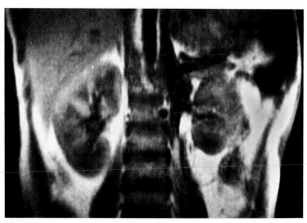

Figure 21–54. *Kidney following infarction.* Coronal (SE 500/28). The left kidney is much smaller than the right and there is absence of corticomedullary differentiation on this T1 weighted image.

within the lumen of a vessel or to slow flow of blood within the vessel. These two entities may be distinguished by observing the signal intensity of the problem area on the second-echo images. Slow flow shows an increase in signal intensity on the second or even echo (even-echo rephasing),[6] whereas thrombus decreases in intensity on the second-echo images.

Sickle Cell Disease

Sickle cell disease is one cause of renal failure in children that does not always have the same nonspecific appearance seen in most children with renal failure. Instead, patients with sickle cell nephropathy who have undergone chronic dialysis may demonstrate decreased signal intensity of the renal cortex compared with the medulla on T1 weighted images, and very low signal intensity of the cortex on T2 weighted images.[124] Although the low signal intensity of the cortex is probably due to hemosiderin deposition in the glomerular epithelium,[124] it is interesting to note that this does not occur in children with thalassemia major and other iron overload states, and so is not simply due to systemic iron overload.

Adrenal Hemorrhage

Adrenal hemorrhage in the perinatal period may be unilateral or bilateral.[125] Unilateral involvement is more frequently right-sided, reportedly accounting for 70 percent of lesions.[126] Affected children present with flank masses, jaundice, and anemia. Rarely, when bleeding is severe, hypotension and shock may occur.[127]

The MR appearances of adrenal hemorrhage[21] are similar to those of hematomas seen elsewhere in the body.[116,117] They present as high-signal-intensity masses totally replacing the adrenal parenchyma on both T1 and T2 weighted images (Fig. 21–55). The main differential diagnosis of adrenal hemorrhage is neuroblastoma presenting in the newborn period.[128–130] This disorder is also discussed in the chapter on the Reticuloendothelial and Endocrine Systems.

IATROGENIC DISORDERS: RENAL TRANSPLANTATION

The role of imaging in the evaluation of a renal transplant lies primarily in the detection and differentiation of complications. The abilities of both ultrasonography[131–136] and renal radionuclide scintigraphy[137–140] to demonstrate anatomic complications and detect functional abnormalities have been extensively evaluated in this regard in both adults and children. More recently, duplex ultrasonography has shown great promise in the early detection of graft rejection because of its ability to evaluate blood flow in transplant kidneys.[141–145]

The imaging of renal transplants by MRI has also been evaluated.[146–152] The appearance of the normal renal allograft is the same as that of a normal kidney. In patients who develop cyclosporine toxicity, the appearance of the renal transplant is unchanged on MR images. By contrast, in acute allograft rejection, swelling of the kidney develops and there is loss of corticomedullary differentiation.[140] The intralobar vessels are frequently less apparent than normal and can no

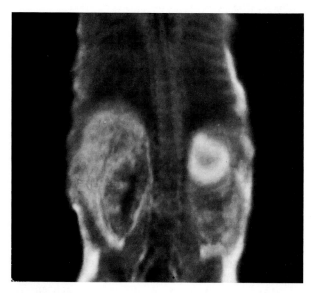

Figure 21–55. *Adrenal hemorrhage.* Coronal image (SE 500/28) shows high-signal-intensity hemorrhage within the left adrenal gland. (From Dietrich RB, Kangarloo H. Pediatric body imaging. In: Stark DD, Bradley WG Jr., eds. Magnetic resonance imaging. St. Louis: CV Mosby, 1988:1434–1452.)

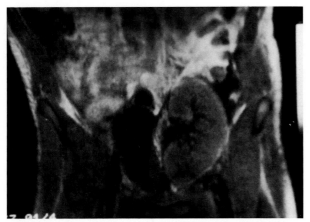

Figure 21–56. *Allograft in early rejection.* Coronal image (SE 500/28) shows loss of corticomedullary differentiation and decreased peri sinus fat. The renal parenchymal vessels cannot be identified peripherally.

longer be identified peripherally (Fig. 21–56).[148] Unfortunately, the kidneys of patients with acute tubular necrosis do not have a specific appearance on MRI but demonstrate a spectrum of different findings. They may appear normal or have a similar appearance to that of kidneys undergoing rejection.

MRI can also demonstrate other complications in transplant patients, such as the presence of hydronephrosis and perinephric fluid collections such as urinomas, lymphoceles, and hematomas.

REFERENCES

1. Moon KL Jr, Hricak H. NMR imaging of the urinary tract. Appl Radiol 1984; January/February:21–30.
2. Hricak H, Crooks L, Sheldon P, Kaufman L. Nuclear magnetic resonance imaging of the kidney. Radiology 1983; 146:425–432.
3. Leung AWL, Bydder GM, Steiner RE, et al. Magnetic resonance imaging of the kidneys. AJR 1984; 143:1215–1227.
4. Dietrich RB, Kangarloo H. Kidneys in infants and children: evaluation with MR. Radiology 1986; 159:215–221.
5. Glazer GM. MR imaging of the liver, kidneys, and adrenal glands. Radiology 1988; 166:303–312.
6. Bradley WG, Waluch V. Blood flow: magnetic resonance imaging. Radiology 1985; 154:443–450.
7. Demas BE, Stafford SA, Hricak H. Kidneys. In: Stark DD, Bradley WG Jr, eds. Magnetic resonance imaging. St Louis: CV Mosby, 1988:1187–1232.
8. Soila KP, Viamonte M, Starewicz PM. Chemical shift misregistration effect in magnetic resonance imaging. Radiology 1984; 153:819–820.
9. Kikinis R, von Schulthess GK, Jager P, et al. Normal and hydronephrotic kidney: evaluation of renal function with contrast-enhanced MR imaging. Radiology 1987; 165:837–842.
10. Bryan PJ, Butler HE, LiPuma IP, et al. NMR scanning of the pelvis: initial experience with a 0.3T system. AJR 1983; 141:1111–1118.
11. Fisher MR, Hricak H, Crooks LE. Urinary bladder MR imaging. Part 1. Normal and benign conditions. Radiology 1985; 157:467–470.
12. Hricak H, Williams RD, Spring DB, et al. Anatomy and pathology of the male pelvis by magnetic resonance imaging. AJR 1983; 141:1101–1110.
13. Heiken IP, Lee JKT. MR imaging of the pelvis. Radiology 1988; 166:11–16.
14. McCarthy S, Fritzsche PJ. Male pelvis. In: Stark DD, Bradley WG Jr, eds. Magnetic resonance imaging. St Louis: CV Mosby, 1988:1233–1264.
15. Hricak H, Dooms GC, McNeal JE, et al. MR imaging of the prostate gland: normal anatomy. AJR 1987; 148:51–58.
16. Lee IKT, Rholl KS. MRI of the bladder and prostate. AJR 1986; 147:732–736.
17. Bryan PJ, Butler HE, Nelson AD, et al. Magnetic resonance imaging of the prostate. AJR 1986; 146:543–548.
18. Phillips ME, Kressel HY, Spritzer CE, et al. Normal prostate and adjacent structures: MR imaging at 1.5T. Radiology 1987; 164:381–385.
19. Hricak H, Marotti M, Gilbert TJ, et al. Normal penile anatomy and abnormal penile conditions: evaluation with MR imaging. Radiology 1988; 169:683–690.
20. Hricak H, Alpers C, Crooks LE, Sheldon PE. Magnetic resonance imaging of the female pelvis: initial experience. AJR 1983; 141:1119–1128.
21. Hricak H. MRI of the female pelvis: a review. AJR 1986; 146:1115–1122.
22. Dietrich RB, Kangarloo H. Pelvic abnormalities in children: assessment with MR imaging. Radiology 1987; 163:367–372.
23. Dietrich RB, Kangarloo H. Pediatric body imaging. In: Stark DD, Bradley WG Jr, eds. Magnetic resonance imaging. St Louis: CV Mosby, 1988:1434–1452.
24. Demas BE, Hricak H, Jaffe RB. Uterine MR imaging: effects of hormonal stimulation. Radiology 1986; 159:123–126.
25. Haynor DR, Mack LA, Soules MR, et al. Changing appearance of the normal uterus during the menstrual cycle: MR studies. Radiology 1986; 161:459–462.
26. McCarthy S, Tauber C, Gore J. Female pelvic anatomy: MR assessment of variations during the menstrual cycle and with use of oral contraceptives. Radiology 1986; 160:119–123.
27. Lee JKT, Gersell DJ, Balfe DM, et al. The uterus: in vitro MR-anatomic correlation of normal and abnormal specimens. Radiology 1985; 157:175–179.
28. Hricak H, Chang YCF, Thurnher S. Vagina: evaluation with MR imaging. Part I. Normal anatomy and congenital anomalies. Radiology 1988; 169:169–174.
29. Dooms GC, Hricak H, Tscholakoff D. Adnexal structures: MR imaging. Radiology 1986; 158:639–646.
30. Sample WF, Lippe BM, Gyepes MT. Gray-scale ultrasonography of the normal female pelvis. Radiology 1977; 125:477–483.
31. Demas B, Thurnher S, Hricak H. The kidney, adrenal gland and retroperitoneum. In: Higgins CB, Hricak H, eds. Magnetic resonance imaging of the body. New York: Raven Press, 1987:373–401.
32. Osathanondh V, Potter EL. Pathogenesis of polycystic kidneys. Arch Pathol 1964; 77:459–512.
33. Grossman H, Rosenberg ER, Bowie JD, et al. Sonographic diagnosis of renal cystic disease. AJR 1983; 140:81–85.
34. Hayden CK, Swischuk LE. The urinary tract. In: Hayden CK, Swischuk LE, eds. Pediatric ultrasonography. Baltimore: Williams & Wilkins, 1987:263–345.
35. Kulkarni MV, Shaff MI, Sandler MP, et al. Evaluation of renal masses by MR imaging. J Comput Assist Tomogr 1984; 8:861–865.
36. Kier R, McCarthy S, Rosenfield N, et al. Undescended testes: evaluation with high field MR imaging. Proceedings of the 5th annual meeting of the Society for Magnetic Resonance Imaging, 1988:61.
37. Kleinteich B, Hadziselimovic F, Hesse V, et al. In: Kongenitale Hodendystopien. Stuttgart: Georg Thieme, 1979.
38. Hricak H, Crooks LE, Sheldon P, Kaufman L. Nuclear magnetic resonance imaging of the kidney. Radiology 1983; 146:425–432.
39. Choyke PL, Kressel NY, Pollack NM, et al. Focal renal masses: magnetic resonance imaging. Radiology 1984; 152:471–477.
40. Marotti M, Hricak N, Fritzche P, et al. Complex and simple

renal cysts: comparative evaluation with MR imaging. Radiology 1987; 162:679–684.

41. Hilpert PL, Friedman AC, Radecki PD, et al. MRI of hemorrhagic renal cysts in polycystic kidney disease. AJR 1986; 146:1167–1172.

42. Lieberman E, Salinas-Madrigal L, Gwinn JL, et al. Infantile polycystic disease of the kidneys and liver: clinical, pathological and radiological correlations and comparison with congenital hepatic fibrosis. Medicine 1971:50:277–281.

43. Glassberg KI, Filmer RB. Renal dysplasia, renal hypoplasia, and cystic disease of the kidney. In: Kelalis PP, King LR, Belman AB, eds. Clinical pediatric urology, 2nd ed. Philadelphia: WB Saunders, 1985:922–971.

44. Hayden CK, Swischuk LE, Smith TN, Armstrong EA. Renal cystic disease in childhood. Radiographics 1986; 6:97–116.

45. Kissane JM. Polycystic disease. In: Kissane JM, ed. Pathology of infancy and childhood, 2nd ed. St Louis: CV Mosby, 1975:586–596.

46. Fellows RA, Leonidas JC, Beatty EC. Radiologic features of "adult type" polycystic disease in the neonate. Pediatr Radiol 1976; 4:87–92.

47. Griscom NT, Vawter FG, Fellers FX. Pelvoinfundibular atresia: the usual form of multicystic kidney; 44 unilateral and two bilateral cases. Semin Roentgenol 1975; 10:125.

48. Beck AD: The effect of intraurinary obstruction on the development of fetal kidney. J Urol 1971; 105:784–789.

49. Felson B, Cussen LJ. The hydronephrotic type of congenital multicystic disease of the kidney. Semin Roentgenol 1975; 10:113–123.

50. Deweerd JH, Simon HB. Simple cysts in children: review of the literature and report of five cases. J Urol 1956; 75:912.

51. Gordon RL, Pollack NM, Popky GL, et al. Simple serous cysts of the kidney in children. Radiology 1979; 131:357.

52. Siegel MJ, McAlister WN. Simple renal cysts in children. J Urol 1980; 123:75.

53. Kissane IM. Congenital malformations. In: Nepinstall RH, ed. Pathology of the kidney. Boston: Little, Brown, 1974:69–119.

54. Banner MP, Pollack NM, Chatten J, Witzleben C. Multilocular renal cysts: radiologic-pathologic correlation. AJR 1981; 136:239–247.

55. Jones DN, Risdon RA, Hayden K, et al. Juvenile nephronophthisis; clinical, radiological and pathologic correlationships. Pediatr Radiol 1973; 1:164–171.

56. Patriquin HB, O'Regan S. Medullary sponge kidney in childhood. AJR 1985; 145:315–319.

57. Mitnick JS, Bosniak MA, Hilton S, et al. Cystic renal disease in tuberous sclerosis. Radiology 1983; 147:85–87.

58. Sato Y, Waziri M, Smith W, et al. Hippel-Lindau disease: MR imaging. Radiology 1988; 166:241–246.

59. Bauer SB. Urodynamic evaluation and neuromuscular dysfunction. In: Kelalis PP, King LR, Belman AB, eds. Clinical pediatric urology, 2nd ed. Philadelphia: WB Saunders, 1985:283–310.

60. Duckett JW, Caldamone AA. Anomalies of the urinary tract: bladder and urachus. In: Kelalis PP, King LR, Belman AB, eds. Clinical pediatric urology, 2nd ed. Philadelphia: WB Saunders, 1985:726–750.

61. Berdon WE, Baker DH, Wigger HJ, Blanc WA. The radiographic and pathologic spectrum of the prune belly syndrome; the importance of urethral obstruction in prognosis. Radiol Clin North Am 1977; 1:83–92.

62. Garris J, Kangarloo H, Sarti D, et al. The ultrasound spectrum of prune-belly syndromes. JCU 1980; 8:117–120.

63. Hricak H, Chun-Fang Chang Y. The female pelvis. In: Higgins CB, Hricak H, eds. Magnetic resonance imaging of the body. New York: Raven Press, 1987:403–431.

64. Cohen MM, Nadler HL. Prenatal disturbances: the sex chromosomes. In: Behrman RE, Vaughan III VC, eds. Nelson textbook of pediatrics, 12th ed. Philadelphia: WB Saunders, 1983:305–311.

65. Shawker TH, Garra BS, Loriaux DL, et al. Ultrasound of Turner's syndrome. J Ultrasound Med 1986; 5:125–130.

66. Dietrich RB, Kangarloo H, Lippe BM, Boechat MI. Role of ultrasonography and magnetic resonance imaging of the Turner syndrome. Proceedings of the 71st scientific assembly and annual meeting of the Radiological Society of North America, 1985:40.

67. Lippe B, Mitchell E, Geffner MD, et al. Renal malformations in patients with Turner syndrome: imaging in 141 patients. Pediatrics 1988; 82:852–856.

68. Allen TD. Disorders of sex differentiation. In: Kelalis PP, King LR, Belman AB, eds. Clinical pediatric urology, 2nd ed. Philadelphia: WB Saunders, 1985:904–921.

69. Togashi K, Nishimura K, Itoh K, et al. Vaginal agenesis: classification by MR imaging. Radiology 1987; 162:675–677.

70. Dewhurst CJ. Congenital malformations of the genital tract in childhood. J Obstet Gynaecol Br Comm 1968; 75:377.

71. Mintz MC, Thickman DI, Gussman D, Kressel HY. MR evaluation of uterine anomalies. AJR 1987; 148:287–290.

72. Wiersma AF, Peterson LF, Justema EJ. Uterine anomalies associated with unilateral renal agenesis. Obstet Gynecol 1976; 47:654–657.

73. Barach B, Falces E, Benzian SR. Magnetic resonance imaging for diagnosis and preoperative planning in agenesis of the distal vagina. Ann Plastic Surg 1987; 19:192–194.

74. Fore SR, Hammond CB, Parker RT, Anderson EE. Urologic and genital anomalies in patients with congenital absence of the vagina. Am J Obstet Gynecol 1975; 46:410–416.

75. Rosenberg HK, Sherman NH, Tarry WF, et al. Mayer-Rokitansky-Küster-Hauser syndrome: US aid to diagnosis. Radiology 1986; 161:815–819.

76. Vainright JR Jr, Fulp CJ, Schiebler ML. MR imaging of vaginal agenesis with hematocolpos. J Comput Assist Tomogr 1988; 12:891–893.

77. Thurnher S, Hricak H, Tanagho EA. Müllerian duct cyst: diagnosis with MR imaging. Radiology 1988; 168:25–28.

78. Vinstein AL, Franken EA. Unilateral hematocolpos associated with agenesis of the kidney. Radiology 1972; 102:625–628.

79. Fritzsche PJ, Hricak H, Kogan BA, et al. Undescended testis: value of MR imaging. Radiology 1987; 164:169–173.

80. Kangarloo N, Gold RH, Fine RN, et al. Urinary tract infection in infants and children evaluated by ultrasound. Radiology 1985; 154:367–373.

81. Leonidas JC, McCauley RGK, Klauber GC, Fretzayas AM. Sonography as a substitute for excretory urography in children with urinary tract infection. AJR 1985; 144:815–819.

82. Hayden CK Jr, Swischuk LE, Fawcett ND, et al. Urinary tract infections in childhood: a current imaging approach. Radiographics 1986; 6:1023–1028.

83. Mason WG Jr. Urinary tract infections in children: renal ultrasound evaluation. Radiology 1984; 153:109–112.

84. Ben-Ami T: Sonographic evaluation of urinary tract infections in children. Semin Ultrasound 1984; 5:19–34.

85. Handmaker H. Nuclear renal imaging in acute pyelonephritis. Semin Nucl Med 1982; 12:246–253.

86. Nasrallah PF, Nara S, Crawford J. Clinical applications of nuclear cystography. J Urol 1982; 128:550–553.

87. Wall SD, Fisher MR, Amparo EG, et al. Magnetic resonance imaging in the evaluation of abscesses. AJR 1985; 144:1217.

88. Brown JJ, van Sonnenberg E, Gerber KH et al. Magnetic resonance relaxation times of percutaneously obtained normal and abnormal body fluids. Radiology 1985; 154:727–731.

89. Terrier F, Revel D, Pajannen H, et al. MR imaging of body fluid collections. J Comput Assist Tomogr 1986; 10:953–962.

90. Strickler GB. Renal parenchymal disease. In: Kelalis PP, King LR, Belman AB, eds. Clinical pediatric urology, 2nd ed. Philadelphia: WB Saunders, 1985:972–991.

91. Marotti M, Hricak H, Terrier F, et al. MR in renal disease: importance of cortical-medullary distinction. Magn Reson Med 1987; 5:160–172.

92. Leichter HE, Dietrich RB, Salusky IB, et al. Acquired cystic kidney disease in children undergoing long-term dialysis. Pediatr Nephrol 1988; 2:8–11.

93. Young JL, Miller RW. Incidence of malignant tumors in U.S. children. J Pediatr 1975; 86:254.

94. Belasco JB, Chatten J, D'Angio GJ. Wilms' tumor. In: Sutpow W, Fernbach D, Vietti T, eds. Clinical pediatric oncology, 3rd ed. St Louis: CV Mosby, 1984.

95. D'Angio GI, Duckett IW Jr, Belasco JB. Tumors: upper urinary tract. In: Kelalis PP, King LR, Belman AB, eds. Clinical pediatric urology, 2nd ed. Philadelphia: WB Saunders, 1985:1157–1189.

96. Miller RW, Fraumeni JF, Manning MD. Association of Wilms' tumor with aniridia, hemihypertrophy, and other congenital malformations. N Engl J Med 1964; 270:922.

97. Sotelo-Avila C, Gonzalez-Crussi DF, Fowler JW. Complete and incomplete forms of Beckwith-Wiedemann syndrome. Their oncogenic potential. J Pediatr 1980; 96:47.

98. Belt TG, Cohen MD, Smith JA, et al. MRI of Wilms' tumor: promise as the primary imaging method. AJR 1986; 146:955–961.

99. Kangarloo H, Dietrich RB, Ehrlich RM, et al. Magnetic resonance imaging of Wilms' tumor. Urology 1986; 28:203–207.

100. Cohen MD, Smith JA, Cory DA, et al. Visualization of major blood vessels by magnetic resonance imaging in children with malignant tumors. Radiographics 1985; 5:441–457.

101. Bar-Ziv J, Hirsch M, Perlman M. Bilateral nephroblastomatosis. Pediatr Radiol 1975; 3:85–88.

102. Franken EA Jr, Yiu-Chiu V, Smith WL, Chiu LC. Nephroblastomatosis: clinicopathologic significance and imaging characteristics. AJR 1982; 138:950–952.

103. Gore RM, Shnolik A. Abdominal manifestation of pediatric leukemias: sonographic assessment. Radiology 1982; 143:207–210.

104. Hartman DS, Davis CJ, Goldman SM, et al. Renal lymphoma: radiologic-pathologic correlation of 21 cases. Radiology 1982; 144:759–766.

105. Timmons JW Jr, Burgert EO Jr, Soule EH, et al. Embryonal rhabdomyosarcoma of the bladder and prostate in childhood. J Urol 1975; 113:694.

106. Hays DM. Pelvic rhabdomyosarcomas in childhood: diagnosis and concepts of management reviewed. Cancer 1980; 45:1810–1814.

107. Fisher MR, Hricak H, Tanagho EA. Urinary bladder MR imaging. Radiology 1985; 157:471–477.

108. Rholl KS, Lee JKT, Heiken JP, et al. Primary bladder carcinoma: evaluation with MR imaging. Radiology 1987; 163:117–121.

109. Buy JN, Moss AA, Guinet C, et al. MR staging of bladder carcinoma: correlation with pathologic findings. Radiology 1988; 169:695–700.

110. Barentsz JP, Lemmens JAM, Ruijs SHJ, et al. Carcinoma of the urinary bladder: MR imaging with a double surface coil. AJR 1988; 151:107–112.

111. Thickman D, Kundel H, Biery D. Magnetic resonance evaluation of hydronephrosis in the dog. Radiology 1984; 152:113–116.

112. London DA, Davis PL, Williams RD, et al. Nuclear magnetic resonance imaging of induced renal lesions. Radiology 1983; 148:167–172.

113. Walther PC, Lamm D, Kaplan GW. Pediatric urolithiasis: a 10-year review. Pediatrics 1980; 65:1068–1072.

114. Berger PE, Kuhn JP. CT of blunt abdominal trauma in childhood. AJR 1984; 142:449–460.

115. Kaufman RA, Towbin R, Babcock DS, et al. Upper abdominal trauma in children: imaging evaluation. AJR 1984; 142:499–460.

116. Hahn PF, Saini S, Stark DD, et al. Intraabdominal hematoma: the concentric-ring sign in MR imaging. AJR 1987; 148:115–119.

117. Unger EC, Glazer HS, Lee JKT, Ling D. MRI of extracranial hematomas: preliminary observations. AJR 1986; 146:403–407.

118. Gomori JM, Grossman RI, Goldberg HI, et al. Intracranial hematomas imaging by high field MR. Radiology 1985; 157:87–93.

119. Belman AB, King LR. The pathology and treatment of renal vein thrombosis in the newborn. J Urol 1972; 107:852.

120. Jobin J, O'Regan S, Demay G, et al. Neonatal renal vein thrombosis. Clin Nephrol 1982; 17:36.

121. Duarante D, Jones D, Spitzer R. Neonatal renal arterial embolism syndrome. J Pediatr 1978; 89:978.

122. Yuasa Y, Kundel HL. Magnetic resonance imaging following unilateral occlusion of the renal circulation in rabbits. Radiology 1985; 154:151–156.

123. Newhouse JN, Brady TJ, Goldman MR, et al. Proton NMR imaging of acute renal vein occlusion. Proceedings of the 1st annual meeting of the Society of Magnetic Resonance in Medicine, 1982.

124. Lande IM, Glazer GM, Sarnaik S, et al. Sickle-cell nephropathy: MR imaging. Radiology 1986; 158:379–383.

125. Snelling EC, Erb IH. Hemorrhage and subsequent calcification of the suprarenal. J Pediatr 1935; 6:22.

126. Johnston JH. Vascular lesions of the adrenal and kidney. In: Rickham PP, Lister J, Irving IM, eds. Neonatal surgery. 2nd ed. St. Paul, MN: Butterworth, 1978:567–575.

127. De Sa DJ, Nicholls S. Haemorrhagic necrosis of the adrenal gland in perinatal infants: a clinicopathological study. J Pathol 1972; 106:133.

128. Cohen MD, Weetman R, Provisor A, et al. Magnetic resonance imaging of neuroblastoma with a 0.15-T magnet. AJR 1984; 143:1241–1248.

129. Schultz CL, Haaga JR, Fletcher BD, et al. Magnetic resonance imaging of the adrenal glands: a comparison with computed tomography. AJR 1984; 143:1235–1240.

130. Dietrich RB, Kangarloo H, Lenarsky C, Feig SA. Neuroblastoma: the role of MR imaging. AJR 1987; 148:937–942.

131. Hricak H, Cruz C, Eyler WR, et al. Acute post-transplantation renal failure: differential diagnosis by ultrasound. Radiology 1981; 139:441–449.

132. Hricak H, Romanski RN, Eyler WR. The renal sinus during allograft rejection: sonographic and histopathologic findings. Radiology 1982; 142:693–699.

133. Fried AM, Woodring JH, Loh FK, et al. The medullary pyramid index: an objective assessment of prominence in renal transplant rejection. Radiology 1983; 149:787–791.

134. Hoddick W, Filly RA, Backman U, et al. Renal allograft rejection: US evaluation. Radiology 1986; 161:469–473.

135. Slovis TL, Babcock DS, Hricak H, et al. Renal transplant rejection: sonographic evaluation in children. Radiology 1984; 153:659–665.

136. Babcock DS, Slovis TL, Han BK, et al. Renal transplants in children: long-term follow-up using sonography. Radiology 1985; 156:165–167.

137. Kim EE, Pjura G, Lowry P, et al. Cyclosporin-A nephrotoxicity and acute cellular rejection in renal transplant recipients: correlation between radionuclide and histologic findings. Radiology 1986; 159:443–446.

138. George EA. Radionuclide diagnosis of allograft rejection. Semin Nucl Med 1982; 12:379–386.

139. Kirschner PT, Rosenthall L. Renal transplant evaluation. Semin Nucl Med 1982; 12:370–378.

140. Singh A, Cohen WN. Renal allograft rejection: sonography and scintigraphy. AJR 1980; 135:73–77.

141. Berland LL, Lawson TL, Adams MB, et al. Evaluation of transplants with pulsed Doppler duplex sonography. J Ultrasound Med 1982; 1:215–222.

142. Rigsby CM, Taylor KJW, Weltin G, et al. Renal allografts in acute rejection: evaluation using duplex sonography. Radiology 1986; 158:375–378.

143. Needleman L, Kurtz AB. Doppler evaluation of the renal transplant. JCU 1987; 15:661.

144. Rifkin MD, Needleman L, Pasto ME, et al. Evaluation of renal transplant rejection by duplex Doppler examination. AJR 1987; 148:759–762.

145. Allen KS, Jorkasky DK, Arger PH, et al. Renal allografts: prospective analysis of Doppler sonography. Radiology 1988; 169:371–376.

146. Hricak H, Terrier F, Demas BE. Renal allografts: evaluation by MR imaging. Radiology 1986; 159:435–441.

147. Geisinger MA, Risius B, Jordan ML, et al. Magnetic resonance imaging of renal transplants. AJR 1984; 143:1229–1234.

148. Baumgartner BR, Nelson RC, Ball TI, et al. MR imaging of renal transplants. AJR 1986; 147:949–953.

149. Winsett MZ, Amparo EG, Fawcett HD, et al. Renal transplant dysfunction: MR evaluation. AJR 1988; 150:319–323.

150. Goldsmith MS, Tanasescu DE, Waxman AD, et al. Comparison of magnetic imaging and radionuclide imaging in the evaluation of renal transplant failure. Clin Nucl Med 1988; 13:250–254.

151. Yap HK, Dietrich RB, Kangarloo H, et al. Acute renal allograft rejection. Transplantation 1986; 43:249–252.

152. Steinberg HV, Nelson RC, Murphy FB, et al. Renal allograft rejection: evaluation by Doppler US and MR imaging. Radiology 1987; 162:337–342.

Reticuloendothelial and Endocrine Systems

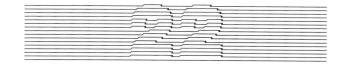

MERVYN D. COHEN, M.B., Ch.B.

NORMAL ANATOMY*

Lymph Nodes

Normal lymph nodes (Fig. 22–1) are seen on MR images as relatively round structures with variable signal intensity on T1 and T2 weighted images. The intensity on T1 weighted images is usually a little less than, equal to, or greater than muscle. There generally is only a small increase in signal intensity on T2, compared with T1, weighted images. Since many lymph nodes are very small, they may not be well visualized on MRI. Visualization is improved if the nodes are surrounded by fat (subcutaneous nodes, retroperitoneal nodes) or by flowing blood and air (mediastinum). The internal structure of lymph nodes is not resolved on MRI.

Ovary

The ovaries are oval, almond-shaped glands with a maximal dimension after puberty of about $3 \times 1.5 \times 1$ cm. In younger prepubertal children they are proportionately smaller. Before puberty the surface of the ovary is smooth; after puberty the surface becomes progressively more irregular as successive corpora lutea degenerate. On MRI the ovaries are best seen on transverse or coronal images. On T1 weighted images they appear homogeneous,[1] with a low to medium signal intensity often similar to that of muscle. On T2 weighted images, particularly at high field strength, the ovary is no longer homogeneous. The stroma increases in signal intensity to about that of fat, while follicles may have a signal intensity even greater than that of fat.[1,2]

Testes

The testes are ovoid structures, usually in the scrotum, but occasionally malpositioned when there is failure of normal descent. The average size after puberty is 3.5×2.5 cm. The testes are extremely well visualized on MRI.[3] Most of the testis is of homogeneous intensity on all pulse sequences. A low-intensity band may be seen at the hilum (mediastinum) of the testis, which is the site of exit of the seminiferous tubules. On T1 weighted images the testes are of medium signal intensity, often greater than that of muscle. On T2 weighted pulse sequences the testes have a very strong signal intensity, usually greater than that of fat (Fig. 22–2). The outer wall of the testis is a thick connective tissue coat called the tunica albuginea. Because of its high collagen content the tunica appears as a low-intensity rim, surrounding most of the testis, on

---

*The pituitary gland is included in the section on the Central Nervous System, and the liver and spleen are covered in detail in the chapter on the Gastrointestinal System.

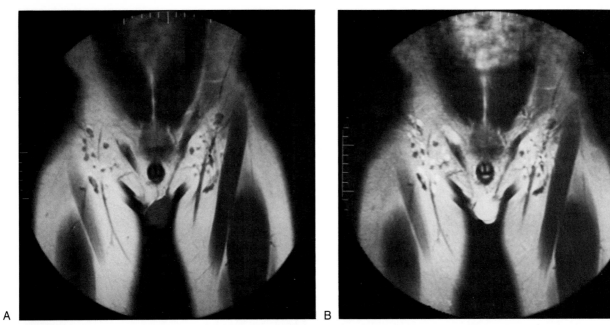

A   B

Figure 22–1. *Normal lymph nodes.* **A, B,** Coronal T1 (800/20) and T2 (2000/80) images through the groin show multiple small lymph nodes lying within the subcutaneous fat. The lymph nodes show little change in signal intensity from T1 to T2 weighting.

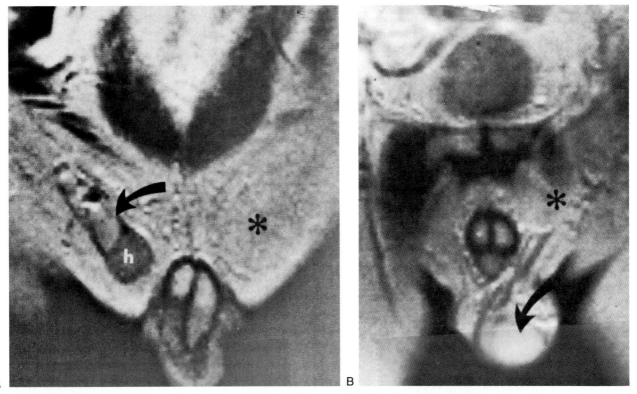

A   B

Figure 22–2. *Undescended testis with atrophy.* **A,** Coronal MR image (2000/60). The right testis (*curved arrow*) is undescended and lies in the inguinal canal. There is a small adjacent hydrocele (h). The testis is very small. Signal intensity from the testis is the same as that of fat (*) but less than normal testis. **B,** Image slightly posterior to **A.** It is the same pulse sequence (2000/60). The left testis (*curved arrow*) is normal and lies in the scrotum. The signal intensity from this testis is greater than that of fat (*). (From Fritzsche PJ, Hricak H, Kogan BA, et al. Undescended testes: value of MR imaging. Radiology 1987; 164:169–173.)

all pulse sequences. Immediately superficial to the tunica albuginea are the layers of the tunica vaginalis, which is a double-layered extension of the peritoneal cavity surrounding most of the testis. There is a very small amount of fluid between the two layers of the tunica vaginalis, and this may be seen as a thin, high-intensity line on T2 weighted images. The epididymis lies posterolateral to the testis with the head lying superiorly. The epididymis stores sperm and is continuous with the ductus deferens. The epididymis is well identified and may be of similar intensity to the testes on T1 weighted images, but is of lower intensity than the testes on T2 weighted images. It is usually possible to separate the head, body, and tail of the epididymis. The spermatic cord is surrounded by a plexus of veins, and slow flow through these veins may produce a strong signal on T2 weighted images.

Adrenal Glands

The adrenal glands lie in the retroperitoneum enclosed, with the kidneys, within the renal fascia.[4,5] Both glands are flattened anteroposteriorly. They vary in size, being about one-third of the size of the kidney at birth and one-thirteenth of renal size in adulthood. The gland grows little during childhood. The right adrenal gland is pyramidal in shape with two limbs; the apex lies superiorly. The gland lies predominantly superior to the right kidney, behind the inferior vena cava, and lateral to the spine. It is inferior to the undersurface of the liver. The left gland is more crescentic in shape, its concavity being adapted to the medial border of the superior pole of the left kidney. It lies lateral to the spine and behind the stomach and pancreas. The adrenal glands are frequently surrounded by fat, which assists their identification on T1 MR images.

On T1 weighted images the adrenal glands are of similar intensity to, or slightly lower intensity than, that of liver. There is a mild increase in signal intensity on T2 weighted images but the glands always remain of lower signal than adjacent fat. It usually is not possible to differentiate the adrenal cortex from the adrenal medulla. On occasion, chemical shift artifact can cause an appearance that mimics the differentiation of cortex and medulla.

Thyroid Gland

The thyroid gland consists of right and left lobes that lie on either side of the trachea, connected by an isthmus that passes in front of the trachea. The size of the thyroid gland is variable. The normal thyroid gland has T1 and T2 relaxation times longer than those of normal muscle.[6] Because of the long T2 relaxation time, thyroid is well seen on T2 weighted images.[7] The appearance of the normal thyroid does not change with a change in the status of thyroid function.[8]

Parathyroid Glands

Parathyroid glands arise from the third and fourth brachial pouches. There are usually four glands but the number can vary between two and six, usually arranged in pairs. The superior pair is the most constant in location and is situated behind the middle of the posterior surface of the lobes of the thyroid gland. The inferior parathyroid glands usually lie close to the inferior surface of the thyroid but can lie some distance inferior to this. In 10 to 15 percent of patients, parathyroid glands are seen in or around the thymus gland. Rarely, parathyroid glands can occur behind the esophagus, around the pharynx, or in the thyroid gland. The glands have a maximal normal size of about $6 \times 3 \times 2$ mm in teenagers; they are smaller in younger children. Normal parathyroid glands may not be identified on MRI.

CONGENITAL ANOMALIES

Polyorchidism

Occasionally one or both of the testes may be duplicated. MRI shows the appearance of these extra testes within the scrotum.[9] Each testis appears normal, with its own tunica and its own epididymis. No treatment is required for this condition.

Turner's Syndrome

In children with Turner's syndrome, MRI is able to show either the absence of ovaries or the presence of abnormal streak gonads.[10]

Undescended Testis

Undescended testis is important because it is one of the most common genitourinary anomalies in male infants;[11-13] the incidence is approximately 3.5 percent at birth. By 1 year of age the incidence has fallen to about 1 percent. The testes normally descend down the inguinal canals at about the seventh fetal month. They follow a fibromuscular band called the gubernaculum testis that lies along the path of the testes, which follow it in its descent (Fig. 22–3).

Undescended testis is clinically extremely important for two reasons. The first is infertility. After the age of about 2 years, the fertility of both the undescended and the opposite normal testis begins to decrease as the testes atrophy (Figs. 22–2, 22–4), and if this is not corrected by the age of puberty, there is almost complete infertility. The second complication is testicular malignancy, which is nine times as common with undescended testis than in normal males. The increased malignancy is believed to be due to a hormonal defi-

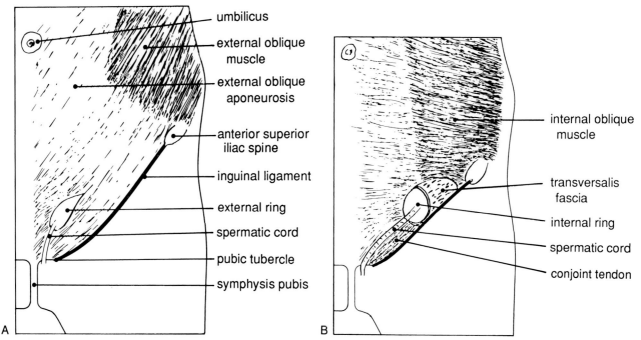

Figure 22–3. *Normal left inguinal canal anatomy.* **A,** The external ring, which is an opening in the external oblique aponeurosis. **B,** The internal oblique muscle, conjoined tendon, transversalis fascia, and internal ring after the external oblique muscle and aponeurosis have been removed. (From Friedland GW, Chang P. The role of imaging in the management of the impalpable undescended testis. AJR 1988; 151:1107–1111.)

ciency that also causes the failure of testicular descent; because of this, surgical placement of the testis in the scrotum does not necessarily decrease the risk of malignancy, but the scrotal testis is better placed for clinical follow-up.

The appropriate treatment of undescended testis is surgery. Because of the high incidence of spontaneous descent in the first year of life, and the increasing risk of infertility after the age of 2 years, surgery is usually performed between the age of 1 and 2 years.

The goal of imaging in the evaluation of patients with undescended testis has two objectives. In young children, imaging is used to locate the testis. In young adults and older men, it is used to screen the testis in order to facilitate early diagnosis of complicating malignancy. Since this is not primarily a pediatric problem, it will not be discussed here further.

Imaging of the undescended testis is still somewhat controversial. Eighty percent of undescended testes are palpable clinically, and in these patients no imaging is required before surgery. The undescended testis may lie high in the scrotum, within the inguinal canal (Fig. 22–4), low in the abdomen, or high in the abdomen. In one study MRI was able to identify 15 of 16 undescended testes.[13] However, these patients had a mean age of 20 years and the success rate may be lower in younger children. In another study MRI was correct in diagnosing absent testes in six of seven patients and in locating undescended testes in five of eight patients.[12] There are several factors that aid in the identification of

an undescended testis. The first of these is knowledge of the most likely location of the ectopic testis. When the testis is low in the abdomen close to the internal inguinal ring, or along the line of the inguinal canal, its location is predictable and helpful. The long axis of the oval undescended testis usually orientates along the direction of descent (Fig. 22–5). The testis usually lies close to the gubernaculum. In most patients the undescended testis has the same signal intensity on T1 and T2 weighted images as a normal testis (Fig. 22–6). In a few patients, however, the testis has a lower signal intensity, which is believed to suggest the presence of atrophy. Visualization of the mediastinum testis (Fig. 22–7), a low-intensity band projecting inward from one surface of the testis, is also helpful in differentiating the testis from, for example, a lymph node or inguinal hernia (Figs. 22–8, 22–9). It is not always seen. Rarely, an undescended testis lies high in the abdomen, and MRI has not been successful in identifying testes in this uncommon location.

Other modalities have been utilized to look for undescended testes. Several reports indicate reasonably good accuracy for computed tomography (CT). Most of these, however, describe older children or adults in whom one would expect a higher success rate than in infants. In addition, most of the successes reported for CT have been with lower abdominal or inguinal testes. Ultrasonography has proved less useful than CT. Abdominal testes are not well visualized by ultrasonography. With inguinal testes, unless the mediastinum tes-

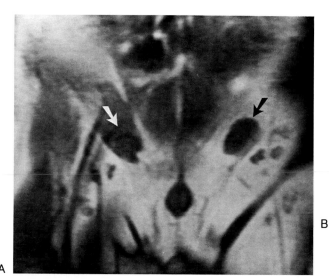

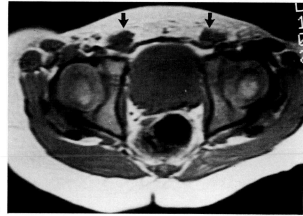

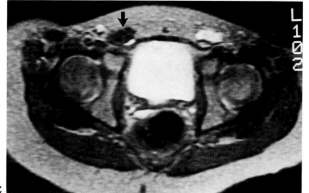

Figure 22–4. *Bilateral nonpalpable undescended testes in a 2-year-old child.* ***A,*** *Coronal image (600/20). Bilateral inguinal testes (arrows) are well seen.* ***B,*** *Transverse image (1700/20). Both testes (arrows) remain hypointense to fat on the spin-density pulse sequence.* ***C,*** *Transverse image (1700/80). The left testis (white arrow) has become hyperintense to fat. The right testis (black arrow) is of low intensity, suggesting atrophy. (From Kier R, McCarthy S, Rosenfield AT, et al. Nonpalpable testes in young boys: evaluation with MR imaging. Radiology 1988; 169:429–433.)*

tis can be identified (and it cannot always be seen), there is difficulty with ultrasound in differentiating an undescended testis from an enlarged inguinal lymph node (Fig. 22–5).

The exact role of imaging in the evaluation of undescended testis is not yet clear, but several conclusions can be drawn. First, undescended testis is a common and important condition that requires surgical intervention. Second, 80 percent of undescended testes are palpable and the surgeon does not require imaging assistance. In the nonpalpable undescended testis, imaging is helpful only if it alters the surgical approach. Unfortunately, the available evidence at the present time suggests that this is seldom so. The surgical approach can be altered in only two ways. First, if imaging demonstrates the presence of a high abdominal testis, this can be approached directly without any surgery being performed in the inguinal area. Second, if imaging can conclusively diagnose the absence of a testis, surgical exploration is unnecessary. Available evidence suggests that imaging is at its weakest in the identification of high abdominal testes or in confident diagnosis of absent testis. Currently, only a few series have been reported evaluating MRI of undescended testes. With larger series of patients or more sophisticated imaging techniques, the role of imaging may increase.

If imaging is used, MRI certainly appears to compare well with other imaging techniques, including CT and ultrasonography. It has the advantage of multiplanar image and the potential of better characterization of testicular tissue by the use of multiple pulse sequences.

MECHANICAL DISORDERS: TESTICULAR TORSION

Early accurate diagnosis of testicular torsion is important because, if untreated, the disorder can lead to infertility. The differential diagnosis is that of acute epididymo-orchitis. Nuclear medicine isotope studies are very helpful in differentiating these two disorders. It is not yet known whether MRI will have any role to play. One obvious problem is the difficulty of finding time on the scanner for acute scanning of patients soon after they present. There are no reports of patients with torsion being studied with MRI. In one experimental study in a rat model, MRI was found to be extremely sensitive for the identification of torsion.[14] Some of the rats showed mild signal decrease a number of hours after the torsion. The most characteristic finding, however, was a whirlpool effect seen in the spermatic cord region; this was due to spiral distortion of the fascial planes around the spermatic cord.

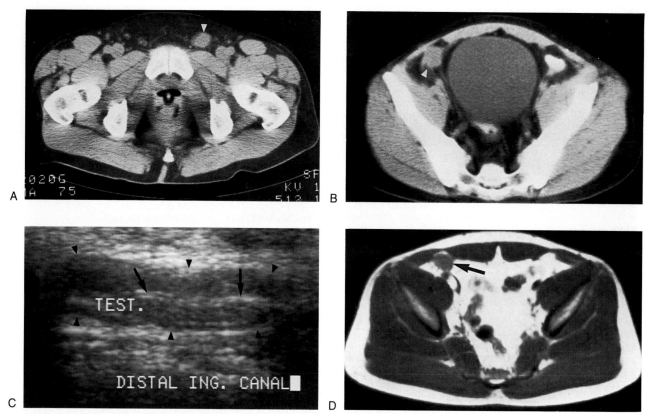

Figure 22–5. *Undescended testes.* ***A, B,*** CT scans in two patients showing undescended testes (*arrowheads*) lying in the inguinal canal. ***C,*** Ultrasound in another patient demonstrates an inguinal testis (*arrowheads*). The testis has a fairly homogeneous echo pattern. The mediastinum testis is visible (*straight arrows*), proving that the structure is testis. ***D,*** Transverse MR image in another patient (600/30). The right testis (*arrow*) is seen just above the internal inguinal ring. (From Friedland GW, Chang P. The role of imaging in the management of the impalpable undescended testis. AJR 1988; 151:1107–1111.)

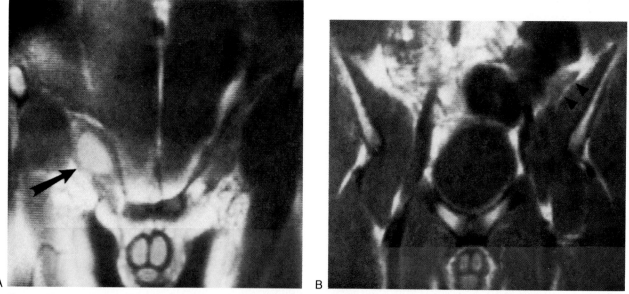

Figure 22–6. *Bilateral undescended testes.* ***A,*** Coronal MR image (1000/30). The right testis (*arrow*) is seen high in the inguinal canal. ***B,*** Coronal image (1000/30) taken 2 cm posteriorly demonstrates a left intra-abdominal testis at the peritoneal border above the inguinal canal (*arrowheads*). The left testis demonstrates atrophy. The signal intensity from this testis is less than that from the right testis. (From Fritzsche PJ, Hricak H, Kogan BA, et al. Undescended testes: value of MR imaging. Radiology 1987; 164:169–173.)

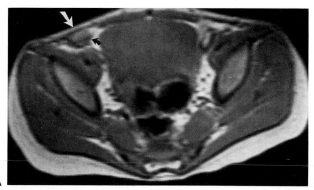
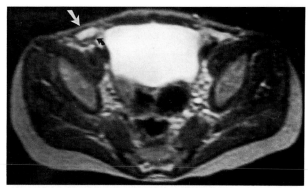

A   B

Figure 22–7. *Undescended testis: demonstration of mediastinum testis in a 2-year-old child with nonpalpable right testis.* ***A,*** Transverse image (1700/20). The undescended testis (*straight arrow*) is identified at the right external ring. A low-signal-intensity band (*curved arrow*) is the mediastinum testis. ***B,*** 1700/80. With the T2 weighting the testis has become a strong signal. The mediastinum testis (*curved arrow*) remains of low signal intensity. Identification of the mediastinum testis helps differentiate undescended testis from an enlarged inguinal lymph node. (From Kier R, McCarthy S, Rosenfield AT, et al. Nonpalpable testes in young boys: evaluation with MR imaging. Radiology 1988; 169:429–433.)

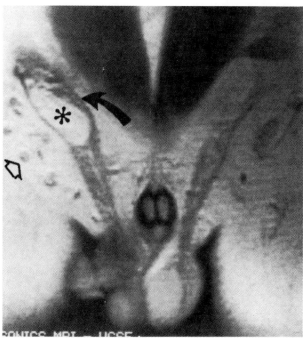
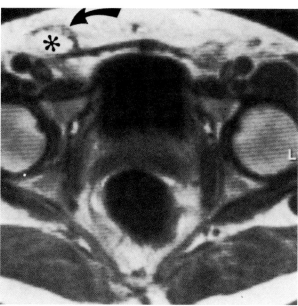

A   B

Figure 22–8. *Inguinal hernia.* ***A,*** Coronal MR image (2000/30). There is a right inguinal hernia (*). The mass is displacing the spermatic cord contents (*curved arrow*). Small inguinal lymph nodes are seen (*open arrow*). ***B,*** Transverse T1 image (500/30). The inguinal hernia mass (*) remains of high signal intensity, indicating that it contains fat. The ductus differens and testicular vessels are displaced anteriorly and medially (*curved arrow*). The demonstration of the ductus and vessels adjacent to the mass is strong evidence in favor of a hernia, rather than undescended testis. (From Fritzsche PJ, Hricak H, Kogan BA, et al. Undescended testes: value of MR imaging. Radiology 1987; 164:169–173.)

TUMORS

Thyroid Tumors

Benign or malignant thyroid tumors are rare in children and have been little studied by MRI.[8] In adults MRI has proved sensitive for the identification of both benign and malignant lesions, bit it has not yet proved good at differentiating benign from malignant or functioning from nonfunctioning nodules. Most thyroid mass lesions have signal intensity consistent with prolonged T1 and T2 relaxation times, compared with normal thyroid tissues. Some tumors may have high intensity on T1 weighted images owing to hemorrhage within them. Some cysts may have high intensity on T1 weighted images that is due either to hemorrhage within them or to the presence of mucoid material with a high protein content.

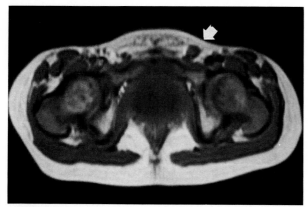
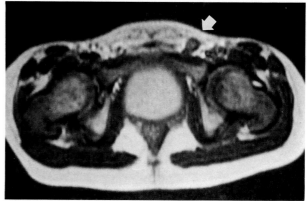

A   B

Figure 22–9. *Undescended testis: lymph node mimics normal testis in a 3-year-old child with no palpable left testis.*
A, B, Transverse spin-density (1500/20) and T2 weighted (1500/80) images. There is a left inguinal soft tissue structure
(*arrow*). The round rather than elongated shape, the absence of demonstration of a mediastinum testis, and the fact that the
lesion is of lower intensity than fat on the T2 weighted image (***B***) all suggest the correct diagnosis of enlarged lymph node
rather than testis. (From Kier R, McCarthy S, Rosenfield AT, et al. Nonpalpable testes in young boys: evaluation with MR
imaging. Radiology 1988; 169:429–433.)

Parathyroid Adenoma and Hyperplasia

Hyperfunction of the parathyroid glands may be due
either to hyperplasia or to a focal adenoma (Figs.
22–10 to 22–12).[8, 15] Little work has been done on these
disorders in children. In adults several early studies
suggest that MRI may be as good as, if not better than,
other modalities including ultrasonography, CT, and
thallium scanning. Most abnormal parathyroid glands
have signal intensity consistent with prolonged T1 and
T2 relaxation, compared with thyroid tissue. This
means that the diseased parathyroids are of lower intensity than thyroid on T1 weighted images and higher
intensity on T2 weighted images. Very occasionally the
abnormal glands do not display high intensity on T2
images.

Adrenal Tumors

Neuroblastoma

Neuroblastoma is the most common solid pediatric
tumor (Figs. 22–13 to 22–17) and the most common
malignancy in the first year of life. It represents between 5 and 15 percent of all pediatric cancers, and
about 500 new cases are seen each year in the United
States. Sixty percent of the tumors present in the first 2
years of life and 85 percent by the age of 10 years.

Neuroblastomas arise from the neural crest. They
are biologically unique tumors in that they can mature
spontaneously into benign ganglioneuromas, and they
exhibit the highest rate of spontaneous regression of
any human malignancy. They are also unusual in that
late relapse can occur; tumor recurrence as late as 15 or
20 years after apparent cure is not uncommon.

Neuroblastomas can be found anywhere along the
sympathetic chain or in the adrenal gland. Approximately two-thirds occur in the abdomen, and of these,

two-thirds arise from the adrenal gland and one-third
from the retroperitoneal sympathetic ganglia. The
chest is the next most common site of the tumor. The
pelvis and neck are unusual locations. The tumors
show varying degrees of differentiation; ganglioneuroma is a benign, mature form of neuroblastoma.

The tumors are staged in four categories. Stage I
tumors are confined to the tissue of origin; stage II

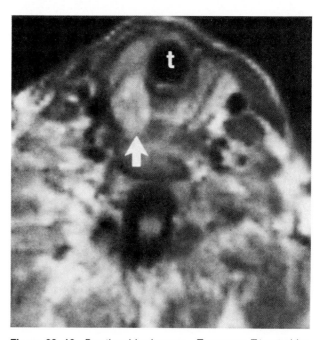

Figure 22–10. *Parathyroid adenoma.* Transverse T1 gated image of the neck shows an adenoma (*arrow*) of moderate signal
intensity lying behind the right lobe of the thyroid. The increase in
signal intensity was due to hemorrhage in the adenoma. t, Trachea.
(From Higgins CB, Aufferman W. MR imaging of thyroid and parathyroid glands: a review of current status. AJR 1988; 151: 1095–
1106.)

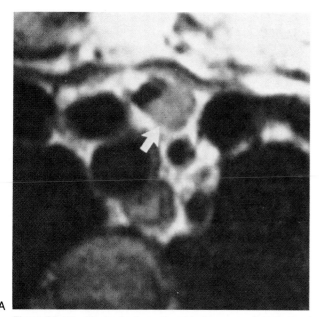
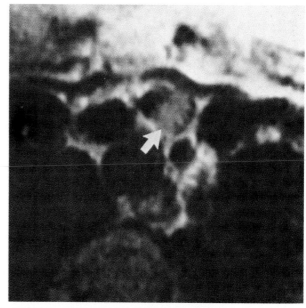

A

B

Figure 22–11. *Mediastinal parathyroid adenoma.* ***A, B,*** Proton density (2000/35) and T2 weighted (2000/70) images of the mediastinum both show a well-defined adenoma (*arrow*). The absence of any increase in intensity on T2 weighted images is atypical of parathyroid adenoma. (From Higgins CB, Aufferman W. MR imaging of thyroid and parathyroid glands: a review of current status. AJR 1988; 151:1095–1106.)

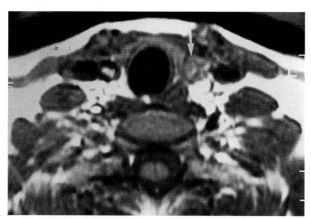
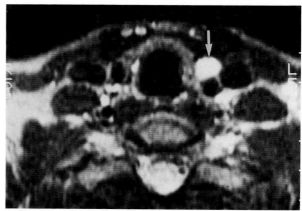

A

B

Figure 22–12. *Parathyroid adenoma.* ***A,*** Transverse neck (500/20). The nodule (*arrow*) is isointensive with thyroid. ***B,*** T2 weighted image (2000/80). The adenoma (*arrow*) is of very strong signal intensity. (From Kier R, Blinder RA, Herfkens RJ, et al. MR imaging with surface coils in primary hyperparathyroidism. J Comput Assist Tomogr 1987; 11:863–868.)

show local regional spread of the tumor without any crossing of the midline; stage III cross the midline; and stage IV tumors have metastases involving the skeleton, distant lymph nodes, or other tissues. Stage IV-S tumors have metastases confined to the liver, skin, or bone marrow and occur in children under the age of 1 year. The tumors are frequently large; gross calcification is present in over 60 percent of cases and microscopic calcification in over 90 percent. Seventy percent of patients have metastases on initial presentation.

Clinically, neuroblastoma may present in a wide variety of ways. The tumors may present as an incidental mass or may cause abdominal pain. Because metastases are so frequently present, the clinical symptomatol-

ogy is often due to the metastatic disease; the children may have bone and joint pain, proptosis from orbital metastases, anemia, weight loss, or even fever. An unusual clinical presentation is myoclonic encephalopathy.[16] These patients present with unusual neurologic clinical symptoms referable to the posterior cranial fossa. Fifty percent of children with this disorder have associated neuroblastoma. The neuroblastoma in these patients is unusual in several ways: (1) most of the tumors are found within the thoracic cavity, rather than the abdomen; (2) the tumors are often fairly mature, and fewer than half of the children have elevated concentrations of catecholamines in the urine; and (3) the clinical symptoms persist in 75 percent of

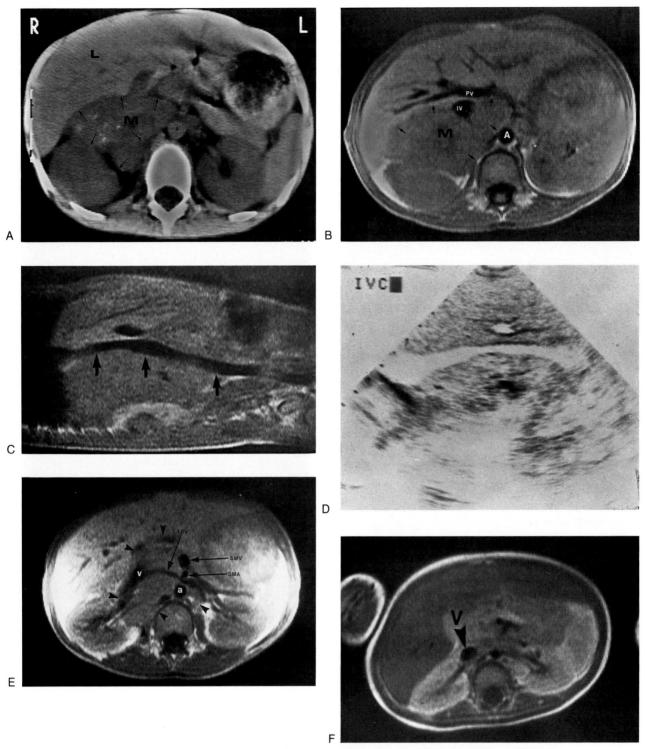

Figure 22–13. *Neuroblastoma in a 2-year-old child with a right upper quadrant mass.* **A,** Transverse CT scan. There is a large calcified right upper quadrant mass (M). The mass is clearly separate from the liver (L). The aorta (A) is well defined but the inferior vena cava is not visualized. **B,** Transverse T1 MR image (500/26). The tumor again is well defined. The calcification seen easily on the CT image is not clearly visualized on MR. The aorta (A), portal vein (PV), and inferior vena cava (IV) are well seen. Note that enlarged retrocaval lymph nodes are displacing the inferior vena cava forward and to the right. The cava is patent. **C,** Sagittal MR image (500/26) shows that the entire inferior vena cava is normal (*arrows*). **D,** Corresponding ultrasound image offers information identical to that of the MR image. **E,** Transverse MR image obtained more inferiorly to **B** (500/26) demonstrates the relationship of tumor-filled lymph nodes (*arrowheads*) to major abdominal vessels. The aorta (a), superior mesenteric artery (SMA), and superior mesenteric vein (SMV) are all displaced slightly by the tumor. The left renal vein (LRV) is completely encased by tumor, which could not be resected without sacrificing the left kidney. The inferior vena cava (V) is displaced forward and to the right. **F,** Transverse MR image (500/26) obtained after 2 months of chemotherapy. There has been marked reduction in tumor size with return of the inferior vena cava (V) to an almost normal position. The advantage of MRI in this patient is its ability to demonstrate the relationship of the tumor to the major vessels.

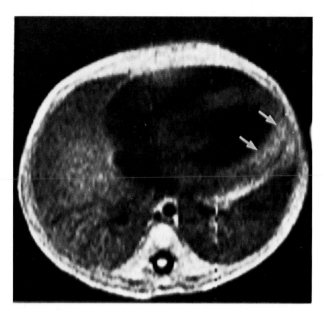

Figure 22–14. *Neuroblastoma.* Transverse image through the heart (500/30) in a 2-year-old boy who presented with congestive cardiac failure from hypertension complicating neuroblastoma. There is marked cardiomegaly. The left ventricular wall (*arrows*) is thickened. There is increased signal in the lung compared with normal, consistent with pulmonary edema.

patients, even after complete resection of the neuroblastoma mass.

In the investigation of patients with suspected neuroblastoma a wide variety of imaging modalities can be used. Plain film radiographs should always be obtained; these frequently show a mass and the presence of calcium. In stage IV-S patients, hepatomegaly may be noticed on the abdominal radiograph. Plain film radiographs should not be used for screening bones for metastases; bone isotope scan is preferable. Ultrasonography should be performed in patients presenting with an unknown isolated abdominal mass; however, if there is already a strong clinical suspicion of neuroblastoma from other information (e.g., bone pain, anemia, calcification on the plain film radiograph), it is better to skip the ultrasound scan and proceed directly to CT or MRI. Ultrasonography does not show the total extent of the tumor, including spread to regional lymph nodes, as well as do other modalities. All patients with neuroblastoma should be studied with CT and/or MRI, because they are excellent imaging tools for studying neuroblastoma. The major advantages of CT are its much greater ability to detect small areas of calcification (Figs. 22–13, 22–15, 22–17) within the tumor, and the fact that it is much less sensitive to motion than MRI. When good quality MR images are obtained (the problems with the motion artifacts are steadily being overcome), MRI offers distinct advantages over CT. The ability of MRI to image in multiple planes (Fig. 22–16) often facilitates definition of the tissue or organ of origin of the tumor, and thus helps with the differential diagnosis (Fig. 22–17).

MRI demonstrates blood vessels more clearly than CT, and this is extremely valuable in determining the surgical resectability of the tumor mass (Fig. 22–13). MRI is also extremely good at identifying or excluding direct extension of neuroblastomas into the spinal canal.

A number of reports have described the MR appearance of neuroblastoma in three fairly large series of patients.[17-19] The MR findings in neuroblastoma are described in detail below.

IDENTIFICATION OF TUMOR. In all reported series, MRI was able to identify all the primary tumors identified by other modalities. In no case were lesions seen on CT not identified by MRI. In many cases the identification of the primary tumor was equivalent to that on CT. In two patients in whom CT showed only a very small localized collection of calcium without any clearly definable associated soft tissue mass, MRI definitely identified a soft tissue tumor.[16,17]

EFFECT OF THE TUMOR ON ADJACENT STRUCTURES. In the abdomen, neuroblastomas frequently cause displacement of blood vessels, and this is well shown by MRI (Figs. 22–16, 22–19). In the chest or neck, neuroblastomas can cause tracheal compression (Fig. 22–20) and this too is easily identified by MRI.[20] Adrenal neuroblastomas displace the kidney in an inferior and sometimes a lateral direction.

TUMOR INTENSITY (Figs. 22–17, 22–18, 22–20). The tumor tissue has a signal intensity consistent with prolonged T1 and T2 relaxation times, appearing of much greater intensity than muscle on T2 weighted images and equal to or less than muscle on T1 weighted images. On inversion recovery pulse sequences the tumors are of much lower intensity than muscle. There is no definite difference between neuroblastomas and ganglioneuromas (Fig. 22–21).

TUMOR MARGINS AND EXTENT. Most neuroblastomas have fairly well defined margins, and the extent of tumor as predicted and defined by MRI correlates well with CT and/or surgery (Figs. 22–16, 22–20). Because the kidney normally has relatively long T1 and T2 relaxation times, it may occasionally prove difficult to distinguish a neuroblastoma from the adjacent kidney.[18,19] In these situations it may be difficult to identify accurately or rule out renal invasion by the tumor. In patients with a moderate amount of perinephric fat, the fat acts as a clear line of demarcation between the tumor and the kidney on T1 weighted images. The use of gadolinium-DTPA as a contrast agent may prove helpful in difficult cases. Occasionally it may be possible to identify clearly true renal invasion by neuroblastoma; secondary hydronephrosis from encasement of the renal hilum can also be seen. Renal invasion may be seen in as many as 10 percent of neuroblastomas. Very rarely the tumor may appear to lie predominantly within the kidney, in which situation it mimics Wilms' tumor.[21] Neuroblastomas frequently spread to local lymph nodes. The margins of neuroblastoma tumor masses are usually well defined on MRI. However, it is usually very difficult to separate primary tumor from tumor in immediately contiguous

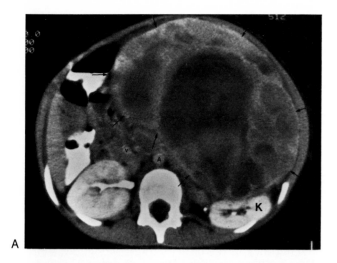

A

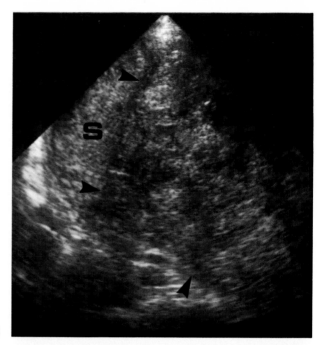

B

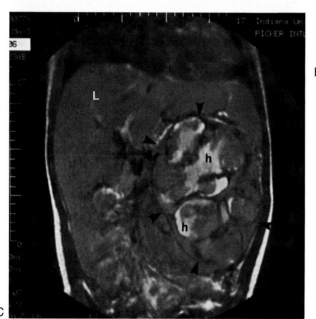

C

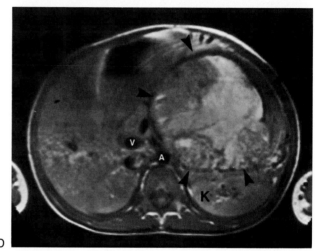

D

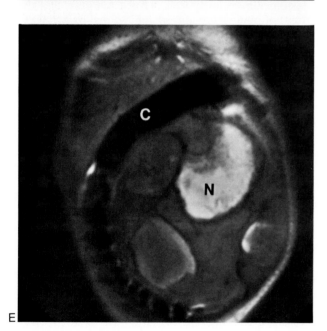

E

Figure 22–15. *Neuroblastoma in an 11-year-old girl with a large abdominal mass.* ***A,*** CT scan showing a large mass lesion (*arrows*) compressing, but clearly separate from, the left kidney (K). The aorta (A) and vena cava (V) can be seen. The mass is of mixed soft tissue, intermediate and of very low intensity. ***B,*** Left longitudinal ultrasound image. The mass (*arrowheads*) consists of mixed high- and low-intensity echoes. It is much less well defined than on the CT scan. The spleen (S) is seen superior to the mass. ***C, D,*** and ***E*** are T1 weighted, spin-density, and T2 weighted images, respectively. ***C,*** Coronal MR image (900/40). The left-sided tumor is well defined (*arrowheads*). High-signal-intensity areas probably represent hemorrhage (h) within the tumor. L, Liver. ***D,*** 2000/20. The mass lesion (*arrowheads*) is again well defined and again is seen to be of mixed high, intermediate, and low signal intensity. The left kidney (K) is seen behind the tumor. The aorta (A) and vena cava (V) are more easily identified than on the CT scan. The vena cava is displaced forward and to the right by large lymph nodes behind it. ***E,*** Coronal (1300/80) MR image obtained through the anterior of the abdomen. The colon (C) is seen draped around the tumor mass. The tumor is mainly of moderate signal intensity. Very-high-intensity signal probably represents liquefied necrotic (N) tumor. Both MRI and CT identify the tumor well. The vessels are a little better imaged with MRI, which also is better able to differentiate hemorrhage from necrosis within the tumor. Ultrasonography does not define the tumor margins well.

lymph nodes; the tumor in the nodes and the primary tumor appear as a conglomerate mass. Neuroblastomas occasionally spread directly through spinal foramina into the spinal canal. In the past, patients with suspected spinal invasion have been studied with myelography. In several patients MRI has very accurately defined spinal extension of neuroblastomas,[19] and it is anticipated that in the future MRI will replace myelography for routine evaluation of these patients. This is a distinct advantage for MRI.

INTERNAL STRUCTURE. Neuroblastomas may be homogeneous or irregular in internal structure. They are more frequently homogeneous than Wilms' tumors, but in over 50 percent of cases some internal irregularity will still be identified, owing to areas of hemorrhage or necrosis within the tumor (Fig. 22–15). Necrotic areas tend to be of lower intensity than soft tissue tumor on T1 weighted images and higher intensity on T2 weighted images. Areas of hemorrhage are usually of strong signal on both T1 and T2 pulse sequences.

TUMOR RESECTABILITY. MRI is extremely helpful in evaluating preoperative surgical resectability of neuroblastomas (Figs. 22–17, 22–19, 22–20). A major factor limiting resection of the primary tumor is encasement of segments of the abdominal aorta, inferior vena cava, renal arteries and veins, celiac artery and branches, and superior mesenteric artery and vein by neuroblastoma (Fig. 22–13). The great vessels can be shown by MRI without the need for contrast agents. MRI has proved very accurate in identifying displacement and encasement of these vessels by tumor. In one study MRI defined vessel involvement better than CT in 14 of 15 patients.[18] Knowledge of direct spread into the spinal canal and into the adjacent kidney is also important in planning surgical resection, and these answers are provided by MRI. In the rare patient with cervical neuroblastoma, MRI has proved extremely accurate in showing anteromedial displacement of the carotid artery and jugular vein, and this information too was helpful in planning surgical resection of the tumor mass.[20]

METASTASES. Tumor spread to local lymph nodes is common (Fig. 22–18). The lymph nodes are enlarged and appear of similar intensity to the primary tumor mass (Fig. 22–17). Spread of tumor to the liver can also be identified. Focal metastases in the liver appear as well-defined regions of signal intensity lower than that of normal liver on T1 weighted images and higher on T2 weighted images. Diffuse infiltrating liver metastases are commonly seen in stage IV-S neuroblastoma (Fig. 22–22) and are also easily identified in the liver. Findings include distortion of the normal smooth course of the portal and hepatic veins, and a very irregular, strong-intensity nodular pattern throughout the liver on T2 weighted images. MRI is also accurate in identifying metastases in more distant sites. In one study MRI demonstrated all metastases seen on other imaging studies, including metastases to bone marrow, intracranial dura, and bone cortex.[19]

Tumor can be accurately identified in bone marrow. It is best seen on T1 weighted images when the normal strong fat intensity signal of bone marrow is replaced by focal or diffuse areas of much lower signal intensity, somewhat similar to that of muscle. On T2 weighted images marrow metastases may be of similar intensity to normal marrow, and therefore not visualized. It is important to remember that MRI is very sensitive for detection of marrow metastasis, but that it is also very nonspecific.

DIFFERENTIAL DIAGNOSIS. Most adrenal neuroblastomas destroy the entire gland, which therefore cannot be identified. The adrenal origin of the tumors is inferred from the position of the tumor. Neuroblastomas must be distinguished from other abdominal tumors. In most cases of neuroblastoma it is possible to identify normal kidneys (apart from displacement) and thereby rule out Wilm's tumor. Small, diffuse, punctate calcifications are fairly characteristic in neuroblastoma and cannot be seen by MRI, which is a disadvantage. In several cases the appearance of the aorta and inferior vena cava has been helpful in distinguishing neuroblastoma from large abdominal retroperitoneal teratomas. Despite their large size, teratomas cause little displacement of the great vessels and never encase them. These are common findings with large neuroblastomas. Another factor strongly suggesting neuroblastoma is the uptake by the primary tumor mass of radiointense isotopes, e.g. MDP (used for bone scanning) or MIBG, which is taken up by neural crest tumors; the presence of bone metastases, marrow metastases, or elevated urine concentrations of catecholamines is a fairly characteristic finding of neuroblastoma. MRI probably cannot distinguish neuroblastoma from ganglioneuroma (Fig. 22–23).

MONITORING THERAPY. MRI can be repeated frequently and safely, and accurately shows change in tumor size in response to chemotherapy or radiation therapy (Fig. 22–13). In most cases a shrinkage of tumor is associated with changes in signal intensity consistent with decreasing relaxation time. In some cases this is seen on both T1 and T2 weighted images,[17] but in others the changes have been seen only on T1 weighted images.[18] It is probable that these changes in signal intensity are not accurate or precise enough to enable one to predict the ultimate outcome and prognosis. In fact, in one series, one patient was identified in whom the tumor shrunk but the signal intensity on T1 weighted images did not alter.[18]

MRI has successfully identified several complications that developed during treatment, including hydronephrosis, thrombosis of the inferior vena cava from a catheter, cerebral infarction, and subdural hematoma.[19]

Several other imaging tools should be mentioned. Bone isotope scanning has a definite role to play in the evaluation of neuroblastoma. MDP bone scan is the method of choice for seeking bone cortical metastases, and technetium sulfur colloid the best for identifying bone marrow metastases. No studies have yet com-

Text continues on page 743.

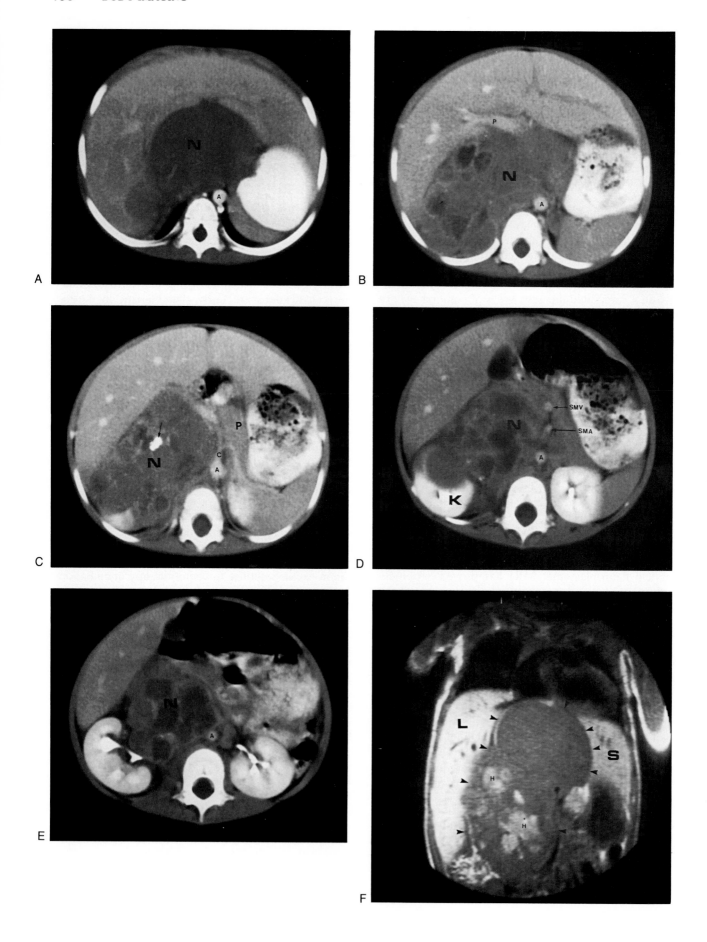

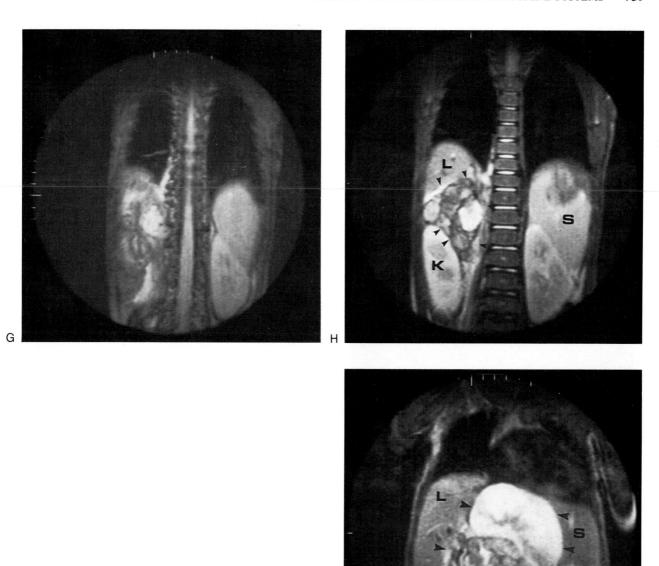

Figure 22–16. *Neuroblastoma: demonstration of a very nonhomogeneous tumor and excellent visualization of vessels on CT with good bolus injection of contrast material, and MRI without contrast injection.* ***A*** *to* ***E,*** Series of transverse CT images after bolus injection of contrast material. The images extend from the level of the superior part of the liver down to its inferior margins. There is a gigantic tumor mass, which is the neuroblastoma (N). Calcification is seen within it (*small arrow*). The mass is of very mixed intensity with areas of soft tissue and low intensity. The tumor lies adjacent to, but does not invade, the portal vein (P). The aorta (A) is partially encased by tumor. The celiac artery (C), superior mesenteric artery (SMA), and superior mesenteric vein (SMV) are displaced and lie adjacent to the tumor. P, Pancreas. Note the apparent invasion of the upper pole of the right kidney (K) by the tumor. This is probably a partial volume artifact. ***F,*** Coronal T1 weighted MR image (300/60) in which the full extent of the tumor is well appreciated. The bilobed tumor is well defined (*arrowheads*). The tumor extends all the way up to the diaphragm. Areas of high signal intensity probably represent hemorrhage (H) in the the tumor. L, Liver; S, spleen. ***G*** *to* ***I,*** Series of coronal T2 weighted MR images (1500/80). The most posterior image shows a very normal spinal canal with no evidence of tumor invasion. More anteriorly the tumor is noted to be of very mixed nonhomogeneous intensity, probably owing to areas of hemorrhage and necrosis within it. The right kidney (K) is rotated, but the upper pole clearly appears normal without any evidence of tumor invasion. L, Liver; S, spleen; arrowheads, tumor.

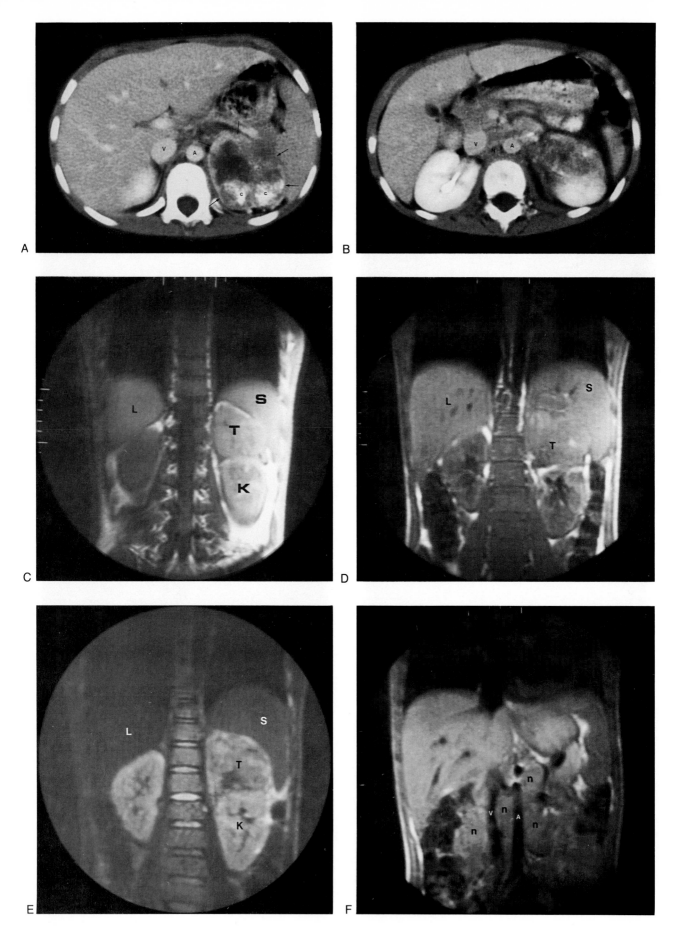

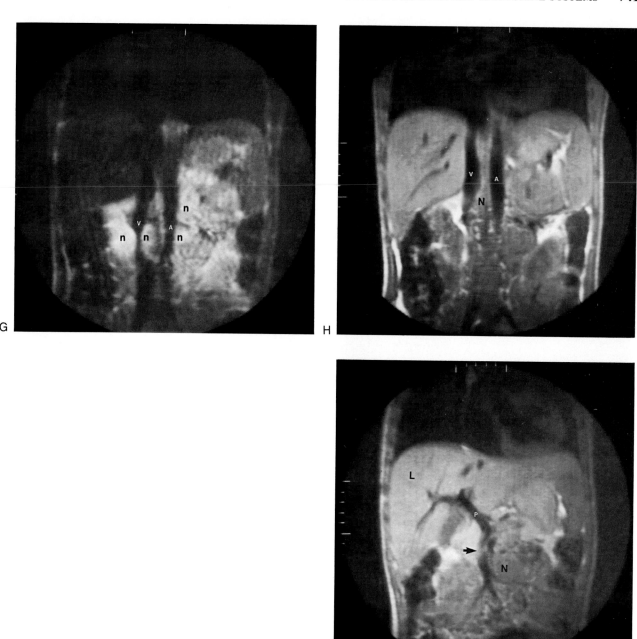

Figure 22–17. *Neuroblastoma: demonstration of features of primary tumor and node metastases.* **A, B,** Transverse CT images. There is a calcified mass in the region of the left adrenal gland (*arrows*). Calcification (C) is seen within the lesion. The aorta (A) and vena cava (V) are well seen. Enlarged lymph nodes (N) separate the aorta and vena cava. **C,** Coronal T1 MR image (500/16), which shows well the origin of the tumor (T) from the left adrenal gland. L, Liver; S, spleen; K, left kidney. **D, E,** Coronal T1 (500/16) and T2 (2000/80) images showing a change in characteristics of the tumor with different pulse sequences. On the T1 weighted image the tumor (T) is of similar intensity to the liver (L) and spleen (S). On the T2 weighted image the tumor (T) is of much higher intensity than the liver (L) or spleen (S) and now of similar intensity to the kidney (K). **F, G,** T1 (500/16) and T2 (2000/80) weighted coronal images to show changes in characteristics of the appearance of nodal metastasis with different pulse sequences. There are multiple enlarged lymph nodes (n) lying between the aorta (A) and vena cava (V) and of similar intensity to the liver. On the T2 weighted image there is marked increase in signal intensity from the nodes (N). **H, I,** More T1 weighted images (500/16) to further demonstrate the ability of MRI to detect nodal metastases. Enlarged lymph nodes (N) are identified between the aorta (A) and inferior vena cava (V) and are also seen to indent and displace the superior mesenteric vein (*arrow*) L, Liver; P, portal vein. Note that the signal intensity of both the primary tumor and the enlarged lymph nodes is consistent with prolongation of T1 and T2 relaxation time compared with most abdominal organs.

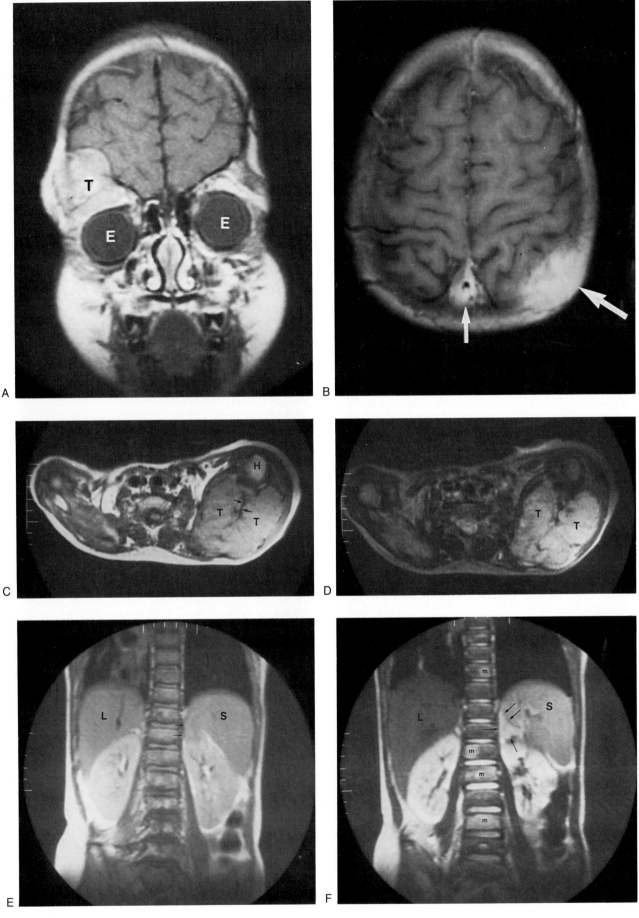

pared the sensitivity of MRI and sulfur colloid for seeking marrow metastases; both appear to be extremely accurate. The advantage of bone marrow scan is that it can survey the entire skeletal system, whereas MRI, because of time restraints, needs to be restricted to selected sites.

Iodine-labeled MIBG is a very sensitive and fairly specific method of studying neuroblastoma. The isotope is taken up by most primary tumors or metastases. However, it does not compete with MRI in the evaluation of the primary tumor mass, because it has poor spatial resolution and therefore has no role to play in defining the resectability of the tumor. Recently, labeled monoclonal antibodies have been utilized; these show strong uptake by tumor and have a potential role in both the diagnosis and treatment of neuroblastoma.[22]

Treatment of stages I, II, and III neuroblastomas consists of surgical resection, with or without chemotherapy and/or radiation therapy. Stage IV tumors are treated initially with chemotherapy; if metastases resolve, the primary tumor is resected. Radiation is used at any time for relief of severe adverse symptoms from metastases. Whole body irradiation and marrow transplant are being evaluated in stage IV patients. Stage IV-S patients often recover with no therapy, or just chemotherapy.

Pheochromocytoma

Pheochromocytomas are rare in children (Figs. 22–24 to Fig. 22–28).[4, 23] Over two-thirds arise in the adrenal gland and the remainder in any location in the neck, chest (Fig. 22–27), abdomen, or pelvis (Fig. 22–29). The tumors are multiple in up to 30 percent of cases; multiple tumors are more frequently found in patients with von Hippel-Lindau disease, multiple endocrine syndromes, and familial pheochromocytomas. Less than 10 percent of the tumors are malignant. They are of moderate size, usually more than 2 cm in diameter at the time of presentation. They are usually well defined. On MRI the tumors show features consistent with long T1 (Fig. 22–24) and very prolonged T2 relaxation times (Figs. 22–25, 22–26). They are of lower

intensity than liver on T1 weighted images and very high intensity on T2 weighted images. This latter finding is fairly characteristic and distinguishes pheochromocytomas from other adrenal tumors. The signal intensity in fact is so high on T2 weighted images that the lesion may mimic a cyst. In some cases ultrasonography or CT is required to differentiate a cyst from a pheochromocytoma. MRI has been found to be equivalent to CT for identification of pheochromocytomas in the adrenal gland,[4] and because of the ability of coronal images to screen large areas of the body, MRI has been better than CT at identifying nonadrenal pheochromocytomas.[4] MIBG isotope scan is also sensitive in identifying the location of pheochromocytomas. This isotope is also taken up by neuroblastoma.

No imaging modalities are able to differentiate between benign and malignant pheochromocytomas from the appearance of the primary lesion. The presence of secondary lesions, e.g., in the liver, strongly suggests malignancy.

Treatment of pheochromocytoma consists of surgical resection.

Other Adrenal Tumors

Other adrenal tumors that can be found include adenomas and, very rarely, carcinomas or metastases (Fig. 22–30). The size of the lesions may vary. Hormone-producing tumors are usually very small.[5] Adrenal adenomas may be classified as functioning or nonfunctioning. Even nonfunctioning adenomas produce hormones but not in excessive amounts. Nonfunctioning adenomas appear of similar intensity to that of normal adrenal gland on all pulse sequences.[4] Some studies have attempted to determine whether MRI can differentiate functioning from nonfunctioning adenomas, and benign from malignant adrenal tumors; it appears that MRI cannot do this accurately. In some series there is a tendency for one group of tumors to appear different from another, but in all series there is always a large group of patients who fall into an indeterminate zone.[5, 23–25]

Compared with other modalities, MRI seems to be

◀ **Figure 22–18.** *Neuroblastoma: MRI demonstration of metastases in a 5-year-old child with a 1-year history of intermittent shoulder pain and a more recent history of diplopia.   **A,** Coronal image through the skull (800/26) with gadolinium-DTPA enhancement. Both eyes (E) are well seen. There is extensive involvement of the roof of the right orbit with epidural extension of the tumor masses (T). **B,** Transverse T1 image (800/26) after gadolinium-DTPA administration. There is a large left posterior occipital calvarial metastasis with epidural extension (large arrow). There is also an enhancing lesion in the superior sagittal sinus (small arrow) believed to be tumor invasion, although not proved histologically. **C,** Transverse T1 image (800/26) through the shoulders. There is massive involvement of the right scapula with a tumor metastasis. The soft tissue component of the tumor (T) is of slightly higher intensity than muscle. The residual bone of the scapula is seen as an irregular low-intensity line (arrow). H, Humeral head. **D,** T2 weighted image at the same level showing marked increase in signal intensity from the soft tissue component of the tumor (T), which is now of stronger signal than muscle and fat. **E, F,** Coronal spin-density (1500/20) and T2 (1500/70) weighted images through the abdomen. The primary tumor (arrows) arises in the left adrenal gland and is very small. It is of similar intensity to liver (L) and spleen (S) on the spin-density image. On the T2 weighted image it is of higher intensity than liver (L) or spleen (S). The tumor retains the shape of the adrenal gland. Note the multiple metastases (m) in the vertebra. They are of slightly decreased intensity on the spin-density image and somewhat difficult to see. They appear of very high intensity on the T2 weighted image.*

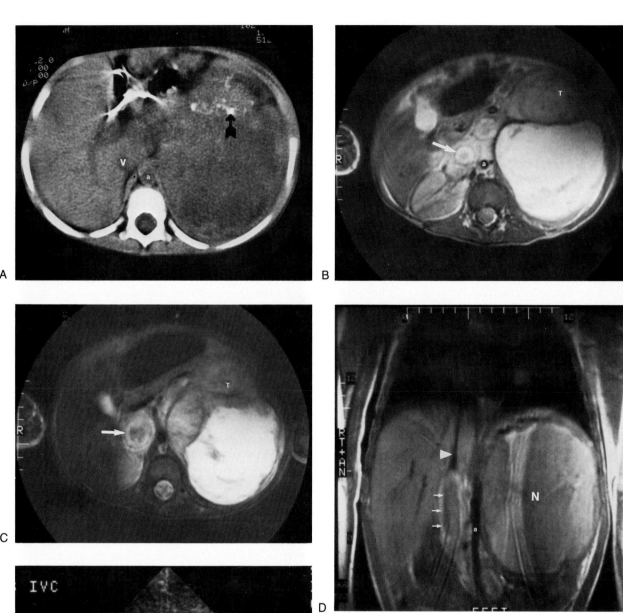

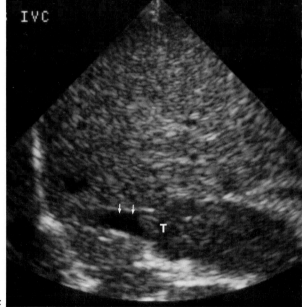

Figure 22–19. *Neuroblastoma: direct invasion of the inferior vena cava.* ***A,*** Transverse CT scan, no intravenous contrast, shows a very large left-sided abdominal mass with anterior calcification (*arrow*). The mass is predominantly of low intensity, suggesting hemorrhage or necrosis. The aorta (a) and vena cava (V) are seen. It is difficult to appreciate tumor in the cava. ***B,*** Transverse T1 spin-density image (2300/30). The tumor is predominantly of high signal intensity, probably representing hemorrhage within it. Soft tissue components of the tumor (T) are of more soft tissue density. The aorta (a) appears normal. A ringlike density, representing tumor, is seen within the inferior vena cava (*arrow*). ***C,*** Transverse T2 weighted image with motion suppression (2300/70). Again the tumor is of mixed very high signal intensity representing blood and moderately strong signal intensity (T). The tumor in the inferior vena cava again is well seen (*arrow*). ***D,*** Coronal T1 weighted image (833/20). A tubular mass of tumor (*arrows*) is seen within the inferior vena cava. The superior part of the inferior vena cava (*arrowhead*) is patent. A, Aorta; N, primary neuroblastoma mass. ***E,*** Longitudinal ultrasound image shows tumor (T) lying within the inferior vena cava. The arrows point to the more superior, patent, part of the superior vena cava.

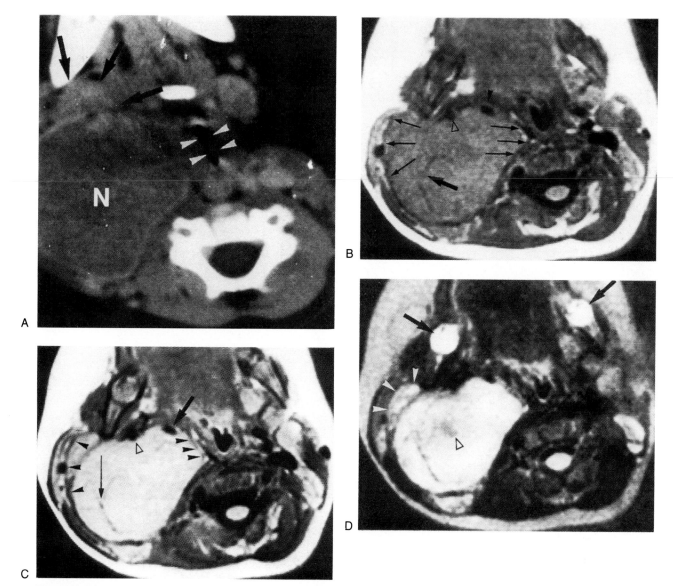

Figure 22–20. *Diagnosis: Cervical neuroblastoma.* ***A,*** Postcontrast CT scan at the level of the floor of the mouth. There is anterior displacement of the submandibular salivary gland (*arrows*) and narrowing of the airway lumen (*arrowheads*) by a large right-sided neuroblastoma (N). ***B,*** Transverse T1 image at the level of the oropharynx (600/22). The tumor intensity is slightly higher than that of muscle. The long arrows demonstrate interfaces between the parotid gland laterally and the pharyngeal muscles medially. The solid arrowhead points to the carotid artery, the open arrowhead to the jugular vein, and the thick arrow to prominent vessels within the tumor mass. ***C,*** Proton density image (3000/22). The thin arrow points to vessels within the tumor, the thick arrow to the carotid artery, the open arrowhead to the displaced jugular vein, and the closed arrowheads to interfaces with the carotid gland and pharyngeal muscle. ***D,*** T2 weighted image (300/95). The tumor is of high intensity. Fluid around developing teeth has very strong signal (*arrows*). (From Casselman JW. Primary cervical blastoma: CT and MR findings. J Comput Assist Tomogr 1988; 12:684–686.)

fairly equivalent to CT for identification of moderate or large lesions, but not as good as CT in identifying lesions less than 1 cm in diameter.[5] One advantage of MRI is that it can differentiate tortuous vessels adjacent to the adrenal gland from small adrenal tumors, especially in patients with portal hypertension. On CT, dilated tortuous vessels occasionally mimic adenomas.[5]

Ovarian Tumors

Ovarian tumors are uncommon in childhood (Fig. 22–31). They are usually benign; less than 30 percent are malignant. They may present with pain, a mass, or secondary effects due to hormone production. Of the tumors, approximately 75 percent are of germ cell origin, 15 percent stromal, and 10 percent epithelial.

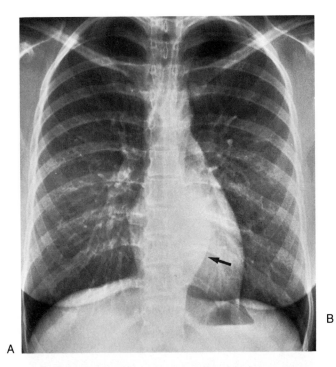

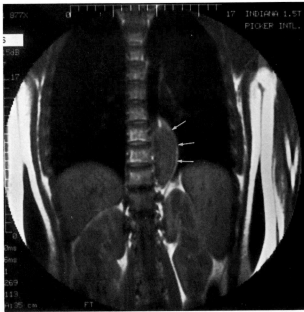

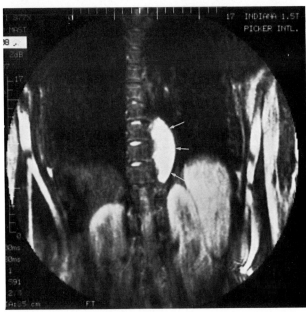

Figure 22–21. *Benign ganglioneuroma in a 15-year-old female with incidental finding of a mass on chest x-ray.* ***A,*** Frontal chest radiograph showing a well-defined soft tissue mass lesion (*arrow*). ***B,*** Coronal T1 MR image. The mass lesion (*arrows*) is seen to lie in the posterior mediastinum adjacent to the spine. Most of the mass is of homogeneous soft tissue intensity. There is a thin rim of high signal intensity along the lateral margin of the mass lesion, the cause of which is unknown. ***C,*** Coronal T2 weighted image (2000/80) obtained with motion suppression technique (MAST). The tumor (*arrows*) is of very high signal intensity, which might suggest the presence of fluid. Histologically the tumor was found to be a soft tissue ganglioneuroma.

Germ cell tumors include dysgerminoma, teratoma, endodermal sinus tumor (yolk sac tumor), embryonal carcinoma, and choriocarcinoma. The dysgerminomas occur before puberty, have a good prognosis, and are occasionally bilateral. Endodermal sinus tumors have aggressive local spread and a poor prognosis; alpha-fetoprotein levels in the blood are elevated with these tumors. Ten percent of teratomas are malignant. Stromal tumors include granulosa–thecal cell tumors and Sertoli and Leydig cell tumors. Estrogen production from these tumors can cause precocious puberty. Most

epithelial tumors are serous cystadenomas or adenocarcinomas.

Many ovarian tumors are complex lesions having both solid and cystic components, and with few exceptions the histology usually cannot be accurately predicted from imaging. MRI of most ovarian masses shows a pelvic mass of variable size and variable signal intensity (Fig. 22–31).

Ovarian teratomas are one of the few lesions in which there are specific findings, enabling an accurate diagnosis to be made by MRI.[2, 26] Ovarian cystic ter-

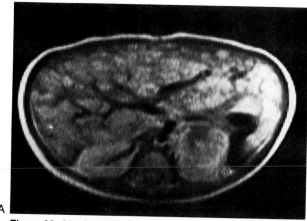
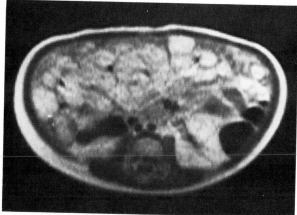

Figure 22–22. *Stage IV-S neuroblastoma.* **A, B,** T1 (500/30) and T2 weighted (1500/60) transverse images of the liver show diffuse replacement of the liver by neuroblastoma.

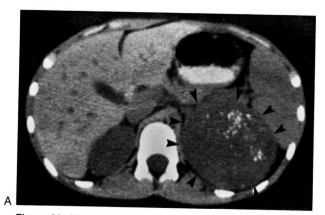
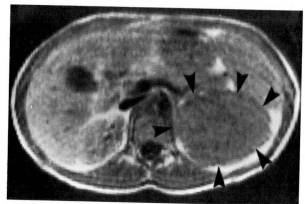

Figure 22–23. *Ganglioneuroma.* **A,** Transverse CT scan showing a well-defined calcified mass (*arrowheads*) in the region of the left adrenal gland. **B,** Transverse MR image (500/30) in which the mass lesion is well seen (*arrowheads*). The calcium cannot be identified. Neither modality differentiates this ganglioneuroma from a neuroblastoma.

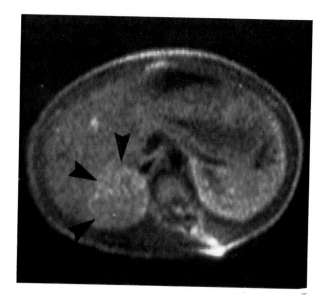

Figure 22–24. *Right adrenal pheochromocytoma in a 13-year-old girl with hypertension.* Transverse T1 image (500/30). There is a large, well-defined right adrenal mass (*arrowheads*) of moderate signal intensity. There are no specific features to differentiate this tumor from other adrenal lesions such as neuroblastoma.

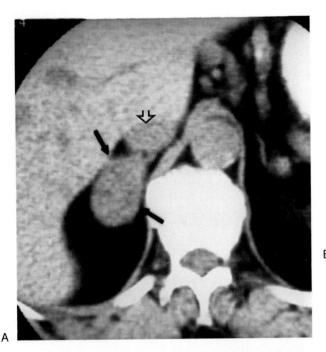

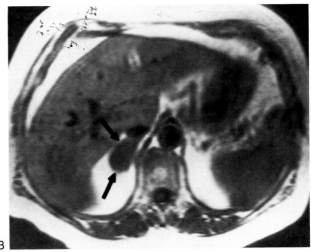

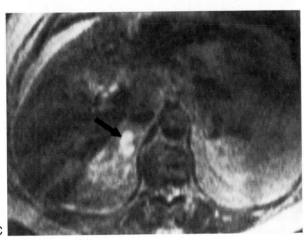

Figure 22–25. *Pheochromocytoma.* ***A,*** Transverse abdominal CT scan shows a 2.5-cm mass (*arrows*) in the right adrenal gland. Open arrow, Inferior vena cava. ***B,*** T1 weighted MR image (300/26) revealing a low-signal-intensity mass (*arrows*) corresponding to the mass seen on the CT scan. ***C,*** Transverse T2 weighted image (250/80) in which the mass (arrow) is of very high signal intensity. This very strong signal is suggestive of pheochromocytoma. (From Doppman JL, Reinig JW, Dwyer AJ, et al. Differentiation of adrenal masses by magnetic resonance imaging. Surgery 1987; 102:1018–1026.)

atomas (dermoid cysts) (Figs. 22–32, 22–33) are composed mainly of a cyst lined entirely or partly by epithelium with sebaceous and sweat glands. Tissues from all three germ layers are present in the lesion. The tumors usually contain a large amount of fat, which is in a fluid state. The signal intensity from the fat is strong on T1 and T2 weighted images and similar to that of subcutaneous fat. Strong chemical shift artifact has been helpful in differentiating cystic ovarian teratomas from other lesions.[26] Several other characteristic features are seen on MR images. Many lesions show layering of gravity-dependent debris within them; this changes with patient position. The interface between the debris, which is mainly hair, and the fatty fluid is not sharply defined. In addition, nodules and protrusions bulge into the cyst. Calcium, which is frequently seen on CT or plain film, is much less commonly identi-

fied on MRI, unless it is a large conglomerate mass or a tooth. The calcium appears of low intensity on all pulse sequences. Hemorrhagic cysts may have a similar strong signal intensity on T1 and T2 weighted pulse sequences, but the layering of debris, the protrusions into the cyst, and the chemical shift artifact all distinguish teratoma.

Benign ovarian cysts (Fig. 22–34) are usually well defined, with low signal intensity on T1 and bright signal on T2 weighted images. Hemorrhage into the cyst may cause a strong signal on T1 images. Polycystic ovaries have a characteristic appearance on T2 weighted images, consisting of multiple peripheral high-signal-intensity cysts surrounding abundant low-intensity central stroma (Fig. 22–35).[2]

Ovarian cyst adenomas and adenocarcinomas (Fig. 22–36) are usually very large cystic lesions with a small

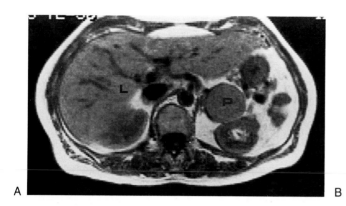

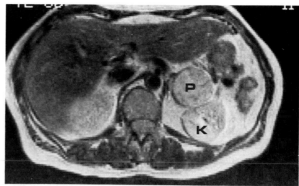

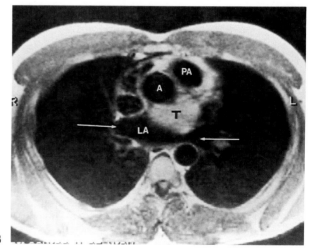

Figure 22–26. *Pheochromocytoma.* ***A,*** Transverse MR image (500/30). There is a well-defined mass lesion (P) lying anterior to the left kidney (K). The pheochromocytoma has a signal intensity less than that of liver (L). ***B,*** T2 weighted image (2000/60). There is a marked increase in the signal intensity from the pheochromocytoma (P). K, Kidney. ***C,*** Transverse MR image (2000/60) through the liver in another patient shows an extremely hyperintense focal lesion (*arrows*) in the right lobe of the liver. This is a metastasis from a pheochromocytoma. The very strong signal from this lesion simulates a hemangioma. (From Quint LE, Glazer GM, Francis IR, Shapiro B, Chenevert TL. Pheochromocytoma and paraganglioma: comparison of MR imaging with CT and I-131 MIBG scintigraphy. Radiology 1987; 165:89–93.)

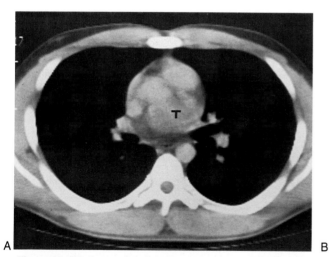

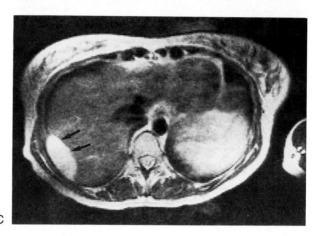

Figure 22–27. *Intrapericardial pheochromocytoma.* ***A,*** Drip infusion transverse CT scan shows a hyperintense tumor (T) that could easily be mistaken for opacified left atrium. ***B,*** Gated MR image shows a well-defined tumor (T) abutting on the left atrium (LA) and posterior to the aorta (A). At surgery a benign pheochromocytoma was identified (without cardiac invasion). PA, Pulmonary artery; arrows, pulmonary veins. (From Quint LE, Glazer GM, Francis IR, Shapiro B, Chenevert TL. Pheochromocytoma and paraganglioma: comparison of MR imaging with CT and I-131 MIBG scintigraphy. Radiology 1987; 165:89–93.)

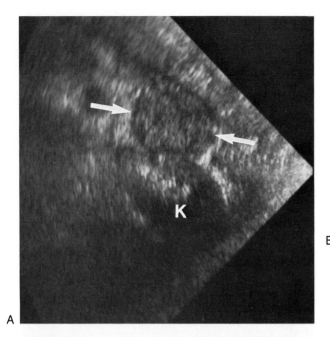

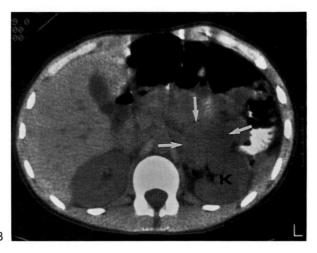

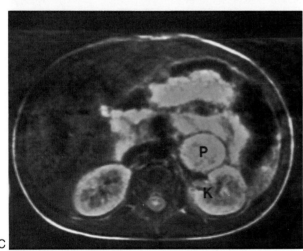

Figure 22–28. *Pheochromocytoma in a 12-year-old male.* The tumor is well seen on three different imaging modalities. **A,** Longitudinal ultrasound showing a well-defined mass lesion (*arrows*) lying anterior to the left kidney (K). **B,** Transverse abdominal CT scan. There is a homogeneous soft tissue mass (*arrows*) lying anterior to the left kidney (K). **C,** T2 weighted transverse MR image (2000/60) also identifies a well-defined pheochromocytoma (P) tumor mass lying anterior to the left kidney (K). The very strong signal intensity on this image is suggestive of pheochromocytoma. Most other adrenal lesions do not have such a high signal intensity on T2 weighted images. The appearance of the lesion on CT and ultrasound is completely nonspecific. MRI defines the lesion precisely.

soft tissue component; identification of this component differentiates these lesions from simple cysts. The mass lesions in both cystadenoma and cystadenocarcinoma appear similar on MRI. The malignancy can only be suspected by the identification of ascites, enlarged lymph nodes, or focal liver lesions.

Testicular Tumors

Testicular tumors are not particularly common in children. They include leukemic infiltration, Leydig cell tumors (Fig. 22–37), seminomas, and embryonal cell carcinoma. MRI has proved sensitive in identifying testicular tumors.[27, 28] In several patients MRI was able to identify tumors not seen on ultrasound images.[27] Although MRI is sensitive, it is found to be fairly nonspecific.[27, 28] It cannot differentiate between the different tumors and in many cases cannot distinguish benign from malignant testicular processes. In addition, MRI has not been shown to be accurate in demonstrating local invasion of testicular tumor through the tunica albuginea.[27] A typical appearance of a testicular tumor is of approximately similar intensity to normal testes on T1 weighted images, with markedly less signal intensity, compared with normal testes, on T2 weighted images. Hemorrhage, which can occur into testicular tumors, alters the homogeneity of the tumor and also the signal intensity. MRI can identify testicular involvement with leukemia even when other imag-

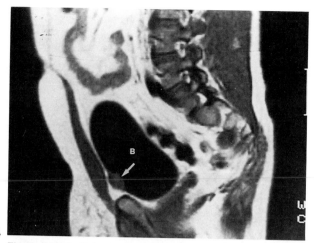

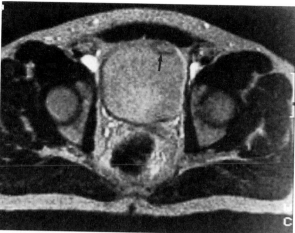

Figure 22–29. *Ectopic pheochromocytoma in a patient with headaches and intermittent hypertension after micturition.* ***A,*** Sagittal T1 MR image (500/16). There is an intramural mass (*arrow*) projecting into the bladder (B). ***B,*** Transverse T2 weighted image (1600/90). The mass lesion (*arrow*) has a similar signal intensity to that of urine in the bladder. The mass was surgically resected. (From Schmedtje JF, Sax S, Pool JL, Goldfarb RA, Nelson EB. Localization of ectopic pheochromocytomas by magnetic resonance imaging. Am J Med 1987; 83:770–772.)

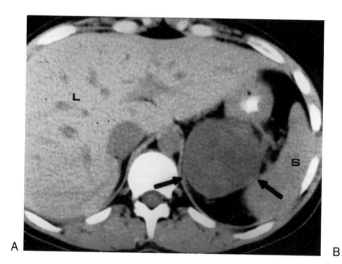

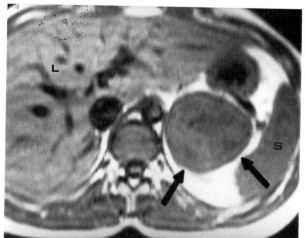

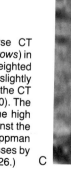

Figure 22–30. *Adrenocortical carcinoma.* ***A,*** Transverse CT scan demonstrates a large, well-defined soft tissue mass (*arrows*) in the region of the left adrenal gland. S, Spleen; L, liver. ***B,*** T1 weighted MR image (300/26). The mass lesion is of signal intensity slightly below that of liver. It is well defined and seen as well as on the CT image. L, Liver; S, spleen. ***C,*** T2 weighted MR image (250/80). The mass has a very high signal intensity. It is believed that the high signal intensity on the T2 image is suggestive evidence against the presence of a benign hyperfunctioning adenoma. (From Doppman JL, Reinig JW, Dwyer AJ, et al. Differentiation of adrenal masses by magnetic resonance imaging. Surgery 1987; 102:1018–1026.)

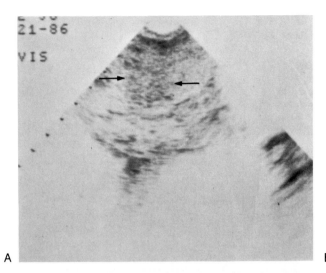

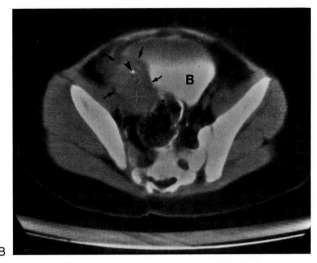

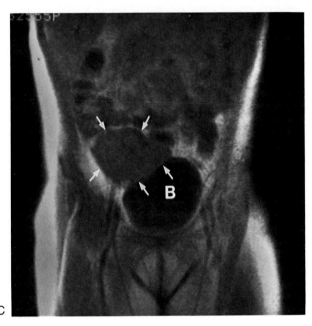

Figure 22–31. *Ovarian hemangioma in a teen-age girl with known renal anomalies.* **A,** Ultrasound shows a poorly defined moderately echogenic mass (*arrows*) in the pelvis. **B,** CT scan shows a soft tissue mass (*arrows*) on the right side of the pelvis, in the location of the right ovary. The mass is predominantly of soft tissue intensity. A small focus of calcium (*arrowhead*) is identified. The mass is indenting the bladder (B). **C,** Coronal T1 weighted MR image (550/32). The margins of the mass lesion (*arrows*) are better defined than with either CT or ultrasound. The mass is of nonspecific appearance with intensity similar to that of muscle. The calcium seen on the CT scan cannot be identified. The mass is seen to be indenting the bladder (B). There are no specific features on any of the images to suggest the actual diagnosis. All three modalities show the mass lesion. MRI misses calcification but defines the margins of the lesion well.

ing modalities are negative. There is a reduction in the normal high signal intensity of the testis on T2 weighted images (Fig. 22–38).

Lymphoma

Both Hodgkin's and non-Hodgkin's lymphoma are relatively common pediatric tumors. Pathologically, Hodgkin's disease is characterized by the identification of Reed-Sternberg cells. Hodgkin's disease is classified into four histologic types:[29, 30] in order of worsening prognosis, these are lymphocyte dominant, nodular sclerosing, mixed cell, and lymphocyte depleted. In children, lymphocyte dominant and nodular sclerosing are by far the most common types. Lymphocyte dominant is characterized by the presence of abundant nor-

mal lymphocytes. The tumor may be diffuse or nodular. Systemic symptoms are present in less than 10 percent of these children. One characteristic of nodular sclerosing disease is that the mediastinal lymph nodes are invariably involved. In Hodgkin's disease the spread is always predictable and is via contiguous node groups. Several pathologic features help in further evaluation of the disorder.[31] For example, the liver and bone marrow are never positive unless the spleen is positive for disease. If pulmonary disease is present, there is always involvement of the hilar lymph nodes. Pleural effusions do not necessarily indicate pleural disease and are due to lymphatic obstruction. Pericardial effusions always indicate direct invasion of the pericardium by tumor.

The pathologic classification of non-Hodgkin's lymphoma is very confused; there are several good re-

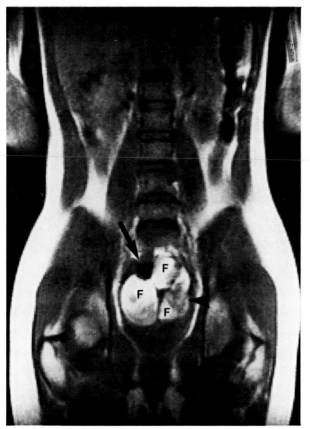

Figure 22–32. *Ovarian teratoma.* Coronal T1 weighted image (500/30). There is a mass lesion anterior to the sacrum. High-intensity areas (F) correspond to the fatty components of the tumor. Moderate-intensity areas correspond to the soft tissue component of the tumor (*arrowhead*). Very-low-intensity areas correspond to densely calcified teeth (*arrow*).

views.[32, 33] Many different classifications have been suggested. Many of the older classifications based only on cell type are now outdated.[32] It is fashionable now to use a more complex classification system based on degree of cell differentiation, distribution of disease in the nodes, size of pathologic cells, cell type, and biologic and cytologic markers. The most widely used classification at the present time is the Working Formulation.[32] From an imaging point of view, the classification is not of great importance.

Clinical presentation of non-Hodgkin's lymphoma is extremely varied and includes enlarged lymph nodes, generalized illness, weight loss and anemia, and focal symptoms referable to almost any organ system. The presentation of Hodgkin's disease is less varied. A common finding is the identification of painless enlarged nodes, frequently in the neck, axilla, or femoral and inguinal regions. Sometimes lymphadenopathy is detected as an incidental finding on chest radiograph. Some patients do present with systemic symptoms, including weight loss, night sweats, pleuritis, and fever.[29]

Hodgkin's disease is classified as follows:
1. Stage I involves one lymph node region.
2. Stage II involves two or more node regions on the same side of the diaphragm, with or without localized disease in one extralymphatic organ.
3. Stage III involves lymph nodes on both sides of the diaphragm, with or without splenic involvement and with or without localized disease in another organ.
4. Stage IV is diffuse disseminated disease involving multiple organs and lymph nodes.

MRI can successfully evaluate many different aspects of lymphomas. These are discussed below.

IDENTIFICATION OF DISEASE. Both Hodgkin's and non-Hodgkin's lymphomas can be well identified by MRI. In one study MRI was able to identify all sites of pathology seen on CT scans in ten of ten children.[34] In this study both modalities missed small positive abdominal lymph nodes. In the mediastinum, enlarged diseased lymph nodes are well defined because of adjacent low-intensity signal from lung and major vessels. In the abdomen, demarcation between fluid or feces in the bowel and pathologic nodes is often not clearly defined. Differentiation of diseased nodes from adjacent organs such as liver, spleen, pancreas, and kidneys is usually very good. Lymphoma can be identified in almost any tissue or organ, including abdominal organs, chest, and bone (Figs. 22–39, 22–40).

LOCAL EFFECTS OF TUMOR. Displacement of vessels by enlarged nodes is well identified (Fig. 22–41).[34] Tracheal narrowing from extrinsic node compression can also be well identified.

FLUID COLLECTIONS. Malignant fluid collections are not uncommon in patients with lymphoma. Ascites and pericardial and pleural effusions are easily identified as regions of very prolonged T1 and T2 relaxation times. It usually is not possible on MRI to differentiate malignant from nonmalignant effusions.

TUMOR INTENSITY. Most lymphomas have long T1 and T2 relaxation times compared with liver, muscle, and normal lymph nodes. However, the appearance of the tumors is not very specific; measurements of T1 and T2 relaxation time cannot always differentiate lymphoma from other disorders (Fig. 22–42) and cannot distinguish between the various histologic subtypes of lymphoma.[34, 35]

SPLEEN AND LIVER INVOLVEMENT IN HODGKIN'S DISEASE. Clinical and other imaging methods are notoriously unreliable for detection of disease in the liver and spleen. For example, identification of splenomegaly carries only a 36 percent sensitivity and a 61 percent specificity for lymphoma.[36] The accuracy of ultrasonography and CT is only between 60 and 75 percent.[36] In another study, ultrasonography and CT were reported as being able to diagnose only one-third of lymphoma in the liver and spleen.[37] There are a number of reports of identification of splenic and liver disease involvement with Hodgkin's disease.[34, 36, 38] At the present time it is probably fair to say that normal MR results do not completely exclude the presence of

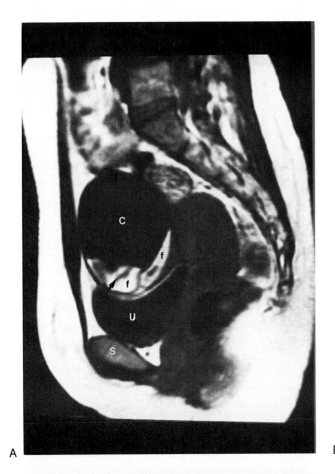

A

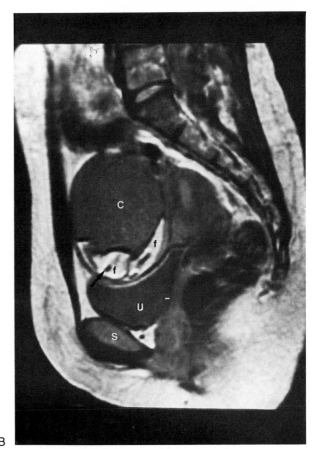

B

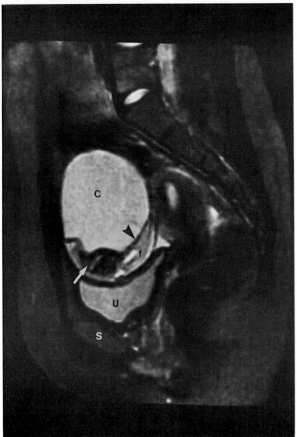

C

Figure 22–33. *Ovarian teratoma in a 16-year-old girl.* **A** to **C,** Three sagittal images of the pelvis with T1 (600/25), spin-density (200/20) and T2 (2000/60) weighting, respectively. Filling most of the pelvis is a very large mass lesion with several clearly defined components. The fluid in the cystic (C) component of the tumor appears black on the T1 weighted image, gray on the spin-density image, and of high signal intensity on the T2 weighted image. The fatty component of the tumor (f) appears of strong signal intensity on all pulse sequences. The calcified component (*arrow*) of the tumor appears of low signal intensity on all pulse sequences. Note the marked chemical shift artifact (*arrowheads*) at the interface of fluid and fat. S, Symphysis pubis; U, urine in the bladder. (From Togashi K, Nishimura K, Itoh K, et al. Ovarian cystic teratomas: MR imaging. Radiology 1987; 162:669–673.)

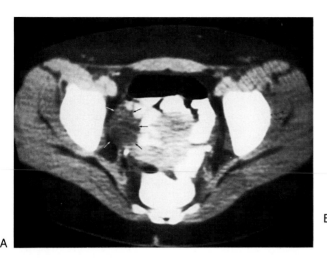

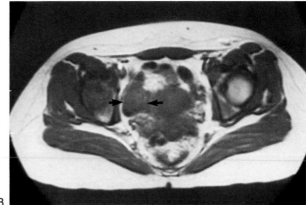

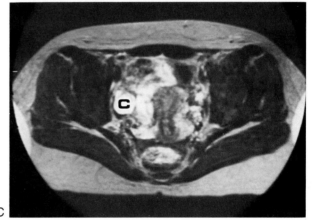

Figure 22–34. *Ovarian cyst in a 14-year-old girl with pelvic pain.* ***A,*** CT scan demonstrates a low-intensity mass lesion (*arrows*) in the region of the right ovary. ***B,*** Transverse pelvic MR image (850/26) also shows a mass lesion (arrows). On this pulse sequence the lesion is of similar intensity to that of adjacent bowel loops, from which it cannot be clearly differentiated. ***C,*** T2 weighted image (2000/90) shows a well-defined mass (C) of very strong signal intensity. The margins are better seen than in ***A*** or ***B.*** Some high-signal-intensity fluid is seen in the bowel loops, but shape and contour are very different from those of the ovarian cyst. At surgery a simple ovarian cyst was excised.

tumor in the liver or spleen.[39] The sensitivity and specificity of MRI may well continue to improve with further refinements in imaging techniques, including improvement of image quality due to improved motion suppression techniques, and the use of selective contrast agents. In one study the detection of splenic involvement with lymphoma was greatly improved with the use of superparamagnetic iron as a contrast agent.[36] This agent turns normal spleen of low intensity in all pulse sequences as it is taken up by reticuloendothelial cells. Lymphomatous spleens either have macrophages replaced by tumor or have the activity of these cells suppressed by the tumor. Lymphoma shows up as increased signal compared with the low-intensity background. In this study precontrast MRI was positive in four of eight patients and postcontrast in eight of eight.

MONITORING THERAPY   (Fig. 22–40). Some reports have described the changes in lymphoma with therapy. In two patients a decrease in size of the tumor mass was associated with increasing intensity of the tumor on T1 weighted images;[34] in a third patient in whom the tumor size did not decrease, there was no change in signal intensity. A persistent mediastinal mass after therapy for Hodgkin's disease is not uncommon. In 17 patients a low signal intensity in residual mediastinal tissue on T2 images suggested the diagnosis of residual fibrotic tumor matrix and the absence of tumor activity.[40] In another report by the same workers, 18 patients with mediastinal Hodgkin's disease all showed decreasing T2 relaxation time and signal intensity on T2 images after therapy.[41] The percentage decrease in tumor size correlated with the decrease in signal intensity ratios between the tumor and fat and also between the tumor and muscle. These workers did not find a change in T1 relaxation time with therapy. Much work still needs to be done on further evaluating the role of MRI in monitoring therapy, but this may provide a unique role for MRI.[42] For example, residual mediastinal masses were seen in as many as 80 percent of Hodgkin's patients following therapy, and although most of these lesions are benign, relapse is twice as likely in these patients as in patients with no residual mass.[42] Webb believes that we cannot dogmatically equate low signal with fibrosis at the present time.[42]

Text continues on page 758.

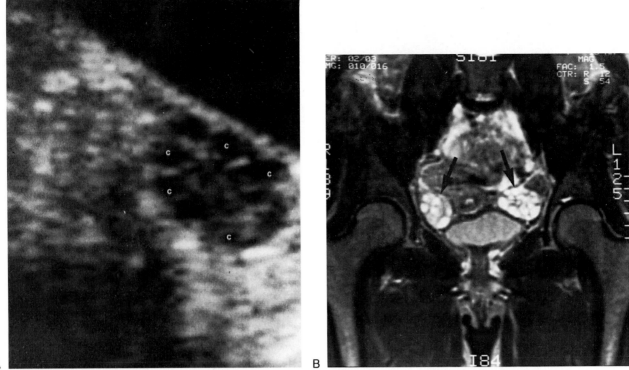

A   B

Figure 22–35. *Polycystic ovaries (Stein-Leventhal syndrome) in a 20-year-old woman with oligomenorrhea.* **A,** Longitudinal sonogram of the right ovary. There are multiple small peripheral cysts (c). **B,** Coronal T2 MR image (2000/70). Both ovaries (*arrows*) are well seen and enlarged. Throughout both of the ovaries there are multiple high-intensity cysts, all less than 1 cm in diameter. (From Mitchell DG, Gefter WB, Spritzer CE, et al. Polycystic ovaries: MR imaging. Radiology 1986; 160:425–429.)

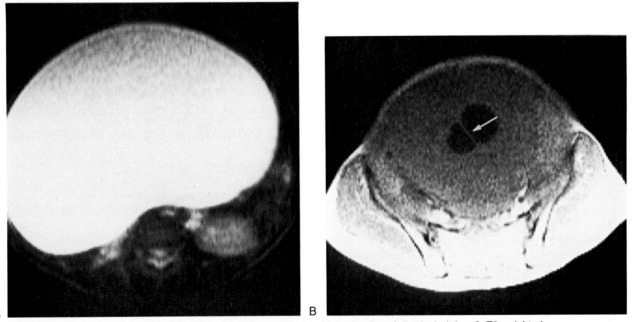

A   B

Figure 22–36. *Ovarian cyst adenocarcinoma in a 13-year-old girl with increasing abdominal girth.* **A,** T2 weighted image (2000/60) shows a giant abdominal mass of very strong signal. At this level the mass appears as a simple cyst. **B,** T1 weighted image (500/30). At this level the giant mass is predominantly a single large cyst and a small bilobed daughter cyst within it. The septa (*arrow*) contain the malignant soft tissue component of this predominantly cystic tumor.

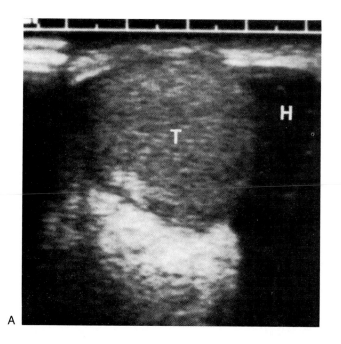

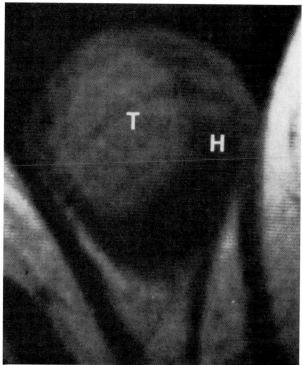

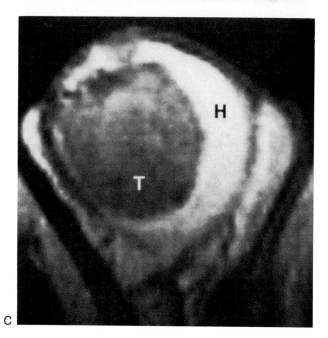

Figure 22–37. *Leydig cell tumor of the testis in a 5-year-old boy.* ***A,*** Ultrasound shows a hydrocele (H). The testis (T) was thought to be a little large for the patient's age, but the echo pattern is normal and no focal abnormality is identified. ***B,*** T1 weighted MR image (500/40). The testis (T) appears enlarged. The hydrocele (H) is of low signal intensity. ***C,*** T2 weighted image (2000/80). The hydrocele (H) is of strong signal intensity. The testis (T) is of much lower signal intensity than normal and shows a very nonhomogeneous pattern. The entire testis was found to be infiltrated with tumor. (From Thurnher S, Hricak H, Carroll PR, et al. Imaging the testis: comparison between MR imaging and US. Radiology 1988; 167:631–636.)

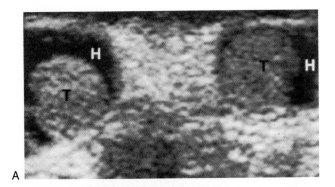

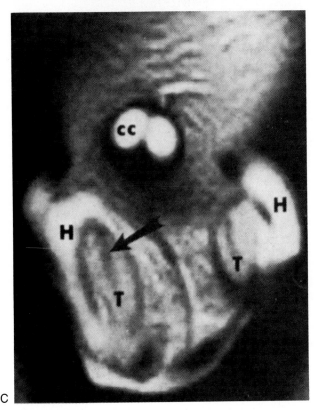

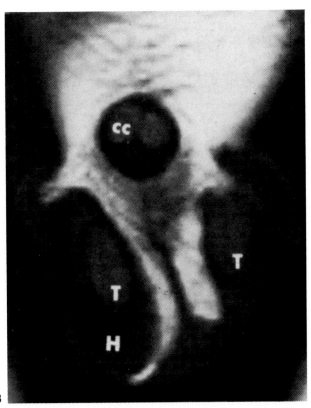

Figure 22–38. *Lymphocytic leukemia.* ***A,*** Transverse sonogram through the scrotum shows both testes (T) surrounded by hydroceles (H). The testes appear normal. ***B,*** T1 weighted MR image (500/40). The signal intensity from the testes (T) is similar to that of the corpus cavernosum (CC). The hydrocele (H) is of low intensity. ***C,*** T2 weighted image (2000/120). The corpora cavernosa (CC) and the hydroceles (H) appear of high signal intensity. The testes (T), which normally also have a very high signal intensity, show a reduction in signal intensity compared with the corpus cavernosum and subcutaneous fat. This is consistent with diffuse leukemic infiltration of the testes. The arrow points to the mediastinum testis. (Thurnher S, Hricak H, Carroll PR, et al. Imaging the testis: comparison between MR imaging and US. Radiology 1988; 167:631–636.)

Cystic Hygroma

These are benign lymphatic tumors that usually are seen in the neck, but can occur at almost any site. They are predominantly cystic and usually show a low internal soft tissue network. Because the internal fluid may be of high protein content, it can appear of strong signal intensity on T1 images. When the protein content is low, signal intensity is low on T1 weighted images. Signal intensity is always high on T2 weighted images. MRI is very helpful for the planning of surgery because it identifies the full extent of the lesions very well (Fig. 22–43).

INFECTION

Infections of most of the endocrine glands are uncommon.

Tubo-ovarian Abscess

Ovarian infection is usually a tubo-ovarian abscess. This has a very inhomogeneous appearance that is nonspecific. There is a mass lesion in the pelvis with low signal intensity on T1 weighted images and bright signal on T2 weighted images; there may a thick rim to the lesion or internal septations.[43]

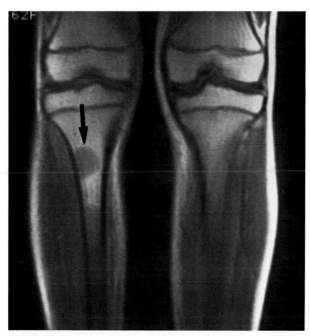

Figure 22–39. *Burkitt's lymphoma with bone involvement in a 13-year-old boy who presented with knee pain.* Spin-density coronal MR image (2000/32). Normal bone marrow appears of strong signal intensity. A well-defined focal mass lesion (*arrow*) is seen localized to the bone marrow of the right proximal tibia. Bone cortex and the overlying soft tissue appear normal. The appearance of the lesion is nonspecific but biopsy was positive for Burkitt's lymphoma. Subsequent investigation also identified enlarged abdominal lymph nodes.

Epididymo-orchitis

Acute epididymitis is the most common intrascrotal infection.[28] It may be diffuse or focal. MRI shows evidence of prolongation of the T2 and T1 relaxation times with increased signal of the epididymis, compared with normal on T2 weighted images. The epididymis is also seen to be swollen. The infection may spread to involve the testis, which is seen as a reduction of the normal very high signal in the testis on T2 weighted images. In two patients MRI proved much more sensitive than ultrasonography in identifying testicular inflammation, which suggests that MRI may have an important role to play in the evaluation of these patients. Testicular inflammation may progress to formation of an abscess. With testicular inflammation the sharp definition of the tunica albuginea is lost. With acute inflammation of both testis and epididymis, several secondary signs may be identified. The scrotal wall may be thickened, and the low-signal-intensity vascular venous plexuses around this spermatic cord may be more prominent, reflecting increased blood flow to the infected area. Enlargement of local lymph nodes may also be identified.

Lymph Nodes

Lymph nodes are often infected following infection of adjacent tissues. Infected lymph nodes may or may not be enlarged. Signal intensity is increased on T2 weighted images compared with normal nodes (Fig. 22–44). The appearance is nonspecific and there are no reports of MRI being able to differentiate tumor from inflammation of lymph nodes; MRI cannot define the causative organism of infected lymph nodes.

VASCULAR DISORDERS: ADRENAL HEMORRHAGE

The diagnosis of adrenal hemorrhage is usually made on the basis of the clinical presentation (Fig. 22–45).[44,45] Clinical signs include palpation of an abdominal mass, jaundice, and anemia. The clinical findings together with the ultrasonographic appearance are usually adequate to make the diagnosis. Ultrasonography shows a low- or mixed-intensity mass lesion in the region of the adrenal gland. Occasionally the distinction between an echogenic adrenal hemorrhage and neuroblastoma cannot be made with certainty by ultrasonography on initial presentation. After a period of 2 to 3 weeks the hemorrhage shrinks, whereas a neuroblastoma does not; serum catecholamine concentrations are elevated only in neuroblastoma. In most patients no treatment is required for adrenal hemorrhage, and spontaneous complete resolution usually occurs within a couple of months. Some residual calcification may or may not be present. In a number of patients adrenal hemorrhage is complicated by renal vein thrombosis, which can extend into the inferior vena cava. The role of MRI in the evaluation of adrenal hemorrhage may be in those individuals in whom there is difficulty in differentiating the hemorrhage from a neuroblastoma, or in confirming the diagnosis of renal vein thrombosis.

On MRI the hemorrhage within the adrenal gland is identified by the presence of a mass lesion, which usually retains the triangular shape of the adrenal gland. This is very helpful in differentiating the hemorrhage from nonadrenal lesions. Because of the presence of subacute blood containing methemoglobin, the hemorrhage appears of very strong signal intensity on T1 and T2 weighted pulse sequences. This is a fairly characteristic appearance and allows accurate differentiation of an adrenal hemorrhage from a neuroblastoma. Hemorrhagic cysts in the region can be distinguished by virtue of the fact that they do not conform to the contour of the adrenal gland. Complicating renal vein or vena caval thrombosis is seen as a linear strong signal in the region where the vessel should be, which persists on multiple pulse sequences in different planes. Associated renal vein thrombosis is seen as enlargement of the kidney with loss of corticomedullary differentiation and a very irregular signal.

Text continues on page 764.

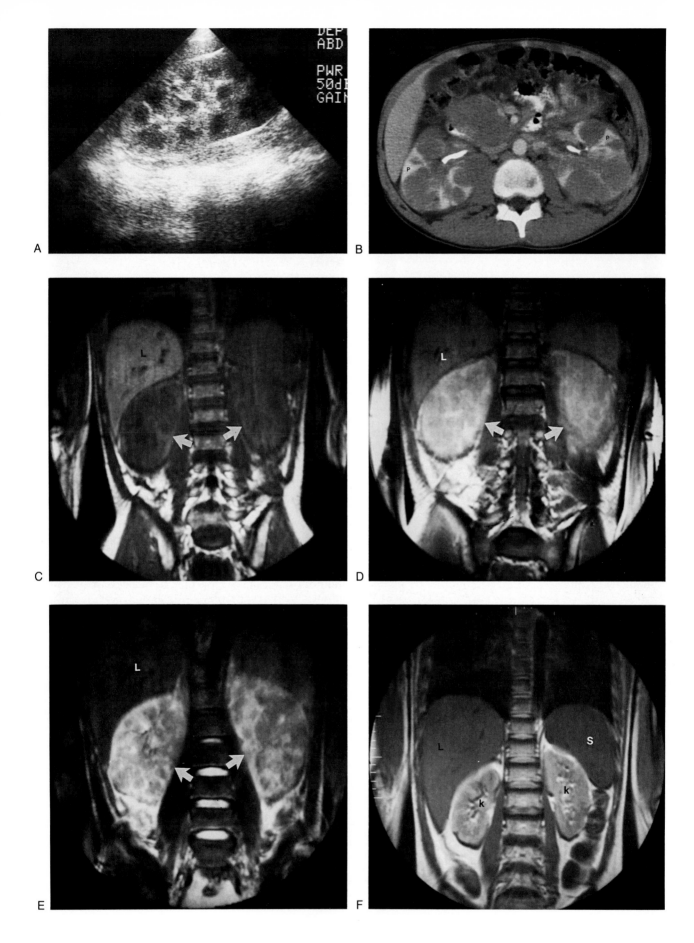

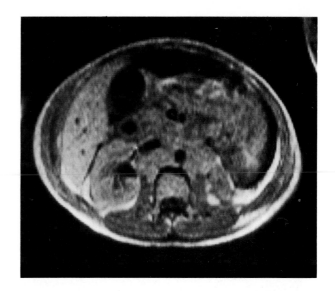

Figure 22–41. *Non-Hodgkin's lymphoma in a 13-year-old girl with weight loss and fatigue.* Transverse T1 weighted MR image (500/30). Massive retroperitoneal lymphadenopathy is identified.

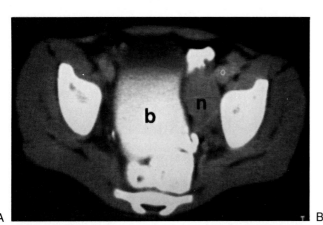

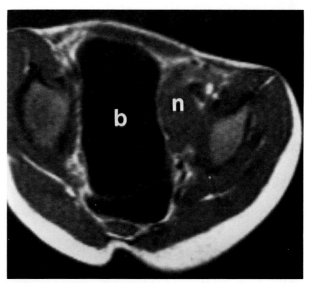

A   B

Figure 22–42. *Lymph node metastases in a 6-year-old boy with known thigh soft tissue malignancy.* **A,** Transverse CT scan. There is a soft tissue lymph node mass (n) in the left pelvis, indenting the bladder (b). **B,** Transverse pelvic MR image (500/30). The appearance is similar to the CT scan. An enlarged node mass (n) is seen to indent the bladder (b). Signal intensity is similar to that of muscle. Both modalities identify the mass well. In neither case is the appearance specific for lymph nodes or tumor.

◀ **Figure 22–40.** *Burkitt's lymphoma with renal involvement in a 13-year-old boy who presented with intussusception due to tumor involvement of mesenteric lymph nodes.* **A,** Longitudinal ultrasound image of the right kidney shows multiple low-echogenicity tumor nodules. **B,** Transverse CT scan after bolus injection of intravenous contrast material. Most of the kidneys are replaced by low-intensity tumor nodules. A small amount of normal-functioning renal parenchyma (P) shows enhancement after contrast injection. **C** to **E,** Three coronal MR images obtained with T1 (500/16), spin-density (2000/20), and T2 (2000/70) weighting, respectively. Both the kidneys (*arrows*) are enlarged. Diffuse abnormality is seen throughout both kidneys with complete lack of corticomedullary differentiation. The renal outlines are smooth. The tumor nodules are particularly ill defined on the T1 weighted images, where they are of slightly lower intensity than more normal kidney. They are best defined in **E,** where they appear of lower signal intensity than normal kidney. L, Liver. **F,** Coronal MR T1 weighted image (500/16) obtained after 3 months of chemotherapy shows both kidneys (k) to be of very normal appearance. S, spleen.

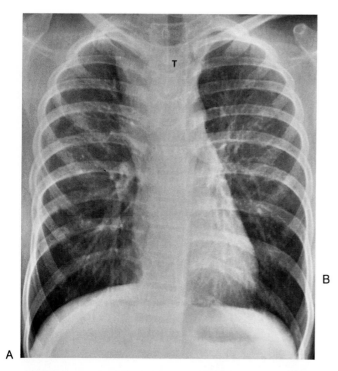

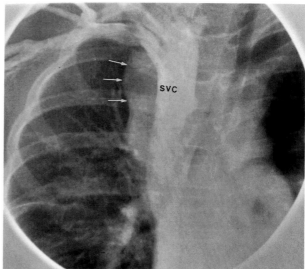

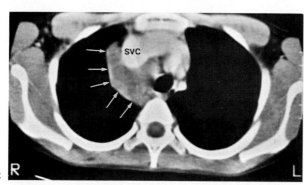

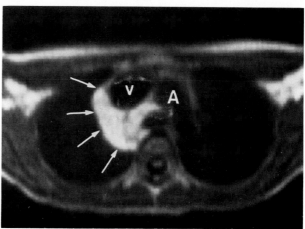

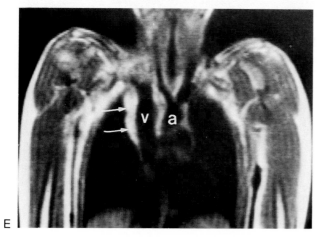

Figure 22–43. *Cystic hygroma (lymphangioma) in a 9-year-old girl who presented with a mediastinal mass. She had had a neck cystic hygroma resected in infancy.* **A,** Chest x-ray shows a right upper mediastinal mass displacing the trachea (T) to the left. **B,** Venogram. The superior vena cava (SVC) is opacified. A soft tissue density mass (*arrows*) is seen lying to the right of the cava. **C,** Transverse CT scan following after injection of contrast medium. There is a mass lesion (*arrows*) lying lateral, posterior, and medial to the superior vena cava (SVC). There are no specific features to suggest the correct diagnosis. The mass is of soft tissue intensity and not fluid. **D, E,** Transverse and coronal T1 weighted MR images (500/30). The mass lesion (*arrows*) is seen as a very sharply defined homogeneous lesion of strong signal intensity. The distribution of the mass is similar to that seen on CT. The coronal image, however, emphasizes the extension of the mass between the superior vena cava (v) and the ascending aorta (A in **D,** a in **E**), which was helpful to the surgeon. The strong signal intensity on the T1 MR images indicates that the mass represents hemorrhage, fat, or mucoid fluid. In the absence of a history of trauma, and because of the uniformity, hemorrhage is unlikely. The CT scan is helpful in indicating that the mass is not fat. With this information, the MR appearance is fairly characteristic of a cystic hygroma.

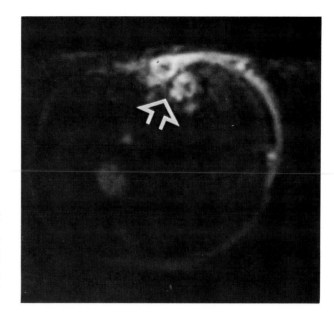

Figure 22–44. *Cat-scratch disease with lymph node involvement in a 16-year-old boy with enlarged epitrochlear lymph nodes.* Transverse T2 MR image (2000/80) through the distal arm shows multiple enlarged lymph nodes (*arrow*) seen as areas of very strong signal intensity. There is a small area of low intensity in the center of two of the larger nodes. The histologic appearance of the nodes was consistent with cat-scratch disease. The etiology of the low-intensity center of two of the nodes is not clear.

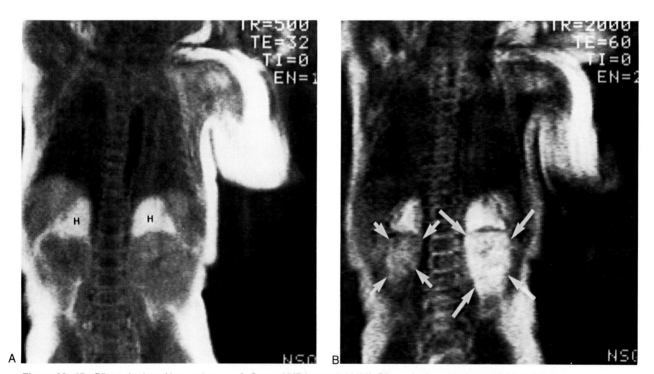

Figure 22–45. *Bilateral adrenal hemorrhage.*   ***A,*** Coronal MR image (500/32). Bilateral adrenal lesions with high signal intensity due to hemorrhage (H). ***B,*** T2 weighted MR image (2000/60) shows an enlarged left kidney (*large arrows*) with a strong signal due to renal vein thrombosis, and a normal right kidney (*small arrows*). The signal intensity from adrenal hemorrhage is still strong. (From Koch KJ, Cory DA. Simultaneous renal vein thrombosis and bilateral adrenal hemorrhage: MR demonstration. J Comput Assist Tomogr 1986; 10:681–684.)

Occasionally, adrenal hemorrhage can be bilateral, and MRI in one case proved extremely accurate in identifying this problem.[44]

In two patients in follow-up studies performed 7, 13, and 24 days after birth, MRI showed rapid improvement with reduction in size of the hemorrhage and reduction in the strong signal intensity on T1 images.[45]

REFERENCES

1. McCarthy S. MRI offers first look into pelvic anatomy. Diag Imag 1987; Aug:100–106.
2. Heiken JP, Lee JKT. MR imaging of the pelvis. Radiology 1988; 166:11–16.
3. Baker LL, Hajek PC, Burkhard TK, et al. MR imaging of the scrotum: normal anatomy. Radiology 1987; 163:89–92.
4. Egglin Tk, Hahn PF, Stark DD. MRI of the adrenal glands. Semin Roentgenol 1988; 23:280–287.
5. Glazer GM. MR imaging of the liver, kidneys, and adrenal glands. Radiology 1988; 166:303–312.
6. Stark DD, Moss AA, Gamsu G, et al. Magnetic resonance imaging of the neck. Part I. Normal anatomy. Radiology 1984; 150:447–454.
7. Stark DD, Clark OH, Moss AA. Magnetic resonance imaging of the thyroid, thymus and parathyroid glands. Surgery 1984; 96:1083–1091.
8. Higgins CB, Aufferman W. MR imaging of thyroid and parathyroid glands: a review of current status. AJR 1988; 151:1095–1106.
9. Baker LL, Hajek PC, Burkhard TK, Mattrey RF. Polyorchidism: evaluation by MR. AJR 1987; 148:305–306.
10. Dietrich RB, Kangarloo H. Pelvic abnormalities in children: assessment with MR imaging. Radiology 1987; 163:367–372.
11. Friedland GW, Chang P. The role of imaging in the management of the impalpable undescended testis. AJR 1988; 151:1107–1111.
12. Kier R, McCarthy S, Rosenfield AT, et al. Nonpalpable testes in young boys: evaluation with MR imaging. Radiology 1988; 169:429–433.
13. Fritzsche PJ, Hricak H, Kogan BA, et al. Undescended testis: value of MR imaging. Radiology 1987; 164:169–173.
14. Landa HM, Gylys-Morin V, Mattrey RF, et al. Detection of testicular torsion by magnetic resonance imaging in a rat model. J Urol 1988; 140:1178–1180.
15. Kier R, Blinder RA, Herfkens RJ, et al. MR imaging with surface coils in primary hyperparathyroidism. J Comput Assist Tomogr 1987; 11:863–868.
16. Ziegelbaum MM, Kay R, Rothner D, Lorig R. The association of neuroblastoma with myoclonic encephalopathy of infants: the use of magnetic resonance as an imaging modality. J Urol 1988; 139:81–82.
17. Cohen MD, Weetman R, Provisor A, et al. Magnetic resonance imaging of neuroblastoma with a 0.15-T magnet. AJR 1984; 143:1241–1248.
18. Fletcher BD, Kopiwoda SY, Strandjord SE, et al. Abdominal neuroblastoma: magnetic resonance imaging and tissue characterization. Radiology 1985; 155:699–703.
19. Dietrich RB, Kangarloo H, Lanarsky C, Feig SA. Neuroblastoma: the role of MR imaging. AJR 1987; 148:937–942.
20. Casselman JW, Smet MH, Van Damme B, Lemahieu SF. Primary cervical neuroblastoma: CT and MR findings. J Comput Assist Tomogr 1988; 12:684–686.
21. Rosenfield NS, Leonidas JC, Barwick KW. Aggressive neuroblastoma simulating Wilms' tumor. Radiology 1988; 166:165–167.
22. Miraldi FD, Nelson AD, Kraly C, et al. Diagnostic imaging of human neuroblastoma with radiolabeled antibody. Radiology 1986; 161:413–418.
23. Doppman JL, Reinig JW, Dwyer AJ, et al. Differentiation of adrenal masses by magnetic resonance imaging. Surgery 1987; 6:1018–1026.
24. Chezmar JL, Robbins SM, Nelson RC, et al. Adrenal masses: characterization with T1-weighted MR imaging. Radiology 1988; 166:357–359.
25. Chang A, Glazer HS, Lee JKT, et al. Adrenal gland: MR imaging. Radiology 1987; 163:123–128.
26. Togashi K, Nishimura K, Itoh K, et al. Ovarian cystic teratomas: MR imaging. Radiology 1987; 162:669–673.
27. Thurnher S, Hricak H, Carroll PR, et al. Imaging the testis: comparison between MR imaging and US. Radiology 1988; 167:631–636.
28. Baker LL, Hajek PC, Burkhard TK, et al. MR imaging of the scrotum: pathologic conditions. Radiology 1987; 163:93–98.
29. Hoppe RT. The contemporary management of Hodgkin disease. Radiology 1988; 169:297–304.
30. Castellino RA. Hodgkin disease: practical concepts for the diagnostic radiologist. Radiology 1986; 159:305–310.
31. Cohen MD, Siddiqui A, Weetman R, et al. Hodgkin disease and non-Hodgkin lymphomas in children: utilization of radiological modalities. Radiology 1986; 158:499–505.
32. Wang Y. Classification of non-Hodgkin's lymphoma. AJR 1986; 147:205–208.
33. Bragg DG, Colby TV, Ward JH. New concepts in the non-Hodgkin lymphomas: radiologic implications. Radiology 1986; 159:289–304.
34. Cohen MD, Klatte EC, Smith JA, et al. Magnetic resonance imaging of lymphomas in children. Pediatr Radiol 1985; 15:179–183.
35. Nyman R, Rehn S, Glimelius B, et al. Magnetic resonance imaging, chest radiography, computed tomography and ultrasonography in malignant lymphoma. Acta Radiol 1987; 28:253–262.
36. Weissleder R, Elizondo G, Stark DD, et al. The diagnosis of splenic lymphoma by MR imaging: value of superparamagnetic iron oxide. AJR 1989; 152:175–180.
37. Nyman R, Rhen S, Ericsson A, et al. An attempt to characterize malignant lymphoma in spleen, liver and lymph nodes with magnetic resonance imaging. Acta Radiol 1987; 28:527–533.
38. Richards MA, Webb JAW, Reznek RH, et al. Detection of spread of malignant lymphoma to the liver by low field strength magnetic resonance imaging. Br Med J 1986; 293:1126–1128.
39. Greco A, Jelliffe AM, Maher EJ, Leung AWL. MR imaging of lymphomas: impact on therapy. J Comput Assist Tomog 1988; 12:785–791.
40. Nyman R, Rehn S, Glimelius B, et al. Magnetic resonance imaging for assessment of treatment effects in mediastinal Hodgkin's disease. Acta Radiol 1987; 28:145–151.
41. Nyman RS, Rehn SM, Glimelius BLG, et al. Residual mediastinal masses in Hodgkin disease: prediction of size with MR imaging. Radiology 1989; 170:435–440.
42. Webb WR. MR imaging of treated mediastinal Hodgkin disease. Radiology 1989; 170:315–316.
43. Fishman-Javitt MC, Lovecchio JL, Stein, HL. Imaging strategies for MRI of the pelvis. Radiol Clin North Am 1988; 26:633–651.
44. Koch KJ, Cory DA. Simultaneous renal vein thrombosis and bilateral adrenal hemorrhage: MR demonstration. J Comput Assist Tomogr 1986; 10:681–683.
45. Brill PW, Jagannath A, Winchester P, et al. Adrenal hemorrhage and renal vein thrombosis in the newborn: MR imaging. Radiology 1989; 170:95–98.

Primary Disorders
of Bone Marrow

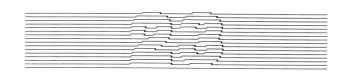

SHEILA G. MOORE, M.D.
GUY H. SEBAG, Med. Doc.

Before the introduction of magnetic resonance imaging (MRI), the radiologist had limited methods of imaging bone marrow. Conventional radiography is relatively insensitive to changes in the bone marrow and requires a loss of trabecular bone before a marrow abnormality can be suspected or detected. Computed tomographic (CT) images of the marrow and CT measured Hounsfield unit values vary depending on the relative amounts of fatty marrow, hematopoietic marrow, and intramedullary trabecular bone. Attenuation of the x-ray beam is greatest in regions with a large amount of trabecular bone (metaphysis, epiphysis, vertebra, and flat bones). When the Hounsfield unit values of the marrow are measured on CT, diaphyseal yellow marrow normally measures -100 HU, while Hounsfield unit values in the metaphyseal and epiphyseal regions are generally positive and approach 100 HU.[1] However, one cannot distinguish hematopoietic marrow from fatty marrow on CT, and recognition of a marrow abnormality can be achieved only with symmetric positioning and meticulous comparison of a marrow abnormality with the normal marrow of the contralateral side. When the marrow from each side is measured and compared, a difference of 20 HU is considered abnormal.[2] Tc-99m diphosphonate radionuclide bone scan reflects bone remodeling and changes in blood flow and metabolism; it images bone cortex primarily. Diffuse marrow disorders such as leukemia, lymphoma, and aggressive tumors often are not appreciated. Tc-99m scintigraphy provides a sensitive physiologic survey of the entire bony skeleton, but there is a lack of specificity and anatomic detail, and no direct evaluation of marrow.

Tc-99m sulfur colloid has also been used to study bone marrow. This colloid is taken up by normal reticuloendothelial cells within the marrow. Replacement of normal marrow by metastases, for example, results in reduction of the uptake of sulfur colloid. Although this technique is sensitive for detection of metastases in tumors such as neuroblastoma, its use has not been widely evaluated in other disorders such as infection or marrow edema.

More precise evaluation of the marrow is now possible with MRI. MR imaging of bone marrow provides excellent spatial resolution and anatomic detail, and for the first time allows visualization and distinction of both hematopoietic (red) and fatty (yellow) marrow. Differences in proton density and T1 and T2 relaxation times allow delineation of pathologic processes on spin-echo MR images. New sequences such as chemical shift and gradient-echo imaging exploit bone marrow chemical shift and magnetic susceptibility as additional parameters of image contrast.

NORMAL BONE ANATOMY, PHYSIOLOGY, AND MR APPEARANCE

It is not the intention of this chapter to provide a comprehensive atlas of normal bone anatomy as depicted by MRI. There are several excellent articles correlating anatomic specimens with MR images.[3–12] However, the normal anatomic distribution of hemopoietic and fatty bone marrow, together with age-related changes in distribution, will be described in detail.

Structure and Function of Marrow

The structure and function of bone marrow have been topics of intense study[13–25] since the first description of blood cell production in the marrow by Neumann in 1868.[2, 26] The bone marrow is the fourth largest organ in the body by weight after bone, muscle, and fat. Active hematopoiesis in the marrow supplies and regulates circulating concentrations of red cells, white cells, and platelet cells that meet the body's demand for oxygenation, immunity, and coagulation. The cell populations in marrow include hematopoietic stem cells, fat cells, and reticulum cells. These cellular elements lie within the cancellous bony matrix of primary and bridging secondary trabeculae, which make up the osseous component of marrow and provide architectural support for the hematopoietic, osteoid, and fatty marrow elements. The vascular anatomy of marrow is complex. In the spine the marrow is supplied primarily by the nutrient artery, which penetrates the medullary cavity on the posterior aspect of the vertebral body near the exit site of the basivertebral vein.[23] In the long bones the nutrient artery runs down the middle of the marrow spaces parallel to the long axis of the bone. The nutrient artery branches toward the endosteal surface of the cortex and coalesces with transosteal vessels (from the periosteum), which ultimately widen to form sinusoids in the endosteal aspect of the bone. This sinusoidal system is complex, branching, and significant as the site of primary hematopoiesis in the marrow.[24] The sinusoids drain into the central venous sinus of the medullary canal and exit through the nutrient foramen. The nerve fibers follow a course similar to those of the nutrient arteries.

In normal adult humans all the erythrocytes, granulocytes, and platelets that circulate in the peripheral blood are produced in the bone marrow. The total weight of erythrocytes and neutrophil granulocytes produced in a lifetime is much greater than the adult body weight. This level of production is possible only because pluripotent stem cells in the marrow are able to differentiate, mature, and amplify their cell numbers during the production of mature cells for release into the circulation. Hematopoiesis is maintained by the sequential activation and proliferation of small numbers of hematopoietic stem cells, which ultimately become exhausted and are replaced.[27] Normal bone marrow function is controlled by several factors, including the microenvironment provided to the hematopoietic cellular component by the marrow stromal cells. This includes fat cells, reticulum cells, fibroblasts, and endothelial cells.[25, 27] The fat cells of the marrow differ from those at other locations in the body in that they are smaller but metabolically similar. The bulk of the lipid in marrow fat cells is triacylglycerol,[27] which contains two distinct components that can be spectroscopically separated.[28] During periods of decreased hematopoiesis the fat cells increase in size and number, and during periods of increased hematopoiesis the fat cells atrophy. Reticulum cells, or macrophages, are found predominantly in hematopoietically active marrow, usually within focal islands of erythroid elements. Two major groups of reticulum cells have been identified, the activated macrophage and the undifferentiated nonphagocytic cell.[21, 25] Both are believed to be components of the marrow stroma.

MR Appearance of Yellow and Red Marrow

Yellow Marrow

MR images of the marrow are a reflection of the diverse components that make up the marrow. Fatty (yellow) marrow has a relatively short T1 relaxation time (approximate range 350 to 500 msec), since most of the fat protons are in the form of hydrophobic CH_2 groups and therefore have an efficient spin-lattice (T1) relaxation. Spin-spin relaxation of fat is less efficient, and consequently the T2 relaxation time is relatively longer than the T2 relaxation time of water.[29, 30] Fatty marrow has a signal intensity greater than that of muscle and similar to that of surrounding subcutaneous fat on T1 weighted spin-echo images. The signal decreases slightly on T2 weighted spin-echo images in concordance with the surrounding subcutaneous fat signal (Fig. 23–1).

Red Marrow

The signal characteristics of hematopoietic (red) marrow differ from those of fatty marrow. In hematopoietic marrow there is increased cellularity, protein, and water. The interaction of these components is complex and at the present time incompletely understood. Protein in general has a long T1 relaxation time owing to the large size of the molecules, while protein in solution causes a shortening of the T1 relaxation time of that solution. The amount of red marrow pro-

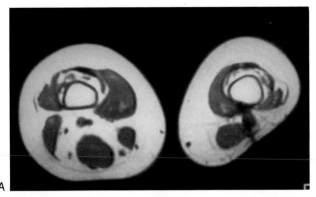
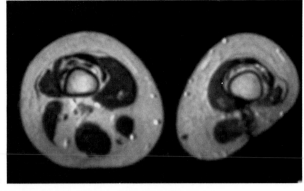

Figure 23–1. *Normal fatty marrow. Transverse images through the middle femora in a 19-year-old female with aggressive fibromatosis.* ***A, B,*** *T1 weighted (800/20) and T2 weighted (2050/80) images show high-signal-intensity fatty marrow. On the T2 image the decrease in signal intensity is commensurate with that of subcutaneous fat. Part of the patient's left thigh was resected as treatment for the aggressive fibromatosis.*

tein that is in solution and its fractional contribution to signal intensity are unclear.[2] The specific contribution of tissue water to the overall signal intensity of hematopoietic marrow is also incompletely understood. Tissue water is thought to exist in three basic states— bound, structural, and bulk, each with its own characteristic relaxation state.[2] Tissues rich in extracellular or free water have relatively longer T1 and T2 relaxation times, while those with greater amounts of intracellular or bound water have comparatively shorter T1 and T2 relaxation times.[29] The relative contribution of each of these components to the overall signal intensity of hematopoietic marrow is unclear; however, depending on the age of the child and the specific anatomic site (e.g., diaphysis of the long bone versus vertebral body), some component of the hematopoietic marrow signal will always be derived from fat. The short T1 and relatively long T2 relaxation times of fat are averaged with the long T1 and long T2 relaxation times of protein and water. Therefore, hematopoietic marrow has a signal intensity that on T1 weighted spin-echo images ranges from low intermediate signal intensity (less than muscle) in the newborn to increased signal intensity (greater than muscle) in the adolescent (Fig. 23–2). On T2 weighted images the signal intensity of hematopoietic marrow increases slightly.

Physiologic Conversion from Hematopoietic to Fatty Marrow

An understanding of the concept of red-to-yellow marrow conversion is central to the interpretation of MR images of the marrow in children. During fetal life, primary hematopoietic activity occurs first in the yolk sac and then, during the second trimester, in the liver and reticuloendothelial system. Hematopoietic activity in the fetal bone marrow begins at 16 to 20 weeks' gestation and continues to increase until birth, when hematopoietic tissue occupies the whole of the bone marrow.[27] Progressive conversion of this hematopoie-

tic marrow to fatty marrow is seen with age (Fig. 23–3). Conversion of hematopoietic to fatty marrow occurs at different rates for different bones and at different rates in the same bone. Conversion occurs first in the hands and feet, and then progressively from the distal to the proximal bones of the extremities. In addition to this distal-to-proximal trend for anatomic site, conversion also occurs at different rates within the same bone, so that marrow converts first in the diaphysis, then in the distal metaphysis, and finally in the proximal metaphysis.

In a landmark 1985 study, Kricun[31] compiled previously reported age-related anatomic data for the conversion of red to yellow marrow as determined by macroscopic examination of the marrow. There is completion of marrow conversion in the phalanges of the feet by 1 year, with microscopic changes of fatty marrow present in more proximal bones at this time. Macroscopic fat is detected in the midshaft of all long bones by 12 to 14 years. The conversion process continues until the adult pattern of macroscopic red marrow remaining in the vertebral bodies, sternum, ribs, pelvis, skull, and proximal shafts of the femora and humeri is reached by the age of 25 years (Fig. 23–4).[31] Microscopic red marrow may also remain in the distal metaphysis of the femora and humeri in adults, but in our experience red marrow is unlikely to be identified on the MR image unless it is macroscopic.[32]

MR Appearance of Marrow Conversion

Although the spectrum of red-to-yellow marrow conversion based on histologic data is known, work is only now being done to define the normal age-related spectrum of red to yellow marrow conversion as reflected on MRI. There is a general trend toward increased-signal-intensity fatty marrow on T1 weighted MR images being seen at an earlier age than would be expected from the anatomic data.[32]

SKULL. Little work has been done on the histologic analysis of marrow conversion in the bones of the skull and face, but it is known that the calvarium and all

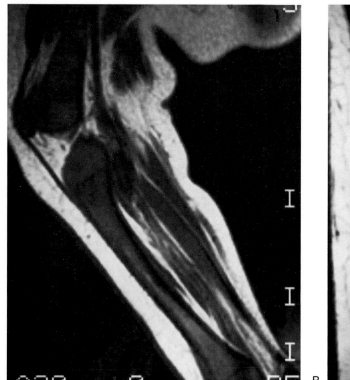
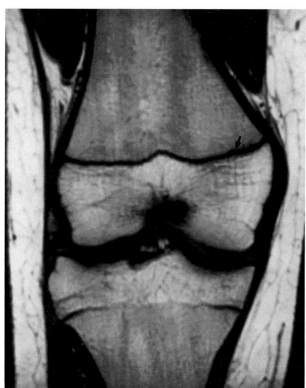

Figure 23–2. *Normal hematopoietic marrow.* ***A,*** T1 weighted (600/20) sagittal image through the distal femur and tibia in a 4-month-old infant. The cartilaginous distal femoral and proximal tibial epiphyses are seen, as is the low to intermediate signal-intensity red marrow of the distal femoral and proximal tibial mataphysis. The tibial diaphysis contains microscopic amounts of yellow marrow, reflected as of slightly increased signal intensity compared with the low to intermediate signal intensity of hematopoietic marrow without fatty elements. ***B,*** T1 weighted (800/20) coronal image through the distal femur and proximal tibia in a normal 14-year-old girl. The femoral and tibial epiphyses are bright-signal-intensity yellow marrow. The physis is seen as a low-signal-intensity line (*arrow*). The signal intensity of the distal femoral and proximal tibial marrow is greater than that of muscle.

facial bones except the maxilla, zygoma, and ethmoid contain some degree of hematopoietic marrow. Okada and colleagues[33] reported the spectrum of red-to-yellow marrow conversion in the clivus and calvaria in 238 patients. The bone marrow in the clivus and calvaria

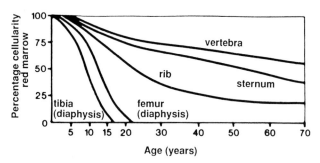

Figure 23–3. *Normal conversion of hematopoietic to fatty marrow.* Relative amounts of macroscopic hematopoietic and fatty marrow in different anatomic sites. The percentage of hematopoietic marrow decreases with age. (Adapted from Kricun ME. Red-yellow marrow conversion: its effect on the location of some bone lesions. Skeletal Radiol 1985: 14:10–19.)

has uniformly low-intermediate-signal-intensity marrow on T1 weighted images in most infants under 1 year of age (Fig. 23–5). Between the ages of 1 and 7 years this low-intermediate-signal-intensity hematopoietic marrow converts to patchy low- and high-signal-intensity marrow on the MR image, so that by the age of 7 years homogeneous low-signal-intensity marrow is seen in neither the clivus nor the calvaria (Fig. 23–6). There is continued conversion of the patchy pattern of marrow in the clivus and calvaria from age 7 until, by age 15, most patients have homogeneous high-signal-intensity fatty marrow (Fig. 23–7). Therefore, a homogeneous low- or low-intermediate-signal-intensity marrow in the skull or near the region of the clivus should be considered abnormal in any child over the age of 7. There is no significant difference in the signal intensity of the clivus between male and female patients at any age. The signal intensity of marrow in the occipital, parietal, and frontal calvaria in male patients tends to be somewhat higher than that of females in the second decade only. Two normal patients in this study had low intermediate signal intensity in the calvaria into the second decade of life, so the MR appearance

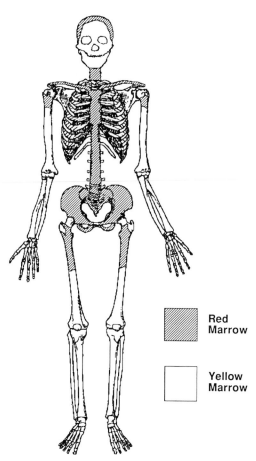

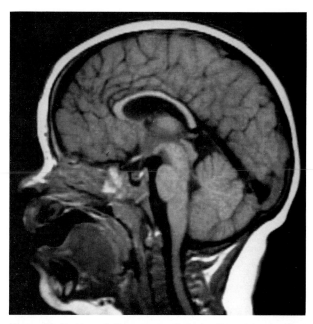

Figure 23–5. *Normal clivus marrow (infant).*   T1 weighted sagittal image through the clivus showing uniform intermediate-signal-intensity marrow in the clivus and calvaria.

Figure 23–4. *Distribution of normal adult marrow.*   Adult pattern of macroscopic red and yellow marrow. Macroscopic red marrow can be seen in the vertebral bodies, flat bones, and proximal metaphyses of the femora and humeri.

Red
Marrow

Yellow
Marrow

of the marrow in normal patients may occasionally lie outside these guidelines. In 4 percent of the patients, fatty marrow was seen in the frontal region of the skull in patients under 1 year of age.

Hematopoietic bone marrow within the skull accounts for approximately 25 percent of all hematopoietic activity at birth and decreases to 12 percent by age 20.[34] Therefore, hematopoietic disorders in children may often be reflected in the MR appearance of the marrow in the skull. In the clivus the proportion of patients with low-signal-intensity marrow decreases to less than 10 percent as early as age 3. Low-signal-intensity marrow in the clivus in children aged 3 to 6 years would therefore be suggestive of a hematopoietic disorder, either infiltration of the clivus by abnormal cells or lack of conversion of hematopoietic to fatty marrow, as would be seen in diffuse infiltrative disorders (Fig. 23–8).

SPINE. The MR appearance of the spine at birth is of low-intermediate-signal-intensity red marrow. The cartilaginous, unossified portions of the vertebral body are seen on MRI as intermediate signal intensity surrounding the lower-signal-intensity red marrow (Fig.

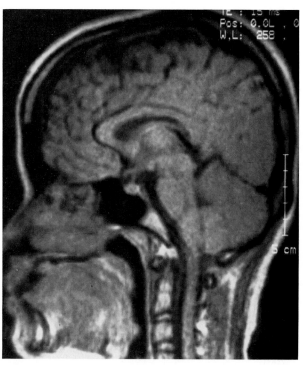

Figure 23–6. *Normal clivus marrow (12-year-old girl).* T1 weighted (500/15) sagittal image of the head. The marrow in the clivus is seen as of patchy intermediate and increased signal intensity.

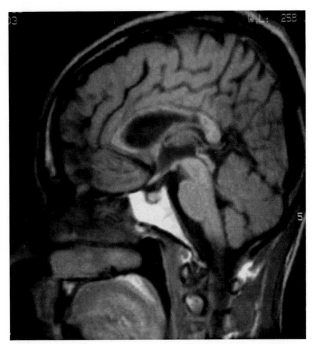

Figure 23–7. *Normal clivus marrow (20-year-old male).* T1 weighted (450/15) sagittal image of the head. The marrow of the clivus is yellow marrow of uniformly increased signal intensity.

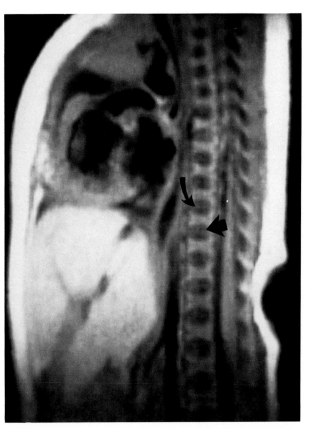

Figure 23–9. *Normal spine marrow in a newborn.* Sagittal T1 weighted (500/15) image through the spine. The cartilaginous, unossified vertebral body can be seen as intermediate signal intensity surrounding the lower-signal-intensity red marrow (*arrow*). The basivertebral vein is seen as a horizontal high-signal-intensity line (*curved arrow*).

23–9). With age the cartilaginous portions of the vertebral column become ossified, and there is a progressive conversion of red to yellow marrow until the adult pattern is reached (Fig. 23–10). In their 1987 study, Hajek and colleagues[35] reported the MR appearance of the spine in 120 patients aged 10 months to 85 years. Localized areas of increased-signal-intensity fatty mar-

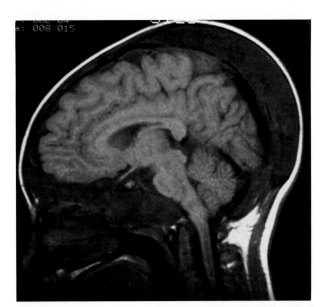

Figure 23–8. *Fibrous dysplasia.* T1 weighted (500/15) sagittal image of the head in a child. The clivus and calvarium are uniformly replaced by low-signal-intensity marrow. Note the gross enlargement of the marrow space.

row, either isolated or multifocal, were seen on both T1 and T2 weighted images within affected vertebral bodies. The changes were usually peripheral and adjacent to the end plates, but a more central position was also seen. Only 13 percent of patients aged 0–10 years manifested this phenomenon, but the incidence increases with age, and focal fatty marrow is seen in up to 93 percent of adult patients over 50 years old. There were no sex differences. Although there are no known histologic differences in the percentage of red versus yellow marrow among the lumbar, thoracic, and cervical vertebral bodies, focal fatty infiltration was more frequent in the lumbar spine.

PELVIS. Preliminary work in the pelvis[36] shows a pattern of red-to-yellow marrow conversion with age, occurring first in the anterior iliac crest and acetabulum (Figs. 23–11*A, B*). The pubic symphysis, posterior iliac crest, and sacral alae maintain varying percentages of intermediate- to high-intermediate-signal-intensity red marrow with age. This pattern of intermediate signal intensity of the posterior aspect of the pelvis, as compared with the anterior aspect, may persist in adults (Fig. 23–11*C*). There may be a great

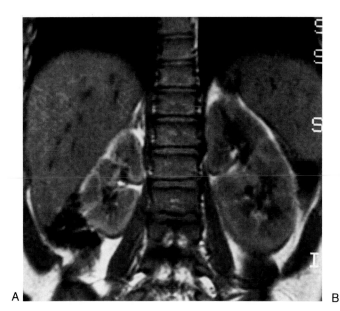

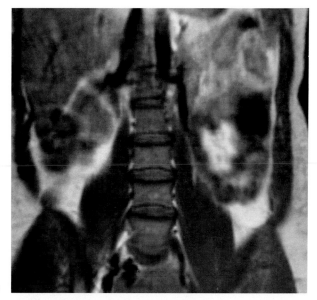

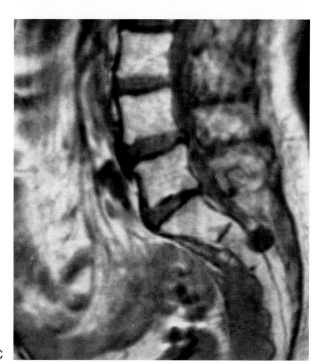

Figure 23–10. *Normal marrow at different ages.* **A,** Coronal T1 weighted (800/30) image through the thoracolumbar spine in a 3-year-old boy with an enlarged left kidney. The marrow signal intensity is of homogeneous intermediate signal intensity only slightly greater than the signal intensity of muscle. **B,** Coronal T1 weighted (800/20) image of the lumbar spine in a young adult patient. Note the intermediate-signal-intensity marrow. **C,** T1 weighted (800/15) sagittal image of the lumbar spine in a 64-year-old patient. Note the increased-signal-intensity marrow.

deal of heterogeneity of the marrow in the pelvis secondary to areas of macroscopic fatty replacement of underlying hematopoietic marrow. A mottled appearance of the pelvic marrow may be normal, especially in adolescents, young adults, and menstruating women; this is due to macroscopic areas of both hematopoietic and fatty marrow. To differentiate normal marrow mottling from focal abnormalities, such as metastases, the T1 weighted images should be compared with the T2 weighted images. If there is a true marrow abnormality, focal areas of low signal intensity on T1 weighted images usually increase in signal intensity and become brighter than normal marrow signal intensity on T2 weighted images. Macroscopically mottled but normal marrow visible on T1 weighted MR images usually becomes more homogeneous on T2 weighted MR images, since the red marrow increases slightly and the yellow marrow decreases slightly in signal intensity. This gives a more overall homogeneous signal intensity without focal areas of bright signal intensity, and can be useful in distinguishing abnormal from macroscopically mottled but normal marrow. How-

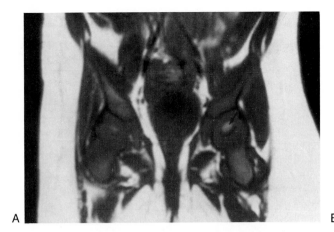

A

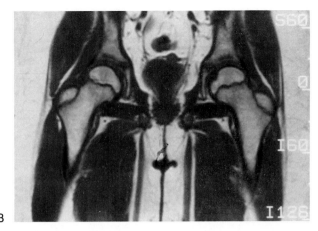

B

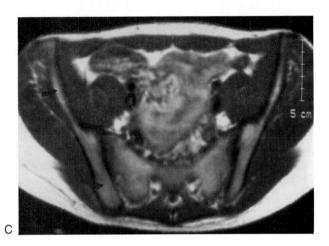

C

Figure 23–11. *Normal pelvis marrow.* **A,** T1 weighted (800/20) coronal image through the pelvis and hips of an 8-month-old boy. The marrow signal intensity of the pelvic marrow is intermediate, similar to that of muscle, except for some slight increase in signal intensity seen in the right iliac crest. The cartilaginous femoral heads are easily identified and are of low to intermediate signal intensity. The ossifying femoral heads can be appreciated, with high-signal-intensity fatty marrow seen (*arrow*). **B,** Coronal T1 weighted (800/30) image through the pelvis and proximal femora in an 11-year-old girl. Compared with the signal intensity of a younger child, the pelvic and proximal femoral marrow is seen as higher intermediate signal intensity, reflecting the increasing percentages of microscopic fatty marrow. **C,** T1 weighted (800/20) transverse image of the pelvis in a healthy 21-year-old female. The signal intensity of marrow in the anterior iliac crest (*arrow*) is slightly higher than that of the posterior iliac crest (*curved arrow*) and portions of the sacrum. This is within the spectrum of normal for pelvic marrow signal intensity.

ever, in patients who have undergone previous chemotherapy, focal marrow lesions with low signal intensity on T2 weighted images may increase only slightly on T2 weighted images and therefore may resemble normal marrow.[35] In these patients, heavily T1 weighted spin-echo images, which exploit the T1 relaxation differences and show focal areas of signal intensity lower than that of normal marrow, are more useful in distinguishing metastatic disease from normal but heterogeneous marrow.

FEMUR. Our study of 77 children[32] elucidated the spectrum of the MR appearance of the femoral marrow with age on T1 weighted images. Low-intermediate-signal-intensity marrow is seen throughout all the bones of the body at birth, including the femur, while the cartilaginous femoral epiphyses are of intermediate signal intensity. There are four recognizable patterns of red and yellow marrow in the femur: infant, childhood, adolescent, and adult. Homogeneous low intermediate signal intensity seen during the first year of life in the diaphysis and proximal and distal metaphysis of the femur is part of the MR infant pattern (Fig. 23–12). Between the ages of 1 and 5 years, the childhood pattern continues with apparent initiation

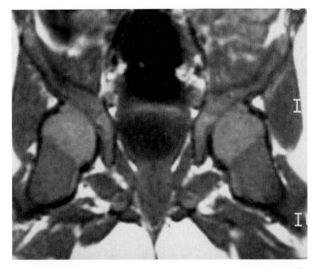

Figure 23–12. *Normal pelvis and femur marrow in a newborn.* T1 weighted (600/20) coronal image of the pelvis and proximal femora. The marrow is of uniformly low signal intensity, which reflects the underlying homogeneous hematopoietic marrow and lack of microscopic fatty marrow. The cartilaginous femoral heads are seen as slightly higher signal intensity. A distinct proximal metaphyseal physis cannot be appreciated. (Figures 23–12 through 23–14 from Moore SG, Dawson KL. Red and yellow marrow in the femur: age-related changes in appearance at MR imaging. Radiology 1990; 175:219–223.)

and near-conversion of diaphyseal red to yellow marrow on MRI (Fig. 23–13). Histologically the diaphyseal marrow at this age still maintains a large proportion of red marrow, and the increased signal intensity from fatty marrow appears to predominate to give an overall MR appearance of ''yellow'' marrow. This appearance is noted at a younger age than would be expected for the anatomic data, and probably reflects the increased sensitivity of MRI to the high signal intensity and short T1 relaxation time of underlying fatty marrow (Fig. 23–14). Between the ages of 6 and 10 years, diaphyseal red-to-yellow marrow conversion appears completed on MRI, and the diaphysis is seen as homogeneous increased signal intensity consistent with yellow marrow. This appearance of complete conversion of red to yellow marrow in the diaphysis by the age of 10 is earlier than would be expected from the anatomic data, and constitutes the MRI childhood pattern of marrow conversion in the femur.

Between the ages of 11 and 15 years, distal metaphyseal red marrow begins to convert to yellow marrow on MRI, with a slightly increased signal intensity of the distal metaphysis compared with the homogeneous intermediate-signal-intensity distal metaphysis seen in the earlier age groups (Fig. 23–15). One may consider this MR pattern of distal metaphyseal red-to-yellow conversion the adolescent pattern. Between the ages of 16 and 20 years this adolescent pattern progresses with the development of patchy distal metaphyseal red marrow on MRI. By 21 to 24 years of age an adult pattern is reached (Fig. 23–16). There appear to be no sex differences or field strength differences (0.38T versus 1.5T) in the observed MR marrow patterns reported in this study. Studies of the other long bones have not been performed, but personal experi-

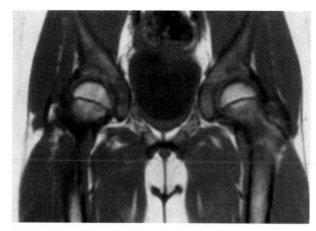

Figure 23–13. *Normal pelvis and femur marrow in a 5-year-old girl.* Coronal T1 weighted (800/20) image through the pelvis and proximal femora. There is increased-signal-intensity fatty marrow in the femoral epiphyses bilaterally as well as in the diaphysis of the femora.

ence shows that at a young age, usually by the age of 5 years, significant amounts of apparently fatty marrow are seen on MRI in the diaphyses of the hands, feet, tibia, fibula, radius, and ulna. The humerus appears to follow a pattern similar to that of the femur. The above guidelines will be useful until larger studies of the long bones can be performed.

Reconversion in Pathologic States

The marrow of the long bones in adult mammals, including humans, is predominantly yellow and forms a large reserve potentially available for the formation of

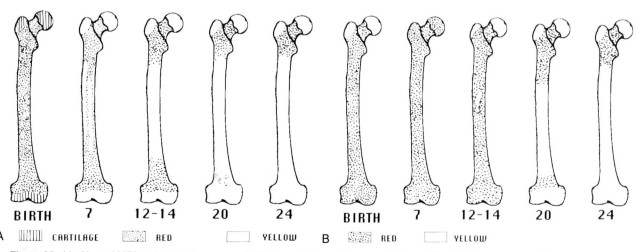

Figure 23–14. *Normal MRI and anatomic marrow distribution.* Schematic representations of the *A,* MR appearance of red and yellow marrow with age and *B,* macroscopic anatomic spectrum for red and yellow marrow with age. At age 7 years one would expect the marrow signal intensity on T1 weighted MR images to reflect the gross, or macroscopic, hematopoietic marrow that is present, but the signal intensity of marrow on MR images is higher than would be expected and more accurately reflects microscopic fatty marrow.

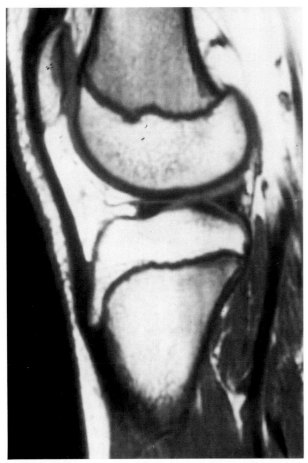

Figure 23–15. *Normal tibia and femur marrow.* Sagittal T1 weighted (800/20) image through the distal femur and proximal tibia in a 13-year-old normal girl. The marrow signal intensity of the hematopoietic distal metaphyseal marrow is intermediate to that of muscle and fat, while the marrow signal intensity of the proximal tibial metaphysis, which has a greater percentage of microscopic fatty marrow and a smaller percentage of hematopoietic marrow at this age, is closer to that of the signal intensity of fat. The increased-signal-intensity fatty marrow in the femoral and tibial epiphyses can be distinguished from the gradations of red marrow present in the two metaphyses.

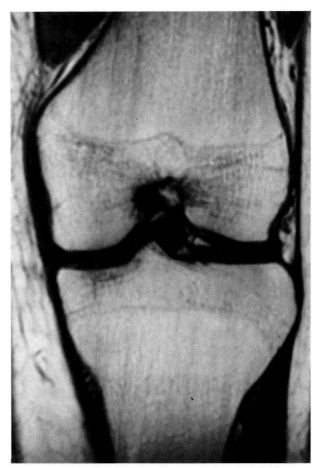

Figure 23–16. *Normal tibia and femur marrow at knee: adult pattern.* T1 weighted (800/20) coronal image through the knee in a 23-year-old male. The physis is closed, and the marrow is of fairly homogeneous increased signal intensity consistent with fatty marrow.

blood cells. This reserve is not used under normal conditions.[24] "Reconversion" of the bone marrow is a term used to describe the conversion of the marrow back to a previous state, i.e., activation of quiescent hematopoietic precursors present in fatty marrow, which results in repopulation of fatty marrow by active hematopoietic cells. Under normal physiologic conditions, regions of marrow that have converted from red to yellow marrow remain as yellow marrow. However, with stress, anemia, or infiltration of the hematopoietic marrow by a neoplastic process, there is reconversion of yellow to red marrow.[31] This generally occurs in a pattern converse to that of red-to-yellow marrow conversion (Fig. 23–17). Since there is residual red marrow in the spine and flat bones throughout life, reconversion occurs first in these regions. In the long bones,

reconversion of marrow is seen first in the proximal metaphyses of the femur and humerus, then in the distal metaphyses of the femur and humerus, and finally in the diaphyses of the femur and humerus. Reconversion also occurs in the proximal, then in the distal, metaphyses, and finally in the diaphyses of the tibia-fibula and/or radius-ulna, but lags behind reconversion in the femur and humerus. Final reconversion of marrow is in the hands and feet.

The impact of MRI on the evaluation of marrow and marrow disease promises to be significant. The marrow should be evaluated on every MR examination for the presence of pathologic infiltrative processes or of the reconversion phenomena. An understanding of the spectrum of normal age-related marrow patterns serves as the foundation for this interpretation and is essential before patterns of marrow reconversion can be recognized. In evaluating the marrow for yellow-to-red reconversion, it is the degree of intermediate signal intensity of the marrow on spin-echo MRI that must be assessed. Marrow in children is seen as either bright-

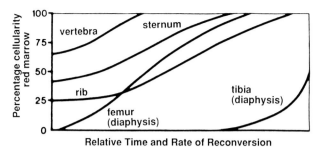

Figure 23–17. *Pattern of marrow reconversion.* Reconversion of yellow to red marrow generally occurs in a pattern converse to that of red-to-yellow-marrow conversion. The marrow in the vertebral bodies responds first, followed by the marrow in the flat bones, and finally the marrow in the metaphyses of the long bones. (Adapted from Kricun ME. Red-yellow marrow conversion: its effect on the location of some bone lesions. Skeletal Radiol 1985; 14:10–19.)

signal-intensity yellow marrow or intermediate- to increased-signal-intensity red marrow, depending on the percentage of yellow marrow within the hematopoietic marrow. The presence of microscopic yellow marrow within hematopoietic marrow results in an overall red marrow signal intensity greater than or equal to muscle but less than fat on T1 weighted MR images obtained after the first year of life. In the newborn period, when there is little to no microscopic yellow marrow within hematopoietic marrow, or in pathologic states in which there has been either extensive reconversion of marrow or replacement of marrow by neoplastic processes (e.g., leukemia or neuroblastoma), the marrow signal intensity is similar to or less than that of muscle on T1 weighted images.

In older children (above the age of 10), homogeneous low-signal-intensity marrow is likely to be abnormal except when confined to symmetric focal areas of expected hematopoiesis (e.g., the proximal metaphysis). When regions of marrow that should be bright-signal-intensity yellow are seen as of intermediate to low signal intensity on MRI, reconversion phenomena,

as well as infiltrative processes, should be considered. In our experience, the lower the signal intensity of the marrow compared with the signal intensity of muscle and the more homogeneous the marrow with advancing age, the more likely it is that an underlying pathologic process exists. The above are general principles gleaned from our experience with pediatric bone marrow imaging, but further study is needed before definite conclusions can be made regarding the spectrum of normal and abnormal marrow and before conversion and reconversion processes can be evaluated.

Normal Epiphysis, Physis, and Cortex

Epiphysis

The cartilaginous epiphyses are seen as intermediate signal intensity on T1 weighted images, and vary from intermediate to bright signal intensity on T2 weighted images, depending on the TR used (Fig. 23–18). The ossification center of the epiphysis is seen initially on T1 weighted images as a small focus of increased signal intensity, primarily fatty marrow, which may be surrounded by a rim of low signal intensity (Fig. 23–11*A*). Until cortical bone is formed around the ossified epiphysis, this low-signal-intensity rim is most likely a consequence of the combined effect of peripheral cartilaginous mineralization and a chemical shift effect. The ossification center of the epiphysis increases in size as the child grows, and remains bright in signal intensity, replacing the intermediate-signal-intensity cartilaginous epiphysis. The ossified epiphysis ultimately assumes the adult size and shape, and fuses with the metaphysis.

In our experience the ossified epiphyses are always of bright signal intensity on both T1 and T2 weighted images, and follow the signal patterns of subcutaneous fat, reflecting underlying fatty marrow. There is histologic evidence that epiphyses contain hematopoietic marrow during early ossification.[25] Despite the presence of some hematopoietic marrow, even developing

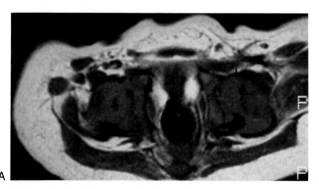

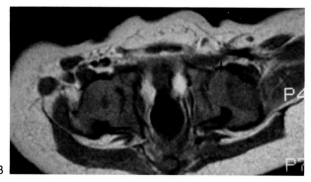

A   B

Figure 23–18. *Normal epiphyses.* Axial images through the acetabulum and cartilaginous femoral epiphyses in a 9-month-old girl. The signal intensity of the cartilaginous femoral epiphysis (*arrow*) at **(A)** TR 800/20 msec is less than that seen at **(B)** TR 2000/20 msec. The femoral epiphyses were not yet ossified, but the region of potential ossification can be appreciated within the right femoral epiphysis.

ossified epiphyses appear on MRI as primarily yellow marrow and are of bright signal intensity on both T1 and T2 weighted images.[32] If the ossified epiphyses are not of bright signal intensity on T1 weighted images, this indicates either conversion of yellow to red marrow, edema, ischemia, sclerosis, or infiltration by a neoplastic process. Subtle heterogeneous low or intermediate signal intensity rarely may be seen as a normal finding within the bright-signal-intensity ossified epiphysis, and may result from partial volume effect of either the cortex or peripheral rim of mineralization of the epiphysis, especially in young patients in whom there is a small volume of ossified epiphyses (Fig. 23–19). Sclerosis within the epiphysis, such as seen in the femoral head representing compressive trabeculae in the weight-bearing axis, is hypointense on both T1 and T2 weighted images.[37] Given that small amounts of hematopoietic marrow may be present within ossifying epiphyses at an early age, the possibility that subtle low to intermediate signal intensity within the bright-signal-intensity ossified or ossifying epiphyses could represent some residual hematopoietic marrow cannot be excluded. However, it is never normal for the entire ossified epiphyses to contain homogeneous low- or intermediate-signal-intensity marrow. If homogeneous replacement of marrow in the epiphysis is seen, further investigation should be instituted to exclude replacement of fatty marrow by hematopoietic cells or infiltrative processes.

Ossified epiphyses develop with increasing age, and a normal ossified epiphysis with yellow marrow eventually replaces the intermediate-signal-intensity cartilaginous epiphysis. The intermediate-signal-intensity cartilaginous epiphyses, especially in newborns, should not be confused with replacement of the yellow marrow of the epiphysis by abnormal infiltrated or hematopoietic marrow (Figs. 23–11A, 23–13).

In young children an ossifying epiphysis that is void of signal intensity on both T1 and T2 weighted images is likely to represent a densely sclerotic epiphysis, and does not represent infiltration of the epiphyseal yellow marrow by hematopoietic marrow or other abnormal

cells. This can be seen in the proximal femoral epiphysis of children with congenital dislocation of the hip (Fig. 23–20). Comparison with plain films shows densely sclerotic epiphyses and helps to distinguish a very-low-signal-intensity sclerotic epiphysis from a low- to intermediate-signal-intensity epiphysis with replacement of the normal yellow marrow by edema, hematopoietic cells, or diffuse infiltrative processes.

Physis

On MRI the physis is not readily apparent at birth or before the development of an ossified epiphysis, but blends with the cartilaginous epiphysis that is adjacent to the metaphysis of the bone being examined (Fig. 23–12). With age and the development of an ossified epiphysis, the physis may be appreciated as a line of low signal intensity that separates the ossified epiphysis from the metaphysis (Figs. 23–11B). The physis decreases in size with age and advancing physeal closure (Figs. 23–15, 23–16). In children a linear chemical shift artifact of low and bright signal intensity may be seen parallel to the physis (Fig. 23–21); this is not seen in the adult physeal scar. A physis may be seen on MRI adjacent to any epiphysis or apophysis, including the greater and lesser trochanters of the femur and the trochlear epiphyses of the humerus (Fig. 23–21).

Cortical Bone

Cortical bone is readily evaluated by MRI[38] and is seen on MR images as a signal void on all pulse sequences surrounding the intermediate- or bright-signal-intensity marrow. This signal void is primarily due to the lack of mobile protons and consequent long T1 and short T2 relaxation times. It is best evaluated on T1

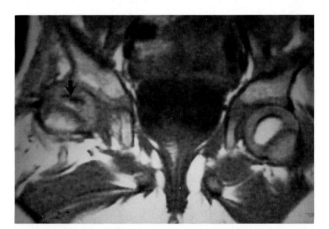

Figure 23–20. *Sclerotic epiphysis.* T1 weighted (600/20) coronal image of the pelvis and hips in a 2-year-old girl with congenital dislocation and persistent subluxation of the right hip. The high-signal-intensity ossifying femoral head can be seen on the left, surrounded by the intermediate-signal-intensity normal epiphyseal cartilage. On the right the femoral epiphysis is subluxed, although the signal intensity of the cartilaginous epiphysis is within normal limits. A low-signal-intensity, sclerotic, ossifying femoral epiphysis is apparent (*arrow*). On radiography, a sclerotic femoral epiphysis with an identical contour and size was appreciated. Note the prominent chemical shift effect superior to the ossifying left femoral epiphysis.

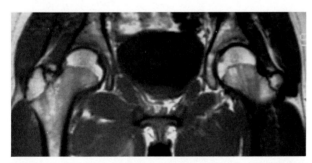

Figure 23–19. *Normal epiphyses (12-year-old girl).* T1 weighted (800/20) coronal image through the pelvis and proximal femora. The ossified femoral epiphyses are clearly bright-signal-intensity fatty marrow, but close scrutiny reveals subtle inhomogeneity within the marrow signal. This can be a normal finding.

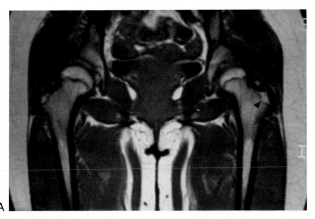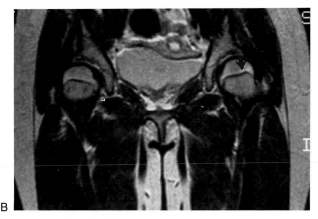

Figure 23–21. *Chemical shift artifact at the physis.* ***A,*** T1 weighted (800/20) and ***B,*** intermediate weighted (1500/70) coronal images through the pelvis and proximal femora in a 14-year-old girl. ***B*** is 1.1 cm anterior to ***A***. A bright-signal-intensity line is seen adjacent to the physis, in the frequency-encoding direction (*arrow*). This represents chemical shift effect from the interface between the high-signal-intensity fatty marrow and the low-signal-intensity cartilaginous physeal plate. The low-signal-intensity physis adjacent to the greater trochanter can be seen (*arrowhead*).

weighted or proton density images.[38] Intermediate signal intensity within the cortical bone is evidence of a pathologic process and is discussed further in the chapter on Tumors of the Musculoskeletal System. There are several pitfalls in evaluating cortical bone. Chemical shift misrepresentation of cortical bone can be especially apparent on images obtained with high-field-strength magnets (1.5T). With a horizontal frequency encoding gradient, apparent thinning of the cortical bone is seen on one side and apparent thickening of the cortical bone on the opposite side of the bone (Fig. 23–22).[39] The position of adipose tissue–related protons is shifted approximately 2 pixels from water-related protons so that the chemical shift artifact is more prominent in bones with fatty marrow. On axial images, partial voluming of marrow and muscle with the cortical bone in areas of rapid tapering of bone, e.g., the femoral neck, may be seen as an intermediate signal intensity within cortical bone, and this should not be confused with pathology.

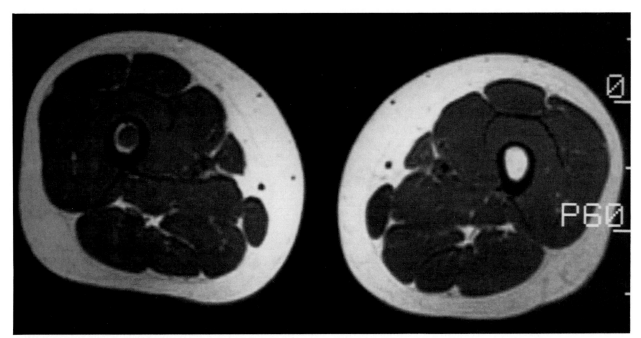

Figure 23–22. *Chemical shift misrepresentation of the cortex.* Axial image through the middle femora in a 15-year-old girl with focal fibrous dysplasia of the right mid femur. The fibrous dysplasia is seen as low signal intensity surrounded by normal higher-signal-intensity yellow marrow. There is a chemical shift misrepresentation of cortical bone, seen here as anterior thinning and posterior thickening of the cortex.

MARROW IMAGING TECHNIQUES

STIR Imaging

Short TI inversion recovery (STIR) imaging of the marrow can increase lesion conspicuity and is gaining favor in the evaluation of pediatric marrow disorders. In STIR imaging, an initial 180-degree radio frequency pulse is followed by a 90-degree pulse and then a second 180-degree pulse. The 90-degree pulse is given at a time when fat protons (T1 relaxation time approximately equal to 300 msec) are at the "null point" at the intersection of the X-, Y-, and Z-axes. Fat protons and protons with a relaxation time similar to that of fat are not flipped into the X-Y plane and do not emit a signal that can be received by the coil. The net effect is that the T1 and T2 contrast is additive in STIR images, and therefore lesion recognition is often enhanced.[40]

The signal from fat, and any tissue with a T1 relaxation time similar to that of fat, is suppressed and seen as very low or black signal intensity on STIR images. Air, fibrosis, calcification, and paramagnetic substances (gadolinium-DTPA and hemorrhage) can also be seen as low signal intensity on STIR images. Muscle is of intermediate signal intensity, and fluid, edema, lymph nodes, and tumor are all bright on STIR imaging. Lesion conspicuity, especially in older children who have a higher percentage of yellow marrow, is increased (Fig. 23–23).[41] Conversely, any tissue with an extremely short T1 relaxation time (much shorter than fat) is also of bright signal intensity. Practically speaking, there are few biologic tissues with a T1 relaxation time significantly shorter than fat, and therefore areas of bright signal intensity on STIR images most likely represent tissues with long T1 and T2 relaxation times.

Our experience with STIR imaging suggests that the normal signal intensity of marrow on STIR images may reflect the percentage of red marrow present. In very young children, the marrow is of intermediate signal intensity on STIR images, while the marrow in teenagers and young adults, except in areas with residual hematopoietic marrow such as the proximal femoral metaphysis, has the suppressed or black signal intensity typical of yellow marrow (Fig. 23–24). The spectrum of signal intensity of the marrow on STIR images is likely to depend on the patient's age and the percentage of hematopoietic marrow present.

Gradient-Echo Imaging

Gradient-recalled echo (GRE) imaging represents a new horizon in the imaging of bone marrow. These fast imaging techniques are based on the use of a partial flip-angle excitation pulse (typically less than 90 degrees) followed by a gradient reversal to refocus the echo and generate the signal. Because the protons are only partially excited, TR values may be markedly

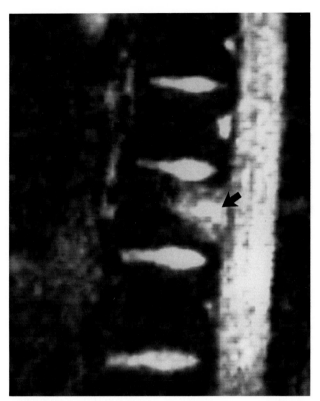

Figure 23–23. *STIR suppression of fatty marrow.* Sagittal STIR (1500/30/TI 100) image through the thoracic spine in a child with metastatic Ewing's sarcoma. Yellow marrow is seen as low signal intensity, discs are seen as bright signal intensity, and the metastatic lesion is seen as bright signal intensity (*arrow*). STIR increases lesion conspicuity.

shortened (20 to 30 msec), and consequently imaging time is proportionally diminished. In order to maximize signal, free induction decay is used for data acquisition.

Factors that influence gradient-echo image contrast include the acquisition technique and bone marrow characteristics. TR, TE, and flip angle can be selected to provide contrast similar to that in spin-echo imaging. However, there are several contrast characteristics of gradient-echo imaging that are distinct from spin echo and that influence the interpretation of marrow signal. Most important is the dependence of signal characteristics on the effective transverse relaxation time (T2*) as opposed to the T2 dependence of spin-echo sequences.[42] On gradient-echo imaging there is no refocusing of local magnetic field inhomogeneities by a 180-degree pulse, and thus dephasing occurs during the entire acquisition time. Gradient-echo imaging is therefore very sensitive to field inhomogeneities arising either extrinsically (magnet or siting factors) or intrinsically (tissue differences in chemical shift frequency or magnetic susceptibility). Second, in contrast to spin-echo imaging in which TR shortening increases the degree of T1 weighting, on gradient-echo imaging

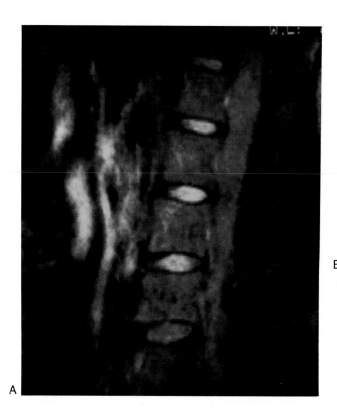

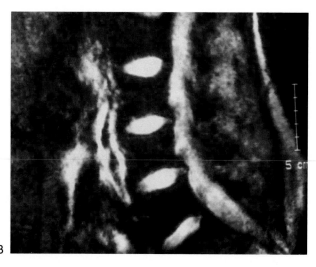

Figure 23–24. *STIR suppression of marrow signal.* STIR (1500/30/TI 100) sagittal image through the spine in *(A)* an 8-year-old child and *(B)* a 23-year-old adult. The signal intensity of the hematopoietic marrow in the child is increased compared with the suppressed signal intensity of the fatty marrow in the young adult.

at TRs below 150 to 200 msec the transverse magnetization remaining from the last pulse is rotated around, setting up the condition of steady state free precession with tissue contrast dependent on T2*/T1 rather than T1 alone. As a consequence, the magnetic susceptibility and chemical shift characteristics of marrow are well demonstrated only by gradient-echo imaging. Since fat contains several spectral components, yellow marrow signal displays a chemical shift–induced amplitude modulation with echo delay at 1.5T.[28] There are two amplitude modulations:

1. A high-frequency modulation with a period of approximately 4 msec related to the chemical shift of 4.1 ppm (260 Hz at 64 MHz resonance frequency) between the vinyl CH protons and the CH_2 moiety of long-chain fatty acid.

2. A low-frequency modulation with a period of approximately 20 msec related to the chemical shift difference between the center CH_2 and $-CH_2-O$ protons of the acid chain.

This phenomenon has important consequences for yellow marrow contrast. Yellow marrow is more intense than muscle on in-phase images, in contrast to out-of-phase images, even though the echo delay between these two images may differ by only 2 msec.[28]

Magnetic susceptibility is an important aspect of marrow contrast on gradient-echo images. It has been shown both in vitro and in vivo at high field strength that marrow in contact with trabecular bone exhibits a shortened T2* and resultant signal loss on gradient-echo images.[43] This T2* effect is increased in regions with a greater amount of trabecular bone (epiphysis, metaphysis, vertebra, short bones) compared with regions that have little trabecular bone (diaphysis), and is increased by increasing TE on a given gradient-echo sequence (Fig. 23–25).[44] This T2* dephasing is most likely due to local field gradients resulting in inhomogeneous susceptibilities where the mineralized matrix interfaces with marrow.

Knowledge of the effect of trabecular bone on gradient-echo images is important for MR analysis of bone marrow, for several reasons. Low signal intensity on gradient-echo images may in fact represent fatty marrow with a high content of trabecular bone, and should not be interpreted as hematopoietic marrow. If one analyzes gradient-echo images of the femur in an older child, the signal intensity of the diaphyseal marrow is different from that of the epiphyseal marrow. This is unexpected, since both contain fatty marrow and on spin-echo images have a similar appearance of increased signal intensity. However, histologic analysis of the marrow shows an increased percentage of trabecular bone in the epiphysis compared with the diaphysis. Since fat and water in contact with trabecular bone exhibit shortened effective transverse relaxation times (T2*), the low signal intensity of epiphyseal marrow on gradient-echo images is likely secondary to the effect of trabecular bone on T2*. The fatty marrow in the diaphyseal region is of bright signal intensity since there is little or no trabecular bone. It appears, therefore, that the signal intensity of the marrow seen on gradient-echo images reflects hematopoietic and fatty marrow

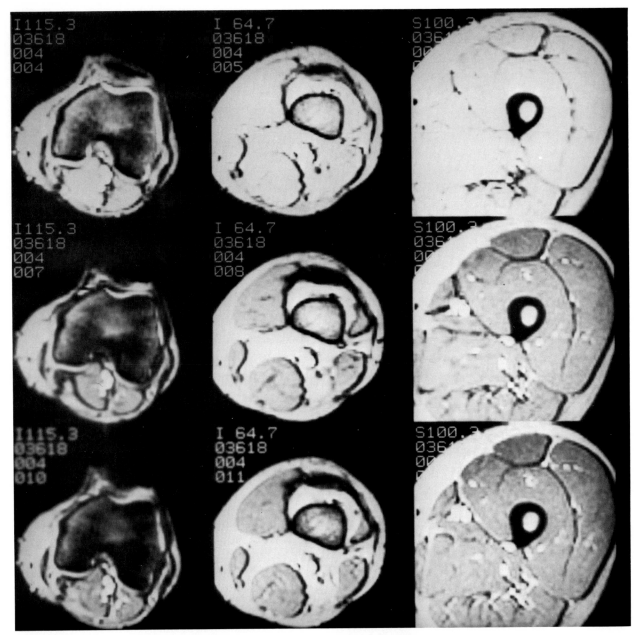

Figure 23–25. *Magnetic susceptibility artifact.*   Gradient-recall-echo images (TR 60, flip-angle 30 degrees) through the femoral epiphysis (*first column*), femoral metaphysis (*second column*), and femoral diaphysis (*third column*) in a normal 28-year-old male. The first transverse row represents images acquired at a TE of 12, the second row at a TE of 16, and the third row at a TE of 20. With increasing TE, there is increasing magnetic susceptibility effect in the trabecular bone-rich epiphysis, whereas no magnetic susceptibility effect on the marrow is seen in the trabecular-poor diaphyseal marrow. (Sebag GH, Moore SG. Effect of trabecular bone on the appearance of marrow in gradient-echo imaging of the appendicular skeleton. Radiology 1990; 174:855–859.)

as well as the magnetic susceptibility and chemical shift characteristics of marrow that are accentuated by gradient-echo imaging.[44]

Image resolution and detection of bone marrow lesions may be improved by decreasing TE and pixel size on a given gradient-echo sequence, or by using a three- or four-dimensional acquisition mode for a fixed TE.[44] Specifically, lesions that are easily seen on gradient-

echo images using a TE of 10 msec are not as readily apparent on gradient-echo images obtained with a TE of 40 msec. It is important to be aware of this effect when using gradient-echo images to evaluate bone lesions.

The decrease in imaging time with gradient-echo acquisition has several benefits. It is highly desirable in the pediatric population and is more cost effective.

Motion artifact is minimized and dynamic MR contrast studies can be performed. Contiguous slices without interslice gaps are quickly obtained. Although the sensitivity of gradient-echo imaging to local field inhomogeneities may be a nuisance in relation to the image quality, it also has some advantage: gradient-echo imaging is more sensitive in detecting small concentrations of paramagnetic substances, calcification, and hemorrhage and is useful in evaluating iron metabolism and hemosiderosis.[42] The most important point to remember in gradient-echo imaging is that hematopoietic versus fatty marrow per se may not be reflected. Rather, gradient-echo images may be useful in the evaluation of bone marrow when it is desirable to determine the amount and effect of surrounding trabecular bone, or in the evaluation of paramagnetic substances.

Chemical Shift Imaging

Because of the different chemical environment, aliphatic protons and water protons have slightly different resonant frequencies. Therefore, as time passes after excitation, fat and water protons dephase relative to each other. This phenomenon, which is the basis of MR spectroscopy, may be exploited to separate the MR signal into a water component and a fat component. Addition and subtraction of in-phase and out-of-phase images will result in the creation of water and fat images.[45] Water and fat images may be either T1 or T2 weighted.[46] In T2 weighted water images (T2 "fat suppression" images) the image contrast is similar to that of STIR, and this leads to improved tissue contrast and better lesion conspicuity, as described previously with the STIR technique. True water images may have some advantage over STIR imaging since a larger number of images can be acquired. The major drawback of this technique is the sensitivity to local field inhomogeneities, and the requirement that the main field inhomogeneities over the field of view be significantly less than the chemical shift between lipid and water.[47] The image contrast on chemical shift imaging is highly variable, depending on the sequence type, the image reconstruction technique (magnitude versus phase), and the composition of the marrow (site, age). The spectrum of normal bone marrow appearance has not been described on chemical shift imaging and requires further study.

Chemical shift imaging can also be used in the quantitative assessment of fat and water fractions in bone marrow in vivo. The respective relaxation times of the fat fraction and the water fraction can also be measured. Rosen and colleagues[48] found in vivo a fat fraction value of 30 percent (range 20 to 40 percent) in the lumbar spine marrow of six healthy adult volunteers. The fat fraction was decreased less than 10 percent in six leukemic patients, and increased more than 50 percent in three patients with aplastic anemia.

EDEMA OF MARROW

Pathophysiology and MR Appearance

Marrow edema is a generalized response either to trauma or to stress of the bone marrow. The stimulus and controlling factors for the initiation of edema are uncertain, but it is known that the amount of extracellular water increases as a result of hypervascularity and hyperfusion.[49] In pediatric patients, bone marrow edema may be the first recognizable MR finding in many conditions, including transient synovitis, trauma, stress, infection, ischemia, tumor, and reflex sympathetic dystrophy. The severity of the hypervascularity and hyperfusion most likely modulates the amount of increased extracellular water, and the MR appearance is a reflection of this increase in extracellular water. The MR features of edema in the bone marrow are nonspecific and consist of a decrease in the marrow signal intensity on T1 weighted spin-echo images, with a commensurate increase in marrow signal intensity on T2 weighted images. The contour of the changes varies and may be either well defined although geographic (Fig. 23–26) or less well defined and feathery in appearance. The signal changes are often fairly homogeneous.

Differential Diagnosis of Marrow Edema

As an imaging modality, MRI is exquisitely sensitive in detecting the presence of marrow edema. This sensitivity is potentially problematic, since we do not always know what degree of importance to give to the marrow edema seen on MRI. One of the difficulties facing the radiologist today is the separation of MRI-diagnosed "transient" marrow edema that requires either no or only conservative treatment from those entities that require immediate and often prolonged treatment. The armamentarium of the physician for differentiating these entities includes the clinical history and examination, radiography, MRI, CT, scintigraphy, ultrasonography, and biopsy. It should be emphasized that prospective studies that definitively compare the accuracy, sensitivity, and specificity of MRI with radiography, scintigraphy, CT, and ultrasonography in the evaluation and differential diagnosis of bone pain and marrow edema have not yet been completed; however, we have found the following guidelines useful.

In our experience, it may be difficult to distinguish marrow edema, such as that seen in stress fracture, osteoid osteoma, infection, or other inflammatory processes, from Ewing's sarcoma or other intramedullary tumor that has not yet affected the cortical bone or surrounding soft tissues (Fig. 23–26). In many of these disorders, the child presents with a nonspecific history of bone pain, which in some cases has been present for months. The plain films may be normal or may show some degree of osteopenia. Bone scan, if

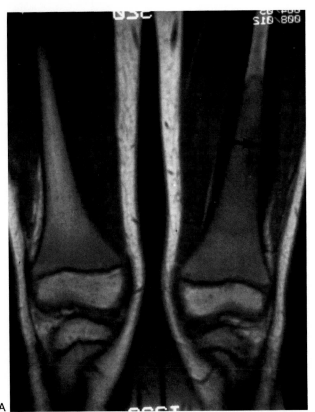
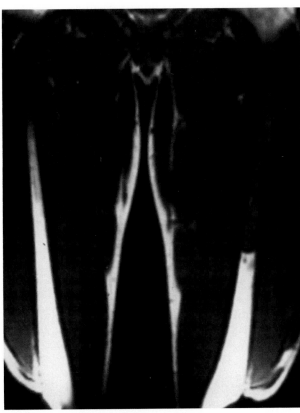

A   B

Figure 23–26. *Differentiation of marrow tumor and edema.* **A,** T1 weighted (800/20) coronal image through the femurs in an 8-year-old girl with an osteoid osteoma of the right femur. The region of the osteoid osteoma is identified (*arrow*) with surrounding well-defined low-signal-intensity marrow edema. This increased on the T2 weighted image. This amount of marrow edema is not unusual for osteoid osteoma. **B,** Low signal intensity in the proximal left diaphyseal shaft on this T1 weighted (800/20) coronal image of the femurs represents intramedullary Ewing's sarcoma. It may be difficult to distinguish diffuse marrow edema from diffuse intramedullary tumor.

performed, often shows increased uptake. A preliminary report[50] attempted to establish guidelines for the interpretation of marrow and soft tissue edema. The investigators found that extensive involvement of the marrow or soft tissues by edema, reflected as decreased signal intensity on T1 weighted images and isointense or increased signal intensity on T2 weighted images, was more often associated with inflammatory processes (such as infection), fracture, or trauma. Edema was present in neoplastic processes but in general was much less extensive than that seen in inflammatory processes. Benign processes, such as an old infarct or enchondroma, are unlikely to be associated with marrow edema. A diffuse marrow abnormality on MRI with extensive soft tissue edema is more likely to represent an inflammatory process than a neoplastic process. This finding may not help, however, in the case of osteoid osteoma, since these lesions have been seen in association with extensive marrow edema without significant soft tissue edema. In cases of stress fractures, Brodie abscesses, or osteoid osteoma, the MR examination can be supplemented with high-reso-

lution, thin-slice CT scanning to identify the cortical lesion. However, if a child presents with bone pain, little or no abnormality on the radiograph, and a diffuse marrow abnormality on the MR scan with a negative CT examination, it may be prudent to perform a biopsy to exclude tumor. This is a decision that requires the clinical acumen of the pediatrician, oncologist, orthopedic surgeon, and radiologist.

Some of the different causes of marrow edema will now be discussed, with emphasis on factors that help to differentiate these disorders.

Idiopathic Marrow Edema

Children with fairly acute pain but without specific symptoms suggesting infection, trauma, or tumor may be found to have transient marrow edema on MRI. The radiographs will be normal or show some mild degree of osteoporosis. The abnormal low signal intensity of the edema may be seen in the epiphysis or both the epiphysis and metaphysis of these children who require nothing more than conservative treatment for complete resolution of their symptoms and MR findings. Such transient marrow abnormalities on MRI are described in three children with hip pain.[51] In these children, low-signal-intensity patterns in the femoral head on T1 weighted images eventually resolved, reverting to the normal marrow signal pattern. The resolution of the signal abnormalities coincided with documented improvement of the clinical condition. Areas of abnormal intermediate signal intensity on T1 weighted images were isointense on initial T2 weighted images and remained isointense on follow-up T2 weighted images. Since the MR changes resolved rapidly and the patients became asymptomatic, these changes were probably due to transient bone marrow edema and not early avascular necrosis. Similar findings of low signal intensity in the femoral epiphysis have been seen in Perthes' disease,[52,53] but there was no evidence of a double line sign on T2 weighted images to confirm actual femoral ischemia. The cause of these transient findings is uncertain. The MR appearance of transient synovitis is unknown, but the initial clinical presentation as well as the resolution of clinical and imaging findings suggested the diagnosis of transient synovitis. However, other diagnoses such as migratory osteoporosis or mild reflex sympathetic dystrophy should also be considered. Similar changes have been described in adults with transient osteoporosis[49,54] and reflex sympathetic dystrophy.[55] The acetabulum as well as the femoral head and the neck may be involved in these entities, and the condition is often accompanied by joint effusion.[49]

Osteonecrosis

A child presenting with bone pain and at risk for the development of infarction, avascular necrosis, or Perthes' disease should have a plain radiograph after physical examination and assessment of the clinical history. When the radiograph is diagnostic for ischemic necrosis or Perthes' disease, further diagnostic imaging workup is not usually warranted, although MRI may play a role in monitoring therapy and in the evaluation of the contralateral femoral head for signs of early disease.

On MRI, a double rim sign or low signal intensity on both T1 and T2 weighted images suggests the diagnosis of avascular necrosis and not "transient" edema. The appearance of acute marrow ischemia in children is not well defined, and it may be difficult to distinguish idiopathic transient marrow edema from ischemia, since "edema" is present in both entities.

A bone scan may or may not aid in distinguishing ischemia from "transient" edema. In children with vascular insufficiency as the cause of the edema, a completely photopenic area in the region of the MR marrow abnormality without a rim of increased signal intensity would confirm the diagnosis of avascular necrosis secondary to vascular insufficiency. Joint fluid is not useful in distinguishing the two, since joint fluid is known to be associated with both entities.

Infection

Infection will be mentioned briefly here as it is another cause of marrow edema. If there is a strong clinical suspicion of infection, imaging procedures other than radiography, if it is positive, are probably unnecessary unless the surgeon wants precise delineation of the extent of infection. In these patients MRI plays an ancillary role in defining the extent of disease and therapeutic staging. Ultrasonography could be used to evaluate the presence of joint fluid, but MRI may be preferable, since abnormalities in the underlying bone marrow and surrounding muscles or fascial planes suggesting osteomyelitis, myositis, or fasciitis may be seen. If infection is suspected and the radiograph is negative, MRI or bone scan may be used effectively to detect abnormality; both are very sensitive. If clinical symptoms point to a specific body region, MRI is preferable because of its superb anatomic resolution. Bone scan is preferred for screening of the entire skeleton.

Trauma–Stress Fracture

Extensive marrow edema may be seen as a result of stress fracture. Prominent intramedullary areas of edema of low signal intensity on T1 weighted images and increased signal intensity on T2 weighted images have been noted in stress fractures within 3 weeks of the onset of symptoms (Fig. 23–27).[56] It is uncertain how long these abnormalities persist.[56,57] The bony sclerosis causes a low-signal-intensity linear line that usually abuts and is perpendicular to the cortex. On high-field-strength systems[56] there is an absence of discernible cortical interruption, and the juxtacortical findings are less prominent than on lower-field-strength systems. Lack of a soft tissue mass, or cortical destruction combined with characteristic extensive intramedullary edema, helps to distinguish stress fracture from tumor. Occasionally the low signal intensity of the sclerotic fracture line may be obscured in MRI because the reactive edema is so pronounced. In these cases, a high-resolution, thin-section CT scan may be required to define the stress fracture. Thin-section, high-resolution CT may be especially necessary around the hip, where small stress fractures of the acetabulum, ilium, and femur may be associated with extensive edema that obscures the hairline fractures on MRI. However, in view of the cost, bone scintigraphy will probably remain the method of choice for screening for stress fracture, if stress fracture is the primary clinical consideration. MRI would be necessary only if clinical evaluation suggested an entity other than stress fracture.

In addition to stress fractures, edema of the marrow may be appreciated in other traumatic or inflammatory lesions of bone. Bony "contusions" have been reported that are of low signal intensity on T1 weighted images and isointense to slightly increased signal intensity on T2 weighted images after traumatic injury to the bone

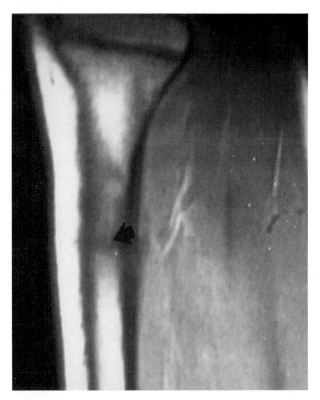

Figure 23–27. *Sagittal T1-weighted (600/20) image of the tibia in an 11-year-old girl with tibial pain.* Stress fracture (*arrow*) is seen as a low signal intensity line perpendicular to the cortex. Low-signal-intensity edema surrounding the stress fracture can be appreciated.

in which a fracture was not sustained (Fig. 23–28) (see the chapter on Miscellaneous Disorders of the Musculoskeletal System).[58, 59] Lesions such as osteoid osteoma may also be associated with extensive marrow edema (Fig. 23–26A). If a diagnosis of osteoid osteoma is suspected, meticulous review of the plain film should be made followed by thin-section CT to assess for cortical abnormality.

Neoplastic Disease

Tumors usually cause an abnormality on the radiograph, although some cases of medullary tumor, especially Ewing's sarcoma, may be difficult to appreciate on the plain film. Both early medullary tumor and marrow edema have homogeneous intramedullary low signal intensity on T1 weighted images, which increases in signal intensity on T2 weighted images. In most cases, biopsy is needed if there is a clinical suspicion of tumor.

In summary, clinical history and plain film radiographs are the most important tools in the evaluation of a child with bone pain who may have marrow edema. The next diagnostic examination should probably be MRI in most cases. If the etiology of a marrow abnormality is uncertain from the clinical history, radiograph, and MR examination, either CT (to evaluate for cortical abnormality or trauma) or bone scan (to screen for avascular necrosis, stress fracture, or osteoid osteoma) may be helpful in determining the cause of the bone pain and marrow edema. The sensitivity of MRI to marrow edema may prove both useful and problematic in the interpretation of marrow MR images, in that

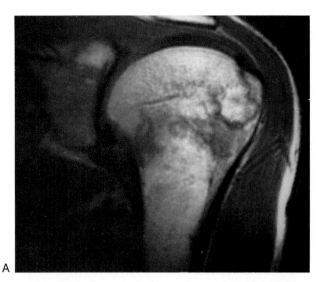

A

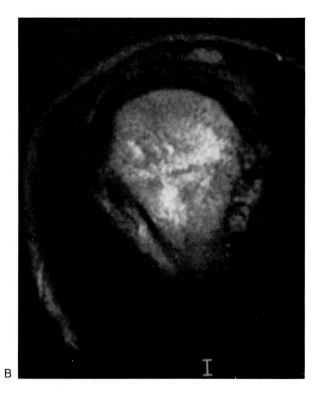

B

Figure 23–28. *Bone contusion.* Sagittal T1 (800/20) **(A)** and T2 (2050/80) **(B)** images of the proximal left humerus in a 17-year-old patient with blunt trauma to the humerus as a result of a skiing accident. On the T1 weighted image, ill-defined low to intermediate signal intensity is noted within the medullary bone. There is heterogeneous increased and intermediate signal intensity on the T2 weighted image. These findings are typical for trabecular microfracture or "bone contusion."

an abnormality may be recognized but, once seen, is difficult to distinguish from other disorders. Further prospective studies correlating MRI, CT, bone scintigraphy, and biopsy are needed before this question can be answered.

HEMATOPOIETIC MALIGNANCIES

Acute Leukemia

Leukemia accounts for more than one-third of all malignancies in children. The onset is often insidious, with low-grade fever, fatigue, and anemia. Patients may present with pancytopenia with or without circulating blast cells, a normal leukocyte count, or marked leukocytosis. Thrombocytopenia is common, and petechiae and bruising may be noted. Hepatomegaly and splenomegaly due to leukemic infiltration may be present. Lymphadenopathy is more common in acute lymphocytic leukemia (ALL) than in acute myelogenous leukemia (AML), and an anterior mediastinal mass is often present in patients with the T-cell variant of ALL. Leukemic cells may infiltrate tissues such as the skin, eye, nasal pharynx, lung, or kidneys. Sanctuary sites include the testicles, the central nervous system (CNS), and to a lesser degree, the ovaries. Soft tissue masses of leukemic cells or chloromas may develop in any location and may occasionally precede detectable involvement in the bone marrow. Bone pain in leukemia is due to increased interosseous pressure from malignant proliferation of leukemic cells in the bone marrow.

MR Appearance of Leukemia

During the early stages of leukemia the marrow cavity is filled with leukemic cells, but there is no bone destruction and the radiographic appearance of the bone is normal.[60] It is the potential of MRI to reflect the underlying cellular structure of the marrow that makes it a useful tool in the evaluation of leukemia (Figs. 23–29 to 23–32). The changes seen in the marrow secondary to leukemia are due to malignant proliferation of cells originally native to bone marrow tissue, rather than malignant proliferation of cells transported from other sites. Therefore, on MRI marrow changes are seen most often in areas that consist primarily of hematopoietic marrow, i.e., spine, iliac crest, proximal femur. In any one bone, leukemic changes are likely to be seen in areas of primarily hematopoietic marrow (the metaphyses), followed by the diaphyses, then the epiphyses.

On T1 weighted MR images, leukemic infiltration of the marrow is seen primarily as homogeneous replacement of the normal marrow by intermediate- to low-signal-intensity leukemic cells (Fig. 23–29). On T2 weighted images the signal intensity increases and may not be appreciated as abnormal on these images alone (Fig. 23–32). The changes are often diffuse, but focal

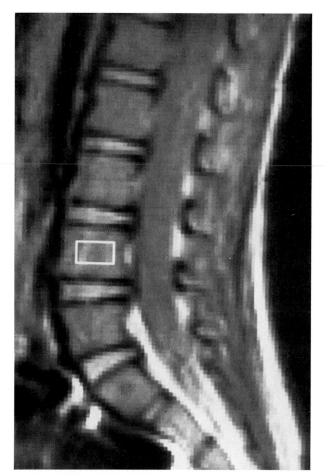

Figure 23–29. *Leukemia.* Sagittal intermediate (2000/30) image through the lumbosacral spine in a 12-year-old patient with newly diagnosed acute lymphocytic leukemia. Diffuse marrow abnormality is noted with homogeneous intermediate-signal-intensity tumor cells infiltrating the marrow. A "region of interest" is drawn in the L4 vertebral body; this can be used to calculate T1 relaxation times. Only the central portion of the vertebral marrow is included, excluding the vertebral cortex, disc, and basivertebral vein complex.

areas of marrow infiltration by leukemia can also be seen (Fig. 23–30). Focal infiltration may be seen in any type of leukemia, but is more common in myelogenous leukemia where chloromas develop in the periorbital tissues and marrow cavities of the long bones and skull. In both diffuse and focal leukemia, leukemic cells may penetrate the overlying cortex and lift the periosteum. This periosteal reaction can be recognized on MRI (Fig. 23–31).

Chemical shift imaging has been performed with success in distinguishing adult patients with leukemia from normal patients.[48, 61] In adults with leukemia, a higher signal on the water fraction image and a lower signal on the fat fraction image is seen than in normal individuals. In the only child reported in the literature,[61] these changes were not as obvious, possibly because pediatric patients have a higher percentage of red marrow and therefore the difference of the water

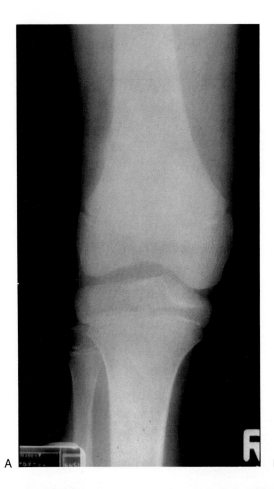

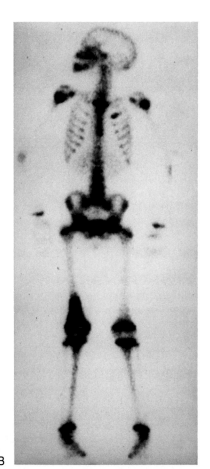

A

B

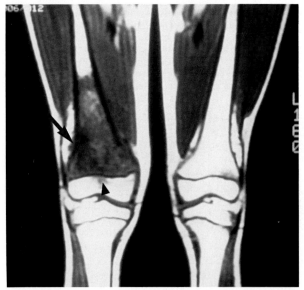

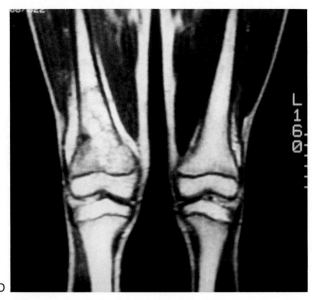

C

D

Figure 23–30. *Adolescent with acute lymphocytic leukemia and right knee pain.* **A,** Radiograph reveals cortical abnormality and periosteal reaction in the lateral distal femur. **B,** Tc-99m bone scan reveals increased activity in the right distal femur. **C,D,** T1 weighted (600/20) **(C)** and T2 weighted (1800/80) **(D)** coronal images through the distal femora. Focal infiltration by leukemic cells can be seen as low to intermediate signal intensity on T1 weighted images and heterogeneous increased signal intensity on T2 weighted images. The cortical breakthrough and periosteal reaction seen on the plain film can be identified (*arrow*). Involvement of the epiphysis is also noted (*arrowhead*). (Courtesy of Dr. Richard Graviss, St. Louis, MO.)

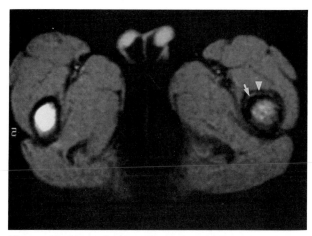

Figure 23–31. *Leukemia.* Transverse STIR (1.5/15/TI 100 [0.38T]) image through the proximal femora in a 4-year-old boy with diffuse marrow disease. Radiography of the left femur showed lifting of the periosteum. This STIR image shows abnormal bright-signal-intensity bone marrow bilaterally. On the left the cortical bone, bright-signal-intensity subperiosteal leukemic infiltrate (*arrow*), and low-signal-intensity lamellated periosteal reaction can be identified (*arrowhead*).

and fat fractions is not as pronounced. Chemical shift imaging may be more useful in the evaluation of older children and adults, in whom there is normally a higher percentage of yellow marrow than in younger children. Further study is necessary in this area.

Preliminary results[63] support the need for further investigation of the use of STIR imaging in the evaluation of leukemia. Anecdotally, children with newly diagnosed leukemia have increased-signal-intensity lumbar vertebral marrow compared with children in relapse or young children with relatively large percentages of hematopoietic marrow. Children with a predominance of hematopoietic marrow in the spine, as well as those in relapse, tend to have intermediate-signal-intensity vertebral marrow.[63] Older children with predominantly fatty vertebral marrow have a much lower signal intensity of the marrow (Fig. 23–24*B*). It is likely, however, that the overlap between children with larger percentages of hematopoietic marrow and those with leukemia may make STIR imaging of the marrow in leukemic children less useful than STIR imaging of the marrow in leukemic adults. Adults have predominantly fatty marrow, even in the spine, with suppressed signal intensity on STIR im-

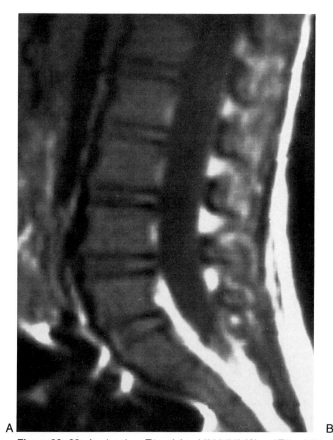

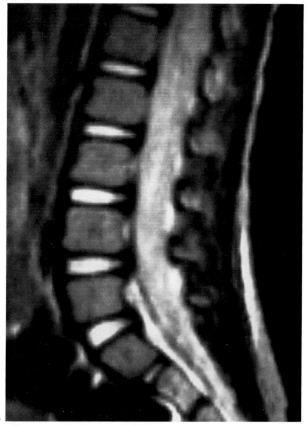

A   B

Figure 23–32. *Leukemia.*   T1 weighted (300/30) *(A)* and T2 weighted (2000/80) *(B)* sagittal images through the spine in a 2-year-old infant with acute lymphocytic leukemia. Marrow signal intensity on the T1 weighted image is low to intermediate, but on the T2 weighted image the signal intensity cannot be appreciated as abnormal.

ages. Increased-signal-intensity leukemic marrow is therefore more readily apparent on STIR images in adults.

The visual analysis of the signal intensity of the marrow alone cannot be used to determine the stage of disease in leukemia.[64] Children with newly diagnosed ALL often have marrow of abnormally low signal intensity, but some of these children and those in relapse may have a marrow signal intensity indistinguishable from that in normal children, especially in the younger age groups in whom normal hematopoietic marrow gives a relatively lower signal intensity.

The relaxation times of normal and leukemic marrow have been measured. Regardless of patient age, the T1 relaxation time of normal marrow is generally between 350 and 650 msec on low,[48, 61, 65] medium,[66] and high[67] field strength magnets, although values as high as 720 msec in infants[68] and 900 msec in adults[69] have been reported. Accurate calculation of T1 relaxation times of vertebral marrow may be difficult, and care must be taken in measuring the regions of interest (Fig. 23–29). If any part of the vertebral cortex, disc, or basivertebral vein complex is included, T1 relaxation time values may be changed by as much as 100 percent.[70] There is controversy regarding the accuracy of T1 relaxation times, and this is an area of investigation. In our experience, we have found consistent and reproducible T1 relaxation times of normal marrow in children ranging from 350 to 650 msec if a carefully prescribed central region of interest in the lumbar vertebral bodies is measured.

Infiltration of the marrow by any abnormal cell including leukemia, metastatic rhabdomyosarcoma, or neuroblastoma causes a prolongation of the T1 relaxation time. There have been several investigations regarding the usefulness of measuring relaxation times of vertebral marrow in assessing leukemia and the stage of disease.[48, 66, 67] In childhood leukemia, the T1 relaxation time of the lumbar vertebral marrow in patients with newly diagnosed ALL is prolonged, with a range of 830 to 1400 msec. This prolongation is statistically significant in comparison with the relaxation time of marrow in normal children (Fig. 23–33).[66] There appears to be a prolongation of T1 relaxation time in the marrow of children in relapse, and while the numbers to date are not sufficient to determine the statistical significance of this prolongation compared with the relaxation time of the marrow in children in remission, the potential for distinguishing these two disease states exists. In no study has a statistically significant difference in T2 relaxation time been found.

The cause of the prolongation of the T1 relaxation time in patients with leukemia is uncertain. Theories include an increased intracellular water content as a result of increased cellularity in the marrow of such patients. However, in vitro studies[71, 72] showed a persistent difference in T1 relaxation time between desiccated samples of leukemic and normal marrow, suggesting that factors other than intracellular water are mediating the prolongation of T1 relaxation time in leukemia. There does not appear to be a consistent relationship between the degree of cellularity, number of blast cells, or fat content of the bone marrow and the quantitative prolongation of T1 relaxation time,[62] although a 1988 report suggests that replacement of fatty marrow by hematopoietic or cellular marrow may play an important role.[48] A significant prolongation of T1 relaxation time in the marrow of patients with polycythemia vera[62] is similar in magnitude to that in the marrow in patients with acute leukemia (690 to 1,390 msec). Both leukemia and polycythemia vera are myeloproliferative disorders characterized by increased cellularity and increased cell turnover. Perhaps some intrinsic factor and/or biochemical structure of these rapidly proliferating cells may contribute to the prolongation of T1 relaxation time. The truth most likely lies in a combination of several factors, and this continues to be an area of investigation.

Indications for MRI in Leukemia

In summary, there are several current and potential indications for MRI in patients with leukemia. If a child presents with clinical symptoms of leukemia, MRI can play a role in the exclusion or confirmation of hematopoietic disease. If the marrow on the MR images is homogeneously low or shows a prolonged T1 relaxation time (greater than 750 msec on midfield-strength magnets), leukemia or another neoplastic disorder may be suspected and a bone marrow biopsy is recommended. If the spin-echo appearance and T1 relaxation time are normal, a biopsy is unlikely to be necessary. MRI may play a role in the near future in the evaluation of the state of disease, whether relapse or remission. MRI is useful in evaluating local areas of bone pain in children to exclude tumor, infection, infarct, or edema. Finally MRI may be useful in evaluating the sequelae of treatment, including steroid-induced avascular necrosis and chemotherapy-induced aplastic anemia, and in monitoring bone marrow transplant patients for engraftment and relapse of disease.

Myeloproliferative Disorders

Children with myeloproliferative disorders are thought to be in preleukemic states. True myeloproliferative disorders are neoplasms of the multipotent hematopoietic stem cell, and include chronic myelogenous leukemia (CML) and polycythemia vera (PV), both of which occur in children, and myeloid metaplasia with myelofibrosis and essential thrombocytosis, neither of which occurs in children. In at least some patients, stem cell involvement includes a progenitor capable of giving rise to lymphocytes as well.

CML occurs at any age, although the peak incidence is in the third and fourth decades. Males and females are equally affected. Clinical findings are characterized by marked splenomegaly and the production of

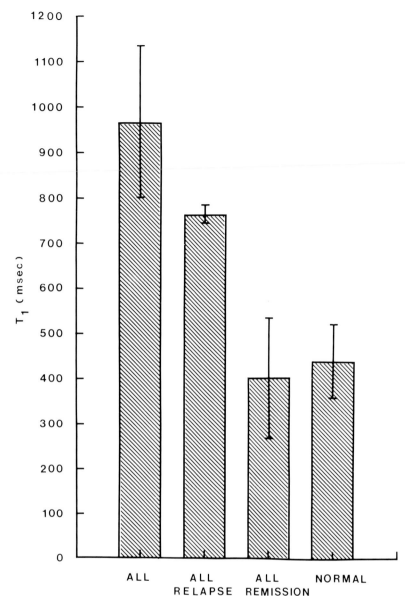

Figure 23–33. *Leukemia* Marrow T1 relaxation times in leukemia. Histogram of mean T1 relaxation time of the vertebral marrow in each of four groups: newly diagnosed acute lymphocytic leukemia, leukemia in relapse, leukemia in remission, and normal age-matched controls. T1 relaxation time is significantly prolonged in children with disease compared with those with no evidence of active disease and age-matched controls. Standard deviation for each measurement is noted. (Moore SG, Gooding CA, Brasch RC, et al. Bone marrow in children with acute lymphocytic leukemia: MR relaxation times. Radiology 1986; 160:237–240.)

increased numbers of granulocytes. The chronic phase of CML in which there is hyperplasia of mature elements in the marrow eventually converts to the more acute blastic phase of CML. In the blastic phase there is replacement of the hyperplastic mature marrow elements by increased numbers of blast cells and promyelocytes.

Polycythemia vera is also characterized by splenomegaly and increased production of myeloid elements, although the disease is dominated by an elevated erythroid population. PV generally begins in middle life and is slightly more common in males, but it is rarely found in children. There is abnormally increased red blood cell production in the absence of peripheral erythropoietin, which is suppressed by the elevated hemoglobin concentration. The abnormal cells in PV

are thought to arise from a pluripotent hematopoietic stem cell and are not regulated by the usual mechanisms. One to 2 percent of patients with PV undergo transformation to acute leukemia, and there is an increased incidence of lymphocytic lymphoma. Fifteen to 20 percent of patients progress to marrow fibrosis.[73]

MR Findings in Myeloproliferative Disorders

On MR examination, diffuse, abnormal, low-signal-intensity marrow is especially prominent on T1 weighted images. This may be most noticeable in areas of the marrow normally occupied by increased-signal-intensity fatty marrow. Reports on work in CML are primarily anecdotal, with few descriptions of the appearance of the disorder in children.[61, 74] In our experience the pattern of abnormality of the marrow in CML differs from that in ALL or AML in that the percentage of marrow affected is likely to be greater. This could be explained by the natural course of CML, which tends to be more long-standing, more insidious in onset, and characterized pathologically in the chronic phase by diffuse myeloproliferation of the marrow (Figs. 23–34, 23–35).

Jensen and associates[62] calculated T1 relaxation times of bone marrow in adult patients with PV. As in acute leukemia there is a two- to threefold increase in the T1 relaxation time of the marrow in patients with PV (range 690 to 1,390 msec) compared with the T1 relaxation time of normal marrow (range 380 to 600 msec). This prolongation of T1 relaxation time is statistically significant. There is no statistically significant difference in T2 relaxation time. The authors felt that increased cellularity and cell turnover may account for at least some of the increase in T1 relaxation time seen in diffuse abnormalities of marrow, and that prolongation of T1 relaxation time is perhaps better correlated with the number of cells in active cycle and cell turnover than with malignancy or cellular infiltration per se.[62]

Lymphoma

Bone lesions in children and adolescents with Hodgkin's lymphoma are infrequent, but when they occur they are usually focal and are seen most frequently in

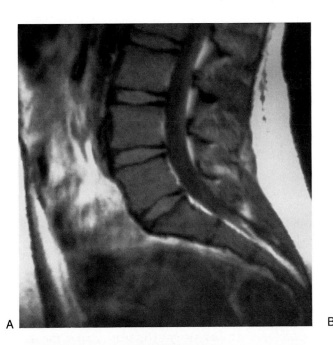

A

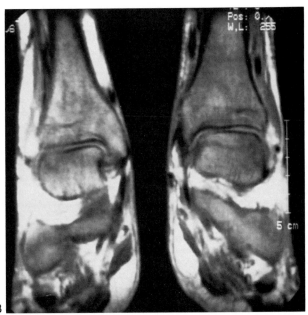

B

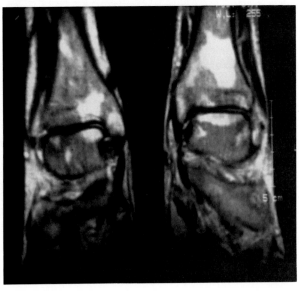

C

Figure 23–34. *Chronic myeloid leukemia in a 19-year-old female.* ***A,*** Sagittal T1 weighted (300/30) image of the lumbar spine shows diffusely homogeneous low signal intensity. Note that the signal intensity of the vertebral body is slightly less than that of the adjacent disc. This is not normal in a person over 1 year of age and should raise the possibility of diffuse hematopoietic disorder. ***B,*** T1 weighted (600/20) coronal image through the ankles in the same patient. Note diffuse homogeneous replacement of bright-signal-intensity fatty marrow by low intermediate signal intensity. The tibia, talus, and forefoot are all involved. ***C,*** T2 weighted (2000/80) image shows well-circumscribed regions of increased signal intensity in tne marrow, consistent with marrow infarct. The marrow infarct was a result of the patient's leukemia.

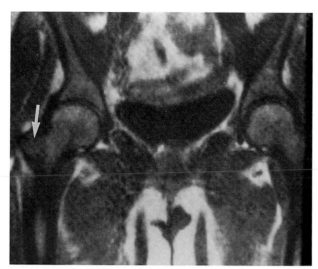

Figure 23–35. *Chronic myeloid leukemia.* Coronal T1 weighted (600/20) image through the hips in a 24-year-old patient. The pelvic marrow, femoral epiphyses, and (right) greater trochanter (*arrow*) show abnormal low to intermediate signal-intensity infiltrated marrow. The ossified epiphyses and trochanter should always be high-signal-intensity fatty marrow, regardless of age.

the spine and pelvis, then in the ribs, femora, and sternum. Lymphocytic (non-Hodgkin's) lymphoma is not uncommon in the pediatric age group, accounting for more than 6 percent of all childhood malignancies,[75] and children often present with marrow changes. Indeed, marrow disease in children and adolescents with lymphoma is one of the more common indications for bone marrow transplantation.

MR Findings in Lymphoma

Since marrow lymphoma behaves more like metastatic disease, MRI may be useful in the detection of focal areas of macroscopic lymphoma, which may cause clinical symptoms but present in patients with negative bone marrow biopsy and negative bone scan.[2,76] On MRI, focal lesions are usually seen as low to intermediate signal intensity on T1 weighted images

and increased signal intensity on T2 weighted and STIR images (Fig. 23–36). The disease may rarely become diffuse and may be indistinguishable on MRI from other diffuse infiltrative neoplastic processes of the marrow. The long bones are rarely involved in Hodgkin's disease. Occasionally, local osteoblasts are stimulated and produce sclerosis of the affected bone, especially in the vertebral body. These lesions tend to be intermediate signal intensity on T2 weighted images, reflecting the sclerotic bone. The T1 weighted images show a more typical low intermediate signal intensity (Fig. 23–37).

The MR findings in the marrow in children with non-Hodgkin's lymphoma are similar to those in Hodgkin's disease,[2] although diffuse disease is more common and may appear similar to that of other diffuse neoplastic marrow disorders, with decreased signal intensity on T1 weighted images and intermediate to increased signal intensity on T2 weighted images (Fig. 23–38). The most common pattern of diffuse disease seen in both Hodgkin's and lymphocytic lymphoma consists of diffuse marrow abnormality punctuated by focal sparing of the marrow, so that several vertebral bodies may appear normal while the remainder are affected. Substantial portions of a diffusely involved long bone may be spared[76] so that macroscopic areas of normal fatty marrow may be appreciated within an underlying milieu of abnormal, low to intermediate signal-intensity marrow. There have been no reports discussing the specific appearance of primary lymphocytic lymphoma of the bone (reticulum cell sarcoma).

Langerhans Cell Histiocytosis

This class of disorders (also known as reticuloendotheliosis or histiocytosis X), although not malignant per se, is characterized by a granulomatous proliferation of the reticulum cells at one or several sites in the reticuloendothelial system. This may occur in the skeleton, spleen, thymus, liver, lymph nodes, or skin. The cause is not established but may relate to previous

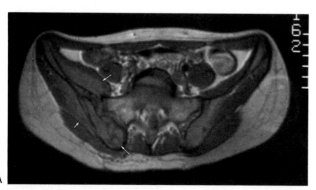

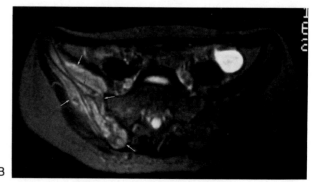

A   B

Figure 23–36. *Hodgkin's lymphoma.* Transverse images through the pelvis in an adolescent. *A,* T1 weighted (800/20) and *B,* T2 weighted (2000/80) images show soft tissue lymphoma (*arrows*) in the right iliac fossa and gluteal region. Soft tissue and marrow involvement is seen as intermediate signal intensity on the T1 weighted image, which becomes bright signal intensity on the T2 weighted image.

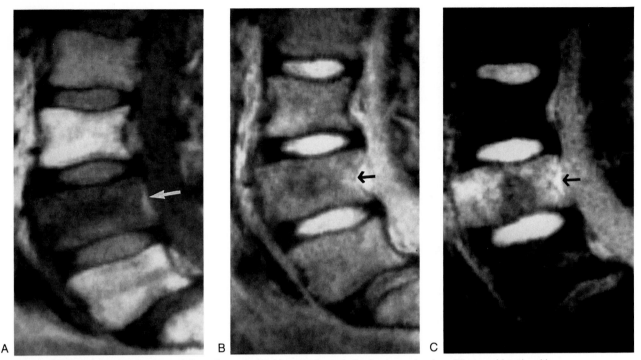

Figure 23–37. *Hodgkin's disease of the spine.*   Sagittal images through the lumbar spine in a 32-year-old male with Hodgkin's lymphoma of the L4 vertebral body *(arrows)*. A focal area of decreased signal intensity is seen on the T1 weighted (330/30) *(A)*, intermediate weighted (2000/30) *(B)*, and STIR (1500/30/TI100 [0.38T]) *(C)* images, representing sclerotic bone. The signal intensity of tumor is decreased in *A*, isointense in *B*, and increased in *C*. Note suppression of the fatty marrow of L2 and L3 in *C*.

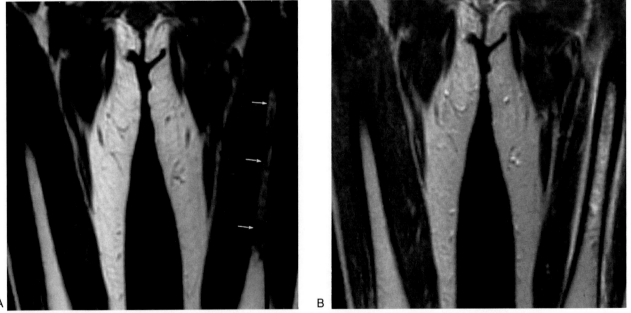

Figure 23–38. *Non-Hodgkin's lymphoma of the left femur.*   T1 weighted (800/20) *(A)* and T2 weighted (2000/80) *(B)* coronal images through the femur in an adolescent male. While a diffuse area of the left femoral diaphysis *(arrows)* is involved by tumor, some underlying normal high-signal-intensity marrow can be seen on the T1 weighted image. The lesion increases in signal intensity on the T2 weighted image, but it does not become diffusely brighter than marrow.

infection. There are three general classes of reticuloses, distinguished by clinical and not pathologic differences.

Letterer-Siwe disease is characterized by generalized proliferation in all parts of the reticuloendothelial system in infants who present with purpuric rash, splenomegaly, hepatomegaly, skeletal defects, and progressive anemia.

In older children, adolescents, and adults the clinical course is more protracted, and granulomatous proliferation of the reticulum cells is more localized. Skeletal lesions are common, whereas cutaneous and lymphatic manifestations are uncommon. This class of disease may be referred to as Hand-Schüller-Christian disease. Lipid may accumulate in the reticulum cells. In the healing stages, fibrous tissue replaces the lipid-laden reticulum cells. Lesions often occur near the base of the skull and orbits, and in some patients are responsible for the exophthalmos and diabetes insipidus once considered cardinal manifestations of this form of reticulosis.[77] Despite the fact that lipid-laden reticulum cells are responsible for the lesions, in the few MR examinations we have seen the lesions are focal, often multiple, and of intermediate signal intensity on T1 weighted images and increased signal intensity on T2 weighted and STIR images (Fig. 23-39). The lipid-laden reticulum cells in these lesions do not appear to show an increased signal intensity on T1 weighted images.

Eosinophilic granuloma tends to be the most benign form of this group of diseases, usually occurring in older children and often limited to bone. There may be single or multiple lesions. The lesions may be difficult to see on plain radiography and usually show no increased activity on MDP bone scan. On MRI, well-defined lesions of low signal intensity on T1 weighted images and increased signal intensity on T2 weighted and STIR images are seen. A low-signal-intensity sclerotic rim may be present, and we have seen subperiosteal new bone with peritumoral edema on both T1 and T2 weighted images (Fig. 23-40). The lesions may enhance after gadolinium-DTPA administration.

In the vertebral body the lesion is seen as a more diffuse infiltration of the entire vertebral body, with signal intensity similar to that of the focal lesions. Epiphyseal lesions have been described.[78]

MRI plays a role in the evaluation of all the reticuloses when a child presents with complaints of bone pain, and plain films do not show a bony lesion. In these cases, bone scan may be either negative or non-

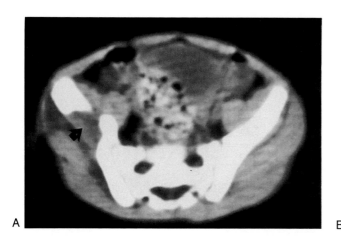

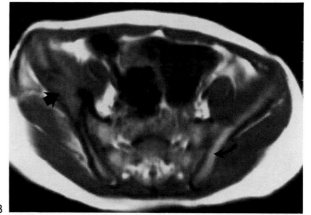

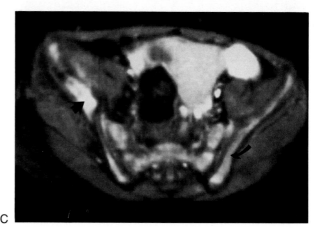

Figure 23–39. *Langerhans cell histiocytosis. Transverse images through the pelvis in a 16-month-old infant.* ***A,*** CT scan shows destruction of the right iliac crest (*arrow*). ***B,*** T1 weighted (600/30) image with intermediate-signal-intensity tumor (*arrow*) replacing bone. Normal marrow contains microscopic fat and has moderate signal (*curved arrow*) even though the marrow is predominantly hematopoietic. ***C,*** Increased-signal-intensity tumor (*arrow*) is easily recognized on the STIR (1500/30/TI100 [0.38T]) image.

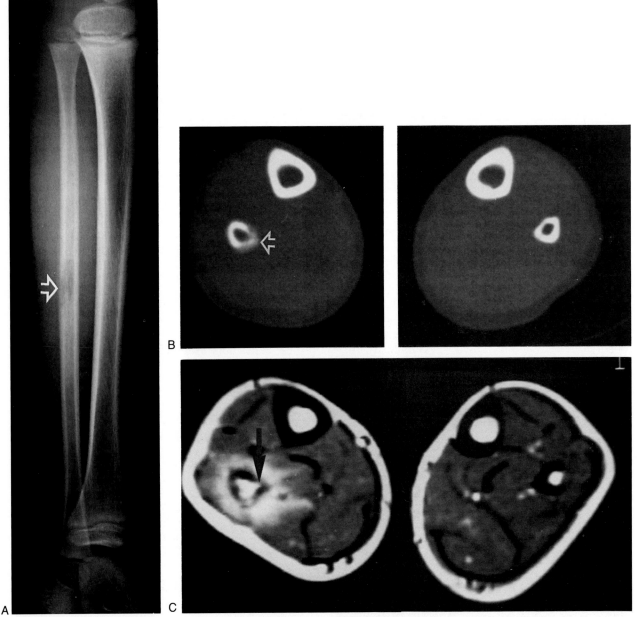

Figure 23–40. *Langerhans cell histiocytosis.* **A,** Radiograph of the right tibia and fibula in a 6-year-old boy. A lytic lesion (*arrow*) is seen in the mid-diaphysis of the fibula. Cortical erosion and periosteal reaction can be appreciated. **B,** Transverse CT scan through the fibular lesion. The cortical abnormality (*arrow*) is appreciated, but neither marrow nor soft tissue abnormality is seen. **C,** Intermediate (1500/20) image through the same region as the CT scan. Cortical erosion by tumor (*arrow*) as well as extensive increased-signal-intensity peritumoral edema is noted. Tumor cells were found in the soft tissues at pathologic evaluation.

specific, and we have often found MRI useful in determining the presence or absence of a medullary or cortical lesion. The appearance of the lesion is not specific, however, and biopsy is usually required to confirm the diagnosis.

Bone Marrow Metastases

The common etiologies of bone metastases in children are neuroblastoma, rhabdomyosarcoma, Ewing's sarcoma, and medulloblastoma. Hematogenous metastases from these tumors involve bone more frequently than other organs, in spite of the relatively low cardiac output to the bone. The vascular nature of red marrow with its dilated sinusoids and looped vessels, as well as the strong affinity of tumor cells for endothelium, account for the high frequency of bony metastases. The distribution of hematogenous metastases is influenced by the vascular anatomy of marrow, with a more common location in the vascular-rich red marrow and a less common location in the vascular-poor yellow marrow. In children, metaphyses of the long bones (especially the most rapidly growing metaphyses) and metaphyseal equivalent areas of the spine and flat bones are the most common sites of metastases, because these have the richest blood supply.[31]

Because metastases grow first in the marrow and then spread to the trabecular and cortical bone, lesions can often be detected on MRI before the appearance of significant bone loss on plain film radiographs. The patchy distribution of bone marrow metastases in solid tumors, especially neuroblastoma, may allow earlier detection of lesions than iliac crest bone marrow aspirate.[79] On T1 weighted images, metastatic lesions exhibit a nonspecific low signal intensity; on T2 weighted images metastatic lesions are usually high in signal intensity (Figs. 23–41, 23–42). This is in contrast to hematologic neoplastic disease (e.g., leukemia and lymphoma) in which the signal on T2 weighted images may become isointense or may increase in signal intensity only minimally. In our experience, metastases usually are well-defined lesions, although the margins may be ill defined if there is a moderate to significant amount of marrow edema associated with the lesion. In some patients, there may be diffuse involvement of the entire marrow of a bone with metastases (Fig. 23–42). In general, metastatic lesions are associated with some marrow or soft tissue edema, but not as much as would be seen with an inflammatory lesion. Therefore, a mild to moderate amount of edema is seen in metastatic lesions, but a moderate to large amount of edema would suggest an inflammatory lesion.[50] Some metastases (such as retinoblastoma and cerebellar medulloblastoma) are known to induce myelofibrosclerosis with osteoblastic reaction and bone production (Fig. 23–43).[80] In these cases a signal loss should be expected on all pulse sequences. The overall sensitivity of MRI for detection of marrow metastases is not yet known.

The appearance of a metastasis on spin-echo images is not specific, and the characteristics of STIR, gradient-echo, and chemical shift imaging and calculated T1 and T2 relaxation times may not be effective in predicting the specific histologic status of a lesion (malignant or benign). However, the sensitivity of MRI in defining the presence and extent of lesions makes it a valuable diagnostic tool in the oncologic setting. Not only does the identification of a metastatic lesion serve to confirm the presence and extent of metastatic disease, but accurate bony and soft tissue margins can be determined to assist in the planning of radiation therapy ports for isolated metastases. The appearance of a lesion on MRI can serve to exclude the diagnosis of metastatic disease and may instead accurately identify ischemia or infection, thereby saving the patient a biopsy or inappropriate and unnecessary therapy (Fig. 23–44). Unfortunately, MRI cannot be used at this time to screen the entire skeleton for metastases.

DISORDERS OF HEMOGLOBIN AND HEMATOPOIESIS

Sickle Cell Anemia

Sickle cell anemia occurs in children who are homozygous for hemoglobin S,[81] and is characterized by anemia associated with acute painful ischemic crises affecting the bones and joints. In the first 2 or 3 years of life, residual hemoglobin F may protect the individual from these crises. In sickle cell anemia the red cells appear normal when fully oxygenated but have elongated, sickle configurations under conditions of reduced oxygen tension. This results in mechanical capillary stasis, because the deformed red cells are unable to traverse small vessels. This leads to obstruction of the vessel and hypoxic damage of tissues distal to the obstruction (primarily bone marrow and bone), with resultant necrosis. Sickle cell trait is found in individuals who are heterozygous for hemoglobin S. Bone

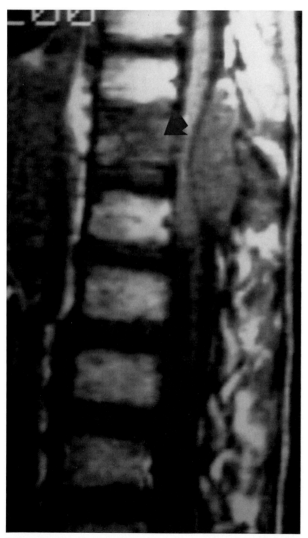

Figure 23–41. *Metastasis from Ewing's sarcoma.* Sagittal image of the spine in a child (1000/30). The vertebral body is replaced by intermediate-signal-intensity tumor (*arrow*). An adjacent subdural metastasis is seen.

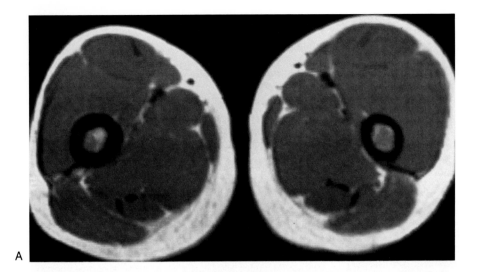

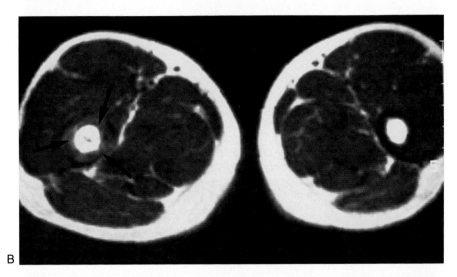

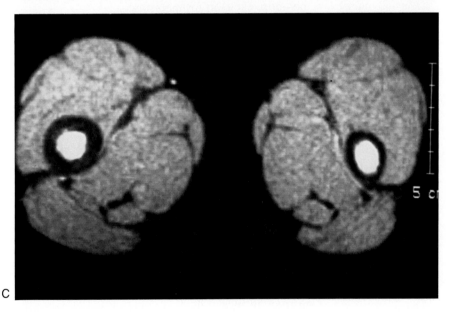

Figure 23–42. *Metastatic neuroblastoma. Transverse images through the femur show diffuse bilateral femoral metastases.* ***A,*** There is decreased signal intensity marrow on the T1 weighted (600/15) image. ***B,*** Increased-signal-intensity marrow is seen on the T2 weighted image (2000/75). Diffuse periostitis is noted in the right femur (*arrows*). ***C,*** STIR image at 0.38T (1500/30/TI 100) accentuates the abnormal increased-signal-intensity marrow with suppression of subcutaneous fat.

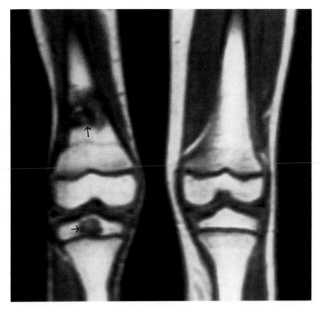

Figure 23–43. *Metastatic medulloblastoma.* Coronal T1 weighted (600/15) image through the femur in a 9-year-old patient. The two well-defined lesions (*arrows*) in the right femoral metaphysis and tibial epiphysis are typical for focal metastatic disease. The signal intensity is intermediate, with focal areas of low to intermediate signal intensity. The focal areas of low to intermediate signal intensity were also seen on T2 weighted images and were due to my-elofibrosclerosis induced by the metastatic tumor.

disease is thought to be rare in individuals with only the trait.

Imaging

Marrow abnormalities on MRI in patients with sickle cell anemia are common and may be considered to fall into one of two categories: (1) marrow changes due to the underlying anemia and (2) marrow changes due to the recurrent marrow ischemia.

Marrow Hyperplasia

The diffuse marrow hyperplasia changes seen in patients with sickle cell anemia relate to the degree of underlying anemia, and are more pronounced in older patients who have had the disease for the longest time and in patients with the most severe anemia. On spin-echo images the signal intensity of marrow reflects the pattern of reconversion of yellow to red marrow, with intermediate-signal-intensity "hematopoietic" marrow seen on T1 weighted images in those areas that should, for the patient's age, contain yellow marrow (Fig. 23–45). Changes are seen first in the spine, flat bones, and skull, and are diffuse. Changes seen in the humerus or femur consist of intermediate-signal-intensity marrow on T1 weighted images in the proximal metaphyses, then in the distal metaphyses, then in the diaphysis, and finally in the epiphysis, indicating an increased population of hematopoietic precursors. This pattern of marrow reconversion is also seen in the forearm and calf, and finally in the hands and feet.

Age-related distribution of red and yellow marrow for sickle cell patients has not been published, but our experience and review of images of such patients published in the literature for other reasons[82, 83] show areas of yellow marrow in these patients. Therefore, normal conversion from red to yellow marrow does take place in early childhood and can be appreciated on MRI images (Fig. 23–46). The intermediate-signal-intensity hematopoietic marrow seen in areas of the bone that should, for the patient's age, contain fatty marrow may therefore represent reconversion of yellow to red marrow as the anemia progresses, and not merely a lack of normal conversion. There is a spectrum of marrow abnormality on MRI in patients with sickle cell anemia ranging from normal marrow patterns (those in the first few years of life) to focal areas of abnormality to more diffuse areas of abnormality that likely relate to the patient's age, the severity of disease, anemia, and other factors such as environment and therapy. As more clinical uses for MRI in the evaluation of patients with sickle cell anemia are found, the establishment of these expected abnormal patterns of red and yellow marrow in these patients will become increasingly important.

Marrow Ischemia and Infarction in Sickle Cell Anemia

The metabolically active hyperplastic hematopoietic marrow in patients with sickle cell anemia requires an increased blood supply to maintain its viability, and the slow sinusoidal circulation in hematopoietic marrow makes the marrow a common place of increased sickling and infarction. Before MRI, bone marrow infarction was diagnosed by conventional radiography and isotope bone marrow scanning. Conventional radiographs show no acute changes, and areas of marrow ischemia are present only on follow-up examinations. Scintigraphic studies do not allow differentiation of acute marrow infarction from chronic marrow infarction. MRI holds promise in the diagnosis of early infarction in patients with sickle cell crisis. Rao and colleagues[82] reported marrow changes in sickle cell disease patients with acute infarction. These infarcts are seen as focal marrow abnormalities of decreased signal intensity on short TR-TE images and increased signal intensity on long TR-TE images (Fig. 23–47). This conversion from low signal intensity on short TR-TE images to high signal intensity on long TR-TE images correlated well with pain and was seen in 12 of 14 patients with painful joints; specific pathologic data were not available to correlate with these changes in signal intensity, but the authors felt they likely represented edema in acute infarction. Three of five patients with painless joints had focal areas of decreased signal intensity on T1 weighted images, with no conversion of these areas to increased signal intensity on T2 weighted images. These areas were thought to represent older infarcts, although the possibility of focal hematopoietic marrow could not be excluded.

The marrow hyperplasia, increased demand for oxy-

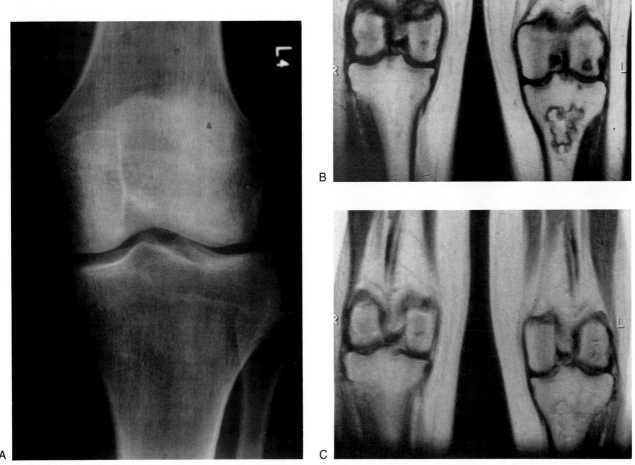

Figure 23–44. *Marrow infarct.* **A,** Radiograph of the left knee in a child with known bony lymphoma and new left knee pain. Subtle sclerosis was seen in the proximal tibial metaphysis. **B,** T1 weighted coronal image through the knees showing a geographic well-defined lesion in the left proximal metaphysis. Low-signal-intensity rim corresponds to sclerotic bone. Central marrow signal intensity is normal. **C,** Longer TR image shows persistent normal marrow signal intensity in the lesion. The findings are consistent with infarct and not tumor.

gen, and vaso-occlusive phenomena that lead to end-organ infarction result in avascular necrosis of the femoral head in 15 to 30 percent of patients with sickle cell anemia. Studies by Rao and colleagues[83] attempt to elucidate the role histologic change in composition of marrow of the femoral epiphysis might play in the development of avascular necrosis of the hip in sickle cell patients. Since the need for increased blood flow to hematopoietic marrow is well known, patients in whom there is conversion of fatty to hematopoietic marrow in the femoral epiphysis (Fig. 23–46) could potentially be at risk for increased incidence of avascular necrosis.

Forty-two percent of the patients with sickle cell anemia studied had mixed hematopoietic and fatty marrow in the femoral epiphyses, 32 percent had primarily fatty marrow, 16 percent had total replacement of the fatty marrow by hematopoietic marrow, and 10 percent had hemosiderotic marrow. Age distribution

was not correlated with marrow replacement or the MR appearance. Avascular necrosis of the femoral epiphysis occurred irrespective of the type of underlying epiphyseal marrow. The most consistent manifestation of avascular necrosis in sickle cell patients was low signal intensity on T1 weighted images in either a ring, band, crescent, or large homogeneous area (Fig. 23–48).[2, 82, 83] The second most common pattern was low signal on T1 and T2 images. Subchondral crescents of low signal on T1 weighted images may also be seen, and although joint fluid may be present, it is rarely increased above the normal range. Recognition of these patterns may be difficult when low- or intermediate-signal-intensity hematopoietic or hemosiderotic marrow is present in the femoral epiphyses as a result of marrow reconversion in patients with sickle cell anemia. The signal intensity on T2 weighted images is most commonly either low or isointense with epi-

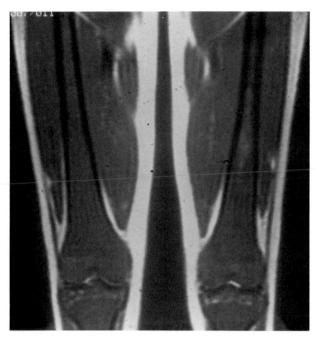

Figure 23–45. *Sickle cell anemia.* Coronal image through the distal femur in a patient with sickle cell anemia. Marrow conversion of increased-signal-intensity fatty marrow to intermediate-signal-intensity hematopoietic marrow can be noted. (Courtesy of Dr. Robert M. Steiner and Dr. Vijay Rao, Philadelphia.)

physeal marrow, although an increased signal intensity may be seen. It is possible that an increase in signal intensity on T2 weighted images signifies a more acute infarct. However, prospective studies with pathologic correlation remain to made.

Despite the general acceptance of MR as the imaging modality of choice in the detection of avascular necrosis, its sensitivity in the detection of early avascular necrosis may actually be less than 50 percent.[84] Although marrow cells, osteocytes, and fat cells die, the length of time required for signal alteration in acute infarction may be several days. It may be necessary to combine MRI with bone scintigraphy to detect early avascular necrosis in patients, like those with sickle cell anemia, who are at high risk for this disorder.[85]

MR Appearance of the Spleen

Patients with sickle cell anemia whose spleens have not completely infarcted may show decreased splenic signal intensity secondary to iron overload in the spleen. The iron deposition causes paramagnetic susceptibility effects, with a resultant T2 relaxation time shortening and decrease in signal intensity. Focal masses of relatively hyperintense splenic tissue represent infarcts or islands of hypertrophied splenic tissue that have less iron deposition than the surrounding tissue.[86]

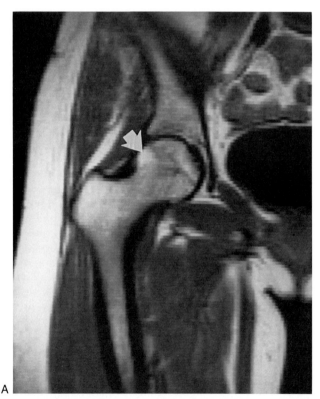

A

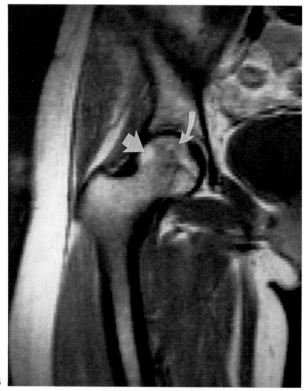

B

Figure 23–46. *Normal red-to-yellow marrow conversion in sickle cell anemia.* Short TR (500/30) *(A)* and long TR (1500/30) *(B)* coronal images through the right femur and iliac bone in a 16-year-old patient. Abnormal intermediate-signal-intensity hematopoietic marrow can be seen in the (normally fatty) femoral epiphysis (*curved arrow*) and in the proximal femoral metaphysis. Normal conversion of hematopoietic marrow to increased-signal-intensity fatty marrow can be seen in the diaphysis and focal areas of the proximal femoral metaphysis (*arrow*) and iliac crest.

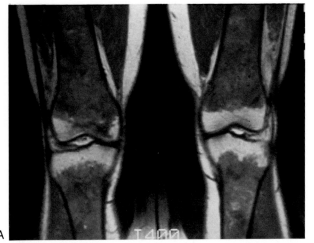 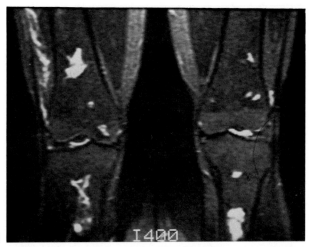

Figure 23–47. *Infarcts in sickle cell disease.* **A,** T1 weighted coronal image with cellular marrow and low-intensity infarcts. **B,** T2 weighted image. Areas of acute infarction have become very bright in intensity. (Courtesy of Dr. Robert M. Steiner and Dr. Vijay Rao, Philadelphia.)

Indications for MRI in Sickle Cell Disease

MRI is likely to become a mainstay in the evaluation of patients with sickle cell anemia. Although not particularly useful in the initial diagnosis of sickle cell anemia, MRI may be useful in the future to assess the severity of disease by monitoring the extent of marrow

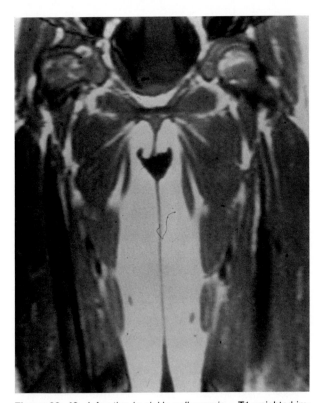

Figure 23–48. *Infarction in sickle cell anemia.* T1 weighted image shows a mixed signal from the right femoral head and proximal femur. (Courtesy of Dr. Robert M. Steiner and Dr. Vijay Rao, Philadelphia.)

reconversion, and identifying large regions of marrow that will no longer be available to the patient for increased hematopoiesis due to underlying large marrow infarcts. MRI also appears to be useful in the assessment of acute marrow ischemia and avascular necrosis. Both of these complications are widespread in sickle cell patients, and may be problematic in these unfortunate children, who may develop drug dependence as a result of treatment for their multiple infarcts. The importance of a diagnostic test that provides an accurate evaluation of acute marrow infarction requiring treatment cannot be sufficiently underscored. This is an important area of research that will certainly have a significant impact on the clinical care of these patients.

One clinical difficulty in patients with sickle cell anemia is distinguishing acute infarction from osteomyelitis. As the infection often occurs in sites of previous infarction,[87] this differentiation may be extremely difficult. Both disorders may present with acute pain and fever. In both there is bone abnormality with adjacent soft tissue abnormality. At the present time it is not known whether MRI will be useful in differentiating these two disorders. Radionuclide scans are currently the best available method for making this distinction.[88] On bone scan, infarction causes focal decreased uptake on MDP bone scan, which is not seen with osteomyelitis: sulfur colloid bone marrow scan shows a defect in uptake with infarction, but remains normal when there is infection.[88]

Sickle cells are paramagnetic and align in a magnetic field (Fig. 23–49).[89] Theoretically, this alignment of cells could enhance vascular occlusion of small capillaries, since the cells would be less compliant. However, it appears that this is only a theoretical risk, since many symptomatic and asymptomatic patients with sickle cell anemia have been imaged without known deleterious effect.[82, 83]

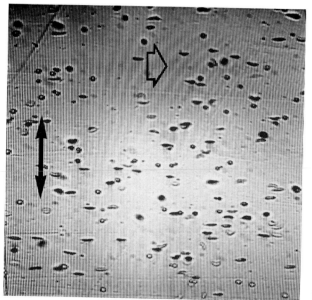 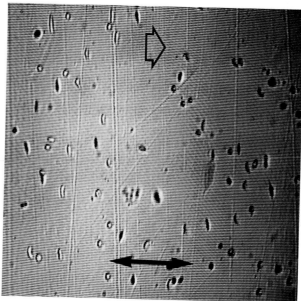

Figure 23–49. *Magnetic field effect on sickle cells. Deoxygenated sickle cells show alignment perpendicular to a magnetic field (0.38T) even when flowing.* ***A,*** Magnetic field is perpendicular to flow. The cell's long axis is parallel to the flow. ***B,*** Magnetic field is parallel to flow. The cell's long axis becomes perpendicular to flow and field direction. (*Open arrow* = direction of flows; *double-headed closed arrow* = direction of magnetic field.) (Brody AS. Induced alignment of flowing sickle cell erythrocytes in a magnetic field. Invest Radiol 1985; 20:560.)

Thalassemia

Seen most frequently in patients of Mediterranean descent, this erythroblastic anemia has strong familial and racial characteristics. The major form of thalassemia is the result of a homozygous state for the gene causing the hemoglobin abnormality, and is characterized by a severe progressive anemia accompanied by splenomegaly, hepatomegaly, and death before adolescence. Pathologically, the marrow is packed with erythroblastic cells that expand the medullary cavity and thin the cortex. The peripheral blood smear shows erythroblastemia. Thalassemia intermedia refers to the homozygous state but one with less prominent clinical manifestations of disease. Thalassemia minor refers to the heterozygous state for the gene causing the hemoglobin abnormality. The clinical and hematologic manifestations are less conspicuous, and life expectancy is prolonged. Extramedullary hematopoiesis occurs more commonly in thalassemia major or intermedia than in thalassemia minor and is most commonly seen as multiple bilateral posterior mediastinal masses originating from the posterior end of the ribs.[90] The hematopoietic tissue overflows the marrow space, destroys the anterior cortex of the posterior part of the rib, and spreads ventrally.[91] Occasionally these masses may be solitary and not associated with the adjacent surface of the rib.

MRI identifies abnormality in patients with thalassemia. In thalassemia major, one sees low to intermediate signal-intensity hematopoietic marrow throughout the medullary cavity on spin-echo MR images (Fig. 23–50). In thalassemia minor, there is conversion of red to yellow marrow in late childhood and early adult life, and while this occurs in the pattern expected for conversion of red to yellow marrow, more red marrow is seen on MRI than one would expect for the patient's age. In addition, there is noted delayed appearance and growth of the ossification centers of the epiphyses, with prominent epiphyseal cartilage remaining late in childhood.

Masses of extramedullary hematopoiesis have a signal intensity similar to that of the adjacent marrow in the thoracic spine and are usually decreased in signal intensity on T1 weighted images. Focal areas of increased signal intensity contribute to overall heterogeneity and probably represent marrow fat.[90] The mass has a sharp margin and may be surrounded by a linear rim of increased signal intensity, which is most likely due to a layer of fat. Since this finding of an increased-signal-intensity rim has not been described in other mediastinal masses,[92] this may represent a characteristic of marrow heterotopia in thalassemia hemoglobinopathy. The MR appearance of focal areas of extramedullary hematopoiesis in the liver, spleen, or lymph nodes has not been described, but one might expect these areas to be focal and well defined since this is the reported appearance on CT.[93]

Patients with thalassemia may have splenomegaly from extramedullary hematopoiesis and systemic iron overload from repeated blood transfusion. Hemolysis initially causes a greater concentration of excess iron in the spleen and reticuloendothelial system than in the liver. With chronic iron overload, iron deposition is

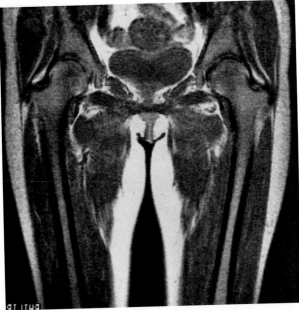

Figure 23–50. *Thalassemia.* Coronal intermediate image (1500/30) through the proximal femora in a young adult with thalassemia, showing diffuse intermediate-signal-intensity hematopoietic marrow in the femur and pelvis. This pattern of red marrow is more extensive than that expected for a young adult, and the intermediate-signal-intensity hematopoietic marrow is never normal in the epiphyses and trochanters.

seen in the liver, spleen, and bone marrow (Fig. 23–51). This iron infiltration shortens the T2 relaxation time and reduces image signal intensity.[86] The decrease in signal intensity is greatest at low tissue iron concentrations, and above tissue concentrations of 2 mg per gram no appreciable additional decrease in signal intensity of the spleen or liver is seen.

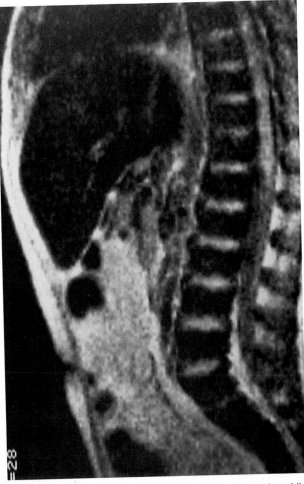

Figure 23–51. *Iron overload.* Sagittal image of the spine in a child with thalassemia and systemic iron overload from repeated blood transfusion. Marked decrease in marrow signal intensity secondary to T2 shortening is seen. (Courtesy of Dr. Charles A. Gooding, San Francisco.)

Spherocytosis

Familial hemolytic anemia (hereditary spherocytosis) is characterized by an abnormality of the cell membrane of the erythrocyte, which becomes spherical and as a consequence easily hemolyzed. The hemoglobin molecule is normal. Compensatory hyperplasia of the bone marrow is seen and relates to the severity of disease. As with other hemolytic anemias, this marrow hyperplasia is characterized on MRI by normal-appearing hematopoietic marrow in regions that should, for the age of the patient, be seen as fatty marrow. Reconversion of the diaphysis and epiphyses from yellow to red marrow is not uncommon.

MARROW DEPLETION

Aplastic Anemia

Aplastic anemia is characterized by acellularity or marked hypocellularity of the bone marrow. This results in pancytopenia with decreased erythroid, my-

eloid, and megaloid precursors. Drugs, viral infections, toxins, and hepatitis have all been associated with the development of aplastic anemia,[94] but the disorder is often idiopathic. Pathologically the marrow is hypocellular with primarily fatty marrow and areas of fibrosis.

There have been several published reports on the MR findings in patients with aplastic anemia.[61, 95–97] The most common pattern seen in untreated aplastic anemia is that of increased signal intensity on both T1 and T2 weighted images (Fig. 23–52). This represents the diffuse replacement of hematopoietic by fatty marrow. It appears that patients being treated for aplastic anemia may develop a heterogeneous pattern in the spine consisting of focal areas of low to intermediate signal intensity within the milieu of increased-signal-intensity fatty vertebral marrow.[95] Percutaneous biopsy of a vertebral body in a patient being treated for aplastic anemia who exhibited this patchy pattern showed hematopoietic tissue within the vertebral marrow. The iliac crest marrow in this same patient did not

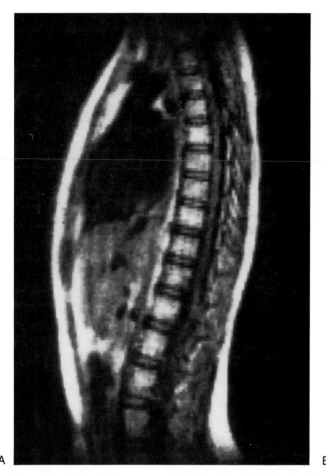
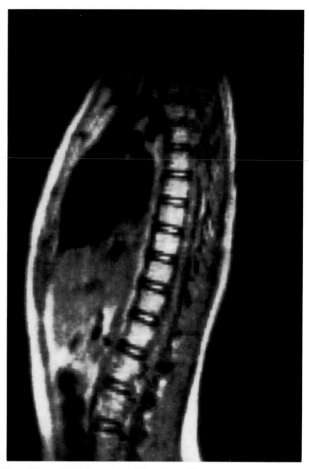

A   B

Figure 23–52. *Aplastic anemia.* ***A,*** Sagittal T1 weighted image (500/20) and ***B,*** sagittal intermediate T2 weighted image (1500/20) of the spine in a 4-year-old boy with aplastic anemia. The signal intensity of the vertebral marrow is abnormally high, consistent with fatty replacement of hematopoietic marrow.

show focal areas of intermediate signal intensity, but rather exhibited a more homogeneous pattern consistent with primarily fatty marrow. The marrow biopsy of the iliac crest showed no hematopoietic precursors. Since vertebral marrow contains a greater percentage of hematopoietic marrow per volume than the flat bones,[16] it is possible that recovery of the marrow may occur first in the vertebral marrow as opposed to the iliac crest marrow. An alternative explanation for the patchy pattern seen on MRI of the marrow in patients with aplastic anemia is that this low to intermediate signal intensity actually represents focal areas of fibrosis, known to occur in aplastic anemia, and does not represent hematopoietic reconstitution. Further studies are needed to answer this important clinical question. The above findings suggest, however, that MRI of the marrow may be useful in identifying areas of hematopoietic marrow, both within the iliac crest and in other marrow spaces in patients being treated for aplastic anemia. Currently, peripheral blood smears and iliac crest bone marrow biopsies are routinely obtained and are the only means available to assess response of the marrow to therapy. MRI may

now play a role in assessment of these patients for response to therapy.

In addition to spin-echo studies, chemical shift evaluation of aplastic anemia before and after treatment has been carried out. McKinstry and colleagues[61] studied three adults and one child with chemical shift imaging before and after treatment for aplastic anemia. Marrow gives a much lower water fraction signal (cellular fraction) on the chemical shift images in patients with aplastic anemia than in control subjects. Patients were followed for 4 to 12 weeks. No patient in this study showed a sustained hematologic response to treatment, and there was little change in the MR appearance of the marrow with treatment. This suggests that MRI may be sensitive to a lack of marrow response to treatment, although further prospective studies must be performed to determine the level of sensitivity of chemical shift imaging to increased cellularity, and therefore to assess the marrow response to treatment of aplastic anemia.

One would expect all pancytopenic anemias to present with a similar appearance of marrow on MRI, specifically diffuse infiltration of the marrow with fatty cells, occasional rests of hematologic cells, and possible areas of fibrosis.

Myelofibrosis

Myelofibrosis is characterized by progressive splenomegaly and a diffuse stromal marrow reaction, with replacement of the normal medullary fat and marrow elements by fibrosis. Myelofibrosis may be the result of myeloproliferative syndromes as well as a sequela of treatment for leukemia, lymphoma, Gaucher's disease, or metastatic carcinoma. Infection may also serve as a causative agent. Although uncommon in childhood, myelofibrosis is most often a result of therapy.

Replacement of the marrow by fibrosis results in either patchy or homogeneous low signal intensity on both T1 and T2 weighted images, depending on the distribution and severity of disease. Some areas of inhomogeneity are presumably secondary to focal areas of preserved marrow fat. Since both malignant and diffuse fibrotic replacement of marrow are seen as low to intermediate signal intensity on T1 weighted images, T2 weighted images are instrumental in distinguishing these two entities. Malignant infiltration of the marrow is seen as intermediate to bright signal intensity on T2 weighted images, while marrow fibrosis remains of low signal intensity.[98] Both myelofibrosis and hemosiderosis are sequelae of disease treatment in children, and it may be difficult to distinguish myelofibrosis from iron deposition in the marrow. However, iron deposition as a result of therapy for disease states such as chronic anemia results in abnormally low signal intensity of viscera as well as of bone marrow. In addition the T1 relaxation time of marrow in hemosiderosis is lengthened fairly quickly with increasing concentrations of iron, and in general usually gives a much lower signal intensity on both T1 and T2 weighted images than does myelofibrosis (Fig. 23–53).

MRI is likely to play an important role in the initial diagnosis and follow-up of marrow depletion states. The child being treated for leukemia or other neoplastic disorders may develop pancytopenia as a result of therapy, and the question will arise of recurrent disease versus a marrow depletion state. It is not difficult to distinguish recurrent disease from aplastic anemia, since the marrow depletion state of aplastic anemia is seen on MRI as increased signal intensity on both T1 and T2 weighted images in regions of the marrow that should normally be hematopoietic. Marrow packed with abnormal cells in recurrent disease is of low to intermediate signal intensity and fairly homogeneous; this can also be distinguished from myelofibrosis, which is typically lower in signal intensity on both T1 and T2 weighted images than recurrent disease and contains prominent areas of inhomogeneity. The T2 weighted images become important in this differential diagnosis, since marrow packed with leukemic or other abnormal cells is usually increased (although not bright) in signal intensity, while the marrow of myelofibrosis remains lower in signal intensity on T2 weighted images.

In addition to the initial diagnosis of marrow depletion states, MRI may play a role in assessing the efficacy of therapy for aplastic anemia. It is likely that areas of regenerating hematopoietic tissue will be seen as intermediate signal intensity on T1 weighted images, and may provide a more sensitive indicator of response to therapy than iliac crest marrow biopsy alone. The role of MRI in assessing the efficacy of treatment in myelofibrosis is uncertain.

ISCHEMIA AND INFARCTION OF MARROW; PERTHES' DISEASE

Not much has been written about the MR appearance of acute and subacute marrow ischemia in children. The appearance is relatively nonspecific and in most cases is independent of the cause of the ischemia. The appearance of marrow infarction in the metaphysis and diaphysis has already been described earlier in this chapter in the section on sickle cell disease. This section will describe the appearance in the epiphyses. Epiphyseal infarction may occur in many bones, but is most common in the femoral head, and in this location the most common disorder is Perthes' disease. For this reason we will use Perthes' disease for illustrative purposes, but it should be borne in mind that identical changes will be found in femoral head osteonecrosis irrespective of the etiology. These other causes include steroid therapy (frequently used in chemotherapy regimens) in pediatric patients, sickle cell anemia, Gaucher's disease, mucopolysaccharidoses, hypothyroidism, Cushing's syndrome, and renal failure. Many of the published reports of ischemic necrosis of the femoral head focus on avascular necrosis of the adult femoral head. It is believed that many of the principles described and discussed in the adult literature are applicable to children.

Pathology and Pathogenesis

The pathogenesis of osteonecrosis is not fully known or understood.[99] It is widely believed that the disorder is due to ischemia. In Perthes' disease it is quite likely that more than one episode of ischemia is required. The ischemia may be caused by a primary deficiency in arterial supply, although recently it has been shown that vascular congestion and edema are an integral part of the pathogenetic mechanism for femoral head osteonecrosis.[99] Insufficient venous drainage from the femoral head can lead to increased intramedullary pressure and decreased marrow perfusion.[100] Fatty marrow is believed to be especially vulnerable to osteonecrosis

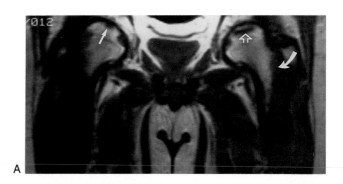

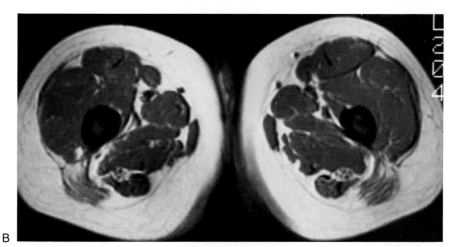

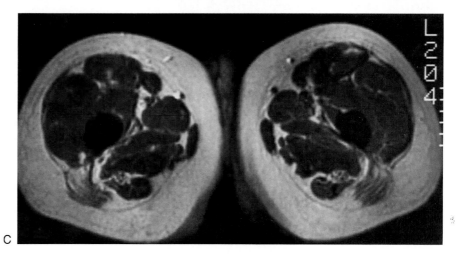

Figure 23–53. *Hemosiderosis in bone marrow.* ***A,*** T1 weighted (800/20) coronal image of the proximal femora in a 24-year-old male with lymphoma treated with multiple transfusions. Marrow hemosiderosis is seen as low to intermediate signal intensity infiltrating the proximal femora bilaterally (*curved arrow*). Note the low-signal-intensity avascular necrosis in the hips. Both focal low-signal-intensity (*arrow*) and crescentic abnormalities (*open arrow*) are seen. ***B,C,*** Spin-density (2000/20) and T2 weighted (2000/80) transverse images show lower-signal-intensity marrow than would be expected with myelofibrosis. This is consistent with hemosiderosis of marrow.

because it has a lower blood supply than hematopoietic marrow.[101]

After the ischemic insult, cellular death begins. Hematopoietic cells are the most sensitive to marrow ischemia and die in the first 6 to 12 hours. Osteoblasts, osteoclasts, and osteocytes show evidence of cellular death by 48 hours. Fat cells, the most resistant cells to ischemia, show evidence of cellular death 2 to 5 days after the ischemic event. Even after death of the fat cells, no change may be seen on MRI because the lipid

in the cells initially persists, and it is the lipid that produces the MR signal.

The body responds to the ischemic insult with inflammation and hyperemia. This is most evident at the interface between viable and necrotic tissue, and is characterized by increased perfusion, the presence of granulation tissue, and a fibroblastic response. After this reactive hyperemic response, there is a permeative ingrowth of the repair tissue into the necrotic zone. Osteoblastic activity deposits new bone on the trabeculae and necrotic tissue. Collapse of trabeculae occurs, and if a sufficiently large area has been involved and weakened a cleft fracture may follow. The final phase is that of osteoclastic removal of the dead collapsed trabeculae, with continued new bone deposition and remodeling.[102] Secondary changes are also seen in the femoral neck, which becomes shortened and widened.[103] Cysts may also develop in the metaphysis.

The MR appearance of the infarction reflects the underlying pathophysiologic process, and the final MR appearance depends on the balance between all the ischemic and repair processes.

Clinical Factors

Perthes' disease occurs most commonly between the ages of 4 and 8 years. It is more common in boys than in girls. Ten percent of the cases are bilateral. When bilateral disease occurs,the stage of the disease is always different in the two hips. The onset of symptoms

is extremely variable;[99, 104] these include limp, pain, and decreased motion of the hip joint. The major thrust of therapy is to maintain as full a range of motion as possible while keeping the femoral head contained within the acetabulum to minimize deformity. The long-term outcome varies from severe deformity of the femoral head to complete recovery. Prognosis is best in younger children, and in patients in whom only part of the femoral head is affected (Fig. 23–54) and in whom marked sclerosis and collapse of the femoral head has not occurred.[105]

Imaging Findings

Plain film radiographs are relatively insensitive in the evaluation of Perthes' disease. Initial necrosis of cells and the hyperemic response produce no changes on the radiograph. A subcortical lucency, seen best in the frog leg lateral view, corresponds to fracture through the necrotic bone. Areas of sclerosis represent new bone deposition on trabeculae or collapse and

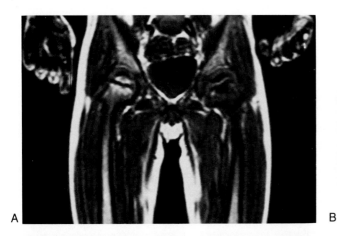

A

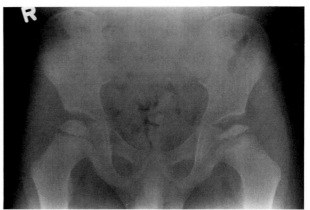

B

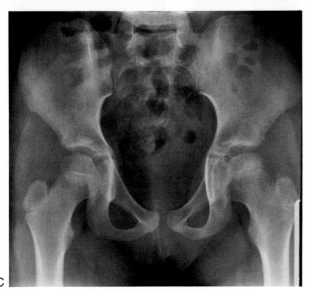

C

Figure 23–54. *Perthes' disease. "Horseshoe" pattern of sparing.* ***A,*** Initial MR image shows persistent normal T1 signal medially and laterally, with a small central area of abnormal low intensity. ***B,*** Corresponding initial radiograph. ***C,*** Follow-up radiograph 21 months later shows complete healing. (From Henderson RC, Renner JB, Shurdwarf MC, Greene WB. An evaluation of MRI in Legg-Perthes' disease. J Pediatr Orthop, in press, 1990.)

compaction of trabeculae (Fig. 23–54). Areas of lucency correspond to regions of osteoclastic removal of dead bone and regions of remodeling with healing.

On MRI, avascular necrosis of the femoral head has a wide variety of appearances (Figs. 23–54, 23–55). These are described in detail later. Some authors have attempted fairly rigid classifications of these different appearances and have tried to correlate each MR appearance with pathologic findings and prognosis. Unfortunately, none of these systems is ideal and there is much overlap; many patients do not fit clearly into a particular classification. There are many causes for the unpredictable appearance and various patterns of abnormality seen on MRI:

1. Avascular necrosis does not follow a predictable course.

2. Repeated episodes of ischemia may occur with varying effect on the tissues.

3. The time pattern and age of the lesions in any particular patient are frequently unknown.

4. Pathologic evaluation is rarely available. A wide variety of pathologic processes are occurring simultaneously and at different rates. These include cell necrosis, reactive hyperemia and cellular infiltration, bone deposition, bone resorption, bone collapse, and hemorrhage.

5. The appearance of the various pathologic processes varies depending on imaging pulse sequences used, magnetic field strength, use of surface coils, and so forth.

As mentioned above, ischemia and necrosis produce a wide variety of different MR signal patterns. On T1 weighted images there may be homogeneous low signal intensity from the femoral head,[99, 106] irregular mixed signal intensity, rings or bands of various thickness and of low signal intensity, or large irregular areas of low signal intensity (Figs. 23–54, 23–55).[106] On T2 weighted images there is variable change, with some, all, or none of the areas of low signal intensity becoming very bright. One pattern believed to be fairly suggestive of the diagnosis of avascular necrosis is the appearance of a low-intensity line with an adjacent high-intensity line seen on T2 weighted images.[110]

The appearance on MRI may be correlated with the underlying pathologic processes. Early in the course of infarction there is often on T1 weighted images a low-intensity ring or band surrounding the infarcted marrow, which still appears of normal intensity (Fig. 23–56). This low-signal ring or band is thought to represent a reactive interface, and is composed of a layer of inflammatory fibromesenchymal tissue that develops at the margin between the viable and infarcted bone.[107, 108] Depending on the age of the infarct, whether subacute or chronic, the signal from the central marrow of the infarct may be decreased (Figs. 23–53, 23–55, 23–57) or isointense (Fig. 23–56) with the marrow signal on T1 images. The bright-signal-intensity rim seen adjacent to a low-intensity area on T2 weighted images may be due to a chemical shift artifact or to the edema (Figs. 23–57). Areas of bone deposition or areas of sclerosis from collapsed trabeculae appear of low signal intensity on both T1 and T2 weighted images. If a fracture has occurred, the fracture cleft may be a gap of low signal intensity on both T1 and T2 weighted pulse sequences. However, the gap may be filled with edema, fluid, or blood and therefore may have high or low signal intensity on T1 or T2 weighted images. A recent study in adult dogs[109] showed a heterogeneous loss of signal intensity on T1 weighted spin-echo images by 7 days after surgical devascularization of the distal femoral epiphysis. This corresponds pathologically to lymphocyte infiltration.

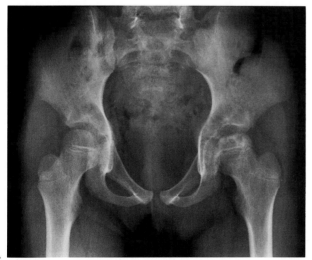
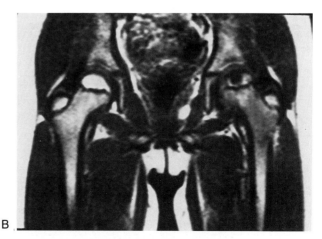

A   B

Figure 23–55. *Legg-Perthes' disease.* **A,** Anteroposterior radiograph showing obvious Legg-Perthes' disease on the left. **B,** MR image with diffuse loss of the normal T1 signal from the left epiphysis, and preservation on the right. (From Henderson RC, Renner JB, Shurdwarf MC, Greene WB. An evaluation of MRI in Legg-Perthes' disease. J Pediatr Orthop, in press, 1990.)

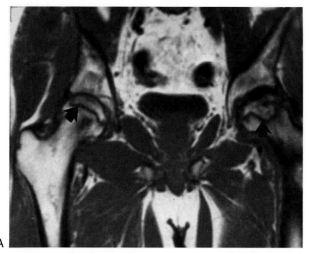

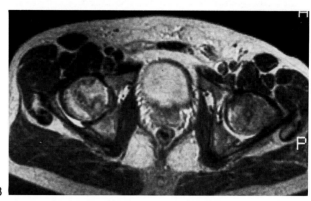

Figure 23–56. *Early infarction of the femoral head.* **A,** Coronal T1 weighted (800/20) image of the hips in a young male undergoing steroid therapy for lymphoma. A well-defined low-signal-intensity line (*arrow*) surrounds the infarcted marrow, which retains a normal increased signal intensity. **B,** Transverse intermediate (1500/80) image through the femoral head shows persistent normal marrow signal intensity.

High signal intensity on T2 weighted images is most likely due to vascular congestion or edema and is a fairly consistent finding in symptomatic avascular necrosis of the femoral head.[99, 110, 111] The mechanism for the increased signal intensity of the marrow in acute osteonecrosis of the femoral head on T2 weighted images is most likely related to free water associated with the vascular congestion. Whether this free water is located in the capillaries and sinusoids, in the interstitial space in the form of edema, or within damaged cells remains to be determined.[104] A characteristic appearance of avascular necrosis consists of a low-signal-intensity rim surrounding the necrotic lesion, with a high-signal-intensity rim inside the low-signal-intensity margin on T2 weighted images.[110] This so-called

double line sign may represent hyperemia or inflammation within the granulation tissue. It does not appear to represent a chemical shift artifact, since reversal of the frequency-encoding gradient direction does not change the appearance of the double line.[107] Some of the patterns seen in the femoral head are strongly suggestive of avascular necrosis. Other patterns, such as a diffuse decrease in signal intensity on T1 weighted images, are more nonspecific. Differential diagnosis includes tumor, infiltration, a large cyst, and storage disorders.[106]

With healing, there is gradual recovery of normal signal on MRI, but this may be delayed for years (Figs. 23–58, 23–59).[105] The role of MRI in the diagnosis and management of patients with avascular necrosis of the

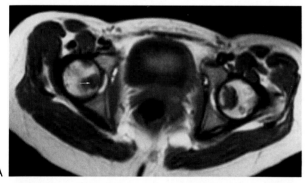

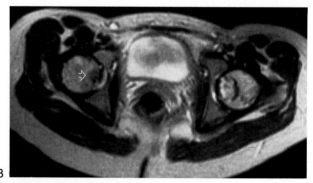

Figure 23–57. *Avascular necrosis of the femoral head.* Transverse images through the femoral head in a young adult with avascular necrosis secondary to steroid therapy. T1 weighted (800/20) **(A)** and T2 weighted (2000/70) **(B)** images. A small, subtle, very-low-signal-intensity line (*arrow*) seen on the right on the T1 image increases on the T2 weighted image (2000/70) (*open arrow*). Edema is the likely explanation. On the T1 weighted image large areas of low-signal infarcted marrow are seen on both sides. On the right there is little increase in signal intensity on the T2 weighted image, whereas marked increase in signal occurs on the left. This difference reflects different ages of the infarct.

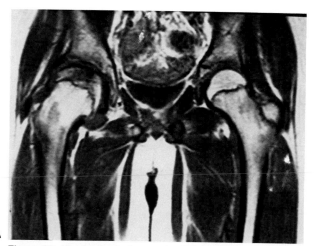
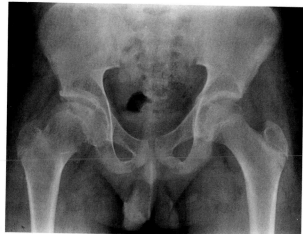

Figure 23–58. *Perthes' disease: healing. Slow return of T1 signal.* **A,** Coronal MR image 4 years after diagnosis of Legg-Perthes' disease shows persistent absence of the normal T1 signal. **B,** Corresponding radiograph shows apparent complete healing. (From Henderson RC, Renner JB, Shurdwarf MC, Greene WB. An evaluation of MRI in Legg-Perthes' disease. J Pediatr Orthop, in press, 1990.)

femoral head has not yet been clearly defined. There is no doubt that MRI can detect abnormality when the plain film radiographs are still normal (MRI may also occasionally be falsely negative).[105] In early disease, MRI is better than plain films for showing the total extent and distribution of abnormality.[105] Whether MRI will ultimately prove more sensitive than bone scan is not known. Another factor, as yet undetermined, is the significance of detection by MRI of early marrow signal abnormality in children presenting with hip pain. Do these children have transient synovitis or do they have early Perthes' disease? Is transient synovitis really an early, mild, self-limiting form of Perthes' disease? Will the early detection of subtle marrow abnormality in patients with hip pain alter management? Once the diagnosis of Perthes' disease has been established, the role of MRI in monitoring therapy is also unknown. Because of the many varied patterns of abnormality identified on MRI, will it prove possible to identify specific patterns that necessitate an alteration in therapy? At the present time there is no conclusive evidence that the pattern of abnormality seen in the femoral head can significantly influence therapy. One aspect of therapy that is universally accepted is the importance of maintaining containment of the femoral head within the acetabulum. In this regard MRI may prove useful because of its explicit ability to detect sphericity of the femoral head and swelling of the articular cartilage of the femoral head and acetabulum in patients with Perthes' disease.[103, 105] This swelling causes lateral displacement of the femoral head. It has been found that the mean increase in thickness of the femoral head articular cartilage ranges from 1.8 to 3.9 mm, depending on the location within the joint.[103] Henderson and associates, in a long-term study of 22 cases of Perthes' disease, concluded that for serial follow-up of the disease process through the natural healing course, plain radiographs were as good as or better than MRI and considerably less costly.[105]

The sensitivity and specificity of MRI for the diagnosis of avascular necrosis of the femoral head are not yet known. Some information is available but further work needs to be done. There are conflicting statements in the literature regarding the sensitivity and specificity of MRI. Many authors have stated that MRI is more sensitive than bone scans. Others have reported the sensitivity of MRI in detecting early avascular necrosis to be no more than 50 percent.[84] Other workers report a sensitivity of 94 percent.[111] Elsig and colleagues reported one case of Perthes' disease with positive MDP and negative MR imaging,[112] and Henderson and associates described one case with positive radiograph and bone scan and normal MRI.[105] The reasons for these discrepancies are many. Very early in avascular necrosis there is ischemia, and it would be expected that imaging studies such as MDP bone scan, which are dependent on flow, would be abnormal very early on. MRI depends on alteration in the signal of the normal fat. The fat cells are the last cells of the bone marrow to die, and even after their death it may take some time before the fat itself is altered. The inflammatory response occurring at the junction of the viable and dead marrow also takes time to develop. This response is often the earliest abnormality detectable on MRI. Therefore, in patients with acute presentation of pain or in the screening of high-risk patients, it may be desirable to combine MRI with bone scintigraphy to maximize the sensitivity of imaging.[85] The choice of imaging techniques is also important; for example, pinhole collimation improves visualization with scintigraphy, and the use of surface coils assists the detection of early abnormality with MRI.[113]

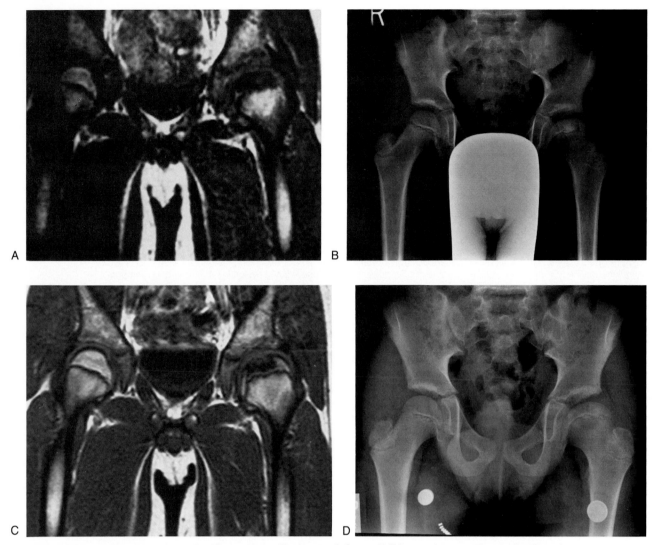

Figure 23–59. *Perthes' disease: healing. Some return of T1 signal.* ***A,*** Coronal MR image shows nearly complete loss of T1 signal. ***B,*** Corresponding radiograph. ***C,*** Follow-up MRI 15 months later (again through the posterior portion of the epiphysis) with some return of T1 signal laterally. ***D,*** Corresponding follow-up radiograph. (From Henderson RC, Renner JB, Shurdwarf MC, Greene WB. An evaluation of MRI in Legg-Perthes' disease. J Pediatr Orthop, in press, 1990.)

METABOLIC DISORDERS

Gaucher's Disease

Infiltration of the marrow occurs in many lysosomal storage diseases. In the lipid storage subclassification, there are several forms of Gaucher's disease that all involve accumulation of glucocerebroside in reticuloendothelial cells of the bone marrow and visceral organs. This accumulation of glucocerebroside is caused by a deficiency of the enzyme glucosylceramidase and cerebroside beta-glucosidase. The most common variety is the "adult" form that may have an onset in childhood. Roentgenographic changes in the skeleton show destruction of bone, reflecting replacement of marrow by cerebroside-laden reticuloendothelial cells. The marrow involvement is patchy or diffuse. Bone

pain, pathologic fractures, osteopenia, reactive sclerosis, bone modeling abnormality, aseptic necrosis of the femoral head, and vertebral collapse may result from this infiltration of the marrow. Splenomegaly and resultant thrombocytopenia are prominent clinical characteristics, and pulmonary infiltrates, pulmonary hypertension, and moderate hepatic dysfunction may be present. Bone marrow transplantation may be considered in the face of life-threatening complications from the disease, and is becoming increasingly more common as a mode of therapy.[115]

MR Findings in Gaucher's Disease

The MR changes seen in lipid storage diseases, specifically Gaucher's disease, have been described.[116, 117] Of the cases reported in the literature, there are 14 children imaged ranging in age from 5 to 17 years.

Several types of MR abnormalities on both medium (0.5T and 0.6T) and high (1.5T) field systems have been described. Infiltration and replacement of the marrow by glucocerebroside-laden cells results in an overall decrease of marrow signal intensity on both T1 and T2 weighted images. The finding of a decreased signal on T2 weighted imaging is unusual for active disease processes. Marrow involvement generally follows the distribution of red marrow and appears to occur first in regions of the marrow normally occupied by hematopoietic marrow (spine, pelvis, proximal femoral metaphysis), then progresses in a proximal to distal manner in the appendicular skeleton. The vertebral marrow demonstrates uniform and widespread abnormality at all levels, with replacement of the normal fatty marrow by low-signal-intensity infiltrated marrow. In the long bones and the flat bones the distribution of abnormality is either patchy or widespread and diffuse (Fig. 23–60). Erlenmeyer flask deformity of the distal femur, both with[116] and without[117] underlying abnormal low-signal-intensity marrow, has been reported. In the report of underlying marrow abnormality,[116] the Erlenmeyer flask appearance of the distal femur was thought to be caused by packing of the marrow with Gaucher cells and subsequent loss of normal remodeling. The epiphyses of the long bones are usually spared even when the adjacent metaphyseal regions are affected, although the epiphyses may be abnormal and of low signal intensity when extensive bone involvement is present.

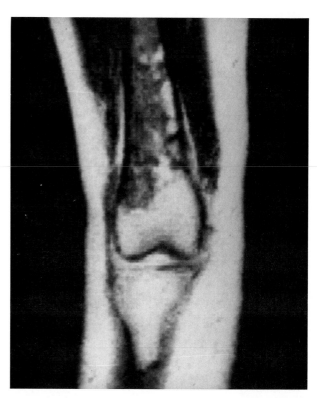

Figure 23–60. *Gaucher's disease.* Coronal T1 weighted (500/20) image through the right femur of a young adult. Patchy but diffuse low to intermediate signal-intensity infiltration of the marrow by glucocerebroside-laden cells is seen. The signal intensity of the infiltrated marrow increased on the T2 weighted images (not illustrated) to slightly more than that of surrounding marrow.

Marrow Infarction in Gaucher's Disease

Patients with Gaucher's disease frequently suffer crises of acute bone pain, most commonly in the hips and knees. These episodes of pain are believed to represent vascular infarction, and there are usually no accompanying radiographic manifestations in the acute phase. In two cases reported by Lanir and associates,[116] acute bone pain was accompanied by increased signal intensity of the marrow on both T1 and T2 weighted images, especially prominent on long TR-TE images. The marrow changes were accompanied by sharply marginated, periosseous, high-signal-intensity soft tissue collections that presumably represented subperiosteal hematoma or fluid collection. This finding resolved with time. Islands of bright signal intensity within the medullary space on T1 weighted images were also reported by Rosenthal and colleagues,[117] corresponding to regions of altered trabecular bone on plain radiographs and CT, and were thought most likely to represent early infarction. It is difficult to explain the increased signal intensity on T1 weighted images by the presence of edema in an early infarct. Since it does not appear that longitudinal studies of these patients were obtained, this increased signal intensity marrow could represent areas of marrow not previously infiltrated by Gaucher cells, and therefore seemingly "increased" in signal intensity as compared with the remainder of the marrow. Alternatively, there

may be a hemorrhagic component to the acute infarct to explain the increased signal intensity on T1 weighted images. This will require further evaluation.

Multiple focal areas of low signal intensity demarcated by sharp, even lower-signal-intensity margins were correlated with the plain film and CT appearance, and thought to represent older infarcts. Patients whose clinical course was complicated by fracture or osteonecrosis were in general older (mean age of 36 years) and had diffuse involvement of the marrow, with no areas of marrow spared. Patients who did not sustain fractures or osteonecrosis often had generalized sparing of the epiphysis as well as the marrow of the distal lower extremities, indicating a less severe stage of disease.

Measurement of T1 and T2 relaxation times of the marrow shows minimal prolongation of T1 relaxation time (marrow values 500 to 700 msec) and shortening of T2 relaxation time (marrow value = 50 msec), with a resultant decrease in signal intensity on both T1 and T2 weighted images.[116] These changes do not appear to be statistically significant.

Indications for MRI in Gaucher's Disease

MRI will continue to be useful in the evaluation of patients with storage diseases, specifically Gaucher's disease. By scanning the primary hematopoietic areas (spine, pelvis, proximal femora, and humeri) with coronal T1 weighted images, one can assess the extent of disease. It is possible that a single T1 weighted MR image of the distal femur and proximal tibia may be used as a screening procedure in patients with Gaucher's disease, since lack of involvement of these areas could indicate a less severe state of disease, whereas patchy involvement could indicate moderate to severe disease, and complete replacement of these marrow regions would indicate severe disease. Any replacement of epiphyses would indicate extensive marrow involvement. In addition to "staging" the degree of marrow affected in Gaucher's disease, MRI will likely play an increasingly important role in the evaluation of these patients for acute marrow infarction and avascular necrosis. The patient population at risk for the complications of fracture and osteonecrosis can potentially be identified with coronal T1 weighted spin-echo imaging, because patients who sustain these complications of Gaucher's disease tend to have diffuse marrow involvement with no areas of normal marrow signal intensity. Precautionary measures could be taken in patients thus identified.

Iron Deposition

Genetic hemochromatosis, an inherited disease known to be associated with an abnormal iron-loading gene linked to the A-locus of the HLA complex on chromosome 6, is an iron storage disorder with an inappropriate increase in intestinal iron absorption. This results in deposition of iron in various organs of the body, especially the liver, heart, pancreas, and pituitary. Acquired hemochromatosis is seen more commonly in children than is genetic hemochromatosis, and is caused by iatrogenic iron overload of the tissues and subsequent tissue injury. The iron overload in children usually occurs in chronic disease, including disorders of erythropoiesis such as thalassemia or sideroblastic anemia, and is the result of increased intestinal iron absorption that is exacerbated by iron therapy and frequent blood transfusions. Deposition of iron in these patients occurs primarily in the organs, particularly the liver, spleen, pancreas, heart, and pituitary, but also in the bone marrow. Hemosiderosis is defined as the presence of stainable iron in tissues (often confined to reticuloendothelial cells), with progression to hemochromatosis only when there is actual iron-induced tissue damage (usually involving organ parenchymal cells) and functional insufficiency of the organs involved.[118]

The deposits of iron in the liver of patients with genetic hemochromatosis are in the form of ferritin and hemosiderin, with deposits of these superparamagnetic compounds first seen in the periportal parenchymal cells. Cirrhosis eventually develops. In contrast, parenteral administration of iron in the form of iron transfu-

sions or iron preparations, the usual inciting factor in pediatric cases of hemosiderosis and acquired hemochromatosis, results in predominantly reticuloendothelial iron overload. This appears to lead to less tissue damage than the iron loading of parenchymal cells seen in genetic hemochromatosis.[118]

MR Findings with Iron Deposition

MARROW. Although the bone marrow is not commonly involved in either the acquired or the genetic forms of hemosiderosis or hemochromatosis,[118] children with acquired hemosiderosis or hemochromatosis are more likely to develop decreased marrow signal intensity, since reticuloendothelial cells of the marrow phagocytose iron. Visceral deposition of iron is seen in both the acquired and genetic forms of hemosiderosis and hemochromatosis.

Ferritin and hemosiderin are superparamagnetic and cause a marked decrease in affected marrow signal intensity on both T1 and T2 weighted images.[119] This may be either focal or diffuse and tends to occur first in areas of marrow with active hematopoiesis (Figs. 23–61, 23–62). The lack of histologic marrow involvement explains the paucity of marrow changes in childhood hemosiderosis or hemochromatosis despite gross involvement of the visceral organs (Fig. 23–63). The marrow signal may be decreased owing to the magnetic susceptibility effect of ferritin and hemosiderin, but it may often be normal. There have been no reports to date correlating the amount of iron deposition in the marrow with a corresponding gradation of decrease in marrow signal intensity.

JOINTS. There are few marrow changes in hemochromatosis, but the joints are commonly involved. Deposits of iron can be seen in synovial cells lining the joints, with calcium pyrophosphate crystals embedded in the synovial tissues. Arthropathy develops in 25 to 50 percent of patients with hemochromatosis, and although it usually occurs in those over 50 years of age, joint changes may occur at any time during the course of the disease. The small joints of the hands, wrist, hips, and knees may show the MR findings of synovitis, subchondral sclerosis, loss of articular cartilage with narrowing of the joint space, and calcification of the synovium. Hemosiderin deposition within the joints in patients with hemophilia has been reported as of low signal intensity on T1 and T2 weighted images and may appear rather thick and bulky.[120]

VISCERA. When low signal intensity on both T1 and T2 weighted images is noted in the liver, spleen, and other organs of a child (Fig. 23–63), a diagnosis of hemochromatosis or hemosiderosis is suggested. Investigation should be made to determine the cause of visceral iron overload, whether genetic hemochromatosis, acquired hemochromatosis, or acquired hemosiderosis. In children with chronic anemia such as in thalassemia or sideroblastic anemia, iron overload secondary to parenteral administration of iron in the form of transfusions or iron preparations is seen pri-

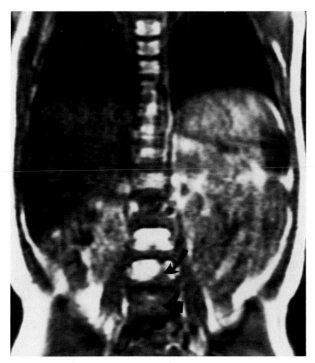

Figure 23–61. *Hemosiderosis.* Coronal T1 weighted (300/20) image through the chest and abdomen in a 4-year-old child with hemosiderosis secondary to transfusion therapy. Focal areas of low signal intensity are seen within the otherwise bright-signal-intensity vertebral marrow. The focal abnormalities involve either part (*curved arrow*) or all (*arrow*) of the vertebral marrow.

marily in the reticuloendothelial system, and therefore both the liver and spleen are of low signal intensity. Because deposition of iron in the reticuloendothelial cells appears to lead to less tissue damage that the iron loading of parenchymal cells that occurs in genetic hemochromatosis, children with acquired hemosiderosis secondary to iron overload often do not exhibit the changes of cirrhosis seen in children with genetic hemochromatosis; i.e., the liver does not exhibit nodularity, inhomogeneity, or a decrease in size.

Most of our knowledge of the effect of iron on MR signal intensity of biologic tissue is derived from studies in the liver. At field strengths of 0.6T and below, spin-echo images show little change in signal intensity of hepatic tissue until iron levels reach 1 mg per gram of liver. Children with hemochromatosis routinely have iron levels greater than 2 mg per gram, and therefore a decrease in hepatic signal intensity often is seen on both T1 and T2 weighted images. At iron levels in excess of 2 mg per gram the liver appears equally dark on T1 and T2 spin-echo images, and therefore the intensity of the liver alone has not been a useful tool in quantitating the degree of iron overload.[119] Dual-energy CT may prove more valuable and accurate than MRI for quantification of liver iron concentrations. There may be a role for spectroscopy in vivo in the quantitative evaluation of tissue iron deposition in hemosiderosis and hemochromatosis.[121]

The causes of selective T2 relaxation enhancement have been previously reviewed.[119] This enhancement is a result of magnetic susceptibility effects on tissue of both ferritin and hemosiderin. The reduction in T2 relaxation is marked, and this results in a decreased (low to black) signal intensity on all spin-echo pulse

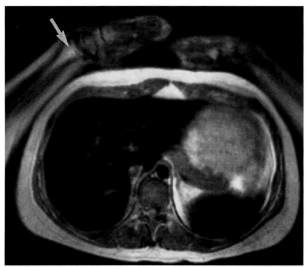
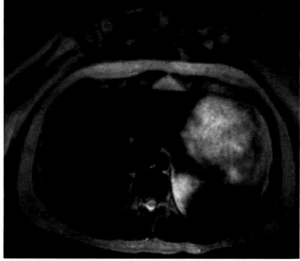

A   B

Figure 23–62. *Hemosiderosis.* **A,** Transverse intermediate weighted (2000/20) image through the abdomen in a 17-year-old girl with hemosiderosis secondary to transfusion therapy. Diffuse decreased signal intensity of the vertebral marrow is seen. Note the normal marrow signal intensity in the distal radius (*arrow*). The hematopoietically active vertebral marrow is usually first affected. In addition to the marrow abnormality, marked decreased signal intensity of both the liver and spleen can be seen. **B,** T2 weighted (2000/80) image shows a further decrease in marrow signal intensity.

sequences; however the decrease in signal intensity of affected organs is most pronounced on T2 weighted spin-echo sequences.

In addition to the liver, decrease in signal intensity is commonly seen in the spleen and pancreas, and less commonly in the endocrine glands (pituitary and heart) in children with hemosiderosis or hemochromatosis.

Of interest, iron deposition is not noted on MRI in the testes despite the fact that testicular atrophy and loss of libido are common manifestations of the disease. Testicular atrophy in hemochromatosis is usually due to the decreased production of gonadotropins secondary to decreased hypothalamic pituitary function, and is not due to direct iron deposition in the testes. Hypothyroidism, hypoparathyroidism, and adrenal insufficiency are rare but have been described; we have seen a case of decreased adrenal signal intensity consistent with iron deposition in the adrenals.

Indications for MRI in Iron Overload

MRI imaging currently plays a role in the evaluation of children with suspected hemosiderosis or hemochromatosis, both in monitoring for the development of hemosiderosis and in the evaluation of specific or-

gans for complications of the disease once the diagnosis has been made. Children can be monitored for the appearance of low-signal-intensity hemosiderin deposition in the marrow. Because chronic liver disease frequently results in increased serum iron levels, MRI can be used to evaluate the liver in children with suspected hemosiderosis or hemochromatosis to determine whether an abnormal serum iron concentration is a secondary result of liver disease, or whether the liver disease is actually caused by excessive iron deposition. If the liver, the marrow, or another organ is imaged and there is decreased signal intensity on T1 and T2 weighted MR images consistent with iron deposition, biopsy may be unnecessary to determine whether the child has sustained iron overload and deposition.

Twenty to 30 percent of patients with hemochromatosis eventually die of hepatoma. MRI can be used to screen children at risk for hepatoma, since tumor cells do not contain excess iron and can easily be distinguished from the low-signal-intensity overloaded liver on MRI (Fig. 23–64). Children with iron deposition in the pancreas may develop diabetes, since pancreatic iron overload can result in pancreatic islet cell atrophy. MRI can be used to determine which children are developing low signal intensity of the pancreas, and

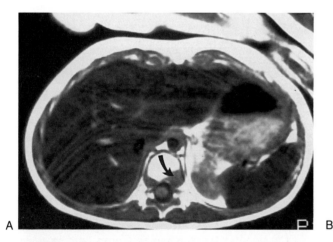

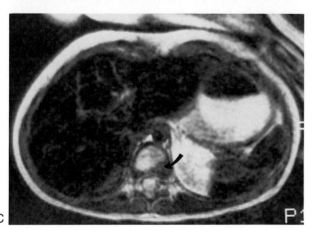

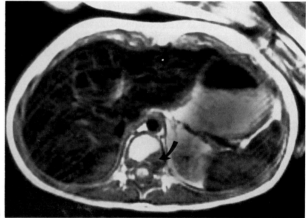

Figure 23–63. *Hemosiderosis.* T1 weighted (250/30) *(A)*, intermediate weighted (2000/20) *(B)*, and T2 weighted (2000/80) *(C)* transverse images through the liver and spleen in a child with hemosiderosis secondary to transfusion therapy for chemotherapy-induced anemia. The child had received only three transfusions, yet a marked decrease in signal intensity of both the liver and spleen is noted. Despite marked involvement of the visceral organs, there was only one small area of focal involvement in the vertebral marrow (*curved arrows*).

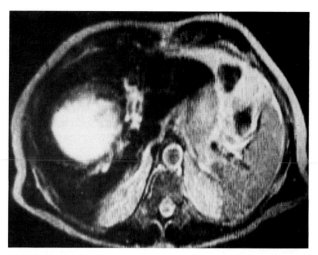

Figure 23–64. *Hemosiderosis.* Transverse T2 weighted image through the liver in a patient with hepatoma thought to be secondary to hemochromatosis. The increased-signal-intensity tumor is easily appreciated when compared with the low-signal-intensity, iron-rich liver. (Stark DD. Liver. In: Stark DD, Bradley WG, eds. Magnetic resonance imaging. St. Louis: CV Mosby, 1988:1033.)

therefore which patients are likely to be at risk for the development of diabetes. The same is true for other organs in the body: children with cardiac iron deposition may develop some degree of cardiac dysfunction, and monitoring of these patients may prove clinically useful in the future. Prospective studies are necessary to determine the accuracy, sensitivity, and specificity of MRI in monitoring organ involvement in hemosiderosis and hemochromatosis.

DEGENERATIVE DISORDERS AFFECTING MARROW

Bone marrow signal changes can be seen in vertebral bodies adjacent to both normal and degenerative discs. In general, it is thought that these marrow changes occur in older rather than younger patients, and 50 percent of adults with a degenerative disc have abnormal bone marrow signal in the marrow adjacent to end plates. While degenerative disc disease in children is uncommon compared with adults, the presence of Scheuermann's disease or degenerative disc disease in child athletes necessitates knowledge of these marrow changes.

The most common MR finding is an area of increased signal intensity on both T1 and T2 weighted pulse sequences that is either bandlike, focal, or mixed bandlike and focal on both sides of the disc. The focal areas of increased signal intensity on both T1 and T2 weighted images most likely represent focal fatty marrow infiltration. Rarely, low signal intensity is seen on both T1 and T2 weighted images corresponding to sclerosis of the end plate. In patients with MR findings other than low-signal-intensity sclerosis on both T1

and T2 weighted images, no focal abnormality will be seen on plain radiographs in the area of MR abnormality.[122] One can also see decreased marrow signal intensity on T1 and relatively high signal intensity on T2 weighted images. In these patients the diagnosis of infection, specifically discitis, must be considered. A desiccated and degenerative disc does not increase significantly in signal intensity on T2 weighted images. The signal intensity of an infected or inflamed disc increases markedly on T2 weighted images despite a flattened and abnormal disc contour. A surrounding soft tissue mass or edema can also suggest a diagnosis of infection or discitis. In patients with low-signal-intensity degenerative discs and increased end-plate signal intensity on T2 weighted images, the latter finding may represent transient edema that could progress to fatty replacement or sclerosis.[122] Further work is required in this area, specifically as it relates to children and their particular response to degenerative disease.

RESPONSE OF MARROW TO THERAPY

Radiation Therapy

Histologic Changes

Several reports have discussed the response of marrow to radiation therapy.[123–126] An understanding of the underlying pathologic changes of the marrow in response to radiation therapy is necessary before MR changes after therapy can be analyzed. Pathologic changes in the spine after radiation therapy include edema, sinusoidal destruction, and lack of hematopoiesis at 1 to 7 days following fractionated radiation of 2,000 to 4,000 rads. At 10 to 14 days, intense hematopoietic activity with persistent edema is seen, while at 1 month, decreased cellularity and increased migration of fat predominate. At 2 months, there is prominent endosteal fibrosis and decreased cellularity, with complete absence of hematopoietic cells at 3 months. The marrow is replaced primarily by fat, with some fibrosis.

The marrow may recover hematopoietic activity with time after fractionated radiation, and may not necessarily remain homogeneous increased-signal-intensity fatty marrow on MRI. After fractionated radiation of 4,000 rads, full histologic recovery of hematopoietic marrow in the vertebral bodies occurs 6 to 9 months after therapy in 27 percent of patients, and an additional 36 percent of patients have partial recovery. Two years after radiation therapy, 55 percent of patients have full recovery of marrow and a full 85 percent have partial recovery.[123] Data suggest that young patients have an increased rate of recovery, while older patients (those over 50 years old) show a reduced rate of recovery.[124, 125] Therefore, intermediate-signal-intensity vertebral marrow after radiation therapy may reflect the reappearance of hematopoietic marrow, and is not surprising in children on the basis of pathophysiologic data. Further studies are necessary both in the pathophysiology of marrow response to radiation therapy in children and in the spectrum of radiotherapy-induced marrow changes on MRI. It is likely that the age of the patient, the total dose delivered, the time course for delivery of dose (days versus weeks), previous chemotherapy, the body part being irradiated, and the patient's overall state of health will all play a role in the cellular response of the marrow to radiation, and the MR appearance of the marrow as a reflection of these varying cellular responses.

MR Findings After Radiation

We have studied the early changes of lumbar spine marrow in response to radiation therapy on 59 serial MR examinations of the lumbar spine to determine the spectrum of "normal" changes in the marrow in response to radiation therapy.[127] There were only two children in the study group (13 and 17 years of age). Patients received paravertebral lymph node radiation for either Hodgkin's disease, seminoma, or prostate carcinoma and had no hematopoietic or marrow disease.

In the first 10 days after institution of fractionated radiation therapy there are no appreciable marrow signal intensity differences on spin-echo T1 weighted MR images compared with pretherapy examinations. At 10 to 14 days, most patients again show no appreciable signal difference in the vertebral marrow, but occasionally a subtle increase in signal intensity on T2 weighted images may be seen in comparison with pretherapy examinations. A more definite increase in signal intensity may be seen on STIR images and reflects the edema present in the marrow at this time (Fig. 23–65). At 3 weeks after therapy either an increase in

central fat or an increase in mottled appearance (Fig. 23–66) is prominent on T1 weighted images.[127] These changes are not as prominent on T2 weighted images, since the fat signal decreases on T2 weighted images, and signal from edema, necrosis, or any residual red marrow increases on T2 weighted images. These changes in signal intensity on T2 weighted images decrease the conspicuity of the differing cellular components, and subtle patterns of inhomogeneity are more difficult to appreciate.

This pattern of increasing homogeneity or increasing central fat that begins 3 weeks after radiation therapy progresses until one of two "late" patterns is seen. There is either a homogeneous increased signal intensity in the vertebral bodies, reflecting yellow marrow (Fig. 23–67),[128, 129] or a second pattern of central increased signal intensity consistent with fatty marrow and a peripheral intermediate signal intensity suggesting hematopoietic marrow.[127]

MRI does play a role in imaging the post-irradiated marrow, primarily to assess for return of disease and the effectiveness of radiation treatment. Knowledge of the chronologic evolution of normal marrow changes both during and after radiation therapy is essential in differentiating normal postradiation change from marrow pathology. No focal marrow lesions or soft tissue edema were identified during the course of radiation therapy; their presence should raise the possibility of metastatic disease or infection. Focal areas of marrow necrosis following radiation therapy that would theoretically be seen as focal low signal intensity on T1 and

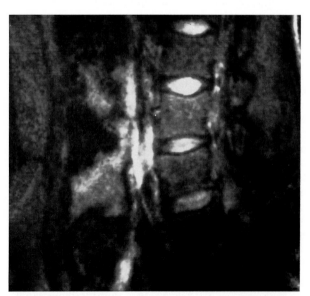

Figure 23–65. *Radiation effect on bone marrow.* STIR (1500/30/TI100 [0.38T]) image of the spine showing increased-signal-intensity marrow in a patient 10 days after radiation therapy. The increased signal intensity reflects postradiation edema.

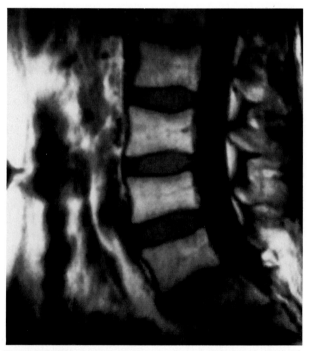

Figure 23–66. *Radiation effect on bone marrow.* Sagittal T1 weighted image of the spine in a patient 3 weeks after radiation therapy. Note the mottled appearance of the vertebral marrow.

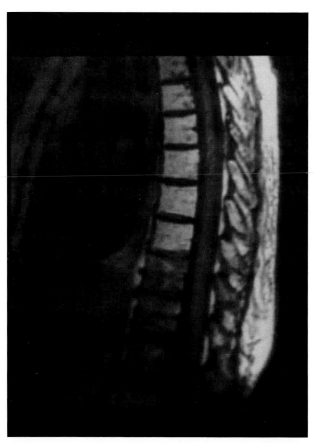

Figure 23-67. *Radiation effect.* Sagittal T1 weighted image of the thoracic and upper lumbar spine in a patient after radiation therapy for Hodgkin's lymphoma. Diffuse increased signal intensity of the vertebral marrow is seen secondary to fatty replacement of hematopoietic marrow as a result of radiation therapy to the thoracic spine.

very bright signal intensity on T2 weighted images were not seen.[127]

Studies exploring the response of marrow lesions to radiation therapy are only now beginning. Anecdotally, transient increases in signal intensity of marrow lesions after radiation and chemotherapy[130] and an increase in marrow edema[131] surrounding these lesions after radiation therapy can be seen. The signal intensity of the lesion may continue to decrease over a period of 4 to 10 weeks, but may remain as a focal area of decreased signal intensity for some time. These focal areas of increased signal intensity correspond to marked areas of necrosis. A report of a focal metastatic lesion from renal adenocarcinoma imaged 2 months after radiation therapy described low signal intensity on both T1 and T2 weighted images.[129] We have seen a similar appearance in irradiated lesions in children. Whether most irradiated bony lesions, if properly treated, will regain isointensity with the remainder of the marrow, and ultimately will be replaced by normal marrow, remains to be seen.

The MR appearance of the marrow following fractionated radiation to the spine has been de-scribed,[127-129] but the MR appearance of the long bones after radiation therapy has not yet been reported. Given the childhood difference in cellular composition of the predominantly hematopoietic spine and flat bones and the predominantly fatty long bones, the pathologic response of marrow to radiation therapy and the resultant changes seen on MRI may be different in the appendicular and axial skeleton. The exact nature of these differences can be elucidated only by further studies. However, we have seen several cases of radiation necrosis of the marrow and soft tissues in the extremities of patients as much as 1 year after radiation therapy for metastatic lesions (Fig. 23-68). Care must be taken to consider radiation necrosis when diffuse abnormalities are seen in the extremities after radiation therapy.

Chemotherapy

Little has been written about the effect of chemotherapy on the MR appearance of the marrow. This may be due to the probable variability of response of the marrow to chemotherapy. In some cases the marrow responds with hypoplasia, resulting in an MR appearance of fatty marrow with increased signal intensity on T1 and T2 weighted images. If the marrow responds with initial congestion and edema followed by fibrosis, the marrow could have either a patchy or more homogeneous fibrotic appearance on MRI with low signal intensity on both T1 and T2 weighted images. We have seen cases of apparent reconversion of yellow to red marrow after chemotherapy (Fig. 23-69), with progressive decrease in marrow signal intensity on MRI from bright to intermediate, consistent with an increase in hematopoietic elements of the marrow and a decrease in fatty elements as a response to chemotherapy. Marrow biopsy after therapy showed no fibrosis. Both diffuse and patchy decreased signal intensity have been reported.[131] An increase in signal intensity of focal bony lesions in the spine after chemotherapy has been reported, consistent with fatty replacement of the metastatic lesion as a response to treatment.[131] At this point, it is wise to recognize that chemotherapy most likely does affect the MR appearance of the marrow, so that changes of the marrow seen in patients who have undergone chemotherapy should not always be attributed to disease. This area requires additional study.

Marrow Transplantation

Marrow transplantation is becoming increasingly used as a form of therapy in the United States. The diseases most amenable to transplantation include hematologic malignancies, especially leukemia and lymphoma. Aplastic disorders, immune deficiency diseases, inborn areas of metabolism, and severe

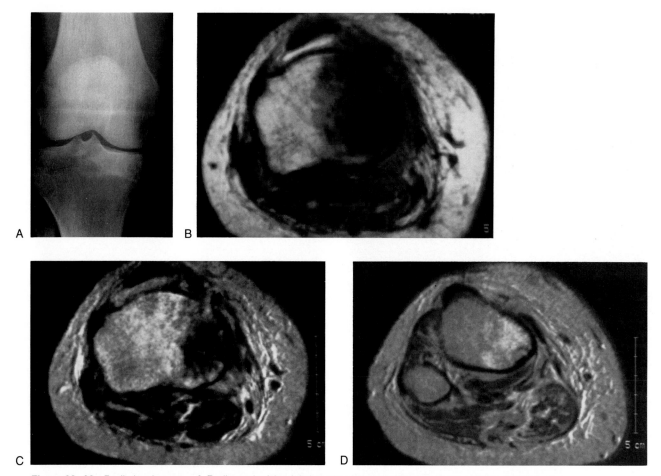

Figure 23–68. *Radiation therapy.* **A,** Radiograph of the right knee in a 56-year-old woman 1 year after radiation therapy to the tibia for metastatic breast carcinoma. Sclerotic bone is noted in the medial tibial epiphysis. **B,** T1 weighted (800/20) transverse image through the proximal tibia shows decreased-signal-intensity marrow. **C,** T2 weighted image shows increased marrow signal intensity consistent with edema and focal decreased marrow signal intensity consistent with sclerosis. Increased signal intensity is noted in the subcutaneous fat and muscle. Biopsy revealed no evidence of tumor, but diffuse edema, thought to be secondary to radiation necrosis, was noted. The previous biopsy site can be appreciated (*arrow*). **D,** T2 weighted (2000/80) image 2 cm distal to the previous image site shows increased-signal-intensity edematous marrow, musculature, and subcutaneous fat consistent with radiation necrosis.

radiation injury are also successfully treated by transplantation. An understanding of the normal appearance of marrow after bone marrow transplantation is important for two reasons. First, a knowledge of the normal pattern of marrow engraftment on MRI is essential so that abnormal patterns can be recognized, especially in patients who often require follow-up MRI for evaluation of the underlying illness (e.g., mediastinal lymph nodes, size of mass). Second, it is possible that MRI may play a role in the evaluation of the success of marrow engraftment and in early diagnosis of nonengraftment and relapse of disease.

Ablation of the marrow is essential before marrow transplantation. This is achieved through either chemotherapy alone or a combination of radiation therapy and chemotherapy. These large doses of chemotherapy and fractionated total body irradiation are de-

signed both to induce immunologic suppression in the recipient and to eliminate any residual cell population. After this pretransplant ablation therapy, bone marrow cells are infused intravenously, and the stem cells "home" into the marrow cavity after a transient residence in the lungs and spleen. They are typically engrafted over the following 3 to 4 weeks.

MR Findings of Transplanted Marrow

SPINE. We have reported characteristic MR marrow changes in the spine in 12 children that occur by 3 months after transplantation.[132] These consist of a peripheral zone of intermediate signal intensity surrounding a central zone of bright signal intensity on T1 weighted images (Fig. 23–70). We have termed these alternating zones of intermediate and bright signal intensity the "band pattern." The band pattern was de-

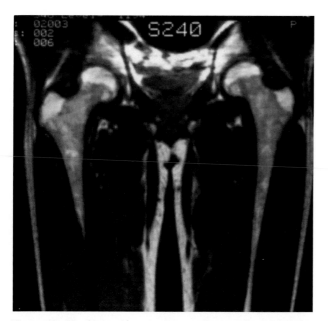

Figure 23–69. *Chemotherapy.* Intermediate weighted (2000/20) coronal image through the pelvis and proximal femora in a 21-year-old patient after chemotherapy for Ewing's sarcoma of the rib. While increased-signal-intensity fatty marrow can be appreciated in the epiphyses, greater trochanters, and acetabulum, intermediate-signal-intensity marrow is seen extending into the femoral diaphysis. This is a more extensive pattern of hematopoietic marrow than would be expected for this patient's age; it may represent chemotherapy-induced conversion of yellow to red marrow.

tected in all but one patient by 90 days after transplantation, and in some individuals as early as 40 days after transplantation.

Pathologic correlation with the band pattern has been made.[132] This peripheral region of intermediate signal intensity corresponds pathologically to a zone of repopulating hematopoietic cells. The central zone of bright signal intensity corresponds pathologically to a central zone of fatty marrow (Fig. 23–70). This pattern of repopulation is most likely a reflection of the unique blood flow and structure of the vertebral body. Vascular sinusoids at the periphery of the vertebral body control blood flow through the marrow cavity and determine the size of the hematopoietic compartment.[24, 133] Blood flow to the peripheral vascular sinusoids is carried by branches of the nutrient arteries, which terminate in capillaries near the endosteal surface of the cortex, anastomose with periosteal capillaries, and then turn back into the marrow to empty into sinusoids. Blood from the sinusoids subsequently empties into venules and the basivertebral vein. We believe this pattern of blood flow determines the distribution of repopulating cells within the vertebral body and is responsible for the band pattern of marrow regeneration seen on MRI in our bone marrow transplant patients. Although the temporal evolution of this pattern may be variable, the appearance of the band

pattern on MRI after marrow transplantation may be considered the normal pattern of marrow engraftment.

After transplantation, loss of the band pattern and appearance of a diffuse low-signal-intensity homogeneous marrow pattern on MRI may herald a relapse of disease, particularly in patients with hematologic malignancy. Further longitudinal studies must be performed to determine whether the vertebral marrow in normal post-transplant patients continues to exhibit the band pattern indefinitely, or whether this pattern changes to a more homogeneous pattern with time.

PELVIS AND FEMORA. The MR appearance after marrow transplantation in the pelvis and proximal femora has been studied in five adults.[74] In these patients a mild but diffusely decreased marrow signal intensity relative to normal marrow was seen, although the signal intensity was greater than the pretransplant images, which showed an overall decrease in signal intensity in these patients with CML. No mention was made of focal areas of fatty versus hematopoietic marrow. However, the focus of this particular study was not to determine the specific appearance of pelvic marrow after transplantation, but rather a more general review of the role of MRI in the evaluation of marrow malignancies. Prospective studies specifically designed to evaluate the pattern of marrow regeneration in bones other than the spine remain to be performed. However, in all likelihood the spine will remain the anatomic site of choice for the evaluation of marrow after marrow transplantation, since it is easy to image and it is a major site of hematopoiesis.

SUMMARY

Magnetic resonance has provided a new opportunity to examine the bone marrow directly without intervention. The indications and algorithms for the MR evaluation of pediatric marrow are evolving. In our experience, MRI is the modality of choice to evaluate bone marrow in children, and should be used in conjunction with the clinical history, physical examination, and plain radiographs. The importance of obtaining plain films before MRI cannot be sufficiently underscored. MRI may be extremely sensitive to marrow changes, but these may be nonspecific. There is no substitution for the 100 years of experience we have gleaned from plain film radiography in the evaluation of bone and marrow lesions. Plain radiographs should be obtained before MRI and must be used to interpret MR findings. To do otherwise does not give the patient the full benefit of the MR examination.

In children complaining of bone pain or with serologic abnormalities suggesting an underlying marrow disorder, either the spine and pelvis (in cases of suspected diffuse marrow disorder) or the specific body part in question should be examined by spin-echo MRI. The roles of STIR, gradient-echo, and chemical shift imaging are not certain at this point, but in all

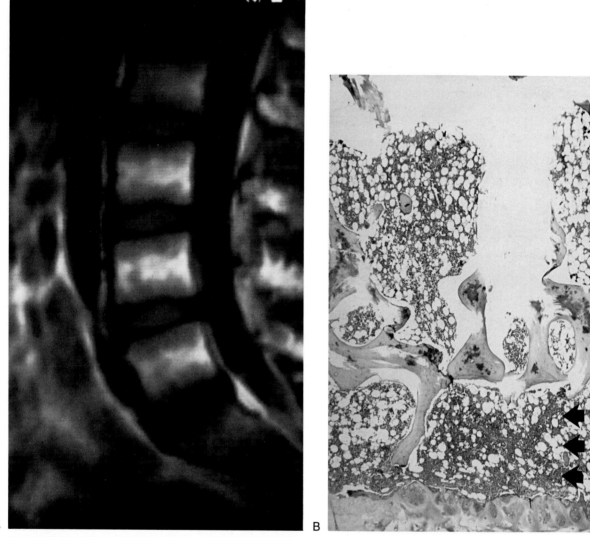

Figure 23–70. *Marrow transplantation.* ***A,*** Sagittal image through the lumbar spine in a child 3 months after marrow transplantation. A peripheral zone of intermediate signal intensity marrow is seen. ***B,*** Histologic section through the vertebral body of a child with a successful marrow transplantation. The peripheral zone of intermediate signal intensity corresponds histologically to repopulation of the vascular sinusoids at the periphery of the vertebral body by hematopoietic cells (*large arrows*). Central fatty marrow is seen. (Stevens SK, Moore SG, Amylon MD. Repopulation of marrow after transplantation: MR imaging with pathologic correlation. Radiology 1990; 175:213–218.)

likelihood these sequences will be useful in the evaluation of musculoskeletal and marrow disease. STIR imaging holds promise as an adjunctive sequence that can increase lesion conspicuity, and in some cases may replace T2 weighted spin-echo images.[41] The combination of spin-echo and STIR images may be used for tissue specificity, especially in instances of fatty lesions that suppress and appear black on STIR sequences. The exquisite sensitivity of STIR imaging to edema promises to make MRI an even more sensitive tool in the detection of marrow abnormalities. However, the specificity of MRI-detected marrow edema is uncertain, and further studies addressing its clinical significance are required. Gradient-echo imaging holds

promise in the evaluation of joints and trabecular bone, but at this time does not appear especially sensitive in the evaluation of red versus yellow marrow. However, in certain bone disorders (osteopenia, reflex sympathetic dystrophy), this sensitivity to changes in trabecular bone may prove useful in the overall analysis of the marrow. Chemical shift imaging of the marrow promises to have an important role in the evaluation of marrow, since the ability to quantify the percentage of fatty as opposed to hematopoietic or abnormal marrow could have important clinical ramifications. The signal intensity of fatty marrow often overrides that of hematopoietic marrow on spin-echo images, making the latter less sensitive to small percentages of red marrow. In the evaluation of disorders such as aplastic anemia, in which the predominant fatty marrow gives an overall increased signal intensity on spin-echo images and does not allow evaluation of early marrow recovery, the more quantitative measurement of hematopoietic marrow on chemical shift images could prove useful in evaluating the efficacy of therapeutic intervention. Fat suppression imaging[134] may also play a role in the evaluation of marrow diseases. It may be the preferred method of chemical shift imaging because linear suppression of lipid signals results in an image with a signal intensity that is linearly related to the water content and does not require subtraction techniques to achieve an image.

Once the clinical history taking, physical examination, radiography, and MR examination have been performed, there are, in our opinion, few reasons to carry out additional imaging studies. If the cortical bone detail obtained on MRI is not adequate for the clinical concern, CT with bone algorithm may be a useful adjunctive examination. In most cases, however, MRI alone, and especially in conjunction with radiography, can adequately evaluate the cortex. In addition, we have found thin-section CT examination more useful in the evaluation of cortical lesions such as osteoid osteoma, since the cortical abnormality on MRI may be subtle and may be missed. If there is any reason to expect multiple bony lesions, a bone scan should be performed in addition to MRI. At the current time, marrow screening via MRI of the entire marrow compartment (cranial vault to toes) is not practical, even in newborns.

It is encouraging that several authors have confirmed the initial observation that T1 relaxation time is significantly increased in patients with acute lymphocytic leukemia. T1 relaxation time prolongation is by itself a nonspecific finding. It appears that any process that diffusely infiltrates the marrow with abnormal cells may cause prolongation of T1 relaxation time. It is important to remember, however, that normal hematopoietic marrow, even with marked cellularity such as that seen in newborns, does not appear to have a T1 relaxation time above 700 msec in either medium- or high-field-strength systems.[66–68,70] MRI may therefore play an important role in the initial screening of marrow for abnormal processes. If a child presents with fever, neutropenia, and malaise, a normal MR appearance and T1 relaxation time of the vertebral marrow precludes the diagnosis of leukemia or any other diffusely infiltrative disorder. The child may still need a bone marrow biopsy to exclude processes such as aplastic anemia, but this depends on clinical factors.

More important, MR evaluation of the marrow, including spin-echo, chemical shift, and fat suppression imaging as well as T1 relaxation times, may prove useful in evaluating therapeutic measures and in distinguishing disease relapse from disease remission. Once a bone marrow biopsy has been performed and the underlying disease state is known (leukemia, lym-phoma, or aplastic anemia), MRI can be used to monitor the state of disease, and can potentially obviate the need for some of the bone marrow aspirates and biopsies currently performed.

FUTURE DEVELOPMENTS

In vivo, high-resolution, volume-selected hydrogen MR spectroscopy of human tibia marrow has been undertaken by Irving and colleagues,[135] using spatial coordinates obtained from MR images. Adult tibial marrow has a hydrogen spectrum-rich fatty acid resonance and is readily distinguished from the spectra of surrounding muscles. Leukemic marrow spectra show marked differences from normal marrow, with an increase in the H_2O peak correlating with infiltration of blast cells and lack of control of neoplastic disease.

Spectroscopy may prove immensely useful in the evaluation of marrow. Spectroscopy of the marrow may allow differentiation between nonspecific edema and edema associated with an underlying neoplastic or infectious process, in that nonspecific edema has a large water peak and no additional metabolic peaks, whereas a neoplastic process has a preponderance of metabolic peaks as well as the water peak. For the first time since the advent of medical imaging, our ability to directly image and spectroscopically analyze bone marrow represents a new opportunity and exciting challenge for the radiologist.

REFERENCES

1. Helms CA, Cann CE, Brunelle FO, et al. Detection of bone-marrow metastases using quantitative computed tomography. Radiology 1981; 140:745–750.
2. Vogler JB, Murphy WA. Bone marrow imaging. Radiology 1988; 168:679–693.
3. Kellman GM, Kneeland JB, Middleton WD, et al. MR imaging of the supraclavicular region: normal anatomy. AJR 1987; 148:77–82.
4. Seeger LL, Ruszkowski JT, Bassett LW, et al. MR imaging of the normal shoulder: anatomic correlation. AJR 1987; 148:83–91.
5. Bunnell DH, Fisher DA, Bassett LW, et al. Elbow joint: normal anatomy on MR images. Radiology 1987; 165:527–531.
6. Middleton WD, Macrander S, Kneeland JB, et al. MR imaging of the normal elbow: anatomic correlation. AJR 1987; 149:543–547.
7. Erickson SJ, Kneeland JB, Middleton WD, et al. MR imaging of the finger: correlation with normal anatomic sections. AJR 1989; 152:1013–1019.
8. Watanabe AT, Carter BC, Teitelbaum GP, et al. Normal variations in MR imaging of the knee: appearance and frequency. AJR 1989; 153:341–344.
9. Beltran J, Noto AM, Mosure JC, et al. Ankle: surface coil MR imaging at 1.5T. Radiology 1986; 161:203–209.
10. Noto AM, Cheung Y, Rosenberg ZS, et al. MR imaging of the ankle: normal variants. Radiology 1989; 170:121–124.
11. Kneeland JB, Marandar S, Middleton WD, et al. MR imaging of the normal ankle: correlation with anatomic sections. AJR 1988; 151:117–123.
12. Beltran J, Noto AM, Herman LJ, Lubbers LM. Tendons: high-field-strength, surface coil MR imaging. Radiology 1987; 162:735–740.

13. Trubowitz S, Davis S. The bone marrow matrix. In: The Human bone marrow: anatomy, physiology, and pathophysiology. Boca Raton, FL: CRC, 1982:43–75.

14. Erslev AJ. Medullary and extramedullary blood formation. Clin Orthop 1967; 52:25–36.

15. Kuntz A, Richins CA. Innervation of the bone marrow. J Comp Neurol 1945; 83:213–222.

16. Piney A. The anatomy of the bone marrow. Br Med J 1922; 2:792–795.

17. Hashimoto M. The distribution of active marrow in the bones of normal adults. Kyushu J Med Sci 1960; 11:103–111.

18. Dunhill MS, Anderson JA, Whitehead R. Quantitative histological studies on age changes in bone. J Pathol Bacteriol 1967; 95:275–291.

19. Custer RP. Studies of the structure and function of bone marrow. I. Variability of the hemopoietic pattern and consideration of method for examination. J Lab Clin Med 1932; 17:951–959.

20. Hashimoto M. Pathology of bone marrow. Acta Haematol 1962; 27:193–216.

21. Biermann A, von Keyserlingk DC. Ultrastructure of reticulum cells in the bone marrow. Acta Anat 1978; 100:34–43.

22. Ben-Ishay Z. Reticulum cells, stem cells and lymphocytes. Isr J Med Sci 1974; 10:1379–1392.

23. deBruyn PPH, Breen PC, Thomas TB. The microcirculation of the bone marrow. Anat Rec 1970; 168:55–68.

24. Sabin FR. Bone marrow. Physiol Rev 1928; 8:191–244.

25. Wolf NS. The haematopoietic microenvironment. Clin Haematol 1979; 8:469.

26. Neumann E. Über die Bedeutung des Knochenmarks für die Blutbildung. Centralblatt Med Wiss 1868; 6:689.

27. Gordon NY, Barrett AJ. Normal haemopoiesis. In: Gordon NY, Barrett AJ, eds. Bone marrow disorders. London: Blackwell Scientific Publications, 1985:3–136.

28. Wehrli FW, Perkins TG, Shimakawa A, Roberts F. Chemical shift–induced amplitude modulations in images obtained with gradient refocusing. Magn Reson Imaging 1987; 5:157–158.

29. Mitchell DG, Burk DL Jr, Vinitski S, Rifkin MD. The biophysical basis of tissue contrast in extracranial MR imaging. AJR 1987; 149:831–837.

30. Wehrli FW, MacFall JR, Shutts D, et al. Mechanisms of contrast in NMR imaging. J Comput Assist Tomogr 1984; 8:369–380.

31. Kricun ME. Red-yellow marrow conversion: its effect on the location of some solitary bone lesions. Skeletal Radiol 1985; 14:10–19.

32. Moore SG, Dawson KL. Red and yellow marrow in the femur: age-related changes in appearance at MR imaging. Radiology 1990; 175:219–223.

33. Okada Y, Aoki S, Barkovich AJ, et al. Cranial bone marrow in children: assessment of normal development with MR imaging. Radiology 1989; 171:161–164.

34. Cristy M. Active bone marrow distribution as a function of age in humans. Phys Med Biol 1981; 26:389–400.

35. Hajek PC, Baker LL, Coobar JE, et al. Focal fat deposition in axial bone marrow: MR characteristics. Radiology 1987; 162:245–249.

36. Dawson KL, Moore SC, Rowland J. Spectrum of appearance of red and yellow marrow in the pelvis with age: magnetic resonance and pathologic correlation. Radiology 1989; 173(P):465.

37. Totty WC, Murphy WA, Ganz WI et al. Magnetic resonance imaging of the normal and ischemic femoral head. AJR 1984; 143:1273–1280.

38. Moore SG. MR precisely evaluates bone tumors: a practical approach to magnetic resonance evaluation of pediatric musculoskeletal tumors. Diagn Imaging 1988; 10:282–289.

39. Dick BW, Mitchell DG, Burk DL, et al. The effect of chemical shift misrepresentation on cortical bone thickness on MR imaging. AJR 1988; 151:537–538.

40. Bydder GM, Young FR. MR imaging: clinical use of the inversion recovery sequence. J Comput Assist Tomogr 1985; 9:659–675.

41. Moore SG. MR imaging evaluation of bone lesions: comparison of inversion recovery and spin echo images. Radiology 1988; 169(P):191.

42. Wehrli FW. Fast-scan imaging: principles and contrast phenomenology. In: Higgins CB, Hricak H, eds. Magnetic resonance imaging of the body. New York: Raven Press, 1987:23–38.

43. Davis CA, Genant HK, Dunham JS. The effects of bone on proton NMR relaxation times of surrounding liquids. Invest Radiol 1986; 6:472–477.

44. Sebag GH, Moore SG. Effect of trabecular bone on the appearance of marrow in gradient-echo imaging of the appendicular skeleton. Radiology 1990; 174:855–859.

45. Brateman L. Chemical shift imaging: a review. AJR 1987: 146:971–980.

46. Szumowski J, Plewes DB. Separation of lipid and water MR imaging signals by chopper averaging in the time domain. Radiology 1987; 165:247–250.

47. Borrello JA, Chenevert TL, Meyer CR, et al. Chemical shift–based true water and fat images: regional phase correction of modified spin echo MR images. Radiology 1987; 164:531–537.

48. Rosen BR, Fleming DM, Kushner DC, et al. Hematologic bone marrow disorders: quantitative chemical shift MR imaging. Radiology 1988; 169:799–804.

49. Wilson AJ, Murphy WA, Hardy DC, Totty WC. Transient osteoporosis: transient bone marrow edema? Radiology 1988; 167:757–760.

50. Harkens KL, Yuh WTC, Katnol MH, et al. Differentiating skeletal neoplasm from non-neoplastic process. Value of MR and Gd-DTPA. Presented at the Annual Meeting of the American Roentgen Ray Society, New Orleans, LA, May 1989.

51. Pay NT, Singer WS, Bartal E. Hip pain in three children accompanied by transient abnormal findings on MR images. Radiology 1989; 171:147–149.

52. Bleumm RG, Flake THM, Ziedses des Plantes BG Jr, Steiner RM. Early Legg-Perthes' disease (ischemic necrosis of the femoral head) demonstrated by MRI. Skeletal Radiol 1985; 14:95–98.

53. Toby EB, Koman LA, Bechtold RE. MRI of pediatric hip disease. J Pediatr Orthop 1985; 5:665–671.

54. Berquist TN, Ehman RL, Richardson ML, et al. Miscellaneous conditions and future potential. In: Berquist TN, ed. Magnetic resonance imaging of the musculoskeletal system. New York: Raven Press, 1987:185–209.

55. Murphy WA, Totty WC. Musculoskeletal magnetic resonance imaging. In: Kressel NY, ed. Magnetic resonance annual. New York: Raven Press, 1986:1–35.

56. Lee JK, Yao L. Stress fractures: MR imaging. Radiology 1988; 169:217–220.

57. Stafford SA, Rosenthal DI, Gebhardt MG, et al. MRI in stress fracture. AJR 1986; 147:553–556.

58. Yao L, Lee JK. Occult intraosseous fracture: detection with MR imaging. Radiology 1988: 167:749–751.

59. Ehman RL. MR imaging of medullary bone. Radiology 1988; 167:867–868.

60. Silverman FN. The bones. In: Silverman FN, ed. Caffey's pediatric x-ray diagnosis. 8th ed. Chicago: Year Book, 1985:895–896.

61. McKinstry CS, Steiner RE, Young AT, et al. Bone marrow in leukemia and aplastic anemia: MR imaging before, during, and after treatment. Radiology 1987; 162:701–707.

62. Jensen KE, Grube T, Thomsen C, et al. Prolonged bone marrow T1-relaxation in patients with polycythemia vera. Magn Reson Imaging 1988; 6:291–292.

63. Moore SG, Parker BR, Northway WH, Zatz LM. Magnetic resonance evaluation of pediatric bone lesions using short T1 inversion recovery. AJR 1988; 151:624.

64. Moore SG, Gooding CA, Ehman R, Brasch RC. Intensity measurement of the marrow in patients with acute lymphocytic leukemia. Book of Abstracts, Society of Magnetic Resonance in Medicine, 4th Annual Meeting, August 1985; 2:1183.

65. Sugimura K, Yamasaki K, Kitagaki H, et al. Bone marrow diseases of the spine: differentiation with T1 and T2 relaxation times in MR imaging. Radiology 1987; 165:541–544.

66. Moore SG, Gooding CA, Brasch RC, et al. Bone marrow in children with acute lymphocytic leukemia: MR relaxation times. Radiology 1986; 160:237–240.

67. Thomsen C, Sorensen PG, Karle H, et al. Prolonged bone marrow T1-relaxation in acute leukemia: in vivo tissue characterization by magnetic resonance imaging. Magn Reson Imaging 1987; 5:251–257.

68. Dooms GC, Fisher MR, Hricak H, et al. Bone marrow imaging: magnetic resonance studies related to age and sex. Radiology 1985; 155:429–432.

69. Nyman R, Rehn S, Glimelius B, et al. Magnetic resonance imaging in diffuse malignant bone diseases. Acta Radiol 1987; 28:199–205.

70. Jenkins JPR, Stehling M, Sivewright G, et al. Quantitative magnetic resonance imaging of vertebral bodies: a T1 and T2 study. Magn Reson Imaging 1989; 7:17–23.

71. Ranade SS, Chaughule RS, Kasturi SR, et al. Pulsed nuclear magnetic resonance studies on human malignant tissues and cells in vitro. Ind J Biochem Biophys 1975; 12:229–232.

72. Ranade SS, Shah S, Advani SH, Kasturi SR. Pulsed nuclear magnetic resonance studies of human bone marrow. Physiol Chem Phys 1977; 9:297–299.

73. Adamson JW. The myeloproliferative diseases. In: Braunwald E, Isselbacher KJ, Petersdorf RG, eds. Harrison's principles of internal medicine. 11th ed. New York: McGraw-Hill, 1987: 1527–1531.

74. Olson DO, Shields AF, Scheurich CJ, et al. Magnetic resonance imaging of the bone marrow in patients with leukemia, aplastic anemia, and lymphoma. Invest Radiol 1986; 21:540–546.

75. Shields AF, Porter BA, Churchley S, et al. The detection of bone marrow involvement by lymphoma using magnetic resonance imaging. J Clin Oncol 1987; 5:225–230.

76. Castellino PA, Parker BR, Non-Hodgkin's lymphoma. In: Parker BR, Castellino PA, eds. Pediatric oncologic radiology. St Louis: CV Mosby, 1977:183.

77. Silverman FN. The bones. In: Silverman FN, ed. Caffey's pediatric x-ray diagnosis. 8th ed. Chicago: Year Book, 1985:899–903.

78. Stern MB, Cassidy R, Mirra J. Eosinophilic granuloma of the proximal tibial epiphysis. Clin Orthop 1976; 118:153–156.

79. Couanet D, Geoffray A, Hartmann O, et al. Bone marrow metastasis in children's neuroblastoma studied by magnetic resonance imaging. Adv Neuroblastoma Res 1988; 2:547–555.

80. Silverman FN. The bones. In: Silverman FN, ed. Caffey's pediatric x-ray diagnosis. 8th ed. Chicago: Year Book 1985:882–886.

81. Bunn HF. Disorders of hemoglobin. In: Braunwald E, Isselbacher KJ, Petersdorf RG, eds. Harrison's principles of internal medicine. 11th ed. New York: McGraw-Hill, 1987:1518–1522.

82. Rao VM, Fishman M, Mitchell DG, et al. Painful sickle cell crisis: bone marrow patterns observed with MR imaging. Radiology 1986; 161:211–215.

83. Rao VM, Mitchell DC, Steiner RM, et al. Femoral head avascular necrosis in sickle cell anemia: MR characteristics. Magn Reson Imaging 1988; 6:661–667.

84. Genez BM, Wilson MR, Houk RW, et al. Early osteonecrosis of the femoral head: detection in high-risk patients with MR imaging. Radiology 1988; 168:521–524.

85. Sebes JI. Diagnostic imaging of bone and joint abnormalities associated with sickle cell hemoglobinopathies. AJR 1989; 152:1153–1159.

86. Stark DD. Biliary system, pancreas, spleen, and alimentary tract. In: Stark DD, Bradley WC, eds. Magnetic resonance imaging. St. Louis: CV Mosby, 1988:1123.

87. Bohrer SP. Bone changes in the extremities in sickle cell anemia. Semin Roentgenol 1987; 22:176–185.

88. Alvai A, Heyman S, Kim HC. Scintigraphic examination of bone and marrow infarcts in sickle cell disorders. Semin Roentgenol 1987; 22:213–224.

89. Brody AS. Induced alignment of flowing sickle erythrocytes in a magnetic field. Invest Radiol 1985; 20:560–566.

90. Papavasiliou C, Trakadas S, Gouliamos A, et al. Magnetic resonance imaging of marrow heterotopia in haemoglobinopathy. Eur J Radiol 1988; 8:50–53.

91. Papavasiliou C, Gouliamos A, Andreou J. The marrow heterotopia in thalassemia. Eur J Radiol 1968; 6:92–96.

92. Gamsu G, Stark D, Webb WR, et al. Magnetic resonance imaging of benign mediastinal masses. Radiology 1984; 151:709–717.

93. Wiener MD, Halvorsen PA, Vollmer RT, et al. Focal intrahepatic extramedullary hematopoiesis mimicking neoplasm. AJR 1987; 149:1171–1172.

94. Thomas ED. Bone marrow transplantation. In: Braunwald E, Isselbacher KJ, Petersdorf RG, eds. Harrison's principles of internal medicine. 11th ed. New York: McGraw-Hill, 1987:1536–1541.

95. Kaplan PA, Asleson RJ, Klassen LW, Duggan MJ. Bone marrow patterns in aplastic anemia: observations with 1.5T MR imaging. Radiology 1987; 164:441–444.

96. Cohen MD, Klatte EC, Baehner R, et al. Magnetic resonance imaging of bone marrow disease in children. Radiology 1984; 151:715–718.

97. Kangarloo H, Dietrich RB, Taira RT, et al. MR imaging of bone marrow in children. J Comput Assist Tomogr 1986; 10:205–209.

98. Lanir A, Aghai E, Simon JS, et al. MR imaging in myelofibrosis. J Comput Assist Tomogr 1986; 10:634–636.

99. Turner DA, Templeton AC, Selzer PM, et al. Femoral capital osteonecrosis: MR finding of diffuse marrow abnormalities without focal lesions. Radiology 1989; 171:135–140.

100. Ficat RP. Idiopathic bone necrosis of the femoral head: early diagnosis and treatment. J Bone Joint Surg 1985; 67B: 3–9.

101. Mitchell DG, Rao VM, Dalinka M, et al. Hematopoietic and fatty bone marrow distribution in the normal and ischemic hip: new observations with 1.5T MR imaging. Radiology 1986; 161:199–202.

102. Lang P, Jergesen HE, Moseley ME, et al. Avascular necrosis of the femoral head: high-field-strength MR imaging with histologic correlation. Radiology 1988; 169:517–524.

103. Rush BH, Bramson RT, Ogden JA. Legg-Calvé-Perthes' disease: detection of cartilaginous and synovial changes with MR imaging. Radiology 1988; 167:473–476.

104. Mitchell DG. Using MR imaging to probe the pathophysiology of osteonecrosis. Radiology 1989; 171:25–26.

105. Henderson RC, Renner JB, Shurdwarf MC, Greene WB. An evaluation of MRI in Legg-Perthes' disease. J Pediatr Orthop 1990, in press.

106. Seiler JG, Christie MJ, Homra L. Correlation of the findings of magnetic resonance imaging with those of bone biopsy in patients who have stage I or II ischemic necrosis of the femoral head. J Bone Joint Surg 1989; 71A:28–32.

107. Mitchell DG, Kresser M. MR images of early avascular necrosis. Radiology 1988; 169:281–282.

108. Ehman RL, Berquist TH, McLeod PA. MR imaging of early avascular necrosis: response. Radiology 1988; 169:282.

109. Brody AS, Strong M, Babikian G, et al. Early avascular necrosis: MRI and histological examination in an animal model. Presented at the Annual Meeting of the Society for Pediatric Radiology, San Antonio, TX, April 1989.

110. Mitchell DG, Rao VM, Dalinka MK, et al. Femoral head avascular necrosis: correlation of MR imaging, radiographic staging, radionuclide imaging, and clinical findings. Radiology 1987; 162:709–715.

111. Coleman BG, Kressel NY, Dalinka MR, et al. Radiographically negative avascular necrosis: detection with MR imaging. Radiology 1988; 168:525–528.

112. Elsig JP, Exner GU, VonSchulthes GK, et al. False negative MRI in early stage of Perthes' disease. J Pediatr Orthop 1989; 9:231–235.

113. Shuman WP, Castagno AA, Baron RL, Richardson ML. MR imaging of avascular necrosis of the femoral head: value of small-field-of-view sagittal surface-coil images. AJR 1988; 150:1073–1078.

114. Markisz JA, Knowles RJR, Altchek DW, et al. Segmental patterns of avascular necrosis of the femoral heads: early detection with MR imaging. Radiology 1987; 162:717–720.

115. Silverman RN. The bones. In: Silverman FN, ed. Caffey's

pediatric x-ray diagnosis. 8th ed. Chicago: Year Book 1985:699–700.

116. Lanir A, Hadar H, Cohen I, et al. Gaucher's disease: assessment with MR imaging. Radiology 1986; 161:239–244.

117. Rosenthal DI, Scott JA, Barranger J, et al. Evaluation of Gaucher's disease using magnetic resonance imaging. J Bone Joint Surg 1986; 68A:802–808.

118. Powell LW, Isselbacher KJ. Hemochromatosis. In: Braunwald E, Isselbacher KJ, Petersdorf RG, eds. Harrison's principles of internal medicine. 11th ed. New York: McGraw-Hill, 1987: 1632–1635.

119. Stark DD. Liver. In: Stark DD, Bradley WC, eds. Magnetic resonance imaging. St. Louis: CV Mosby, 1988:1031–1033.

120. Stoller DW. The knee. In: Stoller DW, ed. Magnetic resonance imaging in orthopaedics and rheumatology. Philadelphia: JB Lippincott, 1989:97–214.

121. Brittenham GM, Farrell DE, Hams JW, et al. Magnetic-susceptibility measurement of human iron stores. N Engl J Med 1982; 307:1671–1675.

122. de Roos A, Kressel H, Spritzer C, Dalinka M. MR imaging of marrow changes adjacent to end plates in degenerative lumbar disk disease. AJR 1987; 149:531–534.

123. Sykes MP, Chu FCH, Wilkerson WG. Local bone marrow changes secondary to therapeutic irradiation. Radiology 1960; 75:919–924.

124. Hill DR, Benak SB, Phillips TL, Price DC. Bone marrow regeneration following fractionated radiation therapy. Int J Radiat Oncol Biol Phys 1980; 6:1149–1155.

125. Sacks EL, Goris ML, Glastein E, et al. Bone marrow regeneration following large field radiation. Influence of volume, age, dose, and time. Cancer 1978; 42:1057–1065.

126. Rubin P, Landman S, Mayer E, et al. Bone marrow regeneration and extension after extended field irradiation in Hodgkin's disease. Cancer 1973; 32:699–716.

127. Stevens SK, Moore SG, Kaplan I. Early and late bone marrow changes after irradiation: MR evaluation. AJR 1990; 154:745–750.

128. Ramsey RG, Zacharias CE. MR imaging of the spine after radiation therapy; easily recognizable effects. AJR 1985; 144:1131–1135.

129. Remedios PA, Colletti PM, Raval JK, et al. Magnetic resonance imaging of bone after radiation. Magn Reson Imaging 1988; 6:301–304.

130. Nolscher HC, Bloem JL, Noon HA, Taminiau AHM. MRS monitoring of patients with bone sarcoma treated with chemotherapy. Poster presentation at the Annual Meeting of the American Roentgen Ray Society, New Orleans, LA, May, 1989.

131. Stoller DW, Genant HK, Lang P. The spine. In: Stoller DW, ed. Magnetic resonance imaging in orthopaedics and rheumatology. Philadelphia: JB Lippincott, 1989:373.

132. Stevens SK, Moore SG, Amylon MD. Repopulation of marrow after transplantation: MR imaging with pathologic correlation. Radiology 1990; 175:213–218.

133. Knopse WN, Blom J, Crosby WH. Regeneration of locally irradiated bone marrow. I. Dose dependent, long-term changes in the rat with particular emphasis upon vascular and stromal reaction. Blood 1966; 28:398–415.

134. Szumowski J, Plewes DB. Fat suppression in the time domain in fast MR imaging. Mag Res in Medicine 1988; 8:345–354.

135. Irving MG, Brooks WM, Brereton IM, et al. Use of high resolution in vivo volume selected 1H-magnetic resonance spectroscopy to investigate leukemia in humans. Cancer Res 1987; 47:3901–3906.

Tumors of the Musculoskeletal System

SHEILA G. MOORE, M.D.
KAREN L. DAWSON, M.B., B.S.

Musculoskeletal tumors account for 11.5 percent of all childhood malignancies. With the advent of new therapies including limb salvage procedures, accurate pretherapy diagnosis and staging, and post-therapy evaluation of these musculoskeletal lesions has become important. Magnetic resonance imaging (MRI) plays a role second only to that of plain film radiography. It is essential to understand the indications, interpretation, advantages, and limitations unique to this modality.

MR evaluation of the musculoskeletal system accounts for a large percentage of the nonneurological MRI currently performed in the United States.[1] The musculoskeletal system in children is well suited to MR investigation for several reasons. There is excellent intrinsic tissue contrast between normal and pathologic processes, and MRI provides excellent images of normal and abnormal bone marrow. Multiplanar images of large anatomic regions can be obtained, and the use of extremity and surface coils allows in-plane spatial resolution of structures smaller than 1 sq mm with high contrast and a high signal-to-noise ratio (SNR). Musculoskeletal lesions are often in anatomic regions essentially unaffected by motion artifact, and in many children swaddling the extremity obviates the need for systemic sedation. Finally, vascular structures and their relationship to the pathologic process being evaluated are easily identified.[2–4]

New advances in imaging techniques such as short TI inversion recovery (STIR), gradient-recalled echo (GRE), and chemical shift promise to increase lesion conspicuity, improve staging, and enhance detection of skip lesions. In addition, mechanically gated rapid imaging techniques (low flip angle gradient-recalled echo imaging) may be useful in assessing the mechanical and anatomic effects of joint motion in children with periarticular pathologic processes.

825

COMPARISON WITH OTHER IMAGING MODALITIES

After clinical and plain film evaluation, a decision must be made regarding the use of MRI, computed tomography (CT), ultrasonography, or bone scintigraphy to study further a lesion of the musculoskeletal system. MRI is often the examination of choice, but there are specific circumstances when CT, ultrasound, or bone scintigraphy is preferable.

Computed Tomography

Compared specifically with CT, MRI has several advantages. Iodinated contrast agents (with the inherent risk of contrast reaction) are not required. Note, however, that the use of specific MR contrast agents (e.g., gadolinium-DTPA) may become important in MRI. The beam-hardening artifact from bone seen on CT can hinder the visualization of soft tissue adjacent to bone. Prostheses may also cause artifacts. Depending on their type, the artifact seen on MRI is less than that seen on CT.[5, 6] Depiction of soft tissue masses on MRI is better than on CT because of the former's ability to manipulate contrast between normal and diseased tissues (Fig. 24–1).

There have been several published reports comparing MR with CT in the evaluation of musculoskeletal tumors.[7–17] In general, MRI is believed to be equal or superior to CT in the evaluation and staging of musculoskeletal tumors (Fig. 24–2), except in the detection of calcification, early cortical bone erosion (Fig. 24–3), and periosteal reaction, in which CT was considered superior to MRI. Recent reports[10, 18] suggest that as our knowledge of the MR appearance of cortical erosion and periosteal reaction increases, the sensitivity and specificity of MRI in the evaluation of corti-

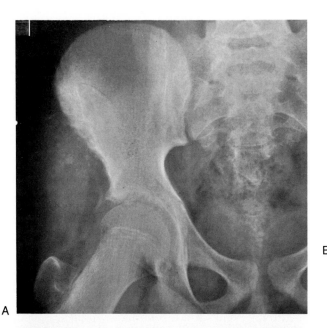

A

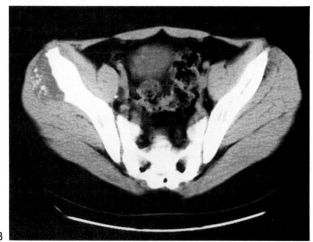

B

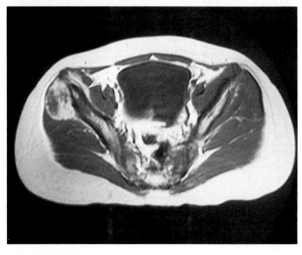

C

Figure 24–1. *Osteogenic sarcoma in an 11-year-old girl with a right pelvic mass.* ***A,*** Pelvic radiograph shows a destructive lesion on the lateral aspect of the right iliac bone with a soft tissue mass containing patchy, speckled calcification. ***B,*** CT scan at the level of the lesion shows a well-defined, calcified soft tissue mass lying lateral to the iliac bone. There is some sclerosis and irregularity in the contour of the iliac bone. ***C,*** Transverse MR image (1300/20) after gadolinium–DTPA administration. Low signal intensity in the bone marrow of the iliac wing indicates tumor invasion. This is better seen than on the CT scan. The lateral soft tissue mass is seen as well as on the CT scan. Note that the speckled calcification is not as clearly identified. In addition the MR image shows a bright signal intensity from soft tissue extension of the tumor (*arrow*) medial to the iliac crest. This is not seen on the CT scan and cannot be appreciated on the plain film radiograph. (Courtesy of Dr. Mervyn D. Cohen, Indianapolis.)

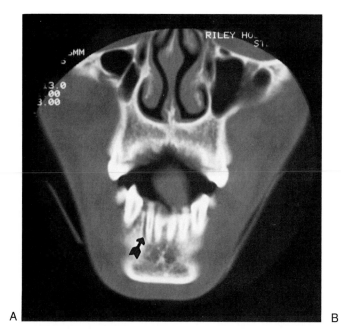

A

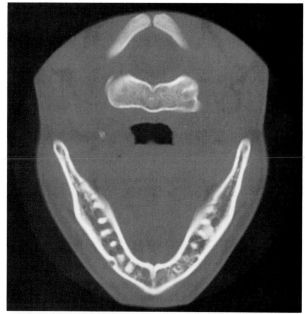

B

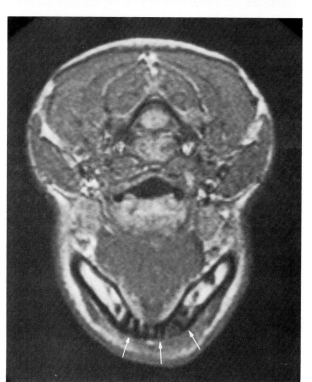

C

Figure 24–2. *Osteogenic sarcoma. MRI shows more extensive tumor than does CT.* **A, B,** Coronal and axial CT images show widening of the periodontal membrane (*arrow*) with no indication of the extent of spread of tumor beyond this location. **C,** MR image (1500/20) shows extensive loss of signal from the bone marrow of the anterior third of the mandible (*arrows*). (Courtesy of Dr. Mervyn D. Cohen, Indianapolis.)

cal bone and periosteal reaction may approach that of CT. Bloem and colleagues[13] reported a comparison of MRI and CT in the evaluation of primary bone sarcoma. MRI had an almost perfect correlation (r = 0.99) with pathologic and morphologic examination, whereas CT had a worse correlation (r = 0.86). For soft tissue extent of tumor and involvement of specific muscle groups, CT had a sensitivity of 71 percent and a specificity of 93 percent, while MR showed a sensitivity of 96 percent and a specificity of 99 percent. In contrast to earlier reports, the authors considered MRI and CT to be equally accurate in demonstrating involvement of cortical bone by tumor. The authors noted one CT study in which the cortex was thought to be invaded by tumor because the density of cortex was identical to that of tumor, whereas MRI correctly exhibited the

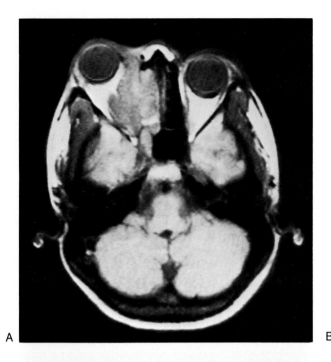

A

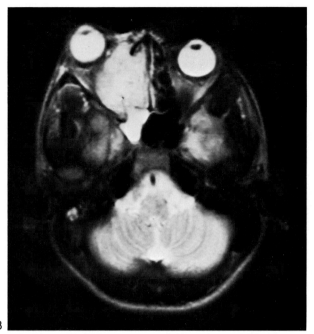

B

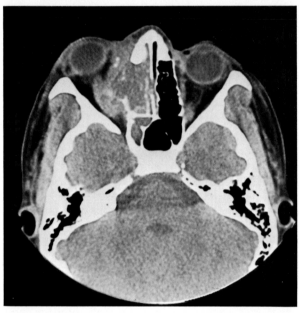

C

Figure 24–3. *Rhabdomyosarcoma of the face.*   CT demonstrates bone destruction. Axial MR images, (800/26) (**A**), (2000/580) (**B**), show a well-defined large mass lesion filling the right ethmoid sinus and extending into the right orbit. The medial wall of the orbit is not defined at all. **C,** CT image also shows the soft tissue tumor mass well. Partial destruction of the medial wall of the right orbit is well defined on the CT scan. (Courtesy of Dr. Mervyn D. Cohen, Indianapolis.)

normal signal void of cortical bone relative to the slightly increased signal intensity of tumor on the T2 weighted sequence. In the evaluation of the neurovascular bundle, MRI was thought to be superior to both CT and angiography, although the difference was not considered significant because confidence limits overlapped to a considerable degree. CT and MRI were felt to be equally accurate in demonstrating or excluding the presence of tumor within major joints, a finding that has been confirmed by other authors.[12, 13, 15]

CT can be used as an adjunct to MRI if subtle cortical erosion or periosteal reaction would influence the differential diagnosis or the treatment of a lesion. Although we believe MRI can provide detailed evaluation of the cortical bone and periosteum, CT remains the modality of choice in the evaluation of subtle cortical or periosteal changes until prospective studies confirm the accuracy of MRI. MRI is generally believed to be superior to CT in the evaluation of the extent of a tumor within the surrounding soft tissues (Fig. 24–1).[7–17] A range of comparative sensitivities and specificities is reported in the literature. One study demonstrated MRI as superior to CT in the evaluation of soft tissues in 89 percent of patients and equal to CT in 11 percent.[12] CT was not reported as superior to

MRI in the evaluation of the soft tissues in any study except in a few anecdotal cases. The accuracy of MRI in the evaluation of soft tissue involvement by osteogenic sarcoma has been reported as approaching 98 percent.[13]

CT has special advantages with tumors of the face (Fig. 24–3) or chest wall. CT is recommended for the evaluation of bone in staging tumors of the nasopharynx, since recognition of subtle erosion of facial bones of the skull base is important clinically. Motion artifact from breathing and head movement in children tends to obscure bony detail on MR images of this region. However, MRI is superior for soft tissue and marrow evaluation of tumor, and for that reason children with nasopharyngeal tumors may need a CT examination for bony detail and an MR examination to further delineate soft tissue, marrow, the spinal canal, and the intracranial extent of tumor. In the evaluation of chest wall masses, CT may be used preferentially or in addition to MRI. Motion artifact in the chest wall often precludes precise MR evaluation of the ribs, particularly if a body coil and larger field of view is used. It is often necessary to use a body coil and larger field of view for the examination, since the presence of mediastinal, hilar, or supraclavicular adenopathy is important in disease staging. Children at our institution who present with a chest wall mass are usually studied first by MRI to assess the soft tissue extent of tumor and exclude adenopathy, and then by CT to evaluate the cortical bone and lung parenchyma. Recently, we have used surface coil MR images to evaluate the bony chest wall with success. However, until such time that high-resolution MR images of the lung parenchyma are feasible, a CT scan is still needed if evaluation of lung parenchyma is necessary. Prospective comparative studies will likely delineate the role of each of these modalities in the evaluation of nasopharyngeal and chest wall masses.

Scintigraphy

Bone scintigraphy is extremely sensitive and the only imaging tool that can provide an overview of the whole skeletal system; it therefore plays an important role in the evaluation of musculoskeletal lesions. At this time it is not feasible to perform total skeleton screening examinations with MRI, and bone scintigraphy should be used when multiple lesions need to be excluded or are suspected. The role of bone marrow sulfur colloid scanning in comparison with MRI is not yet well defined.

Ultrasonography

Although ultrasonography is relatively inexpensive and in widespread use, it is not particularly useful in the evaluation of musculoskeletal tumors. It can be used initially to differentiate solid from cystic lesions

such as Baker's cyst or lymphangioma, and we have occasionally employed it to evaluate cystic lesions that contained complex fluid on MRI and therefore were not characteristically cystic.

IMAGING TECHNIQUES FOR MR EVALUATION OF MUSCULOSKELETAL TUMORS

The MR examination must be tailored to each patient. A complete clinical history and plain film radiography are essential before MRI is performed. The MR appearance and signal intensity of musculoskeletal abnormalities may be nonspecific, and the correct differential diagnosis may be given only by correlation of the MR, radiograph, and clinical findings.

Spin Echo

Transverse T1, proton density, and T2 weighted images are needed for adequate evaluation of musculoskeletal tumors. The examination must be monitored to ensure that the entire extent of the lesion has been imaged. After an initial "localizer" sagittal or coronal scan is performed, T weighted spin-echo images in the transverse plane are obtained. The transverse T1 weighted images should be followed by transverse T2 weighted images at exactly the same level. It is necessary to acquire both T1 and T2 weighted images at the same level in at least one plane so that specific tissue signal characteristics and anatomic regions can be compared from image to image. Although obtaining proton-density and T2 weighted images in one plane and T1 weighted images in a second plane can decrease examination time, we find that this routinely leads to suboptimal signal intensity characterization and error in diagnosis; therefore, this approach is not recommended.

There are several reasons to begin the examination of pediatric musculoskeletal tumors with the transverse images. Experience with interpreting transverse CT images is reassuring to most radiologists and allows greater confidence in the interpretation of images. Transverse images are best for evaluating the local extent of the tumor and its relationship to surrounding structures, and if for some reason the examination is not completed, an adequate evaluation of the tumor can usually be obtained from transverse images alone. Imaging in an orthogonal plane should follow imaging in the transverse plane. These images are beneficial when the anatomy is not clearly seen or is confusing on the transverse images, and can be used to exclude partial volume effects. Sagittal or coronal images may be superior to transverse images in assessing the full longitudinal extent of marrow or soft tissue tumor, physeal or epiphyseal involvement, joint involvement, and the presence of skip lesions.

To determine the best orientation for the orthogonal

plane, the lesion should first be visualized on the transverse image. If a lesion is primarily anterior or posterior, sagittal images should next be obtained. If a lesion is primarily medial or lateral, coronal images are recommended. The contrast of the lesion in comparison with surrounding normal structures, as well as the age of the patient, dictate whether the images in the second plane are T1 or T2 weighted. If the lesion is primarily in the marrow, and the marrow is fatty, T1 weighted images in the second plane will best distinguish bright-signal-intensity marrow from (usually) intermediate-signal-intensity pathology. In an infant or young child with predominantly hematopoietic (red) marrow, T2 weighted images in the second plane are preferable, to increase the conspicuity between the pathologic process and the underlying red marrow. The long T1 relaxation time of many lesions decreases the conspicuity of these lesions compared with red marrow (Fig. 24–4).

If the lesion is primarily muscular, an evaluation of the transverse T1 and T2 weighted images is used to determine which sequence will be required for the

second plane (Figs. 24–5, 24–6). If there is good contrast between the lesion and normal structures on the T1 weighted images, T1 weighted images should be used for the second plane, since these often give greater anatomic detail and require less time to complete (Fig. 24–6). However, if there is little contrast between the lesion and muscle tissue on the T1 weighted images (as is often the case), T2 weighted images in the second plane should be obtained (Fig. 24–5). Alternatively, T1 images with gadolinium-DTPA may be preferred. If the lesion is primarily in the subcutaneous fat (e.g., a hemangioma), T1 weighted images in the second plane can be acquired, since there will usually be good conspicuity between subcutaneous fat with its short T1 relaxation time and musculoskeletal lesions, which frequently have prolonged T1 relaxation times.

T1 weighted images can be acquired with a TR of 600 or 800 msec. Although these are not "true" T1 images, adequate T1 weighting and a sufficient number of slices are usually obtained to evaluate the lesion. T2

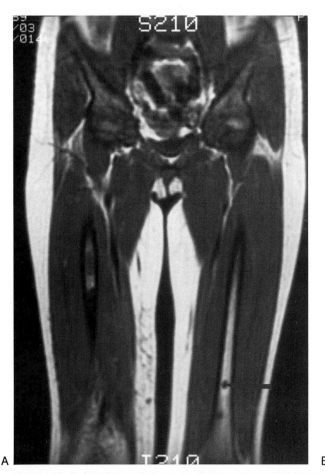 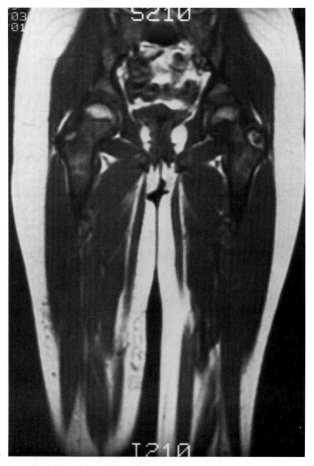

A   B

Figure 24–4. *Imaging techniques to show marrow tumor in an 8-year-old girl with multicentric osteogenic sarcoma.* Coronal T1 weighted images (800/20) of the pelvis and femoral shafts. **A,** Multiple low-signal-intensity foci of tumor are easily recognized within the yellow marrow (*arrow*). **B,** Multiple low-signal-intensity osteogenic sarcoma lesions within the metaphyseal red marrow are not as easily seen as are those within the diaphyseal yellow marrow. The lesions increased in signal intensity on T2 weighted images. (Courtesy of Dr. Charles A. Gooding, San Francisco.)

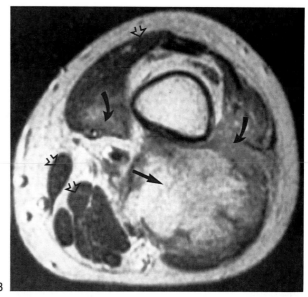

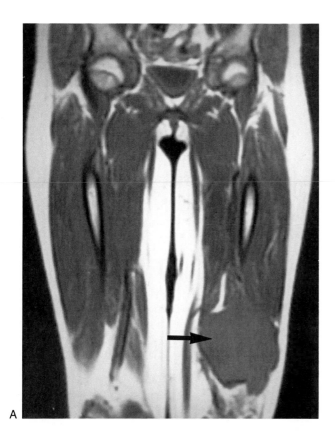

A

B

Figure 24–5. *Imaging techniques to show soft tissue desmoid in the left thigh in a 9-year-old girl.* **A,** T1 weighted coronal image (600/20) of the pelvis and femurs showing an intermediate-signal-intensity mass indistinguishable in signal intensity from muscle (*arrow*). **B,** Orthogonal T2 weighted images were obtained in the transverse plane, with bright-signal-intensity tumor (*arrow*) easily distinguished from surrounding intermediate-signal-intensity muscle. Muscle edema (*curved arrows*) can be seen as increased signal intensity compared with the intermediate-signal-intensity unaffected muscle (*open arrows*).

weighted images should be obtained with a TR of 2000 to 2500 msec. One to two excitations are usually sufficient for the T2 weighted images, while T1 weighted images require two to six excitations. Either a 192 × 256 (medium-resolution) or a 256 × 256 (high-resolution) matrix can be used. Whenever possible we use a 256 × 256 matrix, since this improves spatial resolution and provides for better evaluation of cortical bone and periosteal reaction. A 128 or 192 × 256 matrix usually yields an image of diagnostic quality in a child who is uncooperative or difficult to sedate. The determination of slice thickness and gap depends on the size of the child and the extent of the lesion. For small lesions 5-mm slices are used, while in larger lesions 7- to 10-mm slices may be required. The field of view should be as small as possible and still allow for adequate evaluation of the region.

There are advantages and disadvantages to obtaining images of both extremities during evaluation of pediatric musculoskeletal lesions. The advantage of imaging both limbs is that the normal side is present for comparison, which is particularly useful when evaluating red and yellow marrow. The disadvantage is that the field of view and the coil used must be larger. Both these factors decrease resolution. Once the necessary expertise has been gained by the observer in the evaluation of pediatric musculoskeletal lesions, the extremity with the abnormality should be imaged, using an extremity coil whenever possible.

STIR

Multislice STIR images can routinely be obtained to evaluate pediatric musculoskeletal lesions. STIR imaging can be an important adjunct to spin-echo evaluation of bone lesions[19–21] and could potentially replace T2 spin-echo images. We often use STIR imaging to acquire images in the second (coronal or sagittal) plane, although they may be obtained in the transverse plane if this is considered advantageous. Fat signal and any tissue with a T1 relaxation time similar to fat is suppressed on STIR images, so fatty marrow and subcutaneous fat are of low signal intensity. Cortical bone is also of low signal intensity, whereas muscle and red marrow are of intermediate signal intensity. Tumor, edema, and fluid, with their prolonged T1 relaxation time and therefore increased signal intensity on STIR images, appear conspicuously bright (Fig. 24–7). A TR of 1500 msec, TE of 30 msec, and TI of 100 msec provide good suppression of fat with the use of medium-field-strength magnets (0.35 to 0.5T), while a TI of up to 150 msec may be required on higher-field-strength systems (1.5T).[19]

Gradient Echo

We have recently reported the effect of trabecular bone on gradient-echo images of the marrow in the

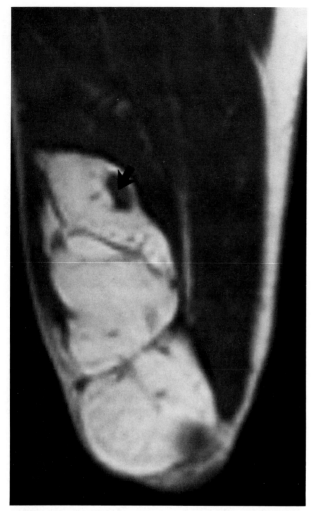

Figure 24–6. *Imaging technique: visualization of fatty tumor.* Coronal image through the anterior thigh of a 19-year-old male with a low-grade liposarcoma. The increased-signal-intensity mass is easily seen compared with the intermediate-signal-intensity muscle of the thigh. Note the multiple septations, focal area of low signal intensity (*arrow*), and irregular contour of the liposarcoma. The focal region of low signal intensity increased in signal intensity on T2 weighted images.

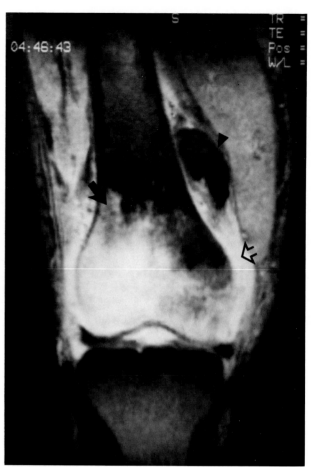

Figure 24–7. *Imaging technique: coronal STIR image (TR 1.5/30/ TI100 msec [0.38T]) through the distal femur in a 19-year-old male with metastatic malignant melanoma.* The increased-signal-intensity tumor and surrounding feathery marrow edema (*arrow*) are seen as bright signal intensity and are conspicuous compared with the suppressed, black-signal-intensity yellow marrow. Muscle is seen as intermediate signal intensity on STIR images. An incidental lipoma (*arrowhead*) is seen in the medial aspect of the thigh adjacent to the femur. Fluid surrounding the distal femur both medially and laterally is bright in signal intensity and easily seen (*open arrow*).

appendicular skeleton.[22] Marrow signal intensity in the metaphysis and epiphysis is markedly decreased as a result of the magnetic susceptibility effect of trabecular bone on marrow signal intensity. Lesion conspicuity is enhanced on these images by loss of trabecular bone in these regions, so that metaphyseal and epiphyseal lesions can be seen as intermediate to increased signal intensity within an underlying milieu of decreased signal intensity on gradient-echo images (Fig. 24–8).[23] The conspicuity of diaphyseal lesions varies, depending on the lesion and the histologic appearance of the underlying marrow, whether red or yellow.[24] Lesion conspicuity is decreased with increasing TE for a given TR and flip angle (Fig. 24–8).[23]

Chemical Shift

There is much work in progress to develop imaging sequences that exploit the chemical shift effect. Chemical shift imaging can generate fat-water images or fat suppression images. The former appears more useful in the evaluation of marrow disease, but fat suppression techniques[25–27] may, like STIR imaging, increase

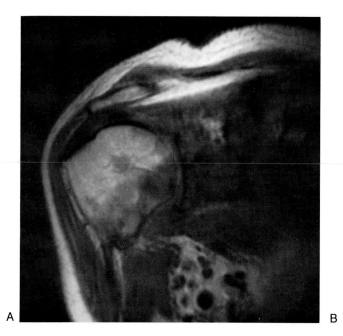

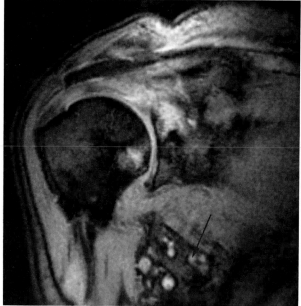

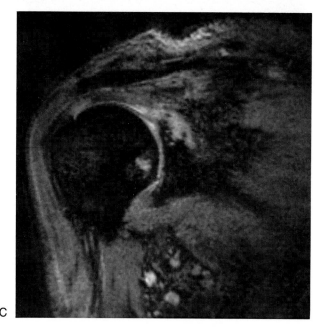

Figure 24–8. *Imaging technique: effect of gradient-echo imaging on the detection of marrow lesions. Coronal images through the proximal humerus in a young woman with metastatic breast carcinoma.* ***A,*** *Proton-density image (1000/20) reveals multiple low-signal-intensity lesions in the epiphysis, most prominent medially. Multiple small nodes are seen in the axilla.* ***B, C,*** *Gradient-echo images at TR60 with a flip angle of 10 degrees. In* ***B*** *the TE is 12 msec. The medial lesion is seen as bright signal intensity secondary to disruption of trabecular bone and loss of the magnetic susceptibility effect of trabecular bone on marrow. The remaining lesions are not well seen on the gradient-echo image alone. In* ***C*** *(TE = 30 msec) the full extent of the lesion is less well seen. Axillary nodes are seen as bright signal intensity (*arrow*).*

lesion conspicuity by decreasing the signal from fatty marrow.

IMAGE ANALYSIS

It is essential that the MR examination be systematically evaluated. Interpretation may be facilitated by hanging the transverse T1 and transverse T2 weighted images for a particular series of slices side by side. The transverse proton density or intermediate images and

STIR images are hung on adjacent boards. Each T2 weighted image should be carefully reviewed, and any bright signal intensity tissue seen on the T2 weighted image should be compared with the same area on the T1 weighted image. This facilitates differentiation of tissue of abnormal high signal intensity (tumor and edema) on T2 weighted images from fat, blood, fluid, or adenopathy. Unless each area of increased signal intensity on the T2 weighted images is compared with the same area on the T1 weighted images, subtle areas of abnormal increased signal intensity may be misinterpreted or missed (Fig. 24–9). The proton-density images are useful when the nature of the suspicious tissue is unclear from analysis of the T2 weighted and T1 weighted images, or to clarify anatomy. The T1 weighted images are again scrutinized for both abnormal signal and anatomic aberration, and any area of abnormality is meticulously compared with the signal intensity on the T2 weighted image. Areas of bright signal intensity on STIR images are compared with the spin-echo images.

The following parameters should be used to evaluate MR images of pediatric musculoskeletal lesions:[3]

1. Location of the lesion (bone or soft tissue).
2. Signal characteristics (intensity and homogeneity of lesion).
3. Extent of marrow disease and edema.
4. Physeal and epiphyseal involvement.
5. Cortical bone involvement (including tumor breakthrough).
6. Periosteal reaction.
7. Joint involvement.
8. Characteristics of primary soft tissue masses.
9. Size and extent of soft tissue mass.
10. Soft tissue edema (extent and differentiation from a mass).
11. Neurovascular involvement.
12. Lymph node involvement.

Each of these must be systematically assessed, and only then can optimal identification and staging of the lesion be achieved.

Location of the Lesion

When evaluating an MR scan with marrow, cortical bone, and soft tissue involvement, criteria can be used in an attempt to determine whether the tumor more likely represents a primary bone tumor or a primary soft tissue tumor. Extensive bony involvement with displacement of juxtacortical muscles probably represents extension of a primary bone tumor into the surrounding soft tissues. If there is replacement, not just displacement, of juxtacortical muscle with extensive bony involvement, an attempt should be made to identify an epicenter of the lesion (marrow, cortex, periosteum, muscle). Evidence from the MR examination should be combined with evidence from the clinical history and radiographs to determine whether the lesion is a primary bony lesion with extension into soft tissues, or a primary soft tissue lesion with extension into the marrow. Even if a large extensive soft tissue mass is seen, a radiographic abnormality typical for primary bone lesion combined with marrow abnormality on MRI and juxtacortical muscular displacement or replacement is more likely to represent a primary bone tumor. Discrete areas of tumor breakthrough (Fig. 24–10) emanating from a marrow lesion are suggestive of a primary bone tumor. On the other hand, if the radiographic findings are not typical for a primary bone tumor, and muscle is replaced by tumor with either edema or little or no bone involvement, a primary soft tissue tumor with extension into the marrow cavity is more likely.

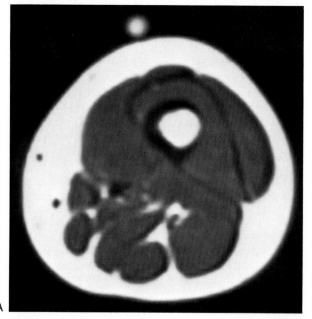
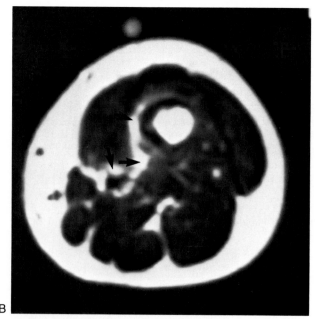

A   B

Figure 24–9. *Image analysis: comparison of T1 and T2 weighted images.* Transverse images through the midfemur in a 10-year-old girl with osteogenic sarcoma: T1 weighted (800/20) (*A*) and T2 weighted (2000/80) (*B*) images through the same plane. On the T2 weighted image, bright signal intensity in the fascial plane separating the vastus intermedius from the vastus medialis could be misinterpreted as fat if this area of increased signal intensity was not meticulously compared with the same area on the T1 weighted image. When compared, edema surrounding the femur, in the fascial plane, and in the neurovascular bundle is obvious (*arrows*).

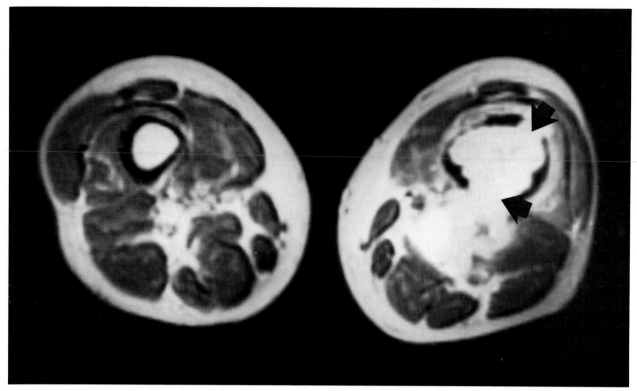

Figure 24–10. *Chondrosarcoma with cortical penetration.* Transverse long TR image (2000/40) of a chondrosarcoma with cortical breakthrough of tumor. The increased signal intensity tumor is clearly seen eroding endosteal bone, breaking through the low-signal-intensity cortical bone, and extending into the surrounding soft tissues *(arrow)*.

Signal Characteristics

Most musculoskeletal lesions show intermediate signal intensity on T1 weighted images and bright signal intensity on T2 weighted images, compared with normal muscle. This is the result of prolonged T1 and T2 relaxation times.[10] However, other signal intensities, on both T1 and T2 weighted images, may be seen in pediatric musculoskeletal lesions. Chronic fibrosis or reactive bone may appear as low signal intensity on both T1 and T2 weighted images.[9] Calcification may also appear as low signal intensity on both T1 and T2 weighted images. It may also be seen as intermediate signal intensity on T1 weighted images, which is slightly brighter on T2 weighted images.[28] This is noted when a protein matrix underlies the calcification, so that the protein matrix, and not the calcium, is visualized on MRI.[28]

Lesions of cartilaginous or neurogenic origin may occasionally have slightly increased signal intensity on T1 weighted images, with further increase in intensities on T2 weighted images.[10, 20, 29] Therefore, a cartilaginous or neurogenic origin may be suggested when slightly increased signal intensity is seen on T1 weighted images. Intermediate signal intensity on T1 weighted images that is decreased on T2 weighted images may represent acute hemorrhage.[20, 30]

As mentioned, high signal intensity on T2 weighted images with decreased signal intensity on T1 weighted images may be seen in most musculoskeletal lesions. Similar signal intensities are seen with edema, fluid (including tumor necrosis), or early fibrosis. An area that is bright on T2 and equally bright on T1 weighted images may represent mucous or subacute hemorrhage.[30] When evidence of blood is seen, hemorrhage into a lesion, recent biopsy, or a primary hemorrhagic tumor (such as telangiectatic osteosarcoma) should be considered. Fat within lesions appears as high signal intensity on T2 weighted images, which increases on T1 weighted images and follows the signal characteristics of subcutaneous fat. Lipoma, liposarcoma, and teratoma should be considered.

Although there are exceptions to the above principles, they provide a useful guideline to the nature of musculoskeletal lesions.

Extent of Marrow Disease and Edema

The extent of marrow involvement can usually be determined on transverse images, although measurement of the length of marrow involvement may be facilitated by sagittal or coronal images. In infants, young children, and children with chronic hematopoietic disorders with marrow expansion (e.g., sickle cell anemia or thalassemia), T2 weighted images may be best for evaluating the extent of marrow involvement, since optimal contrast between the (usually) increased-signal-intensity lesion and intermediate-signal-intensity red marrow can be achieved. In these children, STIR images may be especially helpful, since red marrow is only slightly increased in signal intensity while most tumors are very bright in signal intensity (Fig. 24–11). In older children, the marrow extent of the tumor is usually best appreciated on T1 weighted images, since the long T1 relaxation time, low- or inter-mediate-signal-intensity tumor will contrast well with the short T1 relaxation time, bright-signal-intensity fatty marrow.

In general, a diaphyseal lesion is conspicuous on T1 weighted images in children over the age of 5 years.[31] By the age of 6 or 7 the marrow of the tibia, fibula, radius, and ulna appears yellow on MRI and, regardless of whether the lesion is diaphyseal or metaphyseal, the marrow extent of the tumor will be appreciated as decreased signal on T1 weighted images. Between the ages of 5 and 10 years, distal femoral metaphyseal red marrow begins conversion to yellow marrow,[31] and distal metaphyseal lesions become increasingly conspicuous on T1 weighted images with increasing marrow conversion. There may be persistent red marrow in the proximal femoral metaphysis throughout life, although tumor in this region is normally of lower signal intensity than red marrow on T1 weighted images (Figs. 24–4, 24–12). However, conspicuity in these cases is increased on T2 weighted images.

The position and dimensions of the lesion within the marrow should be recorded. Note should be made of whether the lesion is ill or well defined, whether there is a low-signal-intensity rim (which can correspond to a sclerotic border on plain film), and whether there is surrounding edema.

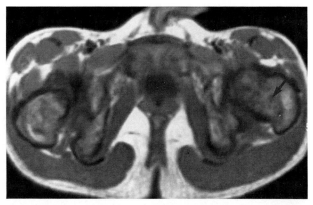

Figure 24–12. *Neuroblastoma metastases to hematopoietic marrow.* Transverse T1 weighted image (600/15) through the proximal femora in a 5-year-old boy with metastatic tumor. The multiple foci of metastatic tumor are seen as low signal intensity (*arrow*), slightly lower than the surrounding intermediate-signal-intensity red marrow.

Evaluation of the marrow for edema may be problematic. There has been little written on the subject, although it is an area of continued interest. Until there are further studies that define the appearance of edema in marrow, the following guidelines may be helpful. Edema of the marrow often appears feathery, with strands of low to intermediate signal intensity on T1 and increased signal intensity on T2 weighted images. Tumor rarely has this appearance. Edema may not be as bright on T2 weighted and STIR images as adjacent tumor (Fig. 24–13). In other instances, however, marrow edema may be extensive, homogeneous, and diffuse. In these patients, it is very difficult to distinguish marrow edema from medullary tumor, such as Ewing's sarcoma. Recent reports on transient edema of the marrow[32, 33] discuss the appearance and resolution of marrow edema.

Our experience suggests that primary bone tumors, specifically Ewing's and osteogenic sarcoma, are not surrounded by extensive marrow edema. Two separate studies correlating the MR appearance with pathologic evaluation[11, 24] show that there is usually only 2 to 3 mm of edema surrounding these primary bone tumors. Extensive edema may be associated with non-neoplastic or inflammatory lesions,[34] and in our experience edema associated with processes such as osteoid osteoma can be homogeneous and difficult to differentiate from tumor. In these patients the clinical history and plain film findings are especially important. STIR imaging, gadolinium-DTPA, other MR contrast agents, and chemical shift imaging may hold promise for future characterization of marrow edema on MRI and accurate differentiation of edema from tumor.

Physeal and Epiphyseal Involvement

The normal physis (growth plate) is seen as a low-signal-intensity line on both T1 and T2 weighted images of varying width separating the metaphysis from

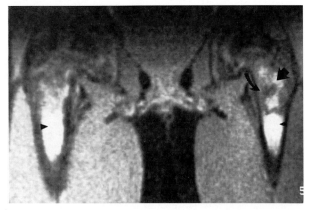

Figure 24–11. *Neuroblastoma metastases to bone marrow.* STIR (TR 1.5/15/TI100 [0.38T]) coronal image through the proximal femora in a 5-year-old boy with metastatic neuroblastoma. Intermediate-signal-intensity red marrow in the proximal left metaphysis was present on the T1 weighted image. Bright-signal-intensity foci of metastatic tumor (*arrow*) are seen within the red marrow (*curved arrow*), which has a slightly increased signal intensity compared with fatty marrow. Diffuse metastatic neuroblastoma replacing the entire marrow cavity is seen in the proximal diaphyses bilaterally (*arrowhead*).

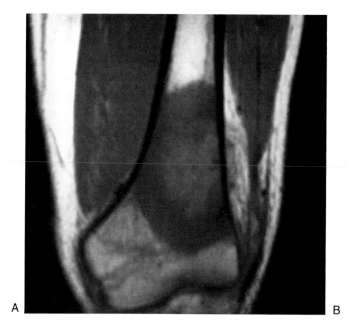

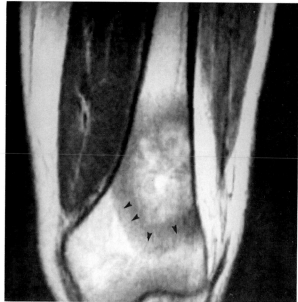

A

B

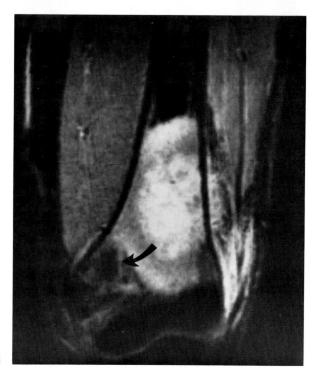

Figure 24–13. *Differentiation of tumor from edema. Coronal MR images through the distal femur in a 10-year-old girl with osteogenic sarcoma.* **A,** T1 weighted image (600/20) intermediate-signal-intensity metaphyseal tumor with a thin rim of surrounding low-intermediate-signal-intensity marrow edema. **B,** T2 weighted image (2000/75). Marrow edema (*arrowheads*) surrounding the tumor has increased in signal intensity compared with the T1 weighted image. **C,** Short TI inversion recovery image (1500/30 TI100). Marrow edema is seen as increased signal intensity on STIR images. Edema is again seen surrounding the tumor, and there are strandlike extensions of edema into the marrow of the medial femoral condyle (*curved arrow*).

C

the epiphysis (Fig. 24–14). With maturation and fusion the physis decreases in size until finally, with fusion, the physis is a thin, low-signal-intensity line on T1 and T2 weighted images. The physeal remnant may still be seen in adults.

The epiphysis begins as a cartilaginous structure, with intermediate signal intensity on T1 and intermediate to increased signal intensity on T2 weighted images. As the cartilaginous epiphysis begins to ossify, a central, high-signal-intensity structure is seen. This

represents the fatty marrow of the ossifying epiphysis. Occasionally, subtle intermediate signal intensity is seen within the epiphysis, especially in very young children. This depends on slice thickness and in most instances represents partial volume averaging of peripheral compressed trabeculae or cortical bone on sagittal or coronal images, or partial volume averaging of the physis on transverse images (Fig. 24–15). Subtle areas of intermediate signal intensity within the ossifying epiphysis may also represent central trabecu-

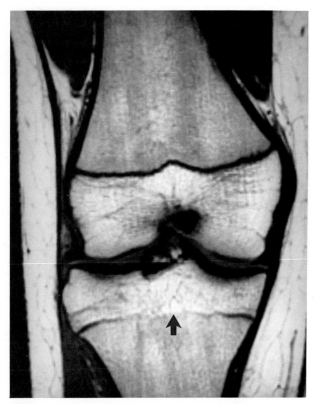

Figure 24–14. *Normal physis (growth plate).* Coronal T1 weighted image (800/20) of the knee in a 14-year-old boy. The normal distal femoral growth plate is seen as a slightly undulating low-signal-intensity line separating the distal femoral metaphysis and distal femoral epiphysis. As the physis closes (tibial physis), it decreases in width and becomes less prominent (*arrow*).

lar bone, since stress lines traverse the epiphysis, particularly in the proximal femur, resulting in increased trabeculation.

In the long bones, invasion of the growth plate by tumor is best seen on T1 weighted coronal or sagittal images (Fig. 24–16). If an intramedullary diaphyseal or metaphyseal tumor stops short of the physis, with normal fatty or red marrow interposed between the physis and tumor, it is unlikely that there is physeal involvement by tumor. In these cases, a low-signal-intensity physis on T1 weighted images, without evidence of intermediate signal within it, may be judged to be normal (Fig. 24–17). If the tumor abuts the physis so that no clear plane of normal marrow can be seen between physis and tumor (Fig. 24–18), it is difficult to exclude microscopic involvement of the physis, although a homogeneous low-signal-intensity physis does make this less likely.

In our experience, an intermediate signal intensity within the physis makes it likely that the physis is invaded by tumor. Care must be taken in evaluating the physis not to mistake partial volume averaging of the physis with surrounding marrow and cortical bone for tumor involvement. Because the physis is not a straight structure but an undulating line, there are times when intermediate signal intensity representing partial volume averaging can be seen in the physis. In these instances, it is helpful to compare coronal and sagittal images. If intermediate signal intensity within the physis on the coronal image is due to partial volume averaging, it will not be seen on the sagittal image. However, if there is involvement of the physis by a pathologic process, intermediate signal intensity within the physis will be seen on both sagittal and coronal images. Practically speaking, we often do not obtain sagittal and coronal T1 weighted images in the same patient. By assessing the coronal or sagittal scout images on the monitor for abnormal signal within or near the physis, the need for an additional imaging plane can be determined at the time of imaging. In addition, proton-density images are usually as good as T1 weighted images in evaluation of the physis. The lack of anatomic detail on T2 weighted images makes these less useful. STIR images are not as helpful in the evaluation of the physis, since both cartilaginous physis and tumor are seen as increased signal intensity.

Determination of epiphyseal involvement by tumor is important when assessing a patient for a limb salvage procedure, since it is less likely that a limb salvage procedure can be performed if the epiphysis is involved. Recent surgical techniques,[35] however, involve replacement of both the epiphysis and the meniscus, enabling these patients to have a limb salvage procedure. To evaluate the epiphysis, one must compare the signal intensity of the epiphysis on T1 weighted and T2 weighted or STIR images. Tumor within the epiphysis is usually seen as intermediate signal intensity on T1 weighted images (Fig. 24–16) and heterogeneous bright signal intensity on T2 weighted and STIR images. It is important to understand the relationship of epiphyseal and physeal involvement. When tumor is seen abutting the physis, but the physis appears uninvolved (Fig. 24–18), the presence or absence of changes in the epiphysis is crucial. Abnormal epiphyseal signal in these patients increases the likelihood of physeal involvement, at least by microscopic tumor,[24] since metaphyseal tumor would have to cross the physis to extend into the epiphysis. If there are no changes in the epiphysis, and the physis appears normal on MRI, both the physis and epiphysis are likely to be free of disease. Indications for a frozen section at the time of surgery to exclude physeal involvement include any abnormal signal intensity within the physis or a normal-signal-intensity physis with adjacent tumor in either the metaphysis, the epiphysis, or both.

Cortical Bone Involvement

There have been several reports assessing the efficacy of MRI and the accuracy of MR and CT in evaluating cortical bone.[9, 12, 13, 17] In early reports, CT was thought to be more accurate than MRI in assessing

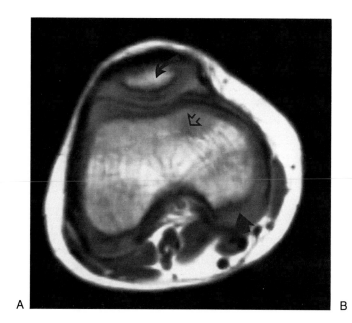

A

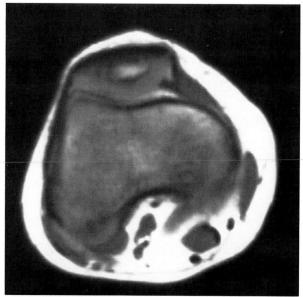

B

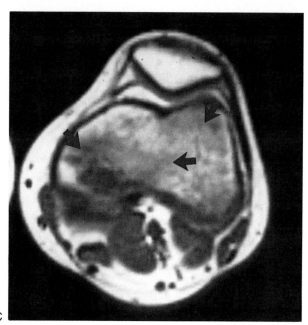

C

Figure 24–15. *Normal appearance of growth plate and adjacent structures: partial volume artifacts. Transverse images through the distal femur in a normal 7-year-old boy.* ***A,*** *The ossifying distal femoral epiphysis containing increased-signal-intensity fatty marrow can be appreciated within the intermediate-signal-intensity cartilaginous epiphysis (arrow). A focal area of low signal intensity in the anteromedial aspect of the epiphysis represents partial volume of the cartilaginous physis (open arrow). The ossifying patella (also containing fatty marrow) (curved arrow) can be seen within the cartilaginous patella.* ***B,*** *The low- to intermediate-signal-intensity cartilaginous physis can be seen on this transverse image just superior to* ***A.*** *This should not be misinterpreted as abnormal marrow (600/20).* ***C,*** *Transverse T1 weighted image (800/20) through the distal femur in an 11-year-old girl. Partial volume averaging of the undulating distal femoral physis imparts a heterogeneous appearance to the distal femoral bone marrow (arrows). This should not be mistaken for a pathologic condition.*

cortical bone. A 1987 study by Wetzel and colleagues reported a 72 percent accuracy rate in the evaluation of cortical bone on MRI.[12] A more recent article by Bloem and colleagues confirmed that "both MR imaging and CT were very accurate in demonstrating involvement of cortical bone."[13] Although no percentages were given, anecdotal note was made of one patient in whom MRI was more sensitive to the invasion of cortical bone than CT, and another in whom both MRI and CT were incorrectly negative in assessing cortical bone involvement. The uncertainty over the efficacy of MRI in evaluating cortical bone most likely reflects early imaging techniques that may not

have allowed detailed evaluation of cortical bone, as well as a lack of knowledge in early MR imaging regarding the criteria for and appearance of cortical bone involvement by tumor. In future studies the accuracy, sensitivity, and specificity of MRI in the evaluation of cortical bone may be seen to approach (or surpass) those of CT.

Cortical bone is usually best evaluated on transverse images. Use of the transverse plane provides the least partial volume averaging artifact. In general, abnormality of cortical bone is seen as intermediate signal intensity within the normally low-signal-intensity cortical bone on T1 weighted, T2 weighted, and STIR im-

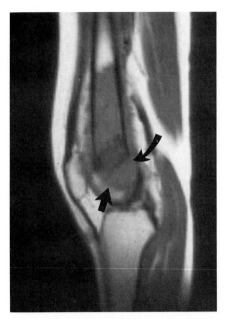

Figure 24–16. *Tumor penetration through the growth plate.* Sagittal T1 weighted image (500/30) through the knee in a 14-year-old girl with osteogenic sarcoma. The low-signal-intensity tumor is sharply demarcated from the normal-signal-intensity yellow marrow (*arrow*). Tumor has broken through the physis, which is no longer identified, and extends into the distal femoral epiphysis (*arrow*). Breakthrough of tumor through the cortex is clearly seen posteriorly (*curved arrow*).

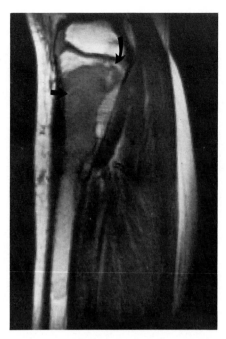

Figure 24–17. *Osteogenic sarcoma with intact growth plate.* Sagittal T1 weighted image (500/30) through the tibia in a 15-year-old male. The tumor is seen as a low-signal-intensity, well-defined lesion within the high-signal-intensity fatty marrow (*arrow*). There is normal high-signal-intensity marrow interposed between the tumor and the low-signal-intensity physis (*curved arrow*).

ages. In our experience, detailed involvement of cortical bone by tumor may often be equally appreciated on proton-density images and T1 weighted images (Fig. 24–19).

In areas of rapid tapering or expansion of bone (e.g., the metaphyseal regions), there may be partial volume averaging of the cortex with muscle or bone marrow lying above or below the cortex on a specific transverse slice. This may result in an appearance suggestive of intermediate signal intensity within the cortical bone (Fig. 24–20). This partial volume averaging effect is more likely with increased slice thickness. In instances of suspected partial volume averaging, the suspicious region of cortex should be examined on the orthogonal plane obtained during the study. If cortical intermediate signal intensity is confirmed on the coronal or sagittal images, the probability of cortical involvement is likely. It may also be helpful to have transverse images of the opposite extremity to compare for partial volume averaging in the same region of the normal extremity.

Intermediate signal intensity within the normally black cortical bone is abnormal, but no prospective studies have specifically addressed the significance of abnormal signal intensity within cortical bone on MRI. If there is tumor in the marrow and a soft tissue mass adjacent to a cortical abnormality, the intermediate signal intensity within cortical bone is likely to represent penetration of tumor through the cortical bone. However, if there is no evidence of adjacent tumor in the marrow and no tumor or soft tissue abnormality in the tissues surrounding this area of abnormal cortical bone signal, it is unlikely that the signal intensity observed within the cortical bone represents tumor. In these instances, artifactual signal intensity within cortical bone should be suspected, and the bone should be scrutinized for rapid tapering (especially in the proximal femoral metaphysis and intertrochanteric regions) or chemical shift artifact. If the abnormal cortical signal intensity is present on both transverse and sagittal or coronal images, but there is no tumor adjacent to this region, other explanations, such as aggressive osteoporosis, periosteal reaction, infection, or other inflammatory processes, should be sought. It is likely that cortical bone signal abnormality may represent a variety of pathologic processes, and it is hoped that prospective studies of cortical bone will elucidate the significance of cortical bone signal abnormality.

In addition to partial volume averaging as a cause of misinterpreted signal within cortical bone, chemical shift artifact may also be problematic (Fig. 24–21).[36] Chemical shift in the frequency encoding direction will cause apparent thickening of the cortex on one side and thinning of the cortex on the opposite side. If a soft tissue mass or marrow tumor is adjacent to the cortical bone that appears thinned, it may give the appearance of erosion of the cortical bone by tumor. In these cases, the frequency encoding direction must be reversed before cortical bone can be accurately evaluated.

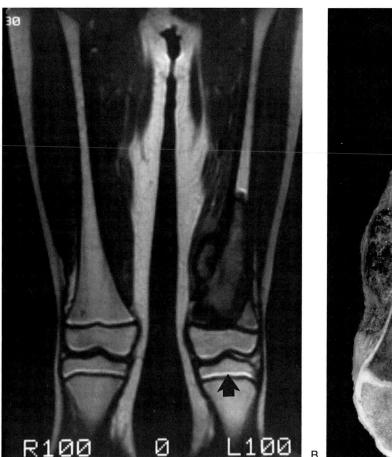

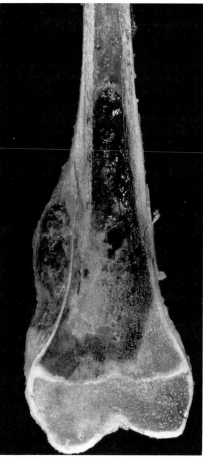

Figure 24–18. *Osteogenic sarcoma with intact growth plate.*   ***A,*** Coronal T1 weighted image (800/15) through the femurs in a 16-year-old boy with osteogenic sarcoma. Tumor is seen abutting the physis, but the physis retains its low signal intensity without evidence of intermediate signal intensity. The epiphysis is unremarkable and there is no evidence of edema. Chemical shift effect is noted adjacent to the physis *(arrow).* ***B,*** Gross specimen shows tumor abutting the physis, without evidence of invasion of the physis.

Until prospective studies can establish uniform criteria for cortical bone abnormality and determine the accuracy, sensitivity, and specificity of MRI in the evaluation of cortical bone, the following guidelines are helpful in evaluating cortical bone in the context of pediatric bone or soft tissue tumors. Endosteal erosion may be recognized on MRI as subtle intermediate signal intensity on T1 weighted images within the endosteal aspect of cortical bone, often with thinning of the very-low-signal (black) cortical bone (Fig. 24–10). The marrow cavity may appear expanded. Permeation of tumor through haversian canals may be appreciated on MRI as intermediate signal intensity extending either partially or completely through the cortical bone (Fig. 24–19). Finally, actual breakthrough of tumor through the cortex into the soft tissues should be recognized. In the most obvious cases of actual tumor breakthrough of cortical bone, solid abnormal tissue signal intensity that is continuous with marrow tumor breaks through the cortex, leaving no remnant of normal cortex, and extends directly into an adjacent soft tissue mass (Fig. 24–10). With permeative spread of tumor,

the intermediate signal intensity within the cortex on T1 weighted images is less pronounced, and there may be some residual cortical bone. The distinction of actual cortical breakthrough from permeative spread of tumor through the cortex is important for two reasons. First, if there is a large defect through the cortex, the overall chance of survival is decreased and amputation is often the preferred method of treatment.[37] Spread of tumor cells associated with pathologic fracture and hematoma formation is responsible for the decreased survival rate in these patients. Second, most surgeons prefer to perform a biopsy through a preexisting cortical defect, if one is present. It is not always possible to distinguish actual tumor breakthrough and pathologic fracture of the cortex from permeative spread of tumor through the cortex on MRI, and plain films must be evaluated in conjunction with the MR examination. In patients in whom cortical breakthrough is suspected on MRI but not obvious on the plain film, CT can be used as an adjunctive modality. However, cortical disruption not seen on the plain film may not be large enough to be clinically significant.

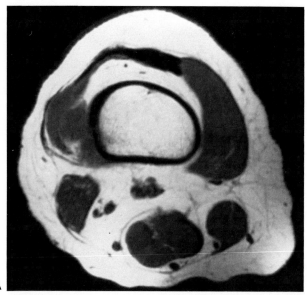
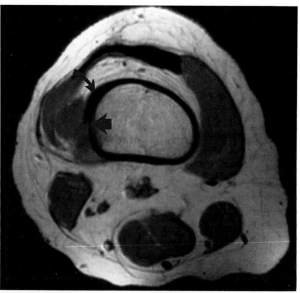

A   B

Figure 24–19. *Osteogenic sarcoma: penetration through the cortex and periosteal reaction.* ***A,*** T1 weighted transverse image (820/20) through the distal femoral metaphysis in a 17-year-old girl. A thin band of tumor is seen intercalating through the cortical bone into the surrounding soft tissues. The image is at the superiormost aspect of the tumor. ***B,*** Proton-density image (2000/20) through the same region, which shows intercalation of tumor to better advantage (*arrow*). Lamellated periosteal reaction is noted anteriorly (*curved arrow*).

Periosteal Reaction

Histology of Periosteum

Evaluation of periosteal reaction by MRI is a relatively new area of investigation. Prospective studies to determine the accuracy, sensitivity, and specificity of MR in this regard are only just beginning, but we have shown[18] that periosteal reaction can be seen and evaluated on MRI.

Before one can adequately evaluate the periosteum on MRI, it is important to understand the pathophysiology of periosteal reaction. Anatomically, the periosteum is an envelope, composed of an outer fibrous layer and an inner cellular or cambium layer, that surrounds the cortical bone and separates it from the surrounding soft tissue. In adults the periosteum is primarily fibrous. However, during normal growth or during reaction to injury, the two distinct layers of periosteum can be distinguished histologically. There is a zone of transition between the two layers in which a change of fibroblasts into preosteoblasts occurs. Subsequent mitosis and cell enlargement create the cambium layer within which osteoid secreting cells emerge.[38] Therefore the periosteum is more accurately thought of as a continuum of cells consisting primarily of fibroblasts that, in response to growth or stimulation, differentiate into a dual layer covering of the bone: the inner layer or cambium consisting primarily of osteoid-secreting cells, and the outer or fibrous layer containing primarily fibroblasts and preosteoblasts.

Appositional activity of the periosteum is not considered "periosteal reaction," but rather as enlargement of the bone shaft during normal growth. Actual "periosteal reaction" is the term used to describe a more vigorous deposition of juxtacortical soft tissue and bone in disease processes. The amount of periosteal new bone relates to the degree of periosteal elevation as well as the level of activity of the process stimulating the new bone. The configuration of periosteal reaction relates to the time course of production and the manner in which the new bone is laid down.[38] Mineralization of the periosteal reaction is necessary before it can be seen on a radiograph or CT scan. This usually requires a period of 10 days to 3 weeks after the initial stimulus, although children exhibit periosteal reaction more quickly than older individuals. It is possible that this reflects the underlying active state of the periosteum in children who are constantly undergoing bone remodeling and growth.

In general, periosteal reaction may be classified as continuous, interrupted, or complex (Figs. 24–22 to 24–24). Continuous periosteal reaction may be accompanied by destruction of underlying endosteal cortex, giving a "shell" appearance. If there is no resorption of endosteal cortex, continuous periosteal reaction is classified as solid, single lamellar, lamellated, or parallel spiculated ("hair on end"). Interrupted periosteal reaction is found when a tumor or another aggressive process breaches a preformed periosteal reaction. Its appearance depends on the type of periosteal reaction invaded (Fig. 24–23). The most common complex periosteal reaction encountered in pediatric musculoskeletal tumors is the sunburst variety.

MR Appearance of Periosteal Reaction

We are only beginning to recognize the spectrum of periosteal reaction that can be appreciated on pediatric musculoskeletal MR examination. The following are

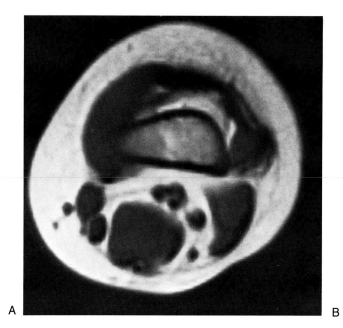

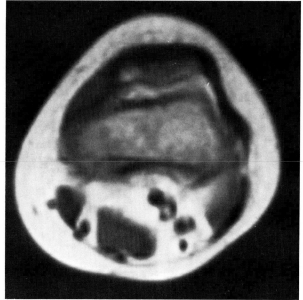

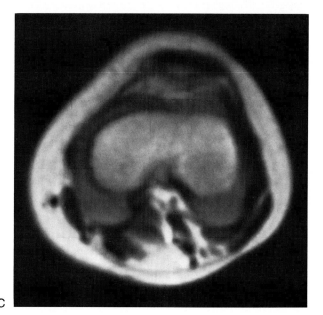

Figure 24–20. *Partial volume artifact. Transverse proton-density images (2000/20) of distal femur in a normal 3-year-old girl.* ***A,*** *Normal low-signal-intensity cortical bone in the proximal metaphysis.* ***B,*** *Apparent intermediate signal intensity within the cortical bone due to partial volume effect from* ***C,*** *the adjacent cartilaginous epiphysis. Intermediate signal intensity from partial volume effect in rapidly tapering or expanding bone is a pitfall in the evaluation of cortical bone.*

guidelines based on preliminary work[18] that should be of some help to the reader in interpreting MR images.

Transverse MR images are more likely to provide the detail necessary for the detection of periosteal reaction than sagittal or coronal images, primarily because the field of view is usually smaller. To recognize periosteal reaction on MRI, the signal intensity external to and adjacent to cortical bone should be observed on T2 weighted images. Knowledge of normal underlying muscle anatomy can be helpful. If normal muscle abuts cortical bone, without interposition of any abnormal or increased signal intensity on T2 weighted images, there is no MR evidence of periosteal reaction. If there is increased signal intensity adjacent to the cortical bone on T2 weighted images, this may represent a fat plane

surrounding the cortical bone, hemorrhage, inflammation, tumor, or periosteal reaction. If there is also increased signal intensity on the T1 weighted images, this most likely represents a normal fat plane. Subacute hemorrhage should also be considered. If the increased signal intensity is seen as intermediate or decreased signal intensity on the T1 weighted image, an inflammatory process, tumor, or periosteal reaction should be suspected.

Periosteal reaction may have a variable appearance on T1 weighted images, but linear areas of very low signal intensity (black or near-black) within the abnormal tissue (representing lamellar bone) are a distinguishing feature. If curvilinear or straight areas of very low signal intensity can be identified on both T1 and T2

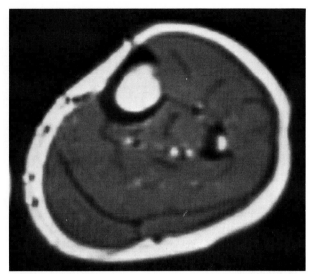

Figure 24–21. *Chemical shift effect in the tibia and fibula.* This causes apparent cortical thinning of the lateral cortex of both bones.

weighted images, a periosteal reaction is likely (Fig. 24–25).

The "shell" type of periosteal reaction is seen in processes where the underlying endosteal surface of the bone is resorbed, either by pressure from impinging growth of a lesion or by the presence of active hyperemia. At the same time, new bone is added to the outer surface of the cortex by periosteal activity. On MRI this "shell" of periosteal new bone is usually not seen, but it may sometimes be seen as a very thin rim of low signal intensity surrounding the abnormal process.

Solid continuous periosteal reaction represents multiple successive layers of new lamellar bone applied to the cortex. The solid periosteal reaction may be created in several ways.[38] There may be slow surface addition of layer after layer of compact lamellar bone, which becomes incorporated and fused. Alternatively, soft tissue spaces between layers of a lamellated reaction may fill in by continued apposition to the lamellae, or an initial woven bone network (produced by the periosteum) may be filled in with an inlay of lamellar bone.

Solid periosteal reaction usually indicates a chronic indolent lesion in the marrow space, cortex, or adjacent soft tissue. Osteoid osteoma, chronic osteomyelitis, eosinophilic granuloma, and large enchondromas may be associated with this type of periosteal reaction. On MRI this may be seen as thickened low-signal-intensity cortical bone. There should be no evidence of intermediate signal intensity within the bone. However, a reported case of Ewing's sarcoma treated with preoperative therapy[13] had a similar appearance on MRI, with viable tumor tissue present within the thickened cortical bone at pathologic examination. Although thickened cortex, without internal signal, most likely represents a chronic indolent lesion, caution

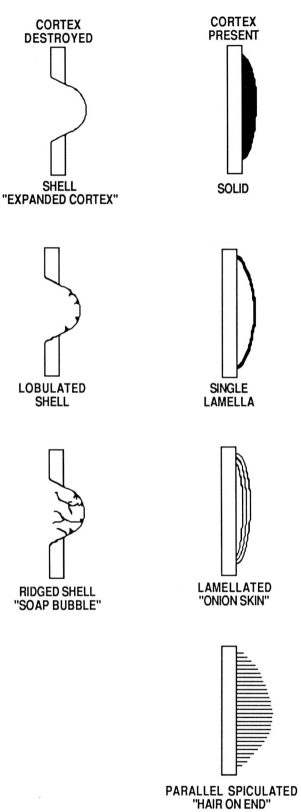

Figure 24–22. *Types of continuous periosteal reaction.* The cortex can be destroyed (first column) or intact (second column). (Adapted from Ragsdale BD, Madewell JE, Sweet DE, et al. Radiologic analysis of solitary bone lesions. Part II: Periosteal reactions. Radiol Clin North Am 1981; 19:749–784.)

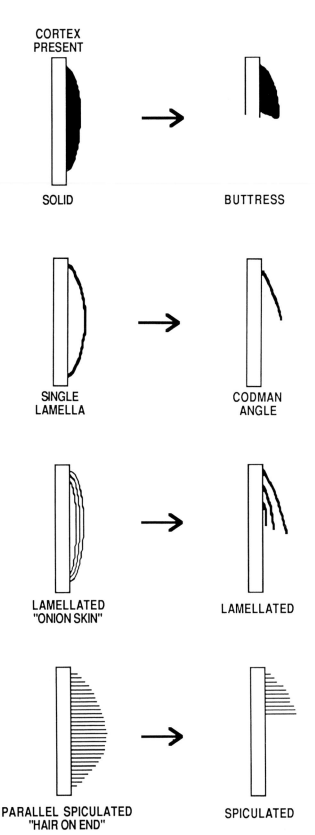

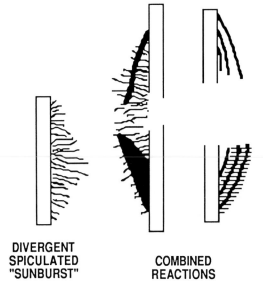

Figure 24–24. *Types of complex periosteal reaction.* (Adapted from Ragsdale BD, Madewell JE, Sweet DE, et al. Radiologic analysis of solitary bone lesions. Part II: Periosteal reactions. Radiol Clin North Am 1981: 19:749–784.)

Figure 24–23. *Types of interrupted periosteal reaction.* (Adapted from Ragsdale BD, Madewell JE, Sweet DE, et al. Radiologic analysis of solitary bone lesions. Part II: Periosteal reactions. Radiol Clin North Am 1981; 19:749–784.)

should be used in interpreting thickened cortical bone on MRI until more studies of the MR appearance of cortical bone have been performed.

A single lamellar periosteal reaction consisting of a single layer of new, lamellar bone is often seen in acute osteomyelitis and in early neoplasms. On MRI, single lamellar periosteal reaction can be appreciated as a thin, often curvilinear, low-signal-intensity line on both T1 and T2 weighted images.[18] The new bone may either surround the entire bone or overlie only a part of it (Fig. 24–25).

"Onion skin" periosteal reaction has classically been associated with Ewing's sarcoma, osteosarcoma, and acute suppurative or syphilitic osteomyelitis. The "onion skin" periosteal reaction is created by concentric planes of lamellar ossification surrounding the cortex.[38] These concentric planes of new bone may be caused by permeation of tumor between layers of lamellated new bone, but "onion skin" periosteal reaction may also be seen in non-neoplastic conditions such as osteomyelitis, hypertrophic pulmonary osteoarthropathy, and stress fracture. It may also be seen as a transient feature of normal growth in infants.

The exact histologic etiology of this layered lamellated periosteal reaction is unknown, but in neoplastic conditions it may be caused by cyclic variation in subperiosteal tumor growth with repeated phases of rapid periosteal elevation and mineralization. In non-neoplastic conditions, the continuous lamellated periosteal reaction may follow "explosive cortical tunneling" caused by active hyperemia.[38] Over time, the layers tend to become thickened and better defined.

On MRI, "onion skin" periosteal reaction can be

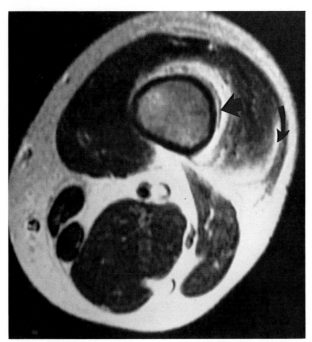

Figure 24–25. *Periosteal reaction with osteogenic sarcoma.* Transverse image (2000/70) through the femoral diaphysis in a 15-year-old girl. Low-signal-intensity, single lamellar periosteal reaction can be identified on the MR image (*arrow*). Increased-signal-intensity tumor fills the marrow cavity. Increased-signal-intensity muscle edema can be identified in the vastus lateralis (*curved arrow*).

seen as alternating areas of intermediate and low signal intensity on T1 weighted images, and alternating areas of intermediate to bright and low signal intensity on T2 weighted images (Fig. 24–26). The concentric rings of low signal intensity on both T1 and T2 weighted images correspond grossly to organized lamellar bone, while the interposing intermediate or bright signal intensity grossly reflects cellular components.[18]

Continuous periosteal reaction characterized by a parallel spiculated appearance is referred to as the "hair-on-end" periosteal reaction. This implies an underlying process that is faster growing than a solid or lamellar reaction. Pathologically, this spiculated reaction is seen as an osseous honeycomb,[38] with tumor cells usually occupying the intervening soft tissue spaces. This pattern of periosteal reaction is often seen in Ewing's sarcoma and in the calvarial reaction associated with severe anemia, such as that in thalassemia. It has also been reported with syphilis, myositis, and Caffey's disease. Parallel spiculated periosteal reaction is seen as intermediate signal intensity in T1 weighted images extending from cortical bone, often appearing as a soft tissue mass. Increased signal intensity is seen on T2 weighted images. The new bone formed is not appreciated as low-signal-intensity bone on T1 and T2 weighted images, unlike the other continuous lamellated periosteal reactions.[18] It is possible that the very thin lamellar bone laid down is not of sufficient volume to be appreciated as signal loss on MRI.

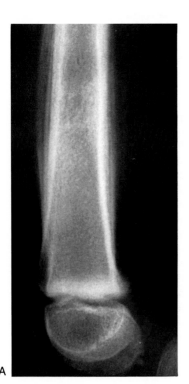

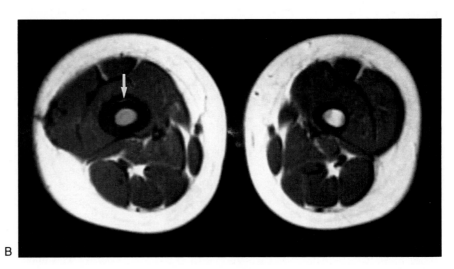

Figure 24–26. *Ewing's sarcoma: onion peel periosteal reaction.* **A,** Lateral radiograph and **B,** transverse long TR image (2000/20) through the femur in a 3-year-old girl with Ewing's sarcoma of the right femoral shaft. "Onion skin" periosteal reaction is seen on the plain film. On MRI this can be identified as concentric rings. Increased signal intensity, representing cellular periosteal reaction and muscle edema, can be seen (*arrow*). Homogeneous intermediate-signal-intensity tumor is seen in the right femoral diaphysis.

Interrupted periosteal reaction is formed when tumor colonizes the soft tissue space within a periosteal reaction, and either denies space for elaboration of new bone in this periosteal reaction or, by direct pressure, stimulates osteoclasts to remove the reactive bone. The type of interrupted periosteal reaction depends on the continuous periosteal reaction present before tumor invasion.[38] The MR appearance of these interrupted reactions reflects the underlying continuous reaction, with abrupt termination of the periosteal reaction by the underlying pathologic process.[18] The interrupted reaction is usually seen at the edge of a lesion on coronal or sagittal images.

Complex periosteal patterns are seen commonly in pediatric bone tumors, especially osteogenic sarcoma. The divergent spiculated, or "sunburst," pattern is a sign of malignant osteoid production. Histologically, the individual "rays" of ossification seen on radiographs or CT commonly represent a combination of sarcoma bone and reactive bone, or sarcoma bone alone.[38] The space between individual rays is usually occupied by cellular tumor and tumor products, often chondroid or myxoid in character. The reactive bone is oldest adjacent to the cortex and is usually the best defined on plain films. On MRI, it is sometimes possible to see this reactive bone as a spiculated "sunburst" pattern of low intermediate signal intensity on T1 and T2 weighted images (although not nearly as low as the continuous lamellated periosteal reactions previously discussed). More commonly, complex periosteal reactions on MRI are seen as an intermediate-signal-intensity soft tissue mass emanating from the cortical bone or medullary cavity of the bone on T1 weighted images, with increasing and usually heterogeneous signal intensity on T2 weighted images. The "sunburst" calcification seen on plain film is not reflected as calcification or ossification of MRI (Fig. 24–27).

An understanding of the histology of the mineralized bone that is a result of periosteal reactions may be important in the interpretation of MR signals. Periosteal reaction results in lamellar bone formation. Cortical bone consists of lamellar bone and represents compact, well-organized mineralized bone with haversian spaces. The structure of lamellar bone is such that protons do not resonate and are not affected at the field strength and radiofrequencies applied during clinical proton magnetic resonance. Therefore, this lamellar bone is seen as black or very low signal intensity on both T1 and T2 weighted images as well as on STIR images. In pediatric bone tumors, the complex periosteal reactions seen are primarily tumor bone. This tumor bone is structurally disorganized, with calcium embedded in a protein matrix, and protons may therefore be more free to process than the protons of lamellar bone. This may result in intermediate or even increased signal intensity of this tumor bone on MRI (Fig. 24–27D).[18, 28] Until we have further knowledge of the specific appearance of tumor bone on MRI, the latter may be seen as less sensitive than CT or plain

radiography to the presence of new bone formation, but in reality may provide important information regarding the structure of calcification seen on plain film.

At this point, the importance of plain film radiography must be stressed. There should be no confusion when evaluating musculoskeletal MR scans for periosteal reaction, since the MR images should never be interpreted without the benefit of a recent plain film examination. Evaluation of periosteal reaction on MRI is in its early stages. One should not try to supplant the 75 years of experience in the evaluation of periosteal reaction on plain film by a few years of experience with MR evaluation of bony lesions.

There are pitfalls in the evaluation of periosteal reaction on MRI.[18] These include partial volume averaging in regions of rapid tapering of bone (Fig. 24–20); partial volume averaging of cartilaginous apophysis seen as intermediate signal intensity adjacent to cortical bone (Fig. 24–28); partial volume averaging of muscle attachments, especially in the posterior and inferior femur; partial volume averaging of the vastus lateralis in the intertrochanteric region; the presence of a soft tissue mass with a fibrous capsule appearing as low signal intensity on T1 and T2 weighted images, thus simulating a lamellated periosteal reaction; the presence of posterior femoral hyperostosis (Fig. 24–29); the presence of normal infantile periostitis; and chemical shift artifact.

Joint Involvement

Although MR criteria for subtle joint involvement have not yet been established, gross extension of tumor into the joint space can be appreciated.[13, 15] Coronal and sagittal MR images of the joint can provide direct evaluation of the tumor as it abuts the joint surface. On transverse images alone it is often difficult to determine the exact presence and intra-articular extent of tumor as it approaches the joint space. This is one of the primary advantages of MRI compared with CT. In studies comparing MRI and CT in the assessment of joint involvement by tumor,[9, 10, 12, 13, 15, 17] MRI was generally thought to be slightly better (7 percent of cases)[17] to significantly better (73 percent of cases)[12] than CT. However, despite these reports, the specific criteria that should be used by the practicing radiologist when evaluating the joint for tumor involvement are somewhat unclear. The following are some practical guidelines to aid in this assessment.

Gross extension of pathologic processes into the joint space can be easily recognized on MRI. When the joint is not clearly involved, the presence or absence of epiphyseal or surrounding soft tissue involvement, and the presence or absence of joint fluid, can aid in evaluating the joint space. If there is no intramedullary or soft tissue tumor abutting the joint space and no joint fluid, joint involvement is unlikely. If epiphyseal involvement by tumor or another pathologic process is

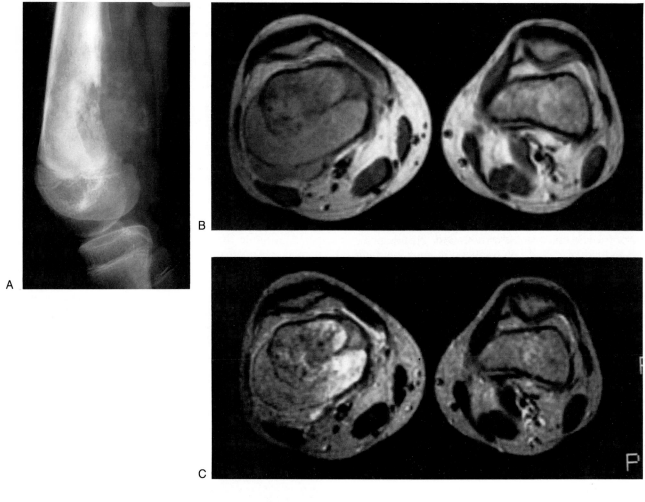

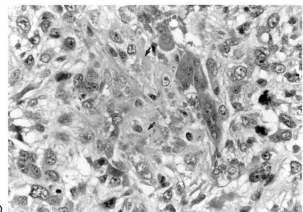

Figure 24–27. *Osteogenic sarcoma with complex periosteal reaction.* ***A,*** Lateral radiograph of the distal femur in an 11-year-old girl. ***B,*** First-echo (2000/20) and ***C,*** second-echo (2000/80) transverse image of the distal femur. The complex periosteal reaction and tumor new bone identified on the plain film are not apparent on the MR image. The calcification/new bone and tumor are seen as an intermediate-signal-intensity, posterior soft tissue mass that increases on T2 weighted images. ***D,*** Tumor new bone, while ossified, is histologically disordered in structure (*arrow*).

seen, the juxta-articular epiphyseal cortical bone is meticulously evaluated on both transverse and coronal or sagittal images. If tumor or another intramedullary or periarticular pathologic process abuts the joint surface, and the cortical bone does not appear black but does appear intermediate in signal intensity, suspicion of microscopic joint involvement from adjacent cortex must be high. The additional finding of a joint effusion increases this level of suspicion. Frozen sections can be obtained at the time of surgery to exclude microscopic invasion of the joint by tumor if this is of clinical importance. If the tumor abuts the joint surface and the cortex is not clearly involved, but is irregular, thinned, or not clearly intact on the images obtained,

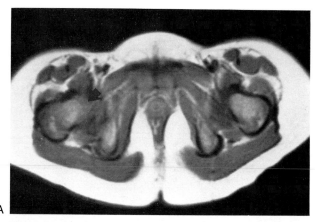
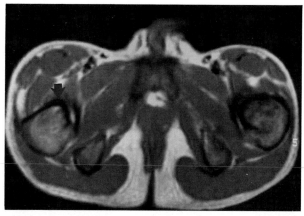

A   B

Figure 24–28. *Pitfall in the evaluation of periosteal reaction.* **A, B,** Transverse images (2000/20) through the inter-trochanteric region in two children showing partial volume effect of the right cartilaginous lesser trochanter (*arrow*). This should not be mistaken for periosteal reaction.

the possibility of microscopic invasion of the joint should be considered. Again, the presence of joint fluid should increase the level of concern, although a joint effusion does not, in itself, confirm microscopic involvement, since sympathetic joint effusions may be seen. When tumor abuts the joint space but is separated from it by normal-appearing cortical bone, involvement of the joint by tumor is less likely (Fig. 24–30). However, until the accuracy, sensitivity, and specificity of specific MR criteria in the diagnosis of joint involvement by tumor are established, the possibility of microscopic involvement of the joint cannot be completely excluded. This is especially true if a joint effusion is noted.

Knowledge of the specific anatomic confines of each joint capsule is essential, since some capsules can extend beyond the level of the physis. In these instances, metaphyseal tumor could theoretically break through the cortex and involve the joint space even in the face of a normal epiphysis, physis, and epiphyseal cortex.

Characteristics of Primary Soft Tissue Masses

Primary soft tissue tumors are readily evaluated by MRI.[3,7,9,12,15,16] Compared with muscle, soft tissue tumors usually have equal or slightly increased signal intensity to muscle on T1 weighted images and increased signal intensity on T2 weighted images. On STIR images the very bright signal intensity of the soft tissue mass increases the conspicuity of the soft tissue tumor as compared with the intermediate-signal-intensity musculature. Primary soft tissue tumors may have either ill- or well-defined margins, and may be either focal or infiltrating; many show a homogeneous high signal intensity on T2 weighted images, but an inhomogeneous mixed high and low signal intensity is also seen. Calcification, hemorrhage, and necrosis may all contribute to tissue inhomogeneity. Demas and col-

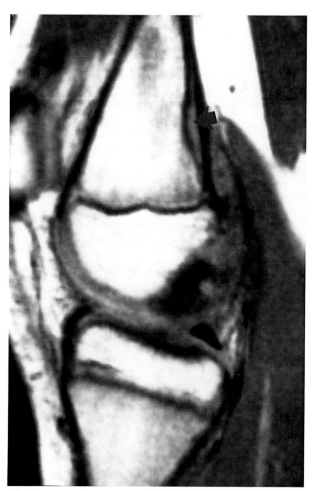

Figure 24–29. *Normal hyperostosis.* Sagittal T1 weighted image (800/30) through the knee in an 11-year-old boy. Posterior cortical hyperostosis is noted (*arrow*).

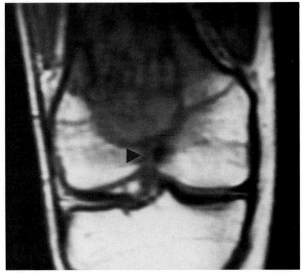

A

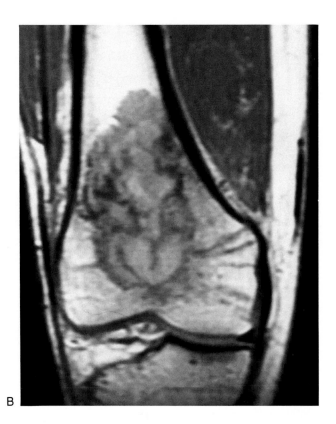

Figure 24–30. *Ewing's sarcoma invading the epiphysis but not the joint. Coronal images through the distal femur in a 17-year-old boy.* **A,** T1 weighted image (800/20) shows tumor, which abuts the joint space (*arrowhead*). There is no joint fluid. **B,** Intermediate weighted image (2000/20) shows a well-defined, heterogeneous lesion with low-signal-intensity linear areas within the tumor that represent reactive bone. The presence of reactive bone makes differentiation of this tumor from osteogenic sarcoma more difficult. The tumor extends through the physis and into the epiphysis.

B

leagues[15] reported on the efficacy of MRI compared with CT in determining the extent of disease in soft tissue sarcomas of the extremities. Tumor dimensions, tumor position in relation to deep fascia, the anatomic compartment and individual muscle involved, neurovascular structures, and underlying bones and joints were evaluated and compared for each modality. The investigators found that MRI and CT were equally accurate in measurement of maximal tumor diameter, detection of tumor depth, and delineation of tumor, neurovascular, osseous, and articular relationships. Evaluation of anatomic compartment and individual muscle involvement was more accurately accomplished with MRI, 23 percent of the MR studies showing tumor involvement of muscles that had appeared normal on CT scans. In most patients, the MR and CT estimates of maximal tumor diameter were within 3 cm of pathologic measurements; 40 percent of the measurements underestimated the extent of tumor and 60 percent equalled or exceeded the dimension of tumor as recorded by the pathologist. No mention was made in the study of the presence of muscle edema or the differentiation of muscle involved by tumor or edema.

Soft Tissue Edema

Differentiation from a Mass

In the evaluation of soft tissue tumors as well as the extension of primary bone tumors into soft tissue on MRI, the following should be considered: the size and position of the mass, the configuration of the abnormal soft tissue, and the effect of the mass on surrounding musculature. Is the abnormal soft tissue nodular and masslike, or is it feathery and conforming to the soft tissue planes? Does the soft tissue mass displace the surrounding normal musculature, or are specific muscle groups actually replaced by tumor, so that the signal intensity of the muscle is increased on T2 weighted and STIR images and the contour of the muscle is either abnormal or enlarged, or both?

The signal intensity and configuration of the abnormal soft tissue noted on MRI are important in distinguishing actual soft tissue mass from soft tissue edema. This becomes a critical question when evaluating postoperative and post-therapeutic (radiation therapy, possibly chemotherapy) fields. There are as yet no well-established criteria enabling the distinction of soft tissue mass from soft tissue edema on MRI, but we use the following criteria with considerable success. Signal abnormality that is masslike in that it displaces normal structures or distorts soft tissue planes, and has a nodular or irregular contour, is likely to represent a discrete soft tissue mass. Obviously, the larger the abnormal region and the more displacement seen, the more likely it is that the abnormality represents a soft tissue mass and not soft tissue edema. However, increased signal intensity on T2 weighted images that is intermediate in signal intensity on T1 weighted images and feathery in appearance, conforms to soft tissue planes, and does not distort surrounding normal structures or musculature is more likely to represent soft tissue edema. An infiltrating neoplastic process, such as juvenile fibromatosis or synovial sarcoma, must also be considered, and these criteria should be used in the appropriate clinical context.

An increase in muscle size and signal intensity on T2 weighted images may represent either replacement of the muscle by pathologic process, or inflammation and edema of the muscle. If the size, contour, and shape of the muscle are normal, and feathery increased signal intensity on T2 weighted images with intermediate signal intensity on T1 weighted images is noted, muscle edema is likely (Fig. 24–31). Either part or all of the muscle may be edematous, and partial or complete edema of adjacent muscles may be seen as well. However, an increase in size and signal intensity of the muscle on T2 weighted images that is associated with a nodular or irregular contour of the muscle is more suggestive of infiltration of muscle by tumor (Fig. 24–32). Distortion of the surrounding soft tissue planes makes this even more likely.

Prospective studies establishing the accuracy, sensitivity, and specificity of MRI in distinguishing muscle tumor from reactive muscle edema have not yet been performed. We do not yet know how sensitive and specific MRI will be in differentiating between microscopic or minimal infiltration of muscle by tumor and reactive muscle edema in a muscle adjacent to tumor. Therefore, interpretation of feathery increased muscle signal as edema must, at this time, be accompanied by the caveat that microscopic tumor involvement of muscle cannot be excluded if a soft tissue mass is seen in the muscles or soft tissues adjacent to the affected muscle. The more removed the muscle is from the primary mass, the more likely the feathery signal changes in the muscle are likely to represent edema, and the less likely to indicate tumor infiltration.

Extent

A recent report has suggested that soft tissue edema is more prevalent and extensive in non-neoplastic musculoskeletal lesions. Comparison of 37 MR examinations with pathologic results showed relatively little soft tissue edema on MR images of malignant bone and soft tissue tumors.[34] Inflammatory lesions, hemorrhage, and other benign processes were, however, accompanied by significantly more extensive edema. This suggests that the presence and extent of edema may relate to the aggressiveness, rate of growth, and chronicity of a musculoskeletal lesion rather than to the aggressiveness of the lesion alone.

Further work is needed in this area, but we believe one possible explanation for the relative lack of edema surrounding many neoplastic tumors, and the presence of extensive soft tissue edema in processes such as hemorrhage, may relate to the chronicity of the lesions. In the early stages of any musculoskeletal lesion, an acute inflammatory reaction is mounted by the body's immune mechanisms. This is characterized by increased blood flow to the region together with acute inflammatory cells. After some time, this acute inflammatory reaction is replaced by a chronic inflammatory reaction with more normal blood flow and a round cell infiltrate. For these reasons, the degree of edema surrounding musculoskeletal lesions seen on MRI may reflect the time the lesion has been present, i.e., acute versus long-standing or chronic, and may be less a reflection of the underlying pathology of the lesion itself than of the body's general response. Until these observations can be studied in a more prospective manner with a larger series of patients, one should be circumspect in attempting to ascribe a differential diagnosis for a musculoskeletal lesion based primarily on the degree of edema appreciated on MRI.

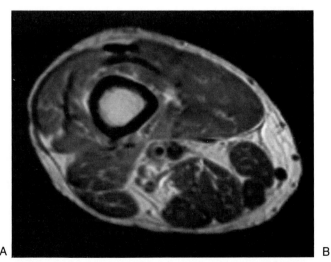
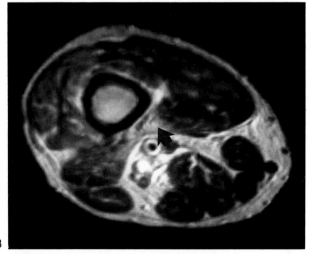

A   B

Figure 24–31. *Muscle edema. Transverse images through the distal femur in a 19-year-old male with malignant melanoma.* ***A,*** Proton-density image (2000/30) shows subtle increased signal intensity in the muscle abutting the posterior femur. ***B,*** T2 weighted image (2000/75) showing increasing signal intensity (*arrow*). The bright signal intensity is feathery, conforms to muscle contour, and does not disrupt fascial planes. This is consistent with muscle edema and not tumor.

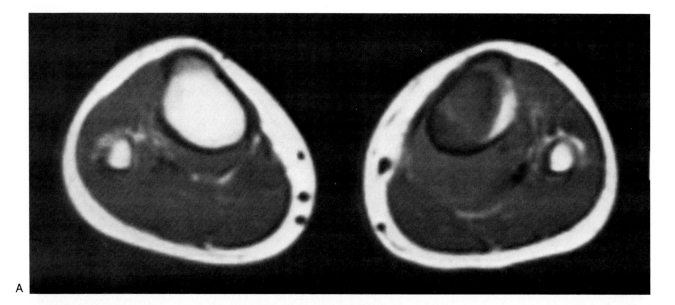

A

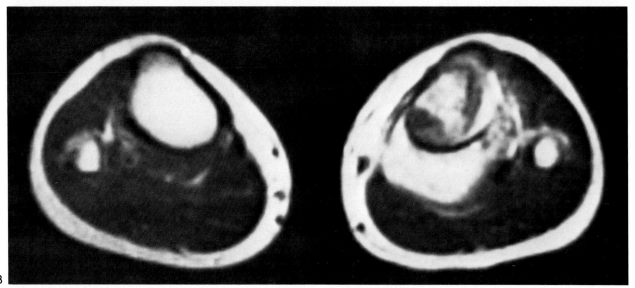

B

Figure 24–32. *Soft tissue tumor.* *A,* T1 weighted (600/20) and *B,* T2 weighted (2000/80) transverse images through the proximal tibia in a patient with osteogenic sarcoma. The soft tissue mass posterior to the tibia is intermediate in signal intensity on T1 weighted images and increases on T2 weighted images. The popliteus muscle is both displaced and replaced by tumor, which is masslike and nodular, consistent with soft tissue mass. Tibial marrow abnormality is also seen.

Neurovascular Involvement

The transverse plane is best for analysis of neurovascular involvement on MRI. Comparison of T1 and T2 weighted images is essential. Displacement of the neurovascular bundle, encasement of the neurovascular bundle by tumor, and signal intensity within large vessels indicating slow or absent flow should be noted. It has been shown that MRI cannot reliably differentiate displacement of vessels by tumor from fixation of vessels by tumor.[10] Therefore, if a neurovascular bundle is displaced or appears encased by tumor, one must assume invasion of the neurovascular bundle by tumor. Surgical inspection of the neurovascular bundle in these cases is strongly recommended. If a mass abuts but does not displace the neurovascular bundle, and there is no evidence of inflammation around the neurovascular bundle (no decreased signal on T1 weighted images and increased signal intensity on T2 weighted images), the likelihood of tumor invasion of the neurovascular bundle is less likely than in cases of abnormal signal surrounding the neurovascular bundle.

When the soft tissue mass is anatomically separate from the neurovascular bundle in question, and the fascial planes surrounding the neurovascular bundle are normal, neurovascular involvement may be confidently excluded. If the soft tissue mass is anatomically separate from the neurovascular bundle but there is associated feathery decreased signal intensity (on T1 weighted images) and increased signal intensity (on T2 weighted images) in the fascial planes surrounding the neurovascular bundle, edema involving the neurovascular bundle is probably present (Fig. 24–9). However, microscopic tumor invasion of the neurovascular bundle cannot be completely excluded in this situation.

Coronal or sagittal images are helpful in assessing blood flow in the large vessels. Given that flow artifacts are common in MRI, correlation of signal abnormalities within vessels on axial images with signal in this same vessel on sagittal or coronal images is recommended. This will decrease the chance of erroneously attributing signal within a vessel to slow flow when in fact it is a flow artifact.

Lymph Node Involvement

The appearance of the surrounding lymph nodes must be noted. Lymph nodes have intermediate signal intensity on T1 and increased signal intensity on T2 weighted images. On STIR images, lymph nodes are of very bright signal intensity (Fig. 24–33). There are presently no criteria for differentiating malignant from hyperplastic or normal nodes on MRI. We use the size criteria established for CT, and nodes greater than 1 to 1.5 cm are considered suspicious. One issue that remains unanswered is whether a different size criteria should be used in pediatric patients, since their body size is smaller. Currently, one can only note the presence and size of nodes and suggest exploration of these nodes during surgery.

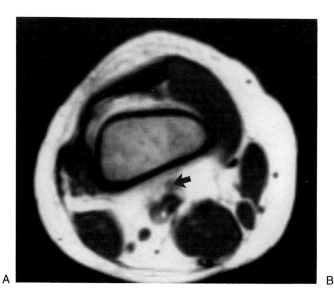

A

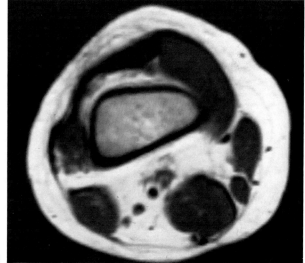

B

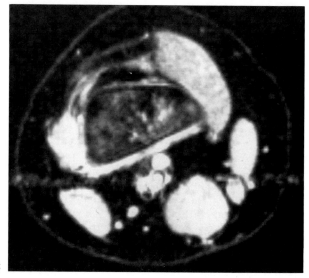

C

Figure 24–33. *Transverse images through the distal femur in a 7-year-old boy with possible osteomyelitis.* **A,** T1 weighted (600/20), **B,** proton-density (2000/30), and **C,** STIR (1.5/30/TI150 [1.5T]) images show a 3-mm popliteal node (*arrow*). An intermediate-signal-intensity node contrasts well with fat on the T1 weighted image, is not well seen on the proton-density image, and appears bright in signal intensity on the STIR image.

MALIGNANT BONE TUMORS

Osteogenic Sarcoma

Osteogenic sarcomas are the most common primary bone tumors in children. They arise primarily from undifferentiated connective tissue of bone that forms neoplastic osteoid and osseous tissue. It is a disease of older children and young adults, 75 percent of cases occurring in patients between the ages of 10 and 25 years. It can occur in any bone of the body, but 86 percent are seen in the long bones (Table 24–1).[39] The most common location is around the knee joint.

The gross histologic appearance depends on the predominant type of tumor tissue present. Osteosarcomas may therefore be classified as osteoblastic, chondroblastic, fibroblastic, or telangiectatic.[29] In addition to the four histologic types of osteogenic sarcoma, these tumors may be either central (diaphyseal, metaphyseal, epiphyseal) or peripheral. (The peripheral lesions, juxtacortical osteogenic sarcoma, are discussed in the next section.) Fifty-two percent of lesions are solely metaphyseal, 30 percent both epiphyseal and metaphyseal, 8 percent both metaphyseal and diaphyseal, 8 percent solely diaphyseal, and 2 percent peripheral.[39]

Pain and swelling of the affected region are the most common early complaints. Systemic signs including weight loss and anemia may be accompanied by rapid growth of the tumor. Osteogenic sarcoma metastasizes relatively early, with metastatic disease seen primarily in the lungs and other long bones. Radiographically, a destructive bone lesion, often with diffuse sclerosis, and a large soft tissue mass with periosteal new bone and tumor bone formation are most commonly seen. In some patients malignant osteoblasts replace bone but produce little or no new bone themselves. In these individuals the tumor consists primarily of primitive osteoid and is categorized as an osteolytic osteogenic

sarcoma (lytic type). This particular class of osteogenic sarcoma is prone to pathologic fracture.

Osteogenic sarcomas most commonly have an origin within the central portion of the metaphysis of a long bone. Local cortical penetration is common, as is elevation of the periosteum, which becomes distended and forms a limiting membrane or barrier to the tumor. The tumor extends deep into the medullary cavity and often terminates in a more or less dome-shaped plug that represents the advancing edge of tumor. This often is not appreciated on plain film. Extension through the physis and into the epiphysis is common. Penetration of the joint capsule to involve the joint space and synovium is unusual but does occur. At pathologic examination the intramedullary spread of tumor is equal in length to, or often greater than, the extraosseous extent of tumor. The extraosseous mass formed in osteogenic sarcoma may eventually encircle the bone.

Osteogenic sarcoma has several appearances on plain film, and a knowledge of these can be helpful in interpreting MR images of this condition. The tumors may be sclerotic or lytic in type.

Sclerotic osteogenic sarcomas may be either purely sclerotic (approximately 10 percent), heavily sclerotic (approximately 45 percent), or moderately sclerotic (approximately 45 percent). The degree of sclerosis seen on plain film reflects the amount of osteoid, tumor bone, and reactive bone. Penetration of the cortex and laminated or spiculated periosteal reaction are prominent features, with rays of periosteal new bone and tumor bone giving a "sunburst" appearance. When the lesions are not homogeneously sclerotic, the sclerosis present may be seen as either single or multiple masses of dense bone or clusters of calcification. In some cases, predominantly sclerotic osteogenic sarcoma contains lytic areas of tumor within coarse strands of dense sclerotic bone. A heterogeneous ground-glass appearance, with an overlay of tiny foci of dense bone or calcific rings, is less common. These scattered foci of bone may not be reflected on MRI, at least not to the degree that large areas of reactive bone would be appreciated.

Lytic osteogenic sarcomas may have nine different patterns on plain film, and the reader is referred to the excellent discussion by Wilner[39] for a complete review. Roentgenographic and histologic changes in the lytic type of osteogenic sarcoma vary from areas of diminished bone density or slight alteration in the trabecular pattern to areas of diminished bone density *and* slight alteration in the trabecular pattern. These changes are usually accompanied by a thin, delicate, laminated periosteal reaction, which is often asymmetric, on one side of the bone, and overlies the medullary lesion. Focal lesions may be surrounded by a zone of hazy sclerosis.

Telangiectatic osteogenic sarcomas often produce a large completely lytic "blowout" pattern of tumor that extends into the soft tissues. This asymmetric, circumscribed type of osteogenic sarcoma is a peripherally

Table 24–1. INCIDENCE OF OSTEOGENIC SARCOMA

Location	Percentage
Skull	<1
Maxilla	3
Mandible	3
Cervical spine	<1
Clavicle	<1
Scapula	1
Humerus	11
Sternum	<1
Rib	1
Thoracic spine	<1
Ilium	7
Other pelvis	1
Hand	<1
Femur	45
Tibia	18
Fibula	3
Foot	<1

Adapted from Wilner D. Radiology of tumor and allied disorders. Philadelphia: WB Saunders, 1982:899.

located, purely lytic lesion primarily limited to the metaphysis, although other portions of the medullary cavity may be invaded. The cortex is destroyed and marginal periosteal reaction is present. A reticular honeycomb pattern of crisscrossing bone is also seen in telangiectatic osteogenic sarcoma.

Osteogenic sarcoma is often a mixture of both lytic and sclerotic processes. The lesions are very heterogeneous in their radiographic appearance, so that large lytic portions may be seen in one segment, permeative patterns in another, and areas of sclerotic bone in another. This leads not only to a variable roentgenographic appearance, but also to a variable appearance on MRI.

MR Appearance of Osteogenic Sarcoma

There have been several studies discussing the appearance of osteogenic sarcoma on MR images.[7, 10, 40, 41] It is not possible at this time to reliably classify an osteogenic sarcoma by tissue type on the basis of the MR appearance, but there are established guidelines that are useful in the evaluation of osteosarcoma. In their 1987 study, Bloem and colleagues[10] studied 53 patients and performed 80 MR examinations of primary lesions of the bone, including 15 osteosarcomas. They reported areas of low signal intensity on both T1 and T2 weighted images in any osteosclerotic tumor, but especially in sclerotic osteosarcomas (Fig. 24–34). This is likely due to the low spin density and short T2 relax-

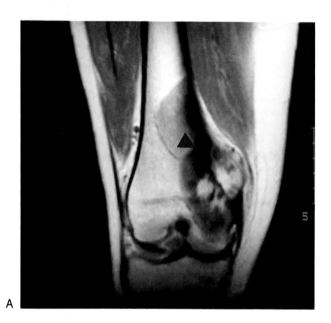

A

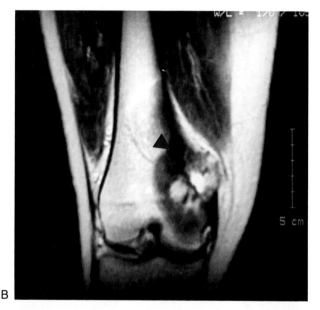

B

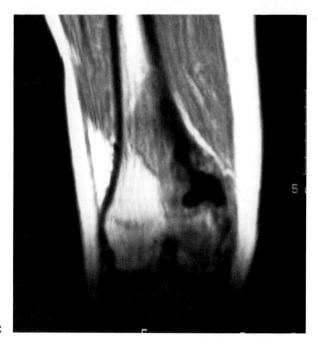

C

Figure 24–34. *Osteogenic sarcoma.* Coronal images through the right femur in a child with osteoblastic sarcoma. Long TR (2000), first- (**A**) and second- (**B**) echo images, which show focal low signal intensity (*arrowhead*) consistent with blastic bone. This is a typical MR appearance of osteogenic sarcoma with well-defined, complex marrow and soft tissue involvement. **C,** TR 2000/20 examination after chemotherapy. The tumor has decreased overall in signal intensity and in the size of the extraosseous component.

ation time of sclerotic bone. Osteolytic tumors were, in general, seen as low to intermediate signal intensity on T1 weighted images and high signal intensity on T2 weighted images (Figs. 24–13, 24–35). This is most likely due to the prolonged T1 and T2 relaxation times of tumor, unencumbered by the presence of sclerotic bone. Depending on the relative predominance of the underlying cell types as well as the presence of necrosis, hemorrhage, and sclerotic bone, osteogenic sarcomas have a homogeneous to markedly heterogeneous appearance on MRI. For instance, an osteolytic osteosarcoma composed almost entirely of primitive osteoid, with little or no new bone formation and no hemorrhage or necrosis, is seen as primarily homogeneous in signal intensity on both T1 and T2 weighted images, whereas a tumor with a large amount of new bone is seen as heterogeneous in signal intensity.

In our experience, the typical osteogenic sarcoma has varying degrees of medullary cavity involvement; it often arises within the central portion of the metaphysis of a long bone (Figs. 24–34, 24–35) and extends into either the diaphysis, the epiphysis, or both the epiphysis and diaphysis. The interface with normal marrow is usually distinct (Figs. 24–13, 24–16, 24–17, 24–34, 24–35), often with a dome-shaped edge that represents the advancing edge of tumor, especially in the diaphysis (Fig. 24–18). A moderate to large soft tissue mass is almost always present (Figs. 24–1, 24–18, 24–27, 24–34 to 24–37) (except with very dense blastic tumors); it is likely to be primarily of intermediate signal intensity on T1 weighted images and increased signal intensity on T2 weighted images, and to have slightly different characteristics compared with the intramedullary portion of tumor.

Osteosarcomas are often associated on MRI with permeation of tumor through the cortical bone in discrete regions (Fig. 24–19, 24–36), with adjacent soft tissue masses of varying size. Intact cortex can be seen interposed between the intramedullary and extramedullary components of the tumor. This is due to cortical penetration by the tumor at a level distant from this region, with soft tissue mass growth occurring outside the confines of the cortex (Fig. 24–35D,E). Metastatic lesions can be appreciated on MRI (Fig. 24–38).

There have been no large prospective studies assessing the accuracy, sensitivity, and specificity of MRI in determining the predominant underlying histologic component of osteosarcoma (osteoblastic, fibroblastic, chondroblastic, or telangiectatic). Osteoblastic osteosarcomas with production of new bone are most likely to be characteristic. However, as mentioned previously, in some cases malignant osteoblasts replace bone but produce little or no new bone themselves, and in these cases of tumors with primarily primitive osteoid, there is not a typical "osteoblastic" appearance. Uncalcified cartilage may have a relatively high signal intensity on T1 weighted images compared with muscle,[10] which could potentially allow preoperative diagnosis of a primarily chondroblastic osteosarcoma. However, only one case has been reported in the literature,[29] and while some areas of the tumor were increased in signal intensity on the T1 weighted image as compared with surrounding musculature, most of the tumor was of intermediate signal intensity, similar to that of muscle. It has been suggested[29] that fibroblastic osteosarcoma is generally characterized by short T1 and T2 relaxation times of fibrous tissue, and would therefore be lower in signal intensity on T2 weighted images than would other types of osteosarcoma. However, there are no images reported in the literature of fibroblastic osteosarcoma and it is likely that, like other cellular tumors (such as liposarcoma) that do not follow the signal characteristics of the underlying benign tissue, fibroblastic osteosarcoma will be more characteristically seen as tumor that is intermediate in signal intensity on T1 and increased in signal intensity on T2 weighted images.

It appears that telangiectatic osteosarcomas have a fairly characteristic appearance on MRI (Fig. 24–39), with high signal intensity on both T1 and T2 weighted images secondary to large blood-filled cavities.[3, 8, 10, 29, 42] (Hemorrhage into a nontelangiectatic osteosarcoma may have a similar appearance.) Fluid-fluid levels and low-signal-intensity septations may be seen. These lesions are potentially difficult to distinguish on MRI from aneurysmal bone cysts. Thus, although sclerotic tumors (particularly sclerotic osteosarcomas), telangiectatic osteosarcomas, and cartilaginous tumors may have some characteristic MR features, our current knowledge suggests that there are in fact no distinguishing differences in appearance and relative signal intensity among most histologic types of osteosarcoma.

As mentioned previously, there is excellent correlation of MRI with gross pathologic specimens in the evaluation of marrow involvement, cortical bone involvement, and soft tissue involvement by tumor, and MRI is the modality of choice in the pretherapeutic staging of osteosarcoma. MRI is more accurate than CT in demonstrating the precise extent of marrow abnormality.[43] Skip lesions and multiple sites of involvement are common in multicentric osteosarcoma, a form of osteosarcoma seen primarily in the younger age group. Skip lesions can best be excluded on either coronal or sagittal MR images, since they usually occur in the bone proximal to the primary tumor.

Well-differentiated osteosarcomas (Fig. 24–40)[44] may be misdiagnosed on plain film alone and confused with benign lesions such as enchondroma or chondroblastoma.[44] MRI may be useful in evaluating these lesions, since cortical erosion, which may or may not be apparent on the plain film, may be readily apparent as irregular thinning of the cortical bone and abnormal intermediate signal intensity within the cortical bone on MRI. More important, any soft tissue mass associated with the lesion will be identified on MRI, allowing appropriate exclusion of more benign processes such as

Text continues on page 860.

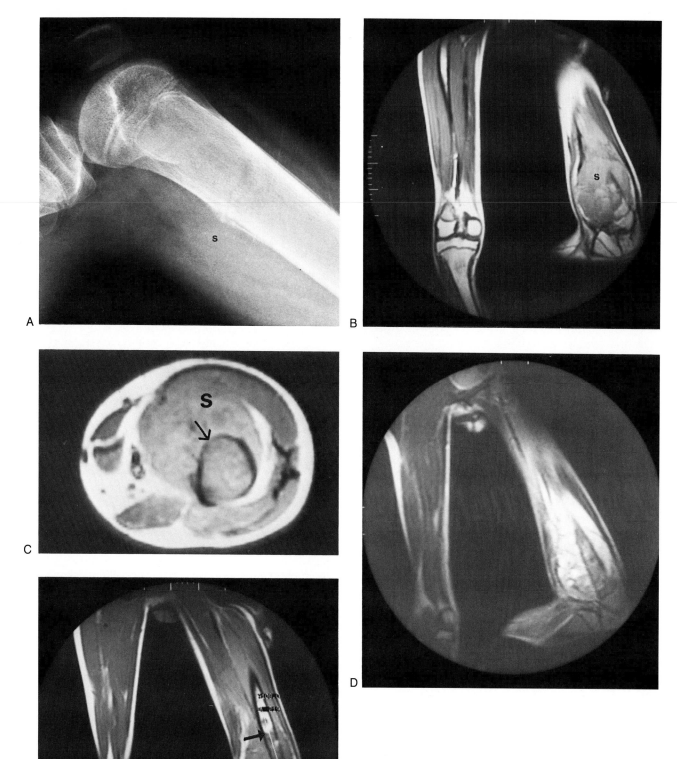

Figure 24–35. *Osteogenic sarcoma of the distal femur.* **A,** Radiograph shows periosteal reaction cloaking the distal femoral metaphysis. A poorly defined soft tissue (S) mass can be seen. **B, C,** Sagittal and transverse T1 weighted MR images (800/26) of the left femur show a well defined soft tissue mass (S) of similar intensity to adjacent muscle. Penetration of the cortex by tumor (*arrow*) can be appreciated as an increase in signal intensity of the normally black cortex. **D,** Sagittal T2 weighted image (2000/80) shows increased signal intensity tumor. **E,** Sagittal T1 weighted image (800/26) shows the extent of the medullary spread of the tumor. There is a sharp demarcation (*arrow*) between low-signal-intensity tumor and high-signal-intensity normal fatty marrow. (Courtesy of Dr. Mervyn D. Cohen, Indianapolis.)

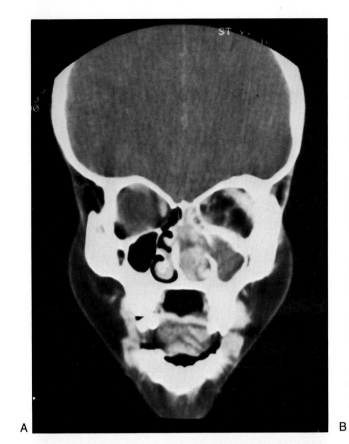

A

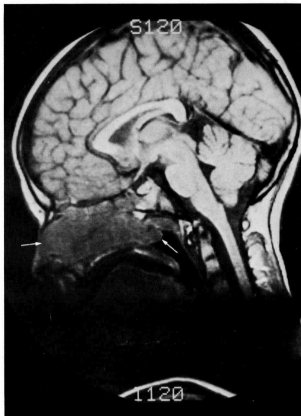

B

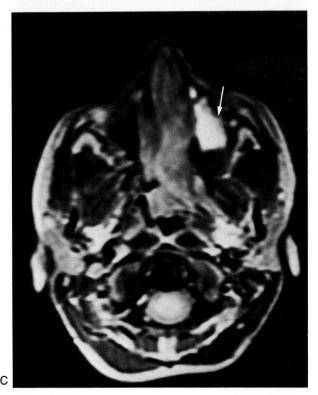

C

Figure 24–36. *Osteogenic sarcoma of the left maxilla.* ***A,*** Coronal CT scan shows a large tumor mass filling the nasal cavity on the left. The nasal septum is displaced to the right. There is destruction of the medial wall of the left maxillary sinus, together with opacification of the sinus cavity. ***B,*** Sagittal midline MR image (600/20) shows the large homogeneous soft tissue tumor mass (*arrow*) filling the nasal cavity. ***C,*** Axial MR image (2000/30). The soft tissue tumor in the nasal cavity is identified. The destruction of the medial wall of the left maxillary antrum is not as well seen as on CT scan. There is bright intensity from the maxillary sinus (*arrow*), which is believed to represent hemorrhagic fluid, not tumor. (Courtesy of Dr. Mervyn D. Cohen, Indianapolis.)

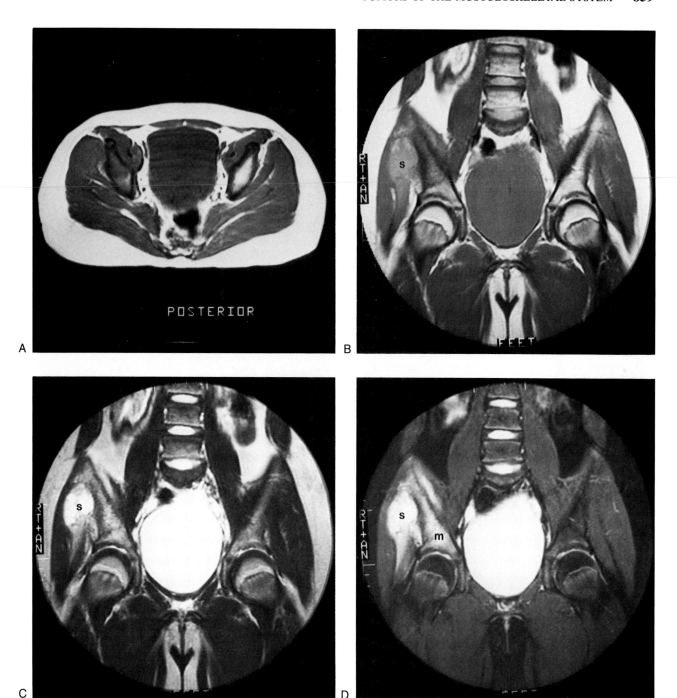

Figure 24–37. *Osteogenic sarcoma of the entire right iliac bone with large adjacent soft tissue mass. Effect of alteration of imaging technique.* ***A,*** T1 weighted axial image (1100/20). The soft tissue tumor is of similar intensity to muscle. ***B,*** Spin-density image (2033/20) shows the soft tissue mass (S) adjacent to the right iliac crest. There is a decrease in signal intensity of the right iliac bone marrow compared with the left. Extension of the tumor into the acetabular marrow cannot be clearly appreciated. ***C,*** T2 weighted image shows marked increase in signal intensity of the soft tissue mass (S). Note increase in right iliac marrow signal intensity, which appears slightly brighter than the marrow signal on the (normal) left side. ***D,*** STIR pulse sequence (2133/30/TI 150) shows both the soft tissue and marrow tumor better than the other pulse sequences. Both the soft tissue tumor (S) and bone marrow tumor (m) are bright signal intensity. Note the normal, suppressed yellow marrow in the left iliac bone and femoral epiphyses. Extension of marrow tumor into the acetabulum is best appreciated on the STIR sequence. (Courtesy of Dr. Mervyn D. Cohen, Indianapolis.)

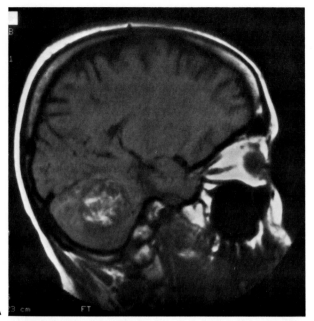

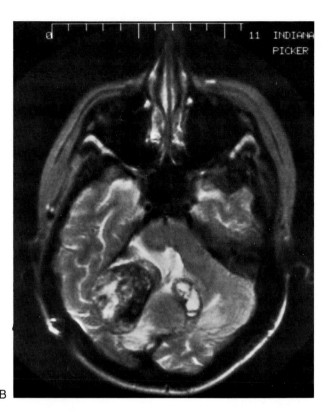

Figure 24–38. *Brain metastasis from osteogenic sarcoma.* ***A, B,*** Sagittal T1 (700/20) and axial T2 (2000/90) images show a large, well-defined mass lesion in the right lobe of the cerebellum. High-intensity regions seen on the T1 weighted image are believed to represent hemorrhage. (Courtesy of Dr. Mervyn D. Cohen, Indianapolis.)

enchondroma or fibrodysplasia, and increasing the level of suspicion for well-differentiated osteosarcoma (Fig. 24–40).

Juxtacortical Osteosarcoma

Juxtacortical osteosarcomas are classified as either parosteal or periosteal osteogenic sarcomas.

Parosteal Osteosarcoma

Parosteal sarcomas arise on the outer surface of the cortical bone from bone-forming connective tissue originating in the periosteum or immediate parosteal connective tissue. Components of all three mesenchymal tissue types (fibrous, cartilage, and bone) can be seen within the tumor. Histologically these tumors range from the completely benign but rare parosteal osteoma, to lesions with minimal evidence of malignancy, to frankly malignant well-differentiated parosteal tumors. They are found almost exclusively in the long tubular bones, with 92 percent in the femur, tibia, and humerus. These tumors grow slowly and tend to occur in the third and fourth decades of life, although parosteal sarcoma has been reported in children as young as 11 years of age.[45]

Even though growth of the tumor is initially slow, the lesion eventually progresses to cortical destruction and medullary invasion. Recurrence and lung metastases are common. Swelling and the presence of a soft tissue

mass are the most common roentgenographic signs. En bloc surgical removal of the tumor is the preferred treatment.

Periosteal Osteosarcoma

Periosteal osteosarcoma is a juxtacortical osteosarcoma with an intraperiosteal site of origin. The tumor is limited to the periphery of the cortex and rarely invades the medullary cavity. Ninety percent occur in the diaphysis of the femur and tibia, while parosteal sarcomas occur more frequently in the metaphyseal region of the long bones, particularly along the posterior aspect of the distal femur. Histologically, periosteal osteosarcoma contains abnormal-appearing cartilage and osteoid intermixed with outer cortex and extending into the soft tissues. This is in contrast to parosteal osteosarcoma, which is predominantly osteogenic, with large amounts of fibroblastic tissue and only small amounts of cartilaginous tissue. The extraosseous mass in periosteal osteosarcoma is usually small, normally no larger than 3 to 4 cm.

Radiologically, there may be complete absence of calcification, a few scattered calcifications, a finely granular appearance, sparse clusters of poorly defined calcification, masses of stippled calcification, striated calcification, or a mixture of the above patterns. Periosteal new bone formation is common and may be striated, spiculated, or lamellated. The outer surface of the cortex shows bony erosion, which may be either smooth or irregular. Cortical thickening often occurs

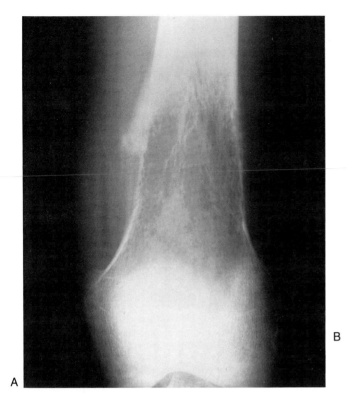

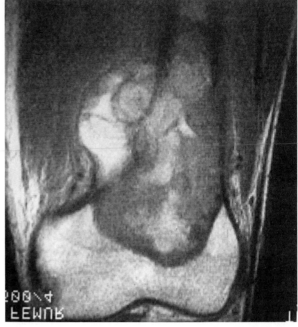

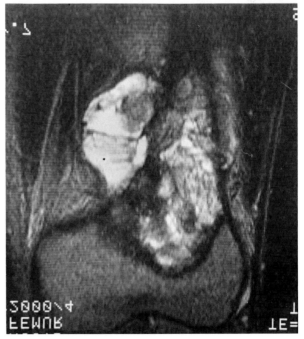

Figure 24–39. *Telangiectatic osteogenic sarcoma of the distal left femur.* ***A,*** Radiograph, and ***B,*** T1 weighted (800/20), and ***C,*** T2 weighted (2000/20) coronal images show complex signal intensity, including hemorrhage. (Courtesy of Dr. Harry K. Genant, San Francisco.)

along the periosteal surface and extends the length of the tumor. The medullary cavity is not involved, which helps to differentiate this condition from parosteal or conventional osteogenic sarcoma.[45, 46]

MR Appearance of Juxtacortical Osteogenic Sarcoma

In juxtacortical tumors the primary role of MR evaluation lies in the assessment of marrow involvement, soft tissue involvement, and the extent of cortical and

periosteal involvement (Fig. 24–41). Accurate staging of the lesion becomes particularly important in assessing a child for a limb salvage procedure. In the assessment of marrow involvement, the marrow adjacent to the juxtacortical tumor is evaluated for low signal intensity on T1 weighted images that increases on T2 weighted images. If this abnormal signal is masslike and well defined within the marrow cavity, tumor invasion is likely. Marrow edema as a result of juxtacortical tumor is potentially seen as intermediate signal inten-

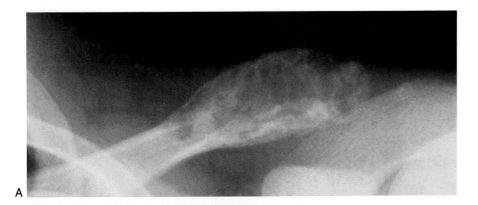

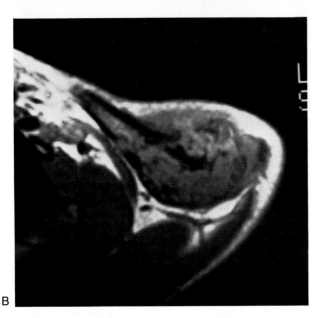

Figure 24–40. *Differentiated osteogenic sarcoma.* **A,** Radiograph reveals a well-defined expansile lesion of the distal left clavicle, with some benign-appearing characteristics. **B,** T1 weighted axial image (800/20) through the clavicle reveals cortical breakthrough and surrounding soft tissue mass suggesting the diagnosis of well-differentiated osteogenic sarcoma, as opposed to the more benign lesions of chondroblastoma or enchondroma.

sity on T1 and increased signal intensity on T2 weighted images, but may be feathery and somewhat less well defined. Even though the marrow appears edematous, marrow involvement is not precluded, and the surgeon must perform a biopsy during surgery to determine whether there is marrow involvement. If there are no marrow changes on MRI, the juxtacortical sarcoma has not invaded the marrow cavity, and a limb salvage procedure can be planned.

Ewing's Sarcoma

Ewing's sarcoma occurs most commonly during the last part of the first decade and the first half of the second decade of life. It is the second most common malignant bone tumor in childhood after osteogenic sarcoma. Histologically, Ewing's sarcoma is characterized by a distinctive small round cell infiltration with a predilection for the shaft rather than the ends of the long bones. The origin of the cell is uncertain, but most authors believe the tumor arises from the marrow reti-

culum stem cells. The tumor is seen frequently in the long bones (50 percent) and the flat bones (40 percent). The femur is most commonly affected, followed by the pelvis, ribs, tibia, humerus, and scapula (Table 24–2). Younger patients present with tumors of the long bones, while involvement of the flat bones is more common in patients over the age of 20; this may relate to the distribution of hematopoietic marrow with age. There is a 2:1 male preponderance.[47]

The growth of Ewing's sarcoma varies considerably and is characterized by an inclination to grow in spurts followed by periods of relative quiescence. Clinical symptoms include pain and usually a soft tissue mass, fever, anemia, and leukocytosis. The combination of mass, fever, and leukocytosis may result in the incorrect diagnosis of osteomyelitis, with treatment by incision and drainage. It is only when frank pus is not obtained in these patients that the lesion is biopsied and the diagnosis of Ewing's sarcoma is made.

Radiographically, Ewing's sarcoma is characterized by osteolysis, cortical erosion, periosteal reaction, and a soft tissue mass. Ewing's sarcoma is classically con-

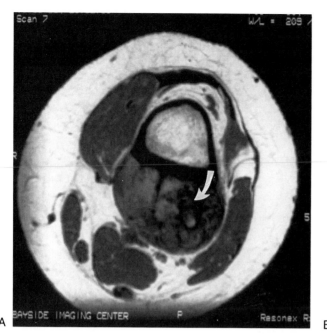
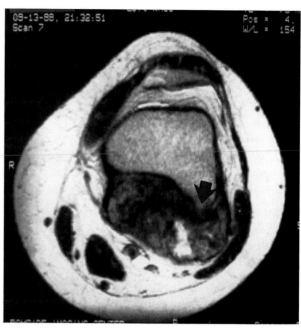

Figure 24–41. *Parosteal osteogenic sarcoma.* Intermediate TR transverse images (1650/75) through the (**A**) middle and (**B**) distal right femur in a 24-year-old patient with a posterior femoral parosteal osteosarcoma. Tumor is seen as a well-defined mass growing from the posterior aspect of the femur. **A,** Proximally, there is thick cortical bone separating the tumor from the marrow cavity. Punctate regions of low signal intensity represent extensive calcification and new bone formation (*curved arrow*). **B,** Inferiorly, erosion through the cortical bone can be seen in the medial posterior aspect of the femur (*arrow*). On T2 weighted images the tumor showed increased heterogeneous signal intensity.

sidered a medullary lesion, but changes in the cortex on plain film may be the dominant finding. The roentgenographic appearance of Ewing's sarcoma in the long bone may depend on the location of the tumor within the bone. The central diaphyseal type of lesion is considered the classic roentgenographic form of Ewing's sarcoma and accounts for up to 50 percent of cases seen. There is a centrally located and symmetrically positioned permeative lesion in the midshaft of the bone, usually involving approximately one-third of the length. Periosteal reaction is often of the laminated type, although half of the cases may also show perpendicular spiculations. A soft tissue mass is often seen. The primary direction of growth is along the medullary shaft.[47] Sclerosis is extremely rare.

The most characteristic feature of the cortical diaphyseal type of Ewing's tumor is the cortical erosion that involves the outer surface of the cortex while the inner surface of the cortex remains intact. These are found at or near the midshaft and, in contrast to the classic or central diaphyseal type, these tumors are asymmetric and involve primarily the cortical bone and not the medullary cavity on plain film. Cortical erosion is saucerized, and at either end of the tumor laminated periosteal action prevails. Widely spaced spicules of periosteal reaction may be seen in the central portion

Table 24–2. INCIDENCE OF EWING'S SARCOMA

Location	Percentage
Skull	2
Maxilla	<1
Mandible	2
Cervical spine	1
Clavicle	3
Scapula	5
Humerus	9
Sternum	<1
Rib	11
Thoracic spine	<1
Lumbar spine	1
Ilium	14
Radius	2
Ulna	1
Sacrum	2
Pubis	3
Ischium	2
Hand	<1
Femur	23
Tibia	9
Fibula	6
Talus	<1
Calcaneus	1
Metatarsal	1
Widespread in bones	6

Adapted from Wilner D. Radiology of tumors and allied disorders. Philadelphia: WB Saunders, 1982:2463.

of the tumor. The extraosseous soft tissue component often contains no evidence of calcification.[47]

The central metaphyseal type of Ewing's tumor is usually pear shaped and symmetric within the metaphysis of the long bone. Growth generally occurs toward the diaphysis. These lesions differ from the classic type of Ewing's sarcoma both in their location and in the diversity of the internal pattern. Sclerotic changes are not infrequent, and the lesions may be primarily sclerotic or may exhibit a mixed pattern of lytic and blastic changes. Periosteal reaction is common and usually is either laminated or spiculated and perpendicular to the bone. An accompanying soft tissue mass is invariably present. The peripheral metaphyseal type is eccentric within the metaphysis and may be mistaken radiographically for osteogenic sarcoma. The appearance of the lesion is variable, either a prominent soft tissue mass with minor cortical erosion; a lytic, eccentrically located metaphyseal process; or an eccentrically located metaphyseal lesion with equal amounts of bone destruction and production.

Primary epiphyseal involvement by Ewing's sarcoma has not been documented, but it is not uncommon for metaphyseal tumor to extend into the epiphysis. The entire epiphysis and metaphysis may be involved. Most tumors are lytic and not especially bone producing, but a great amount of bone production may occasionally be noted.[47]

Cortical involvement in Ewing's sarcoma is common (Fig. 24–42) although not always evident on plain films. Tumor cells may permeate the haversian canals and invade the soft tissues, leaving the cortex either intact, partially destroyed, or completely destroyed (cortical breakthrough). Bone sclerosis is seen in 2 percent of cases of Ewing's sarcoma.[47] Involvement of the soft tissues is almost invariably present, but these soft tissue extensions generally do not show calcification on the plain film. The periosteal reaction seen with Ewing's sarcoma is variable, with two types primarily noted. The parallel or laminated form is seen in almost all cases and varies from the single lamella to multiple lamellated layers or "onion skinning." This reflects the periodic growth of Ewing's sarcoma. Perpendicular spiculation may be seen on plain film in up to half of cases of Ewing's sarcoma. This "hair-on-end" periosteal reaction usually is noted in the center of the tumor, with the lamellated periosteal reaction occurring at the edges of the tumor.

In the flat bones, both diffusely infiltrative and sclerotic (Fig. 24–43) tumors may be seen on plain film. Lamellated periosteal new bone formation is often noted surrounding the tumor. The ilium is the most frequent site of Ewing's sarcoma in the flat bones, and these tumors are invariably associated with a soft tissue mass in the lower abdomen, gluteal region, or groin, or within the pelvis.

Ewing's sarcoma can occur in the ribs and, as mentioned in the section on imaging technique, detailed imaging evaluation of these lesions can be problematic.

On plain film, most rib Ewing's sarcomas are lytic and may cause either expansion or mottling of the bone. Predominantly sclerotic lesions with cortical thickening and obliteration of the medullary cavity have also been reported. Periosteal reaction in rib lesions is relatively insignificant, although irregular lamellation may be seen.

Accurate pretherapy evaluation of Ewing's sarcoma is important, since radiation therapy is the primary method of treatment and it is desirable to limit the port to the smallest effective area possible. In cases in which surgery is recommended, accurate preoperative evaluation is essential to determine the feasibility of resection and the potential for limb salvage.

MR Appearance of Ewing's Sarcoma

Little has been written about the specific signal characteristics of Ewing's sarcoma, although these were mentioned in many papers comparing MRI and CT of primary bone tumors.[8, 10, 12, 14, 29, 40] In general, Ewing's sarcoma appears as intermediate signal intensity on T1 and increased signal intensity on T2 weighted images (Figs. 24–42 to 24–44).[48] The homogeneity or heterogeneity of the lesion depends on the underlying histology: lesions with a large amount of blastic or reactive bone appear heterogeneous (Fig. 24–30), while those composed primarily of homogeneous round cells and no reactive bone appear more homogeneous (Figs. 24–41, 24–42, 24–45). Depending on the stage of presentation and the location of the lesion, the marrow abnormality is either focal or diffuse. The central diaphyseal type of lesion, which accounts for up to 50 percent of Ewing's sarcomas seen, tends to be centrally located and more diffuse in appearance (Figs. 24–42, 24–45). In the past, this has been described as the "classic" MR appearance of Ewing's sarcoma. The metaphyseal type of Ewing's tumor, however, may be either central or peripheral. In our experience, these lesions tend to be well defined, often contain blastic bone, have an adjacent soft tissue mass, and are therefore indistinguishable by MR criteria from osteogenic sarcoma (Fig. 24–30). This appearance of Ewing's sarcoma as a discrete interosseous mass with sharp margins and contiguous areas of cortical bone loss has been recently described.[48]

An extraosseous soft tissue mass is not uncommon with Ewing's sarcoma (Figs. 24–43, 24–44), although in the long bones (Figs. 24–41, 24–45) this does not tend to be as large as those seen with osteogenic sarcoma, in our experience. The soft tissue masses are usually intermediate in signal intensity on T1 and increased in signal intensity on T2 weighted images. They are often more homogeneous in signal intensity than the intramedullary component of Ewing's tumor. This may be due to the lack of calcification and new bone formation seen in the extraosseous component of Ewing's sarcoma. However, the tumor bone formation seen with osteogenic sarcoma, which on plain film appears as calcification and ossification within the ad-

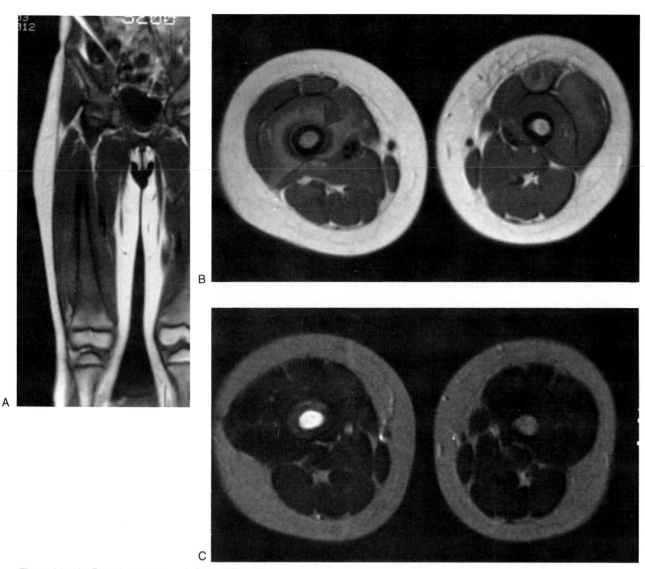

Figure 24–42. *Ewing's sarcoma.*   ***A,*** Coronal T1 weighted image (800/20) through the right femur in a 3-year-old girl with Ewing's sarcoma. Pathologically, the tumor was homogeneous with no evidence of reactive bone. ***B,*** Transverse longer TR image (2000/20) shows homogeneous increased signal intensity marrow tumor. "Onion skin" periosteal reaction is identified. ***C,*** Second-echo transverse image (2000/80) shows bright-signal-intensity tumor within the medullary space.

jacent soft tissue mass, is seen as intermediate signal intensity on T1 and bright signal intensity on T2 weighted images; it therefore gives little heterogeneity to the soft tissue mass associated with osteogenic sarcoma. The homogeneity or heterogeneity of the mass, therefore, may not be helpful in distinguishing Ewing's from osteogenic sarcoma.

Although "onion skin" periosteal reaction may be recognized on MR images of Ewing's sarcoma (Figs. 24–26, 24–42), the cortical erosion and periosteal signals seen most commonly on these images are not particularly characteristic of the tumor. Often the spiculated or "hair-on-end" periosteal reaction seen in these tumors is appreciated only as intermediate signal

intensity on T1 weighted images adjacent to cortical bone.

In our initial experience with MRI of Ewing's sarcoma, we saw primarily extensive marrow tumor. We are seeing increasing numbers of "focal" or smaller Ewing's tumors on MRI, which may be a result of the more routine use of MRI to evaluate bony lesions in children. In the past, only children with fairly extensive disease were referred for MR evaluation. As MRI becomes more readily available, children who show subtle changes on plain film, or who have clinical symptoms of unexplained bony pain on the radiograph, are referred for examination, and the diagnosis of Ewing's sarcoma is being made at an earlier stage.

Text continues on page 868.

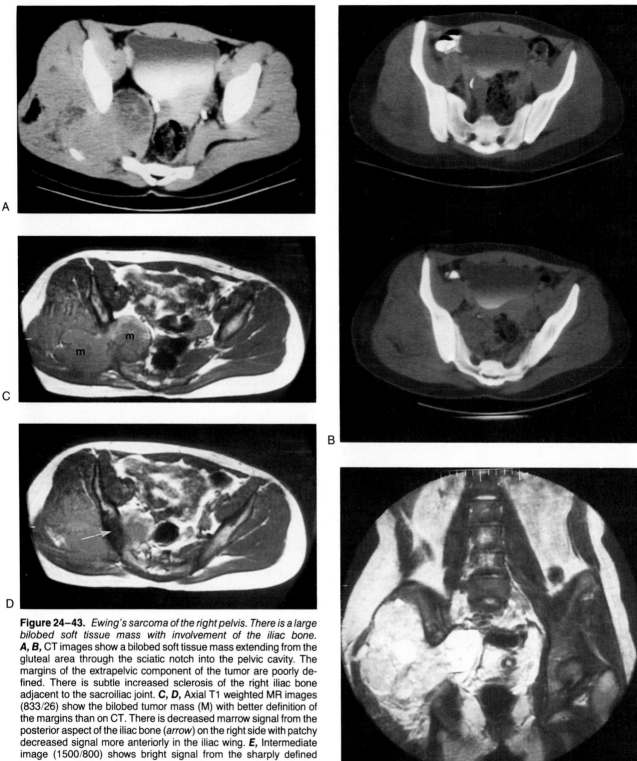

Figure 24–43. *Ewing's sarcoma of the right pelvis. There is a large bilobed soft tissue mass with involvement of the iliac bone.* **A, B,** CT images show a bilobed soft tissue mass extending from the gluteal area through the sciatic notch into the pelvic cavity. The margins of the extrapelvic component of the tumor are poorly defined. There is subtle increased sclerosis of the right iliac bone adjacent to the sacroiliac joint. **C, D,** Axial T1 weighted MR images (833/26) show the bilobed tumor mass (M) with better definition of the margins than on CT. There is decreased marrow signal from the posterior aspect of the iliac bone (*arrow*) on the right side with patchy decreased signal more anteriorly in the iliac wing. **E,** Intermediate image (1500/800) shows bright signal from the sharply defined tumor mass. Both the intra- and extrapelvic components of the lesion are well defined. (Courtesy of Dr. Mervyn D. Cohen, Indianapolis.)

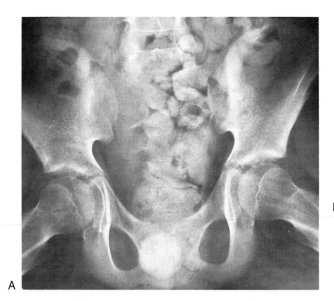

A

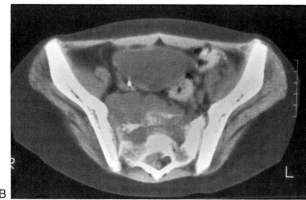

B

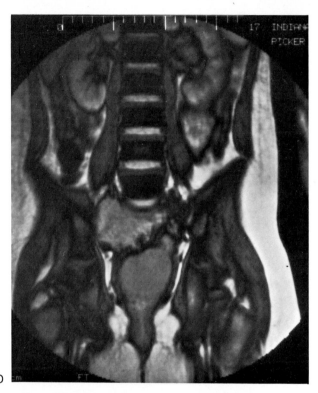

D

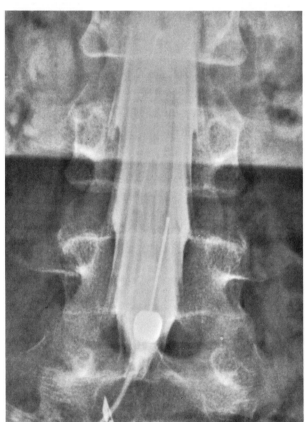

C

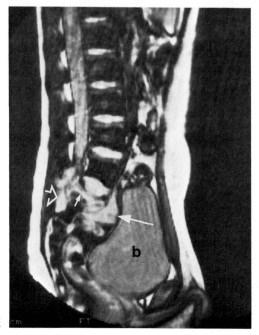

E

Figure 24–44. *Ewing's sarcoma of the sacrum.* ***A,*** Pelvic radiograph shows hazy loss of definition of the right side of the upper two-thirds of the sacrum. ***B,*** Transverse CT scan shows destruction of the sacrum with an adjacent anterior soft tissue mass. There is also a soft tissue abnormality lying within the spinal canal. ***C,*** Myelogram shows obstruction to the flow of contrast at the L5–S1 level. ***D,*** Coronal MR image (1500/30) shows a well defined anterior soft tissue component of the tumor lying in front of the body of the sacrum. ***E,*** Midline sagittal MR image (1500/30) shows the total extent of the tumor well. The bony sacral destruction is not as well seen as on the CT scan. The anterior soft tissue component of the tumor (*long arrow*) is identified. It lies behind the bladder (b) but does not invade the bladder wall. The isthmus of soft tissue tumor permeating through the sacrum is also well-defined (*short arrow*). More posteriorly (*open arrow*) the total extent of the tumor within the spinal canal is accurately defined. The large flaccid bladder is due to neurogenic involvement with tumor invading nerve. (Courtesy of Dr. Mervyn D. Cohen, Indianapolis.)

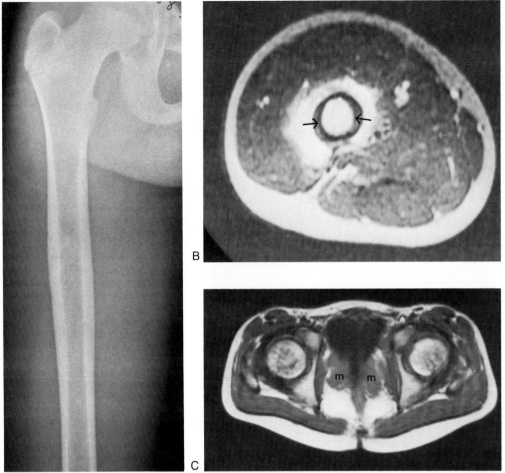

Figure 24–45. *Ewing's sarcoma of the femur.* **A,** Radiograph shows poorly defined thickening of the cortex of the midshaft of the right femur. No definite periosteal reaction is identified. **B,** Transverse T2 weighted image (2000/80) through the area of abnormality in the femur shows a moderately well-defined increased signal intensity soft tissue mass encasing the femur. The medullary space is expanded, and moderate signal intensity (*arrows*) is seen in the cortex. This indicates the presence of tumor tissue within the bone cortex. **C,** Transverse T1 weighted image (700/20) through the pelvis. Multiple lymph node metastases (m) are identified. (Courtesy of Dr. Mervyn D. Cohen, Indianapolis.)

Extraosseous Ewing's sarcoma may be evaluated by MRI (Fig. 24–46). In general, these tumors are seen as a soft tissue mass with intermediate signal intensity on T1 and increased signal intensity on T2 weighted images. The tumors are often homogeneous. Their appearance is very nonspecific. MRI can be used to define the soft tissue extent of tumor, the specific muscle groups involved, involvement of the neurovascular bundle, and involvement of adjacent bony structures. We find CT helpful in cases of extraosseous Ewing's sarcoma that are adjacent to small or flat bones (i.e., ribs or forearm). In these cases, anatomic detail of bony surface may not be sufficient on MRI, and limited CT examination with bone algorithm performed in conjunction with MRI may serve to define bony involvement by these tumors.

Chondrosarcoma

Chondrosarcoma is a malignant tumor of chondrogenic origin that remains essentially cartilaginous throughout its evolution. Although chondrosarcomas may arise in any bone preformed in cartilage, approximately 50 percent are found in the pelvis and upper femur. They can be either primary, arising de novo within a given bone, or secondary, arising from a preexisting cartilaginous lesion. Chondrosarcoma is rare before the age of 20. However, in the pediatric population, secondary chondrosarcomas arising from osteocartilaginous exostoses, enchondroma, chondroblastoma, chondromyxoid fibroma, and unicameral bone cysts are seen. Sarcomatous degeneration of a chondroid lesion is more likely to occur in multifocal than in

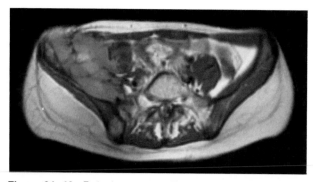
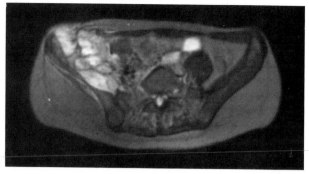

A   B

Figure 24–46. *Ewing's sarcoma. Transverse images through the pelvis in a 15-year-old girl with recurrent extraosseous Ewing's sarcoma.* **A,** Higher intermediate, nodular soft tissue mass is seen cradled by the right iliac crest (2000/20). **B,** On the T2 weighted image (2000/80) the tumor is seen as bright signal intensity.

unifocal disease.[49] Soft tissue chondrosarcoma is rare and generally encountered in the soft parts of an extremity.

Tumors that arise in the interior of a bone are termed central chondrosarcoma, while those that arise on a surface of a bone are designated peripheral chondrosarcoma. Central chondrosarcomas may be either primary or secondary; peripheral chondrosarcomas are likely to be secondary. This classification is preferred by some authors, since it is often difficult to determine whether a central chondrosarcoma is primary or secondary. The MR appearance of cartilage tumors reflects the underlying histology of the neoplasm, and it is thus important to know the various histologic patterns that can occur. Hyaline cartilage is composed of a cellular portion (chondrocyte) and an acellular matrix portion (collagen and mucopolysaccharide). The matrix portion traps water in its interstices and produces high hydrostatic pressure and resultant low compressibility.[50] This low compressibility may result in a lobulated appearance of the tumor, while the increased water content may result in high signal intensity on T2 weighted images. Cartilaginous lesions that are characterized by a primitive cartilage matrix called chondroid, which histologically is distinguishable from hyaline cartilage, include chondroblastoma, clear cell chondrosarcoma, osteosarcoma (chondroid type), and mesenchymal chondrosarcoma. These lesions are often very cellular and contrast histologically with the relatively pure hyaline cartilage of an enchondroma or a well-differentiated chondrosarcoma.

Local pain and evidence of swelling are the most common presenting symptoms. Pain and renewed growth in an area of a known enchondroma or exostosis is often an indication of malignant degeneration and should be evaluated, although the incidence of malignant change of a solitary osteochondroma has been estimated to be less than 1 percent.[51]

Radiographically, these cartilaginous tumors produce a radiolucent lesion with a calcified chondroid matrix seen most commonly as dense rings, floccules, or pinpoint areas of calcium. The cortex often bulges externally and there may be endosteal thinning at the site of the tumor.

MR Appearance of Chondrosarcoma

In general, neoplasms composed of uncalcified cartilage may be either isointense or slightly hyperintense compared with muscle on T1 weighted images, and hyperintense on T2 weighted images. The most typical appearance of a well-differentiated chondrosarcoma on spin-echo images may be seen on T2 weighted images, where homogeneous, diffuse, high-signal-intensity lobules of varying sizes are often separated by thin, low-signal-intensity septa (Fig. 24–47). On T1 weighted images, these lobules are of intermediate signal intensity. Histologically, the lobules are composed of hyaline cartilage, and the septa are composed of fibrous tissue. Many other lesions such as enchondromas and osteochondromas, which are also characterized by a large percentage of hyaline cartilage, have a similar lobulated high-signal-intensity appearance on T2 weighted images.[50] Higher-grade chondrosarcomas, which have an increased cellular component, do not show a homogeneous increased signal intensity on T2 weighted images, but rather reflect the underlying cellular heterogeneity and are seen as a heterogeneous isointense and hyperintense mass (as compared with skeletal muscle) on T2 weighted MR images.

Chondrosarcomas with a chondroid matrix are often very cellular. These lesions may appear isointense to muscle on both T1 and T2 weighted and iso- or hypointense on T2 weighted images, and do not have the lobular appearance seen with hyaline origin tumors.

Malignant degeneration of osteochondroma and enchondroma to chondrosarcoma may be seen on MRI. Features of malignant degeneration include disruption of the medullary space, disruption of the cortex, and extension of tumor into adjacent soft tissues (Fig. 24–47). An enchondroma cartilage cap greater than 1

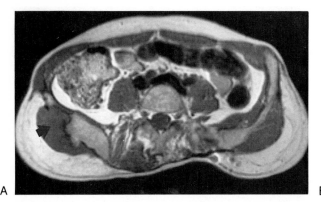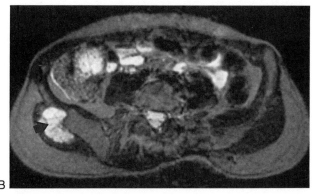

A   B

Figure 24–47. *Chondrosarcoma.* Transverse images through the pelvis in a 21-year-old patient with malignant degeneration of an osteochondroma. The chondrosarcoma (*arrow*) is seen as a large mass invading both soft tissues and bone on (**A**) T1 weighted (800/20) and (**B**) T2 weighted (2000/80) images.

cm in size increases the probability of malignancy.[52] However, the accuracy, sensitivity, and specificity of MRI in the detection of malignant degeneration of these lesions have not yet been prospectively studied.

Neuroectodermal Tumors

Primary neuroectodermal tumors of the peripheral skeleton are rare and histologically resemble neuroectodermal tumors of the peripheral soft tissues and Ewing's sarcoma. They belong to the group of small round cell tumors, which also includes rhabdomyosarcoma, lymphoma, Ewing's sarcoma, and neuroblastoma. These were initially described by Askin and colleagues[53] as tumors of neuroectodermal origin arising from thoracopulmonary soft tissues in children and adolescents. In 1984 these primary neuroectodermal tumors of bone were described and defined by Jaffe and associates.[54] The presence of neurosecretory granules on electron microscopy may be used to distinguish Ewing's sarcoma from neuroectodermal tumor of bone. The age of the patient, male predominance, and length of time between diagnosis and death are similar to those in Ewing's sarcoma.[55] However, metastatic disease is three times more frequent at the time of initial presentation in neuroectodermal tumors than in Ewing's sarcoma.

Radiographically, the lesions are identical to those of Ewing's sarcoma, with poor demarcation of tumor, cortical destruction, periosteal reaction, and soft tissue invasion. There have been no reported series of the MR appearance of neuroectodermal tumor of bone, but we have seen an MR appearance of the chest wall similar to that of Ewing's sarcoma (Figs. 24–48, 24–49). Bony involvement by tumor, especially ribs, may be noted and cortical destruction is common. The lesion is typically located in the chest wall and is characterized by intermediate signal intensity on T1 and increased signal intensity on T2 weighted images. We have seen some heterogeneity of appearance on T2

weighted images, consisting of scattered intermediate-signal-intensity foci on T2 weighted images (Fig. 24–48), which may correspond to fragments of rib within the soft tissue mass. MRI is most useful in these lesions for pretherapeutic staging and follow-up.

Primary Bone Lymphoma

Non-Hodgkin's lymphoma of bone is uncommon in children but can occur during the second decade.[56] The term "non-Hodgkin's lymphoma of bone" is preferred to "reticulum cell sarcoma." These lesions are derived from primitive marrow mesenchyme and present as a single focus in bone without hematopoietic involvement. The clinical course is protracted, and although lesions may be multifocal in older patients, these tumors tend to be solitary in children under 12 years of age.

Radiographically, primary non-Hodgkin's lymphoma of bone appears as a combination of bone destruction and reactive bone formation, with both a permeative and moth-eaten appearance.[44] Soft tissue involvement is common, and periosteal bone formation may be present.

Primary lesions of bone in children and adolescents with Hodgkin's lymphoma are rare but have been reported. Radiographically, these primary lesions appear similar to non-Hodgkin's lymphoma. Hematogenous or lymphatic spread of Hodgkin's lymphoma to bone marrow is more common, and may result in cortical lesions that occur most frequently in the spine, pelvis, ribs, femora, and sternum. The appearance is nonspecific and can be both osteolytic and osteosclerotic. Biopsy is often required for diagnosis.

The MR appearance of these lesions is similar to that noted in other round cell tumors of bone. They are typically of low to intermediate signal intensity on T1 weighted images (Fig. 24–50) and high signal intensity on T2 weighted images. Most commonly the lesions are homogeneous, although inhomogeneity may occur,

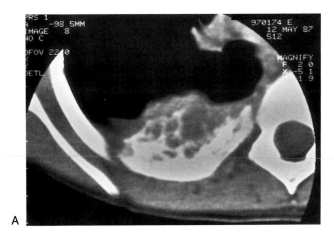

A

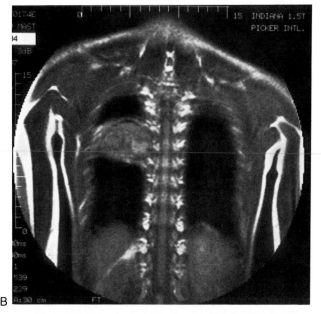

B

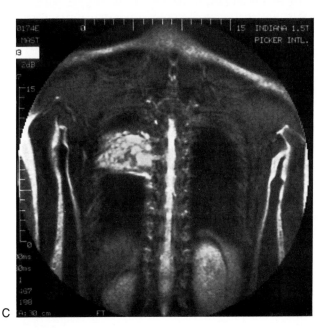

C

Figure 24–48. *Primitive neuroectodermal tumor (Askin's tumor).* ***A,*** CT scan shows marked expansion of the right posterior rib with a large associated soft tissue abnormality. Mottled calcification is seen throughout the soft tissue. The degree of calcification is more than one would expect with Ewing's sarcoma. ***B, C,*** T1 (800/40) and T2 (2000/80) coronal MR images show the abnormality well. The lesion is of moderate intensity, just greater than that of muscle, on the T1 weighted image. On the T2 image there is marked increase in signal intensity with marked heterogeneity seen throughout the tumor mass. (Courtesy of Dr. Mervyn D. Cohen, Indianapolis.)

depending on the degree of osteosclerosis present within the lesion, and is most manifest on T2 weighted images as intermediate-signal-intensity foci within the underlying bright-signal-intensity tumor matrix (Fig. 24–51).

Giant Cell Tumor

Giant cell tumor is typically classified as a benign neoplasm of bone, but there is a strong tendency for recurrence (50 to 60 percent) and degeneration to malignant disease (10 to 15 percent), with metastasis to the lungs a sequela of late disease. There has been confusion over the diagnosis of giant cell tumor in the past since the "giant cell" of these lesions, the osteoclastoma, may be seen in several types of benign neoplastic and non-neoplastic lesions. Although giant cell tumor is virtually nonexistent in infants and exceedingly rare before the third decade of life, recurrent giant cell tumor in the second decade has been reported.

Giant cell tumor has been described in every bone of the body, but is most common at the ends of one of the longer tubular bones, especially the femur or tibia at the knee and radius at the wrist. Fifty percent of cases

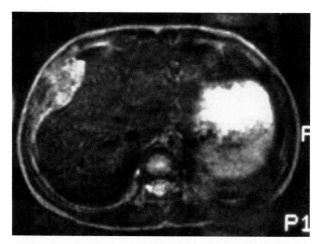

Figure 24–49. *Neuroectodermal tumor.*   T2 weighted transverse image (2000/80) through the chest. Tumor is seen as a heterogeneous increased signal intensity mass involving the right seventh rib.

are seen around the knee. Pain is usually the earliest complaint and may become persistent and severe. Pathologic fracture may be seen.

The roentgenographic appearance is nonspecific and may resemble a primary malignant bone tumor. There are a number of roentgenographic clues to suggest a diagnosis of giant cell tumor in a long bone.

These tumors characteristically occur in the epiphysis of a long tubular bone after the physis has fused. They may be central or eccentric, and although primarily epiphyseal, they may extend into the adjacent metaphysis. The lesion is osteolytic and begins beneath the cortex, with eventual dilatation of the medullary cavity and thinning of the cortical walls. Extension through the articular cartilage into the joint space and into an adjacent bone is rare, but has been reported. Soft tissue extension may occur. Biopsy is usually needed for definitive diagnosis.

Metastasis of giant cell tumor to the lungs has been reported; they usually present as multiple small nodules that remain in the lungs, with no impairment of health and no change in size after treatment. They may disappear spontaneously, but rarely progress to result in death.[57]

MR Appearance of Giant Cell Tumor

The MR appearance of giant cell tumors is interesting. Giant cell tumors of bone are one of the few tumors that can appear of low to intermediate signal intensity on T2 weighted images. These lesions are also of low to intermediate signal intensity on T1 weighted images. Patches of increased signal intensity on T2 weighted images may be seen,[58] most likely reflecting hemorrhage, cyst formation, or cellular elements within the tumor. MRI has been found to be useful in the pre-

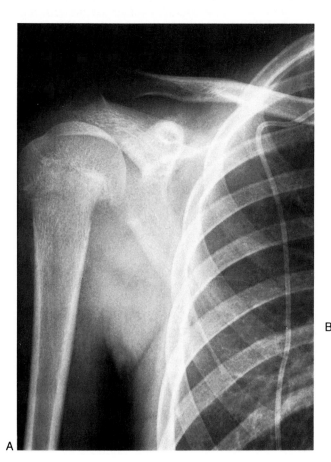

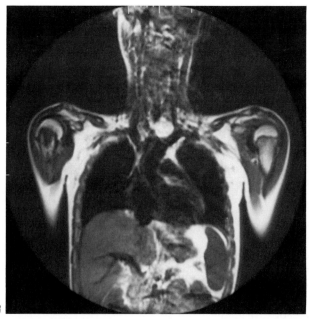

Figure 24–50. *Burkitt's lymphoma of the proximal right humerus with pathologic fracture.* ***A,*** Radiograph shows fracture through the proximal humerus. ***B,*** Coronal T1 weighted image (800/26) shows medial angulation of the proximal right humeral head due to the fracture. There is well-defined homogeneous low signal intensity of the marrow of the proximal metaphysis due to infiltration from Burkitt's lymphoma. (Courtesy of Dr. Mervyn D. Cohen, Indianapolis.)

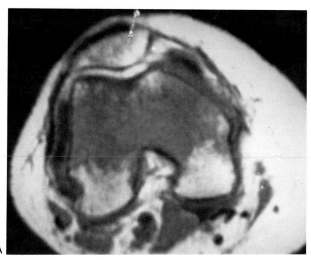
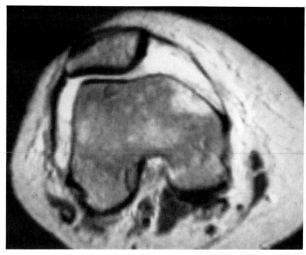

A   B

Figure 24–51. *Lymphoma. Transverse image through the distal femur in a young woman.* **A,** T1 weighted image (600/30) shows intermediate-signal-intensity replacement of the high-signal-intensity fatty marrow by tumor. **B,** T2 weighted image (2000/80) shows heterogeneous increased signal intensity of the marrow lesion. Some regions remain intermediate in signal intensity. Fluid is noted within the joint space.

therapeutic staging of giant cell tumor;[58] it is particularly important to look for joint invasion and soft tissue spread. CT and MRI appear of similar accuracy in determining the intraosseous extent of tumor, but MRI is superior to CT for study of the joints and soft tissues. CT better defines cortical destruction than does MRI. In four cases reported by Herman and colleagues,[58] a thin rim of low signal intensity separated the tumor from the adjacent uninvolved bone marrow. In two additional cases that showed extensive soft tissue spread and more aggressive behavior, this thin rim of low signal intensity was not noted. This was thought to correspond to a rim of reactive bone, and may suggest a less aggressive lesion. These authors also found that the more aggressive lesions showed some increased signal intensity of the intraosseous tumor on T2 weighted images. However, despite some correlation between the presence of a sclerotic rim, areas of tissue inhomogeneity, and the aggressiveness of the lesion, the significance of these MR findings in the evaluation of giant cell tumor is unknown. Further prospective studies are needed to determine the sensitivity and specificity of MRI in predicting the aggressiveness of giant cell tumor.

The absence of fluid levels help distinguish this lesion from aneurysmal bone cyst or telangiectatic osteogenic sarcoma.

A possible role for MRI includes evaluation of the response of giant cell tumor to radiation therapy. It has been suggested that an increasing amount of inhomogeneous low signal intensity within the tumor may correspond to postradiation fibrosis, and therefore a response of the tumor to radiation therapy. A decrease in tumor bulk would also suggest a response of the tumor to radiation. Further studies are needed to assess the role of MRI in the post-therapy evaluation of giant cell tumor.

BENIGN TUMORS AND TUMOR-LIKE BONE LESIONS

Osteochondroma

Osteochondromas (osteocartilaginous exostoses) are one of the most common tumors in the growing skeleton. They are benign bone tumors characterized by cartilaginous, capped bony growths that appear in a variety of sizes and shapes, from slender and bulky to pointed and blunt to sessile and pedunculated. The cartilage cap typically ossifies with maturation of the skeleton. The segment of the shaft from which the exostosis grows is usually widened, but the epiphyseal ossification center is normal. Osteochondromas may be found in any bone that is preformed in cartilage, but are most frequently seen in the metaphyseal portion of the long bones. A single exostosis is termed "solitary osteochondroma," while two or three exostoses in a child with no history of familial exostosis are referred to as "multiple exostoses" or "multiple osteochondromas." When there are exostoses scattered throughout the skeleton, a family history of hereditary multiple exostoses is usually found.

The lesions of both solitary and multiple exostoses are identical radiographically and pathologically; however, the tumor tends to be less extensive in the solitary form. One-third of these lesions are in the distal femur and another one-third are divided equally between the proximal humerus and the proximal tibia. Clinically a child or adolescent presents with a lump on the affected bone that may have been present for many years, without causing symptoms. Clinical symptoms may exist if there is pressure on surrounding nerves or vessels, or if a fracture through the stalk of the osteochondroma causes pain and swelling. In rare instances, osteochondromas occur as a late complication of radiation therapy in children. The most worrisome aspect of osteochondroma is its propensity, on rare occasions, to undergo malignant change, although the overall incidence of malignant change if all osteochondromas are considered is probably less than 0.05 percent. The onset of pain (even if inconstant and not severe) and a sudden spurt of growth of the tumor are reliable evidence that sarcomatous degeneration has occurred. Chondrosarcoma is the most common sarcomatous change, but osteosarcoma has been reported arising in the bone adjacent to an osteochondroma.

Radiographically, malignant transformation of osteochondroma results in an indistinct external surface of the tumor with resorption of calcified areas and small areas of radiolucency in the bony base. The continuity of the cortex of the tumor with that of the host bone may no longer be distinguishable. Tiny areas of calcification may be detected in adjacent soft tissues. With progressive disease a large soft tissue mass containing calcification is seen.[46, 59]

MR Appearance of Osteochondroma

On MRI, osteochondromas are seen as bony growths extending from the metaphyseal region. The marrow signal intensity is normal and of the same signal intensity as the marrow in the shaft. The most characteristic feature of osteochondroma is the cartilaginous cap, which typically ossifies with maturation of the skeleton, marking the end of exostotic growth (Fig. 24–52).[60] Remnants of a quiescent cartilage cap may persist into adult life. On MRI there is continuity of the low-signal-intensity cortex of the osteochondroma with the cortex of the bone from which the lesion arose, just as there is continuity between the marrow of the exostosis and the marrow of the primary bone (Fig. 24–52). The cartilage cap can be identified on MRI, being seen as intermediate (equal to muscle) signal intensity on T1 and increased signal intensity on T2 weighted images. In five cases reported by Lee and associates,[60] a low-signal-intensity zone was seen overlying the cartilaginous cap on both T1 and T2 weighted images. This represented the intact perichondrium (Fig. 24–52).

The identification of the cartilaginous cap and perichondrium is important for several reasons. First, confirmation of the presence of the cartilaginous cap defines the lesion as an osteochondroma and distinguishes it from other juxtacortical lesions such as ossifying hematoma or juxtacortical chondroma. Identification of a smooth and contiguous cartilaginous cap and intact perichondrium suggests a benign lesion. Finally, optimal surgical resection of osteochondroma requires excision of the entire perichondrium. If the perichondrium is incompletely resected, the possibility of tumor recurrence increases. By defining local soft tissue anatomy and delineating the extent of the cartilaginous cap, MRI evaluation facilitates preoperative planning.[60]

MRI is becoming increasingly important in the assessment of malignant degeneration of the cartilaginous cap of an osteochondroma to chondrosarcoma (Fig. 24–47). In general, disruption of the cartilaginous cap and the presence of a soft tissue mass are suggestive of malignant degeneration and should prompt biopsy. Although a review of the published images of osteochondroma reveals no evidence of surrounding marrow or soft tissue edema, it is not known whether there will be significant soft tissue or marrow edema surrounding a chondrosarcoma secondary to osteochondroma. Since soft tissue or marrow edema does not appear to be a companion to osteochondroma, the presence of either of these entities likely warrants further investigation. There has been some suggestion that the degree of thickening of the cartilaginous cap may be suggestive of malignant change. Some authors consider cartilaginous caps thicker than 3 cm as more likely to undergo malignant degeneration,[61] but others feel that both benign osteochondroma and malignant chondrosarcoma may be associated with prominent cartilaginous caps.[62] Since thicker

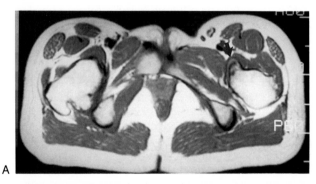
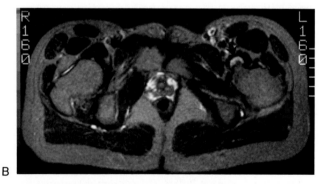

A   B

Figure 24–52. *Osteochondroma. Transverse images of the proximal femora in a 20-year-old woman demonstrating the characteristic MR appearance of an osteochondroma. **A,** TR/TE 1000/20. Mature osteochondroma protruding from the posterior right intertrochanteric region. There is no cartilaginous cap. A second osseous protuberance from the anterior aspect of the left proximal femoral metaphysis is seen with intermediate-signal-intensity cartilage cap. The low-signal-intensity perichondrium (arrow) is intact. **B,** The cartilaginous cap is increased in signal intensity on the T2 weighted image (2000/80). The intact perichondrium (arrow) is again seen.*

cartilaginous caps are generally seen in younger patients, the thickness of the cartilaginous cap, as measured on MRI, is less likely to be useful as a criterion for malignant degeneration in children with osteochondroma.

Varying degrees of mineralization and calcification may be seen within the osteochondroma. Subchondral ossification is likely to be seen as low signal intensity on both T1 and T2 weighted images.[29, 60] The MR appearance of calcification in the cap is uncertain.

Enchondroma

Chondromas are slow-growing benign tumors composed of mature hyaline cartilage. A central chondroma or enchondroma is most common and is centrally located within the medullary cavity of bone. A juxtacortical or periosteal chondroma is rare and develops between the periosteal connective tissue and cortex, eroding the underlying cortical bone. Solitary benign chondromas are common in children and are seen most often in the tubular bones of the limbs, with a predilection for the phalanges and metacarpals of the hand. The tumor usually develops in the metaphysis but eventually extends into the adjacent epiphysis and/or diaphysis. Solitary enchondromas are the most common form of chondroma, but multiple unilateral enchondroma is referred to as Ollier's disease, and multiple enchondromas accompanied by multiple hemangiomas are referred to as Maffucci's syndrome. Enchondromas are usually asymptomatic. Malignant transformation to chondrosarcoma occurs infrequently but has been estimated to occur in as many as 30 percent of patients with Maffucci's syndrome.[63] Malignant degeneration usually occurs during middle life, accompanied by local swelling, mild and constant pain, and change in bone contour. Pathologic fractures that produce pain and swelling often bring the child to the attention of the radiologist.

Radiographically, the lesions are sharply outlined, round or oval, and radiolucent. Cartilaginous calcifications within the lesion are characteristic. In the absence of cartilaginous calcification the enchondroma must be differentiated from other benign lesions or chondrosarcoma. A change in the lesion, calcification in the soft tissues surrounding the lesion, and the presence of a soft tissue mass seen roentgenographically are suspicious for malignant degeneration.[46, 64]

MR Appearance of Enchondroma

On MRI, enchondromas are seen as low to intermediate (less than or equal to muscle) signal intensity on T1 (Fig. 24–53) and increased signal intensity on T2 weighted images.[29, 50, 65] This signal intensity is due to the long T1 and T2 relaxation times of the cartilaginous tissue. Low-signal-intensity bony septations on both T1 and T2 weighted images have been reported,[29, 50] but the presence of these septations is vari-

able. One case report of an enchondroma describes the lesion containing lobules of homogeneous, diffuse high signal intensity, separated by the thin septa of low signal intensity.[50] These lobules were shown to be composed of pure hyaline cartilage, and the septa were composed of fibrous tissue with a cellular component. The subtle calcification seen within an enchondroma on plain films is not reflected on spin-echo MR images.

There has been one report of T2 relaxation times of enchondroma.[65] In a patient with Maffucci's syndrome the T2 relaxation time (using a two-point data fit) was 60 to 65 msec, while the T2 relaxation time of an enchondroma that had undergone malignant degeneration to a chondrosarcoma was 103 to 115 msec. This suggests that, in addition to the finding of a painful soft tissue mass, T2 prolongation may be helpful in distinguishing benign enchondroma from malignant degeneration to chondrosarcoma. Further work is necessary in this area.

Unicameral Bone Cyst

A simple bone cyst is a common condition seen during childhood and adolescence, and although the cause is unknown, it apparently results from a disturbance of growth at the epiphyseal plate.[66] There is a predilection for the metaphyseal region of the bone. All metaphyses in the skeleton may be affected, but the lesion is seen most frequently in the proximal humerus and in the proximal femur (Table 24–3). Eighty percent of simple bone cysts occur between 3 and 14 years of age, with a mean age of 9 years. Males are affected three times as often as females. Patients are usually unaware of any abnormality until the bone fractures, an event that occurs in close to two-thirds of patients with simple bone cysts. Treatment is surgical, with curettage and bone grafting necessary.

Pathologically, this disorder is not a neoplasm but an intramedullary cystic cavity that usually contains clear or amber fluid, although it may also contain blood and clot. The cavity is lined by a thin layer of fibrous tissue. Partial or complete septa may give the cyst a multicameral appearance. Multinucleated giant cells, hemosiderin pigment, and chronic inflammatory cells may be found in the pathologic specimen. Malignancy in a solitary bone cyst has been reported but is extremely rare.[66]

Radiographically, the cyst is clearly medullary in origin, centrally located, and confined to the metaphysis immediately juxtaposed to the epiphyseal line (Fig. 24–54). A thin linear band of sclerotic bone usually demarcates the cyst from normal surrounding medullary bone. During times of active cyst growth, this linear band may reach and blend with the endocortex.[66] In many cases this sclerotic band may be absent and only a sharp distinct margin between normal and destroyed bone is seen. Extension into the epiphysis, although rare, may be seen. During the

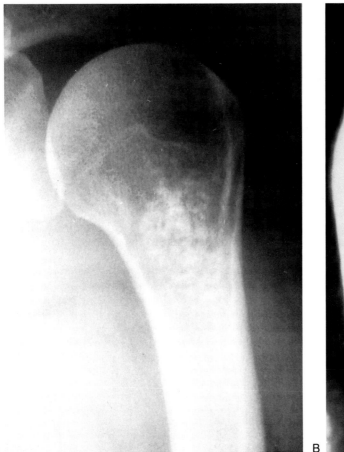

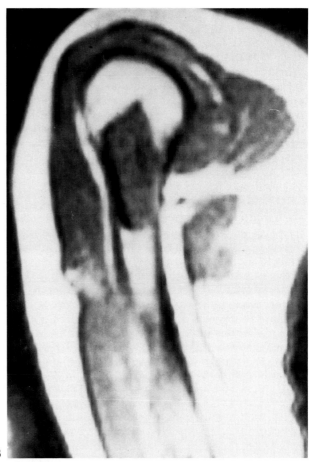

A

B

Figure 24–53. *Enchondroma.* *A,* Radiograph shows punctate, popcorn-like calcification of the proximal metaphysis of the humerus. *B,* Sagittal MR image (1000/20) clearly delineates the intramedullary tumor extension. Visualization of the calcification is inferior to that on the CT image. (Courtesy of Dr. J. Tehranzadeh, Miami.)

latent stage, the cyst appears mid-diaphyseal in location and more oval in shape. Spontaneous fracture through a cyst may be recognized on radiographs and may be accompanied by periosteal reaction, callus formation, and cortical thickening.

Table 24–3. INCIDENCE OF UNICAMERAL BONE CYST

Location	Percentage
Clavicle	<1
Proximal humerus	54
Rib	<1
Distal humerus	2
Proximal ulna/radius	<1
Pelvis	2
Distal radius	2
Distal ulna	1
Proximal femur	23
Hand	<1
Distal femur	3
Proximal tibia	3
Ankle	5
Foot	5

Adapted from Wilner D. Radiology of tumors and allied disorders. Philadelphia: WB Saunders, 1982:925.

MR Appearancve of Unicameral Bone Cyst

The MR appearance of simple bone cysts reflects the stage and contents of the cyst. The lesion is probably metaphyseal if in the active phase of growth and mid-diaphyseal if it has been present for a longer time. The most common appearance is that of a well-defined lesion within the medullary cavity, oval or rounded in shape, and sharply demarcated from normal marrow signal intensity (Fig. 24–54). Depending on the age of the child and the location of the bone cyst, this marrow will be either high-signal-intensity fatty marrow or intermediate-signal-intensity red marrow. A low-signal-intensity rim, corresponding to a thin rim of sclerotic bone, may be seen.[56] Since most simple bone cysts contain serous fluid, the cyst is seen as intermediate to low fluid signal intensity on T1 and homogeneous bright signal intensity on T2 weighted images (Fig. 24–54). However, there is likely to be a broad spectrum of internal signal intensity in unicameral bone cysts, since hemorrhage produces any combination of signal intensity depending on its age and amount and the presence of clot. Simple bone cysts that contain no fluid may be expected to be of intermediate to low signal intensity on both T1 and T2 weighted images,

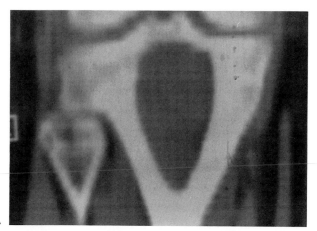

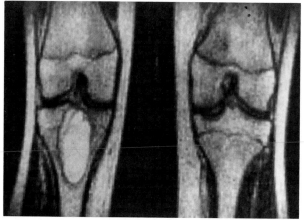

A   B

Figure 24–54. *Unicameral bone cyst.* ***A,*** Reconstructed CT image of the proximal tibia shows a fluid-filled simple bone cyst (c). ***B,*** T2 weighted coronal image (2000/80) through the knees shows the bright-signal-intensity, fluid-filled unicameral bone cyst which is medullary in origin and centrally located, and (in this case) crosses the physis.

although the MR appearance of an "empty" bone cyst has not been described.

Usually, the plain radiograph is sufficient to diagnose a pathologic fracture through a unicameral bone cyst. There is probably little role for MRI preoperatively unless a lesion other than bone cyst is suspected and exclusion of a soft tissue mass is needed. If MRI is performed, the fracture is usually well visualized and a surrounding hematoma may be appreciated (Fig. 24–55). There should be no evidence of periosteal reaction or soft tissue mass on MR images of simple bone cysts unless there has been a complicating factor such as fracture. The presence of periosteal reaction or soft tissue mass on MR examination of a suspected simple bone cyst should suggest other diagnoses.

Aneurysmal Bone Cyst

Aneurysmal bone cyst, a non-neoplastic solitary lesion of bone consisting of a cystic cavity filled with nonendothelium-lined spaces containing blood, has been seen in every bone of the skeleton. Fifty percent occur in the long bones, 30 percent in the spine, and 20 percent equally divided between the flat bones and the short tubular bones (Table 24–4).[67] They are seen most frequently in adolescents, three-fourths of cases occurring below the age of 20. There is a slight female predominance. Unlike simple bone cysts, aneurysmal bone cysts are usually symptomatic, with nondescript pain and swelling. Limitation of motion is a less common symptom. The pathogenesis of aneurysmal bone cyst is a matter of much debate. In the past, aneurysmal bone cyst has been thought to be a variant of giant cell tumor, a result of trauma, a manifestation of solitary dysfibroplasia of bone, or the result of a sudden hemodynamic disturbance. This is the most favored etiology, with the hypothesis that aneurysmal bone cyst is a result of a sudden vascular occlusion of the venous drainage of that segment of bone, or the result

of a development of an arteriovenous shunt. Progressive and enormous dilatation of the sinusoid-like blood spaces in the medullary cavity occurs, leading to a gradual distention of bone and erosion of the cortex. There may be a predisposing lesion that would serve as the nidus for an osseous arteriovenous fistula. This theory is supported in part by a large number of primary benign bone lesions that accompany aneurysmal bone cyst. Treatment includes surgery, irradiation, or arterial embolization. In most patients treated with radiation therapy, sarcomatous change is uncommon, but it may occur in 2 to 6 percent of those who receive a tumor dose of 3,500 rads.[67]

Grossly, aneurysmal bone cyst is a well-circumscribed cavity within the bone that contains communicating cavernous spaces filled with blood. The lesion may be primarily fluid filled, may contain thick connective tissue septa so that it resembles a blood-soaked sponge, or may be predominantly solid and fibrous with few cavities. Microscopically, the most striking feature is the presence of multiple cavernous spaces of varying size that contain blood and are supported by fibrous walls of varying thickness, which often contain bone.[69]

Radiographically, there are four stages of development of aneurysmal bone cyst. These include an initial lytic phase manifested by a well-circumscribed ovoid area of rarefaction. The lesion may be central, eccentric, or parosteal. During the phase of active growth, in which the lesion expands at a rapid rate, there is often rapid destruction of bone and a characteristic subperiosteal "blowout" pattern. The mature stage, or stage of stabilization, is characterized by formation of a distinct peripheral bony shell and internal bony septa and trabeculations. This produces the characteristic roentgenographic "soap bubble" appearance. In the healing phase, there may be progressive calcification and ossification of the cyst, and eventual transformation into a dense bony mass with an irregular structure.

In the tubular bones, there may be several locations

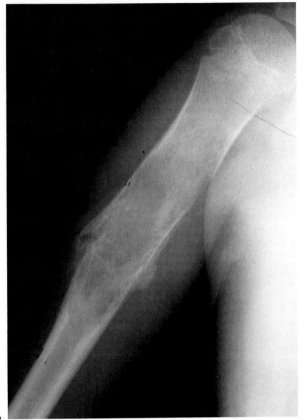

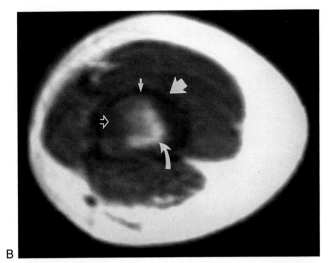

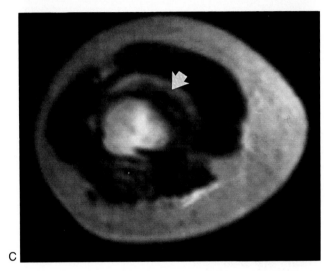

Figure 24–55. *Bone cyst with fracture.* ***A,*** Radiograph of the humerus in a 9-year-old girl demonstrates a pathologic fracture through a diaphyseal unicameral bone cyst. ***B,*** Transverse T1 weighted MR image (600/20) through the lesion. The low- to inter-mediate-signal-intensity component of the lesion (*open arrow*) represents fluid, whereas the high-signal-intensity component reflects hemorrhage associated with pathologic fracture (*curved arrow*). Callus (*small arrow*) and periosteum (*large arrow*) have low signal intensity. ***C,*** T2 weighted image (2000/75) demonstrates the increased-signal-intensity fluid component of the lesion. There is increased signal from the periosteum (*arrow*).

Table 24–4. INCIDENCE OF ANEURYSMAL
BONE CYST

Location	Percentage
Cervical spine	8
Clavicle	
Humerus	10
Thoracic spine	5
Lumbar spine	12
Ulna	6
Radius	2
Sacrum	2
Ilium	3
Pubis	3
Femur	12
Fibula	5
Tibia	15
Tarsus	2
Metatarsus	2

Adapted from Wilner D. Radiology of tumors and allied disorders. Philadelphia: WB Saunders, 1982:1013.

and appearances of aneurysmal bone cyst (Fig. 24–56). The size of the cyst is directly proportional to the age of the lesion. The greatest dimension coincides with the long axis of the bone. The rare parosteal aneurysmal bone cyst has a slightly different appearance, the lesion seeming to arise from the periosteum with minimal erosion of the outer cortex. The bulk of the aneurysmal bone cyst lies in the surrounding soft tissues.

MR Appearance of Aneurysmal Bone Cysts

There have been several reports of the MR appearance of aneurysmal bone cyst.[68–72] The appearance varies, depending on the location of the lesion and the percentage of solid versus fluid content of the aneurysmal bone cyst. However, a fluid-fluid level, or multiple fluid-fluid levels, thought to represent layered uncoagulated blood, appear to be a characteristic MR

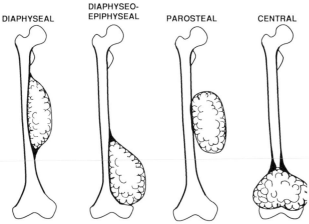

Figure 24–56. Classification of roentgenographic types of aneurysmal bone cyst. (Sherman RS, Soong KY. Aneurysmal bone cyst: its roentgen diagnosis. Radiology 1957; 68:54.)

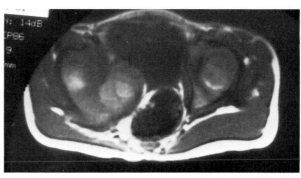

Figure 24–57. *Aneurysmal bone cyst of the pelvis.* MR image (600/20) shows an expanding lesion of the right side of the pelvis. The cortex can be identified around the posterior two-thirds of the lesion but not anteriorly. The presence of multiple horizontal fluid-fluid levels is fairly characteristic of an aneurysmal bone cyst and helps to differentiate this lesion from more malignant bone tumors. (Courtesy of Dr. Mervyn D. Cohen, Indianapolis.)

finding in aneurysmal bone cyst (Figs. 24–57, 24–58). The lesions are typically multiloculated and expansile on MRI, often with a prominent "soft tissue" component. On T1 weighted images, they are usually well demarcated from the surrounding high-signal-intensity fatty marrow (the marrow is usually of high signal intensity since most of these lesions occur in adolescence) and are very heterogeneous in appearance. The internal signal intensity on T1 weighted images includes low signal, intermediate signal, and some high signal intensity (Fig. 24–58). Low signal intensity seems to correspond to fibrous tissue, internal bony

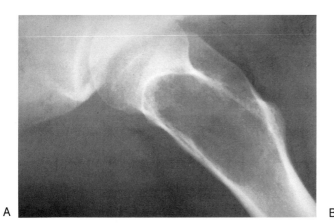

A

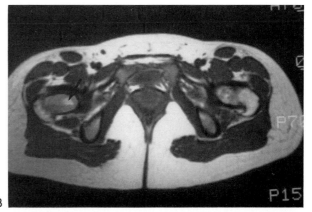

B

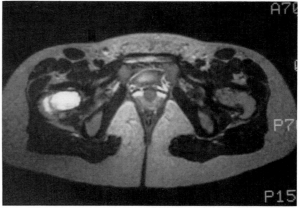

C

Figure 24–58. *Intertrochanteric aneurysmal bone cyst of the right femur in a 15-year-old girl.* **A,** Radiograph of the intertrochanteric expansile lesion. **B,** Transverse proton-density image (2000/20) through the intertrochanteric region shows a fluid-fluid level with some increased-signal-intensity fluid consistent with hemorrhage (*arrow*). **C,** T2 weighted image (2000/80) shows overall increase in signal intensity of the fluid. A persistent fluid-fluid level is seen.

architecture, and hemosiderin. The increased signal intensity seen on T1 weighted images most likely represents hemorrhage (Figs. 24–58, 24–59). On T2 weighted images, this heterogeneity is also prominent, but typically the lesion has more areas of increased signal intensity, since reactive fibrous tissue and especially fluid increase in signal intensity. The lesion remains well demarcated from surrounding normal marrow and there is usually no evidence of marrow edema. However, prospective studies that describe the MR appearance of aneurysmal bone cysts focusing on the mature or stabilization stage of aneurysmal bone cyst, and MR studies during all four phases of aneurysmal bone cysts, particularly the phase of active growth, have not been performed. Until these studies are undertaken, we cannot be certain that there will not be marrow edema surrounding actively expanding lesions. Surrounding soft tissue edema has been reported.[34]

A low-signal-intensity rim corresponding to the presence of reactive bone around the lesion may be seen. However, the thin rim of cortex surrounding the expansile portion of the lesion may or may not be seen. Without plain films, it may therefore be difficult to distinguish an aneurysmal bone cyst from a tumor with a soft tissue mass, since a definite rim of cortical bone

may not be noted on MRI images (Fig. 24–60). This underscores the need for plain films in every patient with a bone lesion or suspected bone lesion undergoing an MR examination. However, the presence of multiple hemorrhagic and serous fluid-fluid levels within cystlike cavities is fairly characteristic of aneurysmal bone cyst on MRI. Differential diagnosis on MRI includes complicated simple bone cyst, hemangioma, and telangiectatic osteogenic sarcoma, all of which can present with hemorrhagic and serous fluid-fluid levels.

MRI can play a role in the diagnosis and evaluation of the rare parosteal aneurysmal bone cyst. In one case (Fig. 24–60) the presence of benign reactive cortical bone surrounding the parosteal lesion and of hemorrhagic fluid-fluid levels on MR examination was sufficient to diagnose parosteal aneurysmal bone cyst in an otherwise radiographically indeterminate lesion.

When it is unclear from the radiograph whether the lesion is an aneurysmal bone cyst, and the MR appearance is not diagnostic, CT examination can be helpful in identifying the thin cortical shell of aneurysmal bone cyst. Fluid-fluid levels can also be appreciated on CT. The sensitivity and specificity of MRI versus CT in identifying these fluid-fluid levels have not been tested. The fluid-fluid levels of aneurysmal bone cyst seen on MRI may have a variety of appearances, with

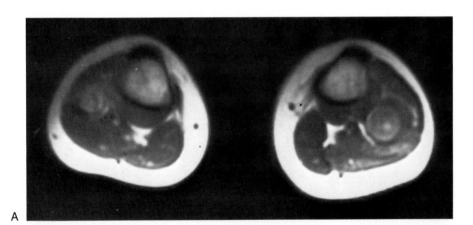

A

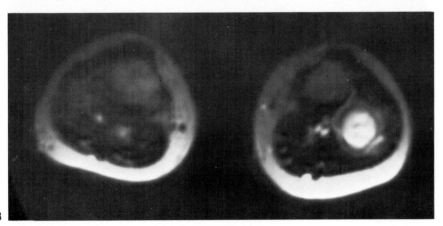

B

Figure 24–59. *Aneurysmal bone cyst of the fibula.* ***A,*** T1 weighted image (800/26) shows expansion of the fibula. Most of the lesion is of moderate intensity. Several small foci of high intensity probably represent hemorrhage. ***B,*** T2 weighted image (2000/90) shows increase in signal from most of the lesion with a small area, centrally, of very low intensity. This could represent either fibrosis or hemosiderin. (Courtesy of Dr. Mervyn D. Cohen, Indianapolis.)

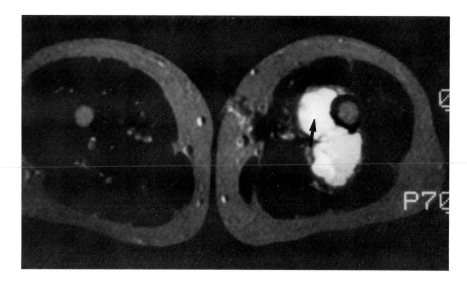

Figure 24–60. *Parosteal aneurysmal bone cyst.* T2 weighted transverse MR image (2000/80) of a femoral parosteal aneurysmal bone cyst. The fluid-fluid level can be appreciated (*arrow*), while the thin rim of cortical bone surrounding the lesion cannot.

the fluid in one cyst appearing as bright signal intensity on both T1 and T2 weighted images, and the fluid in an adjacent cavernous space appearing as low signal intensity on T1 and bright signal intensity on T2 weighted images. Layers within the same cyst may vary in signal intensity: either low signal intensity on T1, bright signal intensity on T2, or bright signal intensity on both T1 and T2 weighted images. When fluid levels of differing signal intensity are seen on T1 weighted images, the dependent layer is usually of bright signal intensity, presumably secondary to T1 shortening by methemoglobin in the more dense blood layer. Since both hemorrhage and fluid increase in signal intensity on T2 weighted images, fluid-fluid levels are less often appreciated on T2 weighted images because the intensity difference between these two layers has decreased.[68] The age of the blood, the presence of proteinaceous fluid, and the degree of solid fibrous tissue and bony tissue all affect the MR appearance of the lesion.

Fibroxanthoma

This term is preferred by the Armed Forces Institute of Pathology[73] to describe histologically similar lesions occurring in the metaphysis of growing long bones.

The fibrous cortical defect is a small lytic lesion filled with fibrous tissue. These lesions are usually less than 2 cm in diameter and are eccentrically located within the metaphysis, with a predilection for the medial femoral condyle. The lesions occur in young children between the ages of 4 and 8 years, although cases in younger children have been reported. There is a slight male predominance. The lesions may rarely be associated with neurofibromatosis and craniofacial dysostosis.[74] They do not require treatment and usually disappear spontaneously.

Persistent lesions that show interval growth are termed "nonossifying fibromas." A nonossifying fi-

broma is a well-defined osteolytic lesion that involves the cortex and medullary cavity of the metaphysis and adjacent diaphysis of the long bone. The lesion is usually 4 cm or more in diameter and often the result of a fibrous cortical defect that has persisted. Seventy percent occur in children between the ages of 10 and 15, and although most occur in the tibia (30 percent in the distal tibia and 20 percent in the proximal tibia), another 20 percent are found in the distal femur. The remaining lesions are found in the fibula, humerus, and flat bones. In the distal femur and proximal tibia the lesion is usually seen in the medial and posterior aspect of the bone, whereas in the distal tibia the lateral and posterior bone is more likely to be involved. Most lesions are asymptomatic, although local pain may develop. The lesions usually heal spontaneously.

Pathologically, the lesions contain foci of fibrous tissue. Each focus may be surrounded by a thin shell of reactive bone or sclerotic spongiosa. The stroma of the fibroxanthoma consists of spindle-shaped fibroblasts.[74] In addition to fibrous stroma, these lesions contain multinucleated giant cells, cholesterol crystals, foam (xanthoma) cells, and red blood cells in hemorrhage.[73]

Radiographically, a fibrous cortical defect is first recognized as subtle loss of the metaphyseal cortex. The margin of the fibrous cortical defect is poorly defined in the early phases, but there may be a thin rim of reactive bone, especially in lesions that have been present for longer periods. The lesion undergoes spontaneous regression and/or extrusion of the defect through the cortex. There may be recurrences.

Radiographically, nonossifying fibromas have a typical appearance. They are usually peripheral and metaphyseal, although if followed, may drift toward the mid-diaphysis. The inner boundary is usually well demarcated by a scalloped sclerotic border, although this feature may be absent. The cortex may be either thin or thickened and sclerotic. The lesion may involve the entire diameter of the long bone. Pathologic fractures are uncommon but do occur. A slight increase in radioactivity on a bone scan is common and corresponds to the often present sclerotic rim.[74]

MR Appearance of Fibroxanthoma

There is no indication for MR imaging of benign fibrous cortical defect. However, it is important to be familiar with the MR appearance of these lesions, since they are common in the pediatric population and may appear as an incidental finding on MRI.

The diagnosis of nonossifying fibroma is usually made from the plain film alone. However, when a lesion is eccentric and has destroyed the cortex, is complicated by a pathologic fracture, is located in an unusual skeletal site, or has extended across the entire diameter of the shaft, there may be a role for MRI in the imaging of nonossifying fibroma.

Fibroxanthomas are seen as loculated heterogeneous lesions with low to intermediate signal intensity on T1 weighted images; they may have increased intensity on T2 weighted images.[8] More commonly, however, the lesions have low signal intensity on T2 weighted images, owing to the presence of minute amounts of hemosiderin (Fig. 24–61).[73] The low-signal-intensity adjacent cortical bone may be thickened, but there is no edema in the surrounding soft tissues or marrow.[72] Nonossifying fibromas are often lobulated and are sharply demarcated from the surrounding normal bone marrow. The lesions are often eccentric and metaphyseal in position, but there should be no soft tissue or periosteal component.[72]

Osteoid Osteoma

Osteoid osteoma, a benign osteoblastic tumor, is characterized by a small reddish-brown nidus less than 1 cm in size. It accounts for 10 percent of all benign tumors. The lesion has been reported in every bone of the skeleton except the sternum and clavicle,[75] but is most common in the femur and tibia (Table 24–5). It occurs most commonly in children, adolescents, and young adults, with 76 percent of the patients being between 5 and 25 years of age. There is a 3:1 male predominance. Clinically, children present with bone pain that is worse at night and improves after aspirin administration. The typical clinical symptoms are found in only about 75 percent of patients; in the remainder, clinical suspicion of the diagnosis may be very low. The pain may be referred to a nearby joint. Swelling of the soft tissues and limitation of joint motion may occur. There may be secondary effects on growth and associated reduction in the size of muscle bulk, because of disuse atrophy. Scoliosis occurs as a result of osteoid osteoma of the spine. Removal of the nidus cures the disease. It is therefore important that imaging accurately identifies the nidus. Radiation therapy has not been particularly useful.

Pathologically, the lesion consists of a central nidus of vascular osteoid tissue,[75] which is capable of bone production. In some patients a central area of calcification is seen within the nidus. The nomenclature is sometimes confused, with the central calcification called "the nidus." This is incorrect and the term "nidus" should be reserved for the whole lesion irre-

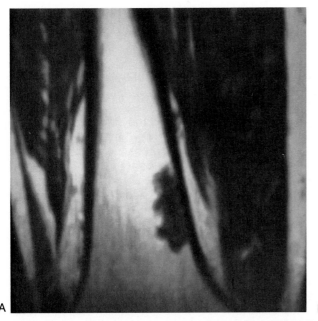 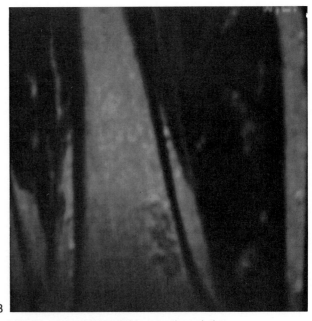

A   B

Figure 24–61. *Fibroxanthoma.* Coronal (**A**) T1 weighted (600/20) and (**B**) T2 weighted (2000/80) images through the femur. A lobulated, well-defined, low-signal-intensity lesion is seen along the medial aspect of the femur, abutting the endosteal surface of the cortical bone. While the signal intensity of the lesion increases on the T2 weighted image, it retains some intermediate signal intensity.

Table 24–5. INCIDENCE OF OSTEOID OSTEOMA

Location	Percentage
Skull	<1
Mandible	<1
Cervical spine	<1
Scapula	<1
Humerus	7
Rib	<1
Thoracic spine	<1
Lumbar spine	5
Ulna	3
Pelvis	3
Carpal	2
Metacarpal	3
Phalanx	5
Femur	27
Patella	<1
Fibula	3
Tibia	29
Talus	2
Calcaneus	2
Metatarsal	2
Phalanx	2

Adapted from Wilner D. Radiology of tumors and allied disorders. Philadelphia: WB Saunders, 1982:146.

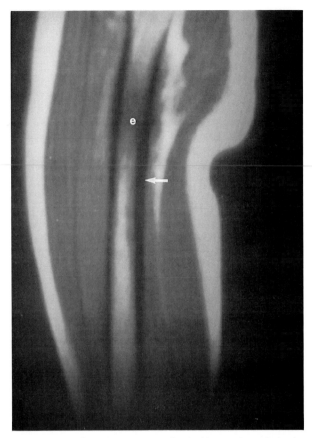

Figure 24–62. *Osteoid osteoma.* Sagittal image through the femur. Low-signal-intensity marrow edema (e) is appreciated. The anterior cortical bone (*arrow*) is thickened but remains low in signal intensity. Extensive marrow edema and thickened low-signal-intensity cortical bone are anecdotally characteristic of osteoid osteoma. The nidus is not seen, and therefore the diagnosis cannot be confirmed.

spective of whether central calcification is present. The nidus stimulates the formation of reactive bone sclerosis in the adjacent bone surrounding the nidus. This sclerotic rim is usually well defined and may be quite large and dense. It may encroach into the marrow cavity.

Radiographically, osteoid osteoma appears as an oval or round radiolucent lesion (the nidus) surrounded by a wide zone of sclerotic bone. The amount of associated reactive bone varies with the age of the child and the location of the lesion. In the long bones the nidus can be seen as a small lucency. It is usually eccentric and does not invade the soft tissues. Whether a nidus is lucent or dense may depend on the age of the lesion, with increased density (calcification) found more commonly late in the disease. The lesion may be associated with intense cortical thickening that may give the bone a fusiform configuration.

MR Appearance of Osteoid Osteoma

On MRI it may be difficult to identify the exact location of the nidus. This relates primarily to the small size of the lesion, and surface coil images can provide a more detailed examination of a smaller region. Osteoid osteoma is often accompanied by extensive marrow edema (Fig. 24–62) seen as decreased signal intensity marrow on T1 weighted images, which increases on T2 weighted images. STIR images can be especially helpful in identifying marrow edema to suggest or support the diagnosis of osteoid osteoma. Low signal can also be seen in the marrow on T2 weighted images owing to encroachment from sclerotic cortex into the marrow space. When searching for osteoid osteoma, we obtain coronal or sagittal STIR images to screen for marrow edema, followed by axial T1 and T2 weighted images through the region of edema or clinical symptoms. Careful scrutiny of the cortical surface of the bone usually reveals the osteoid osteoma (Fig. 24–63).

Since the lesion can be seen in both the spongiosa and the cortex of bone, the nidus is identified either peripherally or centrally on MRI. The sclerotic bone surrounding the nidus is seen as low signal intensity on both T1 and T2 weighted images. The appearance of the nidus can vary and may be seen as of low or intermediate signal intensity on T1 weighted images, increasing on T2 weighted images. In other cases, when the nidus contains a central calcified focus, it may appear of low to intermediate signal intensity on both T1 and T2 weighted images.[72, 76] If the osteoid osteoma is near a joint, and particularly if it is intracapsular, an associated joint effusion may be seen. Synovial hypertrophy may also occur.

The cortex should be carefully examined in cases of suspected osteoid osteoma. There may be marked thickening of cortical bone (Fig. 24–62), which is reactive and retains the low signal intensity seen in benign reactive thickening of cortical bone. This cortical thickening may be especially prominent when the lesion is intramedullary. Cortical osteoid osteoma may be identified as a small focal area of intermediate signal intensity within the cortex on T1 weighted or proton-density images (Fig. 24–63). There should be no surrounding soft tissue mass unless there has been intervention (i.e., biopsy). Edema of the soft tissues may be seen, particularly if the lesion is cortical in origin.

In the evaluation of suspected osteoma, a wide variety of different imaging modalities may be used. Plain film easily identifies the sclerotic reaction in most cases. As noted above, however, this sclerotic reaction may be minimal, particularly when the nidus is located within the confines of a joint or in some of the smaller bones such as the talus. Definitive diagnosis depends on identification of the nidus. The presence of sclerosis alone is not adequate to confirm the diagnosis. In some patients the plain film radiograph is sufficient to identify both the nidus and the surrounding sclerosis. In other patients linear conventional tomography may be all that is required to identify the nidus. As noted above, the nidus may or may not contain a central focus of calcification. A technetium 99m-MDP bone scan is invariably hot in osteoid osteoma and this is a very useful screening test for the disorder, since it has an extremely high sensitivity. In some cases the specific diagnosis may be accurately suggested on the bone scan because the lesion appears very hot with maximal uptake of the radioisotope within the nidus, which is not surprising as the nidus consists of very vascular osteoid tissue. CT scan in some cases identifies a nidus not seen on conventional radiography. In a series of eight patients, CT was more accurate than either plain film radiographs or isotope bone scan in identifying the nidus.[77] On CT the interface between the nidus and the adjacent sclerosis is well defined and smooth. In five of

eight patients a central area of calcification was seen within the nidus.[77] When present, this calcium always had a smooth contour.

MRI can be used to identify an osteoid osteoma, but if there is strong clinical suspicion of osteoid osteoma and the plain films are not diagnostic, thin-slice CT images with bone algorithm reprocessing are probably more useful than MRI. CT is exquisitely sensitive to cortical involvement and may be diagnostic when MRI is only suggestive (Fig. 24–63). On the other hand, an intramedullary osteoid osteoma may be potentially difficult to identify on CT if the nidus is not calcified or ossified, or if the lesion is in an area of already dense bone. Currently, we obtain plain radiographs in children suspected of having an osteoid osteoma. If this is diagnostic, surgical intervention is undertaken. If it is not, and the clinical suspicion is that of osteoid osteoma, we obtain a thin-slice CT scan. If the clinical history suggests tumor as well as osteoid osteoma, we obtain an MR image, which is usually diagnostic and excludes soft tissue mass and other evidence of tumor. If MRI is not diagnostic and the clinical suspicion of osteoid osteoma remains, we obtain a CT scan at that time.

The main consideration and differential diagnosis in osteoid osteoma is chronic osteomyelitis. In the latter disorder there is always abundant bone sclerosis. Focal areas of destruction may mimic the presence of a nidus, and a small sequestrum may be mistaken for a central area of calcification within the nidus. However, it should always be easy to distinguish between these disorders. The interface between the nidus and adjacent bone is always well defined and smooth, and calcification within the nidus is always central. With chronic osteomyelitis, interfaces between areas of bone destruction and sequestrum or sclerotic bone are always irregular, and not nearly as symmetric as in osteoid osteoma.

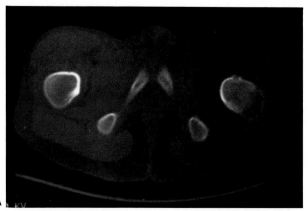
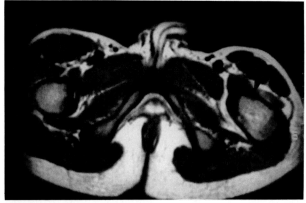

A   B

Figure 24–63. *Oseoid osteoma.* *A,* CT scan (bone windows) reveals anterior femoral intertrochanteric osteoid osteoma (*arrow*). *B,* Intermediate MR scan (2000/30) at the same level reveals the osteoid osteoma within the cortical bone (*arrow*). Increased-signal-intensity edema in the surrounding musculature can be identified.

Osteoblastoma

Benign osteoblastoma, an uncommon neoplasm of bone, occurs primarily in the second decade, although the youngest reported patient is a 3-year-old boy. There is a 2:1 male predominance. Forty percent of osteoblastomas occur in the vertebra and 25 percent in the long bones, primarily the lower extremities. Children most commonly present with pain and mild local tenderness. The pain does not awaken them at night and does not respond to aspirin. There have been reports of rare malignant sarcomatous degeneration.[78] Treatment includes surgical excision, and in cases of extensive vertebral involvement and subsequent cord compression, adjunctive radiation therapy may be required. Recurrence is rare.

Pathologically, the lesions may be quite vascular. There is an underlying loosely fibrillar and highly vascular matrix that alternates with areas of conspicuous osteoid trabeculae. With progression of the lesion the osteoid may calcify and transform into primitive osseous tissue.[78] Osteoid osteoma and osteoblastoma may be indistinguishable histologically, but the number of osteoblasts in osteoblastoma is usually much greater. The size of the nidus, as well as the clinical history, can be used to distinguish the two entities. Lesions with a nidus of less than 1 cm are thought to represent osteoid osteoma; those with a nidus greater than 2 cm, osteoblastoma.

Radiographically, the osteoblastoma is usually lytic and less dense than normal surrounding bone. There may be varying degrees of matrix bone production. With time the lesion expands, erodes, and finally destroys the cortex and produces a soft tissue mass. The bony lesion and soft tissue mass, however, maintain distinct borders, and often a thin, calcific shell of cortical bone can be seen surrounding the lesion. An internal pattern of equal-sized flecks of calcification may be characteristic. Occasionally the lesion may appear as completely lytic. In the spine, benign osteoblastoma is usually confined to the neural arch.

MR Appearance of Osteoblastoma

Of the benign osteoblastomas occurring in long bones, three-fourths occur in the diaphysis and one-fourth in the metaphysis. Location in the epiphysis is rare. Diaphyseal lesions may be central, cortical, or periosteal. Both metaphyseal and epiphyseal lesions can be either central or peripheral. The location of the lesion on MRI reflects the above classification. The amount of underlying ossified bone may vary, depending on the position and age of the lesion, and the MR appearance will reflect underlying stromal matrix, the amount of ossification, and the degree of cellularity. There have been no prospective studies to determine the sensitivity and specificity of MRI in the diagnosis of osteoblastoma, but anecdotal cases have been reported.[29] The central diaphyseal lesions tend to be predominantly lytic and are often quite vascular and

cellular. These osteoblastomas tend to be of intermediate signal intensity on T1 and homogeneous or heterogeneous increased signal intensity on T2 weighted images. The flecks of calcium noted on the plain film will probably not be appreciated as calcification on MRI. Cortical diaphyseal lesions are accompanied by thickened cortical bone and varying degrees of internal ossification. On MRI, cortical thickening that accompanies these cortical lesions is usually low in signal intensity, without evidence of edema or infiltration of the cortical bone as a result of the lesion. One report of periosteal osteoblastoma[79] shows an osteoblastoma arising from the periosteum; on MRI there was evidence of buttressing and thickening of cortical bone, and the lesion was of intermediate signal intensity on T1 and heterogeneous increased signal intensity on T2 weighted images. There was no abnormality of the bone marrow or surrounding soft tissues.

Chondroblastoma

Benign chondroblastoma is a rare primary bone tumor seen in children before epiphyseal closure. The tumor is of chondrogenic origin and is thought to derive from cartilage "germ cells" or cells of the epiphyseal cartilage. The lesion has a predilection for the ends of the larger long bones, with more than 50 percent of chondroblastomas occurring in the bones about the knee or in the proximal femur. The proximal humerus is a third common site (Table 24–6). Seventy percent of the lesions occur during the second decade, with a male to female predominance of 2:1. Referred pain to the joint closest to the lesion is a common presenting complaint. There may be localized swelling and tenderness. Treatment is conservative, usually consisting of curettage and packing of the lesion with cancellous bone chips. Recurrence occurs in 10 to 25 percent of patients but does not necessarily herald malignant degeneration. Malignant degeneration can occur, but often the diagnostic dilemma lies in differen-

Table 24–6. INCIDENCE OF CHONDROBLASTOMA

Location	Percentage
Proximal humerus	17
Scapula	2
Innominate	5
Femur (head & neck)	16
Femur (trochanter)	7
Hand	2
Patella	1
Distal femur	20
Proximal tibia	17
Proximal fibula	1
Tarsus	9
Metatarsus	1

Adapted from Wilner D. Radiology of tumors and allied disorders. Philadelphia: WB Saunders, 1982:455.

tiating a newly diagnosed chondroblastoma from chondrosarcoma and giant cell tumor of bone.

Pathologically, the lesions are well demarcated from surrounding normal bone. Histologically, cartilage, as well as reticulohistiocytes, hemorrhage, and necrosis, may be seen. Chondroblastoma is believed to arise from cartilaginous cells, but there is some support for a reticulohistiocytic origin. At this time it is thought that the tumor cells of chondroblastoma exhibit characteristics of both immature (primitive) and mature cartilaginous cells and that it is a tumor of cartilaginous origin.[80] The cartilage is often very cellular.[81]

In the long bones, an eccentric epiphyseal lesion with complete bone replacement results in a uniformly lucent appearance of the lesion on radiographs. At times an internal pattern of calcific flecks and strands results in a fuzzy and mottled appearance. Faint bony septa and a surrounding sclerotic margin that is smooth and well defined separate the lesion from normal bone. Occasionally, the zone of transition may be ill defined. The cortex may be thin and expanded, and rarely may have the appearance of complete destruction, simulating a giant cell tumor or sarcoma. Lamellated or buttressed periosteal reaction may be seen. Soft tissue swelling may be detected in 50 percent of patients, but a tumor mass is rarely identified.

MR Appearance of Chondroblastoma

The MR appearance of chondroblastoma has been described in a few patients.[4, 9, 29, 72] On MRI the lesions appear as well-defined areas of intermediate to low signal intensity on T1 weighted images, with an increase or a decrease[50] in signal intensity of the cellular chondroid matrix on T2 weighted images (Fig. 24–64). Trabeculations within the lesion may be seen as low signal intensity on both T1 and T2 weighted images. A low-signal-intensity rim, corresponding to a sclerotic margin, may also be seen. It has been sug-

gested that tumors of cartilaginous origin may exhibit a slightly increased signal intensity compared with muscle on T1 weighted images,[10] but in our experience this is not always the case; more commonly, chondroblastoma appears isointense with muscle on T1 weighted images. However, we have seen cases of slightly increased signal intensity of the chondroid matrix compared with muscle on T1 weighted images, so if a lesion does exhibit this characteristic, chondroid matrix tumor should be considered.

Because chondroblastoma can be associated with cortical thinning, disruption, and periosteal reaction, one should not assume the presence of a malignant lesion if loss of cortical bone is identified on MRI. It is possible that the evaluation of surrounding periosteal reaction (i.e., "benign"-appearing periosteal reaction on MRI) as well as lack of signal in surrounding cortical bone (thickened cortical bone is frequently seen in slow-growing lesions on MRI) may be useful in differentiating chondroblastoma from a more malignant lesion. The rare association of chondroblastoma with a soft tissue mass does not allow the use of this criterion to exclude chondroblastoma. MRI does play a role in the preoperative evaluation of chondroblastoma to exclude abnormality of surrounding bone marrow (extensive marrow abnormality suggesting either tumor or marrow edema has not been seen with chondroblastoma); to check for the presence or absence and extent of the soft tissue mass; and in many cases to better evaluate the proximity of the lesion to the joint space.

Further prospective studies are needed to determine the sensitivity and specificity of MRI in the diagnosis and pretherapeutic evaluation of chondroblastoma. However, ill-defined margins of the lesion with the surrounding, extensive marrow edema, and extensive cortical destruction with a large soft tissue mass, are all more suggestive of chondrosarcoma rather than chondroblastoma. It has been suggested[50] that chondrosar-

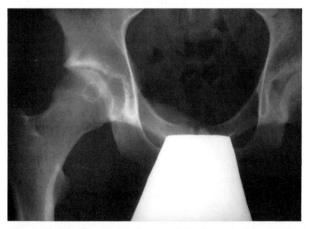
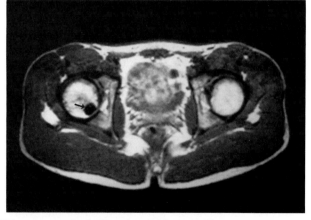

A B

Figure 24–64. *Chondroblastoma.* ***A,*** Radiograph of the proximal right femur in a patient with a chondroblastoma. The lesion is well defined with a thin sclerotic rim. ***B,*** T1 weighted axial image (600/30) through the femoral epiphyses shows the well-defined, low-signal-intensity chondroblastoma (*arrow*). The lesion is easily differentiated from surrounding increased-signal-intensity fatty marrow. The signal intensity of the lesion increased only slightly in T2 weighted images and remained overall intermediate in signal intensity.

coma has a homogeneous increased signal intensity on T2 weighted images and a more lobulated appearance than chondroblastoma, which is seen as a heterogeneous increase in signal intensity on T2 weighted images. However, this report is anecdotal, and prospective studies testing this hypothesis remain to be undertaken.

METASTATIC LESIONS TO BONE

In children, metastatic disease in the bone is seen most commonly with neuroblastoma, rhabdomyosarcoma, medulloblastoma, and the lymphoreticular disorders, including leukemia and lymphoma.[4] Metastatic lesions may also be seen in children with primary osteogenic sarcoma, primary Ewing's sarcoma, and Wilms' tumor (with unfavorable histology). Children may present with bony metastatic disease at the time of diagnosis, or bony metastases may occur later in the course of treatment, when either the surgical, radiation, or chemotherapeutic interventions have been inadequate. The children may be asymptomatic, but commonly present with a complaint of bony pain.

MRI is playing an increasingly important role in the diagnosis of bony metastatic disease, and in distinguishing metastatic disease from other causes of bone pain in the child with cancer, including infection, infarction, and trauma. A child may present with complaints of bone pain, tenderness, and limitation to motion. While plain film radiography is the first imaging modality used, there are cases in which the plain film is either normal or nondiagnostic. Extensive prospective studies to determine the accuracy, sensitivity, and specificity of MRI in the detection and diagnosis of bony metastases have not been performed; however, we have had many patients in whom the plain film results were either nondiagnostic or normal but in whom, because of the child's persistent complaints, MRI was performed. This examination not only revealed a lesion in many cases but also was often able to suggest the correct diagnosis. A bone scan can be used to determine whether an abnormality does exist in an area of pain, as well as to determine the presence of additional bony lesions, but a bone scan can rarely be falsely negative if the lesion is particularly aggressive. In addition, and importantly, metastatic disease often cannot be distinguished from acute ischemic disease, since increased activity is seen in both entities. Although scintigraphy does provide gross anatomic localization of bony abnormality, it does not provide the detailed evaluation of the marrow, cortical bone, periosteum, and surrounding soft tissues afforded by MRI. MRI is thus performed in children with focal symptoms; bone scintigraphy remains the modality of choice for screening the whole skeleton for metastatic disease. We have found little indication for CT in these children, since MRI provides superior anatomic detail and increased sensitivity to metastatic lesions, marrow edema, soft tissue edema, and (in most instances) mar-

row ischemia. However, if the identification of small flecks of calcification or very subtle periosteal reaction is essential, CT will play a role.

MR Appearance of Metastases

In general, the MR appearance of most metastatic lesions in children is similar, and a tissue diagnosis cannot be made from the MR criteria alone. To screen children for metastatic disease in an area of bone pain, a gradient-recalled echo image can be obtained as well as the T1 weighted coronal image. On gradient-echo imaging, lytic areas within bone are seen as bright signal intensity, surrounded by the low-signal-intensity normal marrow (Fig. 24–8). The normal metaphyseal and epiphyseal marrow is of low signal intensity because trabecular bone within the marrow exerts a magnetic susceptibility effect, which results in decreased signal intensity of trabeculated marrow.[22] This magnetic susceptibility effect is also prominent in the vertebral bodies. Depending on the flip angle used, one can enhance T2 contrast on gradient-echo images and therefore increase the signal intensity of metastatic disease (Fig. 24–65). This becomes important in the diaphysis, where there is little trabecular bone and the signal intensity of diaphyseal marrow on gradient-echo images reflects the underlying marrow composition. This allows enhanced contrast of metastatic lesions compared with the diaphyseal marrow signal intensity. Gadolinium–DTPA also enhances metastatic lesions (Fig. 24–66).

After the scout and gradient-echo images, transverse T1 and T2 weighted spin-echo images are obtained through any region of abnormality identified on the scout images and through the area of clinical symptoms. While these sequences are often sufficient to evaluate metastatic disease, a sagittal or coronal T1 weighted or STIR image of the lesion may be taken as indicated. The addition of STIR imaging can be particularly helpful in cases of metastatic disease involving the soft tissues, since bright-signal-intensity tumor on STIR images can be easily seen and lesion conspicuity is greater than on spin-echo images.[19] The examination requires less time than T2 weighted spin-echo images and in most cases has adequate signal-to-noise ratio.

Metastatic disease is seen most commonly as intermediate signal intensity on T1 and increased signal intensity on T2 weighted images. Metastatic lesions are often well defined, although diffuse lesions can also be seen (Figs. 24–67, 24–68). Surrounding marrow edema can be seen, and periosteal reaction may be prominent. A soft tissue component, if present, can be assessed. The total extent of the lesion can be accurately defined in order to plan radiation ports. It is also important to assess the proximity of the metastatic lesion to physeal plates, the epiphysis, and joints.

We have seen multiple cases of medullary infarcts after therapy for malignancy in children. These children present with bone pain and are often thought to have recurrent or metastatic disease. Obviously the distinction among medullary infarct, medullary infec-

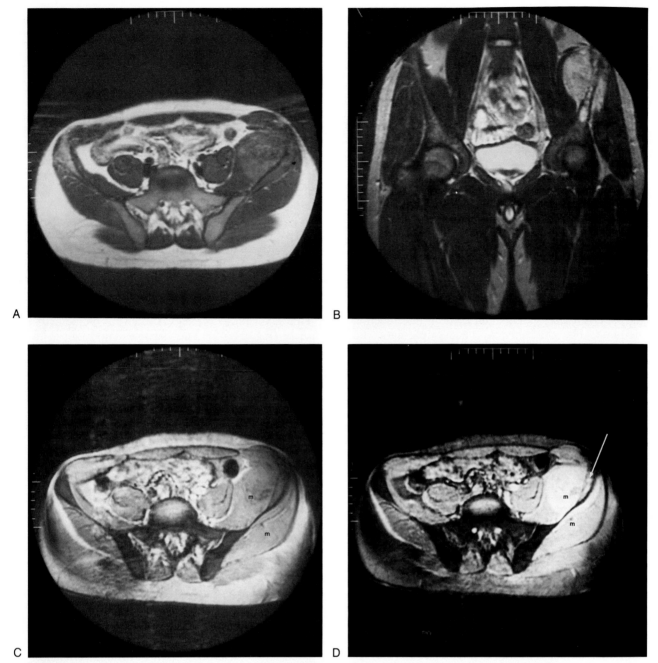

Figure 24–65. *Metastatic Ewing's sarcoma to the pelvis in a teenage boy who had a primary tumor of the scapula several years previously. Effect of imaging technique.* **A,** Transverse T1 weighted image (800/26) shows a poorly defined soft tissue mass on both sides of the left iliac crest, with a slight reduction in signal intensity from the adjacent bone marrow, compared with the opposite side. **B,** Coronal T2 weighted image (2000/80) shows increased signal intensity from both the soft tissue and bone marrow components of the metastasis. **C, D,** Gradient-echo images (500/14) with 90- and 20-degree flip angles. With the 90-degree flip angle the soft tissue mass (m) is well defined but the marrow tumor is less clearly visualized. With the 20-degree flip angle the very bright soft tissue tumor mass (m) is again well seen. The tumor in the bone marrow appears of very strong signal intensity (*arrow*) and is clearly visualized. (Courtesy of Dr. Mervyn D. Cohen, Indianapolis.)

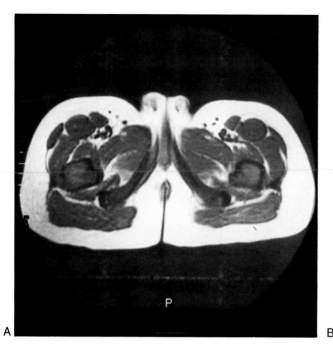

A

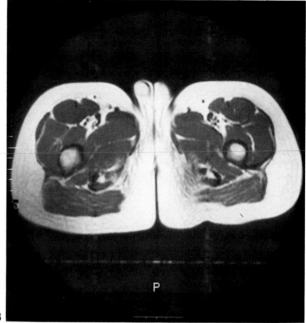

B

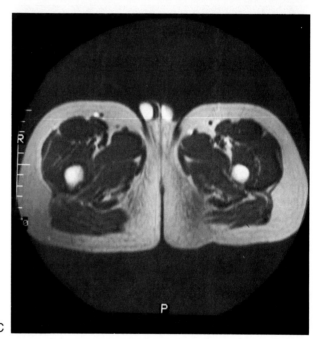

C

Figure 24–66. *Marrow metastases from rhabdomyosarcoma.* **A,** T1 weighted image (800/26) shows homogeneous low signal intensity from the marrow of both proximal femora. **B,** T1 weighted image shows uniform enhancement of the marrow metastasis after gadolinium–DTPA administration. **C,** T2 weighted image (2000/80) obtained before gadolinium–DTPA administration shows very strong signal intensity from the bone marrow metastasis. The signal is stronger than that of subcutaneous fat.

tion, and bony metastases is of significant consequence. Specific criteria for distinguishing these entities are still not clearly known, but in general an ill-defined lesion, especially when present in a metaphyseal or juxta-articular position, exhibiting signal characteristics of edema, may well represent early infarction, infection, or transient ischemia and not meta-

static disease (Fig. 24–69). Inflammatory lesions, particularly infection, are associated with extensive soft tissue and marrow edema. Some marrow edema may be seen with metastatic disease, but it is less pronounced than the marrow and soft tissue edema seen with inflammatory processes such as acute infarction or infection. Older infarcts have a characteristic ap-

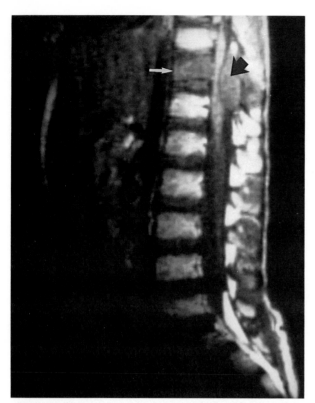

Figure 24–67. *Bone metastasis from Ewing's sarcoma.* Sagittal image through the spine in a 10-year-old boy with metastatic Ewing's sarcoma to the T11 vertebral body (*white arrow*). Intermediate-signal-intensity tumor is seen replacing the vertebral marrow. Posteriorly, tumor is seen compressing the cord (*black arrow*).

pearance and can be easily distinguished from metastatic disease (Fig. 24–70). Most important, MRI has sufficient sensitivity for the detection of metastatic lesions to effectively exclude metastases in the region imaged.

MALIGNANT SOFT TISSUE TUMORS

Rhabdomyosarcoma

Rhabdomyosarcoma represents 10 to 15 percent of all childhood solid tumors. It is a tumor of embryonic mesenchyme in which differentiation of rhabdomyoblasts has occurred.[82] It is an aggressive tumor that can occur in multiple sites and may arise in any part of the body, even in regions where striated muscle is not normally present. The median age of occurrence is 5 years and the presenting symptoms depend on the anatomic site. Of embryonal rhabdomyosarcomas, 35 to 50 percent originate in the head and neck, with the pelvic region the second most common site of occurrence. In the pelvis, the urinary bladder, prostate, vagina, testes and peritesticular tissues, pelvic floor, and perineum are common sites of occurrence.[82] Tumors may arise in the thoracic and abdominal walls, with a predilection for the retroperitoneal space in the abdomen. One-third of cases occur in the extremities and trunk, and arise within the striated muscle. Recurrence is common, as is metastatic disease, which disseminates through hematologic and lymphatic channels. Metastases are found in the lung, lymph nodes, mediastinum, brain, liver, and skeleton. In the skeleton, metastases are most likely to occur in sites of rapid skeletal growth; the metastases, especially in the spine, not uncommonly have an adjacent soft tissue mass. Skeletal metastases occur in 20 percent of cases.[82] Sites include the long bones, pelvis, spine, skull, and ribs. Therapy consists of surgical removal and chemotherapy and radiation therapy in patients with gross or microscopic residual disease.

Grossly, the tumors are solid and may form either a solid or a lobulated mass (the so-called sarcoma botryoides). The "botryoides" morphology is found in hollow viscera such as the bladder, vagina, and com-

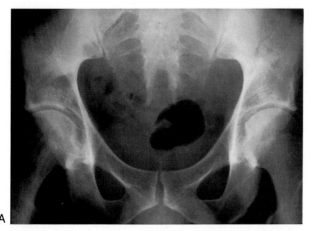

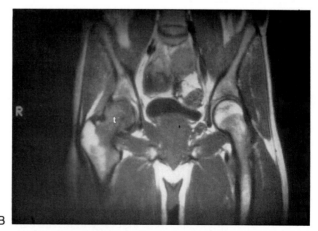

A B

Figure 24–68. *Bone metastasis from melanoma.* **A,** Radiograph and **B,** coronal T1 weighted MR image (500/30) of the pelvis in a 21-year-old man with metastatic melanoma. Although the patient presented with right hip pain and a normal radiograph, MRI shows diffuse replacement of the femoral head and neck marrow by low- to intermediate-signal-intensity tumor (t). The signal intensity of tumor was increased on the T2 weighted image.

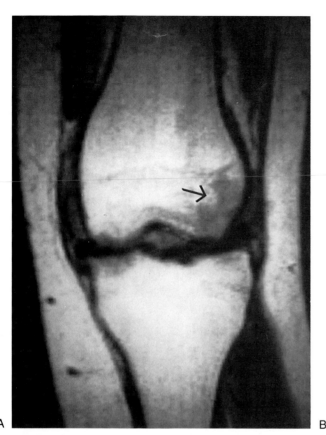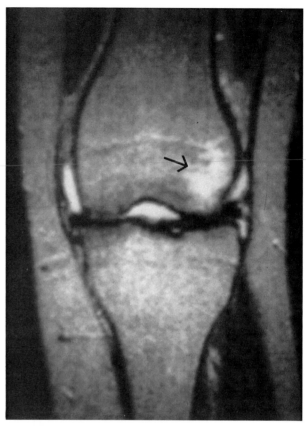

A

B

Figure 24–69. *Acute bone marrow infarct: early infarction in a cancer patient on steroid therapy.* **A,** First-echo (2000/20) and **B,** second-echo (2000/80) images show a juxta-articular, ill-defined, low-signal-intensity region in the lateral left femoral condyle (*arrow*), which increases in signal intensity on the T2 weighted image. A joint effusion is seen. An infarct, and not metastatic disease, was diagnosed.

mon bile duct. Histologically, the tumor consists primarily of small round rhabdomyoblasts, which vary in size and maturation and may or may not contain acidophilic cytoplasm. The tumors usually are fairly homogeneous, although myxoid tissue may predominate with only rare differentiated cells.[82]

Radiologic evaluation is used both in the initial diagnosis of the primary tumor and in the staging of the tumor. Many modalities can be used to identify the tumor mass. The one used for evaluation varies, depending on the site of the tumor. In the extremities, the primary tumor may be identified as a localized or diffuse swelling displacing adjacent soft tissue structures. Displacement of pelvic or colonic structures on intravenous urography or barium enema study may be the only clue to the diagnosis of pelvic and retroperitoneal rhabdomyosarcoma on plain film radiography. CT or MRI can be used to confirm the presence of a primary soft tissue mass that has been suspected on clinical examination or detailed by other imaging modalities.

Metastasis may be identified with many imaging modalities. Bone metastases are hot on bone scans, and on radiographs appear as ill-defined lytic or permeative lesions in the metaphyseal region. Metastatic spread to the lungs is seen on chest radiographs or CT as single,

or more commonly multiple, nodules. Lymph node metastasis causes nonspecific enlargement of lymph nodes seen on ultrasound or CT studies.

MR Appearance of Rhabdomyosarcoma

Little has been written of the MR appearance of rhabdomyosarcoma. It is usually seen as intermediate (equal to muscle) or low signal intensity on T1 (Figs. 24–71, 24–72) and bright signal intensity on T2 weighted images (Figs. 24–72, 24–73).[29, 72, 83] It often has well-defined margins and is relatively homogeneous. It may enhance after gadolinium–DTPA administration (Fig. 24–72). There are no useful MR criteria to distinguish rhabdomyosarcoma from most other soft tissue tumors of childhood. The major role of MRI lies in defining the local extent and staging of the tumor for planning of therapy. Both T1 and T2 weighted images should be taken in all cases, with imaging planes determined by anatomic location. The use of sagittal or coronal images often gives MRI an advantage over CT in defining the total spread of tumor. In different anatomic sites, depending on the adjacent normal tissues, either the T1 or the T2 weighted image will best define the tumor. For example, T2 weighted images are the most useful in the

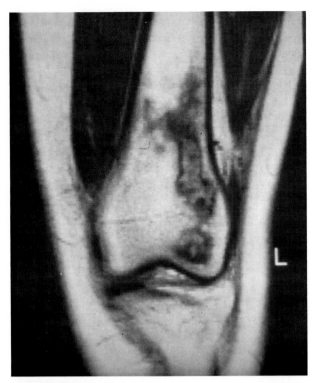

Figure 24–70. *Chronic marrow infarct.* Coronal T1 weighted image (500/30) through the left knee in an adolescent with treated lymphoma and new left knee pain. Bony lymphoma was suspected clinically. MRI reveals geographic, well-defined lesions in the distal femur and juxtacortical region. A low-signal-intensity line circumscribing the lesion represents surrounding sclerotic bone. Marrow signal intensity within the lesion approaches that of normal marrow. On the T2 weighted image the marrow signal intensity within the lesion was isointense with that of normal marrow. This is consistent with an older infarct and not metastatic disease.

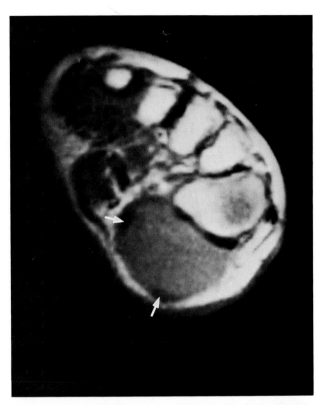

Figure 24–71. *Rhabdomyosarcoma of the foot.* T1 weighted transverse image (800/26) shows a homogeneous, well-defined soft tissue tumor mass (*arrows*). The appearance is nonspecific and there are no diagnostic features to suggest the correct diagnosis. (Courtesy of Dr. Mervyn D. Cohen, Indianapolis.)

limbs, since high-signal-intensity tumor is easily distinguished from intermediate-signal-intensity normal muscle, and exact muscle involvement, violation of tissue planes, and the full extent of the lesion can be appreciated. In the pelvis, retroperitoneum, and body wall, T2 weighted images are also necessary to determine involvement of viscera and musculature. Gadolinium-enhanced T1 weighted images may be most helpful in body regions where motion occurs, degrading T2 weighted images more than the shorter T1 weighted images.

In cases of central nervous system rhabdomyosarcoma, MRI may be preferable to CT in determining the full soft tissue extent of the tumor in the head and neck region and to exclude spread of tumor into the cranial fossa (Fig. 24–72). However, thin-section CT is also needed in cases of rhabdomyosarcoma of the head and neck, since subtle erosion of facial bones (Fig. 24–72) and the base of the skull is not readily appreciated on MRI. As thinner sections become available on MRI, the need for adjunctive CT may be obviated. In the limbs MRI is preferred to CT, because some tu-

mors are isointense with normal muscle on CT. CT is the modality of choice for detection of lung metastases.

Liposarcoma

Liposarcoma, a sarcomatous tumor arising from fatty tissue, may occasionally be seen in infancy or adolescence. In one series of 28 cases, 17 of the 28 occurred in children under 5 years of age. Boys were found to be affected twice as frequently as girls.[84] Given the ratio of one liposarcoma to 120 lipomas, the likelihood of malignant degeneration of lipoma to liposarcoma is rare.[85] Liposarcomas are found in the thigh, buttocks, popliteal region, and retroperitoneum. They can occur in any portion of the extremities, but location in the deep soft tissues is common, whereas location in the subcutaneous tissues is more common for benign lipoma. Depending on the rate of growth and the site of the tumor, children most commonly present with a mass or pain secondary to invasion of surrounding tissues or the neurovascular bundle. Tumors may metastasize but more commonly are locally invasive. Direct extension into bone is uncommon, although erosion of the cortex and scalloping of the cortical contour may be seen.

Pathologically, liposarcoma appears as a grossly nodular mass, apparently encapsulated, with areas of fibrous consistency. The tumor is therefore much firmer than a benign lipoma.[85] Microscopically, the tumors appear well differentiated and consist of myxoid tissue, lipoblasts, and mature fat cells. Poorly differentiated liposarcomas are rich in lipoblasts, connective tissue cells that develop into fat cells. The lipoblasts found in liposarcoma often contain bizarre multinucleated giant cells with vacuolated cytoplasm. In other areas of the tumor, elongated, spindle-shaped lipoblasts may be seen that simulate the cytologic pattern of fibrosarcoma. The more poorly differentiated liposarcomas are fully malignant and have a high rate of recurrence, with frequent metastases.

Radiographically, liposarcoma is seen as a soft tissue mass. The density of the soft tissue mass is variable, depending on the relative amounts of the sarcomatous and fatty elements. The contour is usually irregular, although the pseudoencapsulation often lends a circumscribed appearance to the tumor. Calcification may be seen between fatty lobules, or peripherally with an eggshell pattern. On CT, liposarcomas consist of areas of low and high density. Until the advent of MRI, CT was used to define the extent of the tumor, assess involvement of surrounding soft tissue planes, and assess bone involvement.

MR Appearance of Liposarcoma

Unfortunately, there have been no prospective studies analyzing the MR appearance of liposarcoma; the accuracy, sensitivity, and specificity of MRI in the evaluation of liposarcoma; or the relative value of CT versus MRI in this evaluation. However, several reports[16, 29, 83, 86–88] suggest that some criteria may be useful in the evaluation of liposarcoma by MRI. In general, the MR appearance of liposarcoma reflects the underlying histology of the tumor. Tumors that contain a large percentage of mature fat cells have an MR appearance approaching that of a lipoma (Figs. 24–6, 24–74), with increased (fatty) signal intensity on T1 weighted images, which decreases in an amount commensurate with the subcutaneous fat on T2 weighted images. However, a review of our experience and the cases in the literature suggests that the more aggressive, higher-grade liposarcomas, which contain greater percentages of lipoblasts and connective tissue elements, are seen as intermediate signal intensity on T1 and intermediate to increased signal intensity on T2 weighted images. In a recent report by Kransdorf and associates on soft tissue masses,[83] four liposarcomas were imaged. Of these four, only two showed an MR signal suggesting the presence of fat. It must be hoped that prospective studies correlating the MR appearance of liposarcomas with the underlying histology will enhance our ability to diagnose these lesions on MRI. In reality, however, although the underlying histology of some liposarcomas may be obvious on MRI, a liposarcoma seen as intermediate signal intensity on T1

and increased signal intensity on T2 weighted images cannot be distinguished from many other soft tissue masses, which all appear similar.

Fibrosarcoma

Fibrosarcoma is seen most commonly in young and middle-aged adults, but it does occur in the pediatric population. The soft tissues of the limbs are most frequently involved. The tumor grows slowly and painlessly, so that a large soft tissue mass can be seen at diagnosis. Treatment is primarily surgical with adjunctive chemotherapy. Metastases are seen most frequently in the lungs but occur relatively late in the course of the disease.

Grossly, the tumor is firm, and there is usually no well-defined capsule. The margins are irregular, and extensions of the tumor into the surrounding fascial planes can often be seen.[85] Microscopically, the tumor may be well or poorly differentiated. Well-differentiated tumors contain cellular anaplasia but consist primarily of connective tissue, and in some areas collagen fibers. The poorly differentiated lesions show varying degrees of anaplasia with prominent cellular elements and less connective tissue matrix.

Radiographically, a soft tissue mass can be identified, often with erosion of the adjacent bone cortex, periosteal reaction, and occasionally destruction of cortical bone and invasion of the medullary cavity.

MR Appearance of Fibrosarcoma

The MR appearance of fibrosarcoma is that of most soft tissue tumors, intermediate signal intensity on T1 and high signal intensity on T2 weighted images (Fig. 24–75).[10, 29, 83, 89] The limited experience with fibrosarcoma reported in the literature does not yet show any correlation of the MR appearance with the underlying histology (whether well or poorly differentiated). However, in the cases reported and in our own limited experience, we have not seen cases of fibrosarcoma that remained low in signal intensity on T2 weighted images to any significant degree. Fibrosarcomas can be fairly homogeneous on T2 weighted images, although lesions with underlying necrosis or hemorrhage would appear more heterogeneous. MRI is an excellent tool for staging of fibrosarcoma, with excellent differentiation of tumor from surrounding normal musculature on T2 weighted images. MRI can be used to evaluate involvement of specific muscle groups, adjacent bony involvement, and extension through fascial planes. Since fibrosarcoma tends to be infiltrating, and the signal intensity is similar to that of edema, there may be some difficulty in differentiating edema of the fascial planes from infiltrating tumor. If the increased signal intensity insinuating between fascial planes appears bulky and displaces surrounding musculature, it is likely to represent infiltrating tumor. If, on the other hand, one sees only a feathery increased signal inten-

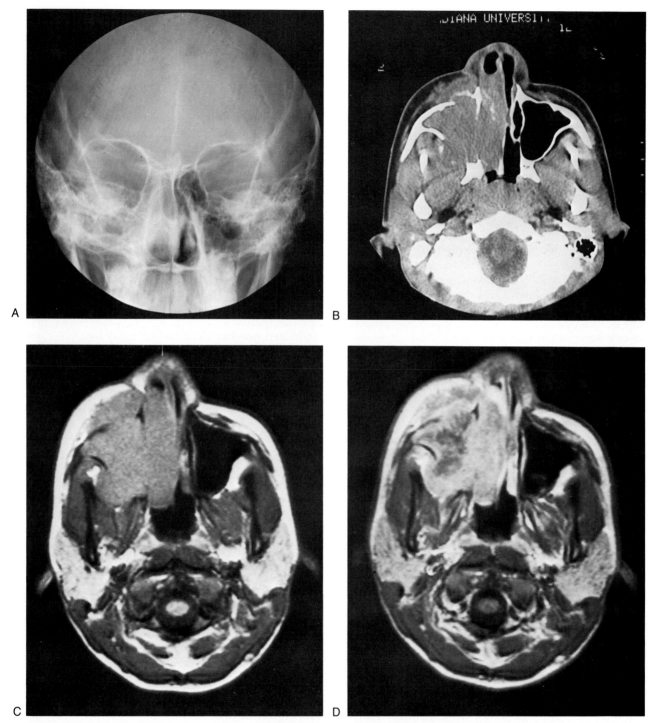

Figure 24–72. *Rhabdomyosarcoma of the face.* ***A,*** Radiograph shows a soft tissue mass in the region of the right maxillary and ethmoid sinuses and right nasal cavity. ***B,*** CT scan shows a large mass lesion filling the right maxillary antrum and the nose. There is partial destruction of all three walls of the sinus. ***C,*** T1 weighted transverse MR image (800/26) shows a well-defined soft tissue mass lesion, homogeneous in appearance. The margins are better defined than on the CT scan. The bony destruction, however, is less well identified. ***D,*** T1 weighted image (800/26) after gadolinium–DTPA administration. There is enhancement of most of the lesion. The enhancement is not uniform, indicating that the tumor is not homogeneous. The reason for the nonuniform enhancement is not known.

Figure continues on following page.

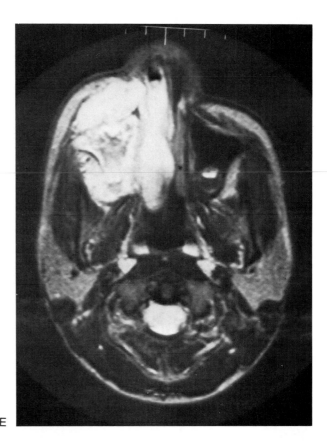

Figure 24–72. Continued.
E, T2 weighted image (2000/80) obtained before gadolinium–DTPA administration. The tumor is bright signal, brighter than on the T1 weighted gadolinium scan. As with the gadolinium image the increase in signal intensity is not uniform and the tumor has a somewhat heterogeneous appearance. The margins of the lesion are much better defined than on the CT scan. Gadolinium–DTPA offers the advantage of improving tumor visualization compared with the nonenhanced image, while giving a better depiction of associated normal anatomy than the T2 weighted image. (Courtesy of Dr. Mervyn D. Cohen, Indianapolis.)

E

sity on T2 weighted images that does not appear bulky, does not invade adjacent muscles, and does not widen the fascial planes or displace adjacent muscles, edema may be more likely. Further work is necessary in this area to determine the reliability of these signs in distinguishing infiltrating tumor from edema.

Angiosarcoma

Primary malignant vascular tumors of bone and soft tissue are rare, making up less than 1 percent of all bone tumors, but they do occur in the pediatric age group. Children with Maffucci's syndrome, or multiple enchondromas and soft tissue cavernous hemangiomas, are certainly at risk for the development of angiosarcoma (hemangio-endothelialsarcoma). Of bone angiosarcomas, 45 percent occur in the long bones, another 26 percent in the flat bones, 11 percent in the facial bones, 10 percent in the vertebral bodies, and 8 percent in the hands and feet.[90] Surgical resection is the treatment of choice, with radiation therapy serving as either an adjunctive or primary form of treatment.

Little has been written on the MR appearance of angiosarcoma. Our experience shows the lesions to be fairly homogeneous, of intermediate signal intensity on T1 and increased signal intensity on T2 weighted images. Both the marrow and soft tissue components

have this appearance. There may be extensive edema (Fig. 24–76). Although the MR appearance is nonspecific, MRI appears to be excellent for staging of these lesions, adequately defining the marrow and soft tissue extent. Since these lesions occasionally are not amenable to surgical resection, accurate definition of tumor margins is important in planning radiation therapy. We have seen one case of angiosarcoma treated by radiation therapy in which the patient developed cystic lesions of the bone after treatment. The lesions in this patient were stable for more than 3 years, and although prospective studies are needed to determine the response of angiosarcoma to radiation therapy, this is one appearance that can be seen (Fig. 24–77).

Hemangiopericytoma

Although primarily a disease of the fourth and fifth decades, hemangiopericytoma can be seen in children and, in fact, has been reported in newborn infants. It is a soft tissue tumor consisting of a rich network of capillaries surrounded by pericytes (specialized contractile cells in the walls of capillaries). It is related to the glomus tumor but does not have the nerve elements seen in that tumor.[90] The patient usually presents with a localized soft tissue mass, which may or may not be painful. Hemangiopericytoma in bone is usually the

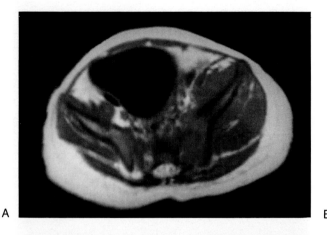

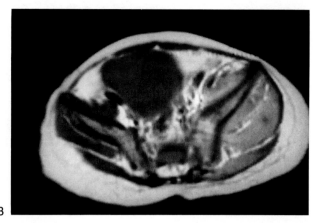

A

B

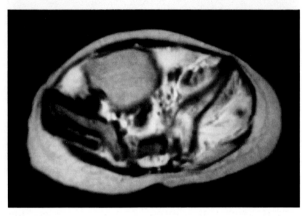

C

Figure 24–73. *Rhabdomyosarcoma. Transverse images through the pelvis in a child with left gluteal rhabdomyosarcoma.* **A,** T1 weighted image (800/20) shows enlargement of the left gluteal and iliac muscles. However, the signal intensity is isointense to that of normal muscle. On longer TR images (**B**) (2000/20) and (**C**) (2000/80), the signal intensity of tumor increases. Increased left iliac marrow signal can be identified (**C**).

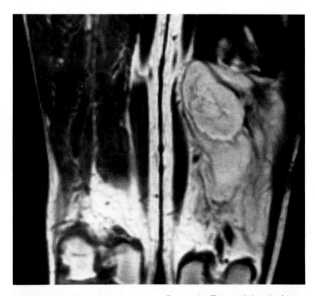

Figure 24–74. *Liposarcoma.* Coronal T1 weighted image (800/20) through the thigh in a 62-year-old patient with an extensive soft tissue liposarcoma. Some regions of tumor show increased signal intensity consistent with fat, but other regions have a more intermediate signal intensity, which increased in signal intensity on the T2 weighted image. The irregular contour, multiple septa, and rapid growth of the tumor are all characteristic of liposarcoma.

result of direct extension of a soft tissue tumor, although in rare cases the tumor may arise directly from bone. The tumor may be self-limited, locally invasive, or aggressive with metastases. The clinical course in patients with tumors that are well circumscribed tends to be self-limited, while the clinical course in patients with infiltrating tumors is usually more aggressive and includes metastatic disease. The radiographic appearance depends on the origin of the tumor; tumors arising primarily in bone appear lytic, while those arising in the soft tissues may cause cortical thickening, periosteal reaction, cortical erosion, cortical destruction, or a medullary lesion. The radiographic appearance depends on the extent of bony involvement.

The MR appearance of hemangiopericytoma depends to some degree on the underlying histology (i.e., whether well defined or infiltrating in appearance) and on the amount of vascularity. In general, the lesion appears as intermediate signal intensity on T1 and increased signal intensity on T2 weighted images. On T2 weighted images of bony lesions, the signal intensity may be either equal to or brighter than surrounding marrow. Serpiginous low-signal-intensity vessels may be seen within the lesion, particularly on T2 weighted images.[91] The MR appearance may not be specific for

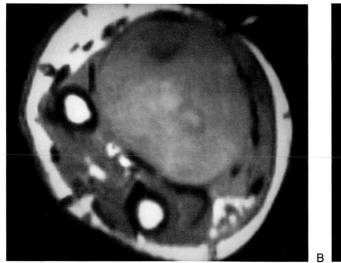
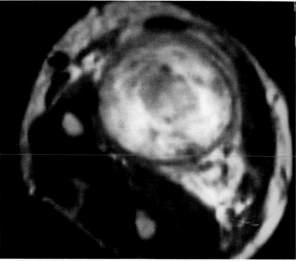

A   B

Figure 24–75. *Fibrosarcoma.* **A,** T1 weighted transverse image (600/20) through the forearm in a patient with malignant degeneration of a neurofibroma to fibrosarcoma. The signal intensity of the soft tissue mass is similar to that of surrounding musculature. **B,** On the T2 weighted image (2000/80) a heterogeneous high-signal-intensity mass is identified.

hemangiopericytoma, but MRI is an accurate tool for pretherapeutic staging of the lesion.

Synovial Cell Sarcoma

Synovial sarcoma, a malignant tumor of epithelioid and spindle cell elements, is a rare soft tissue tumor in children that arises near, but not necessarily from, the synovial lining of joint capsules, tendon sheaths, and bursae. The tumor has been reported in infants, although half of the cases occur in patients between 20 and 40 years of age.[85] Treatment consists of surgical excision followed by radiation therapy. Chemotherapy may be used in an adjunctive role. Metastatic disease, particularly to the lungs, is not uncommon.

Tumors may present either as ovoid, lobulated masses or as diffusely infiltrating tumors. Bone may be invaded. Radiographically, a soft tissue mass is seen, usually near a joint. Calcifications are present in one-third of cases. Fluid may be seen in some tumors. It is usually well loculated.

On MRI, synovial sarcoma most commonly appears as an infiltrating mass, but it can be well defined. There is intermediate signal intensity on T1 (Fig. 24–78) and increased signal intensity on T2 weighted images. Fluid in the tumor has very high signal intensity on T2 weighted images. The tumor has a juxta-articular location, may be separated from the joint capsule by a short distance, or may be invading the joint capsule. Surrounding edema may be seen.[87] MRI can be useful in tracking the synovial sarcoma along tendon sheaths and in assessing invasion of adjacent bone.[92] It may be difficult to appreciate calcifications within the synovial sarcoma on MRI. For this reason, either a plain film or CT should be done as well.

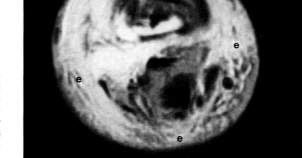

Figure 24–76. *Angiosarcoma.* Transverse T2 weighted image (2050/80) through the distal femora in a 9-year-old girl with right femoral angiosarcoma. An increased-signal-intensity lesion is seen within the marrow. Note the extensive increased-signal-intensity soft tissue edema (e).

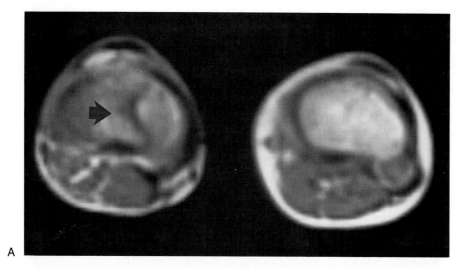

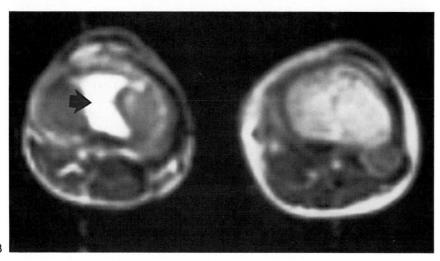

A

B

Figure 24–77. *Cyst following radiation to angiosarcoma. Transverse images through the proximal tibia in a child 2 years after radiation therapy for angiosarcoma.* ***A,*** *T1 weighted (800/20) and* ***B,*** *T2 weighted (2000/80) images. A stable cystic lesion remains in the bone after therapy (arrow).*

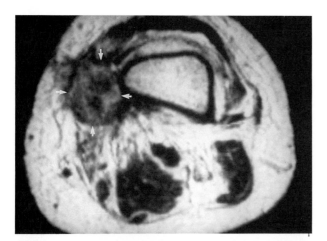

Figure 24–78. *Synovial cell sarcoma.* Transverse long TR image (2000/30) through the distal femur in a patient with synovial cell sarcoma. The lesion is seen as a heterogeneous, low- to intermediate-signal-intensity mass (*arrows*), which is fairly well defined but has some infiltrating components. Signal intensity increased with increasing TE.

BENIGN SOFT TISSUE TUMORS

Lipoma

Lipomas are benign tumors of the soft tissues made up of an accumulation of typical fat cells that may show a variation in cellular pattern from adult cells to small polyhedral fat cells. They may be multiple in 5 percent of cases. They tend to occur on the trunk, proximal upper extremity, and thigh. The patient may present with an asymptomatic mass, although compression of peripheral nerves can result in pain and paralysis. Lipomas are encapsulated but often adherent to the skin, and have a uniform, soft consistency. Rarely, the lipoma does not present as an encapsulated single mass but as a diffuse increase in the adipose tissue, with separation of muscular bundles by thick layers and masses of hyperplastic fat (Fig. 24–79). Radiographically, the tumors appear as a clearly defined radiolucent mass in the soft tissues. The degree of radiolucency depends on the relative amount of ad-

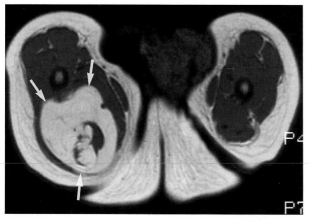
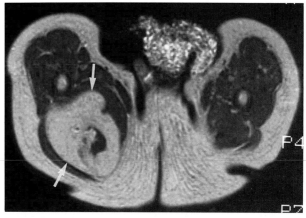

A   B

Figure 24–79. *Lipoma.* **A,** T1 weighted transverse image (800/20) through the proximal femur in a 10-month-old boy reveals a large, increased-signal-intensity lipoma (*arrows*) in the right posterior thigh. The lipoma is infiltrating between muscular bundles. **B,** T2 weighted image (2000/80) shows a decrease in signal intensity of the lipoma (*arrows*) commensurate with that of subcutaneous fat.

ipose and fibrous tissue within the lesion, since these tumors typically contain numerous fibrous septa. Calcification within the mass has been reported. Parosteal lipoma, a deep-seated fatty tumor that arises in or under the periosteum, often causes cortical erosion. In cases of congenital diffuse lipomatosis, hyperplasia of the soft tissues and bones of the affected limb may be seen.

MR Appearance of Lipoma

There have been several reports in the literature of the MR appearance of lipoma and lipomatous tumors.[12, 16, 83, 86, 88, 93] Typically, a lipoma is seen as a well-defined, circumscribed lesion with signal intensity on MR spin-echo images commensurate with that of fat (Figs. 24–79, 24–80), i.e. increased signal intensity on both T1 and T2 weighted images. Septations within the lesion may be prominent but there is typically a lack of edema. Benign lipomas are most commonly seen within the subcutaneous fat, although they may be found in the deep tissue planes (Fig. 24–6, 24–7).

Atypical lipomas are soft tissue tumors that differ from simple lipomas in that they consist of mature fat cells with foci of cellular and connective tissue elements. Pathologically, these lesions may resemble liposarcoma. The MR appearance of three patients with atypical lipoma has been described.[93] Unlike simple lipoma, the MR appearance of these lesions is of areas of typical fat signal intensity and of soft tissue signal intensity, with fairly homogeneous intermediate signal intensity on T1 and increased signal intensity (equal to adipose tissue) on T2 weighted images. Septations within the tumor may be identified as a thin, wispy network of low signal intensity. While the MR appearance of these atypical lipomas would appear to belie the underlying histology (fatty versus cellular), histologic correlation of these lesions with the MR examination has not yet been possible.

In addition to initial diagnosis and pretherapeutic evaluation of lipomatous lesions, MRI can be useful in the post-therapeutic evaluation of the patient. It may be difficult to differentiate atypical lipoma from liposarcoma on the MR appearance alone.

Hemangiomatosis

Hemangioma, a primary neoplasm of either the bone or soft tissue, is a benign and slowly growing tumor arising from newly formed blood vessels.[90] Soft tissue hemangiomas are characterized radiographically by soft tissue density and multiple phleboliths. Hemangiomas may be small and self-limited, or large and invasive. They may be confined to the subcutaneous tissue, to a single muscle, or to bone, or may involve any or all of the tissues of the musculoskeletal system. Clinically, the entire extent of a hemangioma may be apparent on the skin, or the skin lesion may

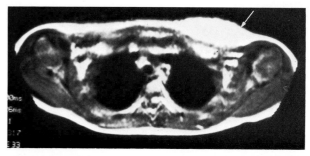

Figure 24–80. *Benign lipoma of the anterior chest wall.* Transverse MR image (1300/26) shows a well-defined, high-intensity mass lesion on the left anterior chest wall. The lesion (*arrow*) is of signal intensity identical to that of the adjacent subcutaneous fat. It is moderately well defined and homogeneous. This is a fairly typical appearance for lipoma. (Courtesy of Dr. Mervyn D. Cohen, Indianapolis.)

represent only a small part of a deep hemangioma. Many deep hemangiomas are not detectable by clinical means.

Pathologically, there are three forms of hemangioma: cavernous, capillary, and mixed. The cavernous hemangioma is characterized by large, thin-walled vessels and sinuses. These vessels are lined by a single layer of endothelial cells. The capillary type consists of fine capillary loops that tend to spread outward in a sunburst pattern. The mixed type have elements of both.[94] Hemangiomas are associated with stroma of fatty or fibrous tissue.

MR Appearance of Hemangioma

There have been several reports describing the MR appearance of hemangioma.[95–101] The spectrum of the MR appearance of extremity hemangioma in 16 patients (mean age 10 years) has recently been reported.[95] In general, the MR image reflects the variable underlying histologic composition of the hemangioma (Fig. 24–81) (densely packed capillary spaces, networks of vascular spaces separated by stroma, adipose tissue, fibrous tissue, calcium, hemosiderin, thrombosis, and hemorrhage).[95, 101] Hemangiomas most often appear heterogeneous and are typically of intermediate signal intensity and serpiginous on T1 weighted MR sequences (Figs. 24–81 to 24–83), while the overall signal intensity is most often increased on T2 weighted images (Figs. 24–82, 24–83). Cases with increased signal intensity on both T1 and T2 weighted images histologically show hemorrhagic change and fatty deposition within the hemangioma.[95, 101] Homogeneous intermediate signal intensity on T1 with homogeneous bright signal intensity on T2 weighted images has also been reported (Fig. 24–84).[100] However, these lesions were small, cavernous, soft tissue hemangiomas with a maximal dimension of less than 2 cm, and may not represent a typical, histologically heterogeneous hemangioma.

There are four criteria that appear helpful in diagnosing hemangioma on MRI.[95] A serpiginous pattern of low to intermediate signal intensity intermixed with areas of intermediate to high signal intensity on either T1 weighted or both T1 and T2 weighted images is highly suggestive of hemangioma (Figs. 24–81 to 24–83, 24–85). Vessels may be seen in the subcutaneous tissues surrounding the lesion (Fig. 24–84), but this appearance is variable, and a lack of feeding vessels in the tissues surrounding the hemangioma does not exclude the diagnosis of hemangioma. The presence of fat and fibrous tissue within a lesion is highly suggestive of hemangioma (Figs. 24–82, 24–83), since few pediatric tumors contain significant amounts of fat. However, the absence of fat does not exclude hemangioma. In general, there is a lack of edema in the tissues surrounding hemangiomas (Fig. 24–85), even when the hemangioma is infiltrating muscle or bone or crossing fascial planes. Soft tissue tumors and inflammatory masses may be associated with edema, and the lack of edema would suggest a more benign process, although recently it has been suggested that some malignant neoplastic processes are not accompanied by edema.[34] Finally, it appears that uninvolved musculature surrounding hemangiomas is either normal or decreased in size (Fig. 24–85). Atrophy or hypoplasia of surrounding musculature suggests a slowly growing process such as hemangioma, and is not usually seen in cases of malignant tumor before therapy, nor with arteriovenous malformations. Primary venous malformations may cause decreased growth by decreasing total perfusion to a limb (Fig. 24–86). Phleboliths, a suggestive finding on radiographs and CT, are not readily identified on MRI.[95] This underscores the need for plain films of any musculoskeletal lesion before MR examination.

MR evaluation of the extent of disease appears accurate, and is the staging procedure of choice in patients with soft tissue masses, including hemangioma.[15, 95, 96] Muscle involvement is best appreciated on T2 weighted images, and subcutaneous fat and intramuscular fat involvement on T1 weighted images. The exact extent of the lesion within muscle, subcutaneous tissue, bone, and fascial planes may be determined on MRI.

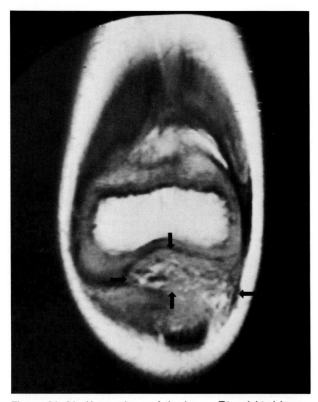

Figure 24–81. *Hemangioma of the knee.* T1 weighted image (800/26) shows a soft tissue lesion (*arrows*) extending into the knee joint, measuring about 2.5 cm in diameter. Within the lesion there are areas of high intermediate and low signal intensity. These correspond to the pathologic specimen, which showed areas of thrombosis, chronic inflammation, and hemosiderin deposition. (Courtesy of Dr. Mervyn D. Cohen, Indianapolis.)

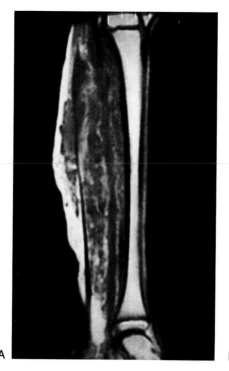
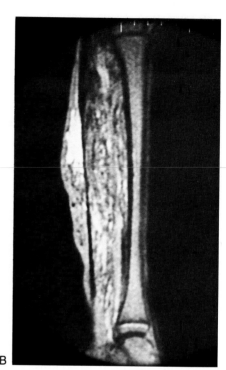

Figure 24–82. *Diffuse hemangioma of the calf: a very large lesion infiltrating most of the subcutaneous fat and muscles of the left calf.* **A,** T1 weighted sagittal image (800/26). The lesion is poorly defined with serpiginous, mixed signal intensity. Note the underlying "fatty" matrix of the lesion. **B,** T2 weighted image (2000/80) with gradient moment nulling. There is a generalized increase in signal intensity throughout the lesion, which remains heterogeneous in appearance. (Courtesy of Dr. Mervyn D. Cohen, Indianapolis.)

Mulliken and Glowacki described two phases of hemangioma: a proliferative phase with high cellular content and an involuting phase with less cellular content.[102] To date, no study of hemangioma has described findings that allow distinction between an involuting and a proliferating hemangioma. There has been some suggestion that the amount of fat within a hemangioma reflects the rate of growth of vertebral hemangiomas,[103] but this was not found to be true in soft tissue hemangiomas.[95]

Juvenile Fibromatosis

Congenital or juvenile generalized fibromatosis is a rare disorder of fibroelastic derivation manifested by locally infiltrating fibrous lesions. The congenital form, usually manifest in the first month of life, is widespread and multiple, with locally infiltrating fibrous lesions involving organs and bones. Although the lesions do not metastasize, they are locally invasive and aggressive, and 80 percent of patients die within the first 4 months of life as a result of involvement of vital organs.[104]

A less aggressive, although potentially fatal, form of the disease has been labeled "aggressive juvenile fibromatosis" or "congenital multiple fibromatosis." These patients show no evidence of visceral involvement, and the fibrous tumors may grow for 3 to 4 months and then regress or remain stable. In other patients the growth of the lesion is relentless and, de-

pending on the site of the lesions, can result in death due to local invasiveness and strangling of vascular structures and normal tissue. If the lesion is in an extremity, amputation may be required to control spread of the disease. The exact factors that determine the aggressiveness of this lesion are unknown.

Pathologically, the lesions are composed of fibroelastic tissue without cellular atypism, mitosis, or pleomorphism. Loss of soft tissue planes is the most common radiographic finding.

MR Appearance of Fibromatosis

There have been anecdotal reports of the MR appearance of juvenile fibromatosis,[7, 29, 72] as well as reports attempting to distinguish malignant from nonmalignant retroperitoneal fibrosis and post-therapeutic fibrosis from tumor recurrence[105, 106] These reports describe the MR appearance of fibromatosis as of low signal intensity on both T1 and T2 weighted images (Fig. 24–87), but many cases of aggressive juvenile fibromatosis imaged at our institution show intermediate signal intensity on T1 and increased signal intensity on T2 weighted images. The lesions appear infiltrating, with some solid masslike components (Fig. 24–88). Desmoid tumors have been reported to be of increased signal intensity on T2 weighted images.[105, 107] MRI appears to be an accurate modality in the pretherapeutic assessment of extent of these lesions, as well as postoperative follow-up evaluations for recurrent fibromatosis.

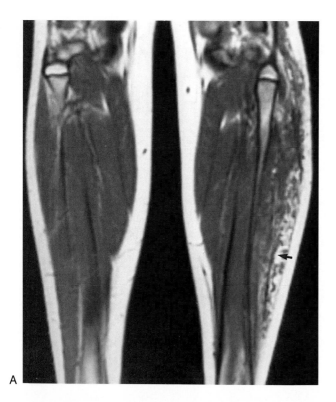

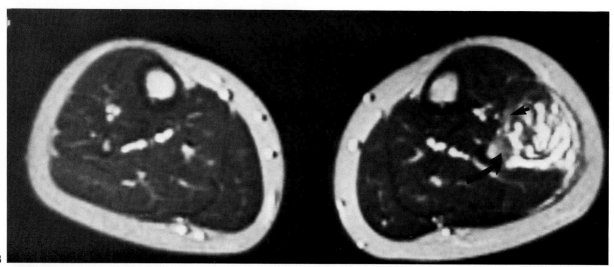

Figure 24–83. *Hemangioma.* **A,** T1 weighted coronal image (800/20) through the calf in an 11-year-old girl with infiltrating hemangioma. An intermediate-signal-intensity serpiginous lesion is seen in the lateral aspect of the left calf. An underlying matrix of high-signal-intensity fat is identified (*arrow*). **B,** Transverse T2 weighted image (2000/80) shows heterogeneous increased signal intensity of the lesion. Invasion of the fibula (*curved arrow*) cannot be excluded. Decreased signal intensity of the fatty matrix, commensurate with that of subcutaneous fat, is identified (*arrow*).

POST-THERAPEUTIC EVALUATION OF MUSCULOSKELETAL TUMORS

With the advent of presurgical adjunctive therapy, the morbidity and mortality rates of most pediatric musculoskeletal tumors have decreased. An imaging tool that allows assessment of this response could make possible more effective use of these adjunctive thera-pies, and for this reason a current focus of radiologic research is the evaluation of MRI in the assessment of the response of musculoskeletal tumors to therapy. Overall, it seems that a decrease in signal intensity of the tumor on T2 weighted images would suggest a response of the tumor to therapeutic interven-tion.[107–111] One study[111] reported the signal intensity of lesions on T2 weighted images following therapy in 60

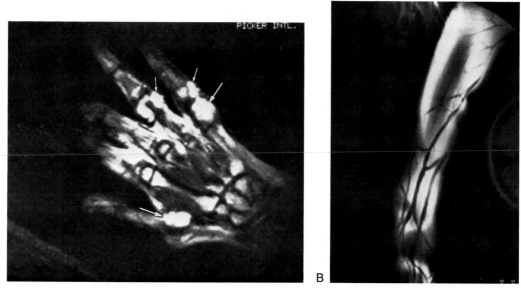

A

B

Figure 24–84. *Multiple hemangiomas of the hand.* **A,** T2 weighted coronal image (1500/80) shows multiple high-intensity lesions (*arrows*), moderately well defined, scattered throughout the hand. **B,** T1 weighted image of the forearm (650/26) shows a marked increase in size of the subcutaneous veins due to increased flow to the hand hemangiomas. (Courtesy of Dr. Mervyn D. Cohen, Indianapolis.)

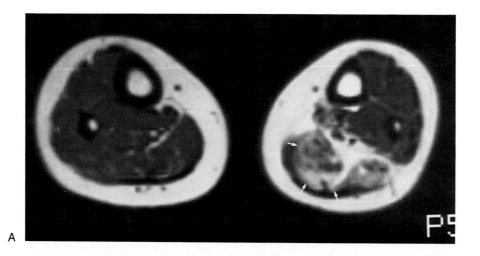

A

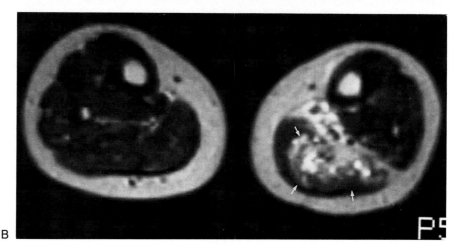

B

Figure 24–85. *Cavernous hemangioma. Transverse images through the calves of a 23-year-old woman with cavernous hemangioma (arrows) of the left calf.* **A,** T1 weighted image (800/20) show a serpiginous intermediate-signal-intensity pattern with atrophy of musculature of the posterior compartment when compared with the right calf. **B,** T2 weighted image (2000/80) shows increased signal intensity of the lesion and lack of surrounding edema.

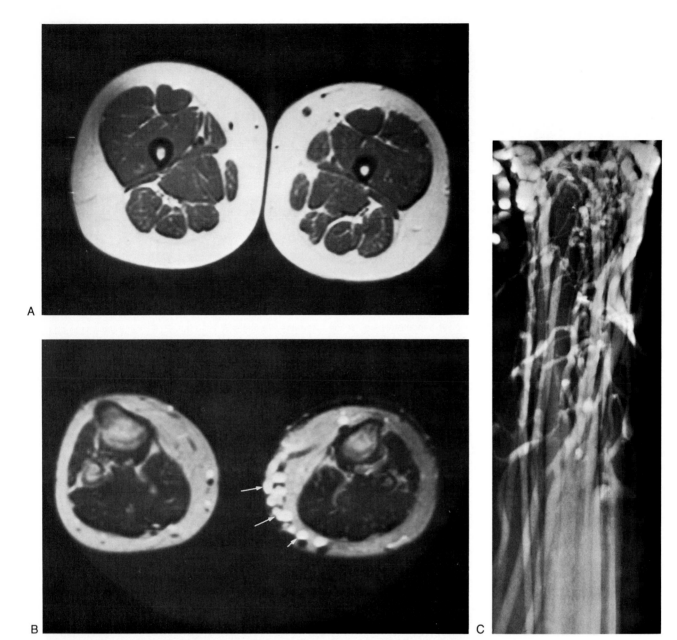

Figure 24–86. *Decreased growth of the left leg as a result of a congenital venous malformation.* **A,** Transverse MR image (2000/20) through the thigh. There is a global decrease in size of the left side compared with the right. **B,** Intermediate weighted image (2000/20) through the calf shows multiple dilated superficial venous channels (*arrows*), the result of a primary venous malformation. **C,** Venogram confirms the presence of the dilated venous channel. An arteriogram showed no arteriovenous malformation. (Courtesy of Dr. Mervyn D. Cohen, Indianapolis.)

patients, 18 with primary tumors of the bone and 42 with primary soft tissue tumors. These patients were imaged after chemotherapy, radiation therapy, and/or surgery. In 20 of the 60, the treated lesion showed low signal intensity on T2 weighted images. Surgical and clinical follow-up revealed residual disease in only 1 of the 20 patients. In the remaining 40 patients, increased signal intensity was noted on T2 weighted images. Of the 30 patients who underwent surgical resection of the lesion, 27 had residual tumor at surgery and 3 had

benign post-therapeutic changes, including edema and cyst formation. The remaining ten patients had either necrosis following radiation therapy (eight patients), dilated veins (one patient), or development of an obvious tumor mass on subsequent MR examinations (one patient).

A second study[109] reported a correlation between a decrease in size and signal intensity on T2 weighted images of the extraosseous component of sarcoma and response to chemotherapy. There was no significant

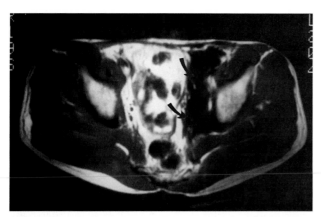

Figure 24–87. *Fibromatosis.* Transverse T2 weighted image (2000/60) through the pelvis in a patient with long-standing fibromatosis. The lesion is of low signal intensity on this image (*curved arrow*). It was also of low intensity on the T1 weighted image.

correlation between decrease in size and signal of the intraosseous component and response to chemotherapy. This suggests that the MR criteria for response of the intraosseous and extraosseous components of musculoskeletal sarcomas may be different, and that decrease in size and signal intensity of the intraosseous portion may not occur despite the histologic response of tumor.

Review of the published reports and images confirms that the accuracy, sensitivity, and specificity of and specific criteria for post-therapeutic MR evaluation of musculoskeletal lesions have not yet been determined. It has been reported that the observance of low signal intensity on T2 weighted images after treatment has a 96 percent sensitivity for indicating the absence of an active neoplasm. When increased signal intensity is seen, the sensitivity for the detection of residual active tumors is 70 percent.[111] These authors reported a 100

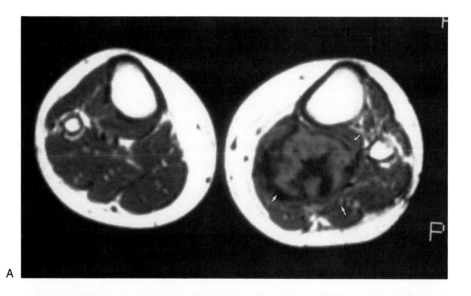

A

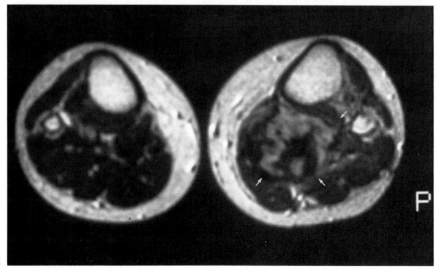

Figure 24–88. *Aggressive fibromatosis seen in transverse images of the calf in an 18-year-old female.* **A,** 800/20. Heterogeneous, predominantly intermediate-signal-intensity calf mass (*arrows*) infiltrating local musculature and fat planes. **B,** 2000/80. On T2 weighted images the tumor (*arrows*) remains heterogeneous in appearance but is predominantly increased in signal intensity.

B

percent accuracy for detection of recurrent tumor, using the criterion of increased signal intensity on T2 weighted images, if patients who receive radiation therapy are excluded, since radiation fibrosis is known to have increased signal intensity.[105, 106, 112] However, many patients with musculoskeletal tumors receive radiation therapy, and therefore a large group of pediatric patients would be excluded. In addition to the problem of increased signal intensity on T2 weighted images as a result of radiation therapy, postoperative fibrosis in the first six months following surgery, or "early" fibrosis, may also be seen as increased signal intensity on T2 weighted images.[105]

Since there appears to be some difficulty in distinguishing between radiation fibrosis, "early" postoperative fibrosis, and recurrent tumor on MRI, we use the following criteria as a practical guide to the post-therapeutic evaluation of pediatric musculoskeletal tumors. First, low signal intensity on both T1 and T2 weighted images is likely to represent post-therapeutic changes and unlikely to indicate residual or recurrent tumor. If the patient has undergone surgery, increased signal intensity in the first 6 months to 1 year may represent postoperative changes, although only if a discrete mass is not present. If a discrete mass or space-occupying increased-signal-intensity lesion is seen on T2 weighted images, this likely represents recurrent tumor and should be biopsied. As a caveat, if the patient is immediately postoperative (first 2 to 3 weeks), this could represent hemorrhage or another acute postsurgical change (Fig. 24–89). The specific signal intensities on T1 and T2 weighted images, as well as the contour of the increased signal intensity, should help in this determination. Conversely, the likelihood that a space-occupying high-signal-intensity mass represents recurrent tumor increases as the time between surgical intervention and the MR examination increases.

Tissue that is feathery and linear and conforms to tissue planes is more likely to represent postoperative change than recurrent tumor (Fig. 24–90). If a patient has undergone radiation therapy, soft tissue edema is not uncommon, and we have anecdotally seen extensive muscle edema in the extremities of patients who received radiation therapy more than 1 year before MRI. We therefore apply the same criteria in post-radiation therapy patients as in postoperative patients: a space-occupying high-signal-intensity mass on T2 weighted images is more likely to represent tumor, while a feathery and diffuse increased signal on T2 weighted images may represent post-radiation inflammation and edema. Obviously the type of underlying neoplastic process must be considered when using these criteria. Synovial sarcoma, aggressive fibromatosis, or some other infiltrating neoplasm is less likely to recur as a space-occupying mass and more likely to recur as an infiltrating process, while rhabdomyosarcoma or Ewing's sarcoma is more likely to recur as a space-occupying mass.

Using the above criteria, we have followed musculoskeletal lesions in children who are clinically stable and do not show physical evidence of recurrent disease by MRI, even in the face of increased signal intensity on T2 weighted images. Each subsequent examination must be meticulously assessed for evidence of increased size or significant change. By using these criteria and the clinical examination, we have been able to avoid frequent post-therapeutic biopsies. However, prospective studies are needed to determine the specific criteria, accuracy, sensitivity, and specificity of MRI in the post-therapeutic evaluation of pediatric musculoskeletal tumors.

Recent reports[108, 110] suggested an expanded role for MRI in the post-therapeutic evaluation of Ewing's sarcoma. These confirm that intraosseous tumor may not change in size[110] or signal intensity[108, 110] after thera-

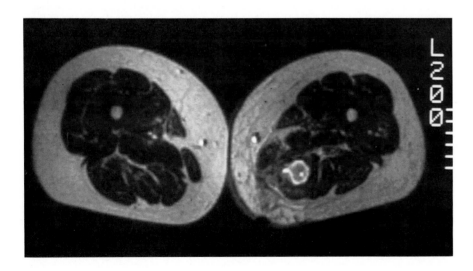

Figure 24–89. *Hemorrhage.* Transverse T2 weighted image (2000/70) shows postoperative hemorrhage in the posteromedial left thigh.

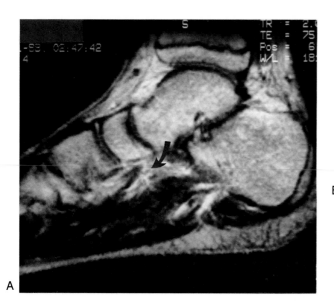

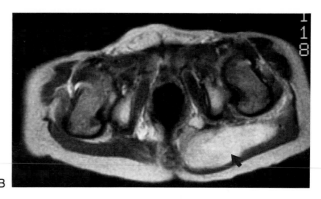

Figure 24–90. *Differentiation of postoperative edema from recurrent tumor.* ***A,*** *Sagittal T2 weighted image (2000/75) through the foot in a boy 4 weeks after removal of tumor. Increased signal intensity from the postoperative edema is feathery and conforms to tissue planes* (*curved arrow*). ***B,*** *Transverse intermediate image (2000/20) through the pelvis in a child with recurrent tumor. The tumor is masslike and distorts surrounding musculature* (*arrow*).

peutic intervention (radiation therapy, chemotherapy) despite the presence of a histologically sterile intramedullary tumor at pathologic evaluation. Therefore, the role of MRI in the post-therapeutic evaluation of intraosseous tumor is unclear. Extraosseous Ewing's sarcoma, however, appears to show a decrease in size or a decrease in overall signal intensity in response to radiation therapy or chemotherapy.[110] A decrease in either size or signal intensity may indicate a response to therapy, but an even higher level of confidence is achieved when the extraosseous extent of Ewing's sarcoma decreases in both size and signal intensity on T2 weighted images.

FUTURE DEVELOPMENTS

There have been several reports describing the utility of gadolinium–DTPA in the evaluation of musculoskeletal lesions.[108, 113–115] In a recent study, static and dynamic MR studies of 69 patients with bone and soft tissue tumors were performed using spin-echo, T1 weighted gadolinium-enhanced, and dynamic gadolinium–DTPA fast low-angle shot imaging (FLASH).[113] Of the 69 patients imaged, 44 had malignant tumors and 25 had benign tumors. The age range of the patients was not given. After intravenous administration of gadolinium–DTPA, the neoplastic tissue exhibited the expected increase in signal intensity within the first 5 minutes. The contrast-to-noise ratio (CNR) between tumor and muscle was approximately 4.5 times higher in the T1 weighted spin-echo images after gadolinium–DTPA administration than in nonenhanced T1

weighted spin-echo images. Comparison of enhanced and nonenhanced T2 weighted spin-echo images showed a 44 percent decrease in the CNR. Only a few benign bone and soft tissue tumors such as lipoma and osteochondroma showed no increase in signal intensity after gadolinium–DTPA administration. While lesion conspicuity compared with surrounding musculature on T1 weighted spin-echo images was enhanced after gadolinium–DTPA administration, the conspicuity of the lesion compared with marrow and subcutaneous tissue was decreased by approximately 40 percent. This was due to an expected increase in signal intensity of the neoplastic tissue on the enhanced images that is then similar in signal intensity to the fatty marrow and subcutaneous fat. It is likely, however, that lesion conspicuity on enhanced T1 weighted spin-echo images would be increased if the patient's underlying marrow were red and therefore intermediate in signal intensity, as is often the case in pediatric patients.

Necrotic, densely fibrous, and sclerotic regions of tumor are all seen as low signal intensity after gadolinium–DTPA administration. To distinguish among these entities, the gadolinium-enhanced T1 weighted spin-echo images are compared with T2 images, with high signal intensity on T2 weighted images seen in necrotic or cystic regions and low signal intensity on T2 weighted images seen in fibrotic, sclerotic regions.

Dynamic studies of the 69 lesions were performed and showed a rapid increase in signal intensity in neoplastic tissue with time. These changes were less pronounced and more gradual in benign tumors. If the tissue enhancement of the FLASH image after gadolinium–DTPA injection is followed over time, the slope of the curve of tissue signal intensity can be calculated as a percentage of the increase of signal intensity over baseline value per minute.[113] These authors found that a slope of 30 percent per minute or higher was associated more frequently with malignant lesions, and a slope of 30 percent per minute or lower was associated more often with benign lesions. The sensitivity for malignant tumors was 84 percent and for benign tumors 72 percent. Much of the overlap was apparently due both to necrotic malignant tumor, which after gadolinium–DTPA had a lower rate of increase of signal intensity, and to aggressive giant cell tumor (classified as benign), which in turn had a higher rate of gadolinium–DTPA contrast uptake.[113]

The use of gadolinium–DTPA holds promise in determining the vascularity of a lesion, the malignant potential of a lesion, and the presence of active (malignant) tissue after therapy, but more work is needed in this area before the role of gadolinium–DTPA in the evaluation of pediatric musculoskeletal tumors can be determined. In one recent study of 27 cases of Ewing's sarcoma (mean age of patients, 14 years) with histologic correlation, it was not possible to differentiate residual tumor from reactive change on MRI, even with gadolinium–DTPA infusion.[108] This is likely due to uptake of the gadolinium–DTPA by reactive tissues that are present in the tumor bed after surgery, radiation, or chemotherapy. One role suggested by several authors for gadolinium–DTPA in the evaluation of pediatric patients is in the elimination of T2 weighted spin-echo sequences by the addition of a gadolinium-enhanced T1 weighted spin-echo sequence, the rationale being that the enhanced tumor can be easily distinguished from the surrounding musculature, as can edema.

However, routine use of only nonenhanced and enhanced T1 weighted spin-echo images in the evaluation of musculoskeletal tumors would not enable distinction of necrotic tissue from sclerotic or fibrotic tissue, and at the present time some T2 weighted imaging is still needed for the complete evaluation of these tumors.

Another area of research is the use of T1 and T2 relaxation times of musculoskeletal tumors for tissue characterization, as well as for the distinction between benign and malignant disease. There have been several reports discussing the relaxation times of musculoskeletal tumors,[17, 86, 116, 117] the most recent of which[116] reports the T1 and T2 relaxation times of 54 primary tumors of the musculoskeletal system. The age range of the patients was not reported. The authors found that musculoskeletal neoplastic disease could, for the most part, be differentiated from normal tissue on the basis of the relaxation time, with prolongation of both the T1 and T2 relaxation values in neoplastic disease. However, the specific histologic type of tissue (benign versus malignant, osteoblastic versus fibroblastic, and so forth) could not be determined on the basis of relaxation times alone, since the ranges of relaxation times for most tumors were similar: approximately 600

to 1500 msec for T1 relaxation time and approximately 40 to 200 msec for T2 relaxation time. Benign lipoma, with a mean T1 relaxation time of 250 msec and a mean T2 relaxation time of 70 msec, was the only musculoskeletal lesion imaged that could be distinguished on the basis of relaxation times alone.

Finally, phosphorus-31 (P-31) MR spectroscopy holds promise in the distinction of benign and malignant musculoskeletal lesions.[107, 118–123] MRI combined with P-31 MR spectroscopy was performed in five children with osteosarcoma. Spectroscopic evaluation showed elevated levels of phosphomonoesters (PME), inorganic phosphate (Pi), and phosphodiesters (PDE) in the osteosarcoma lesions. Both the PME and the PDE peak areas decreased in three of the patients after chemotherapy, while the Pi peak area increased. The remaining two patients were not imaged after therapy. The authors did not find consistent values of phosphorus metabolites to enable characterization of osteosarcoma, but the changes in the PME, PDE, and Pi peaks after treatment were considered statistically significant. Difficulties encountered in spectroscopy of osteosarcomas include decreased resolution of the spectra observed in tumors that are primarily osseous. In general, the larger the soft tissue component of the tumor, the better is the spectral resolution.[119]

A second study of 34 bone and soft tissue lesions (none of which were osteosarcoma) reported the results of phosphorus spectra in 30 of the 34 accessible lesions.[118] P-31 MR spectra were not obtainable in three patients owing to low signal-to-noise ratio (SNR). Biopsy specimen of these three lesions showed hypocellularity, and the low SNR was attributed to this. The spatial resolution varied among the patients, but was similar for both benign and malignant lesions. The P-31 MR spectra of the benign lesions (which included lipoma, hemangioma, myxoma, and desmoid) resembled the P-31 MR spectra of muscle, although the PDE peaks and, in some cases, the PME peaks were larger. In contrast, the P-31 MR spectra of the malignant lesions contained characteristics not found in muscle, including a higher PME-NTP (nucleoside triphosphate) peak ratio and a higher PDE-NTP peak ratio. Therefore, malignant lesions were distinguishable from benign lesions on the basis of significantly higher mean peak ratios of both phosphomonoester- and phosphodiester-to-nucleoside triphosphate. In addition, the peak area ratio of phosphocreatinine NTP was lower and the mean pH was higher.[118] This suggests that P-31 MR spectroscopy may be useful in improving diagnostic specificity, and specifically in distinguishing benign from malignant bone and soft tissue lesions.

There is little doubt that, as we enter the 1990s, magnetic resonance imaging will play the major role in the diagnosis, pretherapeutic evaluation, post-therapeutic evaluation, and surveillance evaluation of pediatric musculoskeletal lesions. The goal in diagnosis is to provide fairly specific tissue information and an accurate assessment of the aggressiveness and malignant potential of a lesion. In pretherapeutic evaluation, the goal is to provide specific information as to the extent of the lesion so that the appropriate therapeutic modality is chosen and, importantly, so that lesions amenable to a limb-salvage procedure, rather than amputation, are identified. In post-therapeutic evaluation, the goal is to provide an accurate assessment of the response of the tumor to the therapeutic intervention, and to predict the efficacy of ongoing therapy. An additional goal is to recognize lesions that are "sterile" after therapy and to distinguish these lesions from those with remaining tumor. Finally, the goal in surveillance examinations is to recognize the earliest stages of recurrent tumor, and to accurately distinguish these earliest stages of recurrence from a post-therapeutic response of normal tissue. If these goals can be met, there is a good chance that the morbidity and mortality rates in children with tumors will be reduced.

REFERENCES

1. Ehman RL, Berquist TH, McLeod RA. MR Imaging of the musculoskeletal system: a 5-year appraisal. Radiology 1988; 166:313–320.
2. Kanal E, Burk DL Jr, Brunberg JA, et al. Pediatric musculoskeletal magnetic resonance imaging. Radiol Clin North Am 1988; 26:211–239.
3. Moore SG. MR precisely evaluates musculoskeletal tumors. Diag Imag 1988; 10:282–289, 439.
4. Parker BR, Moore SG. Approaches to malignant disease in pediatric patients. Radiol Rep 1989; 1:282–312.
5. Shellock FG. MR imaging of metallic implants and materials: a compilation of the literature. AJR 1988: 151:811–814.
6. Mechlin M, Thickman D, Kressel HY, et al. Magnetic resonance imaging of postoperative patients with metallic implants. AJR 1984; 143:1281–1284.
7. Aisen AM, Martel W, Braunstein EH, et al. MRI and CT evaluation of primary bone and soft-tissue tumors. AJR 1986; 146:749–756.
8. Bohndorf K, Reiser M, Lochner B, et al. Magnetic resonance imaging of primary tumours and tumour-like lesions of bone. Skeletal Radiol 1986; 15:511–517.
9. Petersson H, Gillespy T, Hamlin DJ, et al. Primary musculoskeletal tumors: examination with MR imaging compared with conventional modalities. Radiology 1987; 164:237–241.
10. Bloem JL, Bluemm RG, Taminiau AHM, et al. Magnetic resonance imaging of primary malignant bone tumors. Radiographics 1987; 7:425–445.
11. Gillespy T, Manfrini M, Ruggieri P, et al. Staging of intraosseous extent of osteosarcoma: correlation of preoperative CT and MR imaging with pathologic macroslides. Radiology 1988; 167:765–767.
12. Wetzel LH, Levine E, Murphey MD. A comparison of MR imaging and CT in the evaluation of musculoskeletal masses. Radiographics 1987; 7:851–874.
13. Bloem JL, Taminiau AHM, Eulderink F, et al. Radiologic staging of primary bone sarcoma: MR imaging, scintigraphy, angiography, and CT correlated with pathologic examination. Radiology 1988; 169:805–810.
14. Sundaram M, McGuire MN. Computed tomography or magnetic resonance for evaluating the solitary tumor or tumor-like lesion of bone? Skeletal Radiol 1988; 17:393–401.
15. Demas BE, Heelan RT, Lane J, et al. Soft tissue sarcomas of the extremities: comparison of MR and CT in determining the extent of disease. AJR 1988; 150:615–620.
16. Totty WG, Murphey WA, Lee JKT. Soft-tissue tumors: MR imaging. Radiology 1986; 160:135–141.
17. Zimmer WD, Berquist TN, McLeod RA, et al. Bone tumors: magnetic resonance imaging versus computed tomography. Radiology 1985; 155:709–718.
18. Moore SG, Sebag GH, Dawson KL. MR evaluation of cortical bone and periosteal reaction in bone lesions: pathologic and radiographic correlation. Book of Abstracts, Society of Magnetic Resonance in Medicine, 1989; 1:19.
19. Moore SG. MR imaging evaluation of bone lesions: comparison of inversion-recovery and spin-echo images. Radiology 1988; 169(P):191.
20. Bydder GM, Young JR. MR imaging: clinical use of the inversion recovery sequence. J Comput Assist Tomogr 1985; 9:659–675.
21. Porter BA, Shields AF, Olson DO. Magnetic resonance imaging of bone marrow disorders. Radiol Clin North Am 1986; 24:269.
22. Sebag GH, Moore SG. Effect of trabecular bone on the appearance of marrow in gradient echo imaging of the appendicular skeleton. Radiology 1990; 174:855–859.
23. Sebag GH, Moore SG. Gradient echo imaging of abnormal bone marrow in the appendicular skeleton. Radiology 1989; 173(P):141.
24. Moore SG, Berry G, Smith JT, Rinsky LA. Extent of marrow and soft tissue involvement in pediatric bone tumors: magnetic resonance and pathologic correlation. AJR 1989; 153:202.
25. Wood BP, Szumowski J, Totterman S, et al. A method of image enhancement in MR of musculoskeletal and subcutaneous abnormalities of children. AJR 1989; 153:202.
26. Brateman L. Chemical shift imaging: a review. AJR 1987; 146:971–980.
27. Totterman S, Simon J, Szumowski J, et al. PEACH in the detection of musculoskeletal lesions. Book of Abstracts, Society of Magnetic Resonance in Medicine, 1989; 1:284.
28. Scotti G, Scialfa G, Tampieri D, et al. MR imaging in Fahr disease. J Comput Assist Tomogr 1985; 9:790–792.
29. Harms SE, Greenway G. Musculoskeletal system. In: Stark DD, Bradley WG, eds. Magnetic resonance imaging. St Louis: CV Mosby, 1988:1323–1433.
30. Gomori JM, Grossman RI. Mechanisms responsible for the MR appearance and evolution of intracranial hemorrhage. Radiographics 1988; 8:427–440.
31. Moore SG, Dawson KL. Red and yellow marrow in the femur: age-related changes in appearance at MR imaging. Radiology 1990; 175:219–223.
32. Wilson AJ, Murphy WA, Hardy DC, Totty WG. Transient osteoporosis: transient bone marrow edema? Radiology 1988; 167:757–760.
33. Pay NT, Singer WS, Bartal E. Hip pain in three children accompanied by transient abnormal findings on MR images. Radiology 1989; 171:147–149.
34. Harkens KL, Yuh WTC, Kathol MN, et al. Differentiating musculoskeletal neoplasm from nonneoplastic process: value of MR and Gd-DTPA. Book of abstracts, Society of Magnetic Resonance in Medicine, 1989; 1:21.
35. Rinsky L. Limb salvage procedures in epiphyseal lesions. Personal communication, 1989.
36. Dick BW, Mitchell DG, Burk DL, et al. The effect of chemical shift misrepresentation on cortical bone thickness on MR imaging. AJR 1988; 151:537–540.
37. Carnesale PG, Pitcock JA. Tumors. In: Edmonson AS, Crenshaw AH, eds. Campbell's operative orthopedics. St Louis: CV Mosby, 1980:1277–1378.
38. Ragsdale BD, Madewell JE, Sweet DE. Radiologic and pathologic analysis of solitary bone lesions. Part II: Periosteal reactions. Radiol Clin North Am 1981; 19:749–784.
39. Wilner D. Osteogenic sarcoma (osteosarcoma). In: Wilner D, ed. Radiology of tumors and allied disorders. Philadelphia: WB Saunders, 1982:1987–2095.
40. Boyko OB, Cory DA, Cohen MD, et al. MR imaging of osteogenic and Ewing's sarcoma. AJR 1987; 148:317–322.

41. Sundaram M, McGuire MN, Herbold DR. Magnetic resonance imaging of osteosarcoma. Skeletal Radiol 1987; 16:23–29.

42. Harms SE. MRI of the musculoskeletal system. In: Scott WW, Magid D, Tieshman EK, eds. CT of the musculoskeletal system. New York: Churchill Livingstone, 1987:171–206.

43. Gillespy T III, Manfrini M, Ruggieri P, et al. Staging of intraosseous extent of osteosarcoma: correlation of preoperative CT and MR imaging with pathologic macroslides. Radiology 1988; 167:765–767.

44. Ellis JH, Siegel CL, Martel W, et al. Radiologic features of well-differentiated osteosarcoma. AJR 1988; 151:739–742.

45. Wilner D. Juxtacortical sarcoma. In: Wilner D, ed. Radiology of tumors and allied disorders. Philadelphia: WB Saunders, 1982:2096–2031.

46. Silverman FN. The limbs. In: Silverman FN, ed. Caffey's pediatric x-ray diagnosis. Chicago: Year Book, 1985:869–915.

47. Wilner D. Ewing's sarcoma. In: Wilner D, ed. Radiology of tumors and allied disorders. Philadelphia: WB Saunders, 1982:2462–2573.

48. Jones BE, Wood BP, Schwartz C, et al. MR appearances of childhood bone tumors. AJR 1989; 153:202.

49. Wilner D. Chondrosarcoma. In: Wilner D, ed. Radiology of tumors and allied disorders. Philadelphia: WB Saunders, 1982:2170–2280.

50. Cohen EK, Kressel HY, Frank TS, et al. Hyaline cartilage-origin bone and soft tissue neoplasms: MR appearance and histologic correlation. Radiology 1988; 167:477–481.

51. Jaffe HJ. Tumors and tumorous conditions of the bones and joints. Philadelphia: Lea & Febiger, 1958:314.

52. Nurenberg P, Harms SE. Magnetic resonance imaging of musculoskeletal tumors. CRC Crit Rev Diag Imag 1988; 28:331–366.

53. Askin FB, Rosai J, Sibley PK, et al. Malignant small cell tumor of the thoracopulmonary region in childhood: a distinctive clinicopathological entity of uncertain histogenesis. Cancer 1979; 43:2438.

54. Jaffe R, Santamaria M, Yunis EJ, et al. The neuroectodermal tumor of bone. Am J Surg Pathol 1984; 8:885.

55. Rousselin B, Vanel D, Terrier-Lacombe MJ, et al. Clinical and radiologic analysis of 13 cases of primary neuroectodermal tumors of bone. Skeletal Radiol 1989; 18:115–120.

56. Pizzo P, Poplack D. Principles and practice of pediatric oncology. Philadelphia: JB Lippincott, 1989:434.

57. Wilner D. Giant cell tumor. In: Wilner D, ed. Radiology of tumors and allied disorders. Philadelphia: WB Saunders, 1982:783–914.

58. Herman SD, Mesgarzadeh M, Bonakdarpour A, Dalinka MK. The role of magnetic resonance imaging in giant cell tumor of bone. Skeletal Radiol 1987; 16:635–643.

59. Wilner D. Osteochondroma. In: Wilner D, ed. Radiology of tumors and allied disorders. Philadelphia: WB Saunders, 1982:271–386.

60. Lee HK, Yao L, Wirth CR. MR imaging of solitary osteochondromas: report of eight cases. AJR 1987; 149:557–560.

61. Spjut KJ, Dorfman HD, Fechner FE, Ackerman LV. Tumors of bone and cartilage. Washington, DC: Armed Forces Institute of Pathology, 1970:84–110.

62. O'Neal LW, Ackerman LV. Chondrosarcoma of bone. Cancer 1952; 5:551–577.

63. Schwartz HS, Zimmerman NB, Simon MA, et al. The malignant potential of enchondromatosis. J Bone Joint Surg 1987; 69A:269–274.

64. Wilner D. Enchondroma. In: Wilner D, ed. Radiology of tumors and allied disorders. Philadelphia: WB Saunders, 1982:387–437.

65. Unger EC, Kessler HB, Kowalyshyn MJ, et al. MR imaging of Maffucci syndrome. AJR 1988; 150:351–353.

66. Wilner D. Simple (juvenile) bone cyst. In: Wilner D, ed. Radiology of tumors and allied disorders. Philadelphia: WB Saunders, 1982:921–1002.

67. Wilner D. Aneurysmal bone cyst. In: Wilner D, ed. Radiology of tumors and allied disorders. Philadelphia: WB Saunders, 1982:1003–1103.

68. Beltran J, Simon DC, Levy M, et al. Aneurysmal bone cysts: MR imaging at 1.5T. Radiology 1986; 158:689–690.

69. Munk PL, Helms CA, Holt RG, et al. MR imaging of aneurysmal bone cysts. AJR 1989; 153:99–101.

70. Campanna R, Van Horn JR, Biagini R, Ruggieri P. Aneurysmal bone cyst of the sacrum. Skeletal Radiol 1989; 18:109–113.

71. Cory DA, Fritsch SA, Cohen MD, et al. Aneurysmal bone cysts: imaging findings and embolotherapy. AJR 1989; 153:369–373.

72. Moore SG, Stoller DW. Pediatric musculoskeletal magnetic resonance imaging. In: Stoller DW, ed. Magnetic resonance imaging in orthopedics and rheumatology. Philadelphia: JB Lippincott, 1989:23–61.

73. Kransdorf MJ, Utz JA, Gilkey FW, Berrey BH. MR appearance of fibroxanthoma. J Comput Assist Tomogr 1988; 12:612–615.

74. Wilner D. Fibrous defects of bone. In Wilner D, ed. Radiology of tumors and allied disorders. Philadelphia: WB Saunders, 1982:551–611.

75. Wilner D. Osteoid osteoma. In: Wilner D, ed. Radiology of tumors and allied disorders. Philadelphia: WB Saunders, 1982:144–216.

76. Glass RBJ, Poznanski AK, Fisher MR, et al. MR imaging of osteoid osteoma. J Comput Assist Tomogr 1986; 10:1065.

77. Mahboubi S. CT appearance of nidus in osteoid osteoma. J Comput Assist Tomogr 1986; 10:457–459.

78. Wilner D. Benign osteoblastoma. In: Wilner D, ed. Radiology of tumors and allied disorders. Philadelphia: WB Saunders, 1982:217–270.

79. Harms SE, Greenway G. Musculoskeletal system. In: Stark SS, Bradley WG, eds. Magnetic resonance imaging. St Louis: CV Mosby, 1988:1374.

80. Wilner D. Benign chondroblastoma. In: Wilner D, ed. Radiology of tumors and allied disorders. Philadelphia: WB Saunders, 1982:453–510.

81. Cohen EK, Kressel HY, Frank TS, et al. Hyaline cartilage-origin bone and soft-tissue neoplasms: MR appearance and histologic correlation. Radiology 1988; 167:477–481.

82. Wilner D. Other malignant disorders of childhood. In: Wilner D, ed. Radiology of tumors and allied disorders. Philadelphia: WB Saunders, 1982:3408–3418.

83. Kransdorf MJ, Jelinek JS, Moser RP Jr, et al. Soft-tissue masses: diagnosis using MR imaging. AJR 1989; 153:541–547.

84. Kauffman SL, Stout AP. Lipoblastic tumors of children. Cancer 1959; 12:912.

85. Wilner D. Soft tissue tumors. In: Wilner D, ed. Radiology of tumors and allied disorders. Philadelphia: WB Saunders, 1982:3408–3418.

86. Dooms GC, Hricak H, Solitto PA, Higgins CB. Lipomatous tumors and tumors with fatty component: MR imaging potential and comparison of MR and CT results. Radiology 1985; 157:479–483.

87. Stoller DW. The knee. In: Stoller DW, ed. Magnetic resonance imaging in orthopedics and rheumatology. Philadelphia: JB Lippincott, 1989:23–61.

88. Sundaram M, McGuire MN, Schajowicz F. Soft-tissue masses: histologic basis for decreased signal (short T2) on T2-weighted MR images. AJR 1987; 148:1247–1250.

89. Stoller DW, Crues JV. The shoulder. In: Stoller DW, ed. Magnetic resonance imaging in orthopedics and rheumatology. Philadelphia: JB Lippincott, 1989:264–283.

90. Wilner D. Malignant vascular tumors of bone. In: Wilner D, ed. Radiology of tumors and allied disorders. Philadelphia: WB Saunders, 1982:2140–2416.

91. Stoller, Genant HK. The Hip. In: Stoller DW, ed. Magnetic resonance imaging in orthopedics and rheumatology. Philadelphia: JB Lippincott, 1989:215–263.

92. Sundarem M, McGuire MH, Fletcher J, et al. MR imaging of lesions of synovial origin. Skeletal Radiol 1986; 15:133.

93. Bush CH, Spanier S, Gillespy T III. Imaging of atypical lipomas of the extremities: report of three cases. Skeletal Radiol 1988; 17:472–475.

94. Wilner D. Benign tumors and tumorous conditions of bone. In:

Wilner D, ed. Radiology of tumors and allied disorders. Philadelphia: WB Saunders, 1982:662–704.

95. Sebag GH, Moore SG, Parker BR. Magnetic resonance imaging of pediatric musculoskeletal hemangioma. AJR 1989; 153:202.

96. Cohen JM, Weinreb JC, Redman HC. Arteriovenous malformations of the extremities: MR imaging. Radiology 1986; 158:475–479.

97. Yuh WTC, Kathol MN, Sein MA, et al. Hemangiomas of skeletal muscle: MR findings in five patients. AJR 1987; 149:765–768.

98. Kaplan PA, Williams SM. Mucocutaneous and peripheral soft-tissue hemangiomas: MR imaging. Radiology 1987; 163: 163–166.

99. Ross JS, Masaryk TJ, Modic MT, et al. Vertebral hemangiomas: MR imaging. Radiology 1987; 165:165–169.

100. Levine E, Wetzel LH, Neff JR. MR imaging of extrahepatic cavernous hemangiomas. AJR 1986; 147:1299–1304.

101. Cohen EK, Kressel HY, Perosio T, et al. MR imaging of soft tissue hemangiomas: correlation with pathologic findings. AJR 1988; 150:1079–1081.

102. Mulliken JB, Glowacki J. Hemangiomas and vascular malformations in infants and children: a classification based on endothelial characteristics. Plast Reconstr Surg 1982; 69:412–420.

103. Laredo JD, Gilbert F, Assouline E, et al. Fat content: clue for evaluation of aggressiveness in vertebral hemangiomas. Radiology 1988; 169(P):101.

104. Wilner D. Fibromatosis. In: Wilner D, ed. Radiology of tumors and allied disorders. Philadelphia: WB Saunders, 1982: 4031–4035.

105. Ebner F, Kressel HY, Mintz MC, et al. Tumor recurrence versus fibrosis in the female pelvis: differentiation with MR imaging at 1.5T. Radiology 1988; 166:333–340.

106. Glazer NS, Lee JKT, Levitt RG, et al. Radiation fibrosis: differentiation from recurrent tumor by MR imaging. Radiology 1985; 156:721–726.

107. Ross B, Helsper JT, Cox IJ, et al. Osteosarcoma and other neoplasms of bone: magnetic resonance spectroscopy to monitor therapy. Arch Surg 1987; 122:1464–1469.

108. Frouge C, Vanel D, Coffre C, et al. The role of magnetic resonance imaging in the evaluation of Ewing sarcoma. Skeletal Radiol 1988; 17:387–392.

109. Fletcher BD, Lemmi MA, Slade WT, Marina N. MRI signal changes associated with therapy of Ewing sarcoma. AJR 1989; 153:202.

110. Holscher NC, Bloem JL, Nooy MA, et al. The value of MR imaging to monitor the effect of chemotherapy in bone sarcomas. AJR 1990; 154:763–769.

111. Vanel D, Lacombe M-J, Couanet D, et al. Musculoskeletal tumors: follow up with MR imaging after treatment with surgery and radiation therapy. Radiology 1987; 164:243–245.

112. Arrive L, Hricak H, Taveres NJ, Miller TR. Malignant versus nonmalignant retroperitoneal fibrosis: differentiation with MR imaging. Radiology 1989; 172:139–143.

113. Erlemann R, Reiser MR, Peters PE, et al. Musculoskeletal neoplasms: static and dynamic Gd-DTPA-enhanced MR imaging. Radiology 1989; 171:767–773.

114. Pettersson N, Eliasson J, Egund N, et al. Gadolinium-DTPA enhancement of soft tissue tumors in magnetic resonance imaging—preliminary clinical experience in five patients. Skeletal Radiol 1988; 17:319–323.

115. Pettersson N, Ackerman N, Kaude J, et al. Gadolinium-DTPA enhancement of experimental soft tissue carcinoma and hemorrhage in magnetic resonance imaging. Acta Radiol 1987; 28:75–78.

116. Pettersson H, Slone RM, Spanier S, et al. Musculoskeletal tumors: T1 and T2 relaxation times. Radiology 1988; 167:783–785.

117. Reiser M, Rupp N, Heller NJ, et al. MR in the diagnosis of malignant soft tissue tumours. Eur J Radiol 1984; 4:288–293.

118. Negendank WG, Crowley MG, Ryan JR, et al. Bone and soft-tissue lesions: diagnosis with combined H1 MR imaging and P-31 MR spectroscopy. Radiology 1989; 173:181–188.

119. Redmond OM, Stack JP, Dervan PA, et al. Osteosarcoma: use of MR imaging and MR spectroscopy in clinical decision making. Radiology 1989; 172:811–815.

120. Nidecker AC, Muller S, Aue WP, et al. Extremity bone tumors: evaluation by P-31 MR spectroscopy. Radiology 1985; 157:167–174.

121. Ng TC, Majors AW, Meany TF. In vivo MR spectroscopy of human subjects with a 1.4T whole body MR imager. Radiology 1986; 158:517–520.

122. Oberhaensli RD, Bore PJ, Rampling RP, et al. Biochemical investigation of human tumours in vivo with phosphorus-31 magnetic resonance spectroscopy. Lancet 1986; 2:8–11.

123. Semmler W, Gademann G, Bechert-Baumann P, et al. Monitoring human tumor response to therapy by means of P-31 MR spectroscopy. Radiology 1988; 16:533–539.

Infectious, Traumatic, Mechanical, Collagen, and Miscellaneous Disorders of the Musculoskeletal System

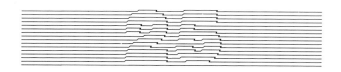

INFECTION

Mervyn D. Cohen, M.B., Ch.B.

Osteomyelitis

Osteomyelitis is a potentially debilitating infection that, if diagnosed early, can be cured with antibiotic therapy and sometimes operative drainage and debridement. Unfortunately the diagnosis is often made late, and complications of delayed or inadequate treatment occur. These include bone deformity, avascular necrosis, and chronic infection with sinus drainage. Pathologically the infection may enter the bone by one of two routes. In most cases the organism is spread in the bloodstream, being carried from a more distant focus of infection; in a few patients it may invade the bone directly. These situations occur following an open fracture, a penetrating wound, or surgery, or in the presence of a foreign body. Osteomyelitis may occur in children who are otherwise healthy, but there is an increased incidence in debilitated patients, e.g., children with leukemia. A large number of bacteria may cause osteomyelitis; staphylococci are by far the most common and account for about 85 percent of cases. *Salmonella* is particularly common in children with sickle cell disease, and *Pseudomonas* is common from penetrating injuries, e.g., from a nail. Osteomyelitis is usually a single focus of infection but can occasionally be multifocal. Multifocal osteomyelitis is most common in children in whom there is an indwelling vascular catheter, especially newborn infants or children in whom native resistance is decreased. Hematogenous osteomyelitis always starts in the spongy part of solid bones. In long bones the infection almost always starts in the metaphysis. This is because the metaphysis has an abundant blood supply and is fed by end arteries ending in abundant slow-flowing capillaries. When infection occurs, there is very early hyperemia with the production of inflammatory fluid. The infection then spreads from the marrow through the cortex to the periosteum. The periosteum in children strips easily and is readily elevated by the spreading infection. Reactive inflammation or direct spread of the infection into the adjacent soft tissues is extremely common.

In children under the age of 1 year the blood vessels frequently cross the growth plate, so that in this age group it is very common for metaphyseal osteomyelitis to spread across the growth plate into the epiphysis and the adjacent joint cavity.

With chronic infection, bone infarction occurs. Areas of dead bone (sequestrum) act as continuing ongoing sources of recurrent infection because, with a very poor blood supply, they cannot be reached with antibiotics. A Brodie's abscess is a well-delineated focus of chronic infection (an abscess) in a region of chronic osteomyelitis.

Clinical Findings

The usual clinical findings in osteomyelitis are pain, local tenderness, fever, elevated blood white blood cell count, and elevated erythrocyte sedimentation rate. The findings are often nonspecific.

Investigations

The diagnosis of osteomyelitis is often difficult. Plain film radiographs are normal in the first few days of the illness (Figs. 25–1 to 25–3). The earliest findings are soft tissue swelling and periosteal elevations. When abnormal, the plain film findings are often nonspecific (Fig. 25–4).[1,2] Nuclear medicine studies are sensitive but miss approximately 10 percent of cases of acute osteomyelitis; positive findings are nonspecific.[2–4] MDP bone scan may not be as sensitive as magnetic resonance imaging (MRI). In one study MRI was positive in six of six patients while bone scan was positive in only five of six patients.[5] The problems with nuclear medicine bone scanning are that accuracy is decreased when patients are already on antibiotics, and there is relatively poor spatial resolution compared with other studies; for example, it may be difficult sometimes to separate soft tissue from bone infection. Indium-labeled white blood cell studies may be positive in osteomyelitis and may be helpful in localizing infection.[3] However, positive findings are nonspecific because the labeled white cells may be taken up by other disorders, e.g., hematomas. They may also be negative in chronic osteomyelitis or in patients who have been on antibiotics. Another disadvantage of some nuclear medicine studies is that they may take a day or longer to perform.

The disadvantages of plain films are that they are not positive for several days, the findings are nonspecific, they are poor at detecting soft tissue abnormality, and in the follow-up of chronic disease they are very poor for evaluating disease status.

There are few reports regarding the use of computed tomography (CT) in the diagnosis of acute osteomyelitis. CT is very sensitive for early detection of bone destruction and periosteal reaction, but probably is not as sensitive as MRI for early detection of abnormality in the bone marrow. In addition, CT is not as sensitive as MRI for identifying inflammation in the adjacent soft tissues.

MR Findings in Acute Osteomyelitis

MRI is extremely sensitive in early identification of acute osteomyelitis (Fig. 25–3). No good studies are yet reported comparing MRI and nuclear medicine for the early detection of osteomyelitis. I strongly believe, however, that MRI will prove to be at least as sensitive as MDP bone scan, if not more so, in the early evaluation of children with suspected acute osteomyelitis. The earliest findings are seen in the bone marrow. On T1 weighted images there is reduction in signal of the normal bone marrow (Figs. 25–1 to 25–3, 25–5). The interface between normal and abnormal marrow is usually poorly defined (Fig. 25–2). On T2 weighted images the marrow may be of normal, or frequently of increased signal intensity. In some reports in the literature these characteristic findings have not been identified and the diseased marrow has been seen to be

Text continues on page 918.

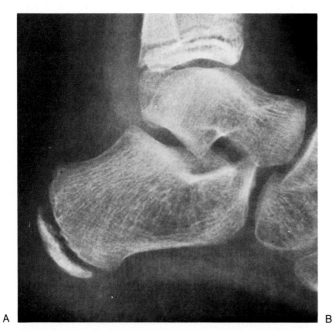
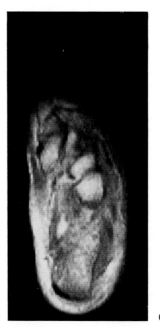
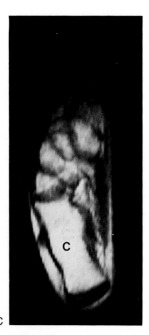

A   B   C

Figure 25–1. *Acute osteomyelitis of the calcaneus in a 10-year-old boy with pain in the heel.* **A,** Plain film radiograph reveals no definite abnormality in the calcaneus. The soft tissues are swollen. **B,** T1 weighted image (500/30). There is patchy loss of signal from almost all of the bone marrow in the calcaneus. There are no margins between normal and abnormal marrow. The outlines of the bones are poorly defined. The soft tissues are swollen and of decreased intensity compared with normal. The interface between muscles and subcutaneous fat is lost and there is patchy decreased signal in the fat due to inflammatory edema. This image was obtained on the same day as **A. C,** The opposite normal foot is shown for comparison. Note the homogeneous strong-intensity signal from the marrow of the calcaneus (C).

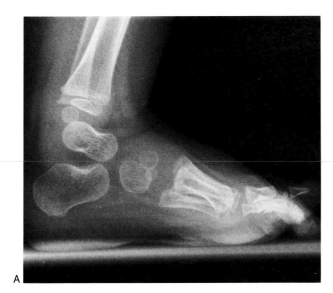

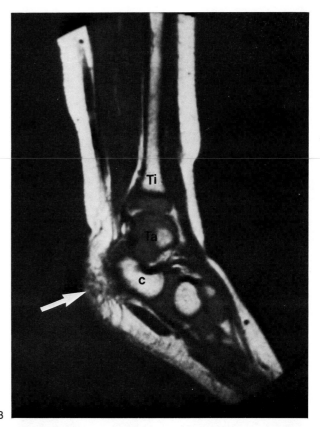

Figure 25–2. *Early calcaneal osteomyelitis in a young child with heel pain.* **A,** Lateral radiograph of the foot is normal. **B,C,** Lateral MR images obtained with T1 weighting (500/16). There is mottled low signal intensity from the fat in the posterior aspect of the heel (*arrow*). There is decreased signal intensity from the posterior half of the calcaneus (in *C*) with poor interface between normal and abnormal bone marrow. These findings are consistent with acute osteomyelitis. Ti, Tibia; Ta, talus; c, calcaneus.

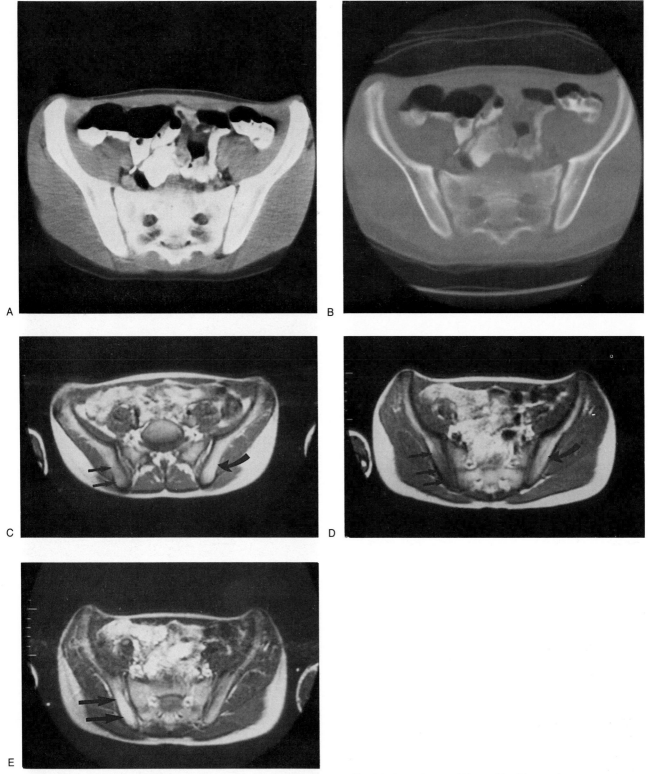

Figure 25–3. *Osteomyelitis of the iliac bone with extension into the sacroiliac joint in a 13-year-old boy with a history of fever and right pelvic and hip pain. Plain film radiographs were normal.* ***A, B,*** Soft tissue and bone windows from a CT scan through the sacroiliac joint. No bone or soft tissue abnormality can be identified. ***C, D,*** Transverse T1 MR images (800/26) through the iliac bones and sacroiliac joint. Moderately extensive decrease in signal intensity in the bone marrow is seen in the posterior part of the right iliac bone (*straight arrows*). Compare this with the uniform strong signal obtained from the opposite side (*curved arrows*). ***E,*** T2 weighted image (2000/80) showing increase in signal intensity (*arrows*) in the posterior aspect of the right iliac bone corresponding to the abnormality seen on the T1 weighted images. The appearance is consistent with the diagnosis of osteomyelitis. In this patient MRI proved very sensitive for demonstration of disease. Even the CT scan was negative.

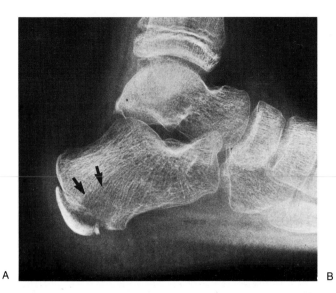

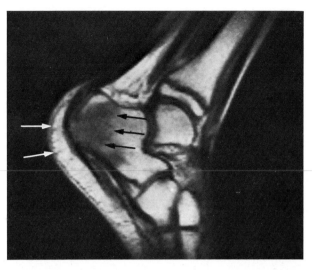

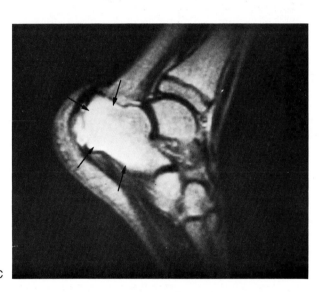

Figure 25–4. *Partially treated chronic osteomyelitis of the calcaneus.* ***A,*** Lateral radiograph. There is a mottled decrease in density in the posteroinferior aspect of the calcaneus (*arrows*). ***B,*** T1 weighted MR image (600/30). There is extensive low signal abnormality affecting about half of the posteroinferior aspect of the calcaneus. The lesion is more extensive than that seen on the plain film radiograph. The margins between the normal and diseased bone marrow are moderately well defined (*black arrows*). There is very minimal patchy irregularity of signal in the overlying fat (*white arrows*). ***C,*** T2 weighted image (2000/120). There is increased signal in the affected area of the calcaneus (*arrows*). The relatively good interface between normal and abnormal marrow, and the very minimal amount of soft tissue abnormality, favor chronic rather than acute osteomyelitis.

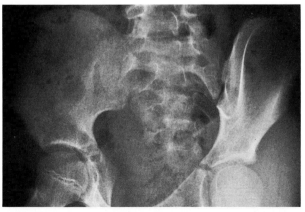

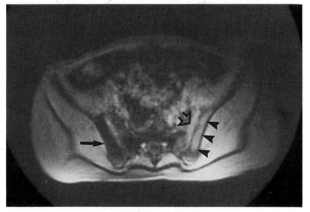

Figure 25–5. *Left sacroiliitis in a 7-year-old boy with a history of fever, left hip pain, and limp.* ***A,*** Plain film radiograph. This oblique view of the sacroiliac joint is normal. ***B,*** Field-echo T2 weighted transverse MR image (500/12), 20-degree tip angle. With this pulse sequence, normal bone marrow appears dark. The normal right iliac bone has a low marrow signal intensity (*black arrow*). There is strong signal intensity from the bone marrow of the left posterior iliac bone (*arrowheads*) and also from the adjacent sacrum (*open arrow*).

isointense with normal marrow on one or other of the pulse sequences.[2,5-7] Some workers have speculated that this may be due to some peculiarity of the disease process in some patients, but I believe it is purely a reflection of the pulse sequences used and that if one uses sequences with strong enough T1 or T2 weighting, one will see the typical findings of low signal on T1 and increased signal on T2 images. In the spine, acute osteomyelitis is diagnosed by identification of decreased signal on T1 weighted images from the vertebral bodies and from the adjacent discs with loss of margins between the disc and the vertebral body.[1] The signal intensity of the diseased structures increases on T2 images (Fig. 25–4). The decrease in signal on T1 weighted images in the marrow of long bones with acute osteomyelitis is usually homogeneous but it may be patchy.[5] In the very early hours of acute osteomyelitis the abnormality is confined to the bone marrow, but it very quickly spreads through the periosteum and causes a reaction in the soft tissues. By the time most patients with acute osteomyelitis are scanned with MRI, increased signal intensity can be identified in the soft tissues on T2 weighted images. This involves the muscle and subcutaneous tissues. Ill-defined decrease in signal in the subcutaneous fat on T1 weighted images reflects extension of the inflammatory process through the muscles into the more superficial tissues (Fig. 25–1). In 35 patients with suspected acute osteomyelitis, MRI was accurate in identifying disease in all 12 patients who were subsequently proved to have osteomyelitis.[4] In 11 of these 12, there was abnormality in the soft tissues as well as the bone marrow.

MR Findings in Chronic Osteomyelitis

In chronic osteomyelitis (Fig. 25–6), areas of bone sclerosis and overgrowth are seen as signal void on all pulse sequences (Fig. 25–7, 25–8). Areas of ongoing infection of the bone marrow are seen as regions of low signal intensity on T1 images, with increase in signal intensity on T2 images (Figs. 25–7, 25–9). The interface between normal and diseased marrow is often quite good (Fig. 25–4). Sinus tracts are identified on T2 weighted images as linear tracts extending from the skin to the bone.[8] Sequestra are seen as small areas of low signal against a background of high signal from the adjacent inflamed soft tissue (Fig. 25–9). Brodie's abscess is seen as a region of very high signal intensity on T2 weighted images against a background of low signal intensity from the dense bone in which the abscess is embedded (Fig. 25–7).[5,8] On T2 weighted images the signal intensity from a Brodie's abscess, because it is fluid, is always greater than that of normal bone marrow. The appearance of an old scar within an area of chronic infection may be difficult to differentiate from a sequestrum. Osteoid osteoma may be differentiated from chronic osteomyelitis by the smooth, uniform cortical thickening with uniform low signal, and the lack of any abscess or significant soft tissue abnormality (Fig. 25–10).

Evaluation of Disease Activity in Chronic Osteomyelitis

In patients with chronic osteomyelitis, it is often extremely difficult to know whether the infection has been completely cured or whether a low-grade infection still persists. In one study of 104 patients Tumeh and colleagues concluded that the identification of a sequestrum was good evidence of ongoing disease activity.[9] In their study they found no correlation between identification of bone erosion, soft tissue swelling, or periosteal reaction with the presence or absence of activity in chronic osteomyelitis. Gallium and MDP isotope scanning have both been used in an attempt to evaluate disease activity.[9,10] MDP has not been found to be helpful. Because remodeling goes on for many years, even after cessation of infection, MDP bone scan may continue to be strongly positive even in the absence of acute infection. The reverse was also found, i.e., that MDP findings may not worsen with infection relapse. On serial studies the intensity of uptake with gallium tends to decrease with the decrease in activity. The problems, however, are that there are still some false results and that the gallium findings lag several months behind clinical findings. The finding of gallium uptake that is much greater than MDP uptake correlates strongly with the presence of ongoing disease activity.[9] However, this is only seen in less than 25 percent of all patients with active chronic osteomyelitis. CT is better than plain film radiography in identifying activity in chronic osteomyelitis.[11] CT is particularly useful for identification of sequestra, and sometimes may also identify the presence of foreign bodies. Unfortunately, CT often reveals only many of the secondary changes of chronic infection, and is not always accurate in identification of chronic activity. There have been no large studies evaluating the role of MRI in determining the activity of chronic osteomyelitis. From some reports it would seem that the presence of areas of tissue of low intensity on T1, with change to high intensity on T2, indicates ongoing active disease. In eight patients with chronic osteomyelitis, MRI prediction of the presence, extent, and location of active areas of chronic osteomyelitis correlated extremely well with subsequent surgical findings.[8]

Differentiation of Acute from Chronic Osteomyelitis

A recent study of 16 patients with osteomyelitis found that MRI was extremely good at differentiating acute from chronic disease.[12] MR abnormality was present in all patients with acute or chronic osteomyelitis and is most readily detected on T1 weighted images. Soft tissue disease is identified in all patients with acute or active chronic osteomyelitis. The margins of the soft tissue abnormality tend to be more sharply defined in chronic osteomyelitis (Figs. 25–7, 25–8, 25–11) and more ill defined in acute osteomyelitis (Fig. 25–7). In addition the extent of soft tissue abnormality tends to be less in patients with chronic osteo-

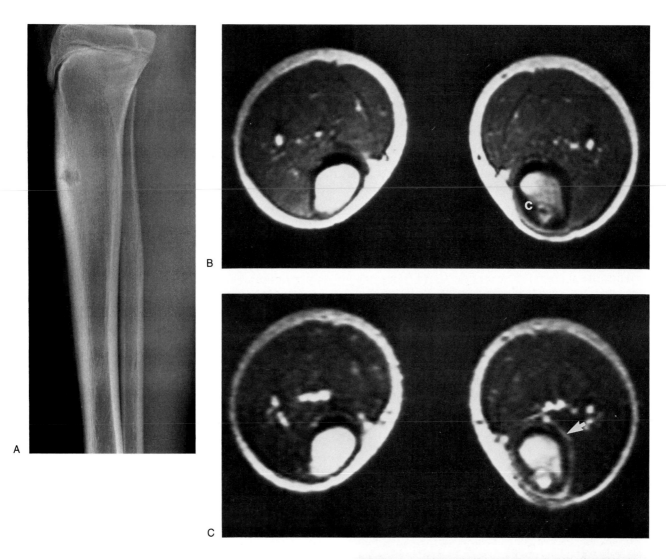

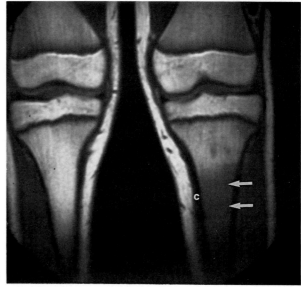

Figure 25–6. *Acute and chronic osteomyelitis in a 13-year-old boy with tibia pain.* ***A,*** Plain film radiograph shows extensive cortical thickening of the anterior aspect of the proximal tibia. A well-defined lucent defect is seen in the center of the cortical thickening. ***B,*** T1 transverse MR image at the level of the cortical lucency (700/26). There is diffuse cortical thickening (c, cortex). There is reduction in signal intensity from most of the marrow. The lucency seen on the radiograph has moderate signal intensity. ***C,*** T2 weighted image (2000/80) at the same level as ***B***. There is strong intensity from the bone marrow and the inflammatory fluid in the hole in the cortex. This change in signal intensity is consistent with infection. Note the thin rim of increased signal in the soft tissues surrounding the tibia (*arrow*). ***D,*** Coronal T1 weighted image (700/26). Note the extensive abnormality in the bone marrow of the left proximal tibia, which appears of low signal intensity (*arrows*). Note also the thickened cortex (c). The appearance of this lesion is consistent with chronic osteomyelitis. Osteoid osteoma would be considered in the differential diagnosis, but the extensive nature of the bone marrow abnormality, and the relative lack of encroachment of cortical thickening into the marrow space, are both very much against this diagnosis.

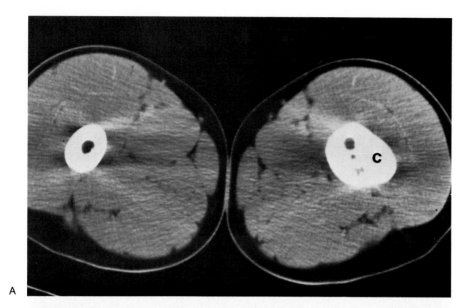

A

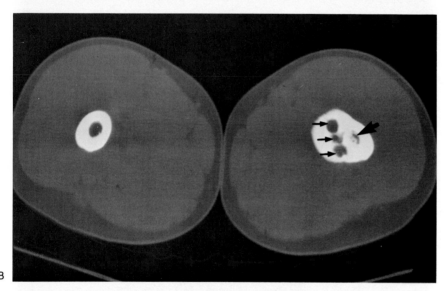

B

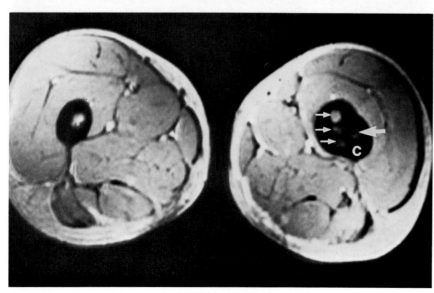

C

Figure 25–7. *Chronic osteomyelitis of the femur in a teenage boy with history of thigh pain.* The total history extended back for over 1 year. He had received no therapy. *A, B,* Soft tissue and bone window transverse CT scans through the middle femur show marked cortical (c) thickening on the left. There is increased signal seen in the bone marrow cavity (*large arrow*) on the left side compared with the opposite normal side. Three other cavitations (*small arrows*) are seen within the markedly thickened cortex, just medial to the bone marrow cavity. No soft tissue abnormality can be appreciated on the CT images. *C,* Transverse T1 weighted field-echo MR image (400/14), 90-degree tip angle. The marked cortical thickening (c) is well defined and of very low signal intensity. The bone marrow cavity (*large arrow*) appears of low signal intensity on this field-echo image. The three more medial cavities (*small arrows*) are of varying intensity.

myelitis. In acute osteomyelitis the bone cortex appears normal, whereas in chronic osteomyelitis it very often appears thickened. Sequestra may be identified on MR images and their presence indicates chronic osteomyelitis. A well-defined interface between diseased and normal marrow is strong evidence of the presence of chronic osteomyelitis (Fig. 25–11). With acute osteomyelitis this interface tends to be much more poorly defined (Fig. 25–2). However, there is some overlap between cases. In summary, chronic osteomyelitis is suggested by a good interface between normal and abnormal bone marrow, cortical thickening with or without sequestrum, and well-defined boundaries to relatively small regions of soft tissue abnormality.

Treatment

In the very early stages of acute osteomyelitis, treatment with antibiotics alone may be adequate. Within a short time, localized edema compresses blood vessels and prevents adequate flow of antibiotics in the blood to diseased areas. Because of this, surgical drainage is often indicated in acute osteomyelitis. It is not yet known whether MRI can differentiate patients requiring surgery from those in whom surgery is not indicated, but it certainly can direct the surgeon to the most appropriate maximally affected region. MRI has not been utilized in any large number of patients to monitor response to therapy, and it is not yet known whether serial MRI can define the best time for stopping therapy.

Text continues on page 924.

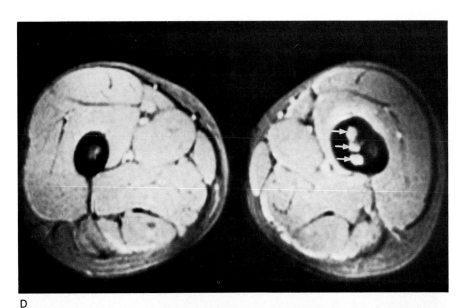

D

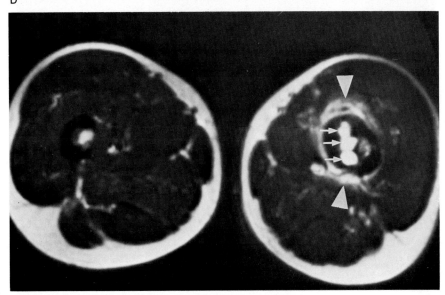

E

Figure 25–7. *Continued.*
D, T2 weighted field-echo pulse sequence at the same level as *B* (400/14), 22-degree flip angle. There is now very strong signal intensity due to infected fluid from the three cavities (*arrows*) lying within the thickened bone cortex. At surgery these all were demonstrated to be abscesses. There is also suspicion of some increased signal in the soft tissues surrounding the femur. *E,* Spin-echo T2 weighted pulse sequence (2000/70) shows strong signal intensity from the three abscess cavities (*arrows*). This also demonstrates the cortical thickening. This image also shows well a small amount of well-defined soft tissue inflammation (*arrowheads*) surrounding the femur. MRI is better than CT at demonstrating the fluid nature of the three cavities in the cortex and also in revealing the presence of soft tissue extension of the inflammatory process. The advantage of the field-echo pulse sequences compared with the spin-echo T2 pulse sequences is that they can be acquired in a much shorter time.

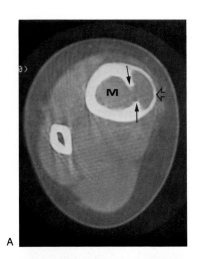

A

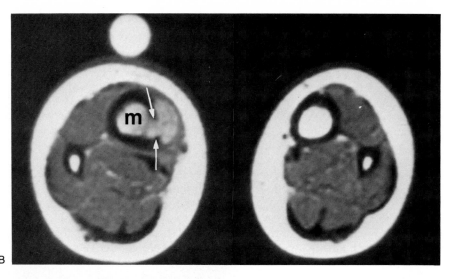

B

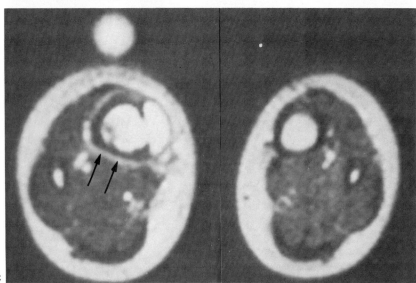

C

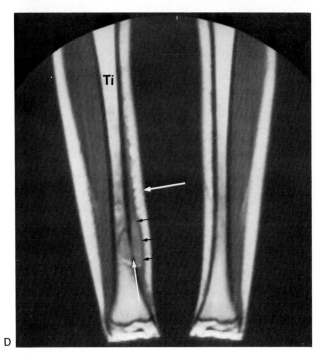

D

Figure 25–8. *Chronic osteomyelitis of the tibia in an 11-year-old girl.* **A,** CT scan. There is a butterfly-type lesion involving the bone marrow (M) extending through a large cortical defect (*small arrows*) into a large subperiosteal collection. The periosteum (*open arrow*) is heavily calcified. **B,** Transverse MR image (800/26) on which the appearance of the abnormality is almost identical to that on the CT scan. The three components of the butterfly lesion are all well seen. The signal intensity is less than that of normal bone marrow and fat. The calcified periosteum is not identified. **C,** Transverse T2 weighted MR image (2000/80) at the same level as **A.** This shows marked increase in signal intensity from the butterfly lesion. This pulse sequence also shows a thin rim of associated inflammation in the soft tissue surrounding the tibia (*arrows*). **D,** Coronal T1 image shows the butterfly lesion well. The isthmus between the marrow and subperiosteal collection is shown by the long arrow. This pulse sequence shows the thickened calcified periosteum (*small arrows*) extremely well. It is of low intensity. It also shows fairly extensive bone marrow abnormality, seen as of lowish signal intensity extending almost halfway up the shaft of the tibia (Ti). Notice also the marked edema in the overlying subcutaneous fat (*curved arrow*). Bone scan and plain film radiographs were also abnormal. MRI was very accurate in defining the total extent of the abnormality.

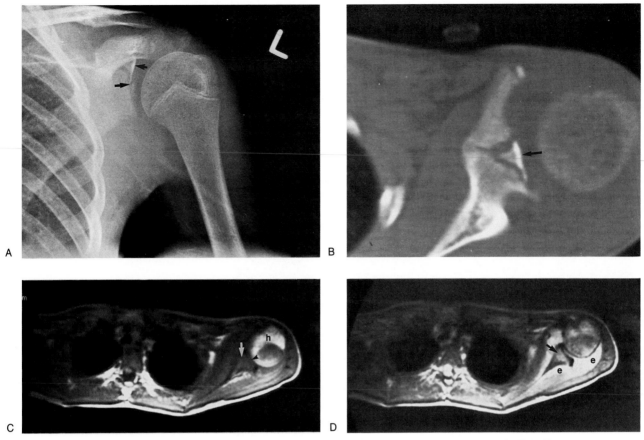

A

B

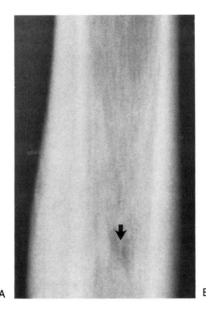

C

D

Figure 25–9. *Chronic osteomyelitis of the shoulder in an 11-year-old girl with a painful left shoulder.* **A,** Plain film radiograph shows sclerosis in the superior aspect of the glenoid (*large arrow*) with a break in the normal smooth margins to the glenoid (*small arrow*). **B,** Transverse CT scan shows a sequestered fragment of bone (*arrow*). **C,** Transverse T1 MR image (700/30) shows a reduction in signal from the glenoid portion of the scapula (*arrow*). The small sequestered fragment can also be identified (*arrowhead*). h, Head of humerus. **D,** T2 weighted image shows increased signal from the infected marrow of the glenoid (*arrow*). There is a large joint effusion (e) of very high signal intensity. The sequestrum is more easily identified on the CT scan. MRI shows the associated inflammation in the bone marrow of the glenoid, and the joint effusion, better than the CT image.

Figure 25–10. *Osteoid osteoma.* **A,** Linear tomogram of the tibia shows marked cortical hyperostosis with a focal lucency consistent with a nidus (*arrow*). **B,** Transverse MR image (1000/30). The cortical thickening (*arrows*) is seen as an increase in thickness of the low intensity from the cortex of the tibia. There is encroachment into the bone marrow space with reduced signal from the marrow of the tibia, compared with the fibula marrow. The nidus is not definitely defined on this image.

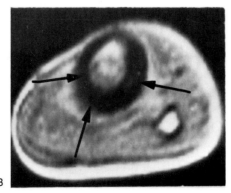

A

B

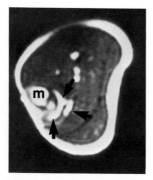

Figure 25–11. *Chronic osteomyelitis of the tibia.* Transverse T2 weighted image (2000/80). Strong signal intensity is identified from the infection within the bone marrow (m) and extending into the soft tissue (*arrows*). The soft tissue component of the infection is well defined. This appearance is consistent with chronic osteomyelitis.

Differential Diagnosis

The MR findings in osteomyelitis are nonspecific, but taken together with an appropriate clinical history are often strongly suggestive of the correct diagnosis. Many disorders, including trauma and tumors, cause a change in signal intensity in the bone marrow similar to that seen with acute infection. Soft tissue abnormality usually is not found with leukemia and is uncommon with marrow metastasis from neuroblastoma, and this finding is often helpful in differentiation. Both of these disorders also usually affect multiple bones, whereas acute osteomyelitis is most commonly focal. Bone tumors involve the bone marrow and the soft tissues. The margins of the soft tissue component of these tumors are frequently much better defined than in acute osteomyelitis, and cortical abnormality is much more evident. A bone fracture may appear similar to acute osteomyelitis, with reduction in signal in the bone marrow on T1 weighted images and increased signal in the soft tissue on T2 weighted images. The correct diagnosis is suggested by the clinical history, plain film radiographs, and the finding of blood (with strong signal on T1 weighted images) within the soft tissues.

Healed Osteomyelitis

With healing of osteomyelitis the soft tissues frequently return to normal. The bone marrow may heal with scarring that appears of low signal on T1 and T2 weighted images or, particularly in children, may return to normal. Occasionally the marrow heals by deposition of fat, which produces an even stronger signal than normal marrow.

Role of MRI in Osteomyelitis

MRI has many roles to play in the evaluation of children with osteomyelitis. It is extremely sensitive for early diagnosis of abnormality. Large studies comparing it with MDP bone scanning have yet to be performed. MRI is more sensitive than bone scan for differentiating soft tissue from bone infection. In pa-

tients with clinical cellulitis, MRI is very accurate in identifying or excluding extension of the soft tissue infection into bone (Fig. 25–12). MRI can accurately direct the surgeon to the precise anatomic region of abnormality for drainage of acute osteomyelitis and more extensive surgical excision of areas of chronic osteomyelitis. MRI can differentiate acute from chronic osteomyelitis and probably will have a significant role to play in evaluating the state of activity within chronic osteomyelitis. The role of MRI in monitoring therapy is not yet known. Its disadvantage is that the findings are not absolutely specific. As indicated previously, many disorders, such as fractures, may appear very similar to acute osteomyelitis on MR imaging. Another disadvantage is that the soft tissue findings in MRI are nonspecific, and it is not able to accurately differentiate inflammatory edema from active bacterial infection within the soft tissue.

Septic Arthritis

This bacterial infection is not uncommon (Fig. 25–9). In infants it is frequently caused by spread from adjacent metaphyseal osteomyelitis that crosses the growth plate and extends into the joint. In these infants the infection is often aggressive, and joint dislocation and bone destruction are common. In older children septic arthritis is often localized to the joint without bone involvement. This is because the infection does not cross the growth plate. In a few joints,

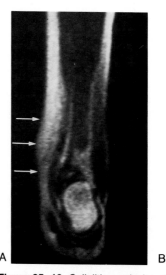
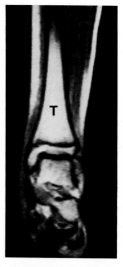

Figure 25–12. *Cellulitis: exclusion of osteomyelitis in a 4-year-old boy with extensive clinical cellulitis around the ankles.* **A,** T2 coronal MR image (1000/60) is obtained in the plane just posterior to the tibia. There is extensive soft tissue swelling with an increase in signal (*arrows*) consistent with cellulitis. **B,** Coronal T1 weighted image (500/30) obtained through the plane of the tibia (T). The bone marrow of the tibia is completely normal, excluding osteomyelitis. MRI is extremely useful in excluding osteomyelitis in these situations.

where the metaphysis is contained within the articular capsule, spread may occur from metaphyseal infection into the joint. These joints include the hip, shoulder, and ankle. *Staphylococcus* is the most common affecting organism, and *Haemophilus* is probably the second most common.

MRI demonstrates the presence of fluid in the joint space. This is seen as low signal intensity on T1 and very high signal intensity on T2 weighted images. There is probably nothing truly specific about this finding that differentiates infection from other causes of joint fluid. In many cases, surrounding inflammation in the soft tissue is seen as of strong signal intensity on T2 weighted images. This finding would support suspicion of infection. The specific role of MRI in detection of septic arthritis and monitoring therapy is not known at this time.

Transient Synovitis

This is a common disorder and probably the most frequent cause of limp in a child. It is a self-limiting and acute inflammation of the hip joint and often follows respiratory infection. There may or may not be a mild pyrexia. The white blood cell count is usually normal. Plain film radiographs may be normal or may show slight widening of the hip joint consistent with a small effusion. MRI is accurate in identification of joint fluid and can exclude abnormality in adjacent soft tissues and bone. The main difficulty in transient synovitis is differentiating it from more serious conditions that might cause limp. The disease requires no treatment. The role of MRI may be first to exclude other disorders in and around the hip joint and to confirm the presence of joint fluid in a patient with suspected transient synovitis. In some patients MRI may not be able to differentiate transient synovitis from early septic arthritis. The absence of elevated white blood cell count, of severe localizing pain to the hip joint, and of involvement of adjacent soft tissues would all be factors strongly favoring the diagnosis of transient synovitis.

Tenosynovitis

MRI shows the accumulation of inflammatory fluid contained within the tendon sheaths (Fig. 25–13). The fluid is of very strong signal on T2 weighted images; the tendons are of low intensity. The margins are sharply defined.

Infected Sinus Tracts

MRI can accurately identify sinus tracts (Figs. 25–14, 25–15). Their inflamed walls appear as tracts (on longitudinal slices) or rings (when imaged transversely) of well-defined high signal on T2 images. Associated foreign bodies may be seen. MRI is useful

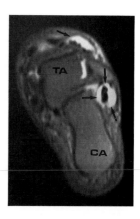

Figure 25–13. *Infected tenosynovitis.* Axial image through the foot (2000/80). The talus (TA) and calcaneus (CA) appear normal. The tendon sheaths of the peroneus and extensor tendons are markedly distended by infected synovial fluid (*arrows*), which appears of very strong signal intensity. The tendons are of very low signal intensity. (From Beltran J, Noto AM, McGhee RB, et al. Infections of the musculoskeletal system: high-field-strength MR imaging. Radiology 1987; 164:449–454.)

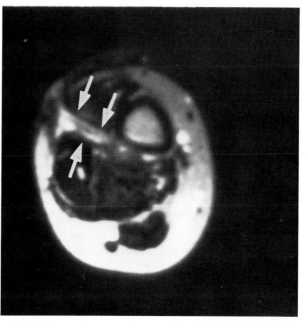

Figure 25–14. *Chronically infected sinus tract with foreign body in a 12-year-old girl with a 6-month history of a chronically draining sinus tract on the lateral aspect of the lower leg.* Transverse T2 weighted image (1500/90). The sinus tract is well defined (*arrows*), extending from the interosseous membrane to the skin surface. There is a very strong signal from the sinus tract representing inflammation. Lying within the sinus tract, and about two-thirds of the length of the whole tract, is a thin linear band of low intensity. This is a piece of wood. At surgery the sinus tract was excised and the presence of the piece of wood was confirmed.

before surgery to define the extent and cause of the tract.

Pyomyositis

Pyomyositis is a bacterial infection of muscles that is common in the tropics but can be seen in children in other areas (Figs. 25–16, 25–17).[13,14] Clinically there is pain, fever, and malaise. There is localized swelling and induration of the affected regions of the body. *Staphylococcus* is the most common affecting organism. MRI is very sensitive for identification of abnormality, and shows decreased signal on T1 and increased signal on T2 weighted images in affected muscle groups. On T2 weighted images the overall appearance of the muscle is nonhomogeneous. The disease is often confined to a single muscle group. In one patient MRI was positive while CT, ultrasonography, and indium-labeled white blood cell studies were all negative.[13]

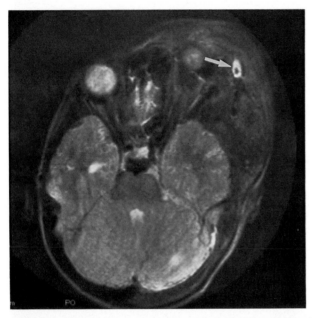

Figure 25–15. *Infected sinus tract in a 10-year-old boy with giant vascular malformation of the left anterior calvarium and face.* After partial resection he developed a chronically draining sinus. MRI was performed to define the extent of the sinus tract. Transverse T2 weighted MR image (2000/90). The giant soft tissue malformation is seen to be of relatively low intensity. The circular sinus tract (*arrow*) is clearly seen as a region of very strong signal intensity. The bright signal is the wall of the tract; the central low signal is its lumen. With serial MR slices it was possible to define the total extent of the sinus tract.

TRAUMA AND MECHANICAL DISORDERS

Paul Berger, M.D.

Imaging of the musculoskeletal system for traumatic injuries has become a major application of magnetic resonance. Initially, when hardware and software were limited and applications were directed toward the central nervous system (CNS), it was felt that MRI was not a good modality for evaluating bone, i.e., it could not detect a skull fracture. Improvements in coil technology and software, and the development of new imaging sequences, have resulted in widespread and simplified application of MRI to musculoskeletal trauma.[15, 16] Fundamental reasons for this increased use are:

1. The unique ability of MRI to delineate subtle abnormalities of medullary bone clearly.[17]

2. The excellent tissue contrast resolution capabilities that MRI possesses, which permit delineation of the anatomy and character of ligamentous abnormalities, far beyond that possible with other modalities.

3. The ability of MRI to image in multiple planes of view, both orthogonal and nonorthogonal.

4. The fact that MRI is a tomographic modality with high contrast and spatial resolution, making possible the depiction of very small structural details.

5. A better understanding of the normal appearance of the structures and tissues of the musculoskeletal system.

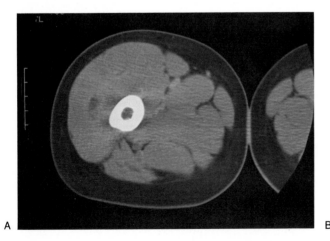
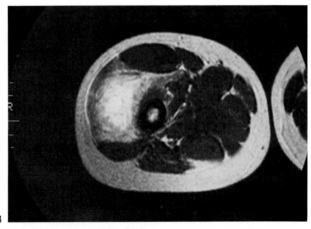

A   B

Figure 25–16. *Pyomyositis.* ***A,*** CT scan shows a small area of low intensity in the right vastus lateralis muscle. ***B,*** T2 weighted transverse MR image (800/80) shows extensive high signal intensity, due to infection and inflammation, involving the entire vastus lateralis muscle. The small area of low intensity seen on the CT scan has very high intensity on the MR image.

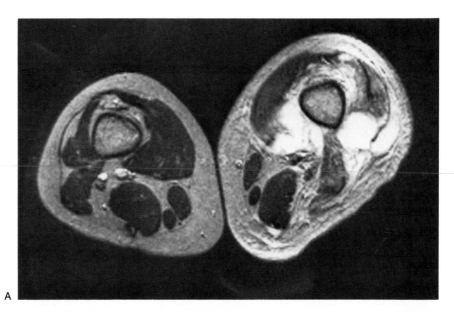

A

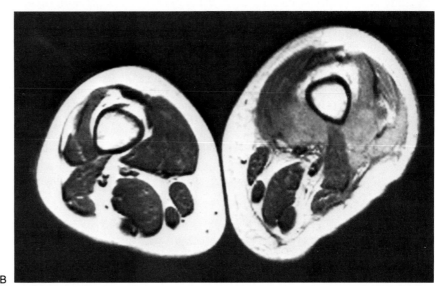

B

Figure 25–17. *Pyomyositis in a 16-year-old girl with a 3-week history of pain and swelling of the left thigh. The disease involves several muscle groups, including the quadriceps and biceps femoris.* **A,** Transverse T2 image (2300/80) shows widespread increased signal intensity in the involved muscle. Several well-marginated abscesses of extremely high signal intensity are also seen. The uninvolved muscles are of low signal intensity. High signal intensity from the anterolateral soft tissues is consistent with subcutaneous edema. **B,** Transverse T1 image (1000/40). The involved muscles are slightly hyperintense compared with the normal muscles. The abscesses show slightly higher signal intensity than other areas. This is due to the presence of proteinaceous material found at surgery. (Yuh WTC, Schnecke AC, Montgomery WJ, Chara S. Magnetic resonance imaging of pyomyositis. Skeletal Radiol 1988; 17:190–193.)

MRI will become a major method for investigating trauma of the musculoskeletal system. This is particularly true of athletic injuries of the soft tissues, ligaments, tendons, and joint cartilaginous structures. MRI will probably prove to be the most sensitive modality for identification and characterization of lesions of these structures. This new sensitivity and visualization of soft tissues should allow the development of new therapeutic regimens for athletic injuries. MRI should be able to differentiate soft tissue edema from hematoma after injury. It should prove valuable in following the response of such injuries to active or passive therapy, and it may prove to be a strong indicator of the best time for an injured athlete to resume rehabilitation and ultimately return to sporting activities.

In the investigation of fractures, MRI will probably have little or no role to play in evaluation of classic bone fractures, which are well identified on plain film radiographs. MRI is proving sensitive in the identification of both stress and occult fractures, but its role in comparison with the bone isotope scan has yet to be clearly defined.

Fractures

Classical Cortical Fractures

The vast majority of fractures involve disruption of the bone cortex. Few classical fractures have been studied with MRI. MRI shows the cortical abnormality as a break in the normal, smooth, low-intensity cortex, which is replaced by areas of varying increased signal intensity. The normal homogeneous high signal in the bone marrow is also replaced by signal of mixed intensity, depending on the degree of edema or hemorrhage present. With fracture healing the appearance of the bone may return completely to normal. However, the signal in the bone marrow may remain of relatively low intensity, presumably owing to fibrosis rather than replacement with normal marrow (Fig. 25–18). Complications of trauma may also be seen, such as early partial fusion of the growth plate (Fig. 25–19). In most cases these fractures are easily diagnosed and categorized by plain film radiographs, which are adequate for planning of therapy. This is particularly true of fractures of the peripheral skeleton. In the spine, conventional radiographs are frequently inadequate for complete demonstration of a fracture and its associated effects. Conventional and computed tomography have provided additional information in these patients. MRI will prove useful in the evaluation of patients with spinal trauma, e.g., for detection of impingement of a bone fragment on the spinal cord. The precise roles of MRI in such matters as patient selection and timing of the study have yet to be defined.

Occult Fractures

As mentioned above, conventional radiology has been the benchmark and standard in the evaluation of bone trauma. However, it has become apparent that MRI commonly reveals occult intraosseous and cortical fractures that are inapparent on plain radiographs.[18–22] There is almost always a good history of acute trauma. One study of 434 unselected and consecutive MR examinations of the knee revealed a 17 percent incidence of intraosseous and/or cortical injuries.[18] All patients in whom plain radiographs were available had been interpreted prospectively as normal.

The appearance of the pathologic changes of occult fractures within the cancellous bone has not been histologically proven, but most authors speculate that there are trabecular microfractures with associated hemorrhage and edema that cause an alteration in marrow signal.[18, 22]

The MR findings of occult bone fractures are of speckled or linear regions of low signal intensity in the marrow on T1 weighted images, with irregular high signal intensity in the same areas on T2 weighted images.[18] The abnormality is usually in the epiphysis but may indent into the metaphysis. Technetium MDP bone scan results often are also abnormal.

Follow-up MR scans (Fig. 25–20) performed in patients with occult bone lesions (bone bruises) demonstrate resolution of the MR findings, often by 3 months or sooner.

Of importance with respect to occult fractures around the knee is the high incidence of associated ligamentous injury. Over 50 percent of patients demonstrating these osseous injuries have associated ligamentous tears, most commonly the anterior cruciate ligament, but also tears of the medial and lateral col-

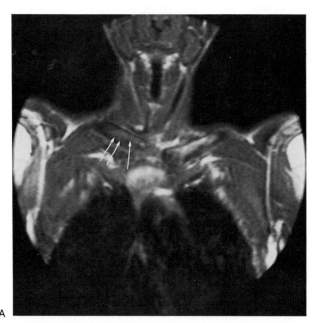
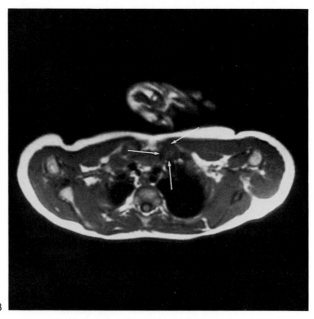

A   B

Figure 25–18. *Healing of clavicle fracture. Two children presented with clavicular mass lesions without a clear history of prior fracture. Both were biopsied and both showed normal callus consistent with healing fracture.* **A,** *Coronal T1 image (700/26) shows a decrease in signal intensity from the medial third of the clavicle, compared with the opposite side (arrows).* **B,** *Transverse T1 image (600/26) in the second patient. There is expansion of the medial end of the left clavicle corresponding to the clinically palpable mass. The expansion is predominantly of low intensity, consistent with abundant callus formation (arrows). The central area of this region contains bone marrow. It is of slightly lower signal intensity than normal marrow on the opposite side.*

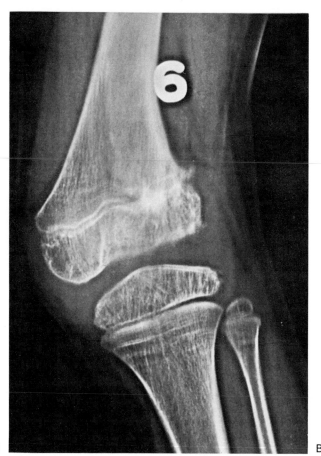
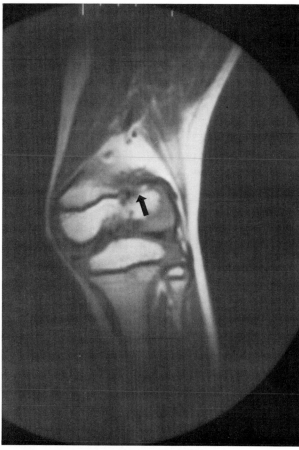

A   B

Figure 25–19. *Growth plate fusion after trauma in an 8-year-old boy with a history of trauma to the distal femur. The study was made to evaluate the extent of fusion of the growth plate.* ***A,*** *Conventional radiograph shows fusion of the lateral part of the growth plate.* ***B,*** *Coronal T1 MR image (700/26). The extent of fusion of the growth plate is well seen and corresponds accurately to the plain film radiograph. The normal growth plate is seen as a well-defined black line between the metaphysis and the epiphysis. In the region of fusion, the growth plate is crossed by high signal due to bone marrow (*arrow*).*

lateral ligaments.[21, 22] Although the knee has been the region most commonly evaluated by MRI in association with trauma, MRI has demonstrated occult fractures in the proximal femur,[20] shoulder,[19, 23] long bones,[24] wrist,[25] and ankle[26] (Fig. 25–21). In these areas the association of soft tissue and ligamentous injuries may also be well delineated.

The clinical significance of these osseous injuries is variable and dependent on the degree of injury and the presence or absence of associated ligamentous tears. At the very least, the MR findings provide an explanation for the pain and show whether there is any associated internal joint derangement. They also may result in a delay in returning to full weightbearing until pain decreases or healing takes place.

The appearance of occult fractures on MRI is nonspecific; the differential diagnosis includes lesions such as osteoid osteoma, infection, osteogenic sarcoma, and stress fractures. Occult fractures are distinguished from stress fractures in that there is often a good history of a single episode of trauma, and involvement is

of the subchondral and epiphyseal areas. Stress fractures, on the other hand, usually have a history of chronic trauma, and rarely a history of acute trauma. They involve the metaphysis and diaphysis rather than the epiphysis, and have more prominent low signal intensity bands on T1 weighted MR images.[27]

Stress Fractures

Stress fractures can occur in both normal and abnormal bones. These types of fractures have been classified as either fatigue or insufficiency type. Fatigue fractures occur when normal bones are subjected to an increased load; they are most commonly seen in the pediatric age group in association with athletics and physical fitness exercises. Insufficiency fractures result from loads applied to bones weakened by underlying disorders such as osteoporosis, osteomalacia, and fibrous dysplasia.

The sensitivity of radiography in the diagnosis of stress fracture is often poor (it is frequently negative early in the disease process) and the differential diag-

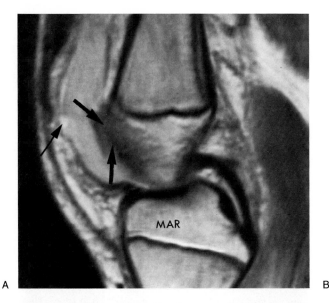

A

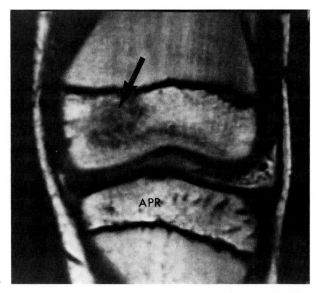

B

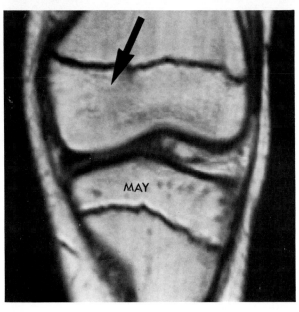

C

Figure 25–20. *Healing of occult cortical and intraosseous injury in a 13-year-old boy who fell off his bicycle.* ***A*** (March), Sagittal T1 weighted image (800/20) shows loss of the normal cortex of the anterior aspect of the medial femoral condyle with diffuse low intensity within the anterior aspect of the condyle (*thick arrows*). Also note the large effusion (*thin arrow*). ***B*** (April), Coronal T1 weighted image (800/20) shows diffuse decreased intensity (*arrow*) persisting within the medial aspect of the epiphysis. ***C*** (May), Abnormal signal within the epiphysis (*arrow*) is now normal.

nosis may be troublesome with stress fractures, which may simulate tumor such as osteogenic sarcoma. Radionuclide scintigraphy is very sensitive but not specific in the diagnosis of stress fractures.

MR imaging of stress fractures shows thick linear bands of low intensity signal on both T1 and T2 weighted sequences that is continuous at some point with the cortex (Fig. 25–22).[21, 27] T1 weighted and intermediate sequences also demonstrate a surrounding area of moderately decreased signal that becomes increased in intensity on T2 weighted sequences. The linear low-intensity band is thought to represent microfractures or bone sclerosis (which may not be identified on a conventional x-ray), and the surrounding area most probably represents some associated edema and/or hemorrhage. There may also be an area of high signal intensity on T2 images in the immediate juxtacortical soft tissues, probably representing edema.

Occasionally, small irregular areas of cortical interruption or subperiosteal high signal may also be seen.[24, 27]

Around the knee, stress fractures may appear similar to occult intraosseous fractures. These may be differentiated when the thick linear band of low intensity is seen on both T1 and T2 weighted sequences. If this is not present, the location of the cancellous abnormality is helpful, being typically subchondral or epiphyseal in occult intraosseous injury (bone bruise) and almost always metaphyseal or diaphyseal in stress fracture. A final differentiating feature may be the history. Although it is unlikely that MRI will prove to be more sensitive than radionuclide scintigraphy for the diagnosis of stress fractures, it may at times be more specific.

With healing, stress fractures often revert to normal on MRI and plain film radiographs. Occasionally, however, there may be excessive periosteal reaction and sclerosis, and on a plain film radiograph the healed stress fracture may be difficult to differentiate from chronic osteomyelitis. The presence of normal signal in the adjacent bone marrow on T1 weighted images distinguishes a chronic healed stress fracture from chronic osteomyelitis.[28]

Classification of Fractures Around the Knee

Attempts have been made to classify the types of osseous injuries occurring around the knee. Lynch and colleagues referred to traumatic lesions as type 1 or 2.[22] Type 1 lesions (Fig. 25–23) on T1 weighted images demonstrate a diffuse, often reticulated signal inten-

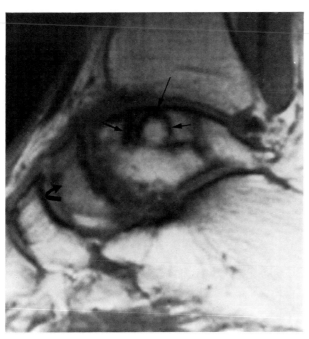

Figure 25–21. *Osteochondral fracture of the talus.* T1 weighted sagittal view (800/20) of the ankle demonstrates linear areas of decreased signal intensity within the superior aspect of the talus (*arrows*). There is also intraosseous injury to the navicular with diffuse decreased signal intensity (*curved arrow*).

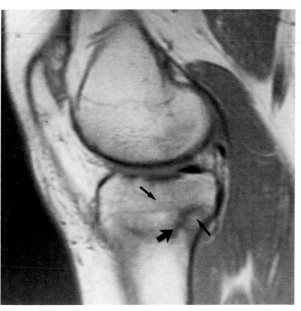

Figure 25–22. *Stress fracture in a patient with knee pain.* Sagittal T1 weighted image demonstrates a thick linear zone of low intensity (*short arrow*) extending horizontally. There is also a diffuse surrounding zone of moderately decreased signal (*long arrows*), most likely representing associated edema and hemorrhage in adjacent cancellous bone. The diagnosis of stress fracture was confirmed on radiographic and clinical follow-up. (Courtesy of Dr. Jerrold Mink, Los Angeles, CA.)

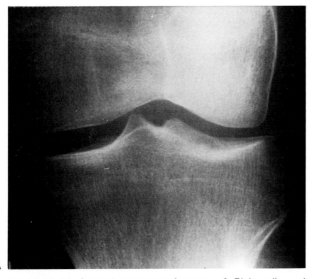

A

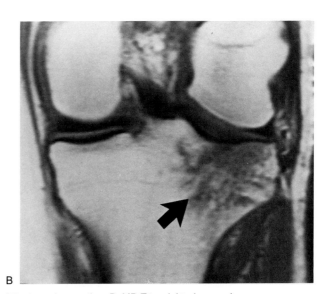

B

Figure 25–23. *Occult intraosseous fracture.* **A,** Plain radiograph of the knee is negative. **B,** MR T1 weighted coronal image (800/20) shows diffuse decreased intensity (*arrow*) in the epiphysis and metaphysis. The cortex of the tibial plateau is intact.

sity loss in the subcortical bone involving the epiphysis and usually a portion of the metaphysis. On T2 weighted images these lesions have increased signal intensity. Type 2 lesions (Fig. 25–24) demonstrate cortical disruption in association with linear or multiple linear areas of decreased signal intensity on both T1 and T2 weighted sequences. Segments of bone or articular cartilage may be depressed or displaced as well. Mink and Deutsch further classified the osseous injury into four types.[21] The type 1 lesions of Lynch were subdivided as either bone bruises or stress fractures, the differentiation often being based on the history and location of the lesion; e.g., if only the metaphysis was involved, a stress fracture was favored. Stress fractures might also show a linear zone of decreased signal intensity within the more amorphous zone of low intensity on T1 weighted images, with this linear area remaining low in intensity on T2 weighted sequences. The type 2 lesions of Lynch were subdivided into tibial plateau and femoral fractures, and osteochondral fractures. The osteochondral fractures have cartilage, and often a small underlying segment of bone, fractured and partially displaced from the site of origin (Fig. 25–25), or they are impacted lesions with the overlying car-

tilage and subchondral bone impacted into the medullary bone. The displaced type occurred most frequently over the inferior pole of the patella and anterior lateral femoral condyle; the impacted type most commonly involved the anterior aspect of the lateral femoral condyle directly over the anterior horn of the lateral meniscus (Fig. 25–24).

Soft Tissue Contusion and Hemorrhage

A common feature of acute musculoskeletal trauma is the presence of contusion and hemorrhage.[29, 30] The appearance of extravascular blood on MR scans is complex and dependent on many factors, including the effects of protein concentration, paramagnetic effects, and spin diffusion effects on the relaxation times of the hematomas.[31, 32] The influence of each of these processes is determined not only by pulse sequence parameters, but also by the magnetic field strength and the cellular content of the hematoma. The intensity of the hematoma depends on a balance of these factors. Ehman and colleagues found the intensity of the central area of 28 hematomas to be extremely variable

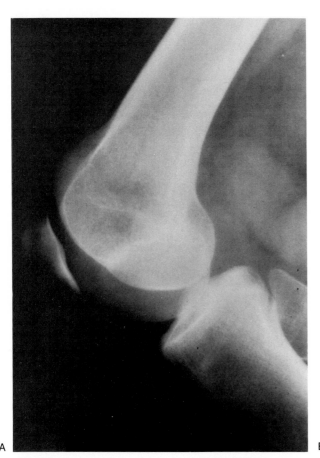

A

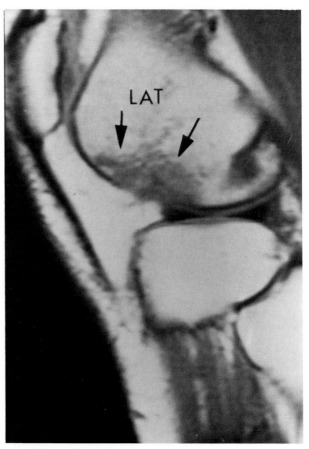

B

Figure 25–24. *Occult intraosseous fracture with cortical disruption.* **A,** Plain radiograph is negative. **B,** MR T1 weighted image (800/20) shows loss of the anterior cortex of the lateral femoral condyle in association with decreased signal within the condyle (*arrows*).

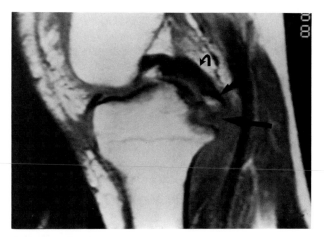

Figure 25–25. *Osteochondral fracture of the proximal tibia.* T1 weighted sagittal view (800/20) demonstrates an avulsion fracture of the posterior tibia (*straight arrows*) at the insertion of the posterior cruciate ligament (*curved arrow*).

relative to the intensity of adjacent muscle and fat.[29] On partial saturation (more T1 weighted) images the hematoma was most commonly isointense with muscle, but often was higher in intensity than muscle. On T2 weighted images the hematoma was usually of higher intensity than muscle and was increased, decreased, or isointense relative to fat intensity. In addition, when plotted over time, there was noted to be great variation in the hematoma intensity, with no temporal pattern identified. Therefore MRI may not be able to determine the age of a soft tissue hemorrhage. However, this may not be of importance since the hemorrhage is usually caused by a well-defined single injury, the date of which is known. There are no reports of the use of MRI to study soft tissue injuries in athletes. Questions that need to be asked are how well MRI can distinguish between edema and hemorrhage, and whether this differentiation matters in terms of therapeutic decisions and long-term prognosis.

Ligament, Tendon, and Meniscal Tears

Tears of the major ligaments and tendons are serious clinical events that require accurate diagnosis. MR imaging, better than any other modality, demonstrates these tendon and ligament injuries.

The most commonly investigated ligaments and tendons are those in the knee. Although clinical examination of the knee is quite good for the diagnosis of injury to the ligaments and menisci, many patients are difficult to evaluate, and a significant level of uncertainty may persist.

For knee imaging, one should use all three imaging planes. The sagittal plane best demonstrates the menisci and cruciate ligaments; the coronal plane the collateral ligaments, chondral surfaces, bones, and periphery of the menisci; and the axial plane the patellofemoral joint. In the knee the most commonly torn ligament is the anterior cruciate (ACL). This runs somewhat obliquely, but with thin sections (3 mm) and with proper external rotation of the knee (approximately 20 degrees), this ligament can almost always be demonstrated on the sagittal images, when intact (Fig. 25–26*A*). When the examination is technically satisfactory, absence of the ACL is indicative of tear (Fig. 25–26*B*). Good technique also demonstrates the infe-

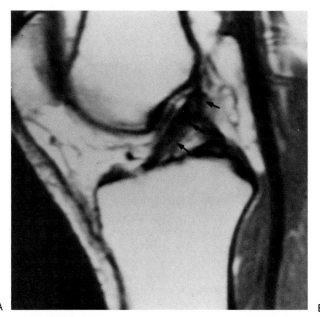

A

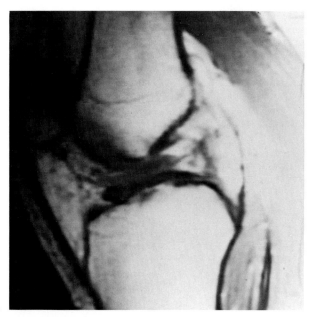

B

Figure 25–26. *Anterior cruciate ligament tear.* **A,** Sagittal T1 weighted image (800/20) demonstrates a normal anterior cruciate ligament (*arrows*). **B,** Sagittal T1 weighted image (800/20) in another patient at the same level shows absence of the anterior cruciate ligament, indicative of a tear.

rior portion of the ligament with tearing at the femoral attachment. In three separate studies the accuracy of diagnosing ACL tears has ranged from 93 to 96 percent.[33-35] Lynch and Mink and their colleagues noted that approximately 50 percent of their patients with bone bruises (occult fractures) also had ACL tears, and of 25 consecutive patients with ACL tears, 92 percent had associated osseous injuries on MRI.[21,22] Lynch noted that 84 percent (16 of 18) of their patients with MR evidence of cortical fracture had associated ligamentous tears, the ACL again being most common.[22]

Moeser and associates, imaging the *intact* anterior cruciate ligament following repair, noted nonvisualiza-

tion of the ligament in 11 of 27 patients and an ill-defined ligament in 10 of 27.[36] In only six of 27 patients was the neoligament well defined; this was thought to be due to the variable appearance of fibrous and fatty tissue investing the neoligament. Thus, MRI may not be satisfactory for the postoperative evaluation of patients who have had ACL repairs.

Tears of the collateral ligaments and posterior cruciate ligament are somewhat easier to diagnose clinically but can also be well demonstrated on MRI (Fig. 25–27). Quadriceps and patellar tendon tears are usually diagnosed clinically, and MRI may be used to reveal associated injuries.

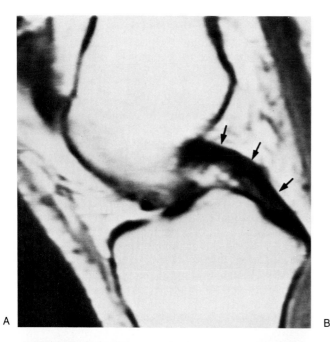

A

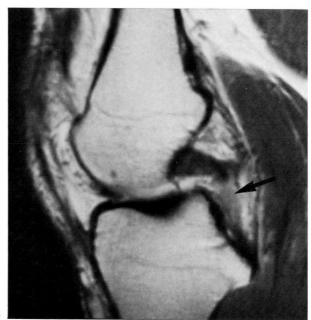

B

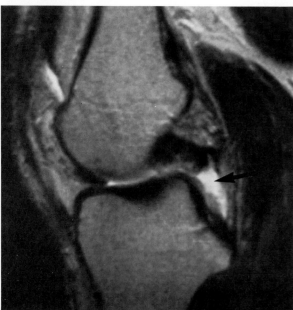

C

Figure 25–27. *Posterior cruciate ligament tear.* **A,** Sagittal T1 weighted sequence (800/20) demonstrates a normal posterior cruciate ligament (*arrows*). **B,** Sagittal intermediate sequence (1800/20) shows increased signal in the region normally occupied by the inferior aspect of the posterior cruciate ligament (*arrow*). **C,** Sagittal T2 weighted sequence (1800/80) shows high-intensity fluid (*arrow*) at the inferior aspect of the torn posterior cruciate ligament.

Meniscal injuries of the knee are well seen on MRI. Since Reicher and colleagues proposed using MRI for evaluation of possible internal derangement of the knee, there has been widespread application of this modality to evaluate the menisci of the knee.[37]

The appearance of the meniscus has been graded as 1, 2, and 3. Grade 1 (Fig. 25–28) shows homogeneous low signal intensity or a very small amount of increased signal within the meniscus, and is thought to be normal.[38] Grade 2 has large, usually linear increased signal within it, but without extension to an articular surface. Stoller and associates showed that this increased signal represents mucinous or myxoid degeneration.[39] In children there sometimes appears to be increased signal within the meniscus simulating grade 2 change. This is not uncommon and may represent a normal appearance rather than myxoid degeneration. The histologic basis for this has not yet been completely evaluated, but it may be due to persistent blood vessels in the menisci of children. A grade 3 meniscus (Fig. 25–29) shows increased signal with extension to the articular surface and is indicative of a tear. Stoller and associates correlated this finding with pathologic material and showed this to be due to fibrocartilaginous separation, i.e., tearing of the meniscus.[39]

Several studies have correlated findings at arthroscopy with MR findings. In experienced hands the overall accuracy in the medial meniscus is 91 to 94 percent and in the lateral meniscus 92 to 96 percent.[33,35,38] The menisci are well visualized on T1 or intermediate sequences but tears are not well seen on T2 weighted images. Gradient-echo sequences have also been used to evaluate the meniscus; the advantages are speed in performance of the examination and the ability to take thinner slices.[40,41] Signal to noise may be compromised in some gradient-echo sequences.

Potential errors and pitfalls in the interpretation of meniscus injuries include volume averaging at the free edge of the meniscus, which could result in false-positive and false-negative interpretations. Thinner slices should decrease this error. Findings mimicking a tear, or a so-called "pseudotear," may be seen near the anterior horn of the lateral meniscus, and are caused by the transverse ligament connecting the two anterior horns or by the lateral inferior geniculate artery simulating a tear. The popliteus tendon behind the posterior horn of the lateral meniscus may also give the appearance of a tear and should not be misinterpreted as such.

MR imaging can also diagnose "bucket-handle" tears (Fig. 25–30) where the meniscus may appear small or a portion may be absent, in conjunction with identifying meniscal tissue or fragments medially located on coronal views.

Meniscal cysts may also be identified as focal soft tissue masses of increased intensity on a T2 weighted sequence (Fig. 25–31).[42] These are often multiseptated and identified as extending anteriorly or laterally from the lateral meniscus, and most commonly medially from the medial meniscus. Meniscal cysts are always associated with underlying horizontal meniscal tears.

A discoid lateral meniscus is recognized by the presence of a complete disc on multiple sagittal images, due to the greater width of the disc. The disc height is also increased.

MRI has proved to be the procedure of choice for evaluating the meniscus and in many centers has completely replaced arthrography.

In the shoulder, MR imaging of rotator cuff tendon tears has drawn the most interest. This is not a common problem in the pediatric age group. MR findings of full-thickness rotator cuff tears include loss of the homogeneous signal void or discontinuity of the rotator cuff tendon, usually the supraspinatus.[23,43] There may

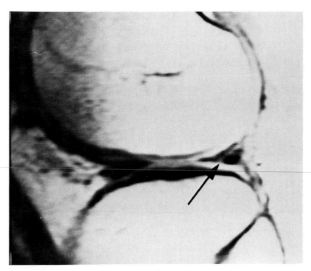

Figure 25–29. *Meniscal tear.* Sagittal T1 weighted sequence (800/20) shows linear increased signal intensity with extension to the inferior articular surface (*arrow*), indicating a tear in the posterior horn of the lateral meniscus.

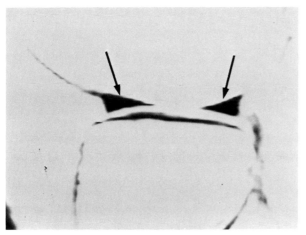

Figure 25–28. *Normal meniscus.* Sagittal T1 weighted sequence (800/20) showing homogeneous low signal intensity in the anterior and posterior horns of the lateral meniscus (*arrows*).

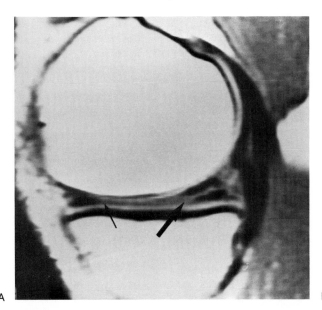

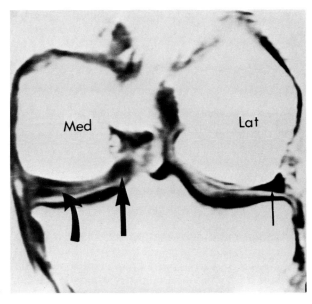

Figure 25–30. *"Bucket-handle" tear of the medial meniscus.* ***A,*** Sagittal T1 weighted image (800/20) shows an extensive tear in the posterior horn (*large arrow*) and anterior horn (*small arrow*). ***B,*** Coronal T1 weighted image (800/20) shows normal lateral meniscus (*small arrow*), a tear in the posterior horn of the medial meniscus (*curved arrow*), and a separate "bucket-handle" fragment (*large straight arrow*) in the intracondylar notch.

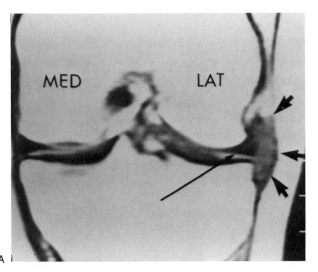

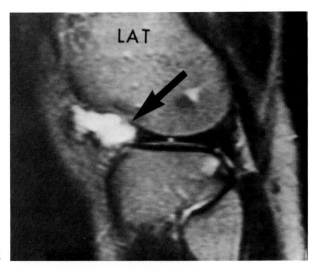

Figure 25–31. *Meniscal cysts.* ***A,*** Coronal T1 weighted image (800/20) shows a linear area of slightly increased signal intensity (*long arrow*) extending to the periphery of the lateral meniscus, and a soft tissue mass of intermediate signal intensity (the meniscal cyst) deep to the iliotibial band (*arrows*). ***B,*** Sagittal T2 weighted sequence (2000/80) showing a high-signal-intensity cyst (*arrow*) extending anteriorly from the anterior horn of the lateral meniscus.

be a small accumulation of fluid on T2 weighted images, seen as a focal area of increased intensity at the very distal aspect of the rotator cuff tendon at its insertion into the humeral head near the greater tuberosity (Fig. 25–32), i.e., at the area of tearing or discontinuity. High-signal-intensity fluid may also be seen in the subdeltoid and subacromial bursae. The true sensitivity and specificity of MRI in the diagnosis of rotator cuff tears are still uncertain.

Imaging of other tendons[44] such as the Achilles[45, 46] and posterior tibial tendons[47] is usually performed with T2 weighted sequences in the transverse axial plane and T1 weighted sagittal images. In the transverse axial plane, both feet and ankles are usually examined simultaneously to compare the clinically involved side with the uninvolved side. The normal tendon is hypointense. Partial tears appear as high-signal intratendinous collections (Fig. 25–33); complete acute tears

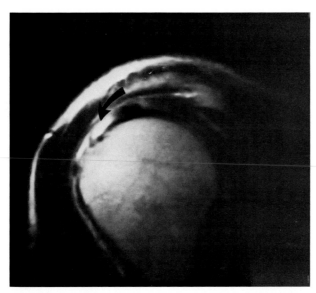

Figure 25-32. *Rotator cuff tendon tear.* Sagittal T2 weighted sequence (1800/80) demonstrates high-signal-intensity fluid (*arrow*) at the distal aspect of the rotator cuff tendon near its insertion into the humeral head, indicating tear and discontinuity.

show tendinous discontinuity. Chronic tendinitis appears as a diffuse thickening of the tendon.[46, 47]

Slipped Capital Femoral Epiphysis

Slipped capital femoral epiphysis can be easily diagnosed on routine radiography. The degree of slippage may be well demonstrated on MRI (Fig. 25-34) along with some abnormal high signal in the physis, which is present early and may be secondary to edema and hemorrhage. However, the MR examination is costly and at present does not appear to offer any additional information that may alter the management of the patient. Until it is shown that MRI can provide information important to the care of these children, it is not recommended for routine evaluation of the slipped capital femoral epiphysis.

Osteochondritis Dissecans

Although ossification variants have been implicated as an etiology for osteochondritis dissecans, trauma may have some role in this entity. The vast majority of cases involve the femoral condyles, the medial condyle being involved four times more frequently than the lateral. Lesions in the dome of the talus have also been referred to as osteochondritis dissecans. The peak age incidence is in the range of 11 to 25 years, and males are much more commonly involved than females. Up to 25 percent of lesions are bilateral.

The lesions of osteochondritis dissecans are classified according to the stability of the affected bone fragment, which may be stable or loose. The loose fragments are further classified as nondisplaced or displaced. The nondisplaced fragments are covered by intact articular cartilage. With fragment displacement, there is disruption of the overlying cartilage.

The management of children with osteochondritis dissecans usually depends on the mechanical stability of the osteochondral fragment, which it is therefore important to evaluate. If the fragment is loose in situ, it may be removed or surgically fixed; if it is displaced, it must be surgically resected; but if the fragment is stable, treatment is conservative.

MRI must be performed in both coronal and sagittal planes to avoid partial volume artifacts. These artifacts vary in each plane, depending on the precise location of the abnormality on the femoral condyle. The affected fragment of bone always shows a decrease in signal on T1 images, with some increase in signal intensity on T2 images. The signal in these fragments is always nonhomogeneous, as is the degree of enhancement on T2 images. The adjacent parent bone demonstrates some areas of low signal intensity on T1 and T2 pulse sequences (these are due to sclerosis and/or fibrosis), and other areas that show low signal intensity on T1 but some increase in signal intensity on T2 pulse sequences (due to reactive edema).

To determine the stability and displacement of the affected fragment, one may use plain film radiographs, bone scan, or magnetic resonance. Unless the fragment is ossified, only MRI will demonstrate a displaced fragment.

Mesgarzadeh and colleagues found that the larger the fragment and the thicker the surrounding sclerotic rim seen on plain film radiographs, the greater was the chance of instability.[48] A lesion larger than 0.8 sq cm with a sclerotic rim more than 3 mm thick is invariably unstable. Very small lesions without significant sclerosis are usually stable. Unfortunately, many lesions are intermediate in size and sclerosis, and therefore cannot be accurately classified on plain film. With radionuclide scintigraphy, the presence of focal hyperemia on a blood-pool image and a high degree of radionuclide accumulation on late-phase images make instability of the fragment more likely. MRI was found to be a sensitive and specific test for differentiating loose from stable osteochondral fragments.[48] A reliable sign of loosening was the presence of fluid on T2 weighted sequences at the interface of the fragment and its parent bone (Fig. 25-35). MRI may also demonstrate directly the displacement of the fragment when present (Fig. 25-36).

MR imaging should be reserved for cases in which results of both radiography and scintigraphy are indeterminate, or in which findings from either modality are strongly suggestive of loosening. MRI can then be performed to confirm the loosening and to evaluate the displacement, size, and location of the fragment.

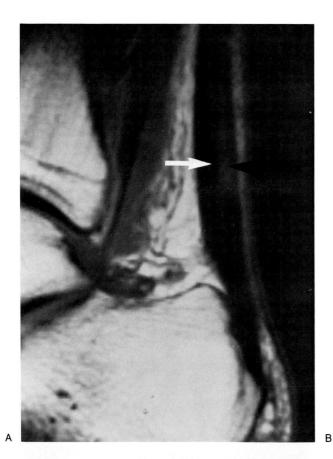

A

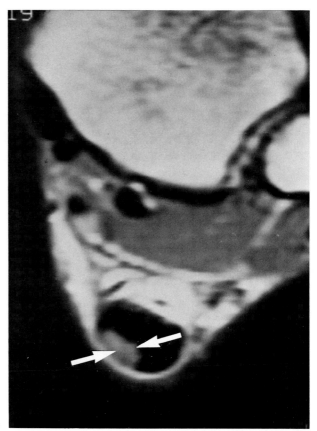

B

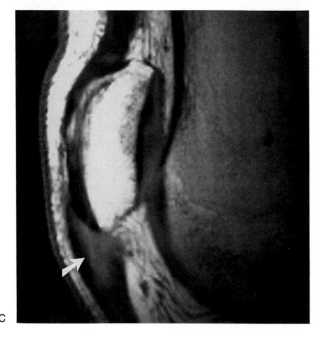

C

Figure 25–33. *Partial tears of the tendons.*   **A,** Achilles tendon tear. Sagittal T1 weighted image (800/20) of the ankle shows some increased signal in the posterior aspect of the Achilles tendon (*arrows*). **B,** This is better demonstrated in the transverse axial plane in a more T2 weighted sequence (1800/60) with a sharply delineated focal area of high intensity posteriorly (*arrows*), indicating a partial tear. **C,** Partial tear of the patella tendon. Coronal image (700/17) shows a focal area of increased intensity (*arrow*) in the patellar tendon.

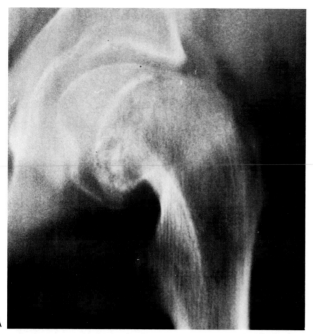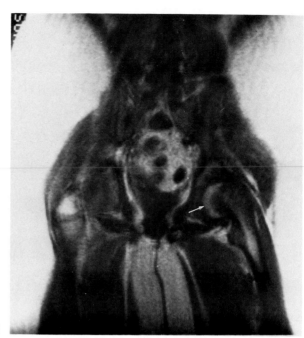

Figure 25–34. *Slipped capital femoral epiphysis.* **A,** Conventional radiograph shows a classic slip of the capital femoral epiphysis of the left hip. **B,** Coronal T1 MR image (500/30) corresponds well with **A.** The slipped epiphysis (*arrow*) is clearly identified.

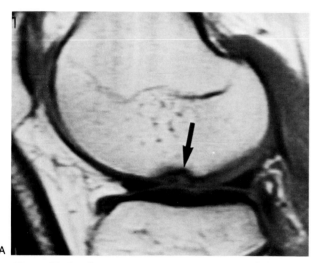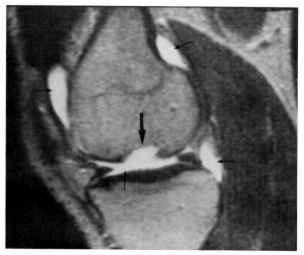

Figure 25–35. *Osteochondritis dissecans.* **A,** Sagittal T1 weighted sequence (800/20) demonstrates chondral and subchondral defect (*arrow*) typical of osteochondritis dissecans. **B,** Sagittal T2 weighted sequence (2000/80) in a different patient demonstrates high-intensity fluid filling the osteochondral defect (*large arrow*), indicating that the osteochondral fragment is displaced. Small arrows show additional areas of effusion.

Foreign Bodies

MRI has been employed to locate foreign bodies accurately. An interesting case illustrates accurate localization of a large metallic bullet fragment that initially could not be found at surgery (Fig. 25–37). There is no artifact from the bullet as one might have anticipated, since the bullet is not ferromagnetic. Bodne and colleagues recorded successful localization of glass or wood foreign bodies in three patients.[49] Both glass and wood are seen as areas of signal void with adjacent inflammation causing an area of strong signal intensity on T2 weighted images. In another patient with a chronically discharging sinus from the muscles of

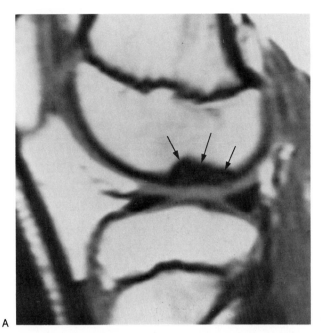 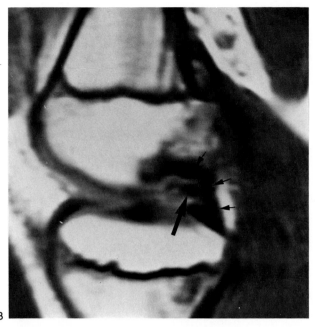

A   B

Figure 25–36. *Osteochondritis dissecans: displaced fragment.* ***A,*** Sagittal T1 weighted sequence (800/20) shows a low-intensity osteochondral defect (*arrows*) in the medial femoral condyle. ***B,*** Sagittal T1 weighted image (800/20) medial to ***A*** shows a loose fragment (*large arrow*) inferior to the posterior cruciate ligament (*small arrows*).

the lower leg, MRI was able to demonstrate the presence of a previously unsuspected wooden foreign body, which was also seen, but not as well, on CT scan (Fig. 25–14). The advantages of MRI are its ability to demonstrate the foreign body, the improved contrast resolution showing changes in the adjacent tissues, its ability to define the extent of the adjacent changes, and the three-dimensional localization of the foreign body and its relationship to adjacent vessels and tendons.

Effects of Exercise

It is important that MR changes after exercise be recognized so that they are not mistakenly attributed to pathology in a patient who is scanned soon after an injury acquired during exercise. Fleckenstein and associates studied humans who exercised selected muscles of the arms and legs under controlled conditions.[50] The exercised muscles demonstrated a decrease in signal intensity on T1 and an increase in signal intensity on T2 images (Fig. 25–38). These changes were distributed throughout the involved muscle. They are believed to be due to an increase in extracellular water content that occurs in response to the exercise. The increased signal intensity on the T2 images improves differentiation of the exercised muscles from adjacent muscles. The finding returns to normal fairly quickly. The amount of change identified on the MR image does not correlate absolutely with the amount of exercise.

Work by McCully and colleagues suggests that MR spectroscopy may have a significant role to play in the evaluation of athletes.[51] These authors studied high-energy phosphorus compounds in the muscles of athletes at rest, during exercise, and after trauma. They also found that strenuous endurance training programs can produce detectable changes in muscle metabolism as seen by an improvement in the muscle metabolism, and that active muscles in endurance-trained athletes demonstrate faster recovery than those in normal controls. In addition, exercise-induced muscle injury, from overtraining, can be detected as an increased inorganic phosphate-to-phosphocreatine ratio in resting muscles.

Dislocations

MRI can easily demonstrate a dislocation or subluxation at almost any joint (Figs. 25–39, 25–40). In many patients, however, this is equally adequately demonstrated by conventional radiography, and the precise role of MRI in the evaluation of dislocation has yet to be determined. This will involve extensive prospective studies comparing MRI with plain film radiography, ultrasonography, CT, and arthrography. It is likely that MRI will have no role in routine evaluation of uncomplicated dislocations. Instead, MRI will play an important role in selected patients in the evaluation of complications such as avascular necrosis, or in deter-

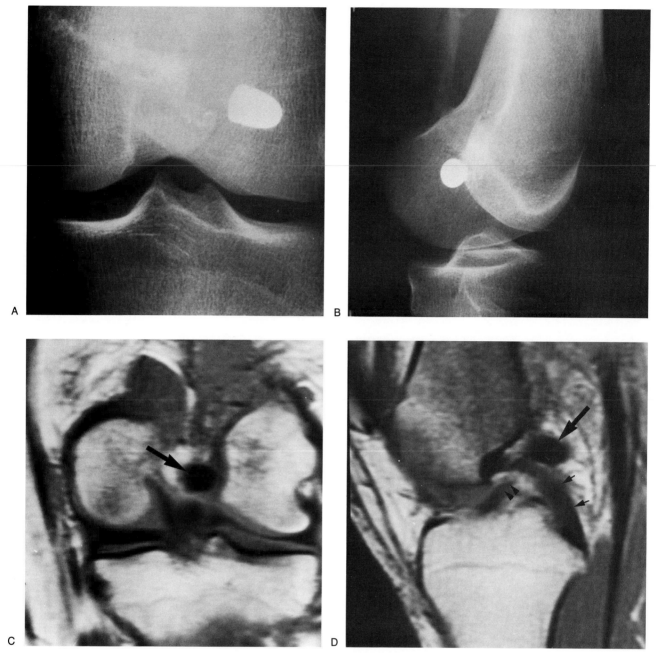

Figure 25–37. *Foreign body localization: gunshot wound to the knee.* ***A, B,*** Anteroposterior and lateral radiographs demonstrate a metallic bullet fragment. The bullet was not found at surgery. Coronal (***C***) and sagittal (***D***) T1 weighted images (800/20) demonstrate the nonferromagnetic bullet (*large arrow*) behind the posterior cruciate (*small arrows*) and anterior cruciate (*arrowheads*) ligaments. Note also the low intensity within the femur, due to edema and hemorrhage within the femur secondary to injury by the bullet.

mining the reason for difficulty in obtaining reduction of a dislocated joint.

A few studies have reported the accuracy of MRI in the evaluation of dislocations. For example, in a series of adults with recurrent anterior dislocation of the shoulder, Kieft and colleagues were able to demonstrate that MRI compared well with CT arthrography or surgery in demonstrating the presence or absence of an associated fracture of the glenoid, disruption of the glenoid labrum, posterolateral impaction fracture of the humeral head, or adjacent soft tissue abnormality.[52] MRI was not as good, however, at demonstrating separation of the capsule from the labrum or glenoid bone.

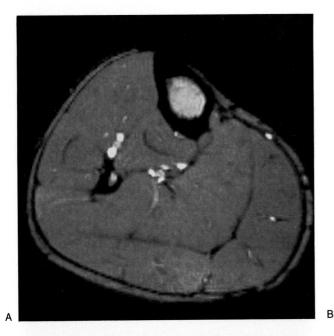

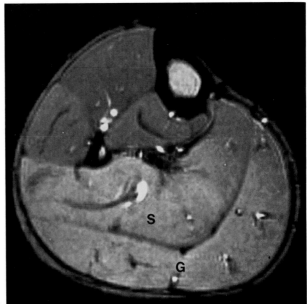

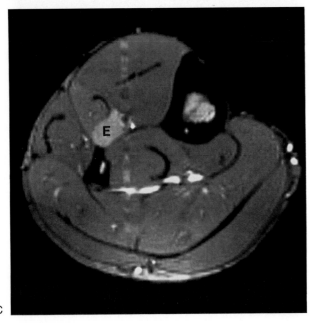

Figure 25–38. *Normal response of skeletal muscle to exercise.* Gradient reversal, partial flip angle images of the proximal calf in a normal human volunteer. **A,** Pre-exercise image shows no difference in the signal intensity between muscle groups. **B,** After plantar flexion, signal intensity increases in the soleus (S) and gastrocnemius (G) muscles. **C,** After extension of the great toe there is increase in signal intensity in the extensor hallucis muscle (E). (Fleckenstein JL, Canhy RL, Parkey RW, Peshock RM. Acute effects of exercise on MR imaging of skeletal muscle in normal volunteers. AJR 1988; 151:231–237; © by American Roentgen Ray Society.)

Congenital Dislocation of the Hip

This is an important and relatively common disorder. Many patients present as newborns with instability of the hip, and in over 95 percent cure is obtained with simple flexion-abduction splinting. These patients are managed successfully by clinical evaluation, with or without plain film radiographs and ultrasound studies. If a congenital hip dislocation is not diagnosed and treated early, relocation of the femoral head becomes progressively more difficult and the role of imaging becomes increasingly important.

There are many imaging methods available for the study of hip dislocations. Conventional radiography is relatively poor in detecting mild subluxation in the first few months of life before ossification of the femoral head epiphysis has started. At any stage it can detect gross dislocation but it cannot define accurately the relationship of the femoral head to the acetabulum in all cases, and it is very poor at demonstrating the femoral head and acetabular cartilage and the adjacent soft tissue. CT provides a tomographic image that occasionally may identify dislocation when the plain film

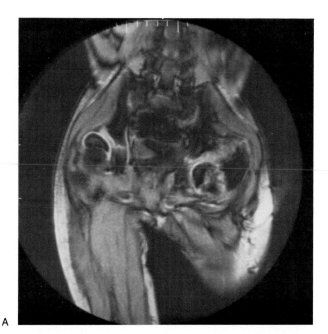

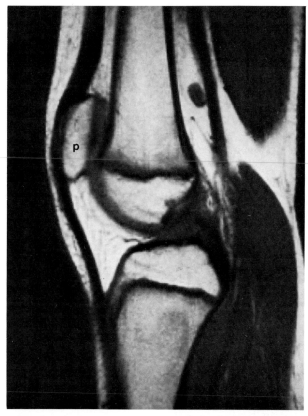

A

B

Figure 25–39. *Subluxation of the right hip in a child with cerebral palsy and coxa vara.* ***A,*** Coronal spin-density (200/20) and ***B,*** field-echo (400/12, 90-degree flip angle) images show upward displacement and lateral subluxation of the right femoral head.

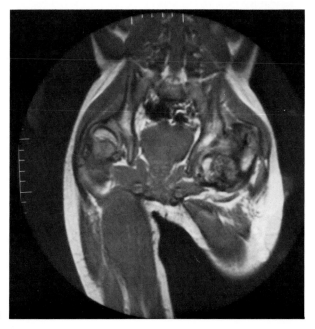

Figure 25–40. *Superior patellar subluxation (patella alta).* Sagittal T1 image (700/17). The patella (p) lies in an abnormally high position, with an increase in the ratio of the length of the patellar tendon relative to the length of the patella. (Courtesy of Curtis W. Hayes, Richmond, VA.)

radiograph appears normal. CT shows the soft tissues only moderately well and the cartilage poorly. Ultrasonography has become widely used to evaluate hip dislocation; it is sensitive for demonstration of early subluxation or dislocation. Its overall value in the evaluation of patients with failed reduction, or in seeking the complications of dislocation, is not known. Arthrog-

raphy is usually reserved for patients in whom there is difficulty in achieving reduction. It is in this area that MRI may have its greatest potential, with the possibility of replacing the need for arthrography. At the present time this is the major indication for performing MRI. There are two reports of the use of MRI to evaluate children with difficulty in achieving hip reduction.[53,54] These authors suggest that the MR images should be performed in the neutral position. MRI has proved excellent at defining the many causes of failed reduction. These include:

1. Infolding of the labrum.
2. Infolding of the capsule.
3. Shortening of the transverse acetabular ligament (this ligament normally bridges the inferior deficit of the limbus at the inferior margin of the acetabulum.)
4. Indentation of the capsule by the iliopsoas muscle. Normally the iliopsoas tendon is flat and not well seen on MRI. In this disorder the tendon becomes rounder and it is easily seen indenting the anterior capsule.
5. Acetabular dysplasia (deformity of the cartilage of the acetabulum).

6. Hypertrophy of the pulvinar (the normal intra-articular fat pad).

In the 34 cases reported in the two series, MRI proved very good at identifying the above abnormalities.[53,54] The only disadvantage of MRI compared with arthrography is that it cannot dynamically view the motion of the femoral head.

Future Applications

Progress continues in hardware and software development, and new sequences and techniques are continually being developed. In addition, coil technology is constantly improving. These factors make it virtually certain that MRI will play a far greater role in the future. Important uses to be developed will be the ability to directly image subtle cartilaginous injuries, and to evaluate vascular integrity in the traumatized limb.

COLLAGEN DISORDER
Philip Stanley, M.D.
Melvin Senac, M.D.

Juvenile Rheumatoid Arthritis

The pathology of rheumatoid arthritis was first described by Charcot in 1853, and this was followed by an account on "childhood inflammatory arthritis" by Cornil in 1864.[55,56] Frederick Still wrote the classic description of juvenile rheumatoid arthritis (JRA) in 1897, which documented the systemic manifestations that may accompany the arthritis.[57]

Juvenile rheumatoid arthritis affects approximately 250,000 children in the United States, with a peak between 1 and 2 years of age.[58] By definition, it is a disease in children under 16 years of age, who have arthritis symptoms lasting for at least 6 weeks and in whom other causes for arthropathy have been excluded. The modern classification of juvenile rheumatoid arthritis in the United States describes systemic, pauciarticular, and polyarticular forms.[59]

As the name indicates, extra-articular manifestations characterize the *systemic* form of juvenile rheumatoid arthritis. The patient may have a fever, rash, and involvement of the heart, liver, and spleen, with enlargement of lymph nodes. Boys and girls are affected equally. Rheumatoid factor (RF) and anti-nuclear antibodies (ANA) are usually absent from the serum.[60] The arthritis can develop at any time, but usually occurs early in the course of the disease. The child complains of pain and morning stiffness with limitations of movement on examination. There is soft tissue swelling with warmth and effusion in the joints. The arthritis is usually polyarticular, affecting small joints of the hand as well as large weight-bearing joints.

Approximately 40 percent of patients in the systemic group have severe progressive joint destruction.

Four or fewer joints are affected in the *pauciarticular* group. This is the most common form, occurring in about 45 percent of patients.[60] Three subtypes are recognized. The first, seen predominantly in girls who are ANA positive, has iridocyclitis, which may lead to blindness, as a common accompaniment. The eye disease bears no temporal relationship to the Activity of the arthritis. The onset of arthritis is either acute or insidious, predominantly involving the large joints of the lower extremity. The second subtype is seen in older boys presenting with heel pain who later develop ankylosing spondylitis. The third subtype involves children without iridocyclitis who are RF negative. This has the best prognosis. Moreover, the arthritis that accompanies this form is less destructive than that seen with the other forms of juvenile rheumatoid arthritis.

In the *polyarticular* form, more than four joints are affected. This type occurs in approximately 25 percent of children with JRA[6] and is more frequent in girls. There may be extra-articular features, but these are not dominant. Large, rapidly growing joints of the knees, hips, wrists, and ankles are first affected, the smaller joints of the hands being later involved. The large joint involvement is usually bilateral but may be unequal. In addition, the cervical spine is involved in about 50 percent of cases. The apophyseal joints are affected with later fusion. The transverse and other ligaments around the odontoid are weakened by rheumatoid granulation tissue. This ligamentous laxity, together with fusion of the posterior elements of the lower cervical spine, can cause C1-C2 subluxation, particularly at the time of intubation with general anesthesia. If there is absence of rheumatoid factor, the outlook is relatively good in this group; only 10 to 15 percent go on to develop progressive joint destruction. However, RF-positive patients, usually an older group, may progress; over 50 percent develop severe destructive arthritis. This subgroup often have extra-articular manifestations.

Independent of the type of arthritis, the pathologic changes are similar although varying in severity.

Pathologic Changes
After Charcot's initial description of the disease in 1853, Weichselbaum (1877) emphasized the inflammation of the synovium seen with "arthritis deformans."[61] This inflammation of the synovium is the first change seen in juvenile rheumatoid arthritis. An as yet unidentified antigen is phagocytosed by type A synovial lining cells.[62] Portions of this antigen diffuse into the synovial fluid where the antigen is bound to B lymphocytes, which are transformed into plasma cells. These produce antibodies, including rheumatoid factor. The subsequent antibody-antigen reaction produces enzymes by activating macrophages and granulocytes. These enzymes (collagenases, elastases, and hydrolases) within the synovium and synovial fluid degrade

the molecular structure of the articular hyaline and meniscal fibrocartilage.

The initial microscopic features of juvenile rheumatoid arthritis consist of edema and swelling of synovium, and perivascular infiltration with lymphocytes, macrophages, and plasma cells. The latter contain eosinophilic inclusions of gammaglobulin (Russell's bodies).[63] As the disease progresses, there is an increase in the inflammation, with hypertrophy and hyperplasia of the synovial cells and thickening of the covering membrane. The synovium has an adherent fibrinous exudate on the surface.[64] The hypertrophic synovium (pannus) later extends over the articular surface, destroying the underlying cartilage by interfering with chondrocytic nutrition and by enzymatic degradation of the matrix. These changes start at the periphery in the synovial recesses where the bone is not covered by articular cartilage, and progress centripetally into the joint. The joint capsule and ligaments may also be destroyed, giving rise to subluxation. In the large joints, such as the knee and hip, ankylosis may occur after extensive destruction of the articular surface.

Radiology

These pathologic changes are reflected in the imaging studies. Plain radiographs, arthrography, and occasionally ultrasound and nuclear radiology studies were the imaging investigations performed for juvenile rheumatoid arthritis in the past. Arthrography, ultrasonography, and to a certain extent nuclear studies have been replaced by MRI.[65] Whereas routine radiographs show osteopenia and periosteal new bone, not apparent on MRI, cartilage can be demonstrated only by injection of contrast material. When radiographs show joint space narrowing, it suggests severe cartilage loss indicative of advanced and usually irreversible disease. Ultrasonography shows fluid and synovial thickening, but the all-important changes in the hyaline and fibrocartilage are not detected. Nuclear studies accurately gauge joint activity and marrow vascularity, but do not demonstrate the cartilage in detail.

MRI has the advantage of demonstrating cartilage and soft tissues noninvasively without irradiation, and has the potential to monitor therapy. Early changes of synovitis and cartilage thinning are not seen on plain radiographs. At this stage of the disease, the process may be halted or reversed with anti-inflammatory therapy. It is important when assessing articular cartilage loss that the observer be familiar with normal appearances in a growing child.[65] In a near-term fetus, the epiphysis is entirely hyaline cartilage. With the development of the epiphyseal ossific center, there is gradual thinning of the hyaline cartilage, so that by early adulthood all that remains of the hyaline cartilage epiphysis is a smooth layer of articular cartilage. Whereas measurements correlating normal articular thickness with age have yet to be developed, certain guidelines have been established. The articular cartilage should be smooth, of uniform thickness, and not associated with a joint effusion.

The articular cartilage has an intermediate signal intensity on both T1 and T2 spin-echo sequences (Fig. 25–41).[66] It has a bright signal on gradient-echo sequences (Fig. 25–41). The fibrocartilaginous structures (menisci and ligaments) are always of low signal intensity, independent of the imaging sequence. The synovium, which is rarely seen in normal joints, is of low signal intensity on T1 and T2 images, although the pannus, which originates from within the synovium, may have a variable signal on T2 weighted images. Cortical bone is dark on T1 and T2 spin-echo sequences. The underlying epiphysis is uniformly bright, with a dark epiphyseal plate. Joint fluid is of low signal on T1 and high signal on T2 weighted images. Tendon sheaths (not studied in this series) may be distended with fluid that has the same characteristics as joint fluid.

The three joints most frequently imaged are described in detail below.

The knee is most often affected in juvenile rheumatoid arthritis, being involved in over 90 percent of patients. The normal knee is illustrated in Figure 25–41 and is to be compared with those showing early changes. The earliest changes visible on MRI are those of synovitis. There may be irregularity or hypertrophy of the synovium. Hypertrophic synovium (pannus) is best seen in the suprapatellar pouch, a linear structure on T1 that may be of low or high signal on T2 weighted images. The high signal probably reflects increased water content secondary to inflammation. The lower signal on T2 within the pannus has been attributed to hemosiderin deposition.[67] Synovial irregularity may be seen in the reflection over the posterior surface of the infrapatellar fat pad (Fig. 25–42).[68] This is usually associated with an effusion. The synovium may enhance after injection of the paramagnetic agent gadolinium-DTPA[69] and this finding is probably indicative of acute synovitis. Local or diffuse loss of hyaline articular cartilage of the femoral and tibial condyle is an early finding followed by hypoplasia or atrophy of the menisci (Fig. 25–43). Synovial cysts (Fig. 25–44) in the popliteal fossa are frequently seen, and Baker's cysts are relatively late manifestations (Fig. 25–45). Later changes include irregularity and erosions of the articular bony cortex (Fig. 25–46). These appear as of low signal on T1 weighted images but have a variable signal on T2, depending on whether there is inflammation or hemorrhage within the adjacent pannus (see above). This may be followed by avascular necrosis (Fig. 25–47), fragmentation of the articular surface, and separation of osteochondral fragments (Fig. 25–48). Abutment and misalignment of the bony articular surfaces, with later ankylosis, occur in advanced disease. It should be noted that MR findings sometimes attributed to avascular necrosis in juvenile rheumatoid arthritis have not always been supported by later examination of an excised specimen.[70] In juvenile rheumatoid arthritis, abnormal signal may be seen in the bone marrow on MR images. Some of the changes seen in the marrow may be due to osteopenia or edema

Text continues on page 950.

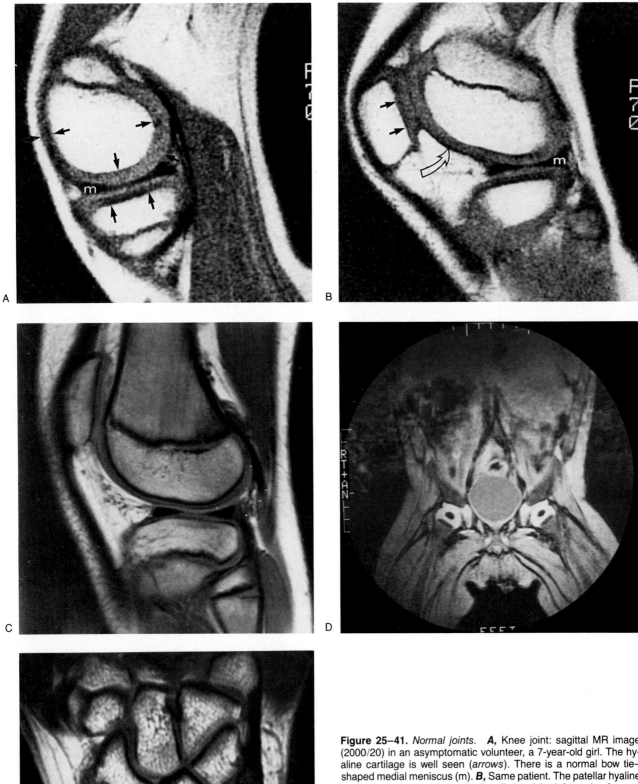

Figure 25–41. *Normal joints.* **A,** Knee joint: sagittal MR image (2000/20) in an asymptomatic volunteer, a 7-year-old girl. The hyaline cartilage is well seen (*arrows*). There is a normal bow tie–shaped medial meniscus (m). **B,** Same patient. The patellar hyaline cartilage (*arrows*) can easily be distinguished from the femoral articular cartilage (*open arrow*). The meniscal cartilage is well shown (m). **C,** Knee joint: sagittal view (SE 2000/20) in a normal 15-year-old boy. Note the smooth articular cartilage covering the femur and tibia. The normal lateral meniscus has a bow tie appearance. **D,** Hip joint: gradient-echo (500/25, 90-degree flip angle). There is a strong signal from the hyaline cartilage of the femoral head and acetabulum. **E,** Normal wrist (600/30). Normal cartilage has an intermediate signal. (From Senac MO, Deutch D, Bernstein BH, et al. MR imaging in juvenile rheumatoid arthritis. AJR 1988; 150:873–878.)

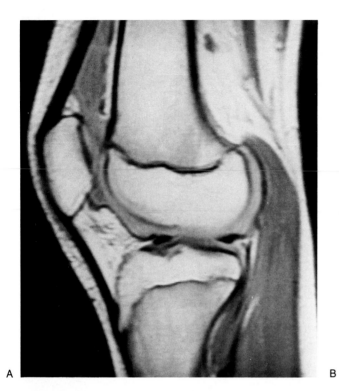

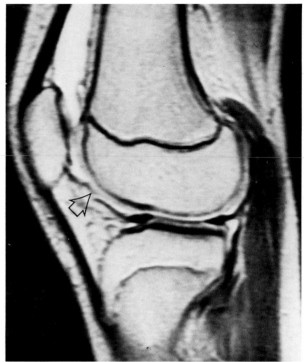

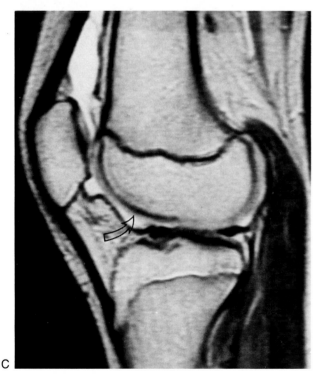

Figure 25–42. *Juvenile rheumatoid arthritis: effusion and cartilage thinning.*   ***A,*** Sagittal view (1000/20) in a 12-year-old girl with moderately severe JRA. It is difficult to distinguish articular cartilage from joint effusion; to do this, either a T2 weighted image or a gradient-echo image is required. ***B,*** Same patient. Sagittal view (2000/60). There is a moderately large effusion that can be distinguished from the articular cartilage, which shows some loss. There is meniscal atrophy and irregularity of the prepatellar fat pad (*arrow*). ***C,*** A more medial sagittal image shows thinned articular cartilage (*arrow*) to better effect. (From Senac MO, Deutch D, Bernstein BH, et al. MR imaging in juvenile rheumatoid arthritis. AJR 1988; 150:873–878.)

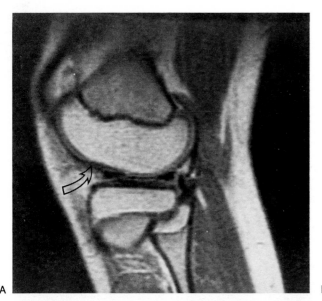

A

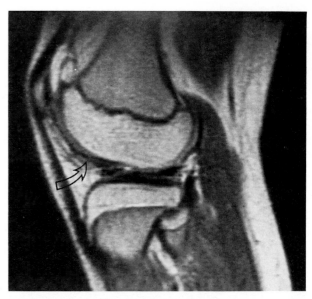

B

Figure 25–43. *Juvenile rheumatoid arthritis: meniscal atrophy and cartilage loss.* **A,** Sagittal image (2000/20) in a 10-year-old girl with moderately severe JRA. There is hypoplasia of the fibrocartilaginous meniscus and diffuse thinning of the hyaline articular cartilage, particularly on the undersurface of the femur (*arrow*) and tibial condyle. **B,** Slightly more medial image showing mild irregularity of the posterior surface of the infrapatellar fat pad indicative of synovitis (*arrow*). (From Senac MO, Deutch D, Bernstein BH, et al. MR imaging in juvenile rheumatoid arthritis. AJR 1988; 150:873–878.)

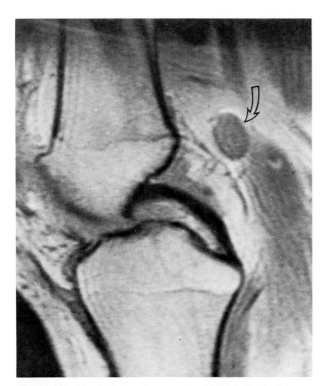

Figure 25–44. *Juvenile rheumatoid arthritis.* Sagittal image (2000/20) shows a popliteal cyst (*arrow*). (From Senac MO, Deutch D, Bernstein BH, et al. MR imaging in juvenile rheumatoid arthritis. AJR 1988; 150:873–878.)

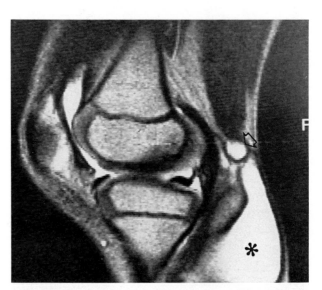

Figure 25–45. *Juvenile rheumatoid arthritis.* Sagittal plane MR image (2500/80). There is a moderate-sized effusion with a small popliteal cyst (*arrow*) and a very large Baker's cyst (*asterisk*). There is good preservation of articular cartilage.

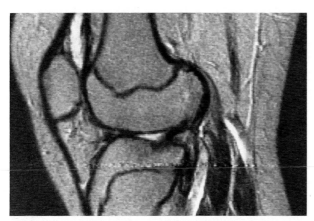

Figure 25–46. *Juvenile rheumatoid arthritis with severe cartilage loss.* Sagittal plane MR image (2500/80) showing an effusion with complete loss of articular cartilage. In addition, there is meniscal atrophy.

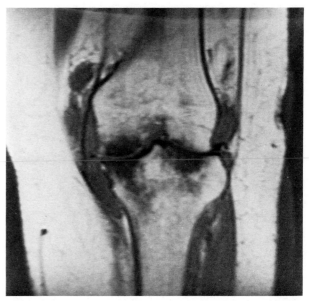

Figure 25–47. *Juvenile rheumatoid arthritis with avascular necrosis.* Coronal MR image (500/20) shows narrowing of the joint space due to loss of hyaline cartilage and meniscal fibrocartilage. There is signal loss in both femoral condyles and upper tibia compatible with avascular necrosis. (From Senac MO, Deutch D, Bernstein BH, et al. MR imaging in juvenile rheumatoid arthritis. AJR 1988; 150:873–878.)

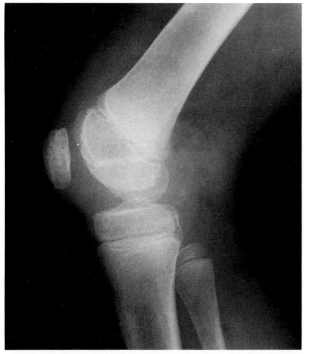

A

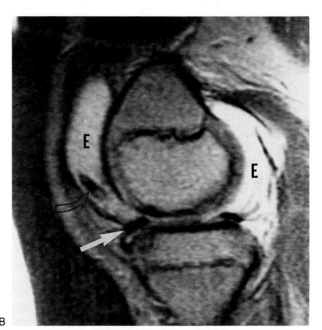

B

Figure 25–48. *Juvenile rheumatoid arthritis with articular fragmentation.* **A,** Lateral radiograph showing knee joint effusion. **B,** Sagittal MR image (2000/60) confirming the effusion (E), but there is also an osteochondral fragment (*open arrow*). There is some loss of articular cartilage and hypoplasia of the menisci (*white arrow*). (From Senac MO, Deutch D, Bernstein BH, et al. MR imaging in juvenile rheumatoid arthritis. AJR 1988; 150:873–878.)

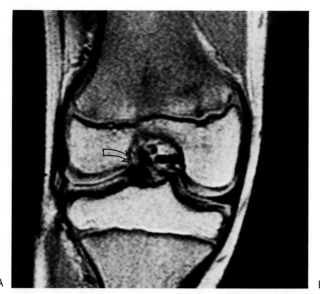

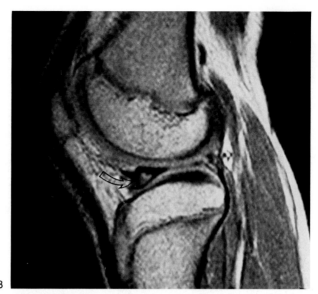

A   B

Figure 25–49. *Juvenile rheumatoid arthritis with meniscal tear.* **A,** Coronal view (2000/30) of a 5-year-old child who had a painful knee. There is a "bucket-handle" tear of the meniscus with anterior infolding of the fragment (*arrow*). There is good preservation of the articular cartilage. The patient's symptoms were attributed to JRA before MRI. **B,** Sagittal projection (2000/30) demonstrating infolding of the fragment (*arrow*).

or an unidentified process that interferes with the normal marrow signal. It is important to appreciate that other derangements of the knee may be found in patients with juvenile rheumatoid arthritis (Fig. 25–49).

Magnetic resonance of the knee is performed with special knee coils. For patients with juvenile rheumatoid arthritis, it is suggested that coronal T1 weighted images be performed, followed by sagittal spin-echo T2 or gradient-echo T2 pulse sequences. Only by use of one of these two techniques in the sagittal plane will it be possible to distinguish between hyaline articular cartilage and joint fluid.

The hip shows changes similar to those of the knee on MRI. The earliest changes are those of synovitis. Whereas the synovial reflections are not well seen on MRI, the presence of synovial fluid, indicative of active synovitis, is easily visible (Fig. 25–50). Irregular loss of hyaline articular cartilage is easily demonstrated on MRI, although routine radiographs are usually normal early in the disease process (Fig. 25–51). Erosions through the cartilage into the bony epiphysis are demonstrated more effectively on MRI. These erosions are probably due to infiltration with hypertrophic synovium rather than avascular necrosis (Figs. 25–52, 25–53). Later changes include fragmentation of the head with osteocartilaginous fragments and ankylosis of the joint. The standard imaging techniques for hips include coronal T1 and sagittal T2 spin-echo or gradient-echo images.

Juvenile rheumatoid arthritis may cause significant abnormalities of *the cervical spine,* which is involved in 25 percent of patients. These children usually are serologically positive. Ligamentous laxity due to synovial

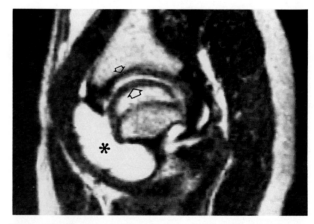

Figure 25–50. *Juvenile rheumatoid arthritis with hip effusion.* Sagittal plane MR image (2000/80). There is a large hip effusion (*asterisk*) with preservation of articular cartilage (*arrows*). The hip effusion is one of the earliest signs of JRA.

hyperplasia affecting the interalar and transverse ligaments, together with apophyseal fusion of the middle and lower cervical spine, may cause atlantoaxial subluxation with cord compression. While the instability and bony fusion may be shown by standard radiographs, the extent of the bone erosions with synovial hyperplasia (pannus) is best demonstrated by MRI (Fig. 25–54). MRI demonstrates indentation of the cord and internal signals within the upper cord and caudal brain stem on T2 weighted images.[71] These signals may represent edema or gliosis. Settling of the

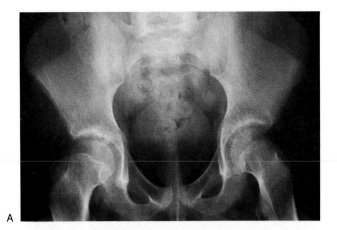

A

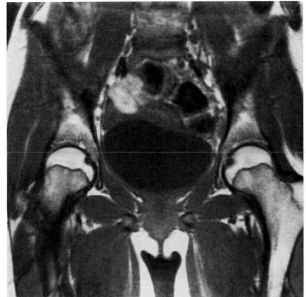

B

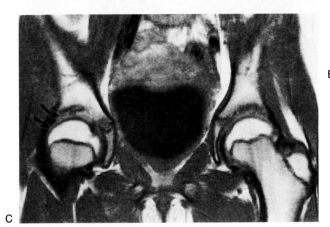

C

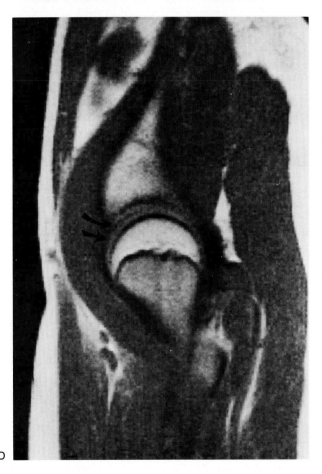

D

Figure 25–51. *Juvenile rheumatoid arthritis with early cartilage loss in the hip.* ***A,*** Anteroposterior view of both hips in an 11-year-old girl with clinical evidence of arthritis in the left hip. The radiograph is normal. ***B,*** Coronal plane MR image (2000/20) shows loss of femoral and acetabular articular cartilage, especially medially. No erosions are seen. ***C,*** Coronal plane MR image (2000/20) of an age-matched volunteer demonstrates normal acetabular femoral head hyaline articular cartilage (*arrows*). ***D,*** Sagittal plane MR image (2000/20) of the same patient as in ***C*** showing the smooth contour of hyaline cartilage covering the femoral head and acetabulum (*arrows*). (From Senac MO, Deutch D, Bernstein BH, et al. MR imaging in juvenile rheumatoid arthritis. AJR 1988; 150:873–878.)

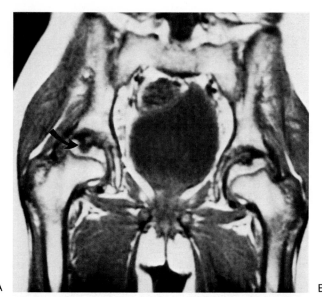
A

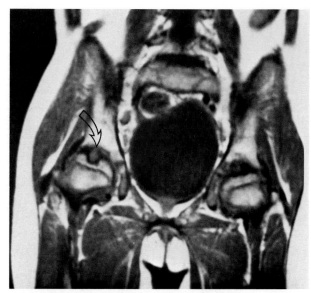
B

Figure 25–52. *Juvenile rheumatoid arthritis with subchondral cyst.* **A,** Coronal MR image (1000/20) shows complete loss of articular cartilage on the right with a subchondral cyst (*arrow*). There are moderately advanced changes on the left, but there is some preservation of acetabular hyaline cartilage. **B,** Coronal MRI. The more anterior image shows pannus within the subchondral cyst on the right (*arrow*). (From Senac MO, Deutch D, Bernstein BH, et al. MR imaging in juvenile rheumatoid arthritis. AJR 1988; 150:873–878.)

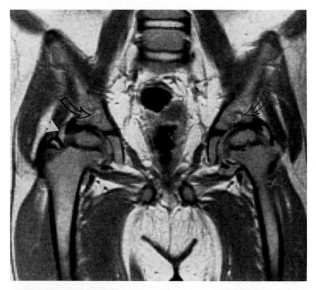

Figure 25–53. *Juvenile rheumatoid arthritis with synovial cyst.* Coronal image (2000/40). There is a small amount of fluid in both hips (*white arrow*) with loss of articular cartilage. There are bilateral synovial cysts of the supra-acetabular regions (*open arrows*).

skull on the upper cervical spine as a result of occipital atlantal joint disease may also be shown. In addition, MRI may be used to demonstrate the compression of the vertebral arteries that can occur in rheumatoid arthritis, although less frequently in children. Usually, T1 axial and T2 sagittal images are performed. To demonstrate instability, sagittal images in flexion and extension are cautiously performed.

Other joints are affected in juvenile rheumatoid arthritis. The ankle is the second most frequently affected joint, being involved in 80 percent of patients with systemic and polyarticular rheumatoid arthritis. In addition, the temporomandibular joint is often involved as are the wrist, hand, and elbow. However, the restraints of time and cost usually restrict imaging to the major joints. Future development will include assessment of activity by gadolinium-DTPA enhancement and demonstration of abnormal joint movement by kinetic MRI, using a nonferromagnetic positioning device. The images may then be viewed on a cine loop format. With kinetic MRI, subtle joint subluxation may be demonstrated that is not apparent clinically. The precise role of MRI in monitoring the response of juvenile rheumatoid arthritis to therapy has yet to be determined.

MISCELLANEOUS DISORDERS

Hemophilia

Sheila Moore, M.D.

Hemophilia is a hemorrhagic disorder caused by deficiency of factor VIII. Musculoskeletal changes in hemophilia are confined primarily to the periarticular region, where repeated episodes of joint hemorrhage cause hemosiderin deposition, fibrous tissue forma-

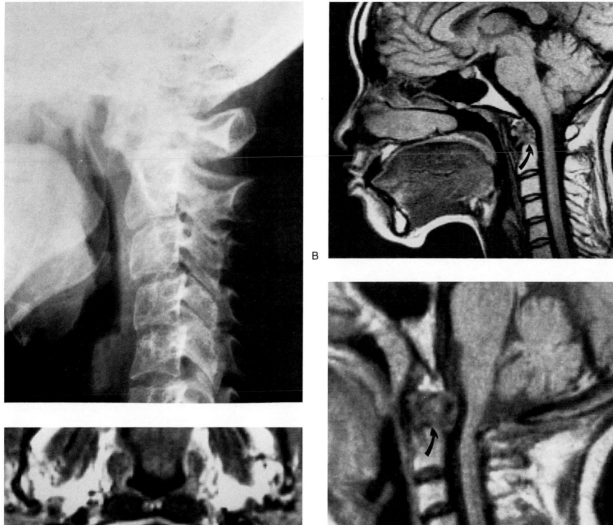

Figure 25–54. *Juvenile rheumatoid arthritis of the cervical spine.* ***A,*** Lateral view of the cervical spine showing forward displacement of C1 on C2. ***B,*** Sagittal MR image (500/40) demonstrates abnormal signal surrounding the dens (*arrow*). There is no cord compression. Abnormal movement may be detected by cautious flexion and extension MRI. ***C,*** Same patient as in ***B***. Axial MR image (500/40) shows rheumatoid granulation tissue around the dens (*arrow*). ***D,*** Sagittal image (1000/40) of another patient with rheumatoid arthritis showing compression of the upper cervical cord by rheumatoid granulation tissue (*arrow*).

tion, loss of articular cartilage, and resultant, often severe, osteoarthropathy. Radiographs of affected joints either are normal or may show varying degrees of joint space loss, spurring, subchondral sclerosis, and intraosseous cysts. The marrow may be involved by intraosseous hemorrhages into the shafts and epiphyses. Subperiosteal hemorrhage is rare, but when the subperiosteal hemorrhage is under tension, pressure atrophy of the underlying cortex occurs.

On MR examination of patients with hemophilic arthropathy, the hemosiderin and fibrous tissue that are deposited as a result of repeated episodes of joint hemorrhage are seen as of low signal intensity on both T1 and T2 weighted spin-echo images (Fig. 25–55).[72,73] The hemosiderin-laden synovial reflections are markedly thickened. Low signal intensity of the synovium, as well as an irregular contour to Hoffa's infrapatellar fat pad, may also be seen.[74]

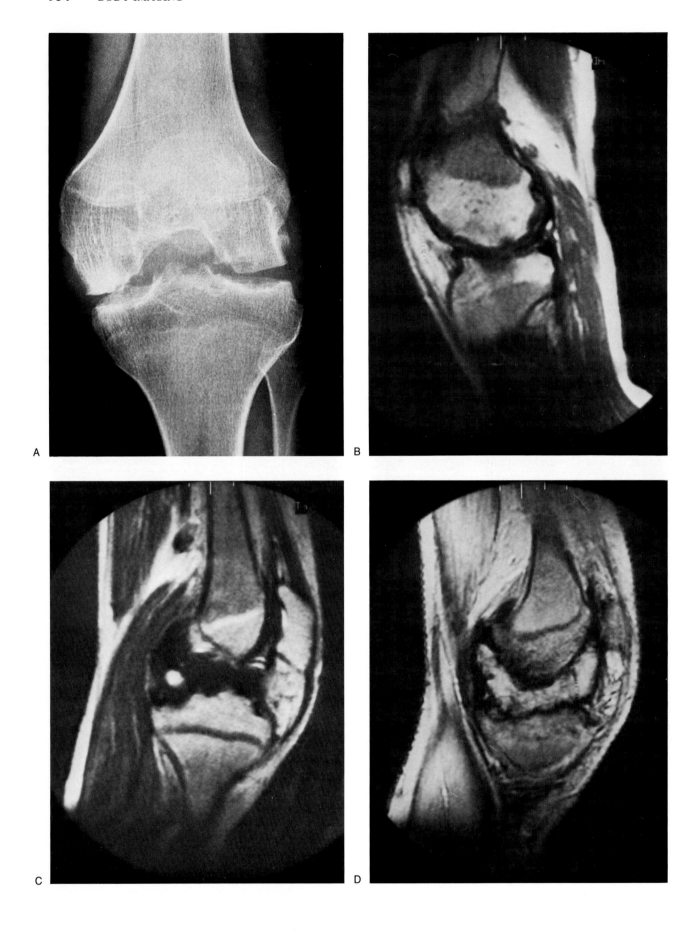

Subchondral and intraosseous cysts or hemorrhage may be identified on both coronal and sagittal MR images (Fig. 25–55). On T1 weighted images, both fluid-filled cysts and areas of sclerosis and fibrosis are of low signal intensity on T1 weighted images. On T2 weighted images the fluid in the subchondral cysts increases in signal intensity, while areas of fibrous tissue remain low in signal intensity. Articular and subchondral abnormalities are found in up to 80 percent of hemophiliac patients. Synovial fluid may be a prominent finding.

Indications for MRI

Indications for MR examination of the musculoskeletal system in patients with hemophilia include imaging of the marrow to assess for intraosseous hemorrhage. MRI is used primarily in the periarticular region, where it may show evidence of hemophilic arthropathy, including hemosiderin deposits, fibrous tissue, cartilaginous erosion, and joint fluid, that cannot be appreciated by radiography. In addition to its use in assessment of arthropathy, MRI is gaining use in the hemophiliac child who presents with acute joint pain. If the patient has a large hemarthrosis, evacuation of hemorrhage is often desirable, both to decrease the arthropathic sequelae of hemophilia and to reduce the risk of infection. Determination of the nature of the fluid can often be made on MRI, since hemorrhage appears complex and often increased in signal intensity on both T1 and T2 weighted images, whereas synovial effusion is seen as of low signal intensity on T1 and of bright signal intensity on T2 weighted images.

Duchenne Muscular Dystrophy

Mervyn D. Cohen, M.B., Ch.B.

This is a disorder of progressive muscle atrophy and patchy muscle necrosis, characterized clinically by progressive muscular weakness. The disease selectively affects certain muscles. For example, in the legs it spares the gracilis, rectus femoris, sartorius, and semitendinosus muscles. Some patients show an apparent pseudohypertrophy of affected muscle groups; this is just an overaccumulation of fat within atrophied muscle. In a study of eight patients with Duchenne muscular dystrophy, it was found that MRI accurately identified patchy replacement of the muscle by fat.[75] It was also found that the amount of fat present correlated well with the clinical staging of the severity of the disease. Abnormality is detected by many modalities other than MRI, but none of them can predict disease severity. For example, gallium shows uptake in affected muscles, but the amount of uptake is not proportional to the stage of the disease. Ultrasonography shows fat in the muscles but cannot quantitate the amount of fat present. The findings on MRI do not reflect a specific disorder in the muscle, but the distribution of the abnormality may suggest the correct diagnosis. The role of MRI seems to be mainly in predicting disease severity by quantifying the amount of fat present or identifying areas for muscle biopsy. The differential diagnosis of fatty replacement of muscle is wide, including many disorders of muscle disuse and also collagen disorders such as polymyositis or dermatomyositis.

Fibrous Dysplasia

Sheila Moore, M.D.

MR Appearance

Fibrous dysplasia is characterized by fibrous displacement of portions of the medullary cavity of a bone. The lesions can be either single (monostotic) or multiple (polyostotic). The cause of fibrous dysplasia is unknown, but it is believed most likely to represent a congenital abnormality of the bone-forming mesenchyme. This results in a replacement of the normal medullary cavity by fibrous tissue and poorly ossified trabeculae. Albright's syndrome is the triad of polyoostotic fibrous dysplasia with ipsilateral café au lait spots and precocious puberty (endocrine dysfunction) in females.

Fibrous dysplasia is thought to have its onset most commonly in childhood, although the actual incidence in infancy is unknown since the abnormality is often unrecognized. Males and females are equally affected and there is no familial tendency. Most patients with monostotic fibrous dysplasia are asymptomatic, but local swelling, especially in superficial bones such as the tibia or clavicle, is not uncommon. Pathologic fracture may often be the first sign of disease. Malignant transformation is rare but occurs more often in polyostotic than in monostotic fibrous dysplasia. Sarcomatous degeneration to osteosarcoma or fibrosarcoma is most common. Chondrosarcoma and giant cell tumor may also occur.

Sexual precocity is noted in approximately one-fifth

◀ **Figure 25–55.** *Hemophilia: chronic changes and acute hemorrhage.* **A,** Radiograph shows extensive overgrowth of the femoral condyles with secondary degenerative changes, including joint narrowing and subchondral sclerosis. **B, C,** Sagittal T1 (850/26) and T2 (2100/90) images show marked joint narrowing. There is extensive cartilage destruction with joint narrowing, the formation of subchondral bone destruction, and cyst formation. Large areas of low signal on both pulse sequences probably represent hypertrophied synovium with hemosiderin deposited within it. **D,** Sagittal image (650/14) obtained 2 weeks later. Clinically the patient had had a hemorrhage into this joint since the previous images were taken. This image shows a new large area of strong signal intensity in the joint: this is the new hemorrhage.

of females with polyostotic disease; only 35 percent have the classic café au lait spots. The precocious puberty seen in Albright's syndrome may be associated with advanced skeletal age. Deformity of the skull may infrequently cause neurologic abnormalities. Sexual precocity in males is mild, when it does occur.

Pathologically, the medullary cavity of bones affected by fibrous dysplasia shows replacement by gray-white fibrous tissue with specules of new bone. The tissue is primarily fibrous, with varying amounts of osseous tissue scattered throughout the fibrous matrix in a disorganized manner. There may be large areas that contain no evidence of osteoid, and other areas with nests of cartilage and multinucleated giant cells.

Radiographically, replacement of the medullary cavity is seen as a radiolucent to homogeneous "ground-glass" density. The density of the lesion depends on the amount of fibrous or osseous tissue deposited within the medullary cavity. The cortex may be thin or thickened and may show endosteal irregularity. Expansion of the bone occurs in the ribs and skull and other long bones, expansion being seen more often when the lesions are radiolucent. Fibrous dysplasia is seen primarily in the metaphysis, although the diaphysis and (rarely) the entire length of the bone may be affected. The bone and medullary cavity not affected by the fibrous replacement remain normal in appearance and composition. The lesions of monostotic and polyostotic fibrous dysplasia differ only in the number of bones involved.

The MR appearance of fibrous dysplasia has been reported both as of low signal intensity on both T1 and T2 weighted images, and as of low signal intensity on T1 and increased signal intensity on T2 weighted images.[76,77] It is likely that there is a spectrum of appearance of fibrous dysplasia on MR images that reflects the underlying histology of the lesion. If the lesion is composed primarily of quiescent fibrous tissue, it is likely to appear of intermediate to low signal intensity on both T1 and T2 weighted images. A large component of reactive or sclerotic bone would also result in low signal intensity on both T1 and T2 weighted images.

If the lesion contains a large cellular component,

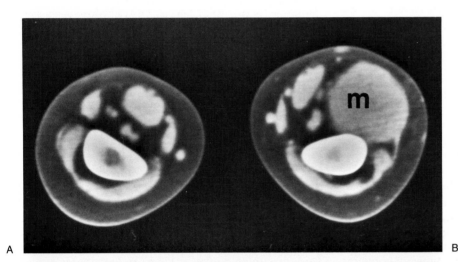

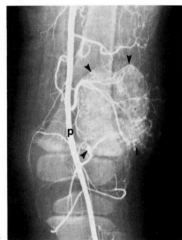

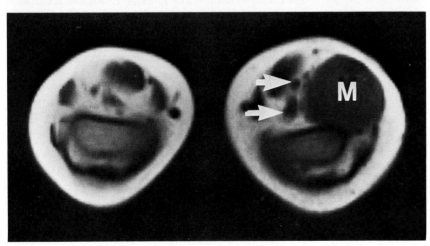

Figure 25–56. *Nodular fasciitis.* ***A,*** CT scan shows a well-defined soft tissue mass (m) in the lateral head of the biceps femoris muscle. The intensity of the lesion is the same as that of adjacent muscle. The femoral blood vessels cannot be differentiated from adjacent muscles or lymph nodes. ***B,*** Angiogram shows the mass lesion (*arrowheads*), which is fairly vascular. The popliteal artery (p) lies to the medial aspect of the mass and curves around it. ***C,*** Transverse T1 MR image (500/26). The mass lesion (M) is well defined and of similar intensity to muscle. Because of flow void the popliteal artery and vein (*arrows*) can be well identified. MRI has the advantage over CT in defining the popliteal vessels. Neither modality shows any features to suggest the final pathologic diagnosis.

intermediate signal intensity on T1 weighted images and high signal intensity on T2 weighted images would be expected. The normal marrow cavity can often be identified, and while the signal intensity of the lesion may increase on T2 weighted images, it can usually be distinguished from the surrounding normal marrow. In my experience, signal can be seen within the cortical bone, presumably secondary to involvement of the cortical bone by the pathologic process. A surrounding soft tissue mass should not be seen. Prospective studies are needed to determine what, if any, MR criteria may be used to distinguish fibrous dysplasia from other pathologic processes.

Fasciitis

Mervyn D. Cohen, M.B., Ch.B.

Eosinophilic Fasciitis

Eosinophilic fasciitis is an idiopathic inflammatory disorder involving the skin and subcutaneous tissues, with marked thickening of the fascia between the fat and muscle. In some ways it resembles scleroderma, but there are no systemic clinical symptoms, and laboratory investigation identifies eosinophilia. Onset of the disorder often follows exercise.

MRI frequently shows more abnormality than does CT. There is a fairly nonspecific, irregular, mottled, soft tissue abnormality and swelling, with low signal intensity compared with normal muscle on T1 and high signal intensity on T2 weighted images. The abnormality is seen to involve the fat and adjacent soft tissue.

Nodular Fasciitis

Nodular fasciitis is a solitary benign localized mass composed of a proliferation of fibrous tissue. The lesions are well defined (Fig. 25–56). Although the MR appearance is somewhat nonspecific, the fibrous and benign nature of the lesion may be suggested by the identification of a lesion that changes little in signal intensity between T1 and T2 weighted images. The intensity of the lesions is similar to or lower than that of muscle. Treatment consists of resection.

REFERENCES

1. Modic MT, Pflanze W, Feiglin DHI, Belhobek G. Magnetic resonance imaging of musculoskeletal infections. Radiol Clin North Am 1986; 24:247–258.
2. Beltran J, Noto AM, McGhee RB, et al. Infections of the musculoskeletal system: high-field-strength MR imaging. Radiology 1987; 164:449–454.
3. McAfee JG, Samin A. In-111 labeled leukocytes: a review of problems in image interpretation. Radiology 1985; 155:221–229.
4. Unger E, Moldofsky P, Gatenby R, et al. Diagnosis of osteomyelitis by MR imaging. AJR 1988; 150:605–610.
5. Tang JSH, Gold RH, Bassett LW, Seeger LL. Musculoskeletal infection of the extremities: evaluation with MR imaging. Radiology 1988; 166:205–209.
6. Bloem HL, Falke THM, Doornbos J. Osteomyelitis in children: detection by magnetic resonance (letter to editor). Radiology 1984; 153:263–264.
7. Fletcher BD, Scoles PV, Nelson AD. Osteomyelitis in children: detection by magnetic resonance. Radiology 1984; 150:57–60.
8. Quinn SF, Murray W, Clark RA, Cochran C. MR imaging of chronic osteomyelitis. J Comput Assist Tomogr 1988; 12:113–117.
9. Tumeh SS, Aliabadi P, Weissman BN, McNeil BJ. Disease activity in osteomyelitis: role of radiography. Radiology 1987; 165:781–784.
10. Alazraki N, Fierer J, Resnick D. Chronic osteomyelitis: monitoring by ^{99m}Tc phosphate and ^{67}Ga citrate imaging. AJR 1985; 145:767–771.
11. Wing VW, Jeffrey RB, Federle MP, et al. Chronic osteomyelitis examined by CT. Radiology 1985; 154:171–174.
12. Cohen MD, Cory DA, Kleiman M, et al. Magnetic resonance differentiation of acute and chronic osteomyelitis in children. Clin Radiol 1990; 41:53–59.
13. Yuh WTC, Schreiber AE, Montgomery WJ, Ehara S. Magnetic resonance imaging of pyomyositis. Skeletal Radiol 1988; 17:190–193.
14. Kauffman LD, Gruber RL, Gerstman DP, Kaell AT. Preliminary observations on the role of magnetic resonance imaging for polymyositis and dermatomyositis. Ann Rheum Dis 1987; 46:569–572.
15. Ehman RL, Berquist TH. Magnetic resonance imaging of musculoskeletal trauma. Radiol Clin North Am 1986; 24:291–319.
16. Reicher MA, Hartzman S, Bassett LW, et al. MR imaging of the knee. I. Traumatic disorders. Radiology 1987; 162:547–553.
17. Ehman RL. MR imaging of medullary bone. Radiology 1988; 167:867–868.
18. Yao L, Lee JK. Occult intraosseous fracture: detection with MR imaging. Radiology 1988; 167:749–751.
19. Berger PE, Ofstein RA, Jackson DW, et al. MRI demonstration of radiologically occult fractures: what have we been missing? Radiographics 1989; 9:407–436.
20. Deutsch AL, Mink JH, Waxman AD. Occult fractures of the proximal femur: MR imaging. Radiology 1989; 170:113–116.
21. Mink JH, Deutsch AL. Occult cartilage and bone injuries of the knee: detection, classification, and assessment with MR imaging. Radiology 1989; 170:823–829.
22. Lynch TCP, Crues JV, Morgan FW, et al. Bone abnormalities of the knee: prevalence and significance at MR imaging. Radiology 1989; 171:761–766.
23. Zlatkin MB, Dalinka MK, Kressel HY. Magnetic resonance imaging of the shoulder. Mag Res 1989; 5:3–22.
24. Stafford SA, Rosenthal DI, Gebhardt MC, et al. MRI in stress fracture. AJR 1986; 147:553–556.
25. Quinn SF, Belsole RJ, Greene TL, Rayhack JM. Advanced imaging of the wrist. Radiographics 1989; 9:229–246.
26. Beltran J, Noto AM, Mosure JC, et al. Ankle: surface coil MR imaging at 1.5T. Radiology 1986; 161:203–209.
27. Lee JK, Yao L. Stress fractures: MR imaging. Radiology 1988; 169:217–220.
28. Castillo M, Tehranzadeh J, Morillo G. Atypical healed stress fracture of the fibula masquerading as chronic osteomyelitis. Am J Sports Med 1988; 16:185–188.
29. Ehman RL, Berquist TH, McLeod RA. MR imaging of the musculoskeletal system: a 5 year appraisal. Radiology 1988; 166:313–320.
30. Dooms GC, Fisher MR, Hricak H. MR imaging of intramuscular hemorrhage. J Comput Assist Tomogr 1985; 9:908–913.
31. Bradley WG, Schmidt PG. Effect of methemoglobin formation on the appearance of subarachnoid hemorrhage. Radiology 1985; 156:99–103.
32. Rubin JI, Gomori JM, Grossman RI. High field MR imaging of extracranial hematomas. AJR 1987; 148:813–817.
33. Jackson DW, Jennings LD, Maywood RM, Berger PE. Magnetic resonance imaging of the knee. Am J Sports Med 1988; 16:29–38.
34. Lee JK, Yao L, Phelps CT, et al. Anterior cruciate ligament tears: MR imaging compared with arthroscopy and clinical tests. Radiology 1988; 166:861–864.
35. Mink JH, Levy T, Crues JY. Tears of the anterior cruciate ligament and menisci of the knee: MR imaging evaluation. Radiology 1988; 167:769–774.

36. Moeser P, Bechtold RE, Clark T, et al. MR imaging of anterior cruciate ligament repair. J Comput Assist Tomogr 1989; 13:105–109.

37. Reicher MA, Bassett LW, Gold RH. High resolution magnetic resonance imaging of the knee joint: pathologic correlations. AJR 1985; 145:903–909.

38. Crues JV, Mink J, Levy TL, et al. Meniscal tears of the knee: accuracy of MR imaging Radiology 1987; 164:445–448.

39. Stoller DW, Martin C, Crues JV, et al. Meniscal tears: pathologic correlation with MR imaging. Radiology 1987; 163:731–735.

40. Tyrrell RL, Gluckert K, Pathria M, Modic MT. Fast three dimensional MR imaging of the knee: comparison with arthroscopy. Radiology 1988; 166:865–872.

41. Haggar AM, Froelich JW, Hearshein DO, Sadasivan K. Meniscal abnormalities of the knee: 3DFT fast scan GRASS MR imaging. AJR 1988; 150:1341–1344.

42. Burk DL, Dalinka MK, Kanal E, et al. Meniscal and ganglion cysts of the knee: MR evaluation AJR 1988; 150:331–336.

43. Zlatkin MB, Iannotti JP, Roberts MC, et al. Rotator cuff tears: diagnostic performance of MR imaging. Radiology 1989; 172:223–229.

44. Beltran J, Noto AM, Herman LJ, Lubbers LM. Tendons: high field strength, surface coil MR imaging. Radiology 1987; 162:735–740.

45. Reinig JW, Dorwart RH, Roden WC. MR imaging of a ruptured Achilles tendon. J Comput Assist Tomogr 1985; 9:1131–1134.

46. Quinn SF, Murray WT, Clark RA, Cochran CF. Achilles tendon: MR imaging at 1.5T. Radiology 1987; 164:767–770.

47. Rosenberg ZS, Cheung Y, Jahss MH, et al. Rupture of posterior tibial tendon: CT and MR imaging with surgical correlation. Radiology 1988; 169:229–235.

48. Mesgarzadeh M, Sapega AA, Bonakdarpour A, et al. Osteochondritis dissecans: analysis of mechanical stability with radiography, scintigraphy, and MR imaging. Radiology 1987; 165: 775–780.

49. Bodne D, Quinn SF, Cochran CF. Imaging foreign glass and wooden bodies of the extremities with CT and MR. J Comput Assist Tomogr 1988; 12:608–611.

50. Fleckenstein JL, Canby RC, Parkey RW, Peshock RM. Acute effects of exercise on MR imaging of skeletal muscle in normal volunteers. AJR 1988; 151:231–237.

51. McCully KK, Kent JA, Chance B. Application of ^{31}P magnetic resonance spectroscopy to the study of athletic performance. Sports Med 1988; 5:312–321.

52. Kieft GJ, Bloem JL, Rozing PM, Obermann WR. MR imaging of recurrent anterior dislocation of the shoulder: comparison with CT arthrography. AJR 1988; 150:1083–1087.

53. Johnson ND, Wood BP, Jackman KV. Complex infantile and congenital hip dislocation: assessment with MR imaging. Radiology 1988; 168:151–156.

54. Bos CFA, Bloem JL, Obermann WR, Rozing PM. Magnetic resonance imaging in congenital dislocation of the hip. J Bone Joint Surg 1988; 70B:174–178.

55. Charcot JM. Etudes pour servir a l'histoire de l'affection décrite sous les noms de goutte asthénique primitive, nodosites des jointures, rhumatisme articulaire chronique (forme primitive), etc. Paris Thèses, No. 44, 1853.

56. Cornil V. Mémoire sur les coïncidences pathologiques du rhumatisme articulaire chronique. CR Soc Biol (Paris), Ser 4, 1864; 3:2–25.

57. Still GF. On a form of chronic joint disease in children. Med Chir Trans 1897; 80:47–59.

58. Butler JL. Juvenile rheumatoid arthritis. In: Ball GV, Koopman WJ, eds. Clinical rheumatology. Philadelphia: WB Saunders, 1886.

59. Calabro JJ. Juvenile rheumatoid arthritis. In: McCarty DJ, ed. Arthritis and allied conditions. Philadelphia: Lea & Febiger, 1985.

60. Brewer EJ, Giannini EH, Person DA. Manifestations of disease. In: Brewer EJ, Giannini EH, Person DA, eds. Juvenile rheumatoid arthritis. Philadelphia: WB Saunders, 1982.

61. Weichselbaum A. Über die senilen Veranderungen der Geienke und deren Zusammenhang mit der Arthritis deformans, Sitzungsb. Kais Adad Wissensch Math-natur Classe Wien 1877; 193:75–76.

62. Bogumil GP, Schwamm HA. Rheumatoid arthritis. In: Bogumil GP, Schwamm HA, eds. Orthopaedic pathology: a synopsis with clinical and radiographic correlation. Philadelphia: WB Saunders, 1984.

63. Bullough PG, Vigorita VJ. Rheumatoid arthritis. In: Bullough PG, Vigorita VJ, eds. Atlas of orthopaedic pathology with clinical and radiographic correlations. Baltimore: University Park Press, 1984.

64. Jaffe HJ. Inflammatory arthritis of undetermined etiology. In: Jaffe HJ, ed. Metabolic, degenerative and inflammatory diseases of bones and joints. Philadelphia: Lea & Febiger, 1972.

65. Senac MO, Deutsch D, Bernstein BH, et al. MR imaging in juvenile rheumatoid arthritis. AJR 1988; 150:873–878.

66. Yulish BS, Lieberman JM, Newman AJ, et al. Juvenile rheumatoid arthritis: assessment with MR imaging. Radiology 1987; 165:149–152.

67. Beltran J, Caudill JL, Herman LA, et al. Rheumatoid arthritis: MR imaging manifestations. Radiology 1987; 165:153–157.

68. Stoller DW. The knee. In: Stoller DW, ed. Magnetic resonance imaging in orthopaedics and rheumatology. Philadelphia: JB Lippincott, 1989.

69. Konig H, Aicher KP. MRI evaluations of cartilage and meniscal disorders of the knee: a comparison with ultrasound, scintigraphy, and CT. Hospimedica 1988; Oct/Nov:49–59.

70. Poznanski AK, Glass RBJ, Feinstein KA, et al. Magnetic resonance imaging in juvenile rheumatoid arthritis. Int Pediatr 1988; 3:304–311.

71. Aisen AM, Martel W, Ellis JH, McCune WJ. Cervical spine involvement in rheumatoid arthritis: MR imaging. Radiology 1987; 165:159–163.

72. Kulkarni MV, Drolshagen LF, Kaye JJ, et al. MR imaging of hemophilic arthropathy. J Comput Assist Tomogr 1986; 10:445.

73. Yulish BS. Hemophilic arthropathy: assessment with MR imaging. Radiology 1987; 164:759.

74. Stoller DW, Genant HK. MR imaging of knee arthritides. Radiology 1987; 165:233.

75. Schreiber A, Smith WL, Ionasescu V, et al. Magnetic resonance imaging of children with Duchenne muscular dystrophy. Pediatr Radiol 1987; 17:495–497.

76. McKenzie DH. The fibromatoses: a clinical concept. Br Med J 1972; 4:277–281.

77. Francis IR, Dorovini-Zis K, Glazer GM, et al. The fibromatoses: CT-pathologic correlation. AJR 1986; 147:1063–1066.

Index